Sixth Edition

Piyush Gupta

Clinical Methods in **Pediatrics**

Sixth Edition

Piyush Gupta

Clinical Methods in
Pediatrics

Piyush Gupta MD FAMS FRCPCH
Professor
Department of Pediatrics
University College of Medical Sciences
and Guru Teg Bahadur Hospital
New Delhi

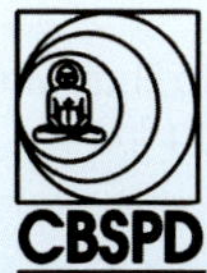

CBS Publishers & Distributors Pvt Ltd

New Delhi • Bengaluru • Chennai • Kochi • Kolkata • Lucknow • Mumbai
Gujarat • Hyderabad • Jharkhand • Nagpur • Patna • Pune • Uttarakhand

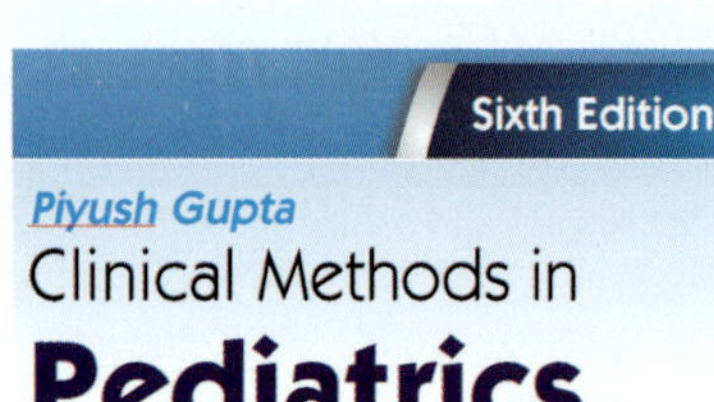

ISBN: 978-93-5466-926-2

Sixth Edition: 2025
Reprint 2025, **2026**[1]
First Edition 2009
Second Edition 2011
Third Edition 2014
Fourth Edition 2017
Fifth Edition 2022
Reprint 2022, 2023, 2024

Published by Satish Kumar Jain and produced by Varun Jain for

CBS Publishers & Distributors Pvt Ltd
4819/XI Prahlad Street, 24 Ansari Road, Daryaganj, New Delhi 110 002, India
Ph: 011-23289259, 23266861 Fax: 011-23243014 Website: www.cbspd.com
e-mail: delhi@cbspd.com

Corporate Office: 204 FIE, Industrial Area, Patparganj, Delhi 110 092, India
Ph: 011-4934 4934 Fax: 011-4934 4935 e-mail: publishing@cbspd.com; publicity@cbspd.com

Branches

- **Bengaluru:** Seema House 2975, 17th Cross, KR Road, Banasankari 2nd Stage, Bengaluru 560 070, Karnataka, India
  Ph: +91-80-26771678/79 Fax: +91-80-26771680 e-mail: bangalore@cbspd.com
- **Chennai:** 7, Subbaraya Street, Shenoy Nagar, Chennai 600 030, Tamil Nadu, India
  Ph: +91-44-26680620, 26681266 e-mail: chennai@cbspd.com
- **Kochi:** 42/1325, 1326, Power House Road, Opp KSEB, Power House, Ernakulum, Kochi 682 018, Kerala, India
  Ph: +91-484-4059061–67 e-mail: kochi@cbspd.com
- **Kolkata:** 147, Hind Ceramics Compound, 1st Floor, Nilgunj Road, Belghoria, Kolkata 700 056, West Bengal, India
  Ph: +91-33-25633055/56 e-mail: kolkata@cbspd.com
- **Lucknow:** Basement, Khushnuma Complex, 7 Meerabai Marg (behind Jawahar Bhawan), Lucknow 226 001, UP, India
  Ph: +91-522-4000032 e-mail: tiwari.lucknow@cbspd.com
- **Mumbai:** PWD Shed, Gala no. 25/26, Ramchandra Bhatt Marg, Next to JJ Hospital Gate no. 2, Opp. Union Bank of India, Noorbaug, Mumbai 400 009, Maharashtra, India
  Ph: +91-22-66661880/89 e-mail: mumbai@cbspd.com

Representatives

• Gujarat • Hyderabad • Jharkhand • Nagpur • Patna • Pune • Uttarakhand

For trade terms please contact customercare@cbspd.com
For general enquiries please contact info@cbspd.com

Printed at Paras Offset Pvt. Ltd., Kundli (Haryana)

to
my students
who remain
my best teachers

Contributing Authors

Aashima Dabas MD
Associate Professor
Department of Pediatrics
Maulana Azad Medical College and
Lok Nayak Hospital
New Delhi
Email: dr.aashimagupta@gmail.com

Anil Agarwal MS MNAMS
Specialist and Head
Department of Pediatric Orthopedics
Chacha Nehru Bal Chikitsalaya
New Delhi
E-mail: anilrachna@gmail.com

Deepika Pandhi MD FAMS
Head, Department of Dermatology and STD
University of Delhi
Director-Professor
Department of Dermatology and STD
University College of Medical Sciences and
Guru Teg Bahadur Hospital
New Delhi
E-mail: deepikapandhi@rediffmail.com

Dheeraj Shah MD FAMS
Director
National Institute of Health and Family Welfare
Delhi; and Director-Professor
Department of Pediatrics
University College of Medical Sciences
New Delhi
E-mail: shahdheeraj@hotmail.com

DK Singh MD
Professor and Head
Department of Pediatrics
Postgraduate Institute of Child Health
Noida, Uttar Pradesh
E-mail: drdksingh1999@gmail.com

Jaya Shankar Kaushik MD DNB MNAMS DM
Additional Professor and Head
Department of Pediatrics
All India Institute of Medical Sciences
Guwahati, Assam
E-mail: jayashankarkaushik@gmail.com

Joseph L Mathew MD PhD
Professor (Pediatric Pulmonology)
Advanced Pediatrics Centre
Postgraduate Institute of Medical Education
and Research, Chandigarh
E-mail: joseph.l.mathew@gmail.com

Lokesh Guglani MD, FAAP
Associate Professor
Division of Pulmonology
Allergy/Immunology, Cystic Fibrosis, and Sleep
Department of Pediatrics
Emory University School of Medicine
Children's Healthcare of Atlanta
Atlanta, Georgia, USA
E-mail: lokesh.guglani@emory.edu

Monica Juneja MD
Director, Professor and Head
Department of Pediatrics
Incharge, Child Development Centre and
Centre of Excellence Early Intervention Centre
(COE-EIC)
Maulana Azad Medical College and
Associated Lok Nayak Hospital
New Delhi
E-mail: drmonicajuneja@gmail.com

Naveen Sankhyan MD DM
Professor and Head
Pediatric Neurology
Department of Pediatrics
Advanced Pediatrics Centre
Postgraduate Institute of Medical Education
and Research, Chandigarh
E-mail: drnsankhyan@yahoo.co.in

Neelima Gupta MS DNB MNAMS
Director-Professor and Head
Department of Otorhinolaryngology
University College of Medical Sciences
and Guru Teg Bahadur Hospital
New Delhi
E-mail: drneelimagupta@gmail.com

Nidhi Bedi MD
Professor
Department of Pediatrics
Faculty of Medicine and Health Sciences
(Formerly Shree Guru Gobind Singh Tricentenary
Medical College Hospital and Research Institute)
SGT University, Gurugram, Haryana
E-mail: drnidhibedi@gmail.com

Payal Gupta MBBS DNB
Consultant
Department of Ophthalmology
Fortis Hospital, Greater Noida
Uttar Pradesh
E-mail: drpayal.pg@gmail.com

Piyush Gupta MD FAMS FRCPCH
Professor
Department of Pediatrics
University College of Medical Sciences
and Guru Teg Bahadur Hospital
New Delhi
E-mail: prof.piyush.gupta@gmail.com

Pooja Dewan MD MNAMS
Director-Professor
Department of Pediatrics
University College of Medical Sciences
and Guru Teg Bahadur Hospital
New Delhi
E-mail: poojadewan@hotmail.com

Prateek Rastogi MS (Orthopaedics)
Assistant Professor
Department of Orthopedics
School of Medical Sciences and Research
Sharda University and associated Hospital
Greater Noida, Uttar Pradesh
E-mail: prateek.rastogi12@gmail.com

Praveen Kumar MD
Director-Professor
Department of Pediatrics
Lady Hardinge Medical College and Associated
Kalawati Saran Children's Hospital
New Delhi
E-mail: pkpaed@gmail.com

Richa Saha MS
Department of Otorhinolaryngology
University College of Medical Sciences
and Guru Teg Bahadur Hospital
New Delhi
E-mail: richadrsaha@gmail.com

Ruchi Rai MD
Professor and Head
Department of Neonatology
Postgraduate Institute of Child Health
Noida, Uttar Pradesh
E-mail: ruchiraialld@gmail.com

S Aneja MD
Ex-Director–Professor and Head
Department of Pediatrics
Lady Hardinge Medical College and
Kalawati Saran Children's Hospital
New Delhi
E-mail: drsaneja@gmail.com

S Srinivasan MD DCH
Ex-Professor and Head
Department of Pediatrics, JIPMER, Puducherry
Professor, MGMCRI Pillayarkuppam, Puducherry
Currently Adjunct Professor
Department of Pediatrics
Mehta Multispeciality Hospital, Chetpet, Chennai, Tamil Nadu
E-mail: srinivasan.renu@gmail.com

Srikanta Basu MD MNAMS FIAP
Director-Professor
Department of Pediatrics
Lady Hardinge Medical College and
Associated Kalawati Saran Children's Hospital
New Delhi
E-mail: srikantabasu@gmail.com

Suvasini Sharma MD DM
Professor, Neurology Division
Department of Pediatrics
Lady Hardinge Medical College and
Associated Kalawati Saran Children's Hospital
New Delhi
E-mail: sharma.suvasini@gmail.com

Swati Kalra MD DNB DPAA
Senior Consultant
Department of Pediatrics
Medanta Hospital
Gurgram, Haryana
E-mail: swatikalra24@gmail.com

Preface to the Sixth Edition

I am overwhelmed by the response received by the last five editions of the book *Clinical Methods in Pediatrics*. This book, first released in 2009 has stood the test of the time, acclaimed by the students and teachers of pediatrics in India and other countries of South Asia. The book has now established itself as the leading text in its category.

In the present edition, two chapters including those pertaining to clinical examination of the newborn and examination of the musculoskeletal system have been completely rewritten. This edition also incorporates the 2024 ICMR recommendations on Recommended Dietary Allowances (RDA), Neonatal Resuscitation Guidelines as adapted by Indian Academy of Pediatrics (IAP) and National Neonatology Forum (NNF). Extended IAP BMI Charts, and IAP Obesity Guidelines 2023; along with National Immunization Schedule for 2024 are also included. All other sections and chapters have been thoroughly updated. We have however, retained the major charms and strengths of the earlier editions: A pleasing 4-color format, student-friendly structure, logical concepts, easy language, and graphical retention. The typesetting is pleasant with better space utilization. Number of figures and photographs have been added to facilitate visualization of clinical examination and its findings.

I thank Mr Satish Kumar Jain (Chairman and Managing Director) and Mr Varun Jain (Director) of CBS Publishers and Distributors Pvt Ltd, New Delhi, for their belief in this project and Mr YN Arjuna (Senior Vice-President, Publishing, Editorial and Publicity) and Ms Ritu Chawla (AGM, Production), for their painstaking efforts in bringing out this edition. This entire exercise would not have been possible without the contributing authors who are the backbone of this venture.

I welcome comments concerning omission and errors, healthy reviews regarding contents, critical thoughts and suggestions for further edition. Critics' reviews, comments and suggestions may be mailed to prof.piyush.gupta@gmail.com.

Piyush Gupta

Preface to the Sixth Edition

Preface to the First Edition

A few years back, one of my brighter students asked me a simple question "... tell me of a book which I can refer to for my needs pertaining to history-taking in pediatrics, assessment of diet and feeding practices, obtaining and interpreting anthropometry, evaluating development, assessing a newborn infant and performing age-specific systemic examination tailored to children." And I started searching for one. Finally, when the search proved futile, I made up my mind to write a book encompassing all these issues. I got a few experts together and with their help in respective sub-specialties of pediatrics, the ball started rolling. This book is the culmination of efforts of many people, the contributors being in the forefront. Only the readers will tell how it has shaped up.

The book is phased into 15 chapters, beginning with the art of communicating with the child and parents. There are plenty of tables, figures and boxes to highlight important information. An elaborate index is provided at the end to facilitate easy retrieval of information. I have endeavored to ensure a consistency in style and minimum of overlap—all eternal headaches for the editor of a multi-authored book. I believe that this book will make a useful contribution to the existing medical literature. The book comes with a promise—the perfect is yet to come!

I thank Mr Satish Jain, Managing Director, CBS Publishers & Distributors, for his overall support and belief in this book. I remain grateful to all the authors for their contributions. They remain the backbone of this venture. I would like to specifically name two of my dear colleagues, Pooja Dewan and Jaya Shankar Kaushik, who helped me at every stage of preparation of this book, in every possible manner. This volume would not have been possible without their dedicated efforts. A near error-free output was fashioned entirely by the efforts of Mr Rajesh Kumar and Sh SS Gehlot. No amount of words can express my gratitude to my wife (Anjali) and children (Payal and Aayush), who gave me unflinching support and allowed me ample time for completing this book.

I welcome comments concerning omissions and errors, healthy reviews regarding content, critical thoughts, and suggestions for further editions. Critics' reviews, comments, and suggestions may please be mailed to prof.piyush.gupta@gmail.com.

Piyush Gupta

Acknowledgments

Typesetting

Jyoti Kaur, Neeraj Sharma, Baljeet Kaur

Secretarial

Anju Kumari

Contents

Chapter

1

Effective Communication with Child and Caretakers

❍ S Aneja ❍ Jaya Shankar Kaushik

Structure

1.1 DEFINING COMMUNICATION

Communication is a process used to exchange information, ideas and feelings and is considered effective when information is clearly understood by both parties.

Communication is, by definition, participatory. It is a two-way process. Talking is the most common way of communication. Other modes of communication include writing, making hand and body gestures, drawing, etc. Communication is essential for building and sustaining relationships, exchanging information and making treatment decision. Four important skills needed for good communication are listed in **Key Box 1**.

Your ability to establish effective communication is determined by whether parents perceive you to be trustworthy and believable. It also depends on few attributes of physician like empathy, caring, competence, expertise, honesty, openness, dedication, and commitment.

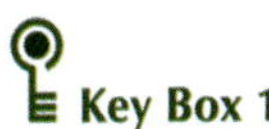

Key Box 1

Essential Skills for Effective Communication

1. Listening and giving attention.
2. Talking and presenting clearly.
3. Discussing and clarifying.
4. Showing appropriate concern and demonstrating empathy.

1.2 IMPORTANCE OF COMMUNICATION SKILLS

Doctors are perceived to be healers, educators, and counselors. Good communication is needed for all these functions. Good communication skills are fundamental to a good patient–doctor relationship. Doctors with good communication skills identify the problems with patients more accurately and have a greater job satisfaction. Their patients are more satisfied with the care and are likely to follow the doctor's instruction and come back for follow-up.

Role of Communication in Pediatric Practice

Communication is essential in healthcare setting at almost every step of the patient care while explaining the medical illness to parents, involving the parents in decision making, or while advising the parents about desired changes in lifestyle of their child. It is also essential prior to obtain informed consent for a procedure or treatment.

How Much Time a Doctor Needs to Spend on Communication

This depends on the type of problem the patient presents with, and the setting in which the patient visit occurs. Considerable time needs to be spent with parents, when eliciting history. Parents of children with chronic diseases or those with life-threatening illness require to be handled with sensitivity and also require ample time of the doctor. The parents may have significant level of distress, and may not be in 'input' mode. In such situations, 2–3 meetings are required with parents.

Time is limited in an emergency room and outpatient setting. The initial communication needs to be short, crisp, and to the point. This may be followed later by a longer session.

Communication with Children and their Parents is Different

You need to be skilled in talking to children ranging from infancy to adolescence as well as to their parents. Be aware of the sensitivity of the child while talking to parents. Simultaneously, attempt to build a rapport with the child and get him involved. The key tasks which require communication skills are highlighted in **Key Box 2**. The stepwise process of communication in pediatric practice is outlined in the next section.

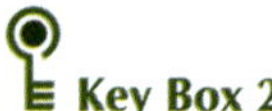

Key Box 2

Key Tasks that Require Effective Communication

1. Eliciting the history.
2. Counseling for promoting child health, e.g. breastfeeding, accident prevention.
3. Instructing to give treatment and checking the understanding.
4. Facilitate decision making, e.g. HIV, genetic counseling.
5. Breaking news, e.g. diagnosis of disability or death.
6. Taking consent.

1.3 PROCESS OF COMMUNICATION

1. Building Rapport with Child and Parents

The first step is to ensure privacy and respect confidentiality. Confidentiality is particularly important for the diseases perceived as stigmatizing in our society. In traditional joint families, with strong family ties, the grandparents and other family members may be involved in decision-making process and in such situations they may be involved in communication process. Mutual trust can be established only if you respect children and their parents. Calling the patient by name rather than 'your child' is a good way of giving respect to the individual. Often the parents are anxious and tense and express their apprehension to the physician. Greet the parents and talk about any local issue so as to help the parents and child to relax. Sit down while talking. Smile appropriately.

2. History-taking

History-taking is the most important skill required in medicine. It is said that nearly 3/4th of all diagnoses can be made by a good history. The key is to use both forms of communication, i.e. verbal and non-verbal.

Nonverbal Communication

Nonverbal communication means showing your attitude through postures, gestures, and expression **(Key Box 3)**. Pay attention and make eye contact with patient when examining the child; and with the mother while talking to her. If the mother is veiled or hesitates to talk to a male doctor, communicate in presence of her husband or an elder.

- Lean forward to indicate attentiveness and nod to indicate understanding.
- Avoid distracting movements, like fidgeting or constantly moving your leg. During the times of epidemics such as COVID, it is good to take appropriate social distancing precautions while examining the child and interacting with parents.
- Smile when you greet the patient. Keep your personal worries and frustrations back home and do not impose them on the child and the parents.
- Do not discriminate one patient from another. Most of the times the patient who is standing in queue outside observes how the doctor was behaving with the previous patient.

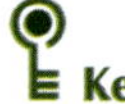

Key Box 3

Methods of Nonverbal Communication

1. Look at the patient and make eye contact.
2. Keep your head at the same level as the parent.
3. Open posture: Facing directly with hands apart on the arms of the chair.
4. Take time. Do not appear hurried.
5. Touch the baby/mother appropriately.
6. Remove barriers, if any, e.g. a large table or a mobile phone.

- Avoid eliciting too many personal information like caste, religious beliefs, etc. unless necessary for medical reasons.
- A mother and child feel comfortable when the doctor displays appreciation of the child. One can probably open the conversation with the child like asking "this shirt looks so good, who got it for you?"

Elicit the Patient's Problem and Concerns

After establishing rapport, you should find the reason for the patient's visit (i.e. presenting complaints). Encourage the patient to be exact about the sequence in which the problems occurred. Ask for the approximate date of key events and about the parent's perception of the problem.

Following techniques are recommended to get correct information:

1. Use open-ended questions.
2. Active listening and appropriate response.
3. Be empathetic and list the problems.
4. Use words that patient/parents understand.

We now discuss these techniques one by one.

A. Use open-ended questions with a few specific close-ended questions

Questions which are answered by 'yes' or 'no' are close-ended questions. These may not yield much information and often do not get to the main concerns.

Close-ended question: *Is fever accompanied with cough?*

Questions which cannot be replied with 'yes' or 'no' are open-ended. The parents have to give a detailed answer to these. Open-ended questions help in eliciting the concerns and parents' perception of the illness.

Open-ended question: *Tell me what all other symptoms are associated with fever?*

However, certain situations demand a leading (close-ended) question. For example, if you ask an 8-year-old child to describe the character of pain and he has difficulty in describing, you may ask whether it is sharp or dull.

B. Active listening

Active listening promotes mutual understanding, increases attention span, and helps the parents to open up. Attentive listening gives you ample time and opportunity to imbibe and understand what the parents told you. Appropriate responses to listening can be both verbal or non-verbal **(Key Box 4)**.

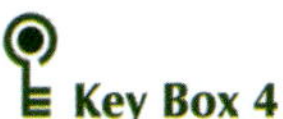
Key Box 4

Active Listening Skills

Nonverbal

Paying attention, nodding head, smiling, eye contact.

Verbal

- Reflecting: Paraphrasing and clarifying
- Affirmations, e.g. I see, I know
- Asking relevant open-ended questions
- Be non-judgemental
- Listen for feelings
- Show empathetic response when required
- Summarize

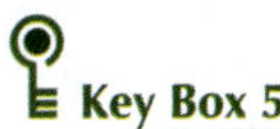
Key Box 5

Do's and Don'ts of Listening

Do's

- Become aware of your own listening habits.
- Concentrate on what the parent/child is saying.
- Listen for the total meaning, including feelings.
- Observe the speaker's non-verbal signals.
- Adopt an accepting attitude.
- Express empathic understanding.
- "Close the loop" of listening by taking appropriate action.

Don'ts

- Don't mistake not talking for listening.
- Don't fake listening.
- Don't interrupt needlessly.
- Don't pass judgment too quickly.
- Don't argue.
- Don't over-react to emotional words.
- Don't give advice unless it is requested.
- Don't use listening as a way of hiding yourself.
- Don't switch topic.

Some Do's and Don'ts of listening are listed in **Key Box 5**.

C. Ways to respond

Respect the child and parents irrespective of social, cultural, and ethnic background or disability. Encourage the patient from time to time. If you want the mother to continue talking, you must look interested and use responses to let her continue talking. Simple responses, such as 'Oh dear', 'do carry on' suggest that doctor is listening. Continuation messages convey to the parents that the doctor needs to know more. The response depends on the situation, and it can be a neutral response such as 'do tell me more about the pain' or an empathizing response such as 'you must have been worried'. Often the parents may have some hidden or unvoiced concerns. Pick up the verbal clues to such concerns and address them.

Sometimes, the mother may say something that you do not understand and would want to have more details. In such cases, it is better to rephrase what she has said and ask her if she meant what you have understood. For example, the mother may say that the child has been having fever for 1 month. You can ask 'do you mean that he/she has been having fever every day for last 1 month'.

The various conversational techniques are summarized below:

i. ***Reflecting***

Parent: I think she does not like the porridge.

Doctor: You think she does not like the porridge.

ii. ***Directing***

Doctor: Tell me what happened next.

iii. ***Clarifying***

Mother: Ankur is feeling giddy.

Doctor: Let me understand what you mean when you said he feels giddy.

iv. ***Empathetic response***

Parent: I was very scared when I saw him having the fit.

Doctor: I can understand you must have felt terribly upset!

D. Praising

Parents are often unsure and lack confidence about child rearing. Praising the parents appropriately at any point of communication helps restore their confidence.

E. Be empathetic

Empathy is being able to put yourself in the patient's or parents' place and able to understand their feelings. Physicians are more effective healers when they engage in the process of empathy.

When you empathize, the parents recognize that you can understand their emotions and develop a trust with you. For example, a mother whose child had a febrile seizure may be extremely anxious about the fever. While you have to reassure the mother about the benign nature of the disorder, you can empathize with her by saying:

"I can see you are feeling scared that he may have a seizure again."

Empathizing with patient or parents' feelings is an important way to get a cordial relationship and should be used appropriately while taking a history or sharing information.

F. List the problem(s)

While eliciting the information, keep on organizing the information so obtained within a diagnostic framework. This often may lead to more relevant questions which you need to ask. It is a good idea to summarize the information and let the parents know what you have understood. This gives them the opportunity to correct any misunderstanding.

G. Use words that the child and parents will understand

Use local terms and try not to use medical jargon. Often a local term may be used for different conditions, e.g. *Peelia* (hindi for jaundice) may be used for anemia as well as jaundice. Tips for history-taking are listed in **Key Box 6**.

Checklist for Communication

Essential 7 elements of communication during a medical encounter were framed by leading experts in medical education in the year 1999. This consensus statement was called **Kalamazoo consensus statement** and is stated in **Key Box 7**.

Key Box 6

Tips for History-taking

1. Ensure privacy and confidentiality.
2. Respect the patient and parents.
3. Use simple language.
4. Listen actively, let the parents talk.
5. Ask open-ended questions.
6. Clarify any ambiguous information.
7. Remain neutral to controversial issues.
8. List the problems and summarize.

Key Box 7

Essential Elements of Communication

1. Build a relationship: Greet the parents and child, make eye contact and show interest
2. Open the discussion by eliciting concerns
3. Gather information by active listening, use open-ended questions, clarify when necessary and continue the conversation for additional information
4. Understanding parents/patient's perspective
5. Share information using simple language that parents can understand
6. Informed/shared decision about treatment plan
7. Summarize and provide closure.

(*Adapted from Kalamazoo consensus statement*)

Media Advances

Face-to-face doctor–patient relationships are slowly getting replaced with advent of mobile phones, media, and the internet which have indeed revolutionized the medical care. Free access to lay websites and social media like personal blogs often mislead the parents. The doctors should be proactive in dispelling the myths and misinformation by giving accurate information. There are portals which offer webcam chat with the patient; or the parents might prefer communication over the telephone. However, there is no replacement for an effective face to face interview and examination. This is especially true for the first few visits. In chronic disorders, communication by telephone or webcam with physician can be encouraged after the initial evaluation.

3. Communicating during Physical Examination

Generally, you would have built rapport with the parents and the child by the time you start examining the child. You may need to ask the parents to undress an infant or a young child. Explain what you are going to do to the child. Children may get upset by seemingly innocuous things like BP apparatus and stethoscope. You must let the child handle the stethoscope or hammer so that the child is not intimidated by these. Keep the child comfortable and warm during the examination. Encourage the mother to undress the baby if required for the examination. Parents often get apprehensive when their baby's clothes are removed by the physician.

When a parent brings the child into your outpatient room, it implies consent for general examination and routine investigation. However, intimate examination including examination of private parts would require verbal expressed consent.

Remember to provide privacy to the child. Examination of a female child by a male physician should be done in the presence of a female attendant. For infants, you will need to explain to mothers what you are going to examine and how she should hold the infant. If the infant is crying and needs to be quiet, ask the mother to quieten the child.

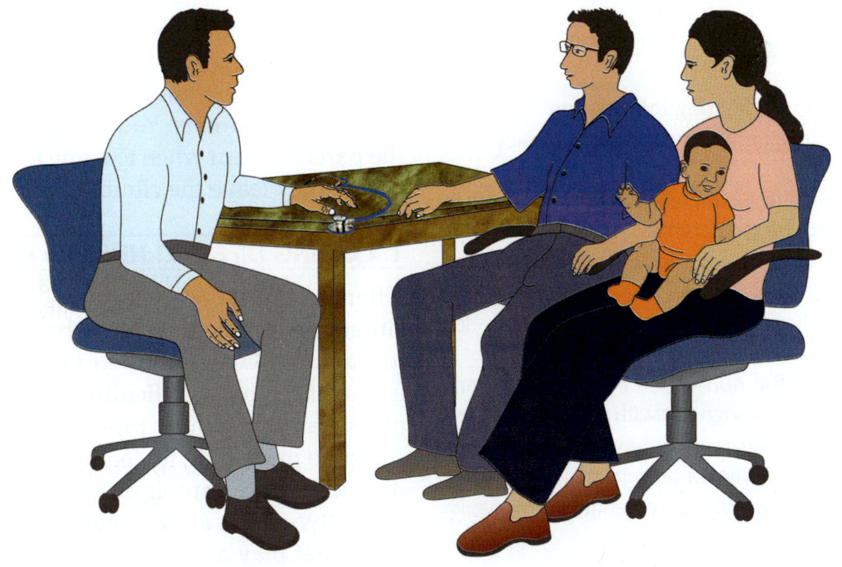

4. Share Information

After history and physical examination, you should inform the parents about your diagnosis and plan of management. A clinician needs to be honest about it. In a chronic disease, sharing of information may require several sessions. Do not be in a hurry to give all the information in a single sitting. State clearly what you think. The disclosed information must include disease or disorder which the child is suffering from, necessity for further testing to confirm the diagnosis, natural course of the disease, problems that may arise in case of non-treatment, available treatment options for the condition, and duration and cost of treatment. Finally, the expected outcome and follow-up plan must be communicated effectively to parents. First explain what you have found and what you think this means **(Key Box 8)**.

- In era of smart phones and internet, many parents wish to know the name of disease so that they can read about it. Parents should be encouraged to seek information from a reliable website and get back for any clarification.
- In contrast, a few parents may not ask any questions. They should be encouraged to do so.

Start with giving important information first and check what has been understood.

Before giving the information, it is a good idea to ascertain what the parents already know. For example, a mother of a child with diarrhea may be asked if she has prepared ORS earlier and how she made it. This helps in reinforcing what she is doing correctly, or rectifying any deficiency. The instruction for giving medication should be clear and specific. It helps if the doctor tells the mother that "I need to give two types of medicines. This tablet is to bring down his fever, and you should give half of this tablet when the patient has high fever. The other is an antibiotic tablet which must be taken twice daily, say at 8:00 AM and 8:00 PM, for next 5 days till Friday this week". Sometimes you may need to demonstrate a skill, e.g. using an inhaler for asthma. It is a good idea to demonstrate it in the clinic and supplement it with written information or a video clip. Finally, before the patient leaves the clinic, check the mother's understanding by asking open-ended checking questions (e.g. how many times you will give the tablets?).

Key Box 8

Steps in Sharing Information

1. Outline the salient aspects of information in your mind.
2. Use words and examples that are likely to be understood by the parents.
3. Take in account the parent's expectations and fears, while talking.
4. Include only as much information that can be handled at one time.
5. Be aware of the non-verbal communi- cation and make them congruent with verbal message.
6. Select a noise free environment especially if the information is complex or important.
7. Get feedback and check if essential points have been understood.

5. Justify Investigations

Explain what tests you want to do and what these entail. Doctors hardly even explain to the parents why investigations are to be done and how these are to be performed. With a flourish of pen, a doctor will send a mother with a child to a strange dark room with gadgets and a stranger inside. Often parents get confused that a child who has rickets has been sent to the X-ray department and the child's hands have been X-rayed. The mother might think that the doctor has misunderstood the ailment.

6. Closure

At the end of interview, you should ask for any other concerns which the parents or the child may have. Summarize the plan agreed upon by the parents. You should also inform the parents about when to come for follow-up before they leave the clinic.

1.4 GIVING DIFFICULT NEWS TO PARENTS

Often, in clinical practice, you will encounter situations where you have to break bad news to parents. Breaking a bad news to parents is one of the most difficult responsibilities of physician in medical practice. A bad news could be pertaining to death, or a child being diagnosed with chronic disease or disability. It is the physician's attitude and communication skills that play a crucial role in how well the

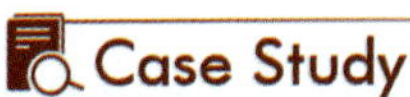

Case Study

Responding Appropriately to Caregivers' Concern

A mother comes to a doctor with her 1-year-old child (Jay). Her complaint is that the child had vomited last night. The doctor examines the child, reassures the mother, gives some instructions as to the diet and writes a prescription. While the doctor is writing the prescription, the mother adds that her mother (child's grandmother) thinks that Jay is not growing well. "Don't worry" says the doctor and asks the next patient to come in.

The real motivation for consulting in this case appears to be anxiety about the child's growth and the vomiting episode is only a precipitating event. In such a case, you should probe further and check why the mother is concerned about growth. If, after detailed history and examination, you find that there is no problem, you should reassure the mother.

An appropriate response in the above example should have been as follows:

Doctor—Why does your mother feel that Jay is not growing well (open question).

Mother—My brother's son was born 2 months later than Jay and he weighs more!

Doctor—I see. I am glad Jay's grandmother is taking interest in Jay's growth. Let us see the growth card (continued conversation and praised).

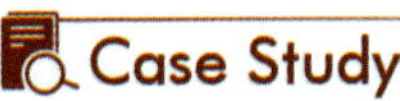

Case Study

Counseling a Parent who Insists on Leaving against Medical Advice (LAMA)

Kiran was admitted 2 days back with bronchopneumonia in your ward. On the 3rd day, you reach the child to examine her. You hear agitated parents say: Doctor, I want to take the child home. How do you handle such a situation?

Inappropriate response

Mother: (in an angry tone) Doctor, I want to take my child home. Please discharge her.

Doctor: (surprised) But she is not well enough to go home.

Mother: It has been 2 days and the child is showing no improvement.

Doctor: It will take another 3–4 days to get alright!! You cannot be so impatient!

Mother: I am not impatient! You would not say this, if it was your child!

Doctor: (in an agitated tone) Do as you please. Sign this form. Take her away. We will not give her any papers......

Appropriate response

Mother: (in an angry tone) Doctor, I want to take Kiran home.

Doctor: I can see you are upset. What is the problem?

Mother: It has been three days. She has been pricked all over and still she is not well.

Doctor: Oh dear! Let me see how she is doing. (examines the child) It seems that she has started taking oral feeds and the fever is much less.

Mother: (no longer angry and pauses)..... Yes. But you see this swelling. (shows the doctor the swelling due to extravasation of IV fluid) It was not there when we came in. She was not letting me touch her arm last night. I kept asking the doctor on night duty, but he never bothered to have a look at the swelling!

Doctor: I am sorry about that. I can understand that you are upset that Kiran is in pain. I will give some medicine to reduce the pain. The swelling should get better in a day. The medicines for pneumonia are working fine and we may discharge Kiran after a couple of days.

Lesson learnt

Parents were more worried about the swelling of hand rather than the lack of improvement which would have been missed unless probed with sensitivity and calm attitude. The doctor acknowledges that the mother is upset and empathized with mother's distress at the child having pain.

Key Box 9

Checklist for Delivering Bad News to Parents (Kaye's model for breaking bad news)

1. ***Preparation:*** Know all the facts, ensure privacy, find out from parents as to who should be present during the session, and introduce yourself.
2. ***What do the parents know?*** Use open-ended questions, statements may make the best questions, use phrases like "How did it all start?"
3. ***Is more information wanted?*** Do not force on them; ask them "Would you like me to explain a bit more?"
4. ***Give a warning shot:*** You may probably say "I'm afraid it looks rather serious".
5. ***Allow denial:*** Allow the patient to control the amount of information they receive.
6. ***Explain if requested:*** Step by step. Detail will not be remembered but the way you explain it will be.
7. ***Listen to concerns*** "What are your concerns at the moment?" Allow time and space for answers.
8. ***Encourage ventilation of feelings:*** Acknowledge the feelings. Be non-judgmental. This is a vital step for patient satisfaction.
9. ***Summarize:*** Outline concerns, plans for treatment, Foster hope.
10. ***Provide with written information/your availability***.

parents are able to cope when they receive the bad news. Kaye's model for delivering bad news to parents is shown in **Key Box 9**.

Generally, a senior member of the team should deliver such news. However, all doctors should master this skill. The basic steps of this task are outlined:

1. Choose the right time and place of conversation

Privacy to the child and parents and undivided attention of the physician is a must for this situation. Turn off your mobile phone. Introduce yourself and ensure that relatives are seated comfortably.

At the outset, physician must be well-prepared and must be aware of the entire medical record; and should also have a thorough knowledge of the condition being discussed.

2. Assess understanding

Assess the parents' understanding of the child's disease by asking them what they have been told of the problem. Often the parents sense a problem, but are unable to express it in words. Share their perceptions in a neutral manner. Correct any misinformation and tailor it to the parental level of understanding. You can start the conversation by saying "It is indeed sad, but I have a bad news to share about your child".

3. Be supportive and empathetic towards the parents

Your tone and manner should be open and available. Your demeanor should reflect your concern, but at the same time you should remain calm. Let the parents express their feelings, and you should empathize with their feelings. Speak compassionately, avoid use of medical jargons, proceed slowly at pace of parental understanding allowing sufficient time for silence and tears.

4. Accept the parents' reaction

How the parents react to the illness or death depends upon their personality, socio-cultural factors, and religious beliefs.

- In traditional Indian society, illness and death used to be generally accepted with stoicism and as will of the God.
- Grief and emotional breakdown are common reactions.
- Many parents may react with denial.
- In some cases, frustration, sadness, and anger associated with illness can lead parents and family members to become suspicious and aggressive.

These emotions are in reaction to the illness of the child and are generally not directed at the physician at a personal level. You will need to learn to accept these different reactions.

5. Empathize with their feelings of grief

You need not agree with all that they say but you can still accept their feelings. For example, a patient has been brought from a nursing home where her diagnosis of the disease was missed, and she died after coming to your hospital. The parents might feel hostile to the referring physician. You can accept their feelings in a neutral manner by saying "I can see that you are upset with care your child got in the nursing home". This means you are accepting that the parents are agitated, but you are not taking sides. It is better not to react to all that the parents say at such a time. Be silent, and take pauses in between conversation. Difficult news takes time to sink. Give time to parents to process any news of chronic or disabling illness. Often you may need to reschedule another visit when parents can ask questions about the illness. It is good to be honest, frank, and compassionate. Avoid using words that create hopelessness. Avoid either being defensive or placing blames on other professional colleagues.

6. Convey information in a simple language

At the end of the meeting, summarize the information provided and ask if the parents have any questions to ask or any other concerns.

Conclusion

Good communication skills are fundamental to a good patient–doctor relationship. The encounter is meaningful and satisfactory when the doctor exhibits good communication skills. It is essential for pediatricians and residents to develop the soft skills of communication before they proceed to eliciting the history and performing examination of the child.

Chapter 2

History-taking in Pediatrics

❍ Jaya Shankar Kaushik ❍ Piyush Gupta

Structure

2.1 OBJECTIVES, PROCESS, AND SEQUENCE OF HISTORY-TAKING

1. Objectives of History-taking

The parents contact the pediatrician for improving, maintaining, or restoring health of their children. As a doctor for the child, you have three tools to arrive at a diagnosis, before remedy can be offered. These three tools are history, examination, and investigations.

History-taking is the most important amongst them, because not only history-taking will guide examination and investigation but also in many cases, history is the only indicator of abnormality. For example, examination and investigation may not provide any evidence of epilepsy and for problems suffered in past. In most cases, history helps to arrive at diagnosis; physical examination and investigation have a complementary role. History-taking also gives an opportunity to build rapport with the child and parents and has some anxiety relieving value. **Key Box 1** summarizes the objectives of history-taking.

Key Box 1

Objectives of History-taking

1. To elicit an accurate account of the symptoms that represent the clinical problem.
2. To help in arriving at a diagnosis.
3. To develop rapport with the child and the parents.

2. Process of History-taking

History-taking is not a mere collection of data concerning health and disease, but the process of getting information is also important. The interview should be a pleasant experience and should help in making a lasting relationship. The interview should end but parents and child should be left with a desire to have another appointment.

Whenever suitable, talk with the child to understand his/her problems, like an individual. History-taking should be in a respectable environment for the child and parents/caregivers.

- Ensure that the history is elicited in an appropriate place. Greet the parents with a gentle smile.
- There should be a seating arrangement for the informants.
- Always introduce yourself and explain, why you want to know about the child's history.
- Always wear decent clothes with an apron and a stethoscope to make an appropriate impression.
- Environment and ambience should exude confidence and comfort both for the child and the parents.

- Ask questions in the language the parents understand.
- Always use open-ended questions for taking the history; it not only helps in diagnosis but also in planning the treatment.
- Follow the standard sequence in obtaining history; this is outlined further in this section.
- The process of history-taking should begin and end as a naturally progressing conversation. Avoid the format of question answer session like a *viva-voce*.
- Try to gather information in the shortest possible time.
- Avoid recording the entire narration. Parents often get apprehensive when they see that their words are being noted down. Prefer to record briefly only at the end of your conversation. This also ensures that flow of ideas is not blocked or distracted.

The essentials of the process of history-taking are summarized in **Key Box 2**.

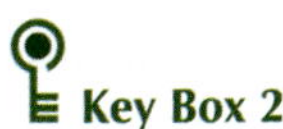

Key Box 2

Process of History-taking

1. *Place* Privacy and without disturbances
2. *Informant* Mother, caretaker or an eyewitness to the event
3. *Setting* Comfortable
4. *Language* Understandable, no ambiguity
5. *Observation* Avoid interpretations
6. *Sequence* From present to past, and individual to family to society.

History-taking in Adolescents

In comparison to adults who can communicate with doctors in privacy and confidentiality, adolescents may not be able to communicate as freely. Certain aspects of history can be elicited only if privacy and confidentiality is maintained, e.g. history of certain problems, like nocturnal enuresis, perianal itching, HIV, thumb sucking, and issues related to sexuality. Girls should be preferably interviewed by a female doctor. If not possible, then in the presence of female nurse.

3. Sequence of History-taking

The history-taking should have a sequence, from present to past including all the events affecting health and disease.

1. ***General information*** Start with the general information and background.
2. ***Presenting complaints*** Brief summary of the complaints with which the child is brought to the health facility, in a numbered chronological sequence.
3. ***History of presenting illness*** Describe the entire course of illness till date, in a narrative format.
4. ***Past illness*** Record all medical illnesses which have occurred till date.
5. ***Personal details*** After obtaining the history of illnesses, i.e. present and past, obtain information on all other important events in the child's life till date.
   a. *Conception to birth and thereafter* Start from the birth; also include important points before and after birth (antenatal, natal, and postnatal history).
   b. *Development* Proceed to enquire how the child achieved maturation of functions after birth (developmental history).
   c. *Immunization* Ask for all vaccinations received from birth till date, or examine the vaccination card, if available.
   d. *Diet and nutritional history* Adequate nutrition is a must for growth and well-being of the child. Enquire about the dietary habits and daily intake of calorie and proteins. Starting from breastfeeding, elicit history of complementary feeding, and the present day dietary intake.
6. ***Family details*** Obtain information about the family including parents and sibs, any illness in the family, consanguinity, etc.
7. ***Social history*** Finally, get to know the social background to which the child belongs.

Logically, history-taking should proceed from present to past, including all the events which have a significant impact on health and disease. For example, if the child presents with fever and seizures, obtain the details of these complaints first and then elicit past history of febrile seizures or any other seizures in the past. The sequence should be such that information is obtained about the sick child first, then the family, and then about the social background to which the patient belongs.

The emphasis on different aspects of history may vary according to age of child, e.g. antenatal and birth history will be more important in newborn and infants; breastfeeding history in first few months of life; development history in pre-school years; performance in school; and effects of peers in school-going children. It also depends on the case being analyzed. For example, in a child with developmental delay, emphasis will be on birth and developmental history.

The 10 steps of history-taking are highlighted in **Key Box 3**.

The usual clinical evaluation consists of history-taking and physical examination, conducted in that order. This is followed by investigations, making diagnosis, and planning management **(Fig. 2.1)**. However, history and examination are not two separate water-tight compartments. In practice, you will find that history and examination may proceed simultaneously. It is also possible that a problem is identified which deserves immediate management even before history and examination are undertaken, e.g. child getting convulsions (needs anticonvulsant), high fever (sponging to bring down the temperature), bleeding (stop bleeding first), respiratory distress, shock, etc. All such situations require management first; details of history should be obtained after or along with concurrent management.

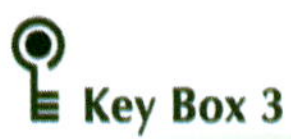

The Sequence: 10 Steps of History-taking

1. General information
2. Presenting or chief complaints
3. History of present illness and treatment history
4. Past history
5. Antenatal, natal and postnatal history
6. Developmental history
7. Immunization history
8. Nutrition and dietary history
9. Family history and pedigree charting
10. Socioeconomic history

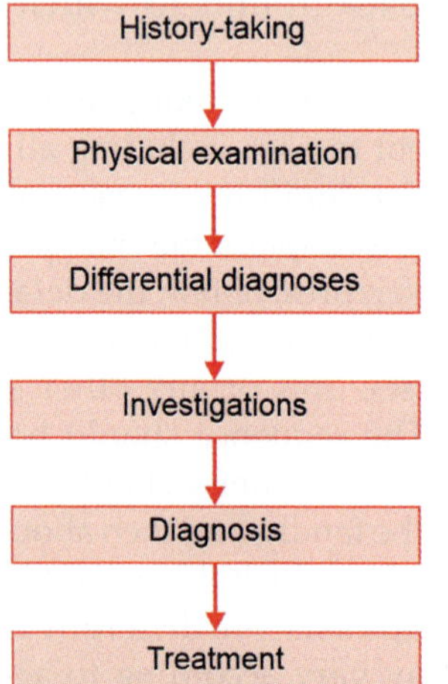

Fig. 2.1: Usual process of managing a patient.

2.2 COMPONENTS OF HISTORY-TAKING

1. Informant and Reliability

The accuracy and reliability of history will depend on the person providing the information. Most of the time it is best to obtain information from the mother; if it is not possible, then from the person involved in care (e.g. grandparents) or the person present at the time of development of problems, e.g. school teacher or colleagues in the school or hostel. However, only the mother can provide accurate account of antenatal, natal, postnatal period, early feeding, developmental and treatment history.

2. General Information

The general information includes name of the child, mother and father, sex, age, date and time of birth (particularly in case of newborn). Also, obtain complete postal address, telephone and mobile numbers **(Key Box 4)**. General information is crucial to establish identity of the individual. Details of address help to identify the child with geographical distribution of diseases and also the family can be contacted, if they fail to report for follow-up. Diseases also have a distribution among castes and religions, so this information is also needed. Also there

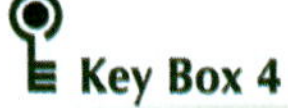

General Information

1. Name
2. Age (date of birth)
3. Sex
4. Complete address
5. Religion/cast (if relevant)
6. Name(s) of the mother and the father
7. Telephone number(s)
8. Date and time of history-taking

Tips for students

- If the child is <1-yr-old, or if you are thinking of an inborn error of metabolism or a genetic disease, then use the phrase "product of consanguineous/non-consanguineous marriage" (as the case may be).
- Always mention the place where the child first reported at, i.e. whether it was an outpatient visit or emergency visit. This may signify the severity of illness at the time of presentation.
- Prefer stating that "child was brought 5 days back to emergency room" rather than mentioning date and time of presentation (so that examiner does not have to calculate!)

Other details like names of father, and mother; and the telephone number may be recorded in your case sheet but they need not be mentioned while you are presenting the case.

are certain social schemes to provide special benefit during sickness, or for those socially deprived or those below poverty line. The general information should include date and time of history-taking, name of informant, and his/her relationship with the child.

3. Presenting or Chief Complaints

These are the complaints for which the child is brought to the hospital. They may be one or more. Record them in patient's/ parent's own words, and in chronological order along with duration of each complaint **(Key Box 5)**. The beginning of acute problems is precise in terms of date and time of appearance of symptom; while in chronic disorders, the beginning of the problems may be vague. When the presenting complaints are more than one, try to identify those, the parents are worried about the most.

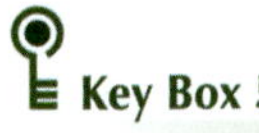

Key Box 5

Presenting Complaints

1. Complaints with duration
2. Chronological order

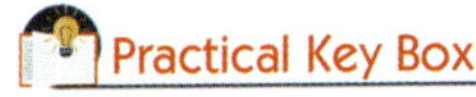

Practical Key Box

I am presenting a case of Naman, 3-yr-old boy, resident of Shahdara, Delhi. The informant is mother and history seems to be reliable. The child was brought to pediatric casualty 6 days back with presenting complaints of....

Number of Chief Complaints

Number of presenting complaints should be kept minimum (maximum 3–4), but should include all major symptoms (important for making a hypothesis). Complaints which after detailed history and examination are found to be medically insignificant may not be included in the presenting complaints (at the discretion of presenter's insight and experience).

Arrange Complaints in the Order of their Appearance

Complaints should be written in chronological order with duration. Chronology of symptoms is important as it gives a clue to the underlying pathophysiological process. Duration should be specific rather than stating a time interval (e.g. 10 days instead of 1–2 weeks). Chief complaint, 'Fever for 10 days', implies that the child was well 10 days back. Fever started 10 days back and is still persisting.

Provide the Status of Complaints till Date

Some important complaints may originate and evolve during the hospital stay, if you are eliciting history in a hospitalized child. Again, they can be included as chief complaints, depending on their merit and importance to the diagnosis and course of the disease. Present the chief complaints and history as on the day you are examining and presenting the case, irrespective of the date of hospitalization.

Example

A child presented 10 days back to the emergency department with chief complaints of abnormal movements (convulsions) and fever. The child was admitted. On day 5 of hospitalization, the parents noticed that the child was not able to move the left side of the body including both upper and lower limbs.

Presenting complaints (as on today):

1. Fever—10 days
2. One episode of abnormal movements—10 days back
3. Inability to move the left half of the body—5 days

Provide the Status of Complaints till Date in a Telegraphic Language

For example, a child was well 10 days back. To start with, he had fever which lasted for

5 days. The child developed a rash over body on 3rd day of fever which lasted for 4 days. As soon as the fever subsided, parents noticed that the child is in altered sensorium which gradually increased and now the child is unconscious and does not respond to verbal commands. The child had 2 episodes of left-sided convulsions 3 days prior to admission and since then he is not moving the left side of the body.

The chief complaints are to be recorded as follows:

	Chief complaints	Duration
1.	Fever lasting for 5 days	10 days back
2.	Rash for 4 days	7 days back
3.	Altered sensorium	5 days
4.	Two episodes of left-sided convulsions	3 days back
5.	Not moving the left half of the body	3 days

This implies that the total duration of illness is 10 days. The illness started with fever which lasted for first five days only. Rash appeared 7 days back and lasted for 4 days. This also depicts that at present there is no fever or rash. This child had 2 episodes of left focal seizures on day 8 of illness, which were followed by neurological weakness of the same side. At present, the child is having altered sensorium (for last 5 days) and is not able to move the left side of the body (for last 3 days).

Include Words to Indicate Character, Nature, and Course of the Complaints

It is desirable that the chief complaints convey an idea about the character of the symptom. This may help in getting to the diagnosis faster. It is better to say "Intermittent high grade fever with chills and rigors for 3 days" (points to malaria as a probable etiology) than simply stating "Fever for 3 days" (you remain clueless!).

Similarly, it is also advantageous, if the symptom is presented to reflect the course and progress of the disease process. For example, to indicate a gradually increasing ascites, chief complaint should be framed as "progressively growing uniform distension of abdomen for 3 months" rather than stating it as "distension of abdomen for 3 months". Also note the word 'uniform' which may help differentiate the swelling due to ascites from that due to a lump or hepatosplenomegaly (which will be localized to a particular region of the abdomen). Another example could be "progressively increasing paleness of the body" instead of saying "paleness" for 3 months.

Chief Complaints for a Chronic Illness

Some diseases begin insidiously and present with full blown disease later with a waxing or waning course (e.g. arthritis leading to valvular heart disease and heart failure); some have long periods of symptom-free interval or remission (e.g. nephrotic syndrome); some diseases are otherwise latent but manifest with acute exacerbations (e.g. bronchial asthma, epilepsy); some diseases are complication of illness in past (paralysis and myocarditis in a child with diphtheria). In all such instances, the chief complaints should be structured so as to convey the overall duration and course of the disease rather than listing only those problems with which the patient has come to you now.

A child with nephrotic syndrome may present to you with generalized swelling over body and decreased urine output for 2 days. However, on further questioning, you get to know that the child has had repeated similar episodes before; these episodes lasted from one week to one month and responded to therapy. The chief complaints in this case will be as follows:

	Chief complaints	Duration
1.	Repeated episodes of generalized swelling of body associated with diminished urinary output lasting for 1–4 weeks, with symptom-free intervals of 2–6 months in between episodes	For 2 years
2.	Generalized swelling of body associated with diminished urinary output	For 2 days

In a child with rheumatic fever, now presenting with heart disease and congestive failure, chief complaints should be presented as follows:

	Chief complaints	Duration
1.	Fever for 3 weeks	6 months back
2.	Migratory pain and swelling in large joints for 2 weeks	6 months back
3.	Palpitation and breathlessness	6 days
4.	Swelling over both feet and diminished urine output	2 days

You would notice that even though fever and joint pains occurred 6 months back and lasted for 1 month; these complaints are included as a part of present history and cited as chief complaints rather than listing them under the history of past illness. This helps in building the hypothesis and making a working diagnosis. The first two complaints point to a rheumatic origin of the heart disease (indicated by the last two complaints). You would have been groping in dark about the etiology had you listed only the complaint numbers 3 and 4 under the chief complaints.

Chief Complaints can be included in Retrospect

This may appear strange, but sometimes it is inevitable. Complaints may be added after the detailed history is taken or even after the physical examination. Sometimes an attendant does not come up with all the symptoms. For example, a mother may complain of progressively increasing pallor of body, swellings in the neck, and fever for 1 month. On physical examination, you notice petechial hemorrhages on limbs and bleeding from gums. You should ask the informant whether they have noticed it. If the answer is yes, ask for how long this has been there. These complaints should then be added to the list of chief complaints as they add to make the hypothesis and frame a diagnosis. Addition of this complaint signifies a bleeding disorder which when clubbed with fever, neck swellings (lymph nodes) and pallor; suggests affliction of reticuloendothelial system with involvement of all 3 cell lines (red cell, white cell, and platelet). Any long-standing complaint of poor activity, lethargy, restlessness, irritability, loss of weight and appetite, loss of interest in play/surroundings should alert you to the possibility of a chronic disease.

Mention any Known Illness Related to Complaints

Any underlying illness of which you are aware after a detailed history or examination, and is of such importance that it has direct understanding of the chief complaints, SHOULD be included in the chief complaints. For example, a 6-year-old child presents with fever for 5 days, vomiting for 2 days, and lethargy for 1 day. This should be modified as follows: *I am presenting a 6-year-old child, a known case of IDDM on insulin now presenting with fever, vomiting and lethargy*. This information clearly indicates that the first possibility is of diabetic ketoacidosis (infectious or other causes to be searched).

Key Box 6 provides some tips for formulating the presenting complaints.

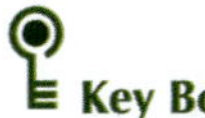

Key Box 6

6 Tips for Formulating Presenting Complaints

1. Describe complaints as described by parents along with their duration.
2. Arrange the complaints in chronological order.
3. Avoid use of medical terms as much as possible.
4. Try to restrict number of complaints to a maximum of 4.
5. Use appropriate phrases to describe the nature of presenting complaints.
6. Revisit your presenting complaint, after you have finished your examination to include retrospectively all significant findings which influence the understanding of illness and formulation of '*hypothesis.*'

4. History of Present Illness

The history of present illness should be an uninterrupted account of problems from beginning to till date, i.e. till the day you are taking, and presenting the history. This, therefore, also includes the time period after hospitalization, if the child is admitted as an in-patient. The course during hospital stay should be in the same flow rather than a separate heading.

The Process

The history should be recorded as paragraphic, orderly detailed description of each of the chief complaints. Remember, every case is

Example: Chief Complaints can be Included in Retrospect

A severely malnourished child presents to you with loose stools for last 3 days.

If we frame the chief complaint as "Loose stools: 3 days", it gives an impression of an acute illness, e.g. acute diarrhea but ignores the nutritional diagnosis.

To obviate the problem, you can ask the informant directly "for how long the child has been losing weight/unable to gain weight?"

Informant tells you that the child is losing weight for last 6 months. On probing further, you may even get to know that the child has lost interest in surroundings and is less interactive. Also, there have been three more episodes of loose motions over last 2 months. Now, the chief complaints will be framed as follows:

1. Progressive loss of weight and appetite: For 6 months
2. Decreased physical activity, increased irritability and loss of interest in play: For 3 months
3. Multiple episodes of loose stools: For 2 months

Inference The child is having a long-standing illness, is losing weight, has a change in behavior, and also having recurrent gastrointestinal infection.

See, how the tenor of your inference has changed!

a mystery, and the challenge is to find the diagnosis. The history should be elicited to obtain clues to help in solving the mystery. Clues can be both positive and negative; these should contribute to a total understanding of the sequential events that have led to the present state of the patient.

Eliciting History

The history starts with the opening line that the patient was apparently well (till the date of onset of the first complaint) when he/she developed (first complaint). This history is best taken and recorded in patient's own words or language. However, some points may be rephrased for clear understanding and to avoid misinterpretation. All parents/patients may not be able to narrate a satisfactory uninterrupted account of their problems; some may be hesitant while others may provide lot of unnecessary information and details. Hence, it is important to modify the course of communication tactfully. Do not include a detailed treatment history in "History of Presenting Illness". A constant active communication is necessary throughout the process of history-taking. Involvement of other people should be strictly avoided as it disrupts the privacy of the patient.

Expand the Chief Complaints

Once a complete history has been taken, each symptom should be analyzed in detail both *qualitatively* and *quantitatively*. While taking the details of particular symptom it is important to insist on observations and NOT on interpretation as it is general tendency of caregivers to mix the two. For example, if a mother of 3 months old child says that her child has pain abdomen, it is her interpretation and not observation. Instead, a history of abdominal distension or excessive crying should be asked.

Each symptom should be assessed under the following headings. Onset (exact date and time of onset), nature of onset (acute, insidious or chronic), duration, frequency, consistency (intermittent, continuous or remittent), severity, evolution (progression, static or regression), aggravating and relieving factors, any diurnal variation, associated symptoms and response to treatment **(Key Box 7)**.

The factors on the basis of which a symptom is analyzed will depend upon the likelihood of the possible cause. For example, fever should be analyzed for duration, type of onset, character, degree and severity, presence of chills and rigors, sweating, association with cough, loose motions, burning micturition, etc. for focus of infections. Also enquire whether the fever has increased, decreased or showing stationary trend.

Similarly, complaint of loose motion should be analyzed for duration, frequency, consistency, volume of each stool, presence of blood, mucus, color, foul smell, relation with

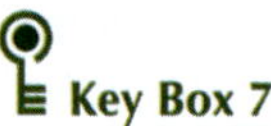

Analysis of Each Symptom

1. Onset—Time and nature
2. Duration, frequency, and consistency
3. Evolution and severity
4. Aggravating and relieving factors
5. Associated symptoms

Practical Key Box

How to Frame Chief Complaints

Problem 1

A 3-month-old infant was brought with fever and cough for 3 days and has not been feeding well. The child is apparently having difficulty in breathing since last evening.

Presenting complaints

1. Fever and cough for 3 days
2. Fast breathing and refusal to feed since last evening

Note that the complaints are described in chronological order; and not used any medical terms. One can club the complaints of similar duration like fever and cough for 3 days. (This restricts the number of presenting complaints to 2 only.)

Problem 2

A 4-year-old boy was brought with fever which was high grade with rigors for last 10 days (afebrile for last 2 days), and an episode of generalized tonic-clonic seizure (GTCS) 4 days back. Following this episode of GTCS, the child remained in unconscious state for next 4 days. Child was brought to you on 10th day of illness.

Presenting complaints

1. High grade fever off and on for 8 days, till 2 days back
2. An episode of abnormal body movement 4 days back
3. Altered sensorium for last 4 days

- *Use of phrase like "off and on" takes care of varying nature of presenting complaints.*
- *We have restricted to 3 complaints and have avoided using medical terms. The word "GTCS" has been replaced with "an episode of abnormal movement".*
- *A common mistake done by many students is in use of words "for" and "since" interchangeably, for stating the duration of complaints. Generally, use 'for' for an approximate duration; and use 'since' for an exact duration. For example: Fever for 1 day OR fever since 1pm yesterday. It is incorrect to say: "fever off and on since 10 days".*

Problem 3

A 5-year-old girl presented 10 days back to emergency department with a generalized tonic-clonic seizure (GTCS) and was admitted. Subsequently, the child continued to have multiple episodes of seizure for next 3 days. Child was in unconscious state for initial 5 days. Parents have now noticed decreased movements (stated as weakness by the parents) of left upper and lower limbs for last 2 days. Frame presenting complaints.

Presenting complaints

1. Multiple episodes of abnormal movement of whole body for 3 days, *starting* 10 days back
2. Altered sensorium *for* initial 5 days, *till* 5 days back
3. Decreased movements of left upper and lower limbs for last 2 days

- *When significant events have happened even after hospitalization; you should present the history as on today (i.e. the day when you saw the patient).*
- *We have included significant events which happened in hospital stay, like multiple episodes of seizure, altered sensorium, and probably (left) hemiparesis.*
- *It is unfair to present this case with presenting complaints of "An episode of abnormal movement 10 days back" alone as it misses refractory seizures, encephalopathy, and evolving hemiparesis which entirely changes our hypothesis.*

Problem 4

A 5-month-old boy was brought with fever, cough, and fast breathing for 5 days; and refusal to feed for the last 2 days. On enquiry, there were two similar episodes in the past at 1½ and 3½ months of age for which the child was hospitalized for 10 days each.

Presenting complaints

1. Three episodes of fever, cough, and fast breathing since the age of 1½ months
2. Fever, cough and fast breathing for 5 days
3. Refusal to feed for last 2 days

- *Any illness in past which appears to be a continuation with the current illness must be included in the presenting complaints.*
- *For instance, if we present the same case as "fever, cough, and fast breathing for 5 days" you might probably think of "pneumonia" alone; whereas with presenting complaints as formulated in our problem, you will think of "recurrent pneumonia" and outline the relevant causes—for example, congenital heart disease.*
- *In this problem, the history of presenting illness would start from age 1½ months. Describe the first episode, and then convey that similar three episodes have occurred since then. Child has now presented with the third episode.*

Problem 5

A 7-year-old girl presented with an episode of generalized tonic-clonic seizures (GTCS) that occurred yesterday evening. There is a history of similar episodes (once in 2 months) since the age of 4 years.

Presenting complaints

1. Multiple episodes of abnormal movement since the age of 4 years [or for last 3 years]
2. An episode of abnormal movement yesterday evening

- *Use word "multiple" when number exceed 3.*
- *Details of seizures like frequency could be mentioned in 'History of present illness'.*
- *Remember we have followed the principles we started with.*

Problem 6

A 1½-year-old boy presented with an episode of focal seizure today morning. Child is developmentally delayed and keeps all four limbs tight. On enquiry, child had delayed cry at birth, developed seizure on 1st day of life, and was admitted in NICU for 15 days. At present, child cannot sit and has not even attained neck holding. He cannot speak as compared to the neighbor's son.

Presenting complaints

1. Inability to sit and speak *till* now (or since birth)
2. Tightening of all 4 limbs noticed by parents *since* the age of 3 months
3. An episode of focal seizures today morning

- *The problems start right from birth. This was followed by developmental delay. Other significant co-morbidities (hypertonia and seizures) are also included.*

---

food, abdominal pain, worm infestation, fluid intake (type and quantity), and frequency and amount of urine. If there was a history of loose motions, obviously you would also want to know whether it was accompanied by fever, vomiting, dehydration, or electrolyte imbalance. Ask following questions to assess dehydration: was the child thirsty or refused fluids, whether urine output diminished or not, were the eyes appeared sunken or not? To confirm or rule out the presence of dyselectrolytemia, ask for the history of convulsions (these would occur, if there is associated hypoglycemia, hypernatremia, hypocalcemia or hyponatremia) and abdominal distension (hypokalemia).

Determine the Inter-relationship between the Symptoms

It is possible that more than one complaint can be because of a single cause (e.g. fever, cough and breathlessness all can be caused

Example: Analysis of Fever

Ask for

1. Onset	Started 8 days back
2. Nature of onset	Sudden, noticed when child woke-up in the morning
3. Duration	Persisting for last 8 days
4. Frequency	2–3 spikes of fever, more in evening hours
5. Character	Intermittent/continuous/remittent
6. Severity	High grade, documented up to 105°F
7. Evolution	Occurring daily for initial 5 days and then child was afebrile for the next 2 days, but again having fever for last 1 day
8. Aggravating or relieving factor	Relieved for 4 hours when given drug (paracetamol)
9. Diurnal variation	More in evening
10. Associated symptoms	Chills/rigors/loose motions

A similar analysis can be done for almost every complaint in the history of present illness.

by a respiratory tract infection). On the other hand, a single complaint may have more than one cause (e.g. generalized edema can be due to malnutrition; or liver, kidney or heart disease). The history of presenting complaints should thus include all information relevant to the possible system(s) involved, e.g. if a child presents with bilateral swelling of legs, then a detailed history of other symptoms related to cardiac, renal, liver and gastrointestinal tract should be obtained.

In a child presenting with fever of 10 days, you will have to search for its focus by obtaining history relevant to almost all systems, i.e. skin (boils, abscess, etc.), GIT (diarrhea, vomiting, constipation, abdominal distension), hepatobiliary (jaundice, pain abdomen, distension), throat (cough, dysphagia, throat pain), larynx (hoarse voice, stridor), trachea (stridor, brassy cough), lower respiratory tract (cough, breathlessness, wheeze), lower urinary tract (burning micturition, frequency, urgency), renal (flank pain with vomiting), CNS (headache, vomiting, neurological weakness, convulsions, altered sensorium), musculoskeletal (joint swelling and pain, myalgia), and reticulo-endothelial system (anemia, swellings suggestive of lymphadenopathy, bleeding from any site and blue patches).

5. Negative History

A negative history is taken to rule in or rule out involvement of a system, identify the nature and etiology of the disease process, assess the severity and complications, and differentiate between the likely diagnostic probabilities.

Negative history does not mean what all is NOT present. Symptoms asked for should be relevant to the history of present illness. For example, it is incorrect to mention negative history of burning micturition in a child presenting with fever and cough for 2 days, since you already have a focus of fever (i.e. in the respiratory tract). Relevant negative history in this example may include: No history of fast breathing, noisy breathing, wheezy sounds from chest, or difficulty of feeding.

Example: Eliciting Negative History

A 2-year-old child is brought with 10–15 episodes of vomiting. Elicit negative history:

1. Rule out involvement of system:
   - *CNS:* No history of head banging/irritability/photophobia
   - *GI tract:* Diarrhea/abdominal distension/constipation
   - *Hepatobiliary system:* High colored urine/yellow eyes
2. For nature and etiology of disease process:
   - *Obstruction* Bilious vomiting
   - *Raised ICT* Projectile vomiting
   - *Upper GI bleed* Blood in vomitus
3. For assessing severity and complications:
   - *Dehydration:* Excessive lethargy, decreased urinary output
   - *Dyselectrolytemia:* Convulsions, altered sensorium
   - *Acidosis:* Fast deep breathing

When a sick child is brought to you, there may be many points related to history which may not be brought up by parents, as they are not considered relevant to present problems. So apart from details of history of present illness, you should make a systematic enquiry for identifying disorders of various organs and systems. It is likely that some positive points may be identified—their details should be obtained, but most of enquiry of system review will remain negative. This negative history will try to help you in excluding disorder of these organs and systems to a great extent.

State all the negative history together at the end. Do not incorporate description of negative history after each and every complaint.

6. Review of Systems

A. General

i. ***Growth and development*** Whether this child is growing and achieving milestones normally in comparison to others of same age or not.

ii. ***Appetite*** How parents describe the appetite of this child. Most of the parents will complain of poor appetite, so it should always be correlated with weight change and activity of child.

iii. ***Sleep*** Whether adequate, recent change, remains sleepy in day.

iv. ***Physical activity*** Normal, decreased, over-active, hyperactive causing disturbance to others.

v. ***Behavior*** Normal, quiet, shy, out-spoken, friendly, quarrelsome particularly with siblings.

vi. ***School*** School performance and relationship with peers, opinion of teachers.

B. Gastrointestinal Tract and Abdomen

Nausea, vomiting, abdominal fullness, diarrhea, constipation, retrosternal or abdominal pain, pain during swallowing or defecation, jaundice, worms in stool, bleeding per rectum.

C. Respiratory System

Cough, dyspnea, stridor, snoring, wheezing, chest pain; family history of tuberculosis, asthma, eczema, pets and smoking.

D. Cardiovascular System

Breathlessness, cyanosis, palpitation, edema over feet, cough, recurrent chest infection, joint pain, pain in right hypochondrium, abdominal distension.

E. Nervous System

Convulsions, loss of consciousness, paralysis, speech problems, vision or hearing problems, abnormal body movements, sensory disturbances, gait abnormalities, bowel and bladder disturbances, pain in neck, abnormal posture, headache, vomit, neck retraction.

F. Urinary System

Change in urinary frequency and amount, color of urine, edema, pain in micturition, flank pain or mass, nocturnal enuresis.

G. Genital System

Age appropriate growth and changes in primary and secondary sex characters; menstruation in girls, pain, discharge and swelling related to genitalia.

H. Blood

Pallor (anemia), fatigue, dyspnea, palpitation, edema, bleeding from various sites (skin, nose, GIT), swelling in neck, groin, etc. (lymph nodes), dietary intake (mainly milk diet will lead to iron deficiency anemia) drugs which may cause bleeding or bone marrow depression, family history of blood disorders, e.g. thalassemia, sickle cell anemia, etc.

I. Miscellaneous

Skin eruption and itching, joint pain and swelling, frequent falls and fluid intake.

> The system review enables to identify involvement of other organs and systems which are either simultaneously affected, or affected due to complication, or affected independently.

7. Past History

Record all major and significant events like illnesses, hospitalization, operation, injuries, etc. **(Key Box 8)**. Avoid accepting diagnosis, it is better to record details of problem experienced and then make your own hypothesis as to most likely diagnosis.

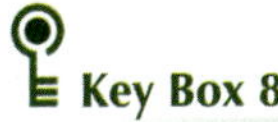

Key Box 8

Past History

1. Prolonged illness
2. Surgery and injuries
3. Hospitalization
4. Diarrhea, dysentery, worm infestation, vomiting, pneumonia, upper respiratory tract infection, malaria, otitis media, urinary tract infections, pertussis, diphtheria, tetanus, tuberculosis, measles, mumps, chickenpox, allergies

This should cover period starting from birth till appearance of present problem. If possible record exact date, duration and place where patient fell ill and received treatment, so if need arises, hospital which treated the child in past could be contacted.

Past history should be relevant. Relevant past history for a 9-year-old child with seizures would be *similar illness in the past, history of measles, and history of head trauma*.

Past history should include elicitation of common problems of childhood and those common in that region, e.g. diarrhea, dysentery, respiratory tract infection, malaria, otitis media, urinary tract infections, pertussis, diphtheria, tetanus, tuberculosis, measles, mumps, and allergies. You should not enquire by the name of the disease; rather ask for the key symptoms, which parents can identify easily. For example, for pertussis, ask for paroxysmal cough, more than 2 weeks duration, posttussive emesis, and whoop; similarly, for measles, ask for maculopapular rash appearing on face below hair line, on third day of fever, and with cough.

8. Drug and Treatment History

You should elicit information regarding various prescribed and self-administered drugs, surgical and dental intervention done, duration of treatment with dates, response to them and any untoward effects, any current therapy and in preceding few days. This is important to plan present therapy to adjust loading doses, e.g. if patient is receiving digoxin or phenobarbitone already, loading dose should not be given. Also enquire whether child is receiving any prophylactic (benzathine penicillin for rheumatic prophylaxis) or suppressive (steroids for nephrotic syndrome) therapy.

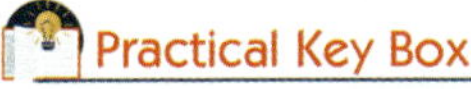

Practical Key Box

"Parents had consulted 2 practitioners prior to their hospital visit. Some oral medications were given, nature of which is not known. Since hospitalization at our center, child has been subjected to blood investigation and a lumbar puncture. Child has been receiving intravenous fluids, and injectable medications thrice a day (nature not known)..."

You should also find out if prescribed drugs were taken in proper doses for adequate duration. If not, ascertain the cause for poor compliance.

Ask for previous prescriptions, packing of partially used or empty containers to identify actual substance taken, because parents may not know generic names of drugs. It is also important to see packing or container of a drug which the child has consumed accidentally or intentionally. **Key Box 9** summarizes the salient points of treatment history.

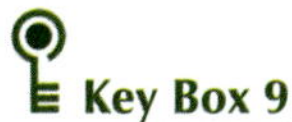

Key Box 9

Drug and Treatment History

1. Prescribed and non-prescribed
2. Amount and duration
3. Habit forming drugs
4. Surgical treatment
5. Adverse events following drug intake
6. Compliance to prescription

9. Antenatal, Natal, and Postnatal History

Events during these periods can affect the fetal growth and development, and neonatal morbidity and mortality. Some of these effects may be permanent.

Antenatal History

History of antenatal period should include information on maternal nutrition (whether diet was adequate and balanced or not), weight gain, illness (tuberculosis, hepatitis, asthma, epilepsy, toxemia of pregnancy, urinary tract infection, cardiac disease, HIV, syphilis, other STD; any obstetric complications, diabetes mellitus and hypertension), and drugs received by mother. Record information about antenatal check-ups, iron-folic acid

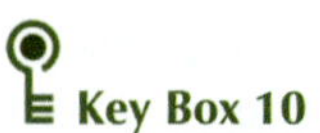

Key Box 10

Antenatal History

- Diet, drugs, and diseases of mother
- Iron and folic acid supplementation
- Tetanus vaccination
- Antenatal check-ups
- Fetal movements and growth

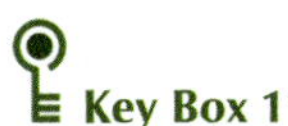

Key Box 11

History Points to be Elicited in Antenatal Period

A. First trimester

Ask for history of

1. Fever with rash (TORCH infection)
2. Swelling in occipital region (occipital adenopathy for rubella)
3. Drug intake
4. Radiation exposure
5. Alcohol/tobacco/substance abuse
6. Bleeding per vaginum

B. Second trimester

Ask for history of

1. Headache, swelling of feet, blurring of vision, documented hypertension (PIH)
2. Polyuria, polydipsia, deranged glucose readings (diabetes mellitus)
3. Fetal movements, bleeding per vaginum, blood transfusion
4. Weight gain

C. Third trimester

Ask for history of

1. Maternal fever
2. Bleeding per vaginum (APH, placenta previa)
3. Leaking per vaginum, foul smelling liqor (chorioamnionitis)
4. Diarrhea/urinary problem (ascending infection)

supplementation and tetanus vaccination. Obtain history of exposure to radiation, any previous abortions and adequacy of fetal movements **(Key Box 10** and **Key Box 11)**.

Birth History

Birth history **(Key Box 12)** should include place and mode of delivery, period of gestation, person conducting the delivery, color of amniotic fluid, duration of labor, particularly of second stage (from rupture of membranes to delivery of newborn), resuscitation required and its details, Apgar score, initiation of breastfeeding within first hour of birth, rooming in, birth weight, maternal fever, drugs given to mother like oxytocin, analgesic, and whether delivery was spontaneous or induced.

Also, ask for any history of instrumentation, time for expulsion of placenta, and whether postpartum period was uneventful. Ask whether there was any apparent birth injury.

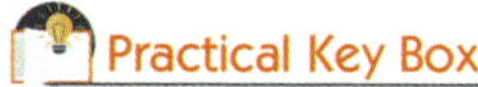

Practical Key Box

"Baby was born to 22-year-old third para mother at 9 months of gestation by vaginal delivery. Antenatal period was supervised; mother had received TT injection and had taken iron, folic acid supplementation for 2 months. Baby was born by vaginal delivery, cried immediately at birth, and weighed 3 kg. Immediate postnatal and neonatal periods were uneventful; breastfeeding was initiated within 2 hours of birth."

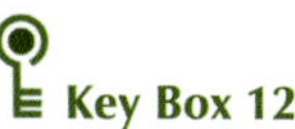

Key Box 12

Natal or Birth History

1. Place and mode of delivery
2. Person conducting the delivery
3. Duration of labor
4. Immediate cry

Postnatal History

Postnatal history **(Key Box 13)** should include details of cry after birth, extent of resuscitation required, time taken after birth to pass urine and meconium, when breastfeeding was started, any prelacteal feeds given, any problem in newborn period like breathing difficulty, poor feeding, jaundice, cyanosis, or seizures. Ask, when did the cord fall? Was

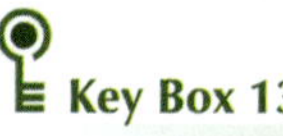

Key Box 13

Postnatal History

1. Birth weight
2. Preterm or full-term or post-term
3. Resuscitation requirement
4. Initiation of breastfeeding
5. Respiratory difficulty, cyanosis, jaundice, feeding difficulty

any treatment sought for any problem in the first month of life?

10. Developmental History

(also *see* Chapter 6)

Developmental history is aimed at assessing the integrity and maturation of central nervous system and special senses by examining the process of acquisition of new skills and behavior. A detailed description of developmental assessment is provided separately also in Chapter 6. Salient points are mentioned below.

Ask for developmental milestones the child has achieved. You should first ask for those milestones which the child should have achieved according to the chronologic age. For example, if the age of child is one year, ask for his ability to stand without support, walking with support, using lip sounds, like *mama, dada*. If a child has achieved milestones expected for his age, there is no need to ask for milestones to be achieved before this age. However, when there is a delay, it is important to record all the milestones in chronological age of appearance.

Developmental milestones should be assessed in all 4 fields, i.e. motor (gross motor, fine motor), adaptive, language, and personal-social fields. Always proceed in a stepwise manner exploring achievements in the four fields, separately. It is possible that development in one field is normal and delayed in the others. You can identify gross delay according to scheme given in **Table 2.1**. If developmental delay is identified in this screening, detailed history and assessment should be done (*see* Chapter 6).

11. Immunization History

The objective of taking immunization history is to ascertain whether the child is fully immunized appropriate for age **(Key Box 14)**. This would help in recommending the missed doses. If the child is vaccinated against a disease, it is unlikely he is suffering from that disease. It is also likely that the current presenting problem is related to recent vaccination, e.g. axillary lymphadenitis following BCG vaccine; mild rash after measles vaccine; and high fever, convulsion and encephalopathy following DPT vaccination.

Obtain immunization history under following headings: Name of vaccine administered, given where, by whom, if any vaccine missing reason for the same, and any adverse events following vaccination. Also see BCG scar. It is better to see the vaccination card and not rely on verbal information as to the dates of vaccination. Also ask if the child has received any newer vaccines, antisera or immunoglobins; apart from routine immunization. Enquire if the child has received oral polio vaccine during pulse polio immunization.

12. Nutrition and Dietary History

Your aim in taking nutritional and dietary history is to find whether the child is getting

Table 2.1: Screening schedule for developmental delay: Upper range

Age (months)	Gross motor	Adaptive	Social skills	Language
3	Some head control, supports weight on forearms	Opens hands spontaneously	Smiles appropriately	Coos, Laughs
6	Sits with support	Transfers objects	Shows likes and dislikes	Babbles
9	Pulls to stand	Pincer grasp	Plays pat-a-cake, peek-a-boo	Imitates sounds
12	Walks with one hand held	Releases object on demand	Comes when called	1–2 meaningful words
18	Walks upstairs with assistance	Feeds from a spoon	Mimics actions of others	At least 6 words
24	Runs	Builds a tower of six blocks	Plays with others	2–3 words sentences

Key Box 14

National Immunization Schedule 2024

Age	Vaccines given
Birth	Bacillus Calmette-Guérin (BCG), Oral Polio Vaccine (OPV)-0 dose, Hepatitis B birth dose
6 weeks	OPV-1, Pentavalent-1, Rotavirus Vaccine (RVV)-1, Fractional dose of Inactivated Polio Vaccine (fIPV)-1, Pneumococcal Conjugate Vaccine (PCV)-1*
10 weeks	OPV-2, Pentavalent-2, RVV-2
14 weeks	OPV-3, Pentavalent-3, fIPV-2, RVV-3, PCV-2*
9–12 months	Measles and Rubella (MR)-1, fIPV-3, JE-1**, PCV-Booster*
16–24 months	MR-2, JE-2**, Diphtheria, Pertussis and Tetanus (DPT)-Booster-1, OPV-Booster
5–6 years	DPT-Booster-2
10 years	Tetanus and adult Diphtheria (Td)
16 years	Td
Pregnant mother	Td-1, Td-2 or Td-Booster***

*PCV in selected states/districts: Bihar, Himachal Pradesh, Madhya Pradesh, Uttar Pradesh (selected districts) and Rajasthan; in Haryana as state initiative

**JE in endemic districts only

***One dose if previously vaccinated within 3 years

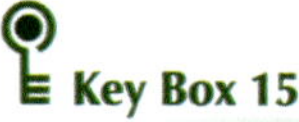

Key Box 15

Nutrition and Dietary History

1. Breastfeeding
2. Complimentary feeding
3. Quality and quantity of feeds
4. Protein and calorie intake per day
5. Diet balanced or not
6. Fast food
7. Vegetarian or mixed
8. Food beliefs, fads, and allergies

adequate and balanced nutrition appropriate for the age. This will help identify nutritional disorders and formulating a diet plan. Collect information appropriate for age **(Key Box 15)**.

Newborns and Infants below 6 Months

Time of initiation of breastfeeding, frequency and duration of feeds, exclusive breastfed or not, feeding directly from breast, or taking expressed breastmilk. Whether started top feeds, and if yes, provide details.

Infants above 6 Months and up to 2 Years

Time of initiation, quality, thickness, frequency, quantity of complementary foods, whether fat/oils added or not, any source of animal protein in diet, who feeds the child, whether breastfeeding continued or not.

From 2 Years Onwards

Collect information for 24-hour dietary intake by recall method. Record all food intake by the child in actual terms from the time he gets up and till he gets back to bed. Also include night feeds, if any. After charting total amount of all types of food consumed, calculate total protein and calories consumed.

Chapter 4 provides a detailed description of obtaining the dietary history in different age groups and provides tools for converting food intake into calories and proteins. Also ascertain whether diet is balanced or not (consuming food from all areas as per the food pyramid (see Chapter 4 for details). Does it have a lot of empty calories, i.e. fast foods and sweet/soft drinks. Also enquire for how long breastfeeding was continued and the period of exclusive breastfeeding. Are there any food fads, belief, food allergy and whether family is vegetarian or non-vegetarian.

At the end of taking dietary history, you should be able to tell how much proteins and calories are deficient or in excess, whether animal protein is included in diet, and whether the diet is balanced or imbalanced (mostly fast foods make diet imbalanced).

13. Personal History

Personal history includes personal information of the child. If a baby book is maintained, have a look. Ask about the child's habits with regard to eating, sleeping, bowels, and micturition, whether he has developed urinary continence by day and night, how parents will describe this child, is he moody, has strong likes and dislikes, does he or she cry a lot, how does this child compare with siblings or friends of the same age.

If of school age, what school does the child go to? Is he a hosteler or day scholar, how he or she is getting on with studies, friends and teachers, is he regular or miss much time from school, if so, why? Ask child if he likes school, friends, teachers and his subjects.

Ask age appropriate habits related to use of tobacco, smoking, and alcohol; particularly in adolescents.

14. Family History and Pedigree Charting

Members of a family share genetic material, receive almost similar nutrition, and are exposed to identical environmental risk factors. Therefore, they have similar chances of remaining healthy or becoming sick. Hence, the family history becomes important.

Ask the age of parents (at the time of birth of this child), their educational status, occupation, income, number of siblings, their age and sex. Find out details of events related to health, illness, nutritional status, and birth order of this child. Health of mother and father and if they are suffering from any disease like diabetes, hypertension, asthma, or ischemic heart diseases, should be noted.

You should elicit history of any close family member suffering from or suffered in recent past with open tuberculosis or received treatment for tuberculosis.

You should avoid asking leading questions like "Is there anyone affected in your family?" This will most often elicit a reply as "No". A better way to ask is "How many sons/ daughters are there? Are they healthy?" This will ensure that parents do not hide the information.

Details of abortions and deaths of children or any close relative and most likely causes should be noted; the cause should be identified on the basis of symptoms preceding death and any medical record available. You should also collect information about type of family, like nuclear or joint, and if joint then details of health and illness of other members of family. Also ask of habits of parents and other members regarding smoking, tobacco chewing, alcohol use. The family history should be complimented with examination of parents and siblings whenever required and possible. Salient points of family history are listed in **Key Box 16**.

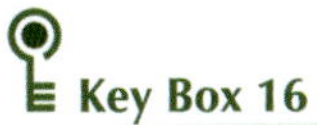

Key Box 16

Family History and Pedigree Charting

1. Type of family
2. Total members with relation
3. Age of mother and father
4. Name, age, and sex of siblings
5. Health and diseases in members
6. Abortion, stillbirths
7. Deaths in close relatives
8. Tuberculosis, diabetes mellitus
9. Obesity, hypertension, heart disease
10. Pedigree up to 3 generations

Consanguinity

Consanguinity ["*con-* (with) *sanguine* (blood) -ity"] refers to the property of being from the same lineage as another person. In that respect, "consanguinity is the quality of being descended from the same ancestor as another person". The products of a consanguineous relationship or marriage are at greater risk of certain genetic disorders, because relatives share a proportion of their genes. Closer is the relation between mother and father, more is the risk of genetic disorder. Degree of consanguineous relationships is categorized as first degree, second degree, or third degree.

The extent to which the risk increases depends on the degree of genetic relationship between the parents; but for relationships between second cousins where the parents only share 1/32rd of their DNA, the risk is less (although still greater than the general population).

- ***First degree relative*** Any relative who is one meiosis away from a particular individual in a family (i.e. parent, sibling, offspring). These are incestuous relationships where the parents share half of their DNA.
- ***Second degree relative*** Any relative who is two meioses away from a particular individual in a pedigree; a relative with

whom one quarter of an individual's genes is shared (i.e. grandparent, grandchild, uncle, aunt, nephew, niece, half-sibling).

Degree of relationship	Percentage of shared genes	Example
First degree	50%	Parents, children and siblings
Second degree	25%	Uncle, aunt, degree nephew, niece and grandparents
Third degree	12.5%	First cousins

- ***Third degree relative*** First cousins, great-grandparents and great-grandchildren; third degree relatives have 1/8th of their genes in common.

Pedigree Charting

A pedigree provides graphic depiction of family. A three generation pedigree should be obtained for every new patient as a screening tool to identify possible inheritable disorders and risk to patient. An extended pedigree may be needed to identify risk of certain disorders. Family history and pedigree charting help to identify inherited disorders, like autosomal dominant (one of the parents is affected phenotypically), autosomal recessive (parents are normal phenotypically, but siblings may be affected), X-linked recessive (only boys are affected) and others. Common symbols used for drawing pedigree charts are depicted in Fig. 2.2.

Pedigrees typical of autosomal recessive, autosomal dominant, and X-linked dominant disorders are depicted in Fig. 2.3.

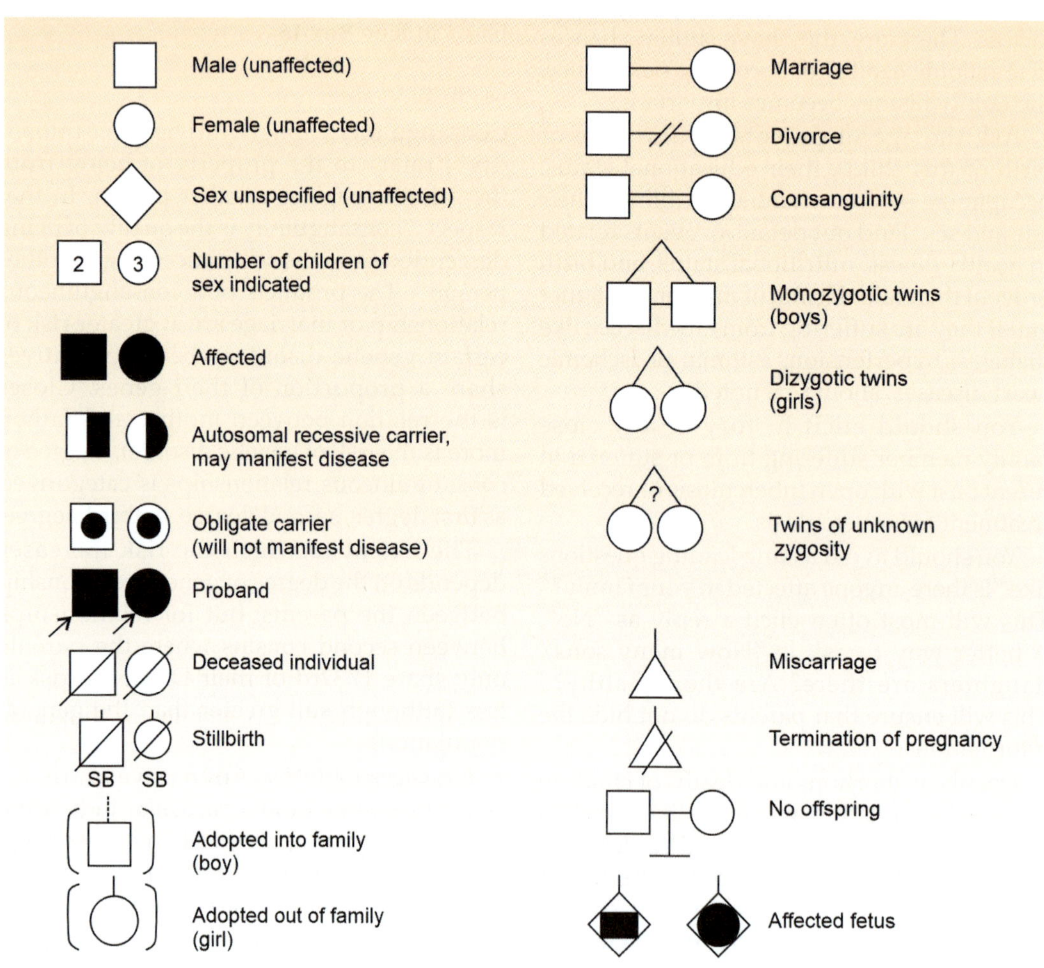

Fig. 2.2: Commonly used symbols in Pedigree charts.

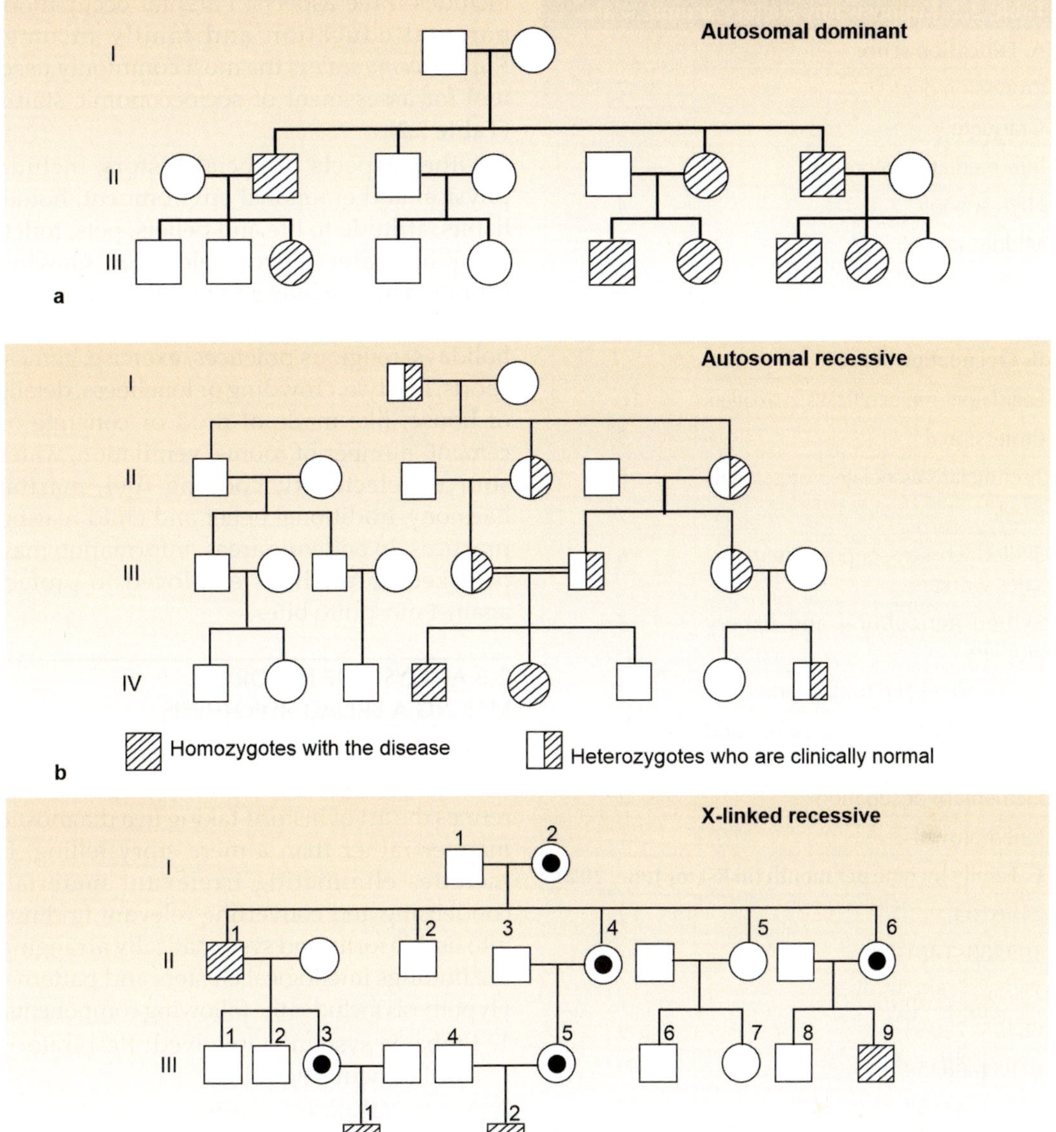

Fig. 2.3: Pedigree charts. (a) Autosomal dominant; (b) Autosomal recessive; (c) X-linked recessive.

Practical Key Box

Child belongs to a nuclear family with 5 living members, residing in a 2-room pukka house. The father is educated up to 8th class, owns a vegetable shop, and earns Rs. 6000/month. Mother is uneducated and is a house maker. The house has 2 living rooms with a separate toilet and bathroom with adequate ventilation. The water supply is by corporation water pipeline.

15. Socioeconomic History

Social history helps in arriving at diagnosis (diseases common in certain groups, like thalassemia in Sindhis and Punjabis, sickle cell anemia in certain tribes), planning of treatment (individual and social resources available), certain practices (head tonsuring, circumcision, dietary habits), and planning with counseling for care of children.

Assessment of the socioeconomic status is an integral part of the socioeconomic history. This

Table 2.2: Kuppuswamy socioeconomic scale

A. Education score	
Profession degree	7
Graduate	6
Intermediate/diploma	5
High school	4
Middle school	3
Primary school	2
Illiterate	1
B. Occupation score	
Legislators, senior officials, managers	10
Professional	9
Technicians/associate professionals	8
Clerk	7
Skilled worker, shop and market sales workers	6
Skilled agricultural and fishery workers	5
Craft and related trade worker	4
Plant and machine operators and assemblers	3
Elementary occupation	2
Unemployed	1
C. Family income per month (in Rs) for June, 2023	
≥146104	12
109580–146103	11
73054–109579	10
68455–73053	9
63854–68454	8
59252–63853	7
54651–59251	6
45589–54650	5
36527–45588	4
21914–36526	3
7316–21913	2
≤7315	1
Total score (A + B + C)	**Socioeconomic class**
26–29	Upper (I)
16–25	Upper middle (II)
11–15	Middle lower middle (III)
5–10	Lower upper lower (IV)
<5	Lower (V)

Radhakrishnan M, et al. Int J Community Med Public Health. 2023 Nov;10(11):4415–4418

includes three aspects: Parental occupation, parental education and family income. *Kuppuswamy scale* is the most commonly used tool for assessment of socioeconomic status **(Table 2.2)**.

Other aspects of social history include physical and emotional environment, home, habits, attitude to life and beliefs, pets, toilet, drinking water source, television viewing (duration of watching and favorite programs), family interests, hobbies, hopes, fears, holidays, religious practices, exercise, games, sports, lifestyle, crowding or loneliness, details of house, like made of mud or concrete or cement, number of rooms, ventilation, water sources, electricity, cooking fuel, marital harmony, traditional belief and child rearing practices. In endemic areas, information may be asked on methods employed to protect against mosquito bites.

2.3 ANALYSIS OF HISTORY: MAKING A BROAD HYPOTHESIS

This is the most crucial exercise which all clinicians should make a habit to practice. It refines the art of history-taking in a diagnostic manner rather than a mere story telling. It includes eliminating irrelevant material, condensing and converting relevant findings into usable form, and systematically arranging the findings into logical clusters and patterns. Hypothesis includes the following components:

1. Probable system(s) involved: Respiratory, cardiac, neurological, etc.
2. *Nature of the disease process:* Acute/chronic/ chronic with acute exacerbation
3. Broad etiology of the disease process: Infectious/malignant/metabolic/immune, etc.
4. Probable site(s) (organ) of involvement
5. Specific etiology of the disease process, i.e. if infectious, whether bacterial, viral, fungal, or protozoal
6. Probable diagnoses
7. Severity of disease process and complications

Hypothesis is to be made at 3 different steps of history-taking. ***First:*** After presenting complaints (you should be able to point out the system involved, nature of disease process, and broad etiology); ***Second:*** After history of

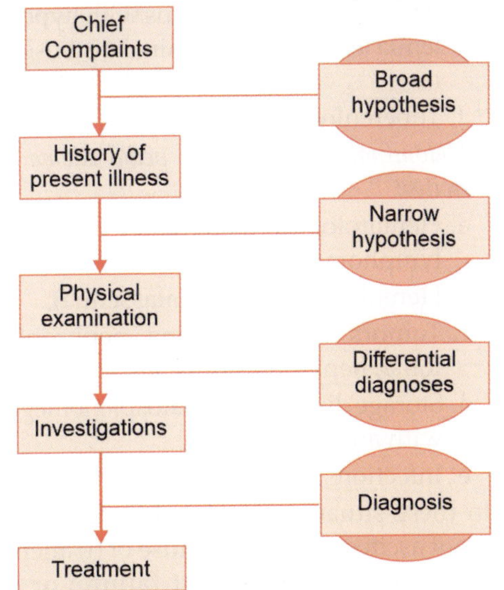

Fig. 2.4: Stepwise interpretation of a case record: Role of hypothesis.

present illness (now you should be able to answer all 7 components of the hypothesis); and *Third:* After complete history and examination (now the hypothesis takes the shape of differential diagnoses). Figure 2.4 provides the evaluation-action tree in clinical practice from obtaining history to treating the patient. Hypothesis making is the most important of these activities and paves the way for making diagnosis, which is essential to treat the patient.

Example 1
A 3-year-old child is brought with the following chief complaints:
1. High grade fever—3 days
2. Generalized tonic-clonic convulsions, one episode, this morning

Broad hypothesis: This child is having involvement of the CNS (because of convulsions). Disease process is acute in nature (short history of 3 days only). Etiology is infective (presenting with fever). Probable diagnoses: Febrile seizures, meningitis, cerebral malaria, cerebritis, etc.

Example 2
A 10-year-old child is brought with the following chief complaint:
1. Fever off and on 20 days

Broad hypothesis: System involvement is not clear. Disease process is chronic in nature (long duration fever of more than 2 weeks). Long duration fever could be because of infection, malignancy, inflammation (collagen vascular/immune etiology) or metabolic cause. A thorough system inquiry is thus needed while eliciting the presenting history.

Example 3
A 6-year-old child is brought with the following chief complaints:

	Chief complaints	Duration
1.	Repeated episodes of generalized swelling of body associated with diminished urinary output lasting for 1–4 weeks, with symptom-free intervals of 2–6 months in between episodes	For 2 years
2.	Generalized swelling of body associated with diminished urinary output	For 2 days

Broad hypothesis: This child is having a chronic disease that is remitting in nature. At present, the child has presented with an acute exacerbation of the illness. Systems involved could be renal, hepatic, or cardiac. Etiology is non-infective in nature.

Example 4
A 12-year-old adolescent is brought with the following chief complaints:

	Chief complaints	Duration
1.	Fever for 3 weeks	6 months back
2.	Migratory pain and swelling in large joints for 2 weeks	6 months back
3.	Palpitation and breathlessness	6 days
4.	Swelling over both feet and diminished urine output	2 days

Broad hypothesis: This child is having involvement of the joints (joint swelling and pain) and cardiovascular system (palpitation). Thus, we are dealing with a multi-system disease of chronic nature. Etiology could be infective, inflammatory, malignant or

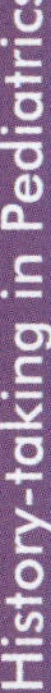

metabolic (because of fever). At present the child has presented with some complications (probably congestive heart failure, myocarditis, pericarditis, renal failure, hepatic failure, etc.). Considering all the presenting complaints, a possibility of rheumatic fever appears likely (it is an inflammatory disease of chronic etiology with recurrences, involve joints and heart, and can present with congestive heart failure during an episode).

Example 5

A 30-month-old girl, product of non-consanguineous marriage presents with following chief complaints:

Chief complaints	Duration
1. Abdominal distension	For 6 months
2. Swelling of feet	For 15 days

Broad hypothesis: With the above presenting complaints, you may make the hypothesis that the child is suffering from a chronic disease (long duration of 3 months) of more likely a non-infectious etiology (as fever is absent). System(s) involved could be hepatobiliary, gastrointestinal, or reticuloendothelial because abdominal distension is suggestive of either organomegaly or ascites. Swelling of legs indicates pedal edema (this could be present because of involvement of liver, kidney or heart). Thus, we are possibly dealing with the case of (i) ascites or hepatosplenomegaly with pedal edema or (ii) abdominal mass(es) with pedal edema. With this in mind, the possible diagnoses can be as follows:

I. *Ascites and/or hepatosplenomegaly with pedal edema:*
   a. Chronic liver disease with or without failure (ascites or hepatosplenomegaly leading to abdominal distension and hypoproteinemia or anemia leading to pedal edema);
   b. Renal disease (nephrotic syndrome presents as anasarca);
   c. Cardiac involvement (right-sided failure presents as hepatomegaly, ascites, pedal edema);
   d. GIT disease, like celiac disease;
   e. Severe malnutrition (kwashiorkor presents with hepatomegaly and pedal edema, severe marasmus with hypokalemia leading to abdominal distension); or
   f. Tuberculosis.

II. *Abdominal mass(es) with pedal edema, no ascites:*
   a. Hematological malignancy (leukemia, lymphoma)
   b. Hemolytic anemia (thalassemia);
   c. Tumors (neuroblastoma, nephroblastoma, hepatoblastoma, etc.)
   d. Storage disorders (hepatosplenomegaly with anemia);
   e. Infections, like tropical splenomegaly.

In these situations, isolated pedal edema without ascites could be because of (i) anemia leading to congestive heart failure; or (ii) hypoproteinemia.

History of presenting complaints described abdominal distension as insidious in onset, generalized to whole abdomen and not lumpy, gradually progressive in course to the present size so that the abdomen appears like a football from distance only. The overlying skin is tight and shiny. The massive distension of abdomen had lead to difficulty in sitting and limitation of physical activity (playing). There is no relation with food or posture. There was no history of jaundice, bleeding from any site or progressive pallor, breathlessness, palpitation, altered bowel and bladder habits, vomiting and decreased appetite. There is no family history of tuberculosis or contact with a patient of tuberculosis.

Narrow hypothesis: As per description of the swelling, we are most likely dealing with a case of massive ascites with pedal edema. Underlying hepatosplenomegaly or other visceromegaly cannot be ruled out at this stage. Presence of massive ascites rules out diseases, like hemolytic anemia, storage disorders and leukemia. Rest of the possibilities still remain.

Examination reveals mild icterus, pallor, generalized edema, massive ascites and small liver (liver span 4 cm). There is no other visceromegaly. Other systems were normal.

Differential diagnosis: Examination is in favor of the first possibility. Most probably this child is having a chronic liver disease which may be now associated with portal hypertension. Physical examination has ruled out a primary cardiac, renal or nutritional disorder. Possibilities, such as lymphoma, neuroblastoma and tuberculosis, still need to be ruled out by investigations.

Diagnosis

His investigations revealed transaminitis, coarse echotexture of liver on ultrasonography, deranged INR, which support the diagnosis of chronic liver disease. Her HBsAg testing was positive, thus reaching a final diagnosis of chronic hepatitis B infection.

2.4 PRESENTING THE HISTORY

You are required to present history either during rounds or while consulting case with your senior, referring case for specialized treatment, or during the examination. Follow the principles given below to make an effective and impressive presentation:

1. Use simple language. While translating information of patient's history in English for writing and presentation, use words which truly reflect meaning of what the informant is saying. If you are unable to find out the actual word(s) conveying its true meaning, tell in informant's words only.
2. Use short sentences. Too long sentence results in loss of continuity and makes the presentation unfocused.
3. History should be presented in a flowing manner just like telling a story, so that listener can develop a visual image of the patient's problem.
4. Speak clearly, slowly, and in a voice which is comfortably audible.
5. Avoid repetitions.
6. Present all the events in a sequence, in a chronological order, give information from present to past of events related to health and disease. First give information about individual patient, then the family, and then about society.
7. Always be ready with the summary of the case to be told in the end.
8. Details of system review and negative history should be brief, precise, and relevant.
9. Keep track of time, nobody has unlimited time to listen you. So stick to time given for presentation.
10. Finally, make a hypothesis detailing what could be the possible conditions in this situation.

Chapter 3

Evaluation of Adolescents

❍ Srikanta Basu ❍ Piyush Gupta

Structure

3.1 IMPORTANCE OF ADOLESCENCE

Definition

Adolescence is a period of transition between childhood and adulthood—a time of profound physical, cognitive, social, and emotional changes. Different cultures recognize these periods of transition differently and it also varies over a period. The precise boundaries are difficult to define, but this period commences with the gradual appearance of secondary sex characteristics at about 10–11 years of age and ending with cessation of body growth at 18–20 years of age. Commonly used definitions for adolescence age are shown in **Key Box 1**.

Conventionally, the adolescent age group is categorized into early (10–13 years), middle (14–17 years) and late adolescent (17 years onwards) age groups. Psychosocial development in each of these categories is described in **Table 3.1**. This development corresponds more to the chronological age than the age at appearance of secondary sexual characteristics. It may happen that an adolescent has achieved all physical growth of puberty but is lagging in psychosocial development.

Key Box 1

Definition of Adolescence

1. WHO defines "Adolescence" as age between 10 and 19 years.
2. Government of India in the National Youth Policy defines adolescence as 13–19 years.
3. "Young people" refers to ages 10–24 years.
4. "Young adults" refers to ages 20–24 years.

Should adolescents be treated differently?

As a clinician, the first question which need to be answered is, "What do I need to know and do differently if I encounter a person aged 14 years, rather than 6 or 23 years?". Moreover, this age group is also heterogeneous, i.e. an 11-year-old is very different from an 18-year-old adolescent. A good understanding of the psychosocial development and common health concerns, issues and diseases is necessary to diagnose and manage health problems and behaviors of the adolescents.

Before we learn to take history and perform clinical examination in this age group, we will discuss briefly about psychosocial development, various health concerns and diseases in adolescents, and factors affecting these, which need to be addressed.

Psychosocial Development

Growth and development during adolescence is a biopsychosocial process characterized by physical, psychosocial and cognitive changes taking place together but at a different pace. These changes may not occur at the same

Table 3.1: Stages of adolescence

Stages	Cognitive development
Early adolescence (10–13 y)	• At this level, they are concrete thinkers: Interested in present, limited thought to future. • There is lack of control of impulsive actions and this may result in risk-taking behavior and experimentation. • Adolescents may set unrealistic academic or vocational goals.
Middle adolescence (14–17 y)	• Abstract reasoning and formal operational thinking begin at this level. They may revert back to concrete thinking at the times of stress. • Feeling of supremacy and immortality increase and this may lead to risk-taking behaviour. • Intellectual ability and creativity further increase and this leads to more realistic choices in carriers and other important life decisions.
Late adolescence (17 y onwards)	• Establishment of abstract reasoning is achieved. Ability to weigh different options develops and decision making becomes more rational and realistic. • Interests about education and vocation are more stable. They develop ability to delay gratification. • Desire for financial independence increase and some may actually attain it.

chronological age in different adolescents and this may cause concern in them. The clinician should be well aware of normal range and variations in these rapid changes so that appropriate counseling can be done and timely referrals can be made.

Adolescence is characterized by gradual change in their thinking capacity which is concrete (short term) in younger adolescents and becomes more abstract (reasoning and future orientation) as the age increases. Concrete thinkers mainly focus on immediate physical world surrounding them, take the word literally and have a little future orientation. During middle and late adolescence, the ability to reason abstractly gradually matures, they learn to handle multiple concepts simultaneously and reach some logical conclusion based on their experience; become more capable of taking another person's perspective and can place themselves and the events in future and accordingly can decide more logically.

These differences have practical implications during counseling adolescents. For example, while counseling a 12-year-old teenager about smoking is more likely to have an impact if we focus more on the immediate consequences of smoking (bad breath, yellow teeth, and decreased exercise performance) rather than on long-term conditions (lung cancer or emphysema). Terms such as cancer or emphysema may be too abstract to have an impact on their decision regarding smoking.

3.2 HISTORY-TAKING IN ADOLESCENTS

Approach to History-taking

Unlike in children, the clinical interview or history taking needs to be flexible. The main aim is to establish a trust between the adolescent and the pediatrician. You have to create an environment (physical as well as attitudinal) where the teenager does not feel threatened and is able to disclose information. You have to devote sufficient time to ensure privacy. Your communication skills are really tested while interviewing adolescents.

- *Communication* is an exchange of information, knowledge, ideas or feelings. In a face to face situation, communication is not just exchange of information. It also conveys one's feelings, by use of gestures, facial expressions, language, and the manner of tone.
- *Counseling* is a person-to-person, two-way communication during which the counsellor provides adequate information to help the adolescent make an informed decision, and then implement it; enables the adolescent to identify his/her problem and possible solutions; helps the adolescents evaluate their feelings and opinions regarding the problem for which help was

Table 3.2: Steps of counseling: The GATHER approach

G—Greet the Adolescent
- Put them at ease, show respect and trust
- Emphasize the confidential nature of the discussion

A—Ask how I can help you
- Encourage them to bring out their anxieties, worries and needs, determine their access to support and help in their family and community
- Find out what steps they have already taken to deal with the situation
- Encourage the person to express their feelings in their own words
- Show respect and tolerance to what they say and do not pass judgement
- Actively listen and show that you are paying attention through your looking
- Encourage them through helpful questions

T—Tell them any relevant information
- Provide accurate and specific information in reply to their questions
- Give information on what they can do to remain healthy. Explain any background information they need to know about the particular health issue
- Keep your language simple, repeat important points and ask questions to check if the important points are understood
- Provide the important information in the form of a leaflet, if possible, that they can take away

H—Help them to make them decisions
- Explore the various alternatives
- Raise issues they may not have thought of
- Careful of letting your own views, values and prejudices influence the advice you give
- Ensure that it is their own decision and not one that you have imposed
- Help them make a plan of action

E—Explain any misunderstanding
- Ask questions to check understanding of important points
- Ask the adolescent to repeat back in his/her own words the key points

R—Return to follow-up/referral
- Plan for a follow-up visit or referral to other agencies if a follow-up visit is not necessary, give the name of someone they can contact if they need help

sought. But it is *not* a method to provide solutions to the adolescent's problems or giving instructions or advise. There are several approaches of counseling and one of the easier to remember approaches is "GATHER" **(Table 3.2)**.

Talking to Adolescents

Some of the basic aspect of good history-taking or communication are described below.

A. Build Rapport

Greet the adolescent, call them by the name, begin the session by allowing the adolescent to talk freely before asking too many questions, express empathy, and make them at ease. Make them feel that you are here to help them, and you will try your best to respond to their needs and problems. Start on time and do not make them wait. It always helps to make a good first impression.

Do not make any negative comments about the adolescent's physical characteristics, e.g. "you look small for your grade." At this age, adolescents are highly anxious about their body image and may suffer from low self-esteem.

Often, pediatricians resort to childish games and gimmicks while establishing rapport with young children. However, while talking to a teenager, do NOT try to behave like a teenager or talk in their 'lingo'. You should not try to parent the adolescent and start preaching in the clinic. Behave like a supportive and mature adult.

B. Maintain Privacy and Confidentiality

Privacy and confidentiality should be clearly spelled in the first meeting itself. It is reassuring for the adolescents to trust the doctor and the system and makes future interactions very congenial and fruitful.

It can go like this: "During this visit, I will ask you some very personal questions to get to know you better. The answers may be sensitive and personal. I promise they will be confidential—that means just between you and me. I will not disclose these to anyone including your parents or teachers, unless you give me permission. The only exception is, if I feel you or anyone have been harmed physically or about to be physically harmed, I am required to take immediate action. What we discuss in this room remains here until you say otherwise".

C. Eliminate Barriers

Avoid judgmental responses of body or spoken language, be impartial. Respect the beliefs, opinions, and diversity or expression regarding the sexuality. Understand and use appropriate terms/expressions while communicating with them about their bodies, dating, and sex and sexuality issues.

D. Active Listening

Show your sincere interest and understanding and give your full attention to the adolescent; avoid movements that might distract the adolescent, listen to problem patiently without being intrusive or taking away her/his control over the issue; give the adolescent some time to think, ask questions, and speak. Periodically repeat what you have heard, confirming that both you and the adolescent have understood (paraphrasing). Clarify terms that are not clear or need more interpretation. Summarize the most relevant information communicated by the adolescent, usually at the end of a topic or session.

E. Ask Appropriate and Effective Questions

Use a tone that shows interest, attention, and friendliness, begin sessions with easy questions, gradually moving up to more difficult/sensitive questions, try not to take notes except in a structured interview that has an established order for special cases.

Adolescents might present with some problem but in reality that they are concerned about some other underlying issue which they may be embarrassed or scared to disclose because they may not be comfortable either with the doctor or the situation they are in. So, one has to go beyond the presenting problem or concern and at times they may not disclose in the first meeting.

F. Provide Information

Speak in a tone and language which the adolescents understand, check their level of understanding and then explain them accordingly using common and simple words avoiding technical terms. Do not overload the adolescent with too much information specially in the first meeting, provide information based on what the adolescent already knows or has heard. Gently correct misconceptions, use audiovisual materials to help the adolescent understand the information and to demonstrate information in more concrete terms. Present all the relevant information; respond to questions as fully and honestly as you can; help them choose and respect their choice even if it is not the one you would have wanted them to make.

3.3 PSYCHOSOCIAL SCREENING

1. HEEADSSS Tool

Once you have obtained the history of presenting complaints, explore whether the adolescent has some other issues to discuss. Like a developmental history in children, psychosocial history is a must know for all the clinicians dealing with adolescents. HEEADSSS is a very useful screening questionnaire used all over the world, and captures almost all the domains affecting the psychosocial development of the adolescent. It focuses on assessment of the **H**ome environment, **E**ducation and employment, **E**ating, peer-related **A**ctivities, **D**rugs, **S**exuality, **S**uicide/depression, and **S**afety from injury and violence; and **S**trength has also been added **(Table 3.3)**.

Administering the HEEADSSS tool is a practical, time-tested, strategy that helps clinicians to explore into the details of the presenting problems and also uncover some

Table 3.3: The HEEADSSS psychosocial interview for the adolescents

Home and environment
- Where do you live?
- Who lives with you?
- What are relationships like at home with parents/siblings?
- To whom are you closest at home?
- Is there anything you would like to change about your family?

Eating (including body image)
- What do you like and not like about your body?
- Have there been any recent changes in your weight?
- Have you done dieting in the last year? How? How often?
- Have you done anything else to try to manage your weight?
- How much exercise do you get in an average day/week?
- What do you think would be a healthy diet?
- How does that compare to your current eating patterns?
- Do you worry about your weight? How often?
- Do you eat in front of the TV/computer?
- Does it ever seem as though your eating is out of control?

Education and employment
- What are your favourite subjects at school? Your least favourite subjects? How are your grades? Any recent changes? Any dramatic changes in the past?
- Have you changed schools in the past few years?
- Are you working? Where? How much?
- Have you ever been suspended/expelled?
- How well do you get along with the teachers/peers at school?
- What are your future education/employment plans/goals?

Activities
- How are your peer relationship? What do you and your friends do for fun? (with whom, where, and when?)
- What do you and your family do for fun (with whom, where, and when)?
- Do you participate in any sports or other activities?
- Do you regularly attend a religious/spiritual congregation or other group, club, or other organized activity?
- Do you have any hobbies? Do you read for fun? What?
- How much time you spend on screen per day? What music do you like to listen to?
- Do you have a job? How many hours a week you work?

Drugs
- Do any of your friends use tobacco/alcohol/other drugs?
- Does anyone in your family use tobacco?
- Do you use tobacco/alcohol/other drugs?
- Is there any history of alcohol or drug problems in your family? Does anyone at home use tobacco?
- Do you ever drink or use drugs when you're alone? (Assess frequency, intensity, patterns of use or abuse, and how youth obtains or pays for drugs, alcohol, or tobacco) (Ask the CRAFFT questions in Key Box 2)

Suicide and depression
- Have you had long periods of time where you felt sad or down more than usual?
- Are you having trouble getting to sleep?
- Have you thought a lot about hurting yourself or someone else?
- Does it seem that you have lost interest in things that you used to really enjoy?
- Do you find yourself spending less and less time with friends?
- Have you ever tried to kill yourself?
- Have you started using alcohol or drugs to help you relax, calm down, or feel better?

Strengths
- What are you good at?
- What do you enjoy doing? What is your life goals?

Sexuality
- Are you in or have you ever been in a romantic relationship?
- Have any of your relationships ever been sexual relationships?
- Are your sexual activities enjoyable?
- What does the term "safer sex" mean to you?
- Are you interested in boys/girls/both?
- Have you ever been forced or pressured into doing something sexual that you did not want to do?
- Have you ever been touched sexually in a way that you did not want?
- Have you ever had a sexually transmitted disease (STD) or worried that you had an STD?

Safety (savagery)
- Have you ever been seriously injured? How?
- Do you always wear a seatbelt in the car?
- Is there any violence in your home?
- Does the violence ever get physical?
- Is there a lot of violence at your school/in your neighbourhood/among your friends?
- Have you ever been physically or sexually abused?

From: Goldenring J and Rosen D, 2004. Getting into adolescent heads: an essential update. Contemporary Pediatrics, 21(1): 64.

issues or factors which are affecting the behavior directly or indirectly (home, school, peer pressure, etc.). It often starts with less threatening issues to more personal and intrusive issues and often helps to build up the trust and rapport. As described under communication, do not strive to get all the information in the first interview. With time and building of trust, further sessions can be arranged and then one can go deeper and develop some kind of intervention plan. You can make a "problem list" which can be explored over time and can be tackled by counseling or therapeutic intervention. The only exception is when you suspect a crisis or impending crisis where you have to intervene immediately.

2. Conducting the Interview

This tool can be used for children more than 10 years and all the initial steps mentioned under good communication should be followed. It is better if you explain the confidentiality issue in front of the teenager and the parents before *asking the parents or other person to leave the room as they are not supposed to be present during the interview*. Before they leave, note any of their concerns and assuring them of further interaction once the interview is over. Rarely, adolescents may request for presence of adults, but it might limit the sensitive information provided by them, and it becomes awkward to exclude them in subsequent visits while the adolescent eventually open up to discuss more private matters. But remember to keep the parents always in the loop for the overall management to succeed. It is not a rigid questionnaire, rather, the order of questioning should be dictated by the common clinical sense and comfort level of both the clinicians and the client.

Another very important aspect, try to find out whom does teen trust at home or outside home to discuss his difficult personal matters. It has been shown that connectivity to a supportive adult (parents, grandparents or any adult) is highly protective against a whole range of health risks and high-risk behaviors. Lastly, also look for positive attributes, i.e. their strengths which can be reinforced to bring about a change in their undesirable behavior to improve the overall outlook.

With practice this interview can be completed in 20–30 minutes. Rarely, when time is less, one can concentrate on only those domains which have a bearing on the immediate problems, e.g. if the adolescent presents with injury after alcohol intake, it is better to go to the drugs section directly. Usually a few minutes are spent with both parents and child together, then with adolescents alone, and lastly addressing the concerns of parents, if any.

3. Tips for Conducting HEEADSSS Questionnaire

There are a few sections in the HEEADSSS questionnaire which are very sensitive and private in nature (sexual activity, drugs, etc.). These are a few practical tips which can help to handle these issues.

A. Start with Non-threatening Issues

Start the clinical interview with issues that are the least sensitive and threatening. First establish the rapport, then ask about his area of interest, friends or even home questions before enquiring them about sexual and reproductive health issues or other sensitive issues.

B. Use the Third Person (Indirect Questions) where Possible

It is often best to ask first about activities of their peers and friends rather than directly about their own activities. So instead of asking directly, "Do you smoke cigarettes?" you could ask, "Do any of your friends smoke?" If the adolescent replies, "Yes", you could then ask, "Have you ever joined them?" This can lead to other questions such as, "How often do you smoke?" or "Youth is a time of sexual exploration. Tell me about your sexual life" which sounds open-ended and nonjudgmental. Don't ask questions which has "yes" or "No" answers, rather ask open-ended ones.

C. Reduce the Stigma around the Issue by Normalising the Issue

An adolescent who has a sexually transmitted infection may feel embarrassed to admit or disclose. One can reduce the stigma around the issue by stating that, "I have treated quite a few teenagers with the same problem you have".

Now, we will discuss how to screen adolescents for a few sensitive issues (drugs, mental health issues—suicide, violence, etc.) in more detail.

3.4 MENTAL HEALTH ISSUES

Mental health disorders are one of the most important non-communicable diseases prevalent in this age group followed by obesity and overweight issues, intentional and unintentional injuries, violence, and alcohol and tobacco abuse. The health risk factors, i.e. physical inactivity, substance abuse, poor nutrition, and risk-taking behavior responsible for these disorders have their origin during childhood and adolescence. The adolescent period is the last opportunity to modify some of these behaviors.

The HEEADSSS approach can help the clinicians assess whether an adolescent is mentally well or ill and, if they are ill, to assess the severity of the illness. Look for warning signs **(Table 3.4)**. Persistence of these symptoms for more than two weeks are important "Red flags" which should alert the clinicians to a possible underlying mental issue.

Drugs and Substance Abuse

Adolescents do not admit taking drugs when asked directly but are willing to tell about

Table 3.4: Warning signs for screening mental health issues

Home	Adolescent has no support at home or anywhere else.
Education	• Adolescent is having trouble at school or work, e.g. problems with school or work, bullying, or problems with teachers or bosses. • Adolescent frequently misses school or work.
Eating	• Adolescent is overweight and has poor eating habits. • Adolescent believes he or she is very overweight, when it is evident that this is not the case. • Adolescent can be obsessive about food, exercise, body weight or shape. • Adolescent is underweight, and from the discussion it appears that financial constraints are contributing to this.
Exercise	• Adolescent participates in no or very little physical activity. • Adolescent is overweight and unfit (e.g. breathless, tired easily walking upstairs). • Adolescent is absorbed or obsessive about exercise and body weight. • Adolescent is undernourished or engages in excessive physical labor.
Activities	• Adolescent has no friends and spends most of the time alone. • Adolescent spends most of the time with people who are 4–5 years older, who affect the behavior negatively.
Drugs	• Adolescent regularly uses legal or illegal substances. • Adolescent has tried illegal substances or has friends who do so. • Substance use is having a negative impact on adolescent's health or ability to function. • Other people have expressed concern about adolescent's substance use.
Sex	• Adolescent is being or has been pressured to have sex. • Adolescent seems at risk for early sexual activity. • Adolescent has had unsafe sex or has had a number of sexual partners. • Adolescent seems upset or worried about his or her sexual orientation.
Safety	• Adolescent is experiencing bullying, violence, sexual harassment or abuse. • Adolescent is withdrawn and unable to talk of experiences, or examination reveals signs of violence.
Suicide and depression	• Adolescent is sad or anxious or feels hopeless most of the time. • Sleep disturbances. • Adolescent talks about hurting or killing themselves or has tried to hurt or kill themselves. • Adolescent frequently uses alcohol or drugs to escape negative feelings. • Adolescent has poor self-esteem and no sense of self-worth.

Key Box 2

CRAFFT Questionnaire for Screening Substance Abuse

1. Have you ever ridden in a CAR driven by someone who was high or had been using drugs or alcohol?
2. Do you ever use alcohol or drugs to RELAX, feel better about yourself, or fit in?
3. Do you ever use drugs or alcohol when you are ALONE?
4. Do you FORGET things you did while using drugs or alcohol?
5. Do your family or FRIENDS ever tell you that you should cut down your drinking or drug use?
6. Have you ever gotten into TROUBLE while using drugs or alcohol?

Two or more "Yes" answers suggest high risk of a serious substance-use problem or a substance-use disorder.

their friends. So, if you ask "Do any of your friends use drugs or alcohol (or get drunk or high)?", they might be more forthcoming. "CRAFFT" questionnaire can be used to screen for substance abuse **(Key Box 2)**.

Suicide

During interactions, most adolescents will admit that they thought about committing suicide but as a clinician you have to decide about the seriousness of ideation, what is their planning or there are some other risk factors or behaviors that are precipitating it. It is also important to remember that teenagers do think about suicide more than we realize and so we should ask this question rather directly and without any hesitation, e.g. "Have you ever felt so bad that you felt like committing a suicide?". Remember, asking about suicidal behavior does not precipitate or trigger it. Any suicidal ideation should prompt a more careful assessment of the patient's suicide risk and must include a referral to a mental health expert. Previous suicide attempts are often a strong risk factor for future attempts and completed suicides.

Violence

Violence, injuries, and abuse are leading causes of distress and death in adolescents. Bullying, domestic violence, school violence, rape, etc. are becoming prevalent in both urban and rural settings. In addition to the immediate effects, violence and abuse can have long lasting physical and psychological effects. **Key Box 3** provides a mnemonic which can help identify adolescents at risk of violence. If violence is suspected, then determine the following:

a. If adolescent was a victim or perpetrator or witness of violence and
b. Nature, context, and location of violence.

Find out motivators or pre-disposing factors for violence. Assess for presence of any mental health illness. Understand the limitations of health services in preventing violence and involve other agencies like Child Line, Child Welfare Committees and police appropriately. Parents should be encouraged to protect and support adolescents in managing their world. Violence and abuse can be prevented and when they occur, they need to be responded to effectively and with sensitivity.

Key Box 3

FISTS Mnemonic to Assess Adolescents at Risk of Violence

F: Fighting

How many fights you had in the last year? Which was the last?

I: Injuries

Have you ever been injured? Have you ever injured someone else?

S: Sex

Has your partner hit you? Have you hit your partner? Have you ever been forced to have sex?

T: Threats

Has someone with a weapon threatened you? What happened? Has anything changed to make you feel safer?

S: Self-defence

What will you do if someone tries to pick a fight? Have you carried weapon in self-defence?

American Medical Association 2002.

Child Abuse

Child abuse is widely prevalent irrespective of caste, religion, socioeconomic status, regional, and other factors. It can be physical, psychological, or sexual. Both adolescent girls and boys can experience all forms of abuse. They can be abused at home as or in the community, and can be perpetrated by family members, as well as other adults and adolescents. In many cases, the perpetrators make the victims feel that they have no option but to accept violence and abuse.

The role and responsibilities of the attending clinician in cases of child abuse are twofold: (*a*) To provide immediate medical care; and (*b*) to ensure the future safety and welfare of the child. Most often we either fail or choose to ignore the second aspect because of lack of knowledge/experience of handling such situations or fear of getting involved in the legal situations. However, by avoiding we invite more problems for ourselves and always carry guilt of not acting in a justified manner to save the life/dignity of the adolescent.

Our immediate goal should be to take care of the medical condition and provide him/her with the best that center can offer. In case of any life-threatening injuries, recent sexual assault or potentially grievous injuries, police has to informed immediately and meanwhile medical care should be continued and if the child needs to be referred best available first aid treatment should be instituted before transporting the child. In other conditions, depending upon the situation, either the family or the caretaker or the child welfare committee of the district or the child helpline (telephone number-1098) or the NGOs dealing with the welfare of the children can be contacted. The cases of sexual abuse should preferably be dealt by the specially trained team. The clinicians should be very well aware of "Protection of Children from Sexual Offences Act 2012 (POCSO)".

3.5 ADOLESCENTS WITH CHRONIC DISORDERS

Increasing numbers of children with chronic disorders are entering adolescent age group. These disorders significantly impact the lives of parents and siblings. Some of the issues like undernutrition, short stature, delayed puberty, and body image issues become more significant due to concurrent chronic disorders and make normal growing up process more troublesome. These adolescents might experience low level of emotional well-being and are at increased risk of behavioral issues, anxiety, stress and depression. Socially, they encounter alienation; and cognitively, there might be a dip in their

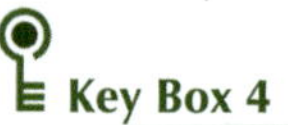

Key Box 4

Dealing Adolescents with Chronic Disorders

1. Ask whether he is aware about his disease and access to treatment modalities
2. Enquire about the difficulties/barriers he is facing as far as adherence to treatment is concerned
3. How is the status in school—school performance, social and sports participation, bullying, etc.
4. Dwell on the mental health issues: Stress, anxiety, depression, etc.
5. Ask about condition at home—relationship with parents, siblings, availability of support system at home

school performance or work output. Families and parents may experience frustration, guilt, anxiety, and stress. The role of the clinicians in handling adolescents with chronic diseases is continued in **Key Box 4**.

3.6 PHYSICAL EXAMINATION IN ADOLESCENTS

Examining the adolescents is a tactful issue and one has to be aware of certain legal implications as well. There is certain examination (e.g. sexual maturity rating) which is sensitive in nature and certain routine precautions are necessary before carrying these examinations in an adolescent.

- If the adolescent is accompanied by a person, reach an agreement as to whether they want this person to be present during the examination or not.
- Inform and explain the adolescent about nature and the purpose of the examination. Specially before the SMR staging and genital examination, explain the procedure in detail.
- Obtain the consent of the adolescent. If the adolescent is below the legal age of being able to give consent, you will need to obtain assent and consent from a parent or guardian. You should not proceed with the examination unless the adolescent agrees.
- Ideally same sex doctor is preferable; if not available, a chaperone (preferably a same gender nurse) should be made available.
- The examination should be done in a room designated for adolescents and ensure privacy, i.e. doors are shut, curtain

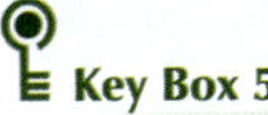

Key Box 5

Physical Examination in Adolescents

- *Anthropometry:* Measure and plot weight and height on IAP growth charts. Calculate and plot the BMI on IAP standard growth charts.
- Measure the blood pressure and plot on the nomogram
- *Skin:* Inspect for acne, acanthosis nigricans, tattoos, signs of abuse or self-inflicted injury
- *Breast:* In girls, assess for SMR and examine breast for breast disorders. In boys observe for breast hypertrophy or gynaecomastia versus another breast pathology
- *Genitalia:*

  Girls: Perform visual inspection for SMR, anatomic and skin abnormalities and signs of STIs (warts, vesicles and abnormal vaginal discharge)

  Boys: Perform visual inspection for SMR, circumcision status, signs of STIs (warts, vesicles and penile vaginal discharge). Examine testicles for abnormalities (hydrocele, hernia, varicocele, and mass, if any).

drawn and no one allowed during the examination.

- Watch for any signs of discomfort or pain during the examination and if necessary, stop the examination.
- Once the history has been taken in detail and rapport and trust has been established, one should proceed with the examination.
- After doing the examination properly explain the findings and its implications.

The physical examination is similar to what you do for younger children. Few pertinent areas which are specific for this age group are given in **Key Box 5**.

3.7 OVERWEIGHT AND OBESITY

A practical way to classify childhood obesity is (a) exogenous/primary/lifestyle obesity and (b) secondary/endogenous obesity. Exogenous obesity accounts for the majority (>90%), of the cases of obesity whereas secondary causes account for <10% of the cases (endocrine causes account for <1% of all cases).

Every overweight or obese child should be evaluated for possible etiology based on the following points in history:

- *Dietary history:* Check by 24-hour recall method of an average day. Check for foods rich in carbohydrates/fat/energy dense foods, large portion sizes and snacking. An increased consumption of JUNCS (junk foods, ultra-processed foods, nutritionally inappropriate foods, caffeinated/coloured/carbonated foods/beverages and sugar-sweetened food and beverages) is usually available.
- *Physical activity:* Sedentary habits, increased non-academic screen time and irregular habits.
- *Family history:* Obesity and associated complications like hypertension, heart disease, eating habits, and behavioral pattern.
- *Drug intake*
- *Development history:* For attainment of milestones, current school performance, developmental disabilities for chromosomal and genetic syndromes associated with obesity.
- *For hypothalamic obesity:* Headache, vomiting, visual disturbances.

Clinical evaluation is summarised in **Table 3.5**.

Screening for Co-morbidities

- *Psychological assessment:* Eating disorder, anxiety, depression, self-esteem, readiness and ability for behaviour change, peer relationship, bullying.
- *Asthma:* Shortness of breath, exercise intolerance.
- *Polycystic ovarian syndrome:* Acne and hirsutism.
- *Obstructive sleep apnea:* Snoring, sleep disruption, morning headaches, day-time somnolence.
- *Slipped capital femoral epiphyses:* Hip, knee, or back pain.
- *Abdominal pain:* Gastroesophageal reflux, constipation, gall bladder disease, non-alcoholic fatty liver disease.
- *Recurrent headache:* Pseudotumor cerebri.

Laboratory Evaluation

The goal of laboratory evaluation is to screen for associated comorbidities and metabolic syndrome (MS). Since exogenous obesity is

Table 3.5: Clinical examination of overweight or obese adolescents*

Parameter	Etiology/co-morbidity
Anthropometry	Weight, height, body mass index, mid-parental height, watch for changing centiles upwards plot on growth chart (IAP Growth Charts 5–18 years). BMI cutoffs (on IAP 2015 BMI charts) of 23rd adult equivalent should be used to define overweight and 27th adult equivalent should be used to define obesity in 5–18 years.
Body fat distribution	Waist circumference, an important predictor of visceral adiposity. In Indian children, waist circumference greater than 70th percentile can be used as a cut-off for identifying children with central adiposity who are at a risk of developing metabolic syndrome.
Pubertal staging for delayed or precocious puberty	Sexual maturity staging by Tanner
Lipomastia and buried penis	Simple obesity
Micropenis, undescended testis	Prader-Willi syndrome
Moon facies, buffalo hump	Cushing syndrome
Blood pressure	Compare with age/sex/height appropriate references
Skin examination	• Acanthosis nigricans—insulin resistance • Acne, hirsutism—PCOS • Violaceous stria—Cushing syndrome • Xanthelasma, skin tags—dyslipidemia • Intertrigo
Hair	Dry, brittle-hypothyroidism
Hepatomegaly	Non-alcoholic fatty liver disease
Skeletal complaints—bowing of legs, limp, limited range of motion, especially in the hip joints	Slipped capital femoral epiphysis, genu valgum, tibia vara

* Indian Academy of Pediatrics Revised Guidelines on Evaluation, Prevention and Management of Childhood Obesity, Indian Pediatrics. December 2023.

3

the most prevalent type of pediatric obesity, testing for secondary causes should only be done in presence of clues on history and examination.

All overweight and obese children ≥10 years of age should be evaluated for hypertension, dyslipidemia, hyperglycemia, metabolic dysfunction-associated steatotic liver disease (MASLD), and other comorbidities in presence of risk factors or waist circumference greater than 70th percentile. As per International Diabetes Federation (IDF), metabolic syndrome can be diagnosed in children aged 10–16 years with the following criteria: Presence of abdominal obesity (waist circumference ≥90th centile for age, gender, and ethnicity) with ≥2 of the following:

- Triglycerides ≥150 mg/dL,
- HDL-cholesterol ≥40 mg/dL,
- Fasting blood glucose ≥100 mg/dL and
- Systolic blood pressure ≥130 mm of Hg; diastolic blood pressure ≤85 mm of Hg (≥95th centile adjusted for age, height, and gender).

Laboratory evaluation according to suspected etiology is summarised in **Table 3.6**.

3.8 ADOLESCENTS, SOCIAL MEDIA, AND SCREEN TIME

Smartphones, laptops, tablets, and social networking sites (Facebook, Twitter, Instagram, etc.) have become an integral part of life of adolescents. Though there are numerous benefits of digital technologies and media but are also fraught with undesirable harmful effects.

Overuse in adolescents must be suspected, identified, and rectified at earliest. This should be a part of history taking in any adolescent examination.

Table 3.6: Suspected etiology and laboratory evaluation of obesity

Exogenous obesity	Fasting lipid profile, alanine aminotransferase (ALT), renal function tests, fasting blood glucose, oral glucose tolerance test, glycosylated hemoglobin (if indicated)
Hypothyroidism	TSH, free thyroxine
Cushing syndrome	Serum or salivary cortisol (11 PM), dexamethasone suppression test, 24-hour urine-free cortisol test
Growth hormone deficiency	Bone age, Insulin-like growth factor-1, Insulin-like growth factor-binding protein-3, growth hormone stimulation test
Pseudohypoparathyroidism	Calcium, phosphorus, parathyroid hormone, X-ray hand
Genetic or monogenic obesity	Specific genetic test (advised by a specialist)
Hypothalamic and pituitary disease	Magnetic resonance imaging (MRI) of brain

Social media use: Three key concepts are important for screening the adolescents for excessive use of social media. These are **Balance** (balance between online and offline time), **Boundaries** (setting limits on the time and sites accessed by adolescents), and **Communication** (parents discussing social media issues with adolescents) **(Key Box 6)**. A few perils of social media that need to be assessed are listed below:

- ***Problematic internet use:*** Internet use that is risky, excessive, or impulsive in nature leading to adverse life consequences, specifically physical, emotional, social, or functional impairment. There are validated scales which can be used in adolescents.
- ***Sexting:*** Refers to sending, receiving, or forwarding sexually explicit messages or pictures over cellphone, computer, or other digital devices. Consequences include embarrassment, regret, or being harassed. This can also have potential legal consequences, which can include prosecution under child pornography status.
- ***Cyberbullying:*** Refers to deliberate use of technology including social media to communicate false, embarrassing, or hostile information about another individual which includes name calling, spreading rumours, pretending to be someone else, sending unwanted pictures or texts, disturbing pictures without consent, making threats. This can lead to depression, anxiety, amongst other consequences.

Ask patients directly about risk behaviours such as sexting and experiences with online harassment or cyber-bulling. After screening they can be appropriately referred to adolescent or mental health experts for remedial action.

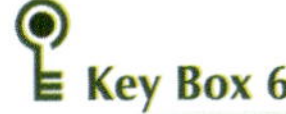

Screening for Screentime and Social Media Use

Balance

- Ask about media and technology use and how much time they spend each day without media.
- Ask about rules, if any, they, or their family use to regulate or monitor media use.

Boundaries

- Ask about their privacy settings on social media sites, and how often they update or check these settings to ensure they are current.

Communication

- Ask about how often they discuss their social media and technology use with their parents, other family member(s), or other adults.

Chapter

4

Assessment of Diet and Feeding Practices

○ Praveen Kumar ○ Piyush Gupta

Structure

4.1 IMPORTANCE AND OBJECTIVES OF THE DIETARY HISTORY

In this chapter, we introduce you to the principles and methods of assessment of diet and feeding practices of a child. Assessment of diet and feeding practices is an integral part of any pediatric clinical case.

Diet is the study of food intake of a person, which varies according to age, sex, and sociocultural status. Nutrients that we obtain through diet have vital effects on physical growth, development, body function, physical activity, and health. Diet is directly or indirectly related to most of the diseases. If you are able to assess diet and feeding practices correctly, this not only helps you in planning treatment, but it also gives you an opportunity to guide and counsel the family in preventing future problems (e.g. malnutrition, obesity).

You need to follow the *evaluation-decision-action* tree **(Fig. 4.1)** to assess, analyze, and advise regarding diet and feeding practices:

A. Evaluate

Evaluation has following four components:

1. Assess food intake—the present intake/pre-morbid status.
2. Calculate calorie/protein content of diet assessed (by converting food constituents into calories and proteins).

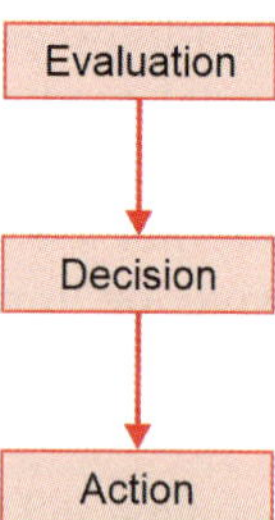

Fig. 4.1: Assessment of diet: The management tree.

3. Assess feeding practices.
4. Assess micronutrient intake.

B. Decide

After evaluation, you will have to decide whether dietary intake is appropriate for the age or not. For this, compare the present dietary intake with recommendations for that age. Based on your decision, the dietary intake and feeding practices in a child could be:

i. Normal—praise and continue same diet;
ii. Feeding problem which needs counseling and follow-up evaluation; or
iii. Inappropriate and needs immediate intervention.

C. Action

You should praise the mother for correct practices; and counsel the mother and family for changes, if dietary intake or practices are not appropriate according to recommendations.

Before we discuss the above steps one by one, you also need to know the following:

1. Nutrient requirements at different ages (calorie, protein, fat, carbohydrate) and recommended daily allowances (RDA) of important micronutrients at different ages.
2. How to calculate the calorie/protein intake:
   - Tools and methods of dietary assessment.
   - Calorie/protein content of common food items.
3. Infant and young child feeding guidelines.

We shall discuss each one of these in the subsequent text.

Determine the Age of the Child

The dietary habits vary according to the age. First determine age of the child because you will have to use different questions and formats according to age. For further discussion, we will categorize our case according to age into three groups:

- 0–6 months
- 6 months–2 years
- More than 2 years

4.2 ASSESSMENT OF DIET AND FEEDING PRACTICES IN INFANTS LESS THAN 6 MONTHS

When you approach a mother with a baby less than 6 months old for assessment of dietary intake, take care of the following:

- *Build rapport:* Greet the mother, introduce yourself, and ask her name and her baby's name. Inform that you will be talking regarding the baby's feeding.
- Make sure the mother is sitting in a comfortable, relaxed position.
- Sit on a chair or stool, or the bed if permissible at same head level and then start interacting with her about infant's feeding.
- Listen patiently to what the mother or caregiver tells.
- Do not interrupt in between.
- Do not be critical even if you identify inappropriate feeding practices or certain hindering factors in the family.

A. Evaluation

1. *Type of feeding:* Ask what feeding the infant is getting—breastfeeding/mixed feeding/animal milk or formula feeding.
2. Try to learn whether colostrum was given or not? If not, try to find out the reason. Also, try to find out about prelacteal feeds and any supplementary fluids given.
3. If breastfed—whether it is exclusive or not? Whether night feeds are given or not? If yes, frequency of night feeds should be noted.
4. *If not breastfed:* Ask which particular milk is being fed (animal/formula milk). What is the dilution? How the baby is being fed—by bottle or by *katori*-spoon?
5. Whether baby is receiving any other food or fluid in addition to breastmilk?
6. Identify barriers to optimal feeding, if any.

Use the format given in **Form (Part A) (Key Box 1)** for recording your observations. After completing **Form (Part A)** you will need to decide whether observation of breastfeeding is required or not? Fill up **Form (Part B) Key Box 2** also, if you have observed the breastfeed.

B. When to Observe a Breastfeed

You need to observe breastfeeding in following situations:

Outpatient settings, e.g. OPD or well-baby clinic

i. If infant's weight is <– 2 SD for that age.
ii. Baby is taking any other feed/drink (other than breastmilk).
iii. If the frequency of breastfeeding is <8 times/day.
iv. If mother reports any problem with breast or difficulty in feeding (pain, fissure, or not enough milk).

Inpatient setting, e.g. postnatal ward or neonatal units

i. All primipara mothers.
ii. Mothers having LSCS.
iii. If baby birth weight <2.5 kg.
iv. Mothers who were separated from babies due to sickness.
v. Any mother reporting any problem in feeding.
vi. History of not able to breastfeed exclusively for 6 months in previous pregnancy.

Key Box 1

Feeding Assessment Form (Part A)
Recording Form for Infants Less Than 6 Months

Name of Mother .... Name of Baby ....
Age (weeks) .... Weight (in grams) .... (WFA) SD score ....

1. When was the first feed given? ....
2. Whether baby received any prelacteal feeds? .... Yes/No
3. How many times breastfeed was given in last 24 hrs? ....
4. How many night feeds were given? ....
5. Does the child receive any other food or drink in addition to breastfeeds? .... Yes/No
6. If yes, which food or drink? ....
7. If animal milk/formula milk—how many times in last 24 hrs? .... and dilution? Yes/No
8. What is being used to feed the child, if baby is receiving feed other than breastfeeds? Cup/Spoon/ Bottle ....
9. How feeding bottle/cup is prepared—Washing .... Yes/No, Boiling .... Yes/No
10. How many times baby is passing urine in 24 hrs? ....
11. What is the color of urine? ....
12. Ask mother if she has any pain during breastfeeding (for sore nipples/breast abscess)? Yes/No

Key Box 2

Feeding Assessment Form (Part B)
Recording Form for Observing Breastfeeding in Less Than 6 months

Observe breastfeeding for 4 minutes

1. Well attached/poorly attached

To check attachment, look for:
- i. Chin touching breast,
- ii. Mouth wide open,
- iii. Lower lip turned outward, and
- iv. More areola visible above than below the mouth.

(All of these signs should be present, if the baby is well attached.)

2. Check position

- Whether infant's head and body is straight or not.
- Whether the baby is facing breast with infant's nose opposite her nipple or not.
- Whether infant's body is close to mother's body or not.
- Whether mother supporting infant's whole body or not.

(The answer to all these questions should be yes, if the positioning is correct.)

3. Is the infant suckling effectively (i.e., slow deep sucks, sometimes pausing)?

Not suckling at all *Not suckling effectively* *Suckling effectively*

4. If baby not suckling effectively or mother complains pain during feeding:
   - Check the baby for ulcer in mouth.
   - Check mother's breast for: i. Flat or inverted nipple; ii. Engorged breasts; and iii. Breast abscess.

Remember the following when you decide to observe breastfeeding

- Take mother's consent to examine baby's feeding.
- Make sure the mother is sitting in a comfortable, relaxed position.
- Then ask her to feed and observe.

Observe breastfeed as per **Form** given in **Key Box 2** and complete it.

C. Decision

Based on your assessment of form (Part A and B), decide whether feeding problem is present or not. You will classify it as feeding problem, if one or more of the following 5 situations are present:

1. If the baby is not exclusively breastfed.
2. If the baby is on animal or formula feeds which is diluted.
3. If the mother is using the bottle for feeding.
4. If the mother is having breast or nipple problem.
5. If the baby is suckling poorly.

D. Action

Counseling

If you have identified feeding problem, you will need to counsel the mother for breastfeeding. Adhere to the following rules of 'non-verbal communication', while you are counseling the mother:

1. Keep yourself at the same head level as that of the mother.
2. Maintain an appropriate distance from her.
3. Maintain eye contact and pay attention.
4. Take time while talking.
5. Remove barriers and use touch appropriately.
6. Give her information according to your specific case.

How to correct attachment: Help the mother by first explaining components of good attachment and positioning and their importance. Then help her to correct herself. Give her suggestions, which you think will help her. Avoid being critical about any point. If she agrees to try your suggestion—advise her to correct position and attachment. You can use doll and breast models to explain her good positioning and attachment. A well-attached baby is shown in **Fig. 4.2**.

Poor attachment can cause pain and damage to the nipples. Infant may not be able to suck breastmilk effectively, which may cause engorgement of the breast. The infant may be unsatisfied after breastfeeds and wants to feed very often or for a very long time. All these problems may improve, if attachment can be improved.

How to correct positioning: Help the mother to position so that she is able to feed in good position. The following signs recognize good positioning:

- Infant's neck is straight or bent slightly back.

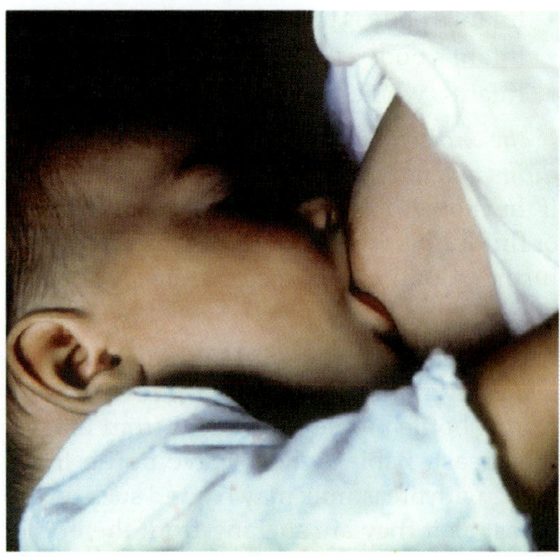

Fig. 4.2: Correct attachment and positioning for breastfeeding. This picture depicts the following signs of correct attachment: (i) Chin touching breast; (ii) mouth wide open; (iii) lower lip turned outwards; and (iv) more areola visible above than below the mouth.

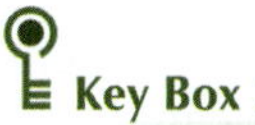

Key Box 3

Optimal Infant and Young Child Feeding (IYCF) Practices

- **Early initiation of breastfeeding** Immediately after birth, preferably within one hour.
- **Exclusive breastfeeding for the first 6 months of life** No other foods or fluids, not even water; but allows infant to receive ORS, drops, syrups of vitamins, minerals and medicines when required.
- **Timely introduction of complementary foods** Start solid, semisolid or soft foods after the age of 6 months (180 days).
- **Continued breastfeeding for 2 years or beyond**
- **Age appropriate complementary feeding for children 6–23 months, while continuing breastfeeding.** Children should receive food from at least 4 out of following 7 food groups (food diversity):
  1. Grains, roots and tubers
  2. Pulses (beans, peas, lentils), nuts and seeds
  3. Dairy products (milk, yogurt, cheese)
  4. Flesh foods (meat, fish, poultry)
  5. Eggs
  6. Vitamin A rich fruits and vegetables and
  7. Other fruits and vegetables
- **Active feeding** for children during and after illness.

- Infant's body is turned towards the mother.
- Infant's body is close to the mother.
- Infant's whole body is supported.

If the mother has started supplementation fluids and not giving exclusive breastfeeding: If the mother has started supplementing feed or fluids, this will decrease her milk secretion further. Counsel her to stop fluid by sharing advantages of exclusive breastfeeds.

If the mother is giving other food and drink and using feeding bottle: The action of sucking from a bottle nipple is different from that on the breast. Babies who receive bottle feeds along with breastmilk may try and suck on the breast as if they are sucking from the bottle. This results in poor milk supply, as nipple sucking does not allow effective milk transfer from the breast to the baby. This is called *nipple confusion*.

The mother should be counseled to stop bottle/top feed, if it is insignificant amount and give breastfeeds frequently. The process has to be slower by reducing the frequency of top feeds gradually; and more frequent breastfeeds, if the amount is significant.

If the mother is feeding less than 8 times per 24 hours or not giving night feeds

It is important to let the mother know that the most effective stimulus for milk secretion is sucking. For maximum milk secretion, she should feed frequently day and night in health and sickness. Night feeding is especially important to increase the milk production. Increasing frequency of feeding needs to be emphasized.

If the mother does not breastfeed at all: If the mother is interested, she may start putting her baby on breast and then gives other milk by cup/spoon. Advise a mother who does not breastfeed at all about choosing and correctly preparing dairy/locally appropriate animal milk without any dilution. Also advise her to feed with a cup and not from a feeding bottle.

In the end, advise her to take care of her health (iron-folic acid tablets and good diet) and tell her about next immunization due for baby. Thank the mother and family members for talking to you.

We are providing two examples of assessment of nutritional intake in infants less than 6 months of age. Case Scenario-1 pertains to a child with NO feeding problem; while Case Scenario-2 is for a child WITH feeding problem.

4.3 ASSESSMENT OF DIETARY INTAKE IN CHILDREN MORE THAN 6 MONTHS

Nutritional intake between 6 months and 2 years is most critical as inappropriate feeding practices at this age are the root cause of malnutrition or obesity. Assessment of diet and its constituents is essential to know nutrients gaps and excess. Assessment aims to find out both quantitative (amount of calories and proteins) and qualitative (food diversity, nature—vegetarian/non-vegetarian, feeding practices) aspects of diet consumed. First obtain 24 hrs diet consumption by recall. This should be followed by probing, further into the dietary history for qualitative assessment.

A. Evaluation

24 Hours Dietary Recall

This is the most common tool used in clinical practice for an individual patient. The parents or patient is asked to recall the actual food and drink consumed in the last 24 hrs. When there is a history of poor appetite, you should take both pre-morbid intake (before the onset of illness) and current intake. It is important to remember that size of utensils and thickness of food prepared varies a lot. Also try to ascertain the size of utensils to know the amount. You can use the format given in **Table 4.1** for this record.

How to Calculate Calorie and Proteins in Diet

The energy values of food items are traditionally expressed in terms of the kilocalorie (kcal) also called "Calorie". Recently 'Joule' has been adopted as the unit of energy internationally.

1 kcal = 4.184 kJ (kilojoules)

However, still Calorie use is more common, and we will be using it for further discussion. The energy in dietary sources is derived from three sources—protein, fat, and carbohydrate.

Fat	9 Cal (kcal) per gram
Protein	4 Cal (kcal) per gram
Carbohydrate	4 Cal (kcal) per gram

4

Case Scenario-1

Dietary Assessment of Rohit, 10-week-old Brought for Immunization

Recording Form (Part-A)

Name of Mother **Kanta** Name of Baby **Rohit**

Age (weeks) **10 weeks** Weight (in grams) **5400 grams** Weight for age SD score > **-2SD**

When was the first feed given? **15 minutes after birth**

Whether baby received any prelacteal feeds? .... Yes/**No**

How many times breastfeed was given in last 24 hrs? **10 times**

How many night feeds were given? **3**

Does the child receive any other food or drink in addition to breastfeeds? Yes/**No**

If yes, which food and drink? **NA** (not applicable)

If animal milk/formula milk—how many times in last 24 hrs? **NA**/dilution ....

What is being used to feed the child, if baby is receiving feed other than breastfeeds? .... Cup/spoon/bottle

How feeding bottle/cup is prepared? By washing .... Yes/No, By boiling .... Yes/No **NA**

How many times baby is passing urine in 24 hrs? **6–7 times**

What is the color of urine? **Colorless**

Ask mother, if she has any pain during breastfeeding? **No**

Decision

After completing Part-A, it was concluded that there is **No feeding problem** in this baby and hence decided that observation of breastfeeding is not required.

- Baby was exclusively breastfed.
- Weight was not low.
- Mother was not having any difficulty in feeding.

Action

Mother was praised for exclusive breastfeeding and counseled for continuing exclusive breastfeeding till 6 months.

Table 4.1: Proforma for 24 hours dietary recall

Time	Food items consumed	Amount (grams)	Calorie (Cal)	Protein (g)
Morning (breakfast)				
Mid-morning (snacks, if any)				
Afternoon (lunch)				
Evening (snacks, if any)				
Dinner				
Pre-sleep (milk/snack, if any)				
Midnight (snack, if any)				

Calorie and protein contents of milk of different types are given in Table 4.2. Nutritive values of cereals, pulses and millets (raw/uncooked) are provided in Table 4.3. Calorie and protein contents of other common food items are depicted in Table 4.4. For certain common cooked foods prepared in Indian kitchen, calories and protein values are provided for cooked items (Table 4.5). Use Tables 4.1–4.5 to calculate calorie and protein of the food item being consumed.

After calculating calorie and protein of these consumed food items, you will need to decide whether it is appropriate for age. For this, compare the intake of your child with the recommended requirement according to age

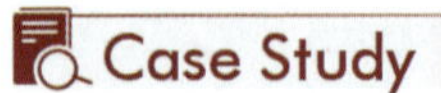

Case Scenario-2

Dietary Assessment of Meena, 14-week-old Admitted with Diarrhea for 5 Days

Recording Form (Part-A)

Name of Mother **Seema** Name of Baby **Meena**

Age (weeks) **14 weeks** Weight (in grams) **3400 grams** WFA SD score **<-2SD**

When was the first feed given? **1 hour after birth**

Whether baby received any prelacteal feeds? **Yes**

How many times breastfeed was given in last 24 hrs? **4 times**

How many night feeds were given? **Once only**

Does the child receive any other food or drink in addition to breastfeeds? **Yes**/No

If yes, which food or drink? **Cow's milk**

If animal milk/formula milk—how many times in last 24 hrs? **4 times** Dilution **2:1**

What is being used to feed the child? .... Cup/Spoon/**Bottle**

How feeding bottle/cup is prepared? By washing .... **Yes**/No, boiling .... **Yes**/No

How many times baby is passing urine in 24 hrs? **8 times**

What is the color of urine? **Colorless**

Ask mother, if she has any pain during breastfeeding. **No**

Decision

4 After completing (Part-A), it was concluded that there is feeding problem in this baby in view of the following: (i) baby was not exclusively breastfed; (ii) low weight; (iii) diluted cow milk (2 : 1); (iv) bottle feeding; (v) prelacteal feeds.

And, hence, it was decided that observation of breastfeeding is required in this baby.

Recording Form (Part-B): Observe breastfeeding for approximately 4 minutes

To check attachment, look for:
- Chin touching breast: **No**
- Mouth wide open: **No**
- Lower lip turned outward: **No**
- More areola visible above than below the mouth: **No**

Well attached/**Poorly attached**

Check position

Whether infant's head and body is straight or not. **No**

Whether the infant's nose is opposite mother's nipple or not? **Yes**

Whether infant's body close to mother's body or not. **No**

Whether mother supporting infant's whole body or not. **No**

Is the infant suckling effectively? **Not suckling effectively**

If baby not suckling effectively, check for ulcer in mouth, and check mother's breast for flat, sore or inverted nipple/engorged breasts/breast abscess **No**

Decision

This child has poor attachment and is not suckling effectively.

Action

Mother was praised for continuing breastfeeding and was counseled for:
- Immediately stopping bottle feeding.
- Stop diluting cow's milk.
- Correcting attachment and positioning.
- Frequent breastfeeds and increased number of night feed.

She was advised to come for follow-up after 2 days. It was planned to counsel her to increase breastfeeds to 8–10 times and gradually stopping cow's milk during follow-up.

Table 4.2: Nutritive value of milk (per 100 grams)

Milk	Calorie (kcal)	Fats (g)	Proteins (g)	Iron (mg)	Calcium (mg)
Buffalo	107	6.6	3.7	0.16	121
Cow	72	4.5	3.3	0.15	118
Goat	72	4.1	3.3	0.10	170
Human	67	4.2	1.1	0.35	35
Skimmed milk powder (cow)	357	0.1	38.0	0	1370
Paneer	258	14.8	18.9	0.9	476
Curd (cow milk)	60	4.0	3.1	0.1	149

Updated from: Indian Food Composition Tables, National Institute of Nutrition, ICMR, 2017.

Table 4.3: Nutritive values of cereals, pulses, millets (per 100 grams)

Food item	Calorie (kcal)	Fats (g)	Proteins (g)	Iron (mg)	Calcium (mg)
Bajra	346	5.4	11.0	6.4	27.3
Bengal gram *dal*	328	5.3	21.6	6.1	46.3
Black gram *dal*	323	1.7	23.1	4.7	55.7
Green gram *dal*	325	1.3	23.9	3.9	43.1
Jowar	332	1.7	10.0	3.9	27.6
Maize (dry)	332	3.8	8.8	2.5	8.9
Peas (dry)	302	1.9	20.4	5.1	75.1
Ragi	320	1.9	7.2	4.6	364.0
Rajma (kidney beans)	296	1.7	19.5	6.1	126.0
Red gram *dal*	330	1.6	21.7	3.9	71.7
Rice raw milled	355	0.5	7.9	0.7	7.5
Soyabean (white)	376	19.4	37.8	8.2	195.0
Wheat (whole)	322	1.5	10.6	4.0	39.4
Wheat, flour (refined)	350	0.8	10.4	1.8	20.4
Wheat, flour (whole)	320	1.5	10.6	4.1	31.0

Updated from: Indian Food Composition Tables, National Institute of Nutrition, ICMR, 2017.

(Table 4.6). Decide whether it is according to the recommendation for the particular age or not.

- A child up to 1 year of age needs 100 kcal/kg/d. Thus, approximately, a 1-year-old healthy child (expected to weigh around 10 kilos) needs 1000 kcal per day.
- Add 100 kcal for every additional year, till puberty. For example, a 5-year-old child will need at least 1000 + 400 = 1400 kcal per day.
- The above calculations are only a crude estimate and reflect the minimum requirements at these ages. *See* **Table 4.6** for exact ICMR recommendations.

History of Feeding Practices and Food-frequency Questionnaire

Although, dietary recall method gives idea about calorie and protein, it is unable to tell us whether diet intake is balanced or not. For this, you need to obtain a proper dietary history and ask questions related to the frequency of consumption of certain food items.

The child or parents are given a list of foods and asked to tell how often each item is consumed per day per week. Ask parents about the frequency of food groups (cereals, pulses, milk and meat products, fruits and vegetables, and fats and sugars) which the

Table 4.4: Nutritive values of other food items (per 100 grams)

Food item	Calorie (kcal)	Fats (g)	Proteins (g)	Iron (mg)	Calcium (mg)
Apple (big)	62	0.6	0.3	0.3	13.7
Banana (ripe)	110	0.3	1.2	0.4	6.8
Bathua leaves	28	0.4	2.5	2.7	211.0
Beans (field)	43	1.0	2.9	1.9	70.9
Bittergourd	21	0.2	1.4	1.1	21.4
Brinjal (eggplant)	27	0.4	1.8	0.4	16.6
Carrot	38	0.5	1.0	0.7	41.1
Cauliflower	23	0.4	2.1	1.0	25.2
Chicken (leg)	382	12.6	19.4	1.3	20.5
Cucumber	20	0.2	0.7	0.5	16.4
Egg (hen) whole	134	13.0	13.3	1.6	50.1
French beans	24	0.3	2.5	1.0	50.0
Goat, meat (shoulder)	187	12.0	20.3	1.5	6.2
Grapes	56	0.3	0.8	0.2	11.2
Guava	32	0.3	1.4	0.3	18.5
Lady finger (okra)	27	0.2	2.1	0.8	86.1
Litchi	54	0.3	1.0	0.8	5.8
Onion	56	0.2	1.8	0.4	21.0
Potato	70	0.2	1.5	0.6	9.5
Pumpkin	24	0.2	0.9	0.3	24.0
Sweet potato	109	0.3	1.3	0.4	27.5
Tapioca	80	0.2	1.0	0.8	25.9
Tomato	20	0.5	0.9	0.3	10.2

Updated from: Indian Food Composition Tables, National Institute of Nutrition, ICMR, 2017.

child is taking in the diet. Also ask whether the child is vegetarian or non-vegetarian. In later case, enquire about the frequency of consumption of such item and the usual portion size. Diet history and food frequency questionnaire usually supplement 24 hrs dietary recall method to know the qualitative aspects of the diet.

Recording form for assessment of diet and feeding practices for a child more than 6 months is provided in **Key Box 4**.

Assessment of Micronutrient Intake

In certain situations, you will also have to assess about micronutrients, e.g. iron in a child with anemia, calcium in presence of signs of rickets, vitamin C in a child with suspected scurvy, and both iron and calcium in adolescents.

Calcium: Calcium is required for formation and maintenance of the skeleton and plays an important role in neuromuscular excitation, blood coagulation, and membrane permeability. Calcium is present in both animal and plant foods. The richest source of calcium among animal foods is milk. Ask for the history of intake of milk, milk products, and egg. Plant foods rich in calcium include amaranth, tapioca, and ragi. Remember that most cereals and millets contain some amount of calcium, but rice is a poor source.

Iron: Cereals, millets, pulses, and green leafy vegetables are rich sources of iron. In addition to these food items, meat particularly organ meat is a rich source of iron. Iron present in meat is also more easily absorbed. Ask whether the family cooks food in iron utensils; this increases the iron content of food.

Table 4.5: Approximate calorific value of some cooked preparation

Preparation	Quantity for one serving	Calories (kcal)	Protein (g)
1. Cereals			
Rice	1 cup	110	2.0
Pulao	1 cup	180	3.8
Phulka/Chapati	1 no.	80	2.4
Paratha	1 no.	150	3.0
Puri	1 no.	80	1.6
Bread (Big)	1 slice	85	2.2
Poha	1 cup	270	5.7
Upma	1 cup	270	8.1
Idli (50 g per piece)	2 nos.	150	6.4
Dosa (plain)	1 no.	125	3.0
Khichdi	1 cup	200	3.5
Porridge	1 cup	220	8.5
Cornflakes with milk	1 cup	220	5.0
Maggi	100 g (per serving = 70–75 g)	413 289	9.2 6.4
2. Pulses			
Plain *dal*	½ cup	100	5.0
Sambar	1 cup	110	5.0
3. Vegetable			
Dry	1 cup	150	1.0
With gravy	1 cup	170	1.0
4. Biscuits			
Fan/puff	1 no.	80	1.4
Good Day	1 no.	50	0.7
Monacco	1 no.	13	0.2
Parle-G/Marigold/Krack Jack	1 no.	30	0.5
Rusk (Britannia)	1 no.	67	1.2
5. Nonvegetarian			
Boiled egg	1 no.	90	6.5
Chicken curry	¾ cup	240	28.0
Mutton curry	¾ cup	260	28.0
Omelette	1 no.	160	6.5
6. Snacks			
Pizza (cheese and tomato) medium	1 slice	200	8.0
Potato chips (salted)	100 g	547	6.6
Samosa (small)	1 no.	200	3.1
Sandwiches (butter 2 tbsp)	2 slices	200	7.0
7. Chutney			
Coconut	1 tbsp	60	0.5
Tomato	1 tbsp	10	0.3
8. Beverage			
Cold drinks	1 bottle (200 mL)	150	-
Fresh lime juice	1 glass	60	-
Lassi (2 tbsp sugar)	1 cup/glass (200 mL)	110	3.1
Squash	1 cup/glass	75	-
Tea (2 tbsp sugar + 50 mL toned milk)	1 cup	75	1.2

1 cup = 1 katori = 1 glass = 200 mL

Source: Dietary Guidelines for Indians. 2nd ed. National Institute of Nutrition, Indian Council of Medical Research; 2011.

Table 4.6: Recommended average requirements of energy and nutrients

Age	Energy (kcal)	Protein (g/day)		Minimum level of total fat (%E)	Calcium (mg/day)			Iron (mg/day)
		EAR	*RDA*		*EAR*	*RDA*	*EAR*	*RDA*
0–6 months	90 cal/kg/d	7	8	40–60	-	300	-	-
6–12 months	80 cal/kg/d	9	10.5	35	-	300	4	6
1–2 years	1110	10	12.3	35	400	500	6	8
3–6 years	1360	13	16	25	450	550	8	11
7–9 years	1700	19.0	23.0	25	500	650	10	15
10–12 years	Boys–2220	26.0	32	25	650	850	12	16
	Girls–2060	27	33	25	650	850	16	28
13–15 years	Boys–2860	36	45	25	800	1000	15	22
	Girls–2400	35	43	25	800	1000	17	30
16–18 years	Boys–3320	45	55	25	800	1000	18	26
	Girls–2500	37	46	25	800	1000	18	32

Source: Indian Council of Medical Research (ICMR);2024.

Estimated average requirement (EAR): EAR refers to the average daily nutrient intake level estimated to meet the requirements of half of the healthy individuals in a particular life stage and gender group. It is used primarily to evaluate populations or groups.

Recommended dietary allowance (RDA): It refers to the daily dietary nutrient intake level that is sufficient to meet the nutrient requirements of nearly all (97–98 percent) healthy individuals in a particular life stage and gender group. This is derived from the EAR as the mean plus 2 standard deviations (SD) of the distribution of requirements. The term is used to primarily evaluate individual diets. The RDA is inappropriate for dietary assessment of groups as it is the intake level that exceeds the requirement of a large proportion of individuals within the group.

Table 4.7: Micronutrients and food sources

Calcium	Milk, cheese, green vegetables, pulses (Bengal gram, horse gram, rajmah), sitaphal, ragi. Bioavailability from cereals is poor because of the presence of phytic acid.
Iron	Liver, meat, seafood, legumes and pulses, enriched grain products, nuts, dried fruits. Food rich in vitamin C increases iron absorption while tannins, phytates decrease it.
Zinc	Seafood, liver, meat, fish
Copper	Seafood, meat, legumes, chocolate
Magnesium	Nuts, seafood, green vegetables

Table 4.7 provides an overview of foods that are rich in calcium, iron, zinc, copper and magnesium. Use it to compare, decide whether micronutrients intake is grossly normal or not. Additional information on the micronutrient content of food groups is provided in **Table 4.8**.

You may use the format given in **Key Box 4** for assessment of diet and feeding practices for a child aged more than 6 months.

How to Calculate Calorie Intake from Breastmilk

This is a common query by the students. The answer is not straightforward. The calorie intake from breastmilk from an individual mother cannot be estimated unless test weighing or some other method is undertaken to determine the intake. Also, the individual breastmilk intake varies a lot from mother to mother and child to child. There are two ways to tackle this:

Key Box 4

Feeding Assessment Form

Recording Form for Assessment of Diet and Feeding Practices for a Child More Than 6 Months

Child's Name: .... Age: .... (in months) Sex: .... Weight: .... (kg)

Relationship with caregiver/attendant: ....

- Was the child exclusively breastfed? If yes, the duration? And if no, the nature and mode of artificial feeding? Does your child take breastfeed now? .... Yes/No ....
  - If yes, how many times in 24 hours? .... times
  - Do you breastfeed during the night? Yes .... No ....
- Any other milk – Yes/No
  If yes then—which milk ....
  - Amount ....
  - Dilution ....
  - By—*Katori*/Spoon/Bottle
- Semi-solid started .... Yes/No
- At what age semi-solids were started? .... months
- Child's Growth Card Availability—Yes .... No ....
  - If available, is the line going well? Yes .... No ....
  - If not available, what is the child's present weight? ....
  - Is child malnourished? Yes .... No ....

In the last week did child eat any

- Pulses — Yes/No. If yes, how many days ....
- Dark green vegetables — Yes/No. If yes, how many days ....
- Eggs/meat/fish/milk products — Yes/No. If yes, how many days ....
- Fruits — Yes/No. If yes, how many days ....
- Fats and sugars including junk foods — Yes/No. If yes, how many days ....

Any difficulty with child's feeding — Yes/No. If yes, list them.

Dietary Recall: List all the foods and drinks consumed in last 24 hours in addition to breastfeeds. Note amount (approx.) of each by showing a suitable katori/glass

Time	*Food items consumed*	*Amount (grams)*	*Calorie (Cal)*	*Protein (g)*
Morning (breakfast)				
Mid-morning (snacks, if any)				
Afternoon (lunch)				
Evening (snacks, if any)				
Dinner				
Pre-sleep (milk/snack, if any)				
Midnight (snack, if any)				

Total Calorie .... **Protein** ....

1. Preferred method: Do not calculate the calorie intake from breastmilk, if the feeding has been going in the usual way (i.e. on demand frequent feeds including night feeds) and just calculate the calorie intake from the complementary foods. These intakes can be compared with the recommended as follows:

The energy needs from complementary foods for infants with "average" breastmilk intake in developing countries (WHO/UNICEF, 1998) are approximately 200 kcal per day at 6–8 months of age, 300 kcal per day at 9–11 months of age, and 550 kcal per day at 12–23 months of age. In industrialized countries, these estimates differ somewhat (130, 310 and 580 kcal/d at 6–8, 9–11 and 12–23 months, respectively) because of differences in average breastmilk intake.

Table 4.8: Food grouping systems

Food group	Main nutrients
Cereals Grains Products	
Rice, wheat, ragi, bajra, maize, jowar, barley, rice-flakes, wheat flour	Energy, protein, invisible fat, vitamin B_1, vitamin B_2, folic acid, iron, fiber
Pulses and Legumes	
Bengal gram, black gram, green gram, redgram, lentil (whole as well as *dhals*), peas, rajmah, soybeans, beans, etc.	Energy, protein, invisible fat, vitamin B, vitamin B_2, folic acid , calcium, iron, fiber
Milk and Meat Products	
Milk, curd, skimmed milk,	Protein, fat
Cheese	Vitamin B_2, calcium
Meat, chicken, liver, fish,	Protein, fat
Egg, meat	Vitamin B_2
Fruits and Vegetables	
Fruits	
Mango, guava, tomato	Carotenoids
Ripe papaya, orange, sweet lime, watermelon, banana	Vitamin C, fiber
Green Leafy Vegetables	
Amaranth, spinach, gogu, drumstick leaves, coriander leaves, mustard leaves, fenugreek leaves	Invisible fats, carotenoids, vitamin B_2, folic acid, calcium, iron, fiber
Other Vegetables	
Carrots, brinjal, lady fingers, capsicum, beans, onion, drumstick, cauliflower, potato	Carotenoids, folic acid, calcium, fiber
Fats and Sugars	
Fats	
Butter, ghee, hydrogenated oils, cooking oils like groundnut, mustard, coconut	Energy, fat, essential fatty acids
Sugar, jaggery	Energy

4

Points to Remember while Assessing Feeding Practices in 6 Months–2 Years Old Children

- Since at this age child starts learning eating, they need help by parents. Many a times child push out food, because they have not learnt the skill of moving food inside or swallow solids. This does not imply that the child is not interested in food.
- Feeding is more successful when it is given in response to child's cues or signals.
- Feeding is more successful when it is given by a person who has a good relationship with the child.
- Feeding is more successful when it is given in suitable feeding situation, i.e. all family members taking meal at same time so child develops interest in feeds, use separate bowl for the child, feed when child is alert and happy.
- If the child is in the initial stages of being given complementary foods, ask what is the consistency of such food (Fig. 4.3).
- Also assess whether foods prepared are safe or not. Talk to the family to know whether following practices are fulfilled or not:
  - Caregiver washes hands and utensils
  - Uses clean and safe water
  - Keeps food at safe temperature and covered
  - Uses freshly prepared foods

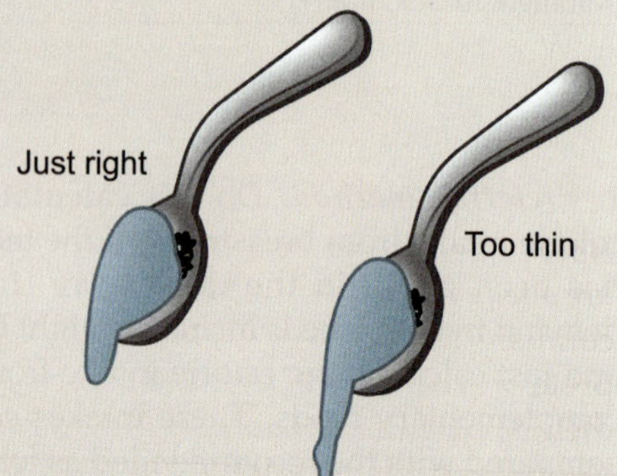

Fig. 4.3: Show this picture to know what is the correct consistency of given food items.

2. Alternative method: Calculate the calorie intake from complementary foods and add to it the average breastmilk intake by a healthy baby of that age as follows:

Among breastfed children in developing countries, average breastmilk energy intake is 413, 379, and 346 kcal/d at 6–8, 9–11 and 12–23 months, respectively (WHO/UNICEF, 1998). The equivalent values for industrialized countries (for breastfed children only) are 486, 375, and 313 kcal/d, respectively. The above guideline is based on children receiving average amounts of breastmilk at each age. If an infant is consuming more or less breastmilk than the average, the amount needed from complementary foods will differ accordingly.

However, both these estimates are based on the assumption that infant is consuming average amount breastmilk. If the breastfeeding is not being given in the usual way, i.e. given only occasionally or only 2–3 feeds, the energy intake would be lower. In that case, it is better to say that the child is consuming so many calories from complementary foods in addition to breastfeeding which is given only 2–3 times in a day.

B. Decision

After taking history, decide:

1. Whether the child is getting adequate calories or not.
2. Whether the child is getting adequate proteins or not.
3. Whether the child is getting recommended food group items or not (if child is not getting any particular food group, you will have to counsel to increase that food item).
4. Whether the child is getting food items with right consistency.
5. Whether the child's growth parameters (weight for age, height for age, weight for height; and body mass index in children >5 years of age) are normal or abnormal.

How to decide whether calories and proteins are adequate in diet: For points 1 and 2 above, compare the present intake of calories and proteins (calculated with the help of 24 hours dietary recall and **Tables 4.1–4.5**) with the recommended intake at that age (calculated as per **Table 4.6**). In case, the present intake is less than the recommended for that age, you also need to calculate the nutrient gap as follows:

Calorie gap: Recommended calories for that age–present intake of calories.

Protein gap: Recommended proteins for that age–present intake of proteins.

How to decide whether the child is getting all food group items: **Table 4.8** lists the various items categorized in main food groups. Relative importance and contribution to diet by the food groups is depicted in **Fig. 4.4**. The dietary habits also vary according to socioeconomic status, customs and traditions. Assessment of diet and its constituents is also essential to know excess or deficiency of different food groups. Ask from the parents regarding relative intake of items from each food group.

Decide whether complementary food is timely, adequate, properly fed and safe. Characteristics of ideal complementary foods are given in **Key Box 5**.

> Finally, you should be able to decide whether the diet and feeding practices of the given child are:
> i. *Normal* Praise and counsel to continue the same diet;
> ii. *Near normal* Need counseling for some changes and follow-up evaluations; or
> iii. *Inappropriate* Need immediate intervention.

Dietary diversity is a proxy for adequate micronutrient density of foods. Dietary

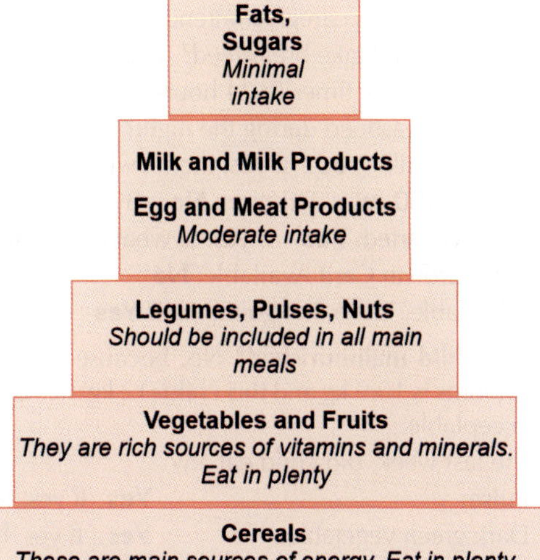

Fig. 4.4: The food pyramid: What should be the optimal food items?

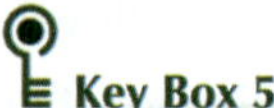

Key Box 5

Characteristics of Ideal Complementary Food

1. **Timely:** Introduced when need for energy and nutrients exceed that provided by breast milk (completes 6 months)
2. **Adequate:** Should provide sufficient energy, protein, and micronutrients (iron, vitamins A, C, etc.)
3. **Properly Fed:** Active feeding method and proper frequency according to age (use feeding guideline table)
4. **Safe:** Should be hygienically prepared, stored and fed
5. **Right consistency:** Soft, easy to digest, which family can afford, easily available, prepared, culturally acceptable
6. **Locally available and culturally acceptable**

diversity in children 2 years and above refers to the child receiving 4 or more of the following food groups:

1. Grains, roots and tubers
2. Legumes and nuts
3. Dairy products (milk, yogurt, cheese)
4. Flesh foods (meat, fish, poultry, etc.)
5. Eggs
6. Vitamin A rich fruits and vegetables
7. Other fruits and vegetables

C. Action

No intervention is required: When nutritional status is normal and assessed diet and feeding practices are normal. Praise parents and advise to continue the same diet.

Needs counseling and follow-up evaluation: You will need to counsel family and the child, if their nutritional status is not normal (undernutrition or obesity), diet is insufficient or excess in any particular food group items.

First praise mother and family for the things they are doing right:

- Give a few relevant information regarding changes you want.
- Suggest changes.
- Check their understanding.

How to Counsel Mother for Complementary Feeding

The process of giving an infant other foods and liquids along with breastmilk is known as complementary feeding. Additional food is required after 6 months of age as breastmilk alone is no longer sufficient to meet the

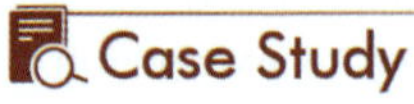

Case Study

Case Scenario-3

An 18 Months Male Child is Brought for Immunization. His Dietary Assessment is as Follows:

Child's Name: **Rohit** Age: **18 months** (in months)

Sex: **M** Weight **12** (kg)

Relationship with caregiver/attendant: **Mother**

Does your child take breastfeed? **Yes**

If yes, how many times in 24 hours? **2** times

– Do you breastfeed during the night? **Yes**

Any other milk: **Yes** If yes, then – which milk? **Mother dairy**

Amount: **250 mL** Dilution: **No** By: **Katori**/spoon/ Bottle

Semisolid started: **Yes** If yes, at what age? **6 months**

Child's Growth Card Available: **No**

– If available, is the line going well? **Yes**

Is the child malnourished? No, because the expected weight (50th percentile of WHO standards) at 18 months is 10.9 kg and this child (12 kg) lies between 75th (11.8 kg) and 90th percentiles (13.1 kg) which is acceptable.

In the last week, did child eat any

– Pulses **Yes.** If yes, how many days? **Daily**

– Dark green vegetables **Yes.** If yes, how many days? **Daily**

– Eggs/meat /fish **Yes.** If yes, how many days? **3**

– Fruits **Yes.** If yes, how many days? **4**

Any difficulty with child's feeding **No.**

Dietary Recall

List all the foods and drinks consumed in last 24 hours in addition to breastfeeds. Note amount (approx.) of each by showing a suitable *katori*/glass. Convert to calories with the help of **Tables 4.1–4.5**.

Meal	Food items consumed	Calorie		Protein	
Breakfast	1. Milk 1 cup (150 mL)	72/100 × 50	= 108	3.3/100 × 50	= 4.9
	2. Sugar 1 tsf (5 g)	4 × 5	= 20		= 0
	3. Bread 1 slice (big)	1 × 85	= 85	2.2 × 1	= 2.2
	4. Butter 1 tsf (5 g)	9 × 5	= 45		= 0
		258 Cal		**7.1 g**	
Snacks	Banana big 1 (80 g)	110/100 × 80	= **88 Cal**	1.2/100 × 80	= **1 g**
Lunch	1. Rice 1 *katori*		= 110		= 2 g
	2. Dal ½ cup		= 100		= 5 g
	3. Ghee 1 tsf (5 g)	9 × 5	= 45		= 0
	4. Vegetable 1 cup		= 150		= 1 g
		405 Cal		**8.0 g**	
Snacks	1. Apple 1 (100 g)		= 60		= 0.3
		60 Cal		**0.3 g**	
Dinner	1. *Chapati* 1	80 × 1	= 80		= 2.4
	2. Ghee 1 tsf (5 g)	9 × 5	= 45		= 0
	3. Dal ½ cup		= 100		= 5.0
	4. Vegetable (1 cup)		= 150		= 1.0
		375 Cal		**8.4 g**	
Bedtime	Milk 100 mL	**72 Cal**		**3.3 g**	

Present intake: 1258 kcal (expected 1110 kcal); and 28.1 g protein (expected 12.5 grams)

Evaluation

1. Whether child is getting adequate calories or not: **Taking adequate calories**
   He is receiving 1258 calories in addition to mother's feed. Requirement for his age is 1110 calories.
2. Whether child is getting adequate proteins or not: **Taking adequate proteins**
   He is receiving more than 20 g proteins in addition to mother's feed. Requirement for his age is approx 13 g.
3. Whether getting all food group items: **He is getting all food group items**
4. Whether right feeding practices are being followed: **Yes**

Decision

Diet and feeding practices in this child are **Normal**.

Action

The child mother duo **needs no intervention**. Parents and child were praised for breastfeeding, and good diet. They were advised to continue same diet.

nutritional requirements of an infant older than 6 months. The term 'weaning' which was earlier used is not used these days because the additional foods complement breastfeed. Breastfeeding should be continued till 2 years or longer and it does not aim to wean from breastfeed **(Table 4.9)**.

Disadvantages of adding foods too soon

- Decrease the intake of breastmilk resulting in a low nutrient diet.
- Increase risk of illness especially diarrhea.

Disadvantages of adding foods too late

- Growth and development slows down.
- Risk of deficiencies and malnutrition.

Substituting breastmilk: A child with severe acute malnutrition or other problems will need urgent attention and hospitalization. Mother is encouraged to breastfeed as much as possible. In addition, these children are managed with special therapeutic diets, i.e. starter (F-75 formula) and catch-up diet (F-100 formula).

Acceptable reasons for substituting the breastmilk with other substitutes are listed in **Key Box 6**.

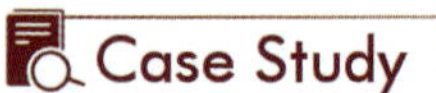

Case Study

Case Scenario-4

A 13 Months Female Child is Brought to OPD for Loose Motion.
Her Dietary Assessment is as Follows:

Feeding Assessment Form

Child's Name: **Rani** Age: **13 months** (in months)

Sex: **F** Weight: **6.7** (kg)

Relationship with caregiver/attendant: **Mother**

Does your child take breastfeed? **Yes**

If yes, how many times in 24 hours? **2** times

Do you breastfeed during the night? **Yes**

Any other milk: **Yes** If yes, then – which milk? **Mother dairy**

Amount **200 mL** Dilution **Yes (1:1)** By – Katori/spoon/ **Bottle**

Semisolid started: **Yes**

- If yes, at what age: **10** months
  Child's Growth Card Available: **No**
- If available, is the line depicting growth is growing upwards? **No**

Is the child malnourished?

4 *Yes; because the expected weight (50th percentile of WHO standards) at 13 months is 9.2 kg and this child (6.7 kg) lies below the 3rd percentiles (7.3 kg).*

In the last week, did child eat any

- Pulses **Yes**
- Dark green vegetables **No**
- Eggs / meat/ fish **No**
- Fruits **Yes**/No. If yes, how many days in a week? **Yes, twice a week**

Any difficulty with child's feeding **Yes**

If yes, list them **Not taking food items from all the food groups**

Dietary recall, evaluation, decision, and action pertaining to Rani (described above) are detailed on the facing page.

Dietary Recall

List all the foods and drinks consumed in last 24 hours in addition to breastfeeds. Note amount (approx.) of each by showing a suitable katori/glass. Convert to calories with the help of **Tables 4.1–4.4**.

Meal	Food items consumed	Calorie	Protein
Breakfast	Milk diluted (1:1) 100 mL	72/2 = 36 Cal	3.3/2 = 1.6 g
	Sugar (5 g)	4 × 5 = 20 Cal	
Snacks	Milk diluted (1:1) 50 mL	72/4 = 18 Cal	3.3/4 = 0.8 g
	Sugar (2.5 g)	4 × 2.5 = 10 Cal	
Lunch	1 *Katori Khichari* 100 g (thin consistency)	= 100 Cal	= 1.8 g
Dinner	*Chapati* 1 (small 20 g)	= 80 Cal	= 2.4 g
	Dal ½ cup	100/2 = 50 Cal	5/2 = 2.5 g
Bedtime	Milk diluted (1:1) 50 mL	72/4 = 18 Cal	3.3/4 = 0.8 g
	Sugar (2.5 g)	4 × 2.5 = 10 Cal	

Present intake: 342 kcal (expected 1110 kcal); and 9.9 g proteins (expected 12.5 g/d)

Evaluation

1. Whether child is getting adequate calories?
   NOT taking adequate calories. There is a ***Calorie gap*** of 1110 – 342 = 768 kcal.
2. Whether child is getting adequate proteins.
   NOT taking adequate proteins. The protein gap is almost 3 g.

3. Whether she is getting all food group items.
   She is not getting adequate green vegetables and fruits.
4. Whether child is getting food items with right consistency.
   No; thin consistency
5. Following feeding problems were identified:
   i. Bottle feeding;
   ii. Diluted milk;
   iii. Delayed introduction of complementary feeds; and
   iv. Inadequate amount and quality of food.
6. Following positive points were also identified: Continued breastfeeding and introduction of complementary feeding.

Decision

The diet and feeding practices in this child are **Not normal** and will **Need intervention**.

Action

Mother was praised for continued breastfeeding and introduction of complementary feeds. Then she was counseled to stop dilution of milk and bottle feeds. She was informed of normal requirement and recommendation for the age. A feeding chart was prepared and she was counseled to adhere to it. She was also advised to come for follow-up and re-checking of dietary intake.

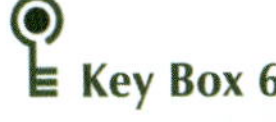

Acceptable Reasons for Using Breastmilk Substitute

Infant conditions

- *Galactosemia:* A galactose-free formula is needed.
- Maple syrup urine disease: A formula free of leucine, isoleucine and valine is needed.
- Phenylketonuria: A phenylalanine-free formula is needed.

Maternal conditions which may justify temporary cessation:

- Herpes simplex virus type 1 infection
- Maternal medications: Antipsychotic or cytotoxic drugs.

Infants for whom breastmilk remains the best feeding option but who may need other food in addition to breastmilk for a limited period

- Risk of hypoglycemia is very high by virtue of impaired metabolic adaptation or increased glucose demand (those who are VLBW, preterm, small for gestational age or who have experienced significant intrapartum hypoxic/ischemic stress)
- And those who are ill and those whose mothers are diabetic, if their blood sugar fails to respond to optimal breastfeeding or breast-milk feeding.

Table 4.9: Feeding recommendations for infants and children (IMNCI)

Up to 6 months	6 to 12 months	12 months to 2 years	2 years and older
• Breastfeed as often as the child wants, day and night, at least 8 times in 24 hours • Do not give any other foods or fluids not even water • Continue breastfeeding, if the child is sick.	• Breastfeed as often as the child wants. • Give at least one *katori* serving* at a time: i. Mashed roti/rice/bread/mixed in undiluted milk. OR ii. Mashed roti/rice/bread mixed in thick dal with added ghee/oil or *khichri* with added oil/ghee. Add cooked vegetables also in the servings. iii. *Sevian/dalia/halwa/kheer* prepared in milk or any cereal porridge cooked in milk. OR iv. Mashed boiled/fried potatoes v. Banana/cheeko/mango/papaya • Keep the child in your lap and feed with your own hands. • Wash you own and child's hands with soap and water every time before feeding.	• Breastfeed as often as the child wants. • Offer food from the family pot. • Give at least 1½ *katori* serving† at a time of: i. Mashed *roti/rice/bread* mixed in *thick dal* with added ghee/oil or *khichri* with added oil/ghee. Add cooked vegetables also in the servings. OR ii. Mashed *roti/rice/bread*/mixed in undiluted milk. OR iii. *Sevian/dalia/halwa/kheer* prepared in milk or any cereal porridge cooked in milk. OR iv. Mashed boiled/fried potatoes. v. Banana/cheeko/mango/ papaya • Ensure that the child finishes the serving • Wash your child's hands with soap and water every time before feeding.	• Give family foods at 3 meals each day. • Also twice daily, give nutritious food between meals, such as banana cheeko/mango/papaya as snacks. • Ensure that the child finishes the serving • Teach your child to wash his/her hands with soap and water every time before feeding.

*3 times per day, if breastfeed; 5 times per day, if not breastfeed.

†5 times per day.

Chapter

5

Anthropometry: Assessment of Growth

❍ Piyush Gupta ❍ Aashima Dabas

Structure

5.1 INTRODUCTION

Definition

The term anthropometry has been derived from Greek language and literally means measurement of humans (*'anthropos'* – human, *'metron'*–measure). It is defined as the study of measurement of the human body in terms of dimensions of the bone, muscle, and adipose (fat) tissue. It is the single most universally applicable, inexpensive, and non-invasive method available to assess the size, proportions, and composition of the human body.

The following steps are required for assessment of growth:

1. Outline the parameters to be assessed for evaluating growth.
2. Identify, select, and use the tools needed for assessment of growth in a particular child.
3. Compare the growth of a child with standard reference values.
4. State, whether the growth in a given child is:
   i. Normal and needs no intervention;
   ii. Borderline, needs follow-up evaluations; or
   iii. Abnormal and needs immediate evaluation.

In this chapter, we introduce you to the principles and actual procedures for assessing and monitoring growth of a child. For assessment of growth, you need to understand certain basic terminologies and the statistical principles involved in the interpretation of anthropometry. The next section of this chapter is devoted to the same.

5.2 STATISTICAL PRINCIPLES IN ASSESSMENT OF GROWTH

A. Measurements

These include age, weight, height, length, arm circumference, etc. However, a measurement alone is of no use unless it is related to another measurement. For example, 'weight of a given child is 10 kg' cannot be interpreted as normal or abnormal, unless the age of this child is also known.

1. Gaussian and Non-Gaussian (Skewed) Distribution

If anthropometric measurements (e.g. weight, height) are obtained in a very large population of healthy children of a given sex and a particular age, and then arranged in a sequence starting from the lowest to the highest, a bell-shaped curve is formed **(Fig. 5.1a)**.

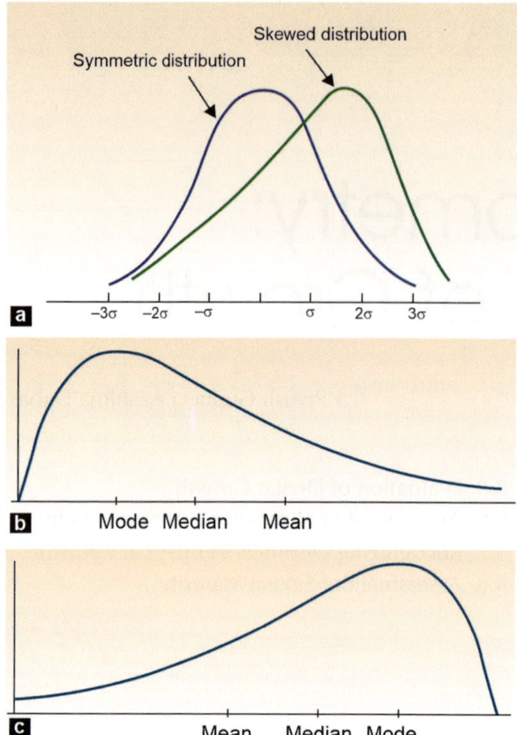

Fig. 5.1: (a) Gaussian (symmetric) and skewed distribution; (b) positively skewed (to the right); (c) negatively skewed (to the left).

This symmetrical curve illustrates a typical *Gaussian (Normal) distribution*, in which maximum values lie around the middle of the curve. The curve tapers off symmetrically on the either side, with fewer observations at both the ends of the curve.

However, most of the anthropometric measurements do not follow a Gaussian distribution, more so if a relatively smaller sample is taken. Such a distribution which is not symmetric on either side of mean is known as *Skewed or Non-Gaussian*. The distribution may be skewed towards right, i.e. positively skewed **(Fig. 5.1b)** or towards left, i.e. negatively skewed **(Fig. 5.1c)**.

2. Mean, Median, and Standard Deviation

Measurement of a parameter in a sample and its recording in a continuous numerical manner can generate several values, the most important of them being mean, median, and standard deviation (SD).

- ***Mean*** (the average) is obtained by dividing the sum of all observations by the number of observations. In a Gaussian distribution, the maximum number of values cluster around the mean, which is the central or representative value of the sample.
- ***Median:*** When data are arranged in ascending or descending order of magnitude, half of the observations are above and the other half below a certain value. This value is known as the median. The Median thus indicates that 50% of observations are above and 50% are below this value. This value thus, in the true sense, lies at the center of the data.

  In a typical Gaussian distribution, the median is expected to be equivalent to the arithmetic mean. However, mean and median are not the same in a non-Gaussian distribution. Since most of the anthropometric parameters in the population follow a non-Gaussian (skewed) distribution; median is considered a better representative of central value as compared to the mean.
- ***Standard deviation*** denotes the degree of dispersion or the scatter of observations away from the mean. It is estimated that 68.3% (approximately two-thirds) of the observations lie within 1 standard deviation (SD) above or below the mean value of the observations. Values within the range of ±2 SD include 95.4% of all values. Values beyond 2 SD are unusual in a normal population. 3 SD around the mean includes 99.7% of all values.

B. Indices

Anthropometric indices (singular *'index'*) are combination of measurements. Weight-for-age, height-for-age, weight-for-height, and body mass index, are some commonly used indices.

For example, *weight-for-age* represents the weight of the index child compared with expected weight of a child of the same age. The expected (reference) weight at a given age is usually represented by the median. Indices can also be expressed in terms of percentiles or Z (standard deviation) score. These terms are discussed below for more clarity.

1. Percentiles

Percentile indicates the position that a measurement would hold in a typical series of

100 arranged in ascending order. The median lies at the center so it is the 50th percentile, on either side of which lie half the observations. Another example is the 85th percentile curve, which denotes that 15 percent of observations are expected to be above and 84% below it.

Percentile location is used to designate where an individual stands with respect to other members of the population. The WHO growth standards show values for 3rd, 5th, 15th, 25th, 50th, 75th, 85th, 95th, and 97th percentiles, corresponding to distances from the average values. One standard deviation above or below the mean coincides with the 84th or 16th percentile curve, respectively. Roughly, 70% of the weight/ height measurements of healthy children at a given age are expected to be between 15th and 85th percentiles. Similarly, 95% of the normal values are expected to be between 3rd and 97th percentile values. Thus, allowable normal range of variation in observations is between 3rd and 97th percentiles, which roughly correspond to ±2 SD.

Example:

- Suppose, a group of 100 children of the same age and sex are arranged in the order of increasing weight. The child on 10th position in this group is the 10th percentile; 9% individuals are below or equal to him and 90% above.
- Thus, a child of a given age, whose weight corresponds to the 10th percentile, weighs the same or more than 10% of the reference population of children of the same age.
- *Median refers to the 50th percentile*. The number of individuals distributed below and above the median is equal.

Remember that a healthy child normally remains and follows the same percentile curve during the entire period of his/her growth.

2. Percent of Median

It is the ratio of a measured value (e.g. weight) to the median value of the reference data for the same age or height, expressed as a percentage.

Example:

Q. The weight of a 4-year-old child is observed to be 12 kg. And the reference weight (median or 50th percentile) at 4 years is 16.3 kg. Calculate percent weight-for-age of this child.

A. (Present weight/expected weight) × 100 = (12/16.3) × 100 = 73.6%.

3. Z (SD)-Score

It represents the deviation of anthropometric measurement from the reference median and is calculated as follows:

$$\frac{\text{Observed value} - \text{Median reference value}}{\text{Standard deviation (SD) of the reference population}}$$

A Z-score value of +1.5 means that the difference between the present (observed) and the expected (reference median value) is 1.5 times of the standard deviation of the reference population. A positive (+) sign of Z-score indicates that the observed value of the measurement/index is more than the reference median. A negative value of Z-score means that the observed value is less than the expected.

Abnormal values usually refer to measurements below –2 *Z*-score (2.3rd percentile) or above +2 *Z*-score (97.7th percentile), relative to the reference median.

Z-score is a method of standardization that helps in comparing values of different variables that are present on different scales. For example, a child having Z-score of –1.5 for height-for-age is below (lesser than) the median to the tune of 1.5 times the SD. If the Z-score of weight-for-age for the same child is –2.5, it means that he/she has a weight which is lesser than the median by a factor of almost 2.5 times of SD. Thus, this child is lagging behind in height as well as weight for his age, but the magnitude of lag is much more for weight than for height.

C. Indicators

An indicator relates to the use or application of an index. Indicator is constructed from the indices, usually in conjunction with a cut-off point. Indicator can thus be used for making an evaluation.

For example, height-for-age (an index) below 90% of the reference median (the cut-off) is an *indicator* of stunting.

Similarly, weight-for-height below 80% and 70% are measures of wasting, and severe wasting, respectively.

5.3 ANTHROPOMETRIC PARAMETERS, TOOLS, AND PROCEDURES

1. Weight

Weight is the best measurement of nutrition and growth and can be easily measured. Before the advent of digital electronic scales, two types of weighing scales were commonly used: Beam balance scales (with moving weights) and the spring balance scales. Of these, beam balancing scales are more accurate. For infants weighing up to 10.0 kg, basket or pan type scale is used **(Fig. 5.2)**. The infant can be placed on the tray, which is supported on a reading frame calibrated for measuring a minimum of 10 g increment. Digital portable weighing scales for infants can measure up to 5 g difference in weight. These should have taring facility to deduct the weight of clothing/diaper, etc. Older children who can climb and stand up on the scale are weighed using the platform scales which usually have a minimum measurable increment of 100 g **(Fig. 5.3)**. All scales need regular calibration with known/standard weights.

Method of Recording the Weight

- Weigh the child in bare minimum clothes and without shoes. Infants should be weighed naked (without diapers) and older children can be weighed with a vest and brief.
- Ensure that the scale is resting on a firm, stable, and even surface or uncarpeted floor.
- Check the zero of the scale before weighing. Calibrate the weight scale at the beginning and at the end of each measurement.
- ***Infants*** Place the infant in a manner so as to distribute the weight evenly about the center of the pan. If a diaper is worn, its weight should be subtracted from the observed weight; because the reference data for infants is based on nude weight.
- ***Children*** Ask them to stand in the center of the platform, with body weight evenly distributed on both feet. Ensure that the child is not holding on to anything.
- A child on follow-up should preferably be weighed on the same scale.
- Read the weight by standing in front of the scale and not from the side.

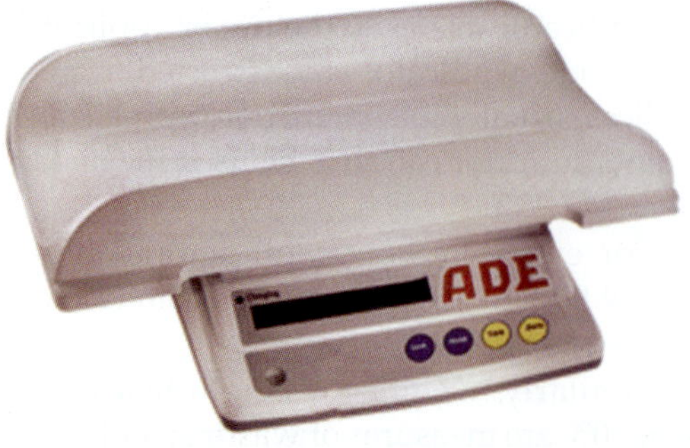

Fig. 5.2: The basket/pan type of weighing scale.

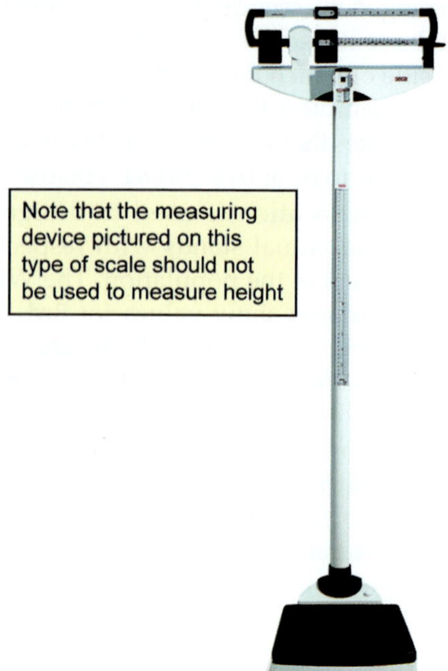

Fig. 5.3: Beam balancing weighing scale.

Normal Pattern of Weight Gain

- An average Indian newborn baby born at full term (40 weeks) gestation weighs 2.9 kg at birth.
- After delivery, 10% of birth weight is lost during first seven days of life. The birth weight is regained after 10 days of life.
- Thereafter, the infant gains at the rate of 20–40 g per day. Approximate daily gain in weight between 0 and 3 years of age is depicted in **Table 5.1**.
- A child doubles, triples, and quadruples the birth weight by 5 months, 1 year, and 2 years, respectively.
- After the second year of life, weight gain occurs at the rate of 2.0–2.5 kg per year, till the onset of puberty.

Table 5.1: Gain in weight, stature, and head circumference in 0–3 years age

Age	Weight gain (grams per day)	Stature gain (cm per month)	Head growth (cm per month)
0–3 mo	30	3.5	2.0
3–6 mo	20	2.0	1.0
6–9 mo	15	1.5	0.5
9–12 mo	12	1.2	0.5
1–3 yr	8	1.0	0.2

- The adolescent acceleration in weight occurs earlier in girls (10–12 years) than in boys (beginning 2 years later).
- The rapid weight gain in girls is greatest in the year before menarche.

Given below are some formulae for a rough and quick calculation of expected weight between the ages of 3 months and 12 years. However, refer to the standard reference growth charts for exact values.

3–12 months	(age in months + 9)/2
1–6 years	2 (age in years) + 8
7–12 years	[7 (age in years) – 5]/2

2. Stature

Stature is ascertained by measuring the length (in children less than 2 years old) or height (in older children).

Measuring the Length

Harpenden's infantometer measures the length of newborns and infants. The tool consists of a horizontal wooden board limited by two vertical planks perpendicular to the two ends (Fig. 5.4). At one end, plank is fixed to the wooden board (headpiece); the other end has a movable vertical plank to adjust to the infant's length (footpiece). There is a calibrated reading strip in the middle of the board on which length of the baby can be read directly. The infantometer is designed to measure lengths between 0 and 100 cm, with a precision of 1 mm. The length is measured by following the steps given below:

Prepare: Undo the braids and remove hair ornaments, as they interfere with positioning of the head. Also remove diapers, as they make it difficult to hold the infant's legs together and straighten them.

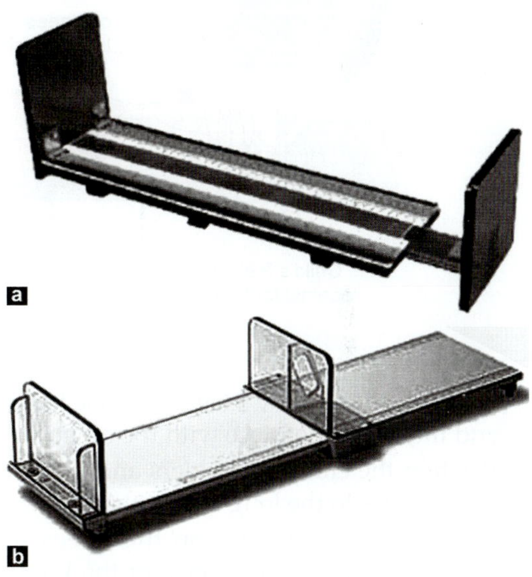

Fig. 5.4: Infantometer (a) and (b).

- You will require an assistant to measure the length with an infantometer.
- Assistant stands at the head end (headpiece).
- Place the child supine on the infant measuring board.
- Ask the assistant to hold the child's head, while you steady the legs (Fig. 5.5).

Position the head end

- Ask the assistant to place the child's head in the Frankfort plane.
- The head is positioned in the Frankfort plane when the crown touches the headpiece and a vertical line from the ear canal to the lower border of the eye socket is perpendicular to the horizontal board (i.e. positioned vertically) (Fig. 5.5).
- Apply gentle traction to bring the head into contact with the fixed headpiece.

Position the foot end

- Stand on one side of the infantometer (the moving board).

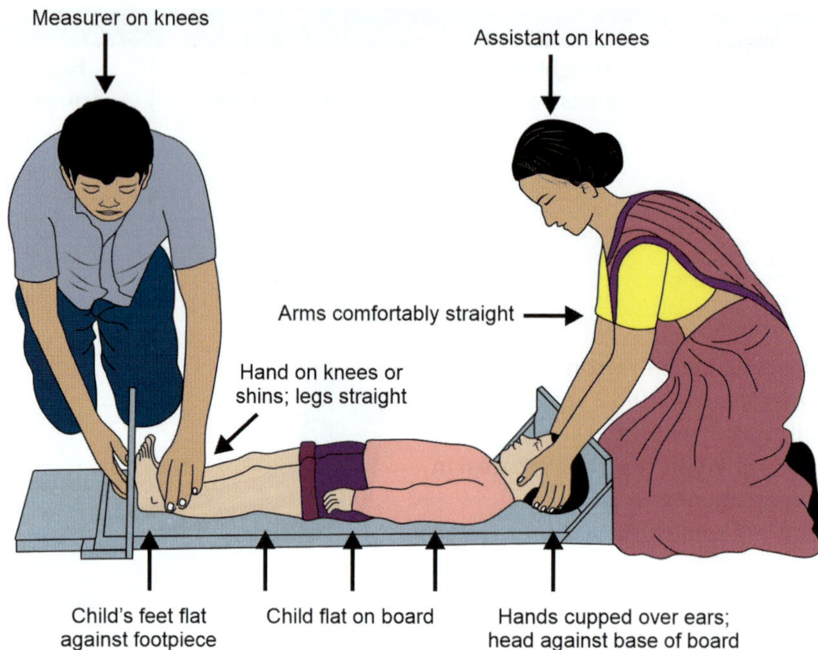

Fig. 5.5: Taking length on an infantometer.

- Hold down the baby's legs with one hand and move the footpiece with the other.
- Position the child's shoulders and hips at right angles to the long axis of the body.
- Apply gentle pressure on the knees to straighten the legs and prevent the knees from flexing.
- Bring the movable footboard to rest firmly against the child's feet with the soles flat on the board and the toes pointing directly upwards.

Record: Record the measurement to the nearest 0.1 cm from the digital counter on the measuring board.

Height

Stadiometer is the instrument used for measuring standing height (Fig. 5.6). The child stands on the wooden plank with the back against the wooden board that is calibrated in cm/inches. Alternatively, the height can also be measured against a flat wall. Child can be placed against this calibrated wall for measuring the stature. A flat board (wooden, metallic, or cardboard) will also be needed to level off the height at head end of the child.

- Remove the hair ornaments, and undo the buns and braids, if any. Remove any footwear.

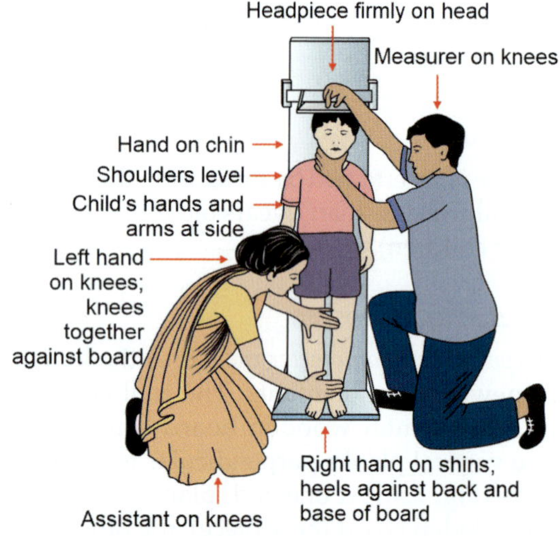

Fig. 5.6: Taking height on a stadiometer.

- Place the child in standing position on the stadiometer or against the wall.
- Ask the child to place the bare feet flat but slightly apart at a 60° angle and confirm that the weight is evenly distributed on both feet.
- Ensure that the back of the head, shoulder blades, buttocks, calves, and heels are touching the vertical board/wall (Fig. 5.7). This can be done by trying to insert a plastic rule at places where these points touch the wall. Inability to insert the rule implies good contact.

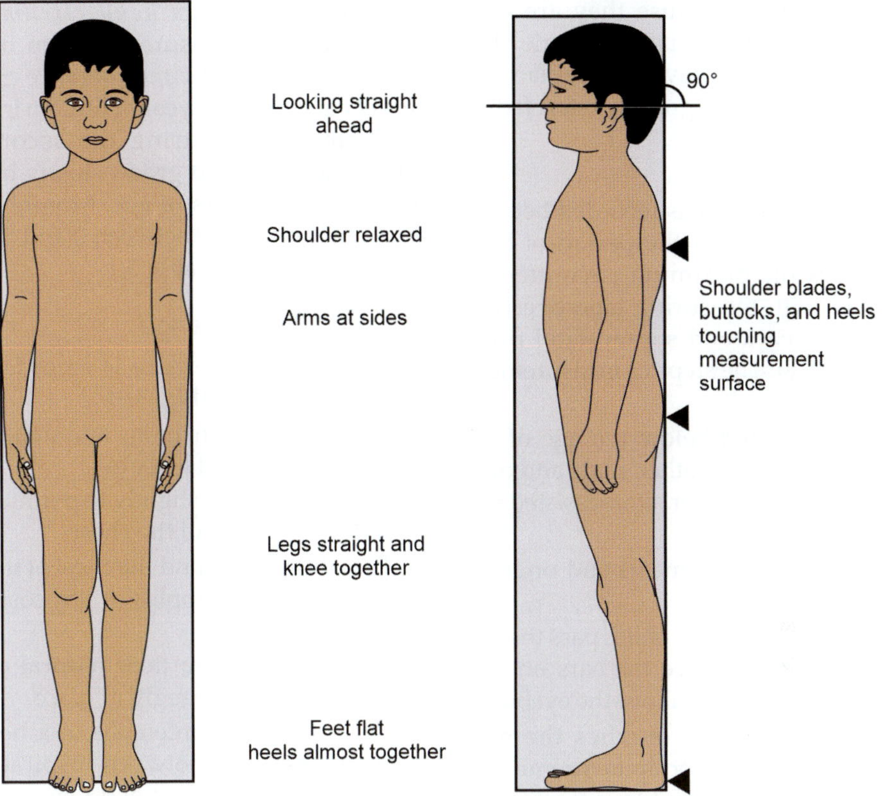

Fig. 5.7: Position for measuring height.

- The arms hang freely by the sides of the trunk with palms facing the thighs.
- Ask the child to look straight ahead.
- Stand on face-to-face level with the child and position the child's head so that a horizontal line drawn from the external auditory meatus to the lower edge of the eye socket runs parallel to the baseboard (i.e. the Frankfort plane positioned horizontally) **(Fig. 5.7)**.
- Because young children have difficulty standing to full stature, a gentle push applied to the tummy may help them stand to full height.
- Ask the child to take a breath, relax the shoulders, and stretch up to be as tall as possible. At the same time, take care so that the heels do not come off the ground.
- The wooden board (headpiece) is moved down to rest firmly on top of the child's head, compressing the hair; keeping it perpendicular to the wall.
- Record the reading to the last completed 1 mm.

Normal Pattern of Gain in Stature

A term newborn measures 50 cm at birth. The length is 75 cm and 90 cm by 1 and 2 years, respectively. Thereafter, till the onset of adolescence, children grow at a rate of 4 to 5 cm per year. Monthly gain in stature between 0 and 3 years of age is depicted in **Table 5.1**.

By 13 years of age, a child triples his birth length. Adolescent spurt of growth in height corresponds closely to weight gain. The following formula can be used for a rough and quick calculation of expected height between the ages of 2 and 12 years.

Expected height = (age in years × 6) + 77

3. Body Circumferences

Circumferences are measured to nearest 0.1 cm with a tape made up of a non-shrinkable, non-stretchable, and flexible material.

WHO used a self-retracting, 0.7 cm wide, flat metal tape with blank lead-in strip (range, 0–200 cm, calibrated to 1 mm) to measure circumferences in its growth study. Metal tapes were chosen because they are more robust and accurate and stay in a single plane around the head. They have to be replaced on a regular basis when the gradings start fading.

A. Head Circumference

The head circumference is recorded between birth to 6 years of age (the period of brain growth). It is the maximum circumference of the head with measuring tape overlying the occiput at back and supraorbital ridges in front (Fig. 5.8). The steps of measurements are as follows:

- An infant or child below the age of two years is held in the mother's lap, and older children could stand or sit unassisted on a footstool.
- Remove the hair ornaments and undo the braids.
- Stand on one side of the child, pass the tape around the head above the ears on each side, and anchor it just above the eyebrows.
- Ensure that the tape overlies the most prominent part of the occipital prominence at the back of the head. Move the tape up and down over the back of the head to locate the maximum circumference of the head.
- The tape should be perpendicular to the long axis of the face and should be pulled firmly to compress the hair, skin, and underlying soft tissues.
- Record the measurement to nearest 0.1 cm by overlapping both the segments of the measuring tape over the temporal region.
- Take 3 such measurements on the same child and select the maximum obtained.

Normal increase in head circumference: At birth, head measures 35.0 cm in a term neonate. The head circumference grows by 10–12 cm in the first year of life. An increment of 2 cm occurs during the second year. Thereafter, the head grows slowly by 0.5 cm per year till 8 years of age. Monthly gain in head circumference between 0 and 3 years of age is depicted in **Table 5.1**.

B. Chest Circumference

The chest circumference is recorded in the following manner (Fig. 5.9):

- Place the infant in the lap and stand in front. The chest should be bare.
- Abduct the arms slightly to permit passage of the tape around the chest.
- Pass the tape around the chest of the infant, at the level of nipples or 4th costosternal joints.
- Lower the arm to their natural position, once the tape is snugly in place.
- Record the circumference in a horizontal plane, midway between inspiration and expiration, to nearest of 0.1 cm.

Chest circumference is less than the head circumference at birth. However, it exceeds the head circumference by one year of age in a well-nourished child.

C. Mid-arm Circumference

Mid-arm circumference (MAC) or mid-upper arm circumference (MUAC) is taken in children between 6 months and 5 years of age.

Position: Ask the child to sit or stand. Position the infant in the mother's lap. Stand on the side facing the arm to be measured.

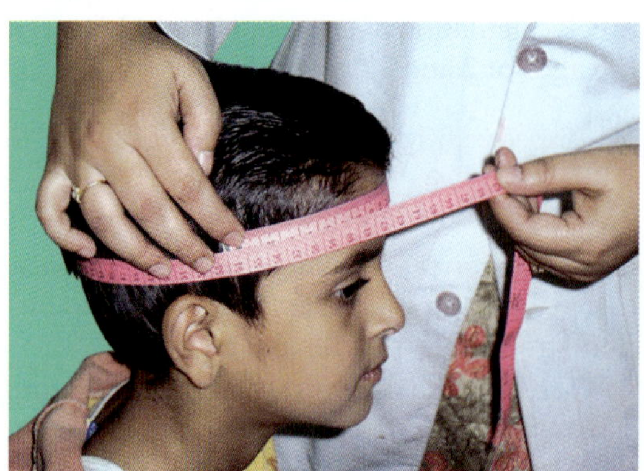

Fig. 5.8: Measuring head circumference.

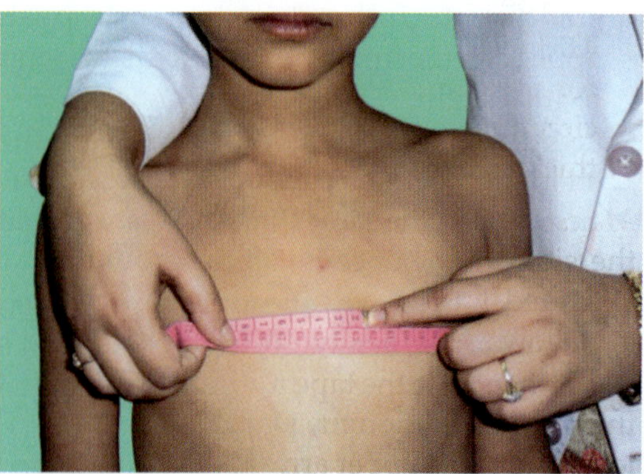

Fig. 5.9: Measuring chest circumference.

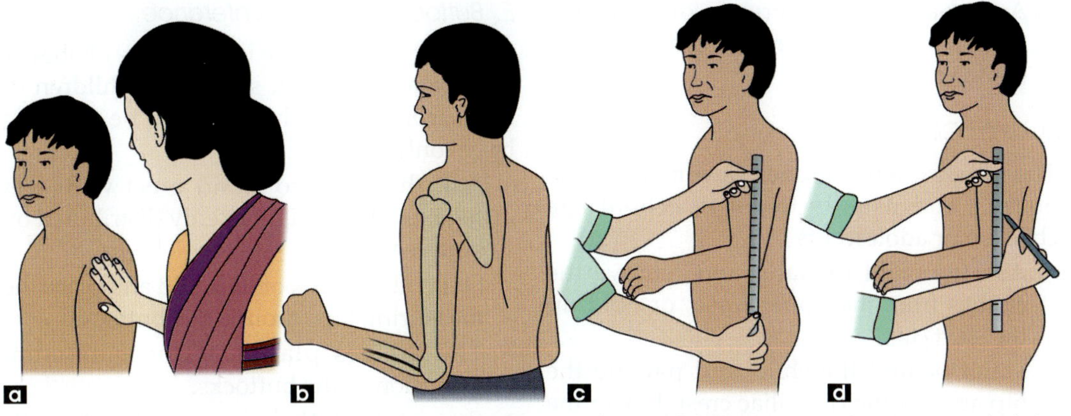

Fig. 5.10: Steps in measuring the mid-arm circumference: (a) and (b) The bony landmarks, (c) and (d) the mid-upper arm point.

Bony landmarks: Palpate and mark the two important bony landmarks, i.e. the acromion process (the most lateral bony protuberance on the back of the shoulder) and the olecranon (the bony structure that stands out when the elbow is bent).

- Palpate the shoulder to find the acromion and mark it with a felt-tip pen **(Fig. 5.10a)**.
- Next, bend the child's forearm by 90 at the elbow, with palm facing up, so that the olecranon stands out at the elbow. Mark this, too **(Fig. 5.10b)**.

Mid-arm point: Find and mark the mid-upper arm point. It is half the distance between the acromion process and the olecranon.

- Place the zero point of the tape on the mark over the acromion process and run it downward along the back of the arm to the other mark at the tip of the elbow, i.e. olecranon **(Fig. 5.10c)**.
- Make a small horizontal mark at the midpoint on the posterior aspect of the arm before the tape is removed **(Fig. 5.10d)**.
- This is the mid-upper arm point, to be used for measurement of the mid-upper arm circumference (MUAC) and triceps skinfold thickness.

Measure: Hang the child's arm freely to the side in a relaxed position, with elbows extended and palms towards the thighs. Do not allow to flex or tighten the muscles.

Now encircle the tape around the arm, over the marked midpoint, perpendicular to the long axis of the upper arm **(Fig. 5.11)**. The tape is again held so that the zero end is held below the measurement value. Ensure that the tape lies flat around the arm, without compressing the skin or underlying tissue; there should be no gap or compression on the inner part of the arm. Record the measurement to nearest of 0.1 cm.

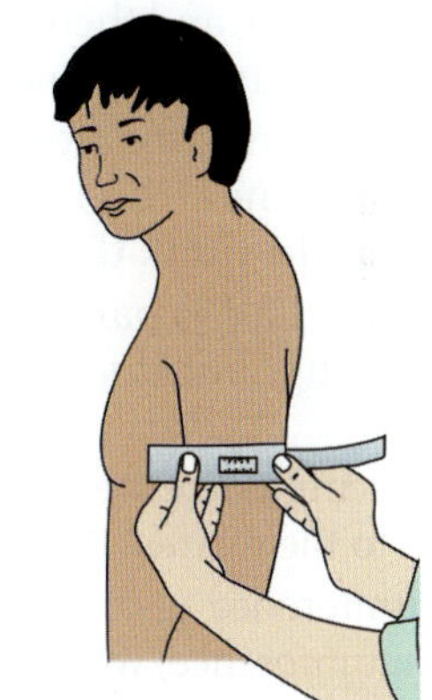

Fig. 5.11: Measuring mid-arm circumference.

- Mid-arm circumference is 9–11 cm at birth in a term neonate.
- It grows to 16 cm by the end of first year of life.
- Thereafter, the mid-arm circumference increases by 0.25 cm per year between 1 and 5 years. Because of a negligible increase in the mid-arm circumference (only 1 cm) between the ages of 1–5 years, it is also known as an age independent anthropometric criteria.
- The normal MUAC is 13.5 cm in children aged 6 months to 5 years.
- A mid-arm circumference of less than 12.5 cm indicates definite malnutrition.

- A mid-arm circumference of less than 11.5 cm indicates severe acute malnutrition (SAM).

D. Waist Circumference

The waist circumference is a measure of obesity and usually taken in school age children or adolescents.

- Ask the child to stand and remove the clothes from the upper torso, or hold up the shirt/top.
- Stand behind the child and palpate the hip area for the right iliac crest. Lower the pants and underclothing slightly to palpate directly on the hip area for the iliac crest.
- Mark a horizontal line at the highest point of the left iliac crest, and then cross this line to indicate the midaxillary line of the body.
- Place the measuring tape around the trunk in a horizontal plane at this level marked on the left side of the trunk **(Fig. 5.12)**.
- Ensure that the tape is parallel to the floor and that is snug, but does not compress the skin.
- Record the measurement at minimal respiration to the nearest 0.1 cm.

Waist circumference is different from the abdominal circumference, which is measured midway between the inferior margin of the last rib and the iliac crest, in a horizontal plane.

E. Buttocks (Hip) Circumference

The hip circumference is a measure of obesity and usually taken in school age children or adolescents. The child should be wearing briefs only.

- Ask the child to stand erect with feet together and weight evenly distributed on both feet.
- Stand at the back of the child and place the measuring tape around the buttocks.
- The tape is placed at the maximum extension of the buttocks.
- Ensure that the plane of the tape is horizontal.
- The tape is held snug against the skin but should not compress the soft tissues.
- Record the measurement from the side, i.e. at thigh, as shown in **Fig. 5.13**.

4. Skinfold Thickness

A skinfold consists of a double fold of skin and subcutaneous fat, excluding the underlying muscle. Measurements of skinfold thickness may be useful in the estimation of muscle mass or of body fat content. In clinical practice, measurements of triceps and subscapular skin-fold thickness generally are sufficient.

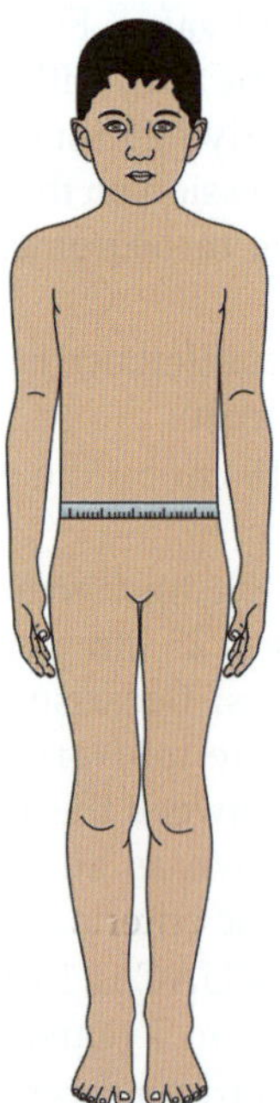

Fig. 5.12: Measuring waist circumference.

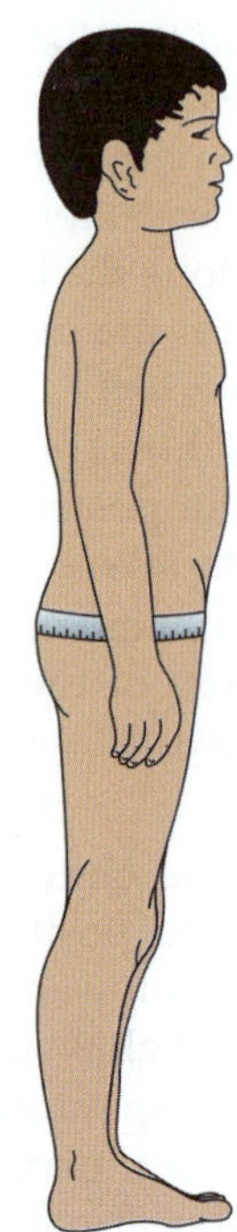

Fig. 5.13: Measuring hip circumference.

Tools for Measuring Skinfolds

The thickness is expressed in mm and is taken using a skinfold caliper (*Lange, Holtain* or *Harpenden*). Measurements are recorded to the nearest 0.5 mm (Lange calipers), 0.2 mm (Holtain calipers), or 0.1 mm (Harpenden calipers) **(Fig. 5.14)**. The caliper should provide a standardized pressure at all jaw openings. WHO used the Holtain/Tanner-Whitehouse skinfold caliper (jaw face area, 35 mm^2; pressure between the jaws, 10 ± 2 g/mm^2; range, 0–40 mm; calibrated to 0.2 mm) to measure skinfolds in children in its growth study.

Process of measurement: The measurements are taken on left side of the body by following the steps mentioned below:

- A young child is unfamiliar with this procedure; therefore, explain the procedure and demonstrate the use of the caliper on the child's palm, before you actually take the reading.
- Grasp the fold of skin and underlying subcutaneous adipose tissue gently between your left thumb and forefingers. Grasp enough skin and adipose tissue to form a distinct fold that separates from the underlying muscle. The sides of the fold should be roughly parallel.
- With your right hand, hold the caliper. Place the jaws of the calipers perpendicular to the length of the fold, and measure the skinfold thickness to the nearest 0.1 mm while the fingers continue to hold the skinfold. The actual measurement is read from the caliper about 3 seconds after the caliper tension is released. All skinfolds are recorded to the nearest 0.1 mm.

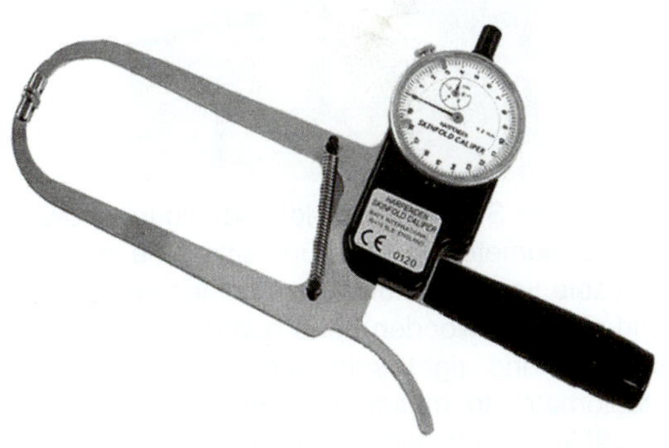

Fig. 5.14: Harpenden skinfold calipers.

A. Triceps Skinfold

Infants are held by their mothers; older children sit or stand.

- Let the left arm hang relaxed at the side or held down by the mother.
- Stand behind the child and pick up the skinfold about 1 cm above the midpoint mark over the triceps muscle, with the fold running downward along the midline of the back upper arm **(Fig. 5.15)**.
- Apply the caliper jaws at right angles to the 'neck' of the fold just below the finger and thumb over the midpoint mark.
- Gently release the caliper handles and allow the jaws to close on the fat fold for two seconds, while maintaining a grip on the skinfold.
- Record the reading to the nearest of 0.5 mm (Lange), 0.2 mm (Holtain), or 0.1 mm (Harpenden).

B. Subscapular Skinfold

Ask the child to sit or stand with shoulders relaxed or gently held down to prevent movement of the scapula.

- Palpate and mark the inferior angle of the left scapula. The measurement point for the subscapular skinfold is located immediately below the inferior angle of the scapula **(Fig. 5.16)**.
- Pick up the skinfold 1 cm below and medial to the subscapular mark. The skinfold should form a line about 45 degrees below

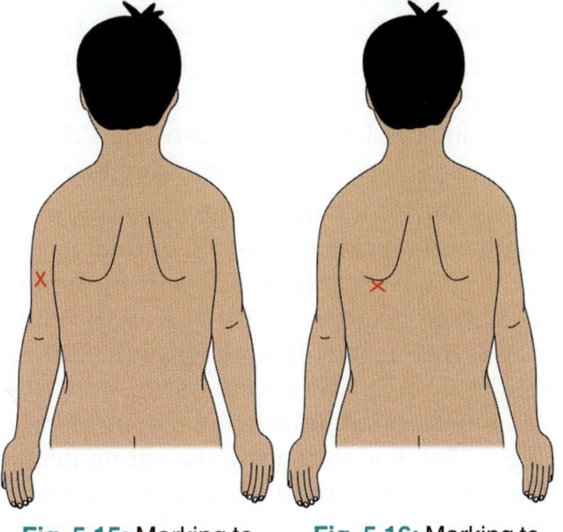

Fig. 5.15: Marking to measure the triceps skinfold.

Fig. 5.16: Marking to measure the subscapular skinfold.

the horizontal extending diagonally toward the left elbow.

- Apply the caliper to the 'neck' of the fold over the mark.
- Place the jaws of the caliper perpendicular to the length of the fold about 1.0 cm lateral to the fingers; the top jaw of the caliper should rest on the mark over the inferior angle of the scapula.
- Record the measurement, as described above for the triceps skinfold.

The proportionate mass of subcutaneous tissue is greatest at about 9 months. It decreases steadily till about 6 years, when it again starts increasing.

5. Body Proportions

Useful body proportions that may help in understanding various growth disturbances include upper segment/lower segment ratio or sitting height, and arm span.

A. Upper and Lower Segment Length and Ratio (Sitting Height)

Lower segment is measured as the length between pubic symphysis and the heel. Upper segment is calculated by subtracting the lower segment length from stature. At birth, head and trunk are relatively large in comparison to rest of the body. As the child grows, the limbs grow more than the trunk and hence body proportions change.

The *ratio of upper segment to lower segment* is 1.7 at birth. It decreases by 0.1 cm per year and by 3–4 years, the ratio is 1:3. Upper segment equalizes the lower segment by 7 to 10 years of age (ratio 1:1). High upper/lower segment ratio for any age indicates short limb dwarfism. US: LS ratio may provide a clue to many pathological conditions **(Key Box 1)**.

Sitting height: It denotes the upper segment length and represents 65–70% of total length in the newborn infant. The sitting height percentage decreases with age as the child grows, due to faster limb growth. Sitting height is best measured using a sitting stadiometer (Holtain) as shown in the picture **(Fig. 5.17a)**. For measuring the sitting height alternately, a flat footstool may be used with the sitting board parallel to the floor level.

- Ask the child to sit erect on the sitting bench of the stadiometer **(Fig. 5.17a)** with his or her back and buttocks in contact with the vertical column of the stadiometer.
- Place the head in the Frankfort horizontal plane. The knees are directed straight ahead with the arms and hands resting at the sides. The legs hang unsupported over the edge of the footstool **(Fig. 5.17b)**.
- Ask the child to sit tall, take a deep breath, and then bring the horizontal board/rule down snugly to the crown of the head with sufficient pressure to compress the hair.

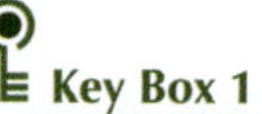

Key Box 1

Diseases with Altered Upper Segment (US) to Lower Segment (LS) Ratio

US:LS ratio for age	Diseases
Normal	Delayed puberty, hypopituitarism, constitutional dwarfism, nutritional dwarfism
Increased	Precocious puberty, achondroplasia, hypothyroidism, chondrodystrophy
Decreased	Mucopolysaccharidoses, hypogonadism, spondyloepiphyseal dysplasia

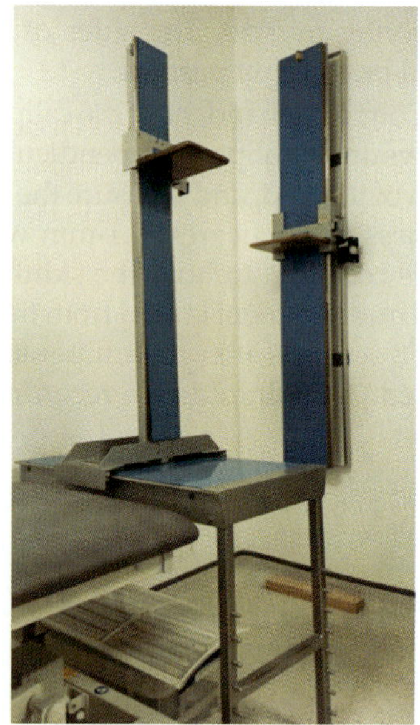

Fig. 5.17a: Stadiometer—left side figure showing the stadiometer to measure sitting height (with movable vertical column across the wooden seat and movable wooden head board on the vertical column) and right side showing wall-mounted stadiometer to measure standing height with a movable wooden head board (permission obtained to reproduce for textbook).

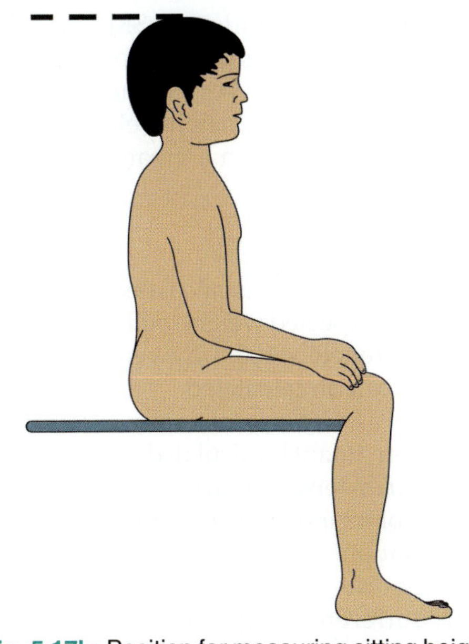

Fig. 5.17b: Position for measuring sitting height.

- Measure the distance between the sitting board of the stadiometer and the horizontal head board to the nearest 0.1 cm.

B. Arm Span

Arm span as compared to the total stature is another useful index. The procedure to measure arm span is as follows (**Fig. 5.18**):

- Ask the child to stand erect against a wall and outstretch both the arms at 90 to the body with palms facing outwards.
- Ensure that the fist should be open.

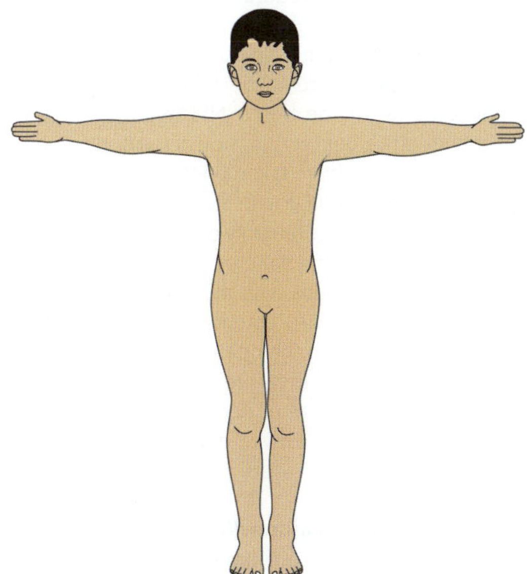

Fig. 5.18: Measuring arm span.

- The arms and the back of palms should also be in contact with the wall.
- Mark the points corresponding to the tips of two middle fingers of opposite hands on the wall with a chalk/pencil.
- Ask the child to move away and then measure the distance between the two points on the wall.

Usually, the difference between arm span and stature is not more than 3 cm. Arm span is less than the stature by 1–2 cm by 10 years of age. Thereafter, arm span exceeds the height but the difference always stays <3–5 cm.

6. Body Mass Index (BMI)

Body mass index (BMI) is calculated as weight/(length/height).^{2} The units for weight and length that are used in calculating BMI are kilogram and meter respectively and thus it is expressed in kg/m^2. It is considered as the most important parameter used for assessment of growth in adolescents and adults. For Asian adults, the normal BMI lies between 18.5 and 23. Adults with BMI between 23 and 26.9 are called *overweight*. *Obesity* in adults is defined as a BMI of more than or equal to 27. Adults with BMI of less than 18.5 are termed to be having *chronic energy deficiency*.

Fixed cut-offs for defining chronic energy deficiency, overweight, and obesity are not applicable for children and adolescents. Therefore, evaluation of BMI in these age groups is carried out by comparison with age-related standard percentile charts. The age and gender-based cutoffs are available as per the IAP growth charts for children aged 5–18 years. A BMI below the 3rd centile is undernutrition, above the orange line but below the red line (cutoff of BMI $\geq$23 kg/m^2 adult equivalent) is overweight and above the red line (cutoff of BMI $\geq$25 kg/m^2 adult equivalent) is obesity. The percentiles for these are different for boys and girls as shown in the box given at the top of next page. In under-five age children, weight for length Z scores (WLZ) serves as a marker to assess nutritional status instead of BMI. A WLZ of >+2 SD indicates overweight and >+3 SD indicates obesity.

The important cutoffs for BMI as per IAP chart for children 5–18 years are summarized as follows:

BMI cutoffs (IAP Growth Charts) for Children 5–18 years old

Classification	Girls	Boys
Underweight	<3rd centile	<3rd centile
Overweight	>75th centile	>71st centile
Obesity	>95th centile	>90th centile

7. Velocity of Growth

Measurement of the velocity of growth or increment in a unit of time is a better tool for early identification of factors affecting growth. The suggested frequency of growth monitoring is every monthly in infancy; once in every three months during second year of life; and once in every 6 months thereafter till 5 years of life. For recording the velocity, you will have to follow-up the child for at least 3–6 months, if the child is less than 2 years; and for 6–12 years in older children.

Velocity of growth can also help in predicting the ultimate adult height. The normal growth velocity curve for height is shown in Fig. 5.19. The growth velocity is maximum during the first year of life in terms of both height and weight. From 2 to 10 years of age, the child continues to grow at a fixed or constant velocity (velocity decreases and is lesser than that during first year). A second growth spurt occurs during puberty. This is known as the *peak height/weight velocity*. Maximum growth velocity occurs at sexual maturity rating (SMR) stage 2–3 in girls and SMR stage 4–5 in boys. The overall growth velocity is lower and occurs earlier (as per chronological age) in girls than boys. The height velocity in boys peaks later to end with a greater final adult height than girls.

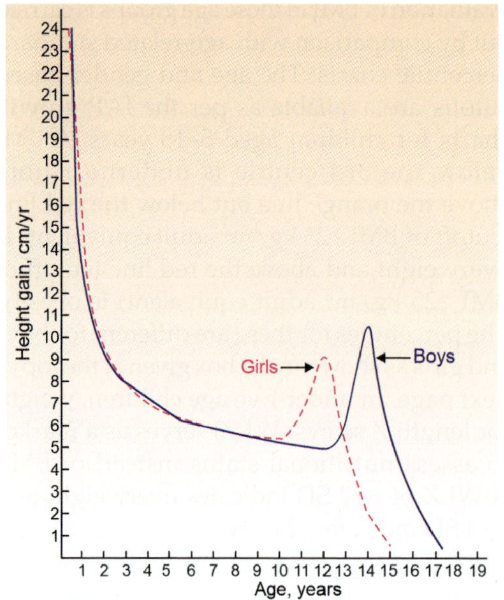

Fig. 5.19: A typical height velocity curve.

8. Derived Indices

- *Percentage weight* is calculated as observed weight/expected weight (50th percentile of the reference) × 100. Likewise, percentage height can be calculated.
- *Ponderal (Rohrer's) index* (PI) for the newborn infant is calculated as birth weight (g)/birth length (cm)^3 × 100. Ponderal index of <2 indicates asymmetrical growth retardation.
- *Waist–hip ratio* is expressed as waist circumference/hip circumference as a decimal fraction. This is a parameter used to assess central adiposity as BMI is not the best measure for assessment of visceral fat (central adiposity).

General Tips for Taking Measurements

1. **Ensure safety.** Performing body measurements on children requires additional safety precautions and monitoring. Children require constant supervision by the technicians. Place all anthropometric equipment out of reach of the smaller children. Hold children carefully to prevent any falls. Keep in mind that babies and small children tend to flip themselves over very quickly.
2. **Inform and take consent.** Explain the body measurement procedures to the parents/older child.
3. **Right or left.** There is no consensus on whether measurements are to be taken on the right or left side of the body. NHANES (US) data obtains all values on right side of the body while measurements were taken on the left side of the body in the WHO Growth Study. We advise you to obtain all measurements on/from the left side of the body for the sake of uniformity, and to enable comparisons with the WHO standards.
4. **Precision.** All measurements, except skinfolds, should be taken to the nearest tenth of a cm or 1.0 mm. Skinfold measurements can be taken to the nearest 0.1 mm, depending on the type of caliper used. However, in the WHO Growth study, all skinfolds were taken to the nearest 0.2 mm.
5. **Recommended measures.** Key Box 2 summarizes the measurements recommended to be taken in different age groups.

Key Box 2

Recommended Anthropometric Measurements for Different Age Groups

Parameter	Newborn	Infant	Children	Adolescent
Age	✓	✓	✓	✓
Sex	✓	✓	✓	✓
Weight	✓	✓	✓	✓
Length	✓	✓		
Height			✓	✓
Sitting height			✓	✓
Head circumference	✓	✓	✓	
Chest circumference	✓	✓		
Mid-arm circumference			✓	
Waist circumference				✓
Hip circumference				✓
Triceps skinfold			✓	✓
Subscapular skinfold			✓	✓
Ponderal index	✓			
Body mass index			✓	✓

5.4 INTERPRETATION OF GROWTH MEASUREMENTS

Once the physical measurements have been taken, the next step is to ascertain whether they are normal or not. For this, you need to compare the observed value with a standard or reference value. Reference values are usually expressed as percentiles.

1. Normal *vs* Abnormal—Percentile, SD, and *Z*-Score

As discussed in the beginning of this chapter, percentile indicates the position that a measurement would hold in a typical series of 100 arranged in ascending order. The median lies at the 50th percentile, on either side of which lie half the observations. The allowable normal range of variation in observations is between 3rd and 97th percentiles, which roughly correspond to ±2 SD (standard deviation).

Usually –1, –2 and –3 *Z*-score correspond to 15.8, 2.28 and 0.13th percentiles; while 1st, 3rd and 10th percentiles correspond to –2.33, –1.88 and –1.29 *Z*-score, respectively. Thus, the 15th percentile and 3rd percentile roughly correspond to –1 SD and –2 SD, respectively.

Conventionally, abnormal values are statistically defined as those below –2 SD (Z) score (2.3rd percentile) or above +2 SD (Z) score (97.7th percentile), relative to the reference median (50th percentile).

2. Growth Charts

The growth charts comprise an X-axis that corresponds to the age in months or years and Y-axis denoting the value of the anthropometric parameter, for example, weight (kg), height (cm), body mass index (kg/m^2), etc. WHO Growth Charts (published in 2006 for children less than 5 years of age) are available for both percentiles and Z-scores, separately (Fig. 5.20). In a standard WHO percentile chart, there are usually 5 percentiles lines corresponding to 3rd, 15th, 50th, 85th and 97th percentiles (from below to above) (Fig. 5.20a). The Z-score charts, however, display curves for median, –2Z, –3Z, 2Z and 3Z-scores (Fig. 5.20b). Abnormal is defined as any discrepancy of more than 2Z-scores in the upper and lower segments. A deviation by more than –3Z-score denotes severe malnutrition.

The WHO Growth Charts have been adopted in many countries including India as a universal global standard, for monitoring growth of children between 0 and 5 years. In 2015, Indian Academy of Pediatrics (IAP) published new revised growth charts for Indian children 5–18 years of age in view of the changing trend in nutritional status of children.

Weight-for-age BOYS

2 to 5 years (percentiles)

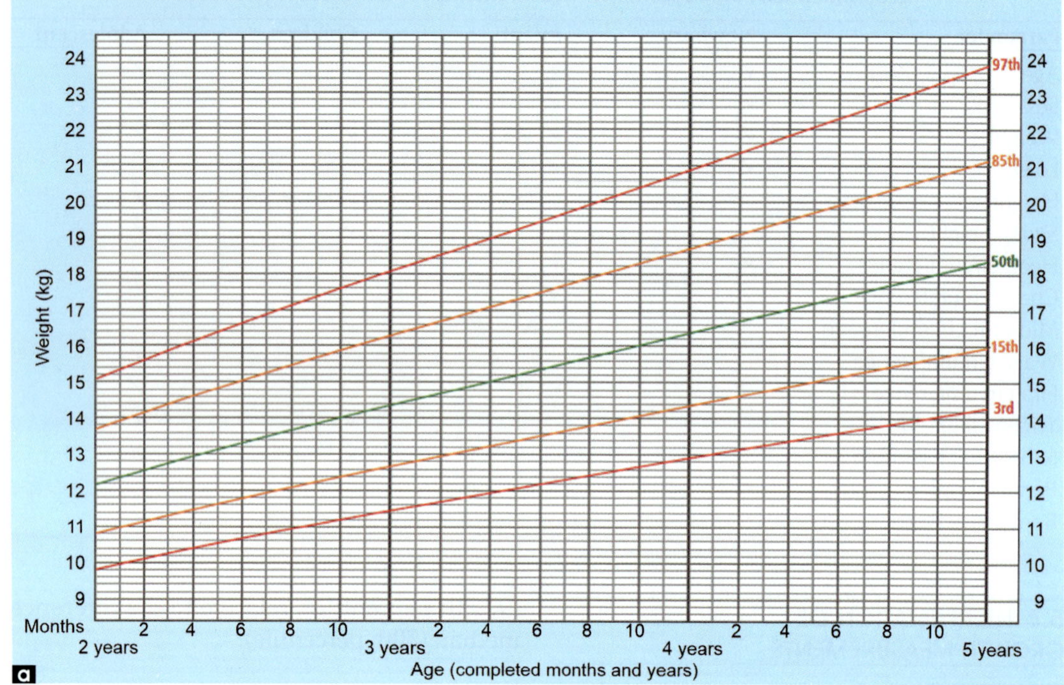

WHO Child Growth Standards

Birth to 2–5 years (Z-scores)

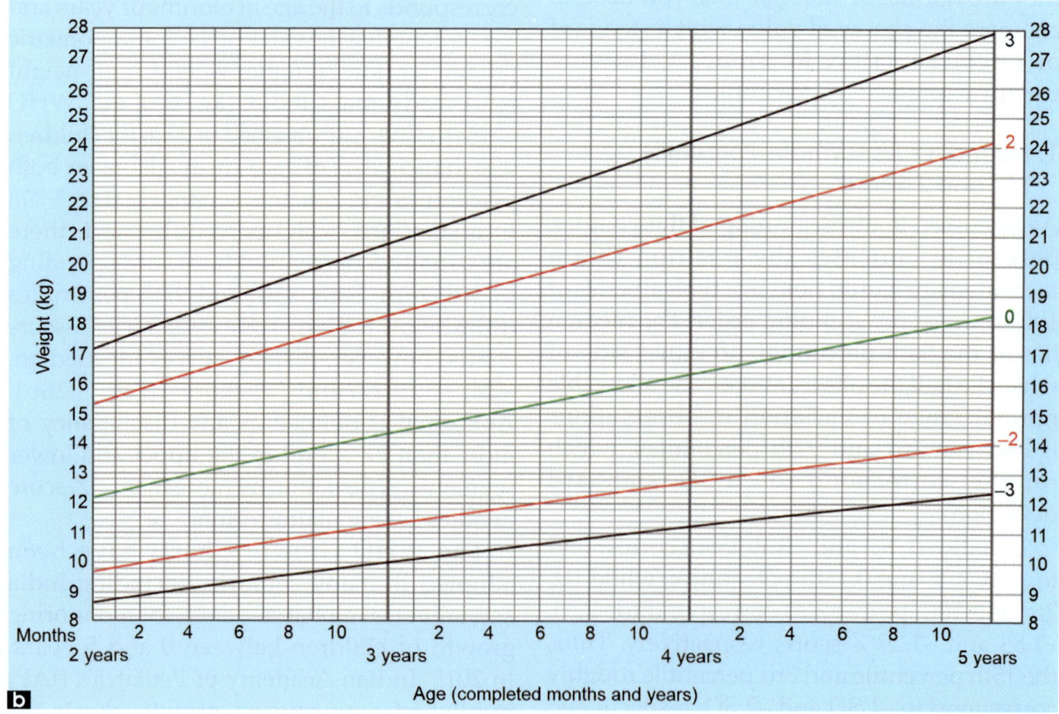

WHO Child Growth Standards

Fig. 5.20: A typical WHO growth chart for weight-for-age for boys 2–5 years of age; for (a) percentiles, and (b) *Z*-scores.

3. Growth References *vs* Growth Standards

Two types of growth charts are available: Growth standards and Growth references.

- *Growth standards* are defined as under the given optimal nutritional and health condition how a population of children should grow.
- *Growth references* are descriptive data that define how children in the population are growing under the best possible state of nutrition and health in a given community. They represent how children are actually growing rather than how they should be growing.

The WHO growth charts published in 2006 for children under the age of 5 years are an example of growth standards. Whereas, the 2015 IAP growth charts are growth references which describe how children in India were actually growing at that point of time.

4. WHO Growth Standards

The new reference growth data generated by the World Health Organization (WHO) are expected to provide a single international standard that represents the best description of physiological growth for all children from birth to 5 years of age. These charts are based on the growth of *exclusively breastfed infants*. The second unique feature of these standards is that it includes children from many of the world's major regions: Brazil (South America), Ghana (Africa), India (Asia), Norway (Europe), Oman (the Middle East) and the USA (North America).

The new standards differ from any existing growth charts in a number of innovative ways.

1. WHO standards are based on longitudinally collected data as opposed to cross-sectional data in previous charts.
2. WHO standards describe 'how children should grow,' as compared to earlier references which simply stated 'how children are growing.'
3. WHO standards make breastfeeding the biological 'norm' and establish the breastfed infant as the normative growth model.
4. WHO standards also include other growth indicators such as the skinfold thickness, and body mass index. These are useful to define obesity and overweight.

These charts have now replaced the National Center for Health Statistics (NCHS)/ Centers for Disease Control (CDC) Growth Charts for assessing the growth of children below 5 years of age.

The WHO growth reference charts and tables are available from the URL *http://www.who. int/childgrowth/standards*. At the end of this chapter, we are providing you with the percentile values of WHO growth standards for the following indices:

a. Weight-for-age [**Table 5.2** (boys: 0–5 yr), Table 5.3 (girls: 0–5 yr)];
b. Length-for-age [**Table 5.4** (boys and girls: 0–2 yr)];
c. Height-for-age [**Table 5.5** (boys and girls: 2–5 yr)];
d. Weight-for-length [**Tables 5.6** and **5.7** (boys and girls: 0–2 yr)];
e. Weight-for-height [**Tables 5.8** and **5.9** (boys and girls: 2–5 yr)];
f. Head circumference for age [**Table 5.10** (boys and girls: 0–5 yr)]; and
g. Body mass index [**Table 5.11** (boys: 0–5 yr), **Table 5.12** (girls: 0–5 yr)].

Percentiles of weight-for-age, height-for-age, and body mass index are tabulated separately for boys and girls 5–18 years age **(Tables 5.13 to 5.18)**. The gender-wise charts for plotting weight, length and head circumference comprehensively on a single chart can be done using the WHO growth charts 0–5 years **(Figs 5.21 and 5.22)**. This helps to plot and interpret all three measures simultaneously.

5. Growth Reference for Indian Children 5–18 Years

Even though growth occurs in a similar manner amongst humans throughout the world, but there do exist some regional variations amongst the pattern of growth due to socioeconomic, geographical and racial differences. The average adult weight and height are also different in different regions of the world because of the same reason. Thus for a particular population, the ideal reference standards would be the ones derived from that population itself. Aggarwal, *et al.* compiled the data based on affluent urban children from all major zones of India, measured between 1989

0 to 5 Years: WHO Boys Length/Height, Weight and Head Circumference Charts
(Z-scores are in Parenthesis)

Name : ________________________________

DOB : ________________________________

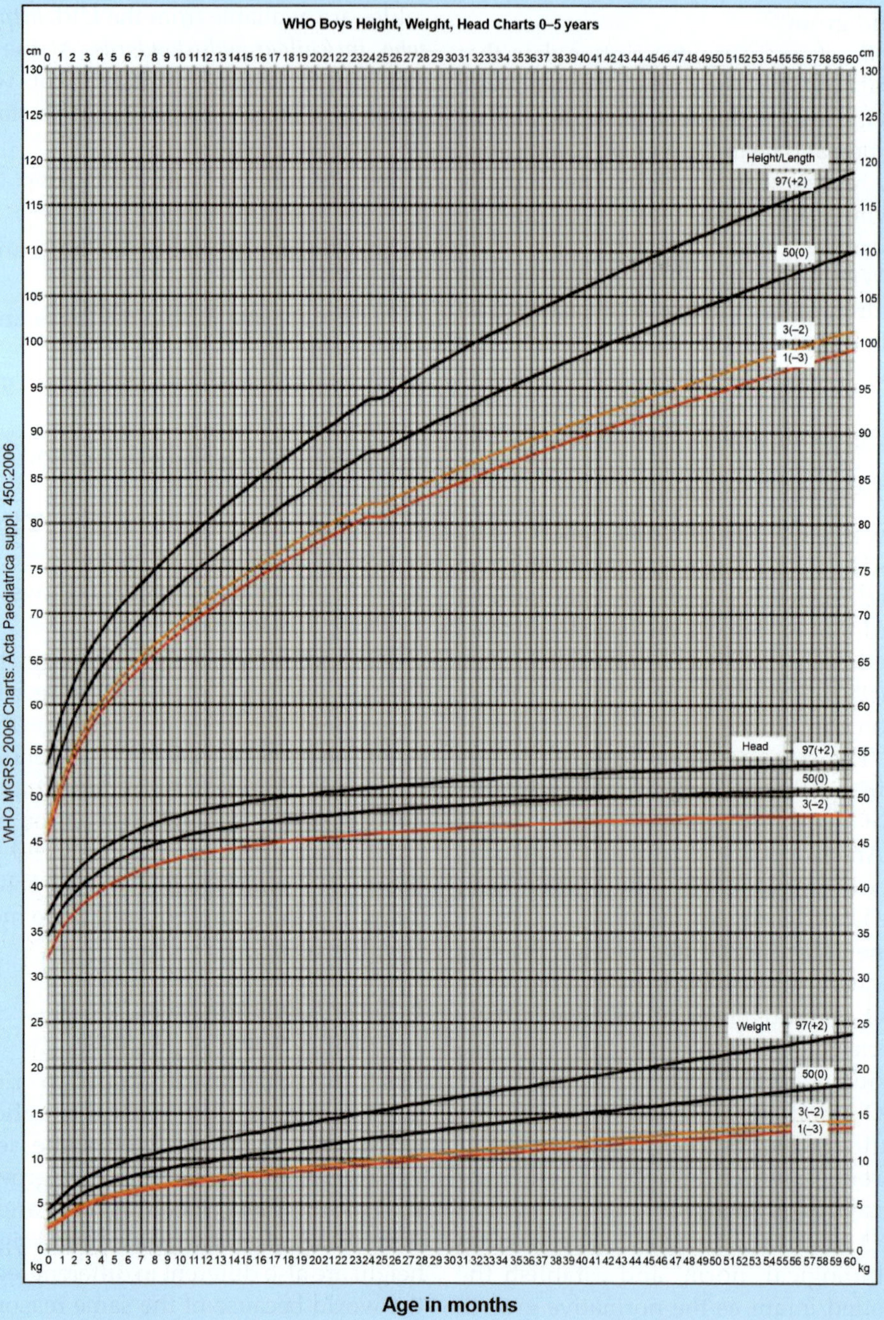

WHO Boys Height, Weight, Head Charts 0–5 years

WHO MGRS 2006 Charts: Acta Paediatrica suppl. 450:2006

Height/Length: 97(+2), 50(0), 3(–2), 1(–3)

Head: 97(+2), 50(0), 3(–2)

Weight: 97(+2), 50(0), 3(–2), 1(–3)

Age in months

Fig. 5.21: Combined WHO growth chart for weight-for-age, length-for-age and head circumference for age in children 0–5 years of age (boys).

0 to 5 Years: WHO Girls Length/Height, Weight and Head Circumference Charts (Z-scores are in Parenthesis)

Name : ________________________

DOB : ________________________

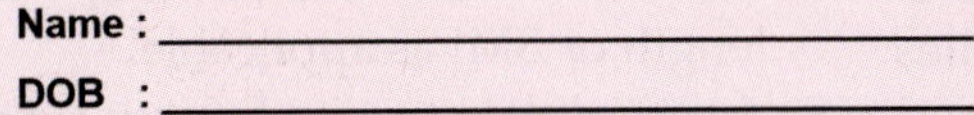

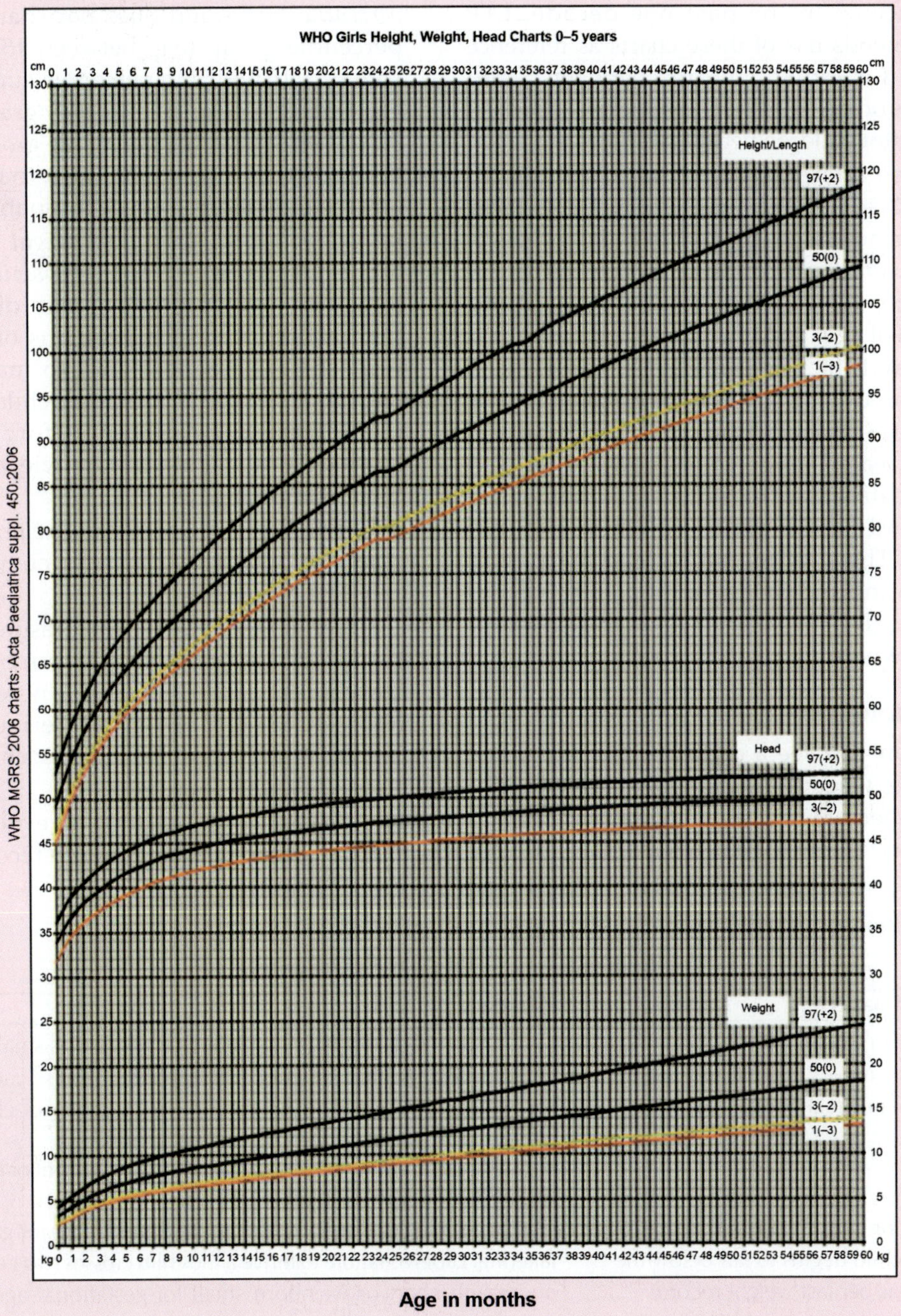

WHO Girls Height, Weight, Head Charts 0–5 years

WHO MGRS 2006 charts: Acta Paediatrica suppl. 450:2006

Height/Length
97(+2)
50(0)
3(–2)
1(–3)

Head
97(+2)
50(0)
3(–2)

Weight
97(+2)
50(0)
3(–2)
1(–3)

cm
kg

Age in months

Fig. 5.22: Combined WHO growth chart for weight-for-age, length-for-age and head circumference for age in children 0–5 years of age (girls).

and 1991. These charts provide information on growth from birth to 18 years of age.

In 2015, Indian Academy of Pediatrics (IAP) published the revised growth charts from data collected from published studies on apparently healthy Indian children and adolescents in the past one decade. IAP recommends use of these charts as reference values for Indian children between 5 and 18 years of age. The WHO charts should be used to monitor children between 0–5 years of age.

These reference curves are provided as Figs 5.23 to 5.26. We suggest using these charts as reference values for children above 5 years of age. One can continue to use the WHO reference values for children between 0 and 5 years of age.

Growth in preterm babies needs to be monitored in special charts to account for prematurity. The INTERGROWTH-21st charts were created using multicentric data of 8 participating sites (including India) to monitor fetal and extrauterine growth in preterm babies. These charts can be used for growth monitoring and follow-up of preterm babies and are given in Chapter 15 on Evaluation of the Newborn.

6. Interpretation

- When you see a child for the first time, assess whether his measurement of weight and height *is less than 3rd or more than 97th percentile* on the corresponding growth chart. If yes, the child may not be growing normally and needs evaluation. Complete the assessment of head circumference and other indicators like MUAC, weight-for-length or BMI as applicable.
- *A normal child remains between 15th and 85th percentile curves* and does not change his percentile group (e.g. between 15th and 25th or 25th and 50th percentile curves) at succeeding ages or change only gradually. A sudden shift in the percentile group (i.e. from a higher to lower or lower to higher) on serial monitoring needs evaluation.
- *In a normal child, height and weight usually follow the same percentile position.* At times, the two parameters may differ in their actual percentile positions on their respective charts, but tend to maintain the same relation throughout childhood. However, these children, before being labeled normal, should be reviewed for growth abnormalities.
- *A normal child stays on or near one percentile curve* or between the same curves on subsequent monitoring.
- Children with weight/height measurements that lie *between 3rd and 15th percentile or between 85th and 97th percentile* need to be followed up and reviewed periodically (infant: monthly for 3–6 months; children: 3 monthly for 1–2 years).

Key Box 3 provides a guide for evaluation of children based on serial growth records.

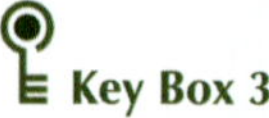

Key Box 3

Interpretation of Serial Growth Monitoring

Growth pattern	Inference
Change in weight centile during early infancy—moves down (catch-down) or moves up (catch-up)	Catch-up growth is physiological in babies born as small-for-gestational-age (birth weight <10th centile); likewise catch-down growth may occur to attain a weight as per a chosen growth centile in babies who are large-for-date. Acute illness can also cause decrease in gain of weight or height and should not be ignored
Weight or height gain begins to slow down (child begins to fall below the centile as per last weight record)	Child needs to be examined and investigated further for growth faltering. Label as failure to thrive if the child crosses two centiles on growth chart or was born small-for-gestational-age and crosses a single centile
Weight or height gain begins to show an upward trend	Be cautious for this pattern of gain in weight—indicative of edema, obesity, or other systemic conditions. Likewise, a jump in height centiles may indicate abnormal skeletal growth (precocious puberty)

5.5 EVALUATION OF DENTAL GROWTH

The deciduous teeth start erupting at 6 months of age and the permanent teeth at about 6 years of age. All the deciduous teeth are replaced by the permanent teeth by the age of twelve years. A child between the age of 6 and 12 years has a mixed dentition. Eruption dates of various human teeth are provided in **Key Box 4**.

Primary dentition: The lower central incisors appear between the ages of 5 and 8 months. The upper central incisors appear a month later and the lateral incisors usually within the next 3 months. The first molar teeth appear around the age of 12 to 15 months, preceding the eruption of canine teeth by 6 months, which appear between the age of 18 and 21 months. The second molars are out at the age of 21 to 24 months.

Permanent teeth erupt in the following order. 1st molar—6 years; central and lateral incisors—6 to 8 years; canines and premolars—9 to 12 years; second molars—12 years; third molars—18 years or later.

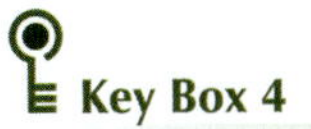

Key Box 4

Sequence of Eruption of Primary and Secondary Teeth

Primary (*Deciduous*) Teeth		
Maxillary	*Eruption*	*Shedding*
Central incisor	7½ months	7–8 years
Lateral incisor	9 months	8–9 years
Canine	18 months	11–12years
First molar	14 months	10–11years
Second molar	24 months	10–12years
Mandibular		
Central incisor	6½ months	6–7 years
Lateral incisor	7 months	7–8 years
Canine	16 months	9–11 years
First molar	12 months	10–12years
Second molar	20 months	11–13years
Eruption of Permanent Teeth		
	Maxillary	*Mandibular*
Central incisor	7–8 years	6–7 years
Lateral incisor	8–9 years	7–8 years
Canine	11–12 years	9–10 years
First premolar	10–11 years	10–12years
Second premolar	10–12 years	11–12years
First molar	6–7 years	6–7 years
Second molar	12–13 years	11–13years
Third molar	13–17 years	13–17years

5.6 ASSESSMENT OF NUTRITION BY ANTHROPOMETRY

The terms 'undernutrition', 'malnutrition', 'protein calorie malnutrition (PCM)', and 'protein energy malnutrition (PEM)' have been widely used to describe abnormal anthropometric measurements. Similarly, anthropometry has been used to signify the duration of undernutrition as being acute, chronic, or acute on chronic. However, there is a need to replace these terms by a more objective terminology based on anthropometric indices with specified cut-offs for indicating abnormal nutritional status. Nowadays, we primarily use three indicators, *viz.* underweight, stunting, and wasting; to describe the severity and duration of undernutrition. **Key Box 5** enlists and describes the utility of a few anthropometric indicators, based on weight and height.

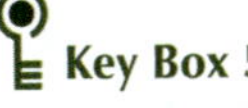

Key Box 5

Height- and Weight-based Anthropometric Indicators for Undernutrition

Indicator	Cut-off	Term	Process
Low height-for-age	85–89% or between –2 to –3 SDS of expected	Stunting	Indicates long-term (chronic) malnutrition
	<85% or below –3 SDS of expected	Severe stunting	
Low weight-for-height	70–79% or between –2 to –3 SDS of expected	Wasting	Indicates acute malnutrition
	<70% or <–3 SDS of expected	Severe wasting	
Low weight-for-age	<80% of expected	Underweight	Implies failure to thrive
High height-for-age	>97th percentile	Tallness	Endocrine disorder

Expected refers to the 50th percentile (median) of the WHO Growth References

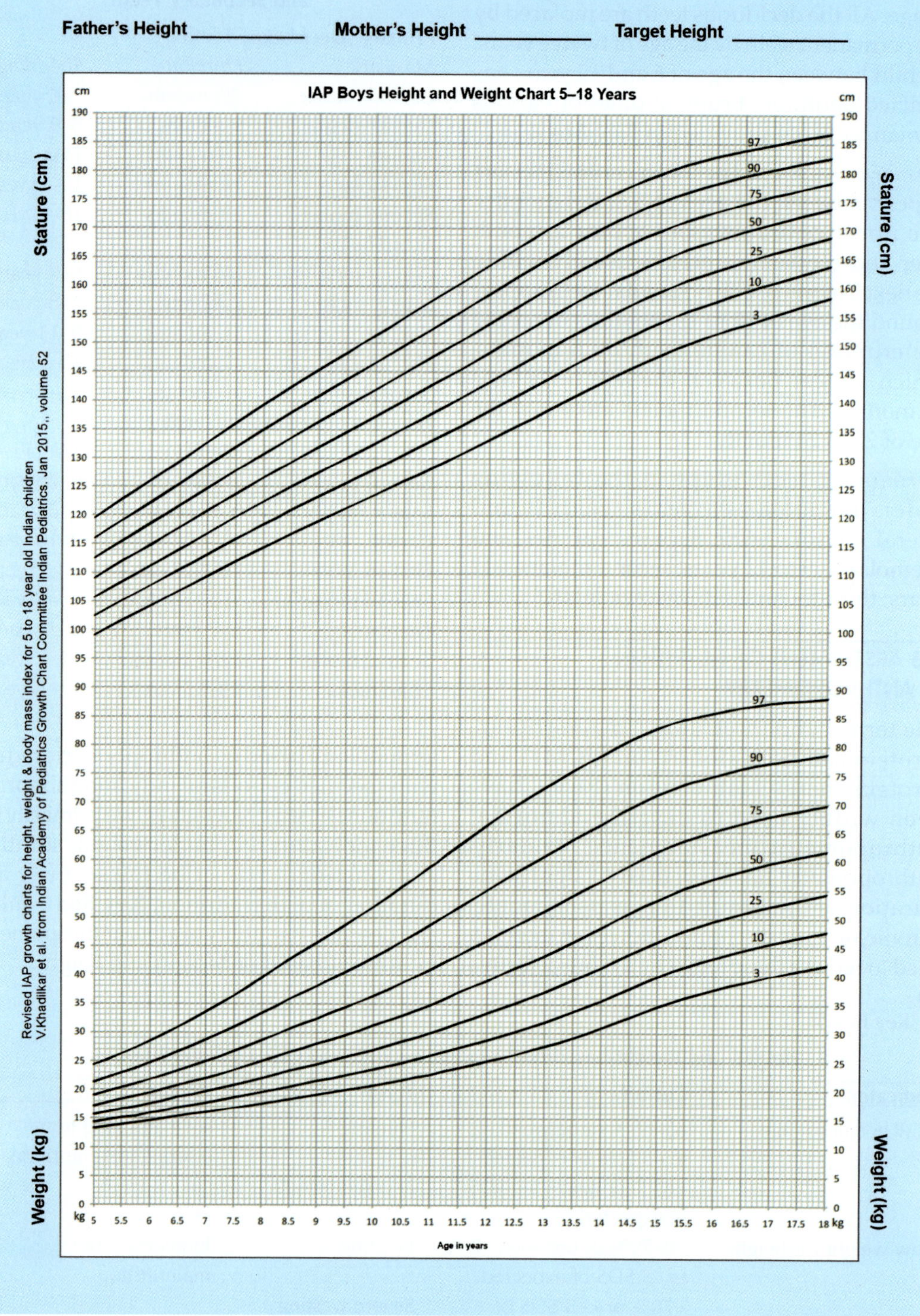

Fig. 5.23: Indian Academy of Pediatrics (IAP) Growth Charts for height-for-age, and weight-for-age (5–18 years) of boys.

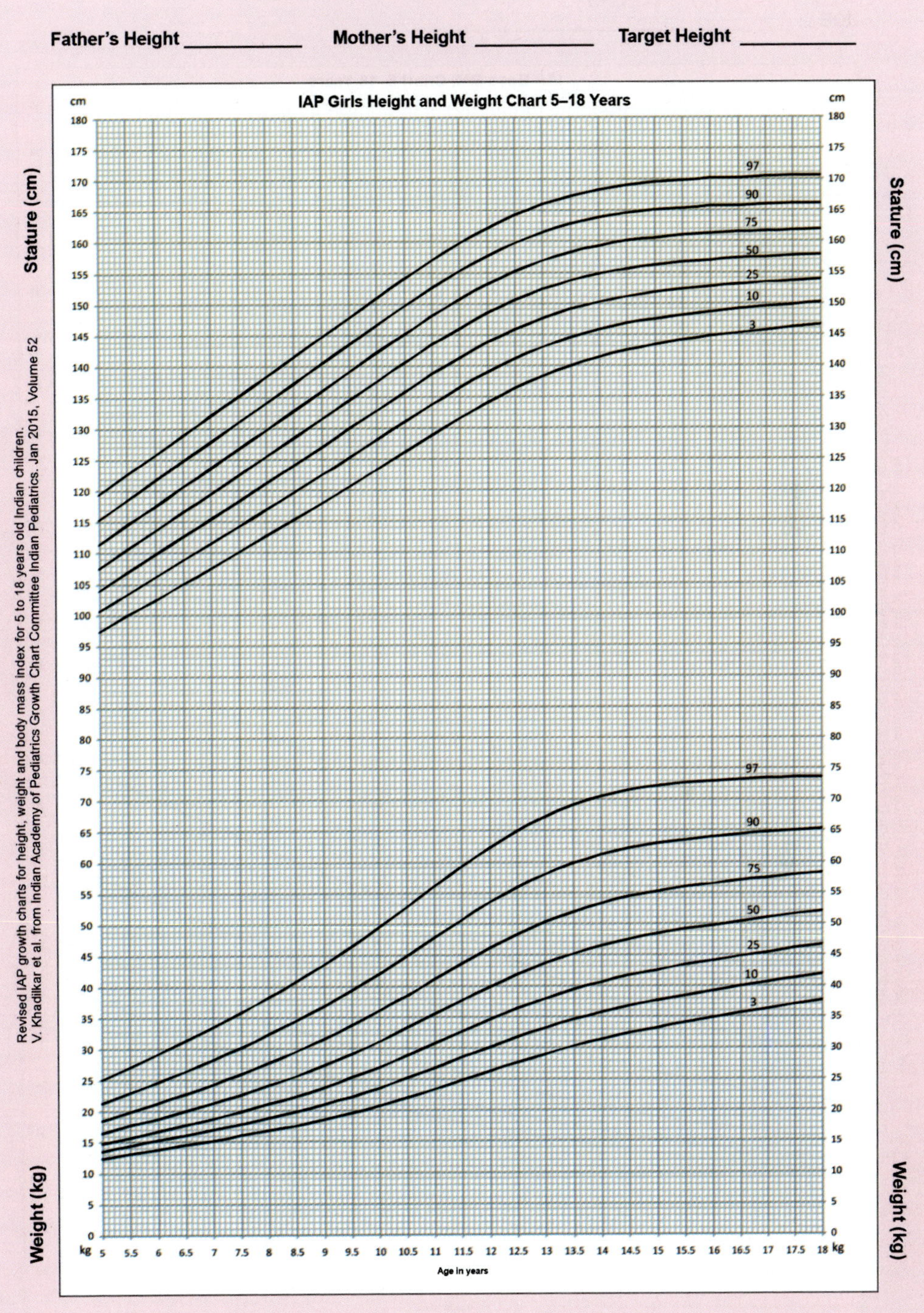

Fig. 5.24: Indian Academy of Pediatrics (IAP) Growth Charts for height-for-age and weight-for-age (5–18 years) of girls.

5 to 18 Years: IAP Boys Body Mass Index Charts

Name : ______________________________

DOB : ______________________________

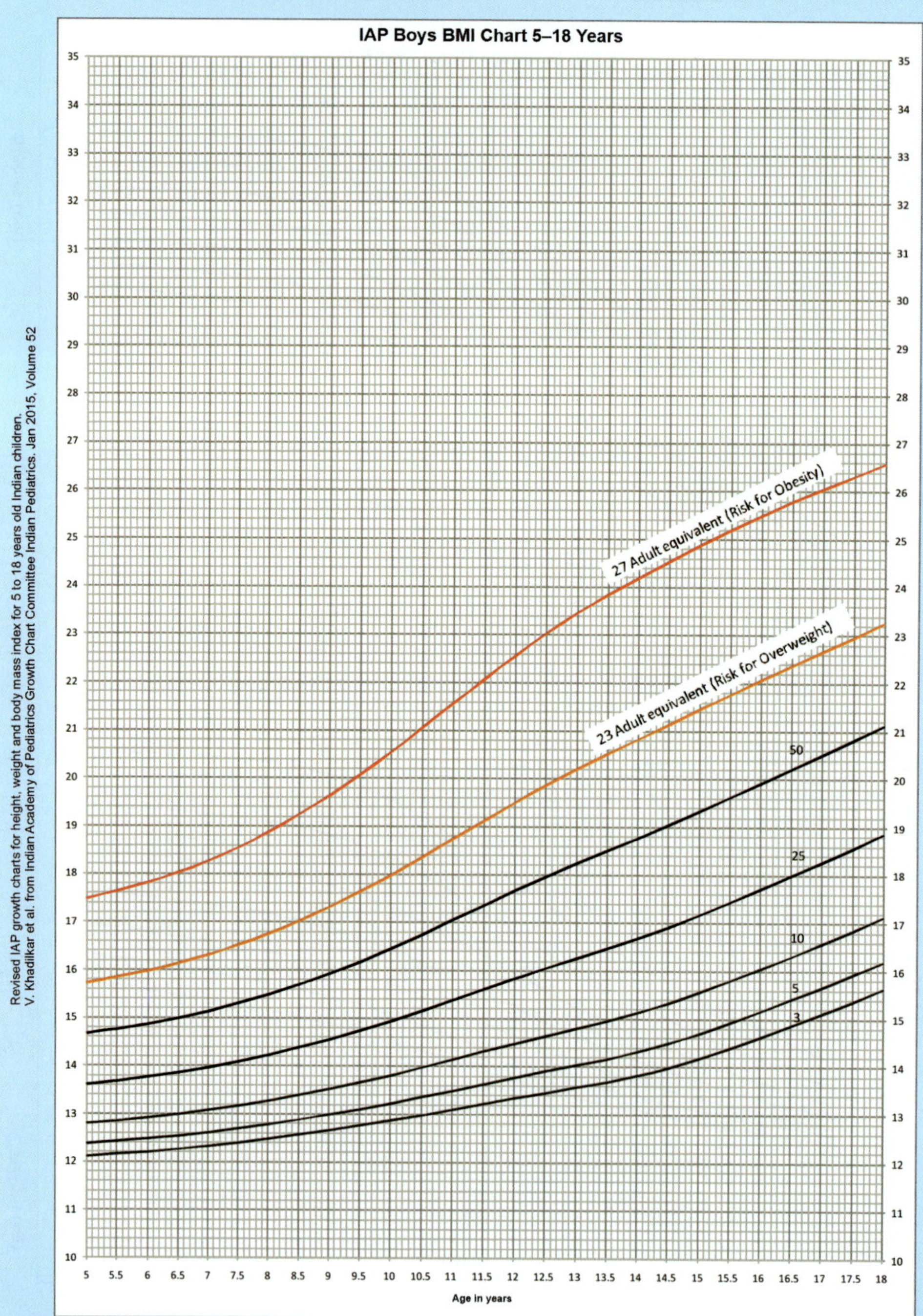

Fig. 5.25: Indian Academy of Pediatrics (IAP) Growth Charts for body mass index (BMI) of boys (5–18 years).

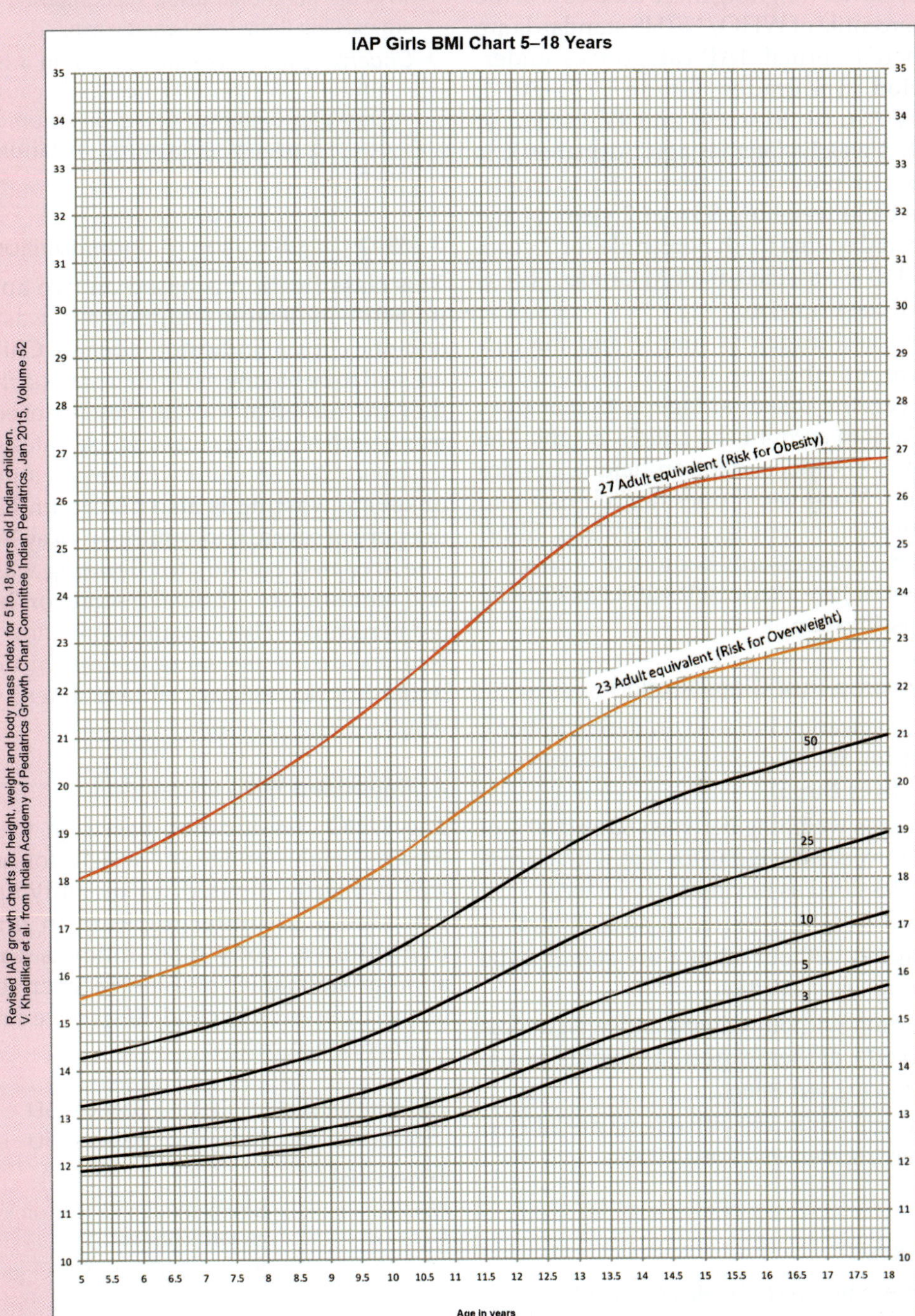

Fig. 5.26: Indian Academy of Pediatrics (IAP) Growth Charts for body mass index (BMI) of girls (5–18 years).

1. IAP (Indian Academy of Pediatrics) Classification of PEM (Protein Energy Malnutrition)

This classification is based on 'weight-for-age'. Children weighing more than 80% of the 50th percentile of WHO/NCHS standards are considered normal. IAP categorizes undernutrition in 4 grades: Grade I (71–80%), II (61–70%), III (51–60%) and IV (≤50%) of expected weight for that age. Alphabet K is postfixed in presence of edema. For example, a male child weighing 8 kg at 2 years of age with pedal edema (50th percentile for 2 years is 12.3 kg) is classified as PEM Grade II (k) as per IAP classification.

IAP classification is simple and the cut-offs are suitable for Indian population. However, the disadvantage is that it does not take into account the child's height. The weight is also dependent on height, besides the built. Moreover, it does not tell us about the duration of energy deprivation. Short children (not necessarily because of nutritional deprivation) are also misclassified as PEM by this classification.

2. Wellcome Trust Classification

This classification is based on deficit in body weight-for-age and presence or absence of edema **(Key Box 6)**.

- Children weighing between 60 and 80% of their expected weight-for-age with edema are classified as having *kwashiorkor*.
- Those weighing between 60 and 80% of expected without edema are stated to be having *undernutrition*.
- Children without edema and weight less than 60% of their expected weight-for-age are having *marasmus*.
- Marasmic children with edema are labeled as having *marasmic kwashiorkor*.

Key Box 6

Wellcome Trust Classification of PEM

Weight-for-age	No edema	Edema
60–80% of expected	Undernutrition	Kwashiorkor
<60% of expected	Marasmus	Marasmic Kwashiorkor

- Presence of *stunting* implies long-term energy deficit, while *wasting* alone indicates acute energy deficit.
- A combination of *wasting and stunting* implies an acute nutritional insult superimposed on a pre-existing (long-term) energy gap.
- *Underweight per se* can result from a lot of conditions: Weight may be less because of energy gap (whether acute or chronic) or a disease process (resulting in failure to thrive).

3. WHO Classification of Undernutrition

This classification is based on two anthropometric indicators (stunting and wasting), and one clinical indicator (edema). Children are said to be having *moderate undernutrition*, if they are stunted or wasted. Presence of edema along with stunting/wasting indicates *severe undernutrition*. A child with severe stunting or severe wasting is also placed under the category of severe undernutrition **(Key Box 7)**. The accepted cut-offs for defining wasting and stunting are '–2 SD (Z) score' or 'below 3rd percentile'. This classification is now used worldwide for assessing the magnitude of undernutrition among children under 5 years of age.

4. BMI-based WHO Classification

The WHO classification based on weight-for-age, height-for-age and weight-for-height was primarily devised for quantifying the prevalence of undernutrition in under-five children. Body mass index is a more appropriate marker of thinness, overweight, or obesity in an older child. Respective cut-offs are mentioned below:

Severe thinness	BMI <–3 SD
Thinness	BMI <–2 SD
Overweight	
0–5 y	BMI or WLZ >+2 SDS on WHO growth charts
5–18 y	BMI >+1SDS on WHO growth charts
Obesity	
0–5 y	BMI or WLZ >+3 SDS on WHO growth charts
5–18 y	BMI >+2 SDS on WHO growth charts

Key Box 7

WHO Classification for Undernutrition

	Moderate undernutrition	Severe undernutrition
Symmetrical edema	No	Yes[a] Edematous malnutrition
Weight-for-height[b, c] *(measure of wasting)*	SD score[b] –2 to –3 (70–79% of expected)[c] ***Wasting***	SD score <–3 (<70% of expected) ***Severe wasting***
Height-for-age *(measure of stunting)*	*SD score[b] –2 to –3* (85–89% of expected)[c] ***Stunting***	*SD score <–3* (<85% of expected) ***Severe stunting***

a. This includes kwashiorkor and marasmic kwashiorkor.

b. SD (Z) score = $\frac{\text{Observed value} - \text{Expected value}}{\text{Standard deviation of reference population}}$

c. Median (50th percentile of WHO standards).

5. Age Independent Anthropometric Indices

Some anthropometric indices do not require consideration of age. These serve as useful one time indicators to assess nutritional status in clinical practice **(Key Box 8)**, where exact age of the child is not known (e.g. orphanages, street children, etc.).

Of these, mid-arm circumference is considered to be the easiest indicator of malnutrition based on a cut-off of 12.5 cm. Recently it has been suggested that MUAC <11.5 cm is a good alternative indicator of *severe acute malnutrition (SAM)*, and thus can serve as a proxy indicator for wasting. Other criteria for diagnosis of SAM include weight-for-height Z-score less than –3 SD, visible severe wasting, and bipedal edema.

6. BMI Quick Screening Tool

A simplified chart in the IAP growth charts allows to screen malnutrition in terms of both thinness and overweight/obesity as shown in **Figs 5.27 and 5.28** for boys and girls, respectively. These charts have only three lines (black, orange and red) and can be used in children 8–18 years of age to simply plot the weight (Y-axis) for a respective height (on X-axis) without the need to calculate the BMI. Any point below the black suggests undernutrition, between black and orange line is normal, above orange suggests overweight and above red line suggests obesity. These charts are incorporated in the revised growth charts as inset on upper left hand corner.

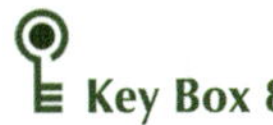

Key Box 8

Age Independent Anthropometric Indices

Name of index	Method to obtain	Normal	Undernourished
Mid-upper arm circumference	Taken between the ages of 1–5 years	>13.5 cm	<12.5 cm
Dugdale's index	$\frac{\text{Weight in kg}}{(\text{Height in cm})^{1.6}} \times 100$	0.88–0.97	<0.79
Rao's index	$\frac{\text{Weight in kg}}{(\text{Height in cm})^{2}} \times 100$	0.15–0.16	<0.14
Kanawati index	$\frac{\text{Mid-arm circumference (cm)}}{\text{Head circumference (cm)}}$	0.32–0.33	≤0.25

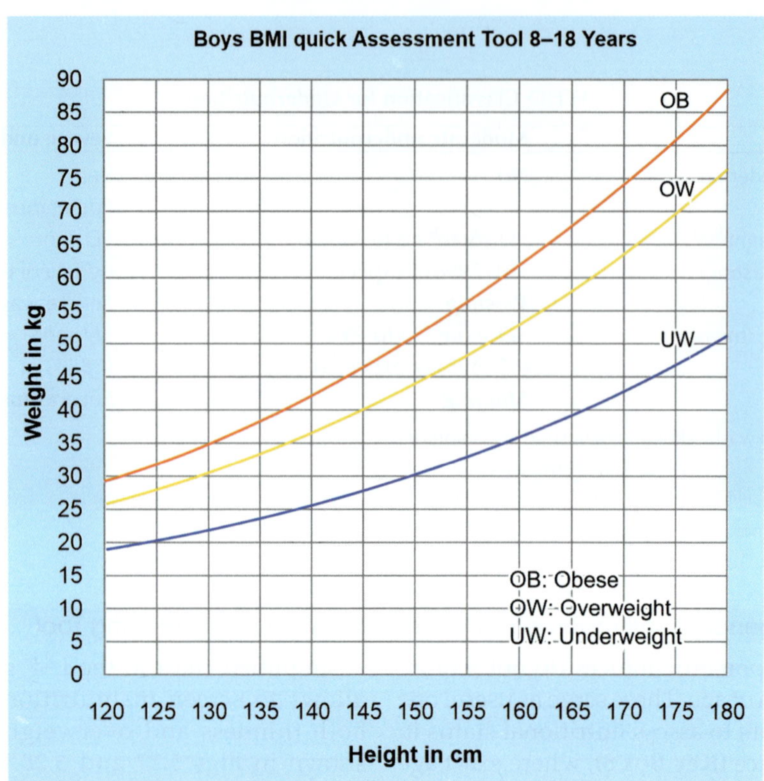

Fig. 5.27: BMI quick assessment tool 8–18 years for boys (*Source:* Khadilkar V, Lohiya N, Chiplonkar S, Khadilkar A. Body Mass Index Quick Screening Tool for Indian Academy of Pediatrics 2015 Growth Charts. Indian Pediatr. 2020;57(10):904–906)

7. Waist Circumference Charts

Waist circumference is a useful marker of central adiposity or visceral fat status. The largest data on normative values has been recently compiled during the Comprehensive National Nutrition Survey (CNNS) across different parts of the country. The percentile based charts are shown below (Fig. 5.29) that can be used.

8. Anthropometry Apps

With easy access to technology to all, the use of apps to calculate and interpret anthropometry has become easier. Separate apps are available for calculating Z-scores based on WHO charts [(**Anthrocal app** for android users: https://play.google.com/store/apps/details?id=appinventor.ai_aditya_mits13.anthroCalc&hl=en&gl=US&pli=1), plotting and interpreting height as per IAP charts (**IAP growth app:** https://play.google.com/store/apps/details?id=com.mindspace.iapgrowthchart&hl=en&gl=US) and using Intergrowth charts (**Intergrowth app:** https://intergrowth21.tghn.org/postnatal-growth-preterm-infants/)].

5.7 RECOGNIZING DISORDERS OF PHYSICAL GROWTH

Physical growth is mostly measured in terms of height and weight. A mother will seek your advice because her child is not gaining weight or height. Most of the time, the child is well and a normal variation. However, it is important to draw a line between normal and abnormal.

For sensitization purposes, we are providing the definitions of some common aberrations in growth and their important causes. *For a detailed description, refer to '**Textbook of Pediatrics**' by Piyush Gupta.*

1. Failure to Thrive (FTT)

Failure to thrive (FTT) in a child implies poor physical growth due to any cause. Though this

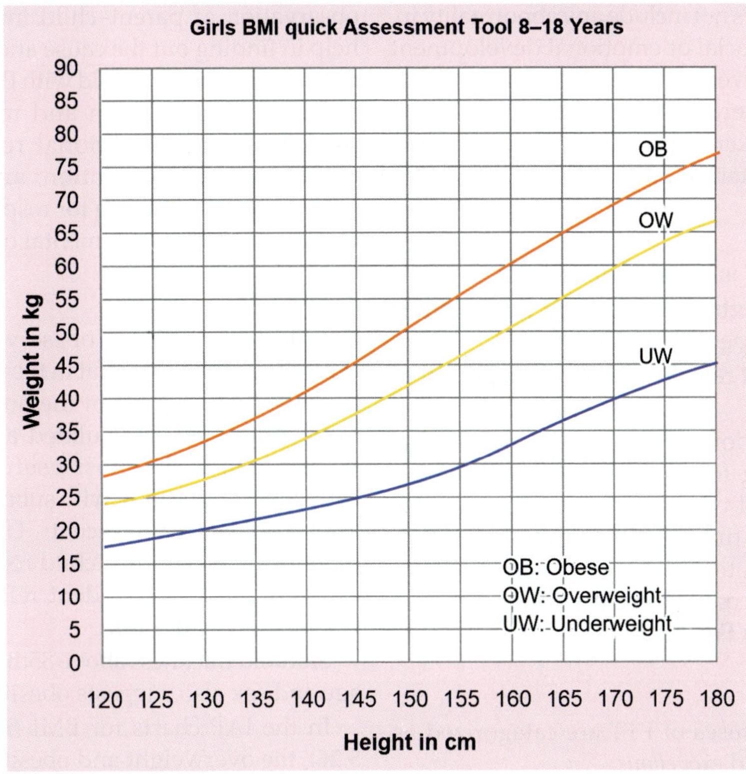

Fig. 5.28: BMI quick assessment tool 8–18 years for girls (*Source:* Khadilkar V, Lohiya N, Chiplonkar S, Khadilkar A. Body Mass Index Quick Screening Tool for Indian Academy of Pediatrics 2015 Growth Charts. Indian Pediatr. 2020;57(10):904–906).

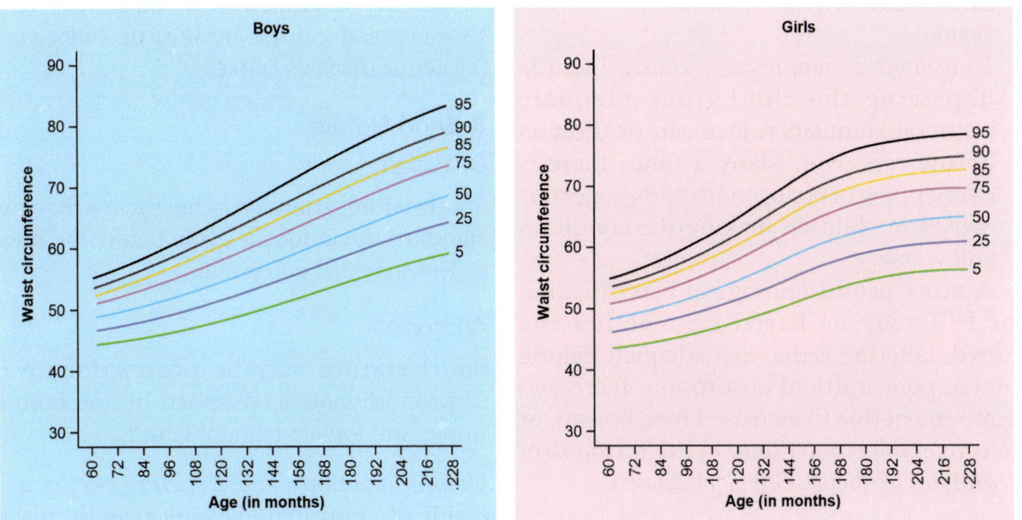

Fig. 5.29: Waist circumference charts for Indian boys and girls (Sarna A, Porwal A, Acharya R, et al. Waist circumference, waist-to-height ratio and BMI percentiles in children aged 5 to 19 years in India: A population-based study. Obes Sci Pract. 2021;7(4):392–404).

term *per se* does not include any abnormality in, intellectual, social or emotional development but FTT can eventually lead to abnormalities in these spheres. Weight being the most objective marker of growth, FTT is also known as 'weight faltering'.

Definition

The term FTT is assigned to a child:

a. Whose weight-for-age at any time point is below 3rd percentile; OR
b. The weight remains static over a period of time; OR
c. There is a downward trend in weight-for-age during follow-up assessment; which has crossed two major growth percentiles in a short time (for example, from 75th percentile to below 25th percentile or from 50th centile to below 15th centile) as depicted in **Fig. 5.30**.

Causes

Classically, causes of FTT are categorized as *endogenous* and *exogenous*.

- *Endogenous causes include organic illnesses* that lead to inability of the child to absorb/ assimilate sufficient nutrients or the current dietary intake is not able to meet the body's increased nutritional demands. These causes can be inborn errors of metabolism; congenital malformations; infections; and disorders of gastrointestinal, hepatobiliary, cardiovascular, renal, endocrine, or nervous systems.
- *Exogenous or non-organic causes* include depriving the child from adequate nutrition, stimulation, love, care or affection by the caregiver. Many a times there is overlapping of endogenous and exogenous causes in children making the condition still worse.

A more useful etiological classification for FTT may be based on whether the growth faltering is due to inadequate calorie intake, poor nutrient absorption, increased requirement due to increased metabolism, or defective utilization (Refer to ***PG Textbook of Pediatrics*** *by Piyush Gupta for details*).

Approach to Management

Complete history, detailed physical examination including anthropometry and careful observation of parent–child interaction will help in finding out the cause and hence guide the management of a child with FTT. Treatment includes identification and managing the primary cause; nutritional rehabilitation; psychological intervention; and follow-up with careful monitoring for response in terms of growth and developmental of the child.

2. Obesity

A child is considered obese when there is excess accumulation of fat in the subcutaneous tissue and other parts of the body. The body mass index (BMI) calculated as Wt/Ht^2 (in kg per m^2), is the most useful index that correlates significantly with subcutaneous and total body fat in adolescents. Use of BMI for monitoring weight in a child requires a set of age and gender-dependent reference charts **(Tables 5.17 and 5.18)**.

Skinfold thickness above 85th percentile for age and sex also suggests obesity.

In the IAP charts for BMI **(Figs 5.25 and 5.26)**, the overweight and obesity cut-offs are not based on centiles, but 'adult equivalent' of BMI 23 (overweight in adults), and 27 (obesity in adults) for Indian population.

Class 2 obesity is defined as ≥120% to <140% of the IAP obesity cutoff values of 27 adult equivalent and *Class 3 obesity* is defined as ≥140% of the IAP obesity cutoff values of 27 adult equivalent.

Obesity occurs due to *exogenous* (due to increased caloric intake) or *endogenous* (systemic disease) causes.

3. Short Stature

Definition

Short stature is defined as height less than two standard deviations (–2 SD) below the mean or less than 3rd percentile.

Approach

Short stature may be proportionate or disproportionate as assessed by the ratio of upper and lower segment length.

Disproportionate short stature occurs as a result of abnormal skeletal growth. Either the limbs or the trunk is short. In short limb dysplasia (e.g. achondroplasia), arm span is less than height and US/LS ratio is high. In short

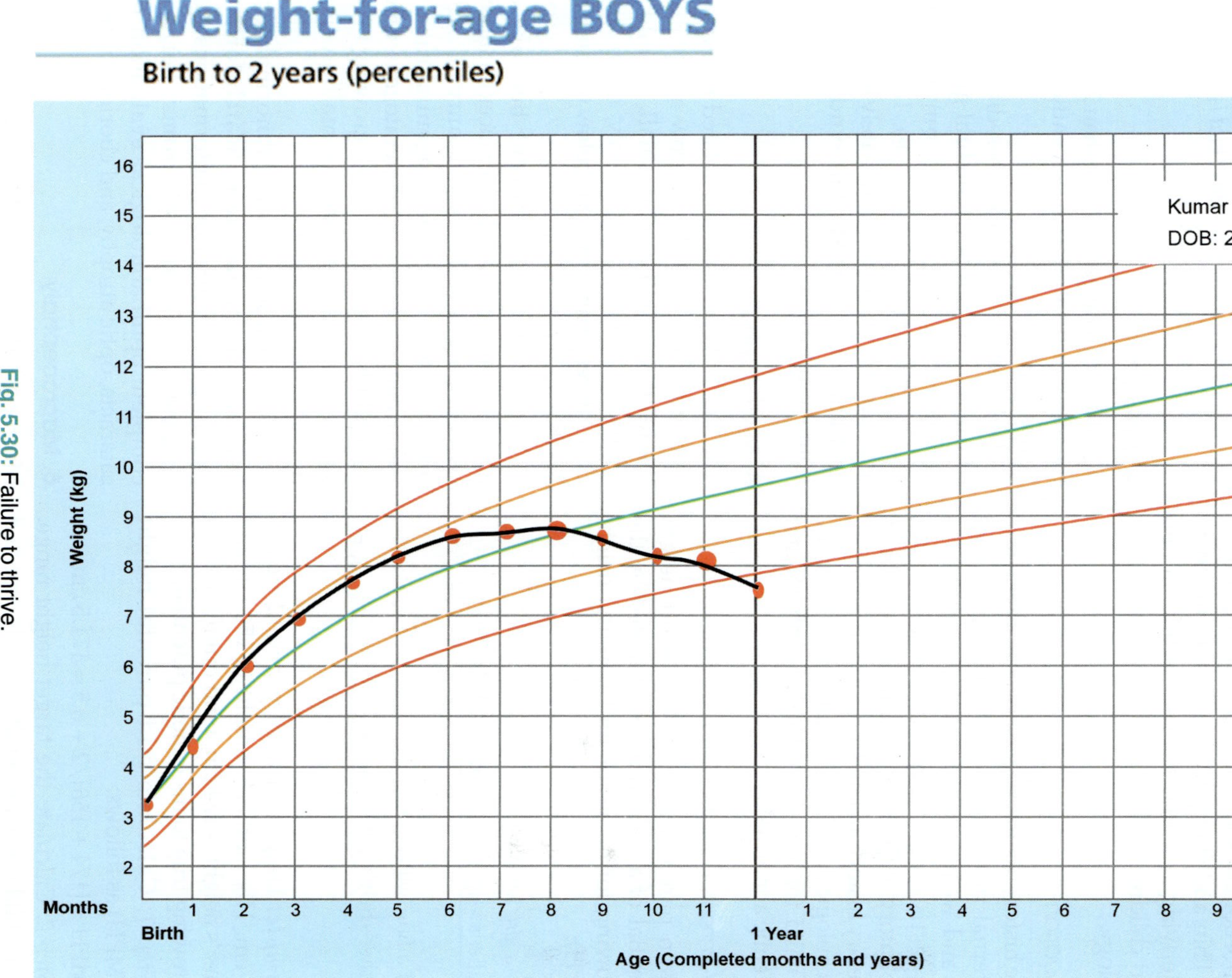

Fig. 5.30: Failure to thrive.

trunk anomalies (e.g. mucopolysaccharidosis), US/LS ratio is decreased and arm span exceeds the height.

Proportionate short stature is more common. This may occur secondary to constitutional delay in growth, chronic infections, malabsorption, congenital heart disease, renal failure, or endocrine malfunctioning. A child with proportionate short stature may be thin or fat. Thin and short children result due to an underlying systemic disorder; while fat and short children are likely to have an endocrine etiology.

Evaluation

Take history of birth regarding any antenatal/maternal problems, record the gestational age and weight at birth. Ask for symptoms suggestive of a chronic cardiac, renal, respiratory, or gastrointestinal disorder. Obtain a dietary history in detail. Enquire about social, psychological, and emotional factors. Examine the child for any sign of dysmorphism and systemic abnormality.

Mid-Parental Height

Obtain parental height. The adult height potential of a child can be estimated by the following formulae for mid-parental height (MPH):

For a girl: MPH (cm) =

$$\frac{\text{Father's height (cm)} + \text{Mother's height (cm)}}{2} - 6.5$$

For a boy: MPH (cm) =

$$\frac{\text{Father's height (cm)} + \text{Mother's height (cm)}}{2} + 6.5$$

Example: Height of a 10-year-old boy is 135 cm. His mother's height is 156 cm and father's height is 174 cm. Find out if the child is growing true to his genetic potential.

- *Step 1:* Calculate mid-parental height (MPH) as follows:
  MPH = [174 + 156]/2 + 6.5 = 171.5 cm
- *Step 2:* Calculate the target height range. The child's own percentile curve is expected to be between 10th and 90th percentile (MPH ±8.5 cm) on the MPH percentile chart. For this child the target height range will be (171.5 ±8.5 cm), i.e. between 163 and 180 cm (plotted in red in Fig. 5.31). Target height range is plotted at 18 years.
- *Step 3:* Plot the present height of the child (135 cm) on the reference growth chart of height-for-age for boys.
- *Step 4:* Observe the present case's height (plotted in blue) is within the acceptable range. It lies in the orange shaded zone, i.e. between 10th and 90th percentile of MPH.
- *Step 5: Interpretation—this child is growing as per his genetic potential.*

4. Tall Stature

A child with a height of more than 2 SD above the mean or beyond 97th percentile is said to be abnormally tall.

This may occur because of hereditary factors (if the parents are tall), cerebral gigantism, acromegaly, and chromosomal abnormality (Klinefelter syndrome). Tall stature associated with disproportionately long limbs is characteristic of Marfan syndrome and homocystinuria.

5. Microcephaly

The size of head is closely related to the size of brain. If brain does not grow adequately, the head size will remain small. A child is labeled as having microcephaly, if the head circumference remains 3 SD below the median for that age (Fig. 5.32).

Microcephaly may occur because of genetic or intrauterine disturbances including chromosomal defects (trisomy 13, 18), intrauterine infections (congenital rubella syndrome), and exposure to teratogens. Once the child is born, insult to the growing brain can be caused by meningitis, malnutrition, hypothermia, and asphyxia.

History of seizure and abnormal tone indicates abnormal brain. Search for any dysmorphic features or malformations that suggest a particular syndrome. Perform complete ophthalmological evaluation for cataracts, optic atrophy, and chorioretinitis.

6. Macrocephaly

Macrocephaly is defined as a head circumference that is >2 SD above the median for that age. It may be caused by increased brain size (megalencephaly), or increased ventricular size (hydrocephalus).

5 to 18 Years: IAP Boys Height and Weight Charts

Father's Height 174 cm, **Mother's Height** 156 cm, **Target Height** 163 cm - 180 cm

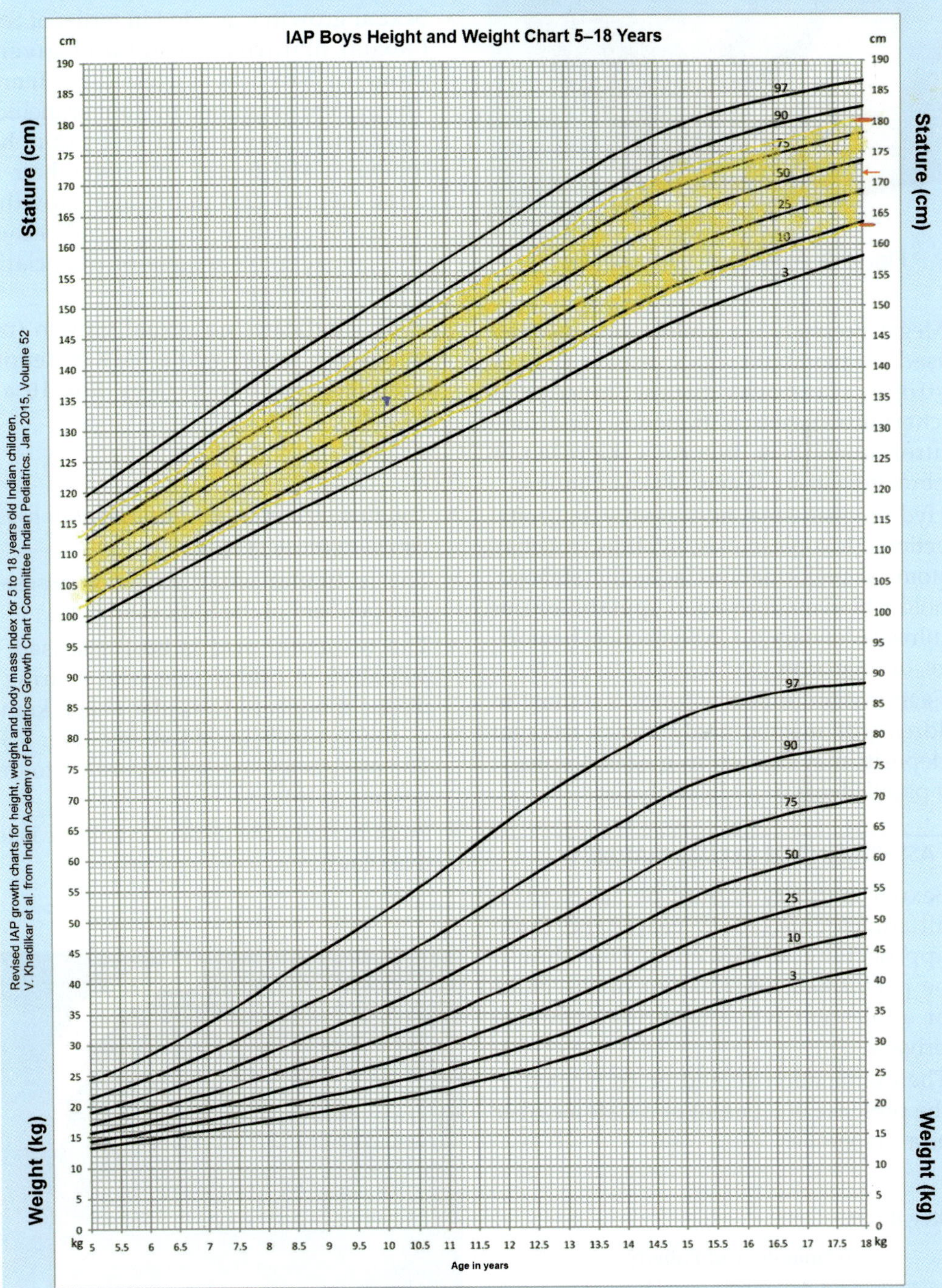

Fig. 5.31: Plotting the mid-parental height.

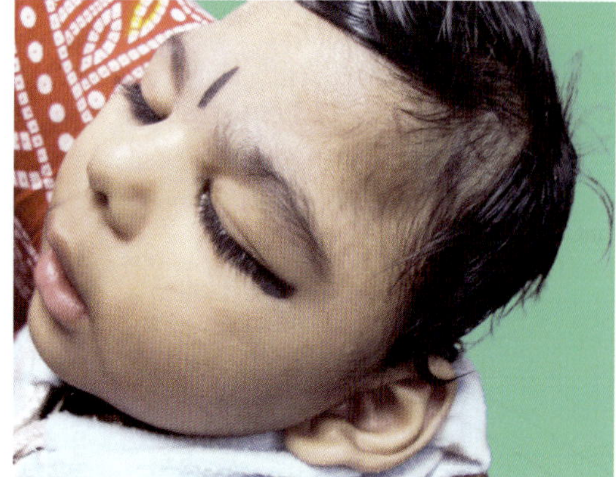

Fig. 5.32: A child with microcephaly.

Megalencephaly is a proliferation disorder caused by metabolic CNS disease (leukodystrophy, Tay-Sachs disease, mucopolysaccharidoses), neurocutaneous syndrome (neurofibromatosis, tuberous sclerosis) or cerebral gigantism. It may also be familial.

Hydrocephalus may be caused by congenital infections (toxoplasmosis, syphilis, rubella), anatomical malformations (aqueduct stenosis, Arnold-Chiari malformation, spina bifida), or acquired secondary to CNS infection, hemorrhage, or infarction.

Examination of ocular fundi is a must in children with macrocephaly: cherry red spot or deposits may be seen in megalencephaly; and papilledema in hydrocephalus.

5.8 ASSESSMENT OF SEXUAL MATURITY

- Sexual maturity should be assessed in all adolescents (10–19 years) and those approaching adolescence. This should be performed after assent of the child or adolescent while ensuring complete privacy.
- The examination should be conducted in the presence of a parent or a staff member as a chaperone.

Key Box 9

Terminology of Puberty

Thelarche: Onset of breast development
Pubarche: Onset of growth of pubic hair
Menarche: Onset of first menstrual period
Gonadarche: Onset of penile/testicular growth in boys and labial growth in girls

- Sexual growth is measured in terms of (i) growth in genitalia, (ii) pubic and axillary hair, and (iii) breast size and contour. Terminology related to pubertal changes is depicted in **Key Box 9**.
- Sexual growth is graded in terms of SMR (sexual maturity rating) and given a rating of 1 to 5 as suggested by Tanner. The system suggested by Tanner includes assessment of genitalia and pubic hair for boys; and breast and pubic hair for girls. Genital and pubic hair growth is treated separately for the male because of a considerable degree of dissociation between the two.
- SMR 1 indicates no sexual growth (prepubescent stage) while SMR 5 denotes complete maturation **(Key Box 10 and Key Box 11)**.

Boys

- The *first sign of sexual maturation in boys is the enlargement of testes.*
- The testicular enlargement is assessed independent of the SMR rating.
- The testicular size is best assessed by palpation in comparison with a string of plastic models of testicular shape known as the Prader's orchidometer (Fig. 5.33). The models are marked according to their volume in mL.
- Prepubertally, the testicular volume is less than 4 mL.

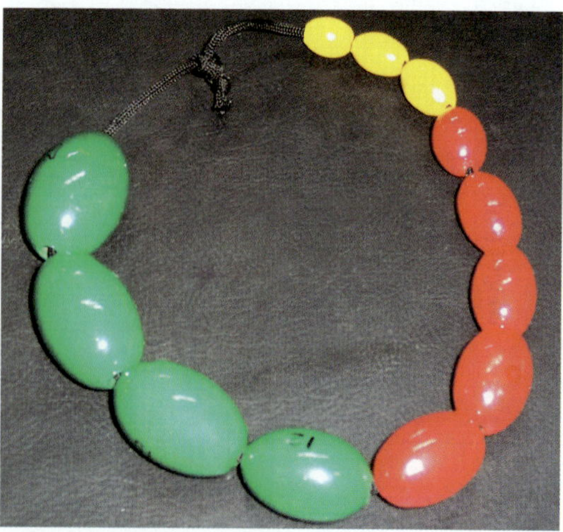

Fig. 5.33: Prader's orchidometer.

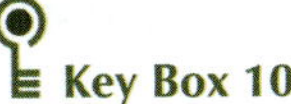

Key Box 10

Tanner Staging for Sexual Maturity Rating (SMR) in Girls

Tanner stage	Breast (B)	Pubic hair (P)
Stage 1	Prepubertal—No breast tissue	Same as abdominal hair
Stage 2	Breast bud appears, enlargement of areola	Sparse hair along labia, minimally pigmented
Stage 3	Further enlargement of breast and areola but contour separation between the two	Darker and coarser hair on mons pubis
Stage 4	A secondary mound is formed by areola and papilla above the level of the breast	Adult type, but limited to mons and labia
Stage 5	Adult breast contour with projection of papilla alone	Adult type, spreads to medial thigh

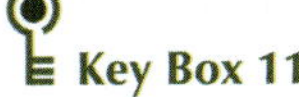

Key Box 11

Tanner Staging for Sexual Maturity Rating (SMR) in Boys

Tanner stage	Genitalia (G)	Testicular volume	Pubic hair (P)
Stage 1	Prepubertal	<4 mL	Same as abdominal hair
Stage 2	Early penile growth, thinning and reddening of scrotal skin	4–10 mL	Sparse growth at the base of penis
Stage 3	Increase in penile length, scrotal thickening and darkening	10–15 m	Darker, coarser, curled hair: Spreads to mons pubis
Stage 4	Increase in penile length and breadth, pigmentation of scrotum	15–20 mL	Adult type, not on thighs
Stage 5	Adult genitalia	>20 mL	Adult type, spreads to medial thigh

- A testicular size of 4 mL signals the onset of puberty.
- Mid-puberty testicular volume is 10–12 mL.
- The maximum volume achieved varies from 20 to 25 mL.
- The mean age of onset of puberty in males is 11.2 years.

Girls

- *Enlargement of breast (thelarche) is the first sign of sexual maturation in females.* This is best assessed by gentle palpation of breast tissue against the chest wall in the supine posture.
- Configuration of breasts and the quantity of pattern of pubic hair and axillary hair along with onset of menarche determines the pubertal status.
- The mean age of onset of puberty in girls is 11 years.
- Menarche usually occurs at breast and pubic hair stage 3 or 4.
- Menarche occurs just after achieving the peak height velocity. Thus, girls gain little in height (max. 5 cm) after they have achieved menarche.

Age and Sequence of Pubertal Changes

There is a wide variability in age of appearance of various stages in sexual development. However, the sequence remains the same. In girls, the interval from first sign of puberty (which is B_2 in 70% cases and PH_2 in 30%) to complete maturity (B_5, PH_5) varies from 1½ to 6 years. Interval from B_2 to menarche averages 2.3 years (range 6 months to 5½ years). In boys, a similar variability occurs.

Early or Precocious Puberty

Sexual precocity is the appearance of sexual characters before the age of 8 years in girls and 9 years in boys. Precocious puberty may be caused by premature activation of the hypothalamic pituitary axis *(central or true precocious puberty)* or due to increased production of sex steroids independent of the hypothalamic pituitary axis *(peripheral or pseudoprecocious puberty)*. Central precocious puberty is characterized by elevated levels of LH and FSH, whereas LH and FSH levels are low (pre-pubertal) in peripheral precocious puberty. About 10–20% of cases of precocious puberty in girls are due to organic causes and 80–90% idiopathic. In boys, most cases (60–80%) of precocity result from organic or pathological causes.

Delayed Puberty

Puberty is delayed, if there is no physical manifestation of sexual maturation in boys (testicular enlargement) and girls (breast enlargement) at a chronological age that is 2 to 2.5 SD above mean age of onset of puberty or at which 99.4% of normal children enter puberty. The cut-off is taken as 13 and 14 years in girls and boys, respectively. In a girl, absence of menarche by the age of 16 years or 5 years after the onset of puberty also indicates pubertal delay. The delay can be constitutional or organic.

Table 5.2: Weight (kg) by age of boys, percentile and Z-scores, 0–5 yr (WHO Standards)

Age		Percentiles							Z (SD) scores					
Year	Month	3rd	15th	25th	50th	75th	85th	97th	$-3Z$	$-2Z$	$-1Z$	$+1Z$	$+2Z$	$+3Z$
	0	2.5	2.9	3.0	3.3	3.7	3.9	4.3	2.1	2.5	2.9	3.9	4.4	5.0
	1	3.4	3.9	4.1	4.5	4.9	5.1	5.7	2.9	3.4	3.9	5.1	5.8	6.6
	2	4.4	4.9	5.1	5.6	6.0	6.3	7.0	3.8	4.3	4.9	6.3	7.1	8.0
	3	5.1	5.6	5.9	6.4	6.9	7.2	7.9	4.4	5.0	5.7	7.2	8.0	9.0
	4	5.6	6.2	6.5	7.0	7.6	7.9	8.6	4.9	5.6	6.2	7.8	8.7	9.7
	5	6.1	6.7	7.0	7.5	8.1	8.4	9.2	5.3	6.0	6.7	8.4	9.3	10.4
	6	6.4	7.1	7.4	7.9	8.5	8.9	9.7	5.7	6.4	7.1	8.8	9.8	10.9
	7	6.7	7.4	7.7	8.3	8.9	9.3	10.2	5.9	6.7	7.4	9.2	10.3	11.4
	8	7.0	7.7	8.0	8.6	9.3	9.6	10.5	6.2	6.9	7.7	9.6	10.7	11.9
	9	7.2	7.9	8.3	8.9	9.6	10.0	10.9	6.4	7.1	8.0	9.9	11.0	12.3
	10	7.5	8.2	8.5	9.2	9.9	10.3	11.2	6.6	7.4	8.2	10.2	11.4	12.7
	11	7.7	8.4	8.7	9.4	10.1	10.5	11.5	6.8	7.6	8.4	10.5	11.7	13.0
1	0	7.8	8.6	9.0	9.6	10.4	10.8	11.8	6.9	7.7	8.6	10.8	12.0	13.3
1	1	8.0	8.8	9.2	9.9	10.6	11.1	12.1	7.1	7.9	8.8	11.0	12.3	13.7
1	2	8.2	9.0	9.4	10.1	10.9	11.3	12.4	7.2	8.1	9.0	11.3	12.6	14.0
1	3	8.4	9.2	9.6	10.3	11.1	11.6	12.7	7.4	8.3	9.2	11.5	12.8	14.3
1	4	8.5	9.4	9.8	10.5	11.3	11.8	12.9	7.5	8.4	9.4	11.7	13.1	14.6
1	5	8.7	9.6	10.0	10.7	11.6	12.0	13.2	7.7	8.6	9.6	12.0	13.4	14.9
1	6	8.9	9.7	10.1	10.9	11.8	12.3	13.5	7.8	8.8	9.8	12.2	13.7	15.3
1	7	9.0	9.9	10.3	11.1	12.0	12.5	13.7	8.0	8.9	10.0	12.5	13.9	15.6
1	8	9.2	10.1	10.5	11.3	12.2	12.7	14.0	8.1	9.1	10.1	12.7	14.2	15.9
1	9	9.3	10.3	10.7	11.5	12.5	13.0	14.3	8.2	9.2	10.3	12.9	14.5	16.2
1	10	9.5	10.5	10.9	11.8	12.7	13.2	14.5	8.4	9.4	10.5	13.2	14.7	16.5
1	11	9.7	10.6	11.1	12.0	12.9	13.4	14.8	8.5	9.5	10.7	13.4	15.0	16.8
2	0	9.8	10.8	11.3	12.2	13.1	13.7	15.1	8.6	9.7	10.8	13.6	15.3	17.1
2	1	10.0	11.0	11.4	12.4	13.3	13.9	15.3	8.8	9.8	11.0	13.9	15.5	17.5
2	2	10.1	11.1	11.6	12.5	13.6	14.1	15.6	8.9	10.0	11.2	14.1	15.8	17.8
2	3	10.2	11.3	11.8	12.7	13.8	14.4	15.9	9.0	10.1	11.3	14.3	16.1	18.1
2	4	10.4	11.5	12.0	12.9	14.0	14.6	16.1	9.1	10.2	11.5	14.5	16.3	18.4
2	5	10.5	11.6	12.1	13.1	14.2	14.8	16.4	9.2	10.4	11.7	14.8	16.6	18.7
2	6	10.7	11.8	12.3	13.3	14.4	15.0	16.6	9.4	10.5	11.8	15.0	16.9	19.0
2	7	10.8	11.9	12.4	13.5	14.6	15.2	16.9	9.5	10.7	12.0	15.2	17.1	19.3
2	8	10.9	12.1	12.6	13.7	14.8	15.5	17.1	9.6	10.8	12.1	15.4	17.4	19.6
2	9	11.1	12.2	12.8	13.8	15.0	15.7	17.3	9.7	10.9	12.3	15.6	17.6	19.9
2	10	11.2	12.4	12.9	14.0	15.2	15.9	17.6	9.8	11.0	12.4	15.8	17.8	20.2
2	11	11.3	12.5	13.1	14.2	15.4	16.1	17.8	9.9	11.2	12.6	16.0	18.1	20.4
3	0	11.4	12.7	13.2	14.3	15.6	16.3	18.0	10.0	11.3	12.7	16.2	18.3	20.7
3	1	11.6	12.8	13.4	14.5	15.8	16.5	18.3	10.1	11.4	12.9	16.4	18.6	21.0
3	2	11.7	12.9	13.5	14.7	15.9	16.7	18.5	10.2	11.5	13.0	16.6	18.8	21.3
3	3	11.8	13.1	13.7	14.8	16.1	16.9	18.7	10.3	11.6	13.1	16.8	19.0	21.6
3	4	11.9	13.2	13.8	15.0	16.3	17.1	19.0	10.4	11.8	13.3	17.0	19.3	21.9
3	5	12.1	13.4	14.0	15.2	16.5	17.3	19.2	10.5	11.9	13.4	17.2	19.5	22.1
3	6	12.2	13.5	14.1	15.3	16.7	17.5	19.4	10.6	12.0	13.6	17.4	19.7	22.4
3	7	12.3	13.6	14.3	15.5	16.9	17.7	19.7	10.7	12.1	13.7	17.6	20.0	22.7
3	8	12.4	13.8	14.4	15.7	17.1	17.9	19.9	10.8	12.2	13.8	17.8	20.2	23.0
3	9	12.5	13.9	14.6	15.8	17.3	18.1	20.1	10.9	12.4	14.0	18.0	20.5	23.3
3	10	12.7	14.1	14.7	16.0	17.4	18.3	20.4	11.0	12.5	14.1	18.2	20.7	23.6
3	11	12.8	14.2	14.9	16.2	17.6	18.5	20.6	11.1	12.6	14.3	18.4	20.9	23.9
4	0	12.9	14.3	15.0	16.3	17.8	18.7	20.9	11.2	12.7	14.4	18.6	21.2	24.2
4	1	13.0	14.5	15.2	16.5	18.0	18.9	21.1	11.3	12.8	14.5	18.8	21.4	24.5
4	2	13.1	14.6	15.3	16.7	18.2	19.1	21.3	11.4	12.9	14.7	19.0	21.7	24.8
4	3	13.3	14.7	15.4	16.8	18.4	19.3	21.6	11.5	13.1	14.8	19.2	21.9	25.1
4	4	13.4	14.9	15.6	17.0	18.6	19.5	21.8	11.6	13.2	15.0	19.4	22.2	25.4
4	5	13.5	15.0	15.7	17.2	18.8	19.7	22.1	11.7	13.3	15.1	19.6	22.4	25.7
4	6	13.6	15.2	15.9	17.3	19.0	19.9	22.3	11.8	13.4	15.2	19.8	22.7	26.0
4	7	13.7	15.3	16.0	17.5	19.2	20.1	22.5	11.9	13.5	15.4	20.0	22.9	26.3
4	8	13.8	15.4	16.2	17.7	19.3	20.3	22.8	12.0	13.6	15.5	20.2	23.2	26.6
4	9	13.9	15.6	16.3	17.8	19.5	20.5	23.0	12.1	13.7	15.6	20.4	23.4	26.9
4	10	14.1	15.7	16.5	18.0	19.7	20.7	23.3	12.2	13.8	15.8	20.6	23.7	27.2
4	11	14.2	15.8	16.6	18.2	19.9	20.9	23.5	12.3	14.0	15.9	20.8	23.9	27.6
5	0	14.3	16.0	16.7	18.3	20.1	21.1	23.8	12.4	14.1	16.0	21.0	24.2	27.9

Table 5.3: Weight (kg) by age of girls, percentiles and *Z*-scores, 0–5 yr (WHO Standards)

Age		Percentiles							*Z* (SD) scores						
Year	Month	3rd	15th	25th	50th	75th	85th	97th	–3*Z*	–2*Z*	–1*Z*	+1*Z*	+2*Z*	+3*Z*
	0	2.5	2.9	3.0	3.3	3.7	3.9	4.3	2.1	2.5	2.9	3.9	4.4	5.0
	0	2.4	2.8	2.9	3.2	3.6	3.7	4.2	2.0	2.4	2.8	3.7	4.2	4.8
	1	3.2	3.6	3.8	4.2	4.6	4.8	5.4	2.7	3.2	3.6	4.8	5.5	6.2
	2	4.0	4.5	4.7	5.1	5.6	5.9	6.5	3.4	3.9	4.5	5.8	6.6	7.5
	3	4.6	5.1	5.4	5.8	6.4	6.7	7.4	4.0	4.5	5.2	6.6	7.5	8.5
	4	5.1	5.6	5.9	6.4	7.0	7.3	8.1	4.4	5.0	5.7	7.3	8.2	9.3
	5	5.5	6.1	6.4	6.9	7.5	7.8	8.7	4.8	5.4	6.1	7.8	8.8	10.0
	6	5.8	6.4	6.7	7.3	7.9	8.3	9.2	5.1	5.7	6.5	8.2	9.3	10.6
	7	6.1	6.7	7.0	7.6	8.3	8.7	9.6	5.3	6.0	6.8	8.6	9.8	11.1
	8	6.3	7.0	7.3	7.9	8.6	9.0	10.0	5.6	6.3	7.0	9.0	10.2	11.6
	9	6.6	7.3	7.6	8.2	8.9	9.3	10.4	5.8	6.5	7.3	9.3	10.5	12.0
	10	6.8	7.5	7.8	8.5	9.2	9.6	10.7	5.9	6.7	7.5	9.6	10.9	12.4
	11	7.0	7.7	8.0	8.7	9.5	9.9	11.0	6.1	6.9	7.7	9.9	11.2	12.8
1	0	7.1	7.9	8.2	8.9	9.7	10.2	11.3	6.3	7.0	7.9	10.1	11.5	13.1
1	1	7.3	8.1	8.4	9.2	10.0	10.4	11.6	6.4	7.2	8.1	10.4	11.8	13.5
1	2	7.5	8.3	8.6	9.4	10.2	10.7	11.9	6.6	7.4	8.3	10.6	12.1	13.8
1	3	7.7	8.5	8.8	9.6	10.4	10.9	12.2	6.7	7.6	8.5	10.9	12.4	14.1
1	4	7.8	8.7	9.0	9.8	10.7	11.2	12.5	6.9	7.7	8.7	11.1	12.6	14.5
1	5	8.0	8.8	9.2	10.0	10.9	11.4	12.7	7.0	7.9	8.9	11.4	12.9	14.8
1	6	8.2	9.0	9.4	10.2	11.1	11.6	13.0	7.2	8.1	9.1	11.6	13.2	15.1
1	7	8.3	9.2	9.6	10.4	11.4	11.9	13.3	7.3	8.2	9.2	11.8	13.5	15.4
1	8	8.5	9.4	9.8	10.6	11.6	12.1	13.5	7.5	8.4	9.4	12.1	13.7	15.7
1	9	8.7	9.6	10.0	10.9	11.8	12.4	13.8	7.6	8.6	9.6	12.3	14.0	16.0
1	10	8.8	9.8	10.2	11.1	12.0	12.6	14.1	7.8	8.7	9.8	12.5	14.3	16.4
1	11	9.0	9.9	10.4	11.3	12.3	12.8	14.3	7.9	8.9	10.0	12.8	14.6	16.7
2	0	9.2	10.1	10.6	11.5	12.5	13.1	14.6	8.1	9.0	10.2	13.0	14.8	17.0
2	1	9.3	10.3	10.8	11.7	12.7	13.3	14.9	8.2	9.2	10.3	13.3	15.1	17.3
2	2	9.5	10.5	10.9	11.9	12.9	13.6	15.2	8.4	9.4	10.5	13.5	15.4	17.7
2	3	9.6	10.7	11.1	12.1	13.2	13.8	15.4	8.5	9.5	10.7	13.7	15.7	18.0
2	4	9.8	10.8	11.3	12.3	13.4	14.0	15.7	8.6	9.7	10.9	14.0	16.0	18.3
2	5	10.0	11.0	11.5	12.5	13.6	14.3	16.0	8.8	9.8	11.1	14.2	16.2	18.7
2	6	10.1	11.2	11.7	12.7	13.8	14.5	16.2	8.9	10.0	11.2	14.4	16.5	19.0
2	7	10.3	11.3	11.9	12.9	14.1	14.7	16.5	9.0	10.1	11.4	14.7	16.8	19.3
2	8	10.4	11.5	12.0	13.1	14.3	15.0	16.8	9.1	10.3	11.6	14.9	17.1	19.6
2	9	10.5	11.7	12.2	13.3	14.5	15.2	17.0	9.3	10.4	11.7	15.1	17.3	20.0
2	10	10.7	11.8	12.4	13.5	14.7	15.4	17.3	9.4	10.5	11.9	15.4	17.6	20.3
2	11	10.8	12.0	12.5	13.7	14.9	15.7	17.6	9.5	10.7	12.0	15.6	17.9	20.6
3	0	11.0	12.1	12.7	13.9	15.1	15.9	17.8	9.6	10.8	12.2	15.8	18.1	20.9
3	1	11.1	12.3	12.9	14.0	15.3	16.1	18.1	9.7	10.9	12.4	16.0	18.4	21.3
3	2	11.2	12.5	13.0	14.2	15.6	16.3	18.4	9.8	11.1	12.5	16.3	18.7	21.6
3	3	11.4	12.6	13.2	14.4	15.8	16.6	18.6	9.9	11.2	12.7	16.5	19.0	22.0
3	4	11.5	12.8	13.4	14.6	16.0	16.8	18.9	10.1	11.3	12.8	16.7	19.2	22.3
3	5	11.6	12.9	13.5	14.8	16.2	17.0	19.2	10.2	11.5	13.0	16.9	19.5	22.7
3	6	11.8	13.1	13.7	15.0	16.4	17.3	19.5	10.3	11.6	13.1	17.2	19.8	23.0
3	7	11.9	13.2	13.9	15.2	16.6	17.5	19.7	10.4	11.7	13.3	17.4	20.1	23.4
3	8	12.0	13.4	14.0	15.3	16.8	17.7	20.0	10.5	11.8	13.4	17.6	20.4	23.7
3	9	12.1	13.5	14.2	15.5	17.0	17.9	20.3	10.6	12.0	13.6	17.8	20.7	24.1
3	10	12.3	13.7	14.3	15.7	17.3	18.2	20.6	10.7	12.1	13.7	18.1	20.9	24.5
3	11	12.4	13.8	14.5	15.9	17.5	18.4	20.8	10.8	12.2	13.9	18.3	21.2	24.8
4	0	12.5	14.0	14.7	16.1	17.7	18.6	21.1	10.9	12.3	14.0	18.5	21.5	25.2
4	1	12.6	14.1	14.8	16.3	17.9	18.9	21.4	11.0	12.4	14.2	18.8	21.8	25.5
4	2	12.8	14.3	15.0	16.4	18.1	19.1	21.7	11.1	12.6	14.3	19.0	22.1	25.9
4	3	12.9	14.4	15.1	16.6	18.3	19.3	22.0	11.2	12.7	14.5	19.2	22.4	26.3
4	4	13.0	14.5	15.3	16.8	18.5	19.5	22.2	11.3	12.8	14.6	19.4	22.6	26.6
4	5	13.1	14.7	15.4	17.0	18.7	19.8	22.5	11.4	12.9	14.8	19.7	22.9	27.0
4	6	13.2	14.8	15.6	17.2	18.9	20.0	22.8	11.5	13.0	14.9	19.9	23.2	27.4
4	7	13.4	15.0	15.8	17.3	19.1	20.2	23.1	11.6	13.2	15.1	20.1	23.5	27.7
4	8	13.5	15.1	15.9	17.5	19.3	20.4	23.3	11.7	13.3	15.2	20.3	23.8	28.1
4	9	13.6	15.3	16.1	17.7	19.6	20.7	23.6	11.8	13.4	15.3	20.6	24.1	28.5
4	10	13.7	15.4	16.2	17.9	19.8	20.9	23.9	11.9	13.5	15.5	20.8	24.4	28.8
4	11	13.8	15.5	16.4	18.0	20.0	21.1	24.2	12.0	13.6	15.6	21.0	24.6	29.2
5	0	14.0	15.7	16.5	18.2	20.2	21.3	24.4	12.1	13.7	15.8	21.2	24.9	29.5

Table 5.4: Length (cm) by age of boys and girls aged 0–2 years (WHO Standards)

Boys	Percentiles							Z (SD) scores					
Age (month)	3rd	15th	25th	50th	75th	85th	97th	–3Z	–2Z	–1Z	+1Z	+2Z	+3Z
0	46.3	47.9	48.6	49.9	51.2	51.8	53.4	44.2	46.1	48.0	51.8	53.7	55.6
1	51.1	52.7	53.4	54.7	56.0	56.7	58.4	48.9	50.8	52.8	56.7	58.6	60.6
2	54.7	56.4	57.1	58.4	59.8	60.5	62.2	52.4	54.4	56.4	60.4	62.4	64.4
3	57.6	59.3	60.1	61.4	62.8	63.5	65.3	55.3	57.3	59.4	63.5	65.5	67.6
4	60.0	61.7	62.5	63.9	65.3	66.0	67.8	57.6	59.7	61.8	66.0	68.0	70.1
5	61.9	63.7	64.5	65.9	67.3	68.1	69.9	59.6	61.7	63.8	68.0	70.1	72.2
6	63.6	65.4	66.2	67.6	69.1	69.8	71.6	61.2	63.3	65.5	69.8	71.9	74.0
7	65.1	66.9	67.7	69.2	70.6	71.4	73.2	62.7	64.8	67.0	71.3	73.5	75.7
8	66.5	68.3	69.1	70.6	72.1	72.9	74.7	64.0	66.2	68.4	72.8	75.0	77.2
9	67.7	69.6	70.5	72.0	73.5	74.3	76.2	65.2	67.5	69.7	74.2	76.5	78.7
10	69.0	70.9	71.7	73.3	74.8	75.6	77.6	66.4	68.7	71.0	75.6	77.9	80.1
11	70.2	72.1	73.0	74.5	76.1	77.0	78.9	67.6	69.9	72.2	76.9	79.2	81.5
12	71.3	73.3	74.1	75.7	77.4	78.2	80.2	68.6	71.0	73.4	78.1	80.5	82.9
13	72.4	74.4	75.3	76.9	78.6	79.4	81.5	69.6	72.1	74.5	79.3	81.8	84.2
14	73.4	75.5	76.4	78.0	79.7	80.6	82.7	70.6	73.1	75.6	80.5	83.0	85.5
15	74.4	76.5	77.4	79.1	80.9	81.8	83.9	71.6	74.1	76.6	81.7	84.2	86.7
16	75.4	77.5	78.5	80.2	82.0	82.9	85.1	72.5	75.0	77.6	82.8	85.4	88.0
17	76.3	78.5	79.5	81.2	83.0	84.0	86.2	73.3	76.0	78.6	83.9	86.5	89.2
18	77.2	79.5	80.4	82.3	84.1	85.1	87.3	74.2	76.9	79.6	85.0	87.7	90.4
19	78.1	80.4	81.4	83.2	85.1	86.1	88.4	75.0	77.7	80.5	86.0	88.8	91.5
20	78.9	81.3	82.3	84.2	86.1	87.1	89.5	75.8	78.6	81.4	87.0	89.8	92.6
21	79.7	82.2	83.2	85.1	87.1	88.1	90.5	76.5	79.4	82.3	88.0	90.9	93.8
22	80.5	83.0	84.1	86.0	88.0	89.1	91.6	77.2	80.2	83.1	89.0	91.9	94.9
23	81.3	83.8	84.9	86.9	89.0	90.0	92.6	78.0	81.0	83.9	89.9	92.9	95.9
24	82.1	84.6	85.8	87.8	89.9	91.0	93.6	78.7	81.7	84.8	90.9	93.9	97.0
Girls	**Percentiles**							**Z (SD) scores**					
Age (month)	**3rd**	**15th**	**25th**	**50th**	**75th**	**85th**	**97th**	**–3Z**	**–2Z**	**–1Z**	**+1Z**	**+2Z**	**+3Z**
0	45.6	47.2	47.9	49.1	50.4	51.1	52.7	43.6	45.4	47.3	51.0	52.9	54.7
1	50.0	51.7	52.4	53.7	55.0	55.7	57.4	47.8	49.8	51.7	55.6	57.6	59.5
2	53.2	55.0	55.7	57.1	58.4	59.2	60.9	51.0	53.0	55.0	59.1	61.1	63.2
3	55.8	57.6	58.4	59.8	61.2	62.0	63.8	53.5	55.6	57.7	61.9	64.0	66.1
4	58.0	59.8	60.6	62.1	63.5	64.3	66.2	55.6	57.8	59.9	64.3	66.4	68.6
5	59.9	61.7	62.5	64.0	65.5	66.3	68.2	57.4	59.6	61.8	66.2	68.5	70.7
6	61.5	63.4	64.2	65.7	67.3	68.1	70.0	58.9	61.2	63.5	68.0	70.3	72.5
7	62.9	64.9	65.7	67.3	68.8	69.7	71.6	60.3	62.7	65.0	69.6	71.9	74.2
8	64.3	66.3	67.2	68.7	70.3	71.2	73.2	61.7	64.0	66.4	71.1	73.5	75.8
9	65.6	67.6	68.5	70.1	71.8	72.6	74.7	62.9	65.3	67.7	72.6	75.0	77.4
10	66.8	68.9	69.8	71.5	73.1	74.0	76.1	64.1	66.5	69.0	73.9	76.4	78.9
11	68.0	70.2	71.1	72.8	74.5	75.4	77.5	65.2	67.7	70.3	75.3	77.8	80.3
12	69.2	71.3	72.3	74.0	75.8	76.7	78.9	66.3	68.9	71.4	76.6	79.2	81.7
13	70.3	72.5	73.4	75.2	77.0	77.9	80.2	67.3	70.0	72.6	77.8	80.5	83.1
14	71.3	73.6	74.6	76.4	78.2	79.2	81.4	68.3	71.0	73.7	79.1	81.7	84.4
15	72.4	74.7	75.7	77.5	79.4	80.3	82.7	69.3	72.0	74.8	80.2	83.0	85.7
16	73.3	75.7	76.7	78.6	80.5	81.5	83.9	70.2	73.0	75.8	81.4	84.2	87.0
17	74.3	76.7	77.7	79.7	81.6	82.6	85.0	71.1	74.0	76.8	82.5	85.4	88.2
18	75.2	77.7	78.7	80.7	82.7	83.7	86.2	72.0	74.9	77.8	83.6	86.5	89.4
19	76.2	78.7	79.7	81.7	83.7	84.8	87.3	72.8	75.8	78.8	84.7	87.6	90.6
20	77.0	79.6	80.7	82.7	84.7	85.8	88.4	73.7	76.7	79.7	85.7	88.7	91.7
21	77.9	80.5	81.6	83.7	85.7	86.8	89.4	74.5	77.5	80.6	86.7	89.8	92.9
22	78.7	81.4	82.5	84.6	86.7	87.8	90.5	75.2	78.4	81.5	87.7	90.8	94.0
23	79.6	82.2	83.4	85.5	87.7	88.8	91.5	76.0	79.2	82.3	88.7	91.9	95.0
24	80.3	83.1	84.2	86.4	88.6	89.8	92.5	76.7	80.0	83.2	89.6	92.9	96.1

Table 5.5: Height-for-age (cm) of boys and girls aged 2–5 years (WHO Standards)

Boys		Percentiles							*Z* (SD) scores					
Year	Month	3rd	15th	25th	50th	75th	85th	97th	–3*Z*	–2*Z*	–1*Z*	+1*Z*	+2*Z*	+3*Z*
2	1	82.1	84.7	85.9	88.0	90.1	91.2	93.8	78.6	81.7	84.9	91.1	94.2	97.3
2	2	82.8	85.5	86.7	88.8	90.9	92.1	94.8	79.3	82.5	85.6	92.0	95.2	98.3
2	3	83.5	86.3	87.4	89.6	91.8	93.0	95.7	79.9	83.1	86.4	92.9	96.1	99.3
2	4	84.2	87.0	88.2	90.4	92.6	93.8	96.6	80.5	83.8	87.1	93.7	97.0	100.3
2	5	84.9	87.7	88.9	91.2	93.4	94.7	97.5	81.1	84.5	87.8	94.5	97.9	101.2
2	6	85.5	88.4	89.6	91.9	94.2	95.5	98.3	81.7	85.1	88.5	95.3	98.7	102.1
2	7	86.2	89.1	90.3	92.7	95.0	96.2	99.2	82.3	85.7	89.2	96.1	99.6	103.0
2	8	86.8	89.7	91.0	93.4	95.7	97.0	100.0	82.8	86.4	89.9	96.9	100.4	103.9
2	9	87.4	90.4	91.7	94.1	96.5	97.8	100.8	83.4	86.9	90.5	97.6	101.2	104.8
2	10	88.0	91.0	92.3	94.8	97.2	98.5	101.5	83.9	87.5	91.1	98.4	102.0	105.6
2	11	88.5	91.6	93.0	95.4	97.9	99.2	102.3	84.4	88.1	91.8	99.1	102.7	106.4
3	0	89.1	92.2	93.6	96.1	98.6	99.9	103.1	85.0	88.7	92.4	99.8	103.5	107.2
3	1	89.7	92.8	94.2	96.7	99.3	100.6	103.8	85.5	89.2	93.0	100.5	104.2	108.0
3	2	90.2	93.4	94.8	97.4	99.9	101.3	104.5	86.0	89.8	93.6	101.2	105.0	108.8
3	3	90.8	94.0	95.4	98.0	100.6	102.0	105.2	86.5	90.3	94.2	101.8	105.7	109.5
3	4	91.3	94.6	96.0	98.6	101.3	102.7	105.9	87.0	90.9	94.7	102.5	106.4	110.3
3	5	91.9	95.2	96.6	99.2	101.9	103.3	106.6	87.5	91.4	95.3	103.2	107.1	111.0
3	6	92.4	95.7	97.2	99.9	102.5	104.0	107.3	88.0	91.9	95.9	103.8	107.8	111.7
3	7	92.9	96.3	97.7	100.4	103.1	104.6	108.0	88.4	92.4	96.4	104.5	108.5	112.5
3	8	93.4	96.8	98.3	101.0	103.8	105.2	108.6	88.9	93.0	97.0	105.1	109.1	113.2
3	9	93.9	97.4	98.9	101.6	104.4	105.8	109.3	89.4	93.5	97.5	105.7	109.8	113.9
3	10	94.4	97.9	99.4	102.2	105.0	106.5	109.9	89.8	94.0	98.1	106.3	110.4	114.6
3	11	94.9	98.5	100.0	102.8	105.6	107.1	110.6	90.3	94.4	98.6	106.9	111.1	115.2
4	0	95.4	99.0	100.5	103.3	106.2	107.7	111.2	90.7	94.9	99.1	107.5	111.7	115.9
4	3	96.9	100.5	102.1	105.0	107.9	109.5	113.1	92.1	96.4	100.7	109.3	113.6	117.9
4	6	98.4	102.1	103.7	106.7	109.6	111.2	115.0	93.4	97.8	102.3	111.1	115.5	119.9
4	9	99.8	103.6	105.3	108.3	111.4	113.0	116.8	94.7	99.3	103.8	112.8	117.4	121.9
5	0	101.2	105.2	106.8	110.0	113.1	114.8	118.7	96.1	100.7	105.3	114.6	119.2	123.9
Girls		**Percentiles**							***Z* (SD) scores**					
Year	**Month**	**3rd**	**15th**	**25th**	**50th**	**75th**	**85th**	**97th**	**–3Z**	**–2Z**	**–1Z**	**+1Z**	**+2Z**	**+3Z**
2	1	80.4	83.2	84.4	86.6	88.8	90.0	92.8	76.8	80.0	83.3	89.9	93.1	96.4
2	2	81.2	84.0	85.2	87.4	89.7	90.9	93.7	77.5	80.8	84.1	90.8	94.1	97.4
2	3	81.9	84.8	86.0	88.3	90.6	91.8	94.6	78.1	81.5	84.9	91.7	95.0	98.4
2	4	82.6	85.5	86.8	89.1	91.4	92.7	95.6	78.8	82.2	85.7	92.5	96.0	99.4
2	5	83.4	86.3	87.6	89.9	92.2	93.5	96.4	79.5	82.9	86.4	93.4	96.9	100.3
2	6	84.0	87.0	88.3	90.7	93.1	94.3	97.3	80.1	83.6	87.1	94.2	97.7	101.3
2	7	84.7	87.7	89.0	91.4	93.9	95.2	98.2	80.7	84.3	87.9	95.0	98.6	102.2
2	8	85.4	88.4	89.7	92.2	94.6	95.9	99.0	81.3	84.9	88.6	95.8	99.4	103.1
2	9	86.0	89.1	90.4	92.9	95.4	96.7	99.8	81.9	85.6	89.3	96.6	100.3	103.9
2	10	86.7	89.8	91.1	93.6	96.2	97.5	100.6	82.5	86.2	89.9	97.4	101.1	104.8
2	11	87.3	90.5	91.8	94.4	96.9	98.3	101.4	83.1	86.8	90.6	98.1	101.9	105.6
3	0	87.9	91.1	92.5	95.1	97.6	99.0	102.2	83.6	87.4	91.2	98.9	102.7	106.5
3	1	88.5	91.7	93.1	95.7	98.3	99.7	103.0	84.2	88.0	91.9	99.6	103.4	107.3
3	2	89.1	92.4	93.8	96.4	99.0	100.5	103.7	84.7	88.6	92.5	100.3	104.2	108.1
3	3	89.7	93.0	94.4	97.1	99.7	101.2	104.5	85.3	89.2	93.1	101.0	105.0	108.9
3	4	90.3	93.6	95.1	97.7	100.4	101.9	105.2	85.8	89.8	93.8	101.7	105.7	109.7
3	5	90.8	94.2	95.7	98.4	101.1	102.6	106.0	86.3	90.4	94.4	102.4	106.4	110.5
3	6	91.4	94.8	96.3	99.0	101.8	103.3	106.7	86.8	90.9	95.0	103.1	107.2	111.2
3	7	92.0	95.4	96.9	99.7	102.4	103.9	107.4	87.4	91.5	95.6	103.8	107.9	112.0
3	8	92.5	96.0	97.5	100.3	103.1	104.6	108.1	87.9	92.0	96.2	104.5	108.6	112.7
3	9	93.0	96.6	98.1	100.9	103.7	105.3	108.8	88.4	92.5	96.7	105.1	109.3	113.5
3	10	93.6	97.2	98.7	101.5	104.4	105.9	109.5	88.9	93.1	97.3	105.8	110.0	114.2
3	11	94.1	97.7	99.3	102.1	105.0	106.6	110.2	89.3	93.6	97.9	106.4	110.7	114.9
4	0	94.6	98.3	99.8	102.7	105.6	107.2	110.8	89.8	94.1	98.4	107.0	111.3	115.7
4	3	96.2	99.9	101.5	104.5	107.5	109.1	112.8	91.2	95.6	100.1	108.9	113.3	117.7
4	6	97.6	101.5	103.1	106.2	109.2	110.9	114.7	92.6	97.1	101.6	110.7	115.2	119.8
4	9	99.1	103.0	104.7	107.8	111.0	112.6	116.6	93.9	98.5	103.2	112.5	117.1	121.8
5	0	100.5	104.5	106.2	109.4	112.6	114.4	118.4	95.2	99.9	104.7	114.2	118.9	123.7

Table 5.6: Weight (kg) for length (cm) for boys 0–2 years (WHO Reference Data) percentiles and *Z* (SD) scores

Length (cm)	Percentiles											Standard deviation (SD) *Z*-scores					
	1st	3rd	5th	15th	25th	50th	75th	85th	95th	97th	99th	–3SD	–2SD	–1SD	+1SD	+2SD	+3SD
45.0	2.0	2.1	2.1	2.2	2.3	2.4	2.6	2.7	2.9	2.9	3.0	1.9	2.0	2.2	2.7	3.0	3.3
45.5	2.1	2.1	2.2	2.3	2.4	2.5	2.7	2.8	2.9	3.0	3.1	1.9	2.1	2.3	2.8	3.1	3.4
46.0	2.1	2.2	2.3	2.4	2.5	2.6	2.8	2.9	3.0	3.1	3.3	2.0	2.2	2.4	2.9	3.1	3.5
46.5	2.2	2.3	2.3	2.5	2.5	2.7	2.9	3.0	3.1	3.2	3.4	2.1	2.3	2.5	3.0	3.2	3.6
47.0	2.3	2.4	2.4	2.5	2.6	2.8	3.0	3.1	3.2	3.3	3.5	2.1	2.3	2.5	3.0	3.3	3.7
47.5	2.3	2.4	2.5	2.6	2.7	2.9	3.0	3.1	3.3	3.4	3.6	2.2	2.4	2.6	3.1	3.4	3.8
48.0	2.4	2.5	2.6	2.7	2.8	2.9	3.1	3.2	3.4	3.5	3.7	2.3	2.5	2.7	3.2	3.6	3.9
48.5	2.5	2.6	2.6	2.8	2.9	3.0	3.2	3.3	3.5	3.6	3.8	2.3	2.6	2.8	3.3	3.7	4.0
49.0	2.6	2.7	2.7	2.9	2.9	3.1	3.3	3.4	3.6	3.7	3.9	2.4	2.6	2.9	3.4	3.8	4.2
49.5	2.6	2.7	2.8	2.9	3.0	3.2	3.4	3.5	3.8	3.8	4.0	2.5	2.7	3.0	3.5	3.9	4.3
50.0	2.7	2.8	2.9	3.0	3.1	3.3	3.5	3.7	3.9	4.0	4.1	2.6	2.8	3.0	3.6	4.0	4.4
50.5	2.8	2.9	3.0	3.1	3.2	3.4	3.6	3.8	4.0	4.1	4.2	2.7	2.9	3.1	3.8	4.1	4.5
51.0	2.9	3.0	3.1	3.2	3.3	3.5	3.8	3.9	4.1	4.2	4.4	2.7	3.0	3.2	3.9	4.2	4.7
51.5	3.0	3.1	3.2	3.3	3.4	3.6	3.9	4.0	4.2	4.3	4.5	2.8	3.1	3.3	4.0	4.4	4.8
52.0	3.1	3.2	3.3	3.4	3.5	3.8	4.0	4.1	4.4	4.5	4.6	2.9	3.2	3.5	4.1	4.5	5.0
52.5	3.2	3.3	3.4	3.6	3.7	3.9	4.1	4.3	4.5	4.6	4.8	3.0	3.3	3.6	4.2	4.6	5.1
53.0	3.3	3.4	3.5	3.7	3.8	4.0	4.3	4.4	4.6	4.7	4.9	3.1	3.4	3.7	4.4	4.8	5.3
53.5	3.4	3.5	3.6	3.8	3.9	4.1	4.4	4.5	4.8	4.9	5.1	3.2	3.5	3.8	4.5	4.9	5.4
54.0	3.5	3.6	3.7	3.9	4.0	4.3	4.5	4.7	4.9	5.0	5.3	3.3	3.6	3.9	4.7	5.1	5.6
54.5	3.6	3.8	3.8	4.0	4.2	4.4	4.7	4.8	5.1	5.2	5.4	3.4	3.7	4.0	4.8	5.3	5.8
55.0	3.7	3.9	4.0	4.2	4.3	4.5	4.8	5.0	5.3	5.4	5.6	3.6	3.8	4.2	5.0	5.4	6.0
55.5	3.9	4.0	4.1	4.3	4.4	4.7	5.0	5.1	5.4	5.5	5.8	3.7	4.0	4.3	5.1	5.6	6.1
56.0	4.0	4.1	4.2	4.4	4.6	4.8	5.1	5.3	5.6	5.7	5.9	3.8	4.1	4.4	5.3	5.8	6.3
56.5	4.1	4.3	4.3	4.6	4.7	5.0	5.3	5.4	5.7	5.9	6.1	3.9	4.2	4.6	5.4	5.9	6.5
57.0	4.2	4.4	4.5	4.7	4.8	5.1	5.4	5.6	5.9	6.0	6.3	4.0	4.3	4.7	5.6	6.1	6.7
57.5	4.4	4.5	4.6	4.8	5.0	5.3	5.6	5.8	6.1	6.2	6.5	4.1	4.5	4.9	5.7	6.3	6.9
58.0	4.5	4.6	4.7	5.0	5.1	5.4	5.7	5.9	6.2	6.4	6.6	4.3	4.6	5.0	5.9	6.4	7.1
58.5	4.6	4.8	4.9	5.1	5.3	5.6	5.9	6.1	6.4	6.5	6.8	4.4	4.7	5.1	6.1	6.6	7.2
59.0	4.7	4.9	5.0	5.2	5.4	5.7	6.0	6.2	6.6	6.7	7.0	4.5	4.8	5.3	6.2	6.8	7.4
59.5	4.8	5.0	5.1	5.4	5.5	5.9	6.2	6.4	6.7	6.9	7.2	4.6	5.0	5.4	6.4	7.0	7.6
60.0	5.0	5.1	5.2	5.5	5.7	6.0	6.3	6.5	6.9	7.0	7.3	4.7	5.1	5.5	6.5	7.1	7.8
60.5	5.1	5.3	5.4	5.6	5.8	6.1	6.5	6.7	7.1	7.2	7.5	4.8	5.2	5.6	6.7	7.3	8.0
61.0	5.2	5.4	5.5	5.8	5.9	6.3	6.6	6.8	7.2	7.4	7.7	4.9	5.3	5.8	6.8	7.4	8.1
61.5	5.3	5.5	5.6	5.9	6.1	6.4	6.8	7.0	7.4	7.5	7.8	5.0	5.4	5.9	7.0	7.6	8.3
62.0	5.4	5.6	5.7	6.0	6.2	6.5	6.9	7.1	7.5	7.7	8.0	5.1	5.6	6.0	7.1	7.7	8.5
62.5	5.5	5.7	5.8	6.1	6.3	6.7	7.0	7.3	7.6	7.8	8.1	5.2	5.7	6.1	7.2	7.9	8.6
63.0	5.6	5.8	5.9	6.2	6.4	6.8	7.2	7.4	7.8	8.0	8.3	5.3	5.8	6.2	7.4	8.0	8.8
63.5	5.7	5.9	6.0	6.3	6.5	6.9	7.3	7.5	7.9	8.1	8.4	5.4	5.9	6.4	7.5	8.2	8.9
64.0	5.8	6.0	6.2	6.5	6.6	7.0	7.4	7.7	8.1	8.2	8.6	5.5	6.0	6.5	7.6	8.3	9.1
64.5	5.9	6.1	6.3	6.6	6.8	7.1	7.6	7.8	8.2	8.4	8.7	5.6	6.1	6.6	7.8	8.5	9.3
65.0	6.0	6.3	6.4	6.7	6.9	7.3	7.7	7.9	8.3	8.5	8.9	5.7	6.2	6.7	7.9	8.6	9.4
65.5	6.1	6.4	6.5	6.8	7.0	7.4	7.8	8.1	8.5	8.7	9.0	5.8	6.3	6.8	8.0	8.7	9.6
66.0	6.2	6.5	6.6	6.9	7.1	7.5	7.9	8.2	8.6	8.8	9.1	5.9	6.4	6.9	8.2	8.9	9.7
66.5	6.3	6.6	6.7	7.0	7.2	7.6	8.1	8.3	8.8	8.9	9.3	6.0	6.5	7.0	8.3	9.0	9.9
67.0	6.4	6.7	6.8	7.1	7.3	7.7	8.2	8.4	8.9	9.1	9.4	6.1	6.6	7.1	8.4	9.2	10.0
67.5	6.5	6.8	6.9	7.2	7.4	7.9	8.3	8.6	9.0	9.2	9.6	6.2	6.7	7.2	8.5	9.3	10.2
68.0	6.6	6.9	7.0	7.3	7.5	8.0	8.4	8.7	9.2	9.3	9.7	6.3	6.8	7.3	8.7	9.4	10.3
68.5	6.7	7.0	7.1	7.4	7.7	8.1	8.5	8.8	9.3	9.5	9.8	6.4	6.9	7.5	8.8	9.6	10.5
69.0	6.8	7.1	7.2	7.5	7.8	8.2	8.7	8.9	9.4	9.6	10.0	6.5	7.0	7.6	8.9	9.7	10.6
69.5	6.9	7.1	7.3	7.6	7.9	8.3	8.8	9.1	9.5	9.7	10.1	6.6	7.1	7.7	9.0	9.8	10.8
70.0	7.0	7.2	7.4	7.7	8.0	8.4	8.9	9.2	9.7	9.9	10.3	6.6	7.2	7.8	9.2	10.0	10.9
70.5	7.1	7.3	7.5	7.8	8.1	8.5	9.0	9.3	9.8	10.0	10.4	6.7	7.3	7.9	9.3	10.1	11.1

(Contd...)

Table 5.6: Weight (kg) for length (cm) for boys 0–2 years (WHO Reference Data) percentiles and *Z* (SD) scores (*Contd...*)

Length (cm)	Percentiles											Standard deviation (SD) *Z*-scores					
	1st	3rd	5th	15th	25th	50th	75th	85th	95th	97th	99th	–3SD	–2SD	–1SD	+1SD	+2SD	+3SD
71.0	7.2	7.4	7.6	8.0	8.2	8.6	9.1	9.4	9.9	10.1	10.5	6.8	7.4	8.0	9.4	10.2	11.2
71.5	7.3	7.5	7.7	8.1	8.3	8.8	9.3	9.6	10.1	10.3	10.7	6.9	7.5	8.1	9.5	10.4	11.3
72.0	7.4	7.6	7.8	8.2	8.4	8.9	9.4	9.7	10.2	10.4	10.8	7.0	7.6	8.2	9.6	10.5	11.5
72.5	7.5	7.7	7.9	8.3	8.5	9.0	9.5	9.8	10.3	10.5	11.0	7.1	7.6	8.3	9.8	10.6	11.6
73.0	7.5	7.8	8.0	8.4	8.6	9.1	9.6	9.9	10.4	10.7	11.1	7.2	7.7	8.4	9.9	10.8	11.8
73.5	7.6	7.9	8.0	8.4	8.7	9.2	9.7	10.0	10.6	10.8	11.2	7.2	7.8	8.5	10.0	10.9	11.9
74.0	7.7	8.0	8.1	8.5	8.8	9.3	9.8	10.1	10.7	10.9	11.4	7.3	7.9	8.6	10.1	11.0	12.1
74.5	7.8	8.1	8.2	8.6	8.9	9.4	9.9	10.3	10.8	11.0	11.5	7.4	8.0	8.7	10.2	11.2	12.2
75.0	7.9	8.2	8.3	8.7	9.0	9.5	10.1	10.4	10.9	11.2	11.6	7.5	8.1	8.8	10.3	11.3	12.3
75.5	8.0	8.2	8.4	8.8	9.1	9.6	10.2	10.5	11.0	11.3	11.7	7.6	8.2	8.8	10.4	11.4	12.5
76.0	8.0	8.3	8.5	8.9	9.2	9.7	10.3	10.6	11.2	11.4	11.9	7.6	8.3	8.9	10.6	11.5	12.6
76.5	8.1	8.4	8.6	9.0	9.3	9.8	10.4	10.7	11.3	11.5	12.0	7.7	8.3	9.0	10.7	11.6	12.7
77.0	8.2	8.5	8.7	9.1	9.4	9.9	10.5	10.8	11.4	11.6	12.1	7.8	8.4	9.1	10.8	11.7	12.8
77.5	8.3	8.6	8.7	9.2	9.5	10.0	10.6	10.9	11.5	11.7	12.2	7.9	8.5	9.2	10.9	11.9	13.0
78.0	8.4	8.7	8.8	9.3	9.5	10.1	10.7	11.0	11.6	11.8	12.3	7.9	8.6	9.3	11.0	12.0	13.1
78.5	8.4	8.7	8.9	9.3	9.6	10.2	10.8	11.1	11.7	12.0	12.4	8.0	8.7	9.4	11.1	12.1	13.2
79.0	8.5	8.8	9.0	9.4	9.7	10.3	10.9	11.2	11.8	12.1	12.5	8.1	8.7	9.5	11.2	12.2	13.3
79.5	8.6	8.9	9.1	9.5	9.8	10.4	11.0	11.3	11.9	12.2	12.7	8.2	8.8	9.5	11.3	12.3	13.4
80.0	8.7	9.0	9.1	9.6	9.9	10.4	11.1	11.4	12.0	12.3	12.8	8.2	8.9	9.6	11.4	12.4	13.6
80.5	8.7	9.1	9.2	9.7	10.0	10.5	11.2	11.5	12.1	12.4	12.9	8.3	9.0	9.7	11.5	12.5	13.7
81.0	8.8	9.1	9.3	9.8	10.1	10.6	11.3	11.6	12.2	12.5	13.0	8.4	9.1	9.8	11.6	12.6	13.8
81.5	8.9	9.2	9.4	9.9	10.2	10.7	11.4	11.7	12.3	12.6	13.1	8.5	9.1	9.9	11.7	12.7	13.9
82.0	9.0	9.3	9.5	10.0	10.2	10.8	11.5	11.8	12.5	12.7	13.2	8.5	9.2	10.0	11.8	12.8	14.0
82.5	9.1	9.4	9.6	10.1	10.3	10.9	11.6	11.9	12.6	12.8	13.3	8.6	9.3	10.1	11.9	13.0	14.2
83.0	9.2	9.5	9.7	10.1	10.4	11.0	11.7	12.0	12.7	13.0	13.5	8.7	9.4	10.2	12.0	13.1	14.3
83.5	9.3	9.6	9.8	10.3	10.6	11.2	11.8	12.2	12.8	13.1	13.6	8.8	9.5	10.3	12.1	13.2	14.4
84.0	9.4	9.7	9.9	10.4	10.7	11.3	11.9	12.3	12.9	13.2	13.7	8.9	9.6	10.4	12.2	13.3	14.6
84.5	9.5	9.8	10.0	10.5	10.8	11.4	12.0	12.4	13.1	13.3	13.9	9.0	9.7	10.5	12.4	13.5	14.7
85.0	9.6	9.9	10.1	10.6	10.9	11.5	12.2	12.5	13.2	13.5	14.0	9.1	9.8	10.6	12.5	13.6	14.9
85.5	9.7	10.0	10.2	10.7	11.0	11.6	12.3	12.7	13.3	13.6	14.1	9.2	9.9	10.7	12.6	13.7	15.0
86.0	9.8	10.1	10.3	10.8	11.1	11.7	12.4	12.8	13.5	13.7	14.3	9.3	10.0	10.8	12.8	13.9	15.2
86.5	9.9	10.2	10.4	10.9	11.2	11.9	12.5	12.9	13.6	13.9	14.4	9.4	10.1	11.0	12.9	14.0	15.3
87.0	10.0	10.3	10.5	11.0	11.4	12.0	12.7	13.1	13.7	14.0	14.6	9.5	10.2	11.1	13.0	14.2	15.5
87.5	10.1	10.4	10.6	11.2	11.5	12.1	12.8	13.2	13.9	14.2	14.7	9.6	10.4	11.2	13.2	14.3	15.6
88.0	10.2	10.6	10.7	11.3	11.6	12.2	12.9	13.3	14.0	14.3	14.9	9.7	10.5	11.3	13.3	14.5	15.8
88.5	10.3	10.7	10.9	11.4	11.7	12.4	13.1	13.5	14.2	14.4	15.0	9.8	10.6	11.4	13.4	14.6	15.9
89.0	10.4	10.8	11.0	11.5	11.8	12.5	13.2	13.6	14.3	14.6	15.2	9.9	10.7	11.5	13.5	14.7	16.1
89.5	10.5	10.9	11.1	11.6	11.9	12.6	13.3	13.7	14.4	14.7	15.3	10.0	10.8	11.6	13.7	14.9	16.2
67.0	6.4	6.7	6.8	7.1	7.3	7.7	8.2	8.4	8.9	9.1	9.4	6.1	6.6	7.1	8.4	9.2	10.0
90.0	10.6	11.0	11.2	11.7	12.1	12.7	13.4	13.8	14.6	14.9	15.4	10.1	10.9	11.8	13.8	15.0	16.4
90.5	10.7	11.1	11.3	11.8	12.2	12.8	13.6	14.0	14.7	15.0	15.6	10.2	11.0	11.9	13.9	15.1	16.5
91.0	10.8	11.2	11.4	11.9	12.3	13.0	13.7	14.1	14.8	15.1	15.7	10.3	11.1	12.0	14.1	15.3	16.7
91.5	10.9	11.3	11.5	12.0	12.4	13.1	13.8	14.2	15.0	15.3	15.9	10.4	11.2	12.1	14.2	15.4	16.8
92.0	11.0	11.4	11.6	12.2	12.5	13.2	13.9	14.4	15.1	15.4	16.0	10.5	11.3	12.2	14.3	15.6	17.0
92.5	11.1	11.5	11.7	12.3	12.6	13.3	14.1	14.5	15.2	15.5	16.1	10.6	11.4	12.3	14.4	15.7	17.1
93.0	11.2	11.6	11.8	12.4	12.7	13.4	14.2	14.6	15.4	15.7	16.3	10.7	11.5	12.4	14.6	15.8	17.3
93.5	11.3	11.7	11.9	12.5	12.8	13.5	14.3	14.7	15.5	15.8	16.4	10.7	11.6	12.5	14.7	16.0	17.4
94.0	11.4	11.8	12.0	12.6	12.9	13.7	14.4	14.9	15.6	16.0	16.6	10.8	11.7	12.6	14.8	16.1	17.6
94.5	11.5	11.9	12.1	12.7	13.1	13.8	14.5	15.0	15.8	16.1	16.7	10.9	11.8	12.7	14.9	16.3	17.7
95.0	11.6	12.0	12.2	12.8	13.2	13.9	14.7	15.1	15.9	16.2	16.9	11.0	11.9	12.8	15.1	16.4	17.9
95.5	11.7	12.1	12.3	12.9	13.3	14.0	14.8	15.3	16.0	16.4	17.0	11.1	12.0	12.9	15.2	16.5	18.0

(Contd...)

Table 5.6: Weight (kg) for length (cm) for boys 0–2 years (WHO Reference Data) percentiles and *Z* (SD) scores (*Contd..*)

Length (cm)	Percentiles											Standard deviation (SD) *Z*-scores					
	1st	3rd	5th	15th	25th	50th	75th	85th	95th	97th	99th	–3SD	–2SD	–1SD	+1SD	+2SD	+3SD
96.0	11.8	12.2	12.4	13.0	13.4	14.1	14.9	15.4	16.2	16.5	17.2	11.2	12.1	13.1	15.3	16.7	18.2
96.5	11.9	12.3	12.5	13.1	13.5	14.3	15.1	15.5	16.3	16.7	17.3	11.3	12.2	13.2	15.5	16.8	18.4
97.0	12.0	12.4	12.6	13.2	13.6	14.4	15.2	15.7	16.5	16.8	17.5	11.4	12.3	13.3	15.6	17.0	18.5
97.5	12.1	12.5	12.7	13.4	13.7	14.5	15.3	15.8	16.6	17.0	17.6	11.5	12.4	13.4	15.7	17.1	18.7
98.0	12.2	12.6	12.8	13.5	13.9	14.6	15.5	15.9	16.8	17.1	17.8	11.6	12.5	13.5	15.9	17.3	18.9
98.5	12.3	12.7	13.0	13.6	14.0	14.8	15.6	16.1	16.9	17.3	18.0	11.7	12.6	13.6	16.0	17.5	19.1
99.0	12.4	12.8	13.1	13.7	14.1	14.9	15.7	16.2	17.1	17.4	18.1	11.8	12.7	13.7	16.2	17.6	19.2
99.5	12.5	12.9	13.2	13.8	14.2	15.0	15.9	16.4	17.2	17.6	18.3	11.9	12.8	13.9	16.3	17.8	19.4
100.0	12.6	13.0	13.3	13.9	14.4	15.2	16.0	16.5	17.4	17.8	18.5	12.0	12.9	14.0	16.5	18.0	19.6
100.5	12.7	13.2	13.4	14.1	14.5	15.3	16.2	16.7	17.6	17.9	18.7	12.1	13.0	14.1	16.6	18.1	19.8
101.0	12.8	13.3	13.5	14.2	14.6	15.4	16.3	16.8	17.7	18.1	18.8	12.2	13.2	14.2	16.8	18.3	20.0
101.5	12.9	13.4	13.6	14.3	14.7	15.6	16.5	17.0	17.9	18.3	19.0	12.3	13.3	14.4	16.9	18.5	20.2
102.0	13.0	13.5	13.8	14.5	14.9	15.7	16.6	17.2	18.1	18.5	19.2	12.4	13.4	14.5	17.1	18.7	20.4
102.5	13.2	13.6	13.9	14.6	15.0	15.9	16.8	17.3	18.3	18.6	19.4	12.5	13.5	14.6	17.3	18.8	20.6
103.0	13.3	13.8	14.0	14.7	15.2	16.0	17.0	17.5	18.4	18.8	19.6	12.6	13.6	14.8	17.4	19.0	20.8
103.5	13.4	13.9	14.1	14.8	15.3	16.2	17.1	17.7	18.6	19.0	19.8	12.7	13.7	14.9	17.6	19.2	21.0
104.0	13.5	14.0	14.3	15.0	15.4	16.3	17.3	17.8	18.8	19.2	20.0	12.8	13.9	15.0	17.8	19.4	21.2
104.5	13.6	14.1	14.4	15.1	15.6	16.5	17.4	18.0	19.0	19.4	20.2	12.9	14.0	15.2	17.9	19.6	21.5
105.0	13.7	14.2	14.5	15.3	15.7	16.6	17.6	18.2	19.2	19.6	20.4	13.0	14.1	15.3	18.1	19.8	21.7
105.5	13.9	14.4	14.6	15.4	15.9	16.8	17.8	18.4	19.4	19.8	20.6	13.2	14.2	15.4	18.3	20.0	21.9
106.0	14.0	14.5	14.8	15.5	16.0	16.9	18.0	18.5	19.6	20.0	20.8	13.3	14.4	15.6	18.5	20.2	22.1
106.5	14.1	14.6	14.9	15.7	16.2	17.1	18.1	18.7	19.7	20.2	21.0	13.4	14.5	15.7	18.6	20.4	22.4
107.0	14.2	14.8	15.0	15.8	16.3	17.3	18.3	18.9	19.9	20.4	21.2	13.5	14.6	15.9	18.8	20.6	22.6
107.5	14.4	14.9	15.2	16.0	16.5	17.4	18.5	19.1	20.1	20.6	21.4	13.6	14.7	16.0	19.0	20.8	22.8
108.0	14.5	15.0	15.3	16.1	16.6	17.6	18.7	19.3	20.3	20.8	21.7	13.7	14.9	16.2	19.2	21.0	23.1
108.5	14.6	15.2	15.5	16.3	16.8	17.8	18.8	19.5	20.5	21.0	21.9	13.8	15.0	16.3	19.4	21.2	23.3
109.0	14.7	15.3	15.6	16.4	16.9	17.9	19.0	19.6	20.8	21.2	22.1	14.0	15.1	16.5	19.6	21.4	23.6
109.5	14.9	15.4	15.7	16.6	17.1	18.1	19.2	19.8	21.0	21.4	22.3	14.1	15.3	16.6	19.8	21.7	23.8
110.0	15.0	15.6	15.9	16.7	17.2	18.3	19.4	20.0	21.2	21.6	22.6	14.2	15.4	16.8	20.0	21.9	24.1

Table 5.7: Weight (kg) for length (cm) for girls 0–2 years (WHO Reference Data) percentiles and *Z* (SD) scores

Length (cm)	Percentiles											Standard deviation (SD) *Z*-scores					
	1st	3rd	5th	15th	25th	50th	75th	85th	95th	97th	99th	–3SD	–2SD	–1SD	+1SD	+2SD	+3SD
45.0	2.0	2.1	2.1	2.2	2.3	2.5	2.6	2.7	2.9	2.9	3.1	1.9	2.1	2.3	2.7	3.0	3.3
45.5	2.1	2.2	2.2	2.3	2.4	2.5	2.7	2.8	3.0	3.0	3.2	2.0	2.1	2.3	2.8	3.1	3.4
46.0	2.1	2.2	2.3	2.4	2.5	2.6	2.8	2.9	3.1	3.1	3.3	2.0	2.2	2.4	2.9	3.2	3.5
46.5	2.2	2.3	2.3	2.5	2.6	2.7	2.9	3.0	3.2	3.2	3.4	2.1	2.3	2.5	3.0	3.3	3.6
47.0	2.3	2.4	2.4	2.6	2.6	2.8	3.0	3.1	3.3	3.3	3.5	2.2	2.4	2.6	3.1	3.4	3.7
47.5	2.4	2.4	2.5	2.6	2.7	2.9	3.1	3.2	3.4	3.4	3.6	2.2	2.4	2.6	3.2	3.5	3.8
48.0	2.4	2.5	2.6	2.7	2.8	3.0	3.2	3.3	3.5	3.5	3.7	2.3	2.5	2.7	3.3	3.6	4.0
48.5	2.5	2.6	2.7	2.8	2.9	3.1	3.3	3.4	3.6	3.7	3.8	2.4	2.6	2.8	3.4	3.7	4.1
49.0	2.6	2.7	2.7	2.9	3.0	3.2	3.4	3.5	3.7	3.8	3.9	2.4	2.6	2.9	3.5	3.8	4.2
49.5	2.7	2.8	2.8	3.0	3.1	3.3	3.5	3.6	3.8	3.9	4.1	2.5	2.7	3.0	3.6	3.9	4.3
50.0	2.7	2.8	2.9	3.1	3.2	3.4	3.6	3.7	3.9	4.0	4.2	2.6	2.8	3.1	3.7	4.0	4.5
50.5	2.8	2.9	3.0	3.2	3.3	3.5	3.7	3.8	4.0	4.1	4.3	2.7	2.9	3.2	3.8	4.2	4.6
51.0	2.9	3.0	3.1	3.2	3.4	3.6	3.8	3.9	4.2	4.3	4.4	2.8	3.0	3.3	3.9	4.3	4.8
51.5	3.0	3.1	3.2	3.4	3.5	3.7	3.9	4.0	4.3	4.4	4.6	2.8	3.1	3.4	4.0	4.4	4.9
52.0	3.1	3.2	3.3	3.5	3.6	3.8	4.0	4.2	4.4	4.5	4.7	2.9	3.2	3.5	4.2	4.6	5.1
52.5	3.2	3.3	3.4	3.6	3.7	3.9	4.2	4.3	4.6	4.7	4.9	3.0	3.3	3.6	4.3	4.7	5.2
53.0	3.3	3.4	3.5	3.7	3.8	4.0	4.3	4.4	4.7	4.8	5.0	3.1	3.4	3.7	4.4	4.9	5.4
53.5	3.4	3.5	3.6	3.8	3.9	4.2	4.4	4.6	4.9	5.0	5.2	3.2	3.5	3.8	4.6	5.0	5.5
54.0	3.5	3.6	3.7	3.9	4.0	4.3	4.6	4.7	5.0	5.1	5.3	3.3	3.6	3.9	4.7	5.2	5.7
54.5	3.6	3.7	3.8	4.0	4.2	4.4	4.7	4.9	5.2	5.3	5.5	3.4	3.7	4.0	4.8	5.3	5.9
55.0	3.7	3.9	3.9	4.1	4.3	4.5	4.8	5.0	5.3	5.4	5.7	3.5	3.8	4.2	5.0	5.5	6.1
55.5	3.8	4.0	4.0	4.3	4.4	4.7	5.0	5.2	5.5	5.6	5.8	3.6	3.9	4.3	5.1	5.7	6.3
56.0	3.9	4.1	4.2	4.4	4.5	4.8	5.1	5.3	5.6	5.8	6.0	3.7	4.0	4.4	5.3	5.8	6.4
56.5	4.0	4.2	4.3	4.5	4.7	5.0	5.3	5.5	5.8	5.9	6.2	3.8	4.1	4.5	5.4	6.0	6.6
57.0	4.1	4.3	4.4	4.6	4.8	5.1	5.4	5.6	5.9	6.1	6.3	3.9	4.3	4.6	5.6	6.1	6.8
57.5	4.3	4.4	4.5	4.8	4.9	5.2	5.6	5.7	6.1	6.2	6.5	4.0	4.4	4.8	5.7	6.3	7.0
58.0	4.4	4.5	4.6	4.9	5.0	5.4	5.7	5.9	6.2	6.4	6.7	4.1	4.5	4.9	5.9	6.5	7.1
58.5	4.5	4.6	4.7	5.0	5.2	5.5	5.8	6.0	6.4	6.5	6.8	4.2	4.6	5.0	6.0	6.6	7.3
59.0	4.6	4.8	4.9	5.1	5.3	5.6	6.0	6.2	6.6	6.7	7.0	4.3	4.7	5.1	6.2	6.8	7.5
59.5	4.7	4.9	5.0	5.2	5.4	5.7	6.1	6.3	6.7	6.9	7.2	4.4	4.8	5.3	6.3	6.9	7.7
60.0	4.8	5.0	5.1	5.4	5.5	5.9	6.3	6.5	6.9	7.0	7.3	4.5	4.9	5.4	6.4	7.1	7.8
60.5	4.9	5.1	5.2	5.5	5.6	6.0	6.4	6.6	7.0	7.2	7.5	4.6	5.0	5.5	6.6	7.3	8.0
61.0	5.0	5.2	5.3	5.6	5.8	6.1	6.5	6.7	7.2	7.3	7.6	4.7	5.1	5.6	6.7	7.4	8.2
61.5	5.1	5.3	5.4	5.7	5.9	6.3	6.7	6.9	7.3	7.5	7.8	4.8	5.2	5.7	6.9	7.6	8.4
62.0	5.2	5.4	5.5	5.8	6.0	6.4	6.8	7.0	7.4	7.6	8.0	4.9	5.3	5.8	7.0	7.7	8.5
62.5	5.3	5.5	5.6	5.9	6.1	6.5	6.9	7.2	7.6	7.8	8.1	5.0	5.4	5.9	7.1	7.8	8.7
63.0	5.4	5.6	5.7	6.0	6.2	6.6	7.0	7.3	7.7	7.9	8.3	5.1	5.5	6.0	7.3	8.0	8.8
63.5	5.5	5.7	5.8	6.1	6.3	6.7	7.2	7.4	7.9	8.0	8.4	5.2	5.6	6.2	7.4	8.1	9.0
64.0	5.6	5.8	5.9	6.2	6.4	6.9	7.3	7.5	8.0	8.2	8.5	5.3	5.7	6.3	7.5	8.3	9.1
64.5	5.7	5.9	6.0	6.3	6.6	7.0	7.4	7.7	8.1	8.3	8.7	5.4	5.8	6.4	7.6	8.4	9.3
65.0	5.8	6.0	6.1	6.5	6.7	7.1	7.5	7.8	8.3	8.5	8.8	5.5	5.9	6.5	7.8	8.6	9.5
65.5	5.9	6.1	6.2	6.6	6.8	7.2	7.7	7.9	8.4	8.6	9.0	5.5	6.0	6.6	7.9	8.7	9.6
66.0	6.0	6.2	6.3	6.7	6.9	7.3	7.8	8.0	8.5	8.7	9.1	5.6	6.1	6.7	8.0	8.8	9.8
66.5	6.1	6.3	6.4	6.8	7.0	7.4	7.9	8.2	8.7	8.9	9.3	5.7	6.2	6.8	8.1	9.0	9.9
67.0	6.1	6.4	6.5	6.9	7.1	7.5	8.0	8.3	8.8	9.0	9.4	5.8	6.3	6.9	8.3	9.1	10.0
67.5	6.2	6.5	6.6	7.0	7.2	7.6	8.1	8.4	8.9	9.1	9.5	5.9	6.4	7.0	8.4	9.2	10.2
68.0	6.3	6.6	6.7	7.1	7.3	7.7	8.2	8.5	9.0	9.2	9.7	6.0	6.5	7.1	8.5	9.4	10.3
68.5	6.4	6.7	6.8	7.2	7.4	7.9	8.4	8.6	9.2	9.4	9.8	6.1	6.6	7.2	8.6	9.5	10.5
69.0	6.5	6.7	6.9	7.3	7.5	8.0	8.5	8.8	9.3	9.5	9.9	6.1	6.7	7.3	8.7	9.6	10.6
69.5	6.6	6.8	7.0	7.3	7.6	8.1	8.6	8.9	9.4	9.6	10.0	6.2	6.8	7.4	8.8	9.7	10.7
70.0	6.7	6.9	7.1	7.4	7.7	8.2	8.7	9.0	9.5	9.7	10.2	6.3	6.9	7.5	9.0	9.9	10.9
70.5	6.7	7.0	7.1	7.5	7.8	8.3	8.8	9.1	9.6	9.9	10.3	6.4	6.9	7.6	9.1	10.0	11.0

(Contd...)

Table 5.7: Weight (kg) for length (cm) for girls 0–2 years (WHO Reference Data) percentiles and *Z* (SD) scores (*Contd...*)

Length (cm)	Percentiles											Standard deviation (SD) *Z*-scores					
	1st	3rd	5th	15th	25th	50th	75th	85th	95th	97th	99th	–3SD	–2SD	–1SD	+1SD	+2SD	+3SD
71.0	6.8	7.1	7.2	7.6	7.9	8.4	8.9	9.2	9.8	10.0	10.4	6.5	7.0	7.7	9.2	10.1	11.1
71.5	6.9	7.2	7.3	7.7	8.0	8.5	9.0	9.3	9.9	10.1	10.5	6.5	7.1	7.7	9.3	10.2	11.3
72.0	7.0	7.3	7.4	7.8	8.1	8.6	9.1	9.4	10.0	10.2	10.7	6.6	7.2	7.8	9.4	10.3	11.4
72.5	7.1	7.4	7.5	7.9	8.2	8.7	9.2	9.5	10.1	10.3	10.8	6.7	7.3	7.9	9.5	10.5	11.5
73.0	7.2	7.4	7.6	8.0	8.3	8.8	9.3	9.6	10.2	10.4	10.9	6.8	7.4	8.0	9.6	10.6	11.7
73.5	7.2	7.5	7.7	8.1	8.3	8.9	9.4	9.7	10.3	10.6	11.0	6.9	7.4	8.1	9.7	10.7	11.8
74.0	7.3	7.6	7.8	8.2	8.4	9.0	9.5	9.9	10.4	10.7	11.2	6.9	7.5	8.2	9.8	10.8	11.9
74.5	7.4	7.7	7.8	8.3	8.5	9.1	9.6	10.0	10.5	10.8	11.3	7.0	7.6	8.3	9.9	10.9	12.0
75.0	7.5	7.8	7.9	8.3	8.6	9.1	9.7	10.1	10.7	10.9	11.4	7.1	7.7	8.4	10.0	11.0	12.2
75.5	7.6	7.8	8.0	8.4	8.7	9.2	9.8	10.2	10.8	11.0	11.5	7.1	7.8	8.5	10.1	11.1	12.3
76.0	7.6	7.9	8.1	8.5	8.8	9.3	9.9	10.3	10.9	11.1	11.6	7.2	7.8	8.5	10.2	11.2	12.4
76.5	7.7	8.0	8.2	8.6	8.9	9.4	10.0	10.4	11.0	11.2	11.7	7.3	7.9	8.6	10.3	11.4	12.5
77.0	7.8	8.1	8.2	8.7	9.0	9.5	10.1	10.5	11.1	11.3	11.8	7.4	8.0	8.7	10.4	11.5	12.6
77.5	7.9	8.2	8.3	8.8	9.1	9.6	10.2	10.6	11.2	11.4	11.9	7.4	8.1	8.8	10.5	11.6	12.8
78.0	7.9	8.2	8.4	8.9	9.1	9.7	10.3	10.7	11.3	11.5	12.1	7.5	8.2	8.9	10.6	11.7	12.9
78.5	8.0	8.3	8.5	8.9	9.2	9.8	10.4	10.8	11.4	11.7	12.2	7.6	8.2	9.0	10.7	11.8	13.0
79.0	8.1	8.4	8.6	9.0	9.3	9.9	10.5	10.9	11.5	11.8	12.3	7.7	8.3	9.1	10.8	11.9	13.1
79.5	8.2	8.5	8.7	9.1	9.4	10.0	10.6	11.0	11.6	11.9	12.4	7.7	8.4	9.1	10.9	12.0	13.3
80.0	8.3	8.6	8.7	9.2	9.5	10.1	10.7	11.1	11.7	12.0	12.5	7.8	8.5	9.2	11.0	12.1	13.4
80.5	8.3	8.7	8.8	9.3	9.6	10.2	10.8	11.2	11.9	12.1	12.7	7.9	8.6	9.3	11.2	12.3	13.5
81.0	8.4	8.8	8.9	9.4	9.7	10.3	10.9	11.3	12.0	12.2	12.8	8.0	8.7	9.4	11.3	12.4	13.7
81.5	8.5	8.8	9.0	9.5	9.8	10.4	11.1	11.4	12.1	12.4	12.9	8.1	8.8	9.5	11.4	12.5	13.8
82.0	8.6	8.9	9.1	9.6	9.9	10.5	11.2	11.6	12.2	12.5	13.1	8.1	8.8	9.6	11.5	12.6	13.9
82.5	8.7	9.0	9.2	9.7	10.0	10.6	11.3	11.7	12.4	12.6	13.2	8.2	8.9	9.7	11.6	12.8	14.1
83.0	8.8	9.1	9.3	9.8	10.1	10.7	11.4	11.8	12.5	12.8	13.3	8.3	9.0	9.8	11.8	12.9	14.2
83.5	8.9	9.2	9.4	9.9	10.2	10.9	11.5	11.9	12.6	12.9	13.5	8.4	9.1	9.9	11.9	13.1	14.4
84.0	9.0	9.3	9.5	10.0	10.3	11.0	11.7	12.1	12.8	13.1	13.6	8.5	9.2	10.1	12.0	13.2	14.5
84.5	9.1	9.4	9.6	10.1	10.5	11.1	11.8	12.2	12.9	13.2	13.8	8.6	9.3	10.2	12.1	13.3	14.7
85.0	9.2	9.5	9.7	10.2	10.6	11.2	11.9	12.3	13.0	13.3	13.9	8.7	9.4	10.3	12.3	13.5	14.9
85.5	9.3	9.6	9.8	10.4	10.7	11.3	12.1	12.5	13.2	13.5	14.1	8.8	9.5	10.4	12.4	13.6	15.0
86.0	9.4	9.8	9.9	10.5	10.8	11.5	12.2	12.6	13.3	13.6	14.2	8.9	9.7	10.5	12.6	13.8	15.2
86.5	9.5	9.9	10.1	10.6	10.9	11.6	12.3	12.7	13.5	13.8	14.4	9.0	9.8	10.6	12.7	13.9	15.4
87.0	9.6	10.0	10.2	10.7	11.0	11.7	12.5	12.9	13.6	13.9	14.5	9.1	9.9	10.7	12.8	14.1	15.5
87.5	9.7	10.1	10.3	10.8	11.2	11.8	12.6	13.0	13.8	14.1	14.7	9.2	10.0	10.9	13.0	14.2	15.7
88.0	9.8	10.2	10.4	10.9	11.3	12.0	12.7	13.2	13.9	14.2	14.9	9.3	10.1	11.0	13.1	14.4	15.9
88.5	9.9	10.3	10.5	11.0	11.4	12.1	12.9	13.3	14.1	14.4	15.0	9.4	10.2	11.1	13.2	14.5	16.0
89.0	10.0	10.4	10.6	11.2	11.5	12.2	13.0	13.4	14.2	14.5	15.2	9.5	10.3	11.2	13.4	14.7	16.2
89.5	10.1	10.5	10.7	11.3	11.6	12.3	13.1	13.6	14.4	14.7	15.3	9.6	10.4	11.3	13.5	14.8	16.4
90.0	10.2	10.6	10.8	11.4	11.8	12.5	13.3	13.7	14.5	14.8	15.5	9.7	10.5	11.4	13.7	15.0	16.5
90.5	10.3	10.7	10.9	11.5	11.9	12.6	13.4	13.8	14.6	15.0	15.6	9.8	10.6	11.5	13.8	15.1	16.7
91.0	10.4	10.8	11.0	11.6	12.0	12.7	13.5	14.0	14.8	15.1	15.8	9.9	10.7	11.7	13.9	15.3	16.9
91.5	10.5	10.9	11.1	11.7	12.1	12.8	13.7	14.1	14.9	15.3	15.9	10.0	10.8	11.8	14.1	15.5	17.0
92.0	10.6	11.0	11.2	11.8	12.2	13.0	13.8	14.2	15.1	15.4	16.1	10.1	10.9	11.9	14.2	15.6	17.2
92.5	10.7	11.1	11.3	12.0	12.3	13.1	13.9	14.4	15.2	15.6	16.3	10.1	11.0	12.0	14.3	15.8	17.4
93.0	10.8	11.2	11.5	12.1	12.5	13.2	14.0	14.5	15.4	15.7	16.4	10.2	11.1	12.1	14.5	15.9	17.5
93.5	10.9	11.3	11.6	12.2	12.6	13.3	14.2	14.7	15.5	15.9	16.6	10.3	11.2	12.2	14.6	16.1	17.7
94.0	11.0	11.4	11.7	12.3	12.7	13.5	14.3	14.8	15.7	16.0	16.7	10.4	11.3	12.3	14.7	16.2	17.9
94.5	11.1	11.5	11.8	12.4	12.8	13.6	14.4	14.9	15.8	16.2	16.9	10.5	11.4	12.4	14.9	16.4	18.0
95.0	11.2	11.6	11.9	12.5	12.9	13.7	14.6	15.1	16.0	16.3	17.0	10.6	11.5	12.6	15.0	16.5	18.2
95.5	11.3	11.8	12.0	12.6	13.0	13.8	14.7	15.2	16.1	16.5	17.2	10.7	11.6	12.7	15.2	16.7	18.4
96.0	11.4	11.9	12.1	12.7	13.2	14.0	14.9	15.4	16.3	16.6	17.4	10.8	11.7	12.8	15.3	16.8	18.6
96.5	11.5	12.0	12.2	12.9	13.3	14.1	15.0	15.5	16.4	16.8	17.5	10.9	11.8	12.9	15.4	17.0	18.7

(*Contd...*)

Table 5.7: Weight (kg) for length (cm) for girls 0–2 years (WHO Reference Data) percentiles and *Z* (SD) scores (*Contd...*)

Length (cm)	Percentiles											Standard deviation (SD) *Z*-scores					
	1st	3rd	5th	15th	25th	50th	75th	85th	95th	97th	99th	–3SD	–2SD	–1SD	+1SD	+2SD	+3SD
97.0	11.6	12.1	12.3	13.0	13.4	14.2	15.1	15.6	16.6	16.9	17.7	11.0	12.0	13.0	15.6	17.1	18.9
97.5	11.7	12.2	12.4	13.1	13.5	14.4	15.3	15.8	16.7	17.1	17.9	11.1	12.1	13.1	15.7	17.3	19.1
98.0	11.8	12.3	12.5	13.2	13.6	14.5	15.4	15.9	16.9	17.3	18.0	11.2	12.2	13.3	15.9	17.5	19.3
98.5	11.9	12.4	12.7	13.3	13.8	14.6	15.5	16.1	17.0	17.4	18.2	11.3	12.3	13.4	16.0	17.6	19.5
99.0	12.0	12.5	12.8	13.5	13.9	14.8	15.7	16.2	17.2	17.6	18.4	11.4	12.4	13.5	16.2	17.8	19.6
99.5	12.2	12.6	12.9	13.6	14.0	14.9	15.8	16.4	17.4	17.8	18.5	11.5	12.5	13.6	16.3	18.0	19.8
100.0	12.3	12.7	13.0	13.7	14.1	15.0	16.0	16.5	17.5	17.9	18.7	11.6	12.6	13.7	16.5	18.1	20.0
100.5	12.4	12.9	13.1	13.8	14.3	15.2	16.1	16.7	17.7	18.1	18.9	11.7	12.7	13.9	16.6	18.3	20.2
101.0	12.5	13.0	13.2	14.0	14.4	15.3	16.3	16.9	17.9	18.3	19.1	11.8	12.8	14.0	16.8	18.5	20.4
101.5	12.6	13.1	13.4	14.1	14.5	15.5	16.4	17.0	18.0	18.5	19.3	11.9	13.0	14.1	17.0	18.7	20.6
102.0	12.7	13.2	13.5	14.2	14.7	15.6	16.6	17.2	18.2	18.6	19.5	12.0	13.1	14.3	17.1	18.9	20.8
102.5	12.8	13.3	13.6	14.4	14.8	15.8	16.8	17.4	18.4	18.8	19.7	12.1	13.2	14.4	17.3	19.0	21.0
103.0	13.0	13.5	13.7	14.5	15.0	15.9	16.9	17.5	18.6	19.0	19.9	12.3	13.3	14.5	17.5	19.2	21.3
103.5	13.1	13.6	13.9	14.6	15.1	16.1	17.1	17.7	18.8	19.2	20.1	12.4	13.5	14.7	17.6	19.4	21.5
104.0	13.2	13.7	14.0	14.8	15.3	16.2	17.3	17.9	19.0	19.4	20.3	12.5	13.6	14.8	17.8	19.6	21.7
104.5	13.3	13.9	14.1	14.9	15.4	16.4	17.4	18.1	19.1	19.6	20.5	12.6	13.7	15.0	18.0	19.8	21.9
105.0	13.5	14.0	14.3	15.1	15.6	16.5	17.6	18.2	19.3	19.8	20.7	12.7	13.8	15.1	18.2	20.0	22.2
105.5	13.6	14.1	14.4	15.2	15.7	16.7	17.8	18.4	19.5	20.0	20.9	12.8	14.0	15.3	18.4	20.2	22.4
106.0	13.7	14.3	14.6	15.4	15.9	16.9	18.0	18.6	19.7	20.2	21.1	13.0	14.1	15.4	18.5	20.5	22.6
106.5	13.9	14.4	14.7	15.5	16.0	17.1	18.2	18.8	20.0	20.4	21.4	13.1	14.3	15.6	18.7	20.7	22.9
107.0	14.0	14.5	14.8	15.7	16.2	17.2	18.4	19.0	20.2	20.6	21.6	13.2	14.4	15.7	18.9	20.9	23.1
107.5	14.1	14.7	15.0	15.8	16.4	17.4	18.5	19.2	20.4	20.9	21.8	13.3	14.5	15.9	19.1	21.1	23.4
108.0	14.3	14.8	15.1	16.0	16.5	17.6	18.7	19.4	20.6	21.1	22.1	13.5	14.7	16.0	19.3	21.3	23.6
108.5	14.4	15.0	15.3	16.2	16.7	17.8	18.9	19.6	20.8	21.3	22.3	13.6	14.8	16.2	19.5	21.6	23.9
109.0	14.6	15.1	15.5	16.3	16.9	18.0	19.1	19.8	21.0	21.5	22.5	13.7	15.0	16.4	19.7	21.8	24.2
109.5	14.7	15.3	15.6	16.5	17.0	18.1	19.3	20.0	21.3	21.8	22.8	13.9	15.1	16.5	20.0	22.0	24.4
110.0	14.9	15.4	15.8	16.7	17.2	18.3	19.5	20.2	21.5	22.0	23.0	14.0	15.3	16.7	20.2	22.3	24.7

Table 5.8: Weight (kg) for height (cm) for boys 2–5 years (WHO Reference Data) percentiles and *Z* (SD) scores

Height (cm)	Percentiles											Standard deviation (SD) *Z*-scores					
	1st	3rd	5th	15th	25th	50th	75th	85th	95th	97th	99th	–3SD	–2SD	–1SD	+1SD	+2SD	+3SD
65.0	6.2	6.4	6.5	6.8	7.0	7.4	7.9	8.1	8.5	8.7	9.1	5.9	6.3	6.9	8.1	8.8	9.6
65.5	6.3	6.5	6.6	6.9	7.1	7.6	8.0	8.2	8.7	8.9	9.2	6.0	6.4	7.0	8.2	8.9	9.8
66.0	6.4	6.6	6.7	7.1	7.3	7.7	8.1	8.4	8.8	9.0	9.3	6.1	6.5	7.1	8.3	9.1	9.9
66.5	6.5	6.7	6.8	7.2	7.4	7.8	8.2	8.5	8.9	9.1	9.5	6.1	6.6	7.2	8.5	9.2	10.1
67.0	6.6	6.8	6.9	7.3	7.5	7.9	8.4	8.6	9.1	9.3	9.6	6.2	6.7	7.3	8.6	9.4	10.2
67.5	6.7	6.9	7.0	7.4	7.6	8.0	8.5	8.7	9.2	9.4	9.8	6.3	6.8	7.4	8.7	9.5	10.4
68.0	6.8	7.0	7.1	7.5	7.7	8.1	8.6	8.9	9.3	9.5	9.9	6.4	6.9	7.5	8.8	9.6	10.5
68.5	6.8	7.1	7.2	7.6	7.8	8.2	8.7	9.0	9.5	9.7	10.0	6.5	7.0	7.6	9.0	9.8	10.7
69.0	6.9	7.2	7.3	7.7	7.9	8.4	8.8	9.1	9.6	9.8	10.2	6.6	7.1	7.7	9.1	9.9	10.8
69.5	7.0	7.3	7.4	7.8	8.0	8.5	9.0	9.2	9.7	9.9	10.3	6.7	7.2	7.8	9.2	10.0	11.0
70.0	7.1	7.4	7.5	7.9	8.1	8.6	9.1	9.4	9.9	10.1	10.5	6.8	7.3	7.9	9.3	10.2	11.1
70.5	7.2	7.5	7.6	8.0	8.2	8.7	9.2	9.5	10.0	10.2	10.6	6.9	7.4	8.0	9.5	10.3	11.3
71.0	7.3	7.6	7.7	8.1	8.3	8.8	9.3	9.6	10.1	10.3	10.7	6.9	7.5	8.1	9.6	10.4	11.4
71.5	7.4	7.7	7.8	8.2	8.4	8.9	9.4	9.7	10.2	10.5	10.9	7.0	7.6	8.2	9.7	10.6	11.6
72.0	7.5	7.8	7.9	8.3	8.5	9.0	9.5	9.8	10.4	10.6	11.0	7.1	7.7	8.3	9.8	10.7	11.7
72.5	7.6	7.8	8.0	8.4	8.6	9.1	9.7	10.0	10.5	10.7	11.1	7.2	7.8	8.4	9.9	10.8	11.8
73.0	7.7	7.9	8.1	8.5	8.7	9.2	9.8	10.1	10.6	10.8	11.3	7.3	7.9	8.5	10.0	11.0	12.0
73.5	7.8	8.0	8.2	8.6	8.8	9.3	9.9	10.2	10.7	11.0	11.4	7.4	7.9	8.6	10.2	11.1	12.1
74.0	7.8	8.1	8.3	8.7	8.9	9.4	10.0	10.3	10.9	11.1	11.5	7.4	8.0	8.7	10.3	11.2	12.2
74.5	7.9	8.2	8.4	8.8	9.0	9.5	10.1	10.4	11.0	11.2	11.7	7.5	8.1	8.8	10.4	11.3	12.4
75.0	8.0	8.3	8.4	8.9	9.1	9.6	10.2	10.5	11.1	11.3	11.8	7.6	8.2	8.9	10.5	11.4	12.5
75.5	8.1	8.4	8.5	9.0	9.2	9.7	10.3	10.6	11.2	11.4	11.9	7.7	8.3	9.0	10.6	11.6	12.6
76.0	8.2	8.5	8.6	9.0	9.3	9.8	10.4	10.7	11.3	11.6	12.0	7.7	8.4	9.1	10.7	11.7	12.8
76.5	8.2	8.5	8.7	9.1	9.4	9.9	10.5	10.8	11.4	11.7	12.1	7.8	8.5	9.2	10.8	11.8	12.9
77.0	8.3	8.6	8.8	9.2	9.5	10.0	10.6	10.9	11.5	11.8	12.3	7.9	8.5	9.2	10.9	11.9	13.0
77.5	8.4	8.7	8.9	9.3	9.6	10.1	10.7	11.0	11.6	11.9	12.4	8.0	8.6	9.3	11.0	12.0	13.1
78.0	8.5	8.8	8.9	9.4	9.7	10.2	10.8	11.1	11.7	12.0	12.5	8.0	8.7	9.4	11.1	12.1	13.3
78.5	8.5	8.8	9.0	9.5	9.7	10.3	10.9	11.2	11.9	12.1	12.6	8.1	8.8	9.5	11.2	12.2	13.4
79.0	8.6	8.9	9.1	9.5	9.8	10.4	11.0	11.3	12.0	12.2	12.7	8.2	8.8	9.6	11.3	12.3	13.5
79.5	8.7	9.0	9.2	9.6	9.9	10.5	11.1	11.4	12.1	12.3	12.8	8.3	8.9	9.7	11.4	12.4	13.6
80.0	8.8	9.1	9.3	9.7	10.0	10.6	11.2	11.5	12.2	12.4	12.9	8.3	9.0	9.7	11.5	12.6	13.7
80.5	8.9	9.2	9.3	9.8	10.1	10.7	11.3	11.6	12.3	12.5	13.0	8.4	9.1	9.8	11.6	12.7	13.8
81.0	8.9	9.3	9.4	9.9	10.2	10.8	11.4	11.8	12.4	12.6	13.1	8.5	9.2	9.9	11.7	12.8	14.0
81.5	9.0	9.3	9.5	10.0	10.3	10.9	11.5	11.9	12.5	12.8	13.3	8.6	9.3	10.0	11.8	12.9	14.1
82.0	9.1	9.4	9.6	10.1	10.4	11.0	11.6	12.0	12.6	12.9	13.4	8.7	9.3	10.1	11.9	13.0	14.2
82.5	9.2	9.5	9.7	10.2	10.5	11.1	11.7	12.1	12.7	13.0	13.5	8.7	9.4	10.2	12.1	13.1	14.4
83.0	9.3	9.6	9.8	10.3	10.6	11.2	11.8	12.2	12.9	13.1	13.6	8.8	9.5	10.3	12.2	13.3	14.5
83.5	9.4	9.7	9.9	10.4	10.7	11.3	12.0	12.3	13.0	13.3	13.8	8.9	9.6	10.4	12.3	13.4	14.6
84.0	9.5	9.8	10.0	10.5	10.8	11.4	12.1	12.5	13.1	13.4	13.9	9.0	9.7	10.5	12.4	13.5	14.8
84.5	9.6	9.9	10.1	10.6	10.9	11.5	12.2	12.6	13.3	13.5	14.1	9.1	9.9	10.7	12.5	13.7	14.9
85.0	9.7	10.1	10.2	10.7	11.1	11.7	12.3	12.7	13.4	13.7	14.2	9.2	10.0	10.8	12.7	13.8	15.1
85.5	9.8	10.2	10.3	10.9	11.2	11.8	12.5	12.8	13.5	13.8	14.3	9.3	10.1	10.9	12.8	13.9	15.2
86.0	9.9	10.3	10.5	11.0	11.3	11.9	12.6	13.0	13.7	13.9	14.5	9.4	10.2	11.0	12.9	14.1	15.4
86.5	10.0	10.4	10.6	11.1	11.4	12.0	12.7	13.1	13.8	14.1	14.6	9.5	10.3	11.1	13.1	14.2	15.5
87.0	10.1	10.5	10.7	11.2	11.5	12.2	12.9	13.2	13.9	14.2	14.8	9.6	10.4	11.2	13.2	14.4	15.7
87.5	10.2	10.6	10.8	11.3	11.6	12.3	13.0	13.4	14.1	14.4	14.9	9.7	10.5	11.3	13.3	14.5	15.8
88.0	10.3	10.7	10.9	11.4	11.8	12.4	13.1	13.5	14.2	14.5	15.1	9.8	10.6	11.5	13.5	14.7	16.0
88.5	10.5	10.8	11.0	11.5	11.9	12.5	13.2	13.6	14.4	14.6	15.2	9.9	10.7	11.6	13.6	14.8	16.1
89.0	10.6	10.9	11.1	11.7	12.0	12.6	13.4	13.8	14.5	14.8	15.4	10.0	10.8	11.7	13.7	14.9	16.3
89.5	10.7	11.0	11.2	11.8	12.1	12.8	13.5	13.9	14.6	14.9	15.5	10.1	10.9	11.8	13.9	15.1	16.4
90.0	10.8	11.1	11.3	11.9	12.2	12.9	13.6	14.0	14.8	15.1	15.6	10.2	11.0	11.9	14.0	15.2	16.6
90.5	10.9	11.2	11.4	12.0	12.3	13.0	13.7	14.1	14.9	15.2	15.8	10.3	11.1	12.0	14.1	15.3	16.7
91.0	11.0	11.3	11.5	12.1	12.4	13.1	13.9	14.3	15.0	15.3	15.9	10.4	11.2	12.1	14.2	15.5	16.9
91.5	11.0	11.4	11.6	12.2	12.5	13.2	14.0	14.4	15.2	15.5	16.1	10.5	11.3	12.2	14.4	15.6	17.0
92.0	11.1	11.5	11.7	12.3	12.7	13.4	14.1	14.5	15.3	15.6	16.2	10.6	11.4	12.3	14.5	15.8	17.2
92.5	11.2	11.6	11.8	12.4	12.8	13.5	14.2	14.7	15.4	15.7	16.3	10.7	11.5	12.4	14.6	15.9	17.3

(Contd...)

Table 5.8: Weight (kg) for height (cm) for boys 2–5 years (WHO Reference Data) percentiles and *Z* (SD) scores (*Contd...*)

Height	Percentiles											Standard deviation (SD) *Z*-scores					
(cm)	1st	3rd	5th	15th	25th	50th	75th	85th	95th	97th	99th	−3SD	−2SD	−1SD	+1SD	+2SD	+3SD
93.0	11.3	11.7	11.9	12.5	12.9	13.6	14.4	14.8	15.6	15.9	16.5	10.8	11.6	12.6	14.7	16.0	17.5
93.5	11.4	11.8	12.0	12.6	13.0	13.7	14.5	14.9	15.7	16.0	16.6	10.9	11.7	12.7	14.9	16.2	17.6
94.0	11.5	11.9	12.1	12.7	13.1	13.8	14.6	15.0	15.8	16.1	16.8	11.0	11.8	12.8	15.0	16.3	17.8
94.5	11.6	12.0	12.2	12.8	13.2	13.9	14.7	15.2	16.0	16.3	16.9	11.1	11.9	12.9	15.1	16.5	17.9
95.0	11.7	12.1	12.4	12.9	13.3	14.1	14.9	15.3	16.1	16.4	17.1	11.1	12.0	13.0	15.3	16.6	18.1
95.5	11.8	12.2	12.5	13.1	13.4	14.2	15.0	15.4	16.2	16.6	17.2	11.2	12.1	13.1	15.4	16.7	18.3
96.0	11.9	12.3	12.6	13.2	13.6	14.3	15.1	15.6	16.4	16.7	17.4	11.3	12.2	13.2	15.5	16.9	18.4
96.5	12.0	12.4	12.7	13.3	13.7	14.4	15.2	15.7	16.5	16.9	17.5	11.4	12.3	13.3	15.7	17.0	18.6
97.0	12.1	12.5	12.8	13.4	13.8	14.6	15.4	15.9	16.7	17.0	17.7	11.5	12.4	13.4	15.8	17.2	18.8
97.5	12.2	12.7	12.9	13.5	13.9	14.7	15.5	16.0	16.8	17.2	17.9	11.6	12.5	13.6	15.9	17.4	18.9
98.0	12.3	12.8	13.0	13.6	14.0	14.8	15.7	16.1	17.0	17.3	18.0	11.7	12.6	13.7	16.1	17.5	19.1
98.5	12.4	12.9	13.1	13.8	14.2	14.9	15.8	16.3	17.2	17.5	18.2	11.8	12.8	13.8	16.2	17.7	19.3
99.0	12.5	13.0	13.2	13.9	14.3	15.1	15.9	16.4	17.3	17.7	18.4	11.9	12.9	13.9	16.4	17.9	19.5
99.5	12.7	13.1	13.3	14.0	14.4	15.2	16.1	16.6	17.5	17.8	18.5	12.0	13.0	14.0	16.5	18.0	19.7
100.0	12.8	13.2	13.5	14.1	14.5	15.4	16.2	16.7	17.6	18.0	18.7	12.1	13.1	14.2	16.7	18.2	19.9
100.5	12.9	13.3	13.6	14.2	14.7	15.5	16.4	16.9	17.8	18.2	18.9	12.2	13.2	14.3	16.9	18.4	20.1
101.0	13.0	13.4	13.7	14.4	14.8	15.6	16.5	17.1	18.0	18.4	19.1	12.3	13.3	14.4	17.0	18.5	20.3
101.5	13.1	13.6	13.8	14.5	14.9	15.8	16.7	17.2	18.2	18.5	19.3	12.4	13.4	14.5	17.2	18.7	20.5
102.0	13.2	13.7	13.9	14.6	15.1	15.9	16.9	17.4	18.3	18.7	19.5	12.5	13.6	14.7	17.3	18.9	20.7
102.5	13.3	13.8	14.1	14.8	15.2	16.1	17.0	17.6	18.5	18.9	19.7	12.6	13.7	14.8	17.5	19.1	20.9
103.0	13.4	13.9	14.2	14.9	15.3	16.2	17.2	17.7	18.7	19.1	19.9	12.8	13.8	14.9	17.7	19.3	21.1
103.5	13.6	14.0	14.3	15.0	15.5	16.4	17.3	17.9	18.9	19.3	20.1	12.9	13.9	15.1	17.8	19.5	21.3
104.0	13.7	14.2	14.4	15.2	15.6	16.5	17.5	18.1	19.1	19.5	20.3	13.0	14.0	15.2	18.0	19.7	21.6
104.5	13.8	14.3	14.6	15.3	15.8	16.7	17.7	18.2	19.2	19.7	20.5	13.1	14.2	15.4	18.2	19.9	21.8
105.0	13.9	14.4	14.7	15.4	15.9	16.8	17.8	18.4	19.4	19.9	20.7	13.2	14.3	15.5	18.4	20.1	22.0
105.5	14.0	14.5	14.8	15.6	16.1	17.0	18.0	18.6	19.6	20.1	20.9	13.3	14.4	15.6	18.5	20.3	22.2
106.0	14.2	14.7	15.0	15.7	16.2	17.2	18.2	18.8	19.8	20.3	21.1	13.4	14.5	15.8	18.7	20.5	22.5
106.5	14.3	14.8	15.1	15.9	16.4	17.3	18.4	19.0	20.0	20.5	21.3	13.5	14.7	15.9	18.9	20.7	22.7
107.0	14.4	14.9	15.2	16.0	16.5	17.5	18.5	19.1	20.2	20.7	21.5	13.7	14.8	16.1	19.1	20.9	22.9
107.5	14.5	15.1	15.4	16.2	16.7	17.7	18.7	19.3	20.4	20.9	21.7	13.8	14.9	16.2	19.3	21.1	23.2
108.0	14.7	15.2	15.5	16.3	16.8	17.8	18.9	19.5	20.6	21.1	22.0	13.9	15.1	16.4	19.5	21.3	23.4
108.5	14.8	15.3	15.6	16.5	17.0	18.0	19.1	19.7	20.8	21.3	22.2	14.0	15.2	16.5	19.7	21.5	23.7
109.0	14.9	15.5	15.8	16.6	17.1	18.2	19.3	19.9	21.1	21.5	22.4	14.1	15.3	16.7	19.8	21.8	23.9
109.5	15.1	15.6	15.9	16.8	17.3	18.3	19.5	20.1	21.3	21.7	22.7	14.3	15.5	16.8	20.0	22.0	24.2
110.0	15.2	15.8	16.1	16.9	17.5	18.5	19.7	20.3	21.5	22.0	22.9	14.4	15.6	17.0	20.2	22.2	24.4
110.5	15.3	15.9	16.2	17.1	17.6	18.7	19.9	20.5	21.7	22.2	23.1	14.5	15.8	17.1	20.4	22.4	24.7
111.0	15.5	16.1	16.4	17.2	17.8	18.9	20.1	20.7	21.9	22.4	23.4	14.6	15.9	17.3	20.7	22.7	25.0
111.5	15.6	16.2	16.5	17.4	18.0	19.1	20.3	20.9	22.1	22.6	23.6	14.8	16.0	17.5	20.9	22.9	25.2
112.0	15.7	16.3	16.7	17.6	18.1	19.2	20.5	21.1	22.4	22.9	23.9	14.9	16.2	17.6	21.1	23.1	25.5
112.5	15.9	16.5	16.8	17.7	18.3	19.4	20.7	21.4	22.6	23.1	24.1	15.0	16.3	17.8	21.3	23.4	25.8
113.0	16.0	16.6	17.0	17.9	18.5	19.6	20.9	21.6	22.8	23.4	24.4	15.2	16.5	18.0	21.5	23.6	26.0
113.5	16.2	16.8	17.1	18.1	18.7	19.8	21.1	21.8	23.1	23.6	24.6	15.3	16.6	18.1	21.7	23.9	26.3
114.0	16.3	17.0	17.3	18.2	18.8	20.0	21.3	22.0	23.3	23.8	24.9	15.4	16.8	18.3	21.9	24.1	26.6
114.5	16.5	17.1	17.5	18.4	19.0	20.2	21.5	22.2	23.5	24.1	25.2	15.6	16.9	18.5	22.1	24.4	26.9
115.0	16.6	17.3	17.6	18.6	19.2	20.4	21.7	22.4	23.8	24.3	25.4	15.7	17.1	18.6	22.4	24.6	27.2
115.5	16.8	17.4	17.8	18.7	19.4	20.6	21.9	22.7	24.0	24.6	25.7	15.8	17.2	18.8	22.6	24.9	27.5
116.0	16.9	17.6	17.9	18.9	19.5	20.8	22.1	22.9	24.3	24.8	25.9	16.0	17.4	19.0	22.8	25.1	27.8
116.5	17.1	17.7	18.1	19.1	19.7	21.0	22.3	23.1	24.5	25.1	26.2	16.1	17.5	19.2	23.0	25.4	28.0
117.0	17.2	17.9	18.3	19.3	19.9	21.2	22.5	23.3	24.7	25.3	26.5	16.2	17.7	19.3	23.3	25.6	28.3
117.5	17.4	18.0	18.4	19.4	20.1	21.4	22.8	23.6	25.0	25.6	26.7	16.4	17.9	19.5	23.5	25.9	28.6
118.0	17.5	18.2	18.6	19.6	20.3	21.6	23.0	23.8	25.2	25.8	27.0	16.5	18.0	19.7	23.7	26.1	28.9
118.5	17.7	18.4	18.7	19.8	20.4	21.8	23.2	24.0	25.5	26.1	27.3	16.7	18.2	19.9	23.9	26.4	29.2
119.0	17.8	18.5	18.9	20.0	20.6	22.0	23.4	24.2	25.7	26.3	27.5	16.8	18.3	20.0	24.1	26.6	29.5
119.5	17.9	18.7	19.1	20.1	20.8	22.2	23.6	24.5	26.0	26.6	27.8	16.9	18.5	20.2	24.4	26.9	29.8
120.0	18.1	18.8	19.2	20.3	21.0	22.4	23.8	24.7	26.2	26.8	28.1	17.1	18.6	20.4	24.6	27.2	30.1

Table 5.9: Weight (kg) for height (cm) for girls 2–5 years (WHO Reference Data) percentiles and *Z* (SD) scores

Height	Percentiles											Standard deviation (SD) *Z*-scores						
(cm)	1st	3rd	5th	15th	25th	50th	75th	85th	95th	97th	99th	–3SD	–2SD	–1SD	+1SD	+2SD	+3SD
65.0	5.9	6.1	6.3	6.6	6.8	7.2	7.7	8.0	8.4	8.6	9.0	5.6	6.1	6.6	7.9	8.7	9.7
65.5	6.0	6.2	6.4	6.7	6.9	7.4	7.8	8.1	8.6	8.8	9.2	5.7	6.2	6.7	8.1	8.9	9.8
66.0	6.1	6.3	6.5	6.8	7.0	7.5	7.9	8.2	8.7	8.9	9.3	5.8	6.3	6.8	8.2	9.0	10.0
66.5	6.2	6.4	6.5	6.9	7.1	7.6	8.1	8.3	8.8	9.0	9.4	5.8	6.4	6.9	8.3	9.1	10.1
67.0	6.3	6.5	6.6	7.0	7.2	7.7	8.2	8.5	9.0	9.2	9.6	5.9	6.4	7.0	8.4	9.3	10.2
67.5	6.4	6.6	6.7	7.1	7.3	7.8	8.3	8.6	9.1	9.3	9.7	6.0	6.5	7.1	8.5	9.4	10.4
68.0	6.4	6.7	6.8	7.2	7.4	7.9	8.4	8.7	9.2	9.4	9.8	6.1	6.6	7.2	8.7	9.5	10.5
68.5	6.5	6.8	6.9	7.3	7.5	8.0	8.5	8.8	9.3	9.5	10.0	6.2	6.7	7.3	8.8	9.7	10.7
69.0	6.6	6.9	7.0	7.4	7.6	8.1	8.6	8.9	9.4	9.7	10.1	6.3	6.8	7.4	8.9	9.8	10.8
69.5	6.7	7.0	7.1	7.5	7.7	8.2	8.7	9.0	9.6	9.8	10.2	6.3	6.9	7.5	9.0	9.9	10.9
70.0	6.8	7.0	7.2	7.6	7.8	8.3	8.8	9.1	9.7	9.9	10.3	6.4	7.0	7.6	9.1	10.0	11.1
70.5	6.9	7.1	7.3	7.7	7.9	8.4	8.9	9.3	9.8	10.0	10.5	6.5	7.1	7.7	9.2	10.1	11.2
71.0	6.9	7.2	7.4	7.8	8.0	8.5	9.0	9.4	9.9	10.1	10.6	6.6	7.1	7.8	9.3	10.3	11.3
71.5	7.0	7.3	7.4	7.9	8.1	8.6	9.2	9.5	10.0	10.3	10.7	6.7	7.2	7.9	9.4	10.4	11.5
72.0	7.1	7.4	7.5	7.9	8.2	8.7	9.3	9.6	10.1	10.4	10.8	6.7	7.3	8.0	9.5	10.5	11.6
72.5	7.2	7.5	7.6	8.0	8.3	8.8	9.4	9.7	10.3	10.5	11.0	6.8	7.4	8.1	9.7	10.6	11.7
73.0	7.3	7.6	7.7	8.1	8.4	8.9	9.5	9.8	10.4	10.6	11.1	6.9	7.5	8.1	9.8	10.7	11.8
73.5	7.4	7.6	7.8	8.2	8.5	9.0	9.6	9.9	10.5	10.7	11.2	7.0	7.6	8.2	9.9	10.8	12.0
74.0	7.4	7.7	7.9	8.3	8.6	9.1	9.7	10.0	10.6	10.8	11.3	7.0	7.6	8.3	10.0	11.0	12.1
74.5	7.5	7.8	8.0	8.4	8.7	9.2	9.8	10.1	10.7	10.9	11.4	7.1	7.7	8.4	10.1	11.1	12.2
75.0	7.6	7.9	8.0	8.5	8.7	9.3	9.9	10.2	10.8	11.1	11.5	7.2	7.8	8.5	10.2	11.2	12.3
75.5	7.7	8.0	8.1	8.6	8.8	9.4	10.0	10.3	10.9	11.2	11.7	7.2	7.9	8.6	10.3	11.3	12.5
76.0	7.7	8.0	8.2	8.6	8.9	9.5	10.1	10.4	11.0	11.3	11.8	7.3	8.0	8.7	10.4	11.4	12.6
76.5	7.8	8.1	8.3	8.7	9.0	9.6	10.2	10.5	11.1	11.4	11.9	7.4	8.0	8.7	10.5	11.5	12.7
77.0	7.9	8.2	8.4	8.8	9.1	9.6	10.3	10.6	11.2	11.5	12.0	7.5	8.1	8.8	10.6	11.6	12.8
77.5	8.0	8.3	8.4	8.9	9.2	9.7	10.4	10.7	11.3	11.6	12.1	7.5	8.2	8.9	10.7	11.7	12.9
78.0	8.0	8.4	8.5	9.0	9.3	9.8	10.5	10.8	11.4	11.7	12.2	7.6	8.3	9.0	10.8	11.8	13.1
78.5	8.1	8.4	8.6	9.1	9.4	9.9	10.6	10.9	11.6	11.8	12.3	7.7	8.4	9.1	10.9	12.0	13.2
79.0	8.2	8.5	8.7	9.2	9.4	10.0	10.7	11.0	11.7	11.9	12.5	7.8	8.4	9.2	11.0	12.1	13.3
79.5	8.3	8.6	8.8	9.2	9.5	10.1	10.8	11.1	11.8	12.1	12.6	7.8	8.5	9.3	11.1	12.2	13.4
80.0	8.4	8.7	8.9	9.3	9.6	10.2	10.9	11.2	11.9	12.2	12.7	7.9	8.6	9.4	11.2	12.3	13.6
80.5	8.5	8.8	9.0	9.4	9.7	10.3	11.0	11.4	12.0	12.3	12.8	8.0	8.7	9.5	11.3	12.4	13.7
81.0	8.6	8.9	9.1	9.5	9.8	10.4	11.1	11.5	12.2	12.4	13.0	8.1	8.8	9.6	11.4	12.6	13.9
81.5	8.6	9.0	9.2	9.6	9.9	10.6	11.2	11.6	12.3	12.6	13.1	8.2	8.9	9.7	11.6	12.7	14.0
82.0	8.7	9.1	9.3	9.7	10.1	10.7	11.3	11.7	12.4	12.7	13.2	8.3	9.0	9.8	11.7	12.8	14.1
82.5	8.8	9.2	9.4	9.9	10.2	10.8	11.5	11.9	12.5	12.8	13.4	8.4	9.1	9.9	11.8	13.0	14.3
83.0	8.9	9.3	9.5	10.0	10.3	10.9	11.6	12.0	12.7	13.0	13.5	8.5	9.2	10.0	11.9	13.1	14.5
83.5	9.0	9.4	9.6	10.1	10.4	11.0	11.7	12.1	12.8	13.1	13.7	8.5	9.3	10.1	12.1	13.3	14.6
84.0	9.1	9.5	9.7	10.2	10.5	11.1	11.8	12.2	13.0	13.3	13.8	8.6	9.4	10.2	12.2	13.4	14.8
84.5	9.2	9.6	9.8	10.3	10.6	11.3	12.0	12.4	13.1	13.4	14.0	8.7	9.5	10.3	12.3	13.5	14.9
85.0	9.3	9.7	9.9	10.4	10.7	11.4	12.1	12.5	13.2	13.5	14.1	8.8	9.6	10.4	12.5	13.7	15.1
85.5	9.4	9.8	10.0	10.5	10.9	11.5	12.2	12.7	13.4	13.7	14.3	8.9	9.7	10.6	12.6	13.8	15.3
86.0	9.5	9.9	10.1	10.6	11.0	11.6	12.4	12.8	13.5	13.8	14.4	9.0	9.8	10.7	12.7	14.0	15.4
86.5	9.6	10.0	10.2	10.8	11.1	11.8	12.5	12.9	13.7	14.0	14.6	9.1	9.9	10.8	12.9	14.2	15.6
87.0	9.7	10.1	10.3	10.9	11.2	11.9	12.6	13.1	13.8	14.1	14.8	9.2	10.0	10.9	13.0	14.3	15.8
87.5	9.9	10.2	10.4	11.0	11.3	12.0	12.8	13.2	14.0	14.3	14.9	9.3	10.1	11.0	13.2	14.5	15.9
88.0	10.0	10.3	10.5	11.1	11.4	12.1	12.9	13.3	14.1	14.4	15.1	9.4	10.2	11.1	13.3	14.6	16.1
88.5	10.1	10.4	10.6	11.2	11.6	12.3	13.0	13.5	14.3	14.6	15.2	9.5	10.3	11.2	13.4	14.8	16.3
89.0	10.2	10.5	10.8	11.3	11.7	12.4	13.2	13.6	14.4	14.7	15.4	9.6	10.4	11.4	13.6	14.9	16.4
89.5	10.3	10.6	10.9	11.4	11.8	12.5	13.3	13.8	14.6	14.9	15.5	9.7	10.5	11.5	13.7	15.1	16.6
90.0	10.4	10.8	11.0	11.5	11.9	12.6	13.4	13.9	14.7	15.0	15.7	9.8	10.6	11.6	13.8	15.2	16.8
90.5	10.5	10.9	11.1	11.7	12.0	12.8	13.6	14.0	14.9	15.2	15.9	9.9	10.7	11.7	14.0	15.4	16.9
91.0	10.6	11.0	11.2	11.8	12.1	12.9	13.7	14.2	15.0	15.3	16.0	10.0	10.9	11.8	14.1	15.5	17.1
91.5	10.7	11.1	11.3	11.9	12.3	13.0	13.8	14.3	15.1	15.5	16.2	10.1	11.0	11.9	14.3	15.7	17.3
92.0	10.8	11.2	11.4	12.0	12.4	13.1	14.0	14.4	15.3	15.6	16.3	10.2	11.1	12.0	14.4	15.8	17.4

(Contd...)

Table 5.9: Weight (kg) for height (cm) for girls 2–5 years (WHO Reference Data) percentiles and *Z* (SD) scores (*Contd...*)

Height	Percentiles											Standard deviation (SD) *Z*-scores					
(cm)	1st	3rd	5th	15th	25th	50th	75th	85th	95th	97th	99th	–3SD	–2SD	–1SD	+1SD	+2SD	+3SD
92.5	10.9	11.3	11.5	12.1	12.5	13.3	14.1	14.6	15.4	15.8	16.5	10.3	11.2	12.1	14.5	16.0	17.6
93.0	11.0	11.4	11.6	12.2	12.6	13.4	14.2	14.7	15.6	15.9	16.6	10.4	11.3	12.3	14.7	16.1	17.8
93.5	11.1	11.5	11.7	12.3	12.7	13.5	14.4	14.9	15.7	16.1	16.8	10.5	11.4	12.4	14.8	16.3	17.9
94.0	11.2	11.6	11.8	12.4	12.8	13.6	14.5	15.0	15.9	16.2	16.9	10.6	11.5	12.5	14.9	16.4	18.1
94.5	11.3	11.7	11.9	12.6	13.0	13.8	14.6	15.1	16.0	16.4	17.1	10.7	11.6	12.6	15.1	16.6	18.3
95.0	11.4	11.8	12.0	12.7	13.1	13.9	14.8	15.3	16.2	16.5	17.3	10.8	11.7	12.7	15.2	16.7	18.5
95.5	11.5	11.9	12.1	12.8	13.2	14.0	14.9	15.4	16.3	16.7	17.4	10.8	11.8	12.8	15.4	16.9	18.6
96.0	11.6	12.0	12.3	12.9	13.3	14.1	15.0	15.6	16.5	16.9	17.6	10.9	11.9	12.9	15.5	17.0	18.8
96.5	11.7	12.1	12.4	13.0	13.4	14.3	15.2	15.7	16.6	17.0	17.8	11.0	12.0	13.1	15.6	17.2	19.0
97.0	11.8	12.2	12.5	13.1	13.6	14.4	15.3	15.8	16.8	17.2	17.9	11.1	12.1	13.2	15.8	17.4	19.2
97.5	11.9	12.3	12.6	13.3	13.7	14.5	15.5	16.0	16.9	17.3	18.1	11.2	12.2	13.3	15.9	17.5	19.3
98.0	12.0	12.4	12.7	13.4	13.8	14.7	15.6	16.1	17.1	17.5	18.3	11.3	12.3	13.4	16.1	17.7	19.5
98.5	12.1	12.6	12.8	13.5	13.9	14.8	15.7	16.3	17.3	17.7	18.4	11.4	12.4	13.5	16.2	17.9	19.7
99.0	12.2	12.7	12.9	13.6	14.1	14.9	15.9	16.4	17.4	17.8	18.6	11.5	12.5	13.7	16.4	18.0	19.9
99.5	12.3	12.8	13.0	13.8	14.2	15.1	16.0	16.6	17.6	18.0	18.8	11.6	12.7	13.8	16.5	18.2	20.1
100.0	12.4	12.9	13.2	13.9	14.3	15.2	16.2	16.8	17.8	18.2	19.0	11.7	12.8	13.9	16.7	18.4	20.3
100.5	12.5	13.0	13.3	14.0	14.5	15.4	16.4	16.9	17.9	18.3	19.2	11.9	12.9	14.1	16.9	18.6	20.5
101.0	12.7	13.1	13.4	14.1	14.6	15.5	16.5	17.1	18.1	18.5	19.4	12.0	13.0	14.2	17.0	18.7	20.7
101.5	12.8	13.3	13.5	14.3	14.7	15.7	16.7	17.2	18.3	18.7	19.5	12.1	13.1	14.3	17.2	18.9	20.9
102.0	12.9	13.4	13.7	14.4	14.9	15.8	16.8	17.4	18.5	18.9	19.7	12.2	13.3	14.5	17.4	19.1	21.1
102.5	13.0	13.5	13.8	14.5	15.0	16.0	17.0	17.6	18.7	19.1	19.9	12.3	13.4	14.6	17.5	19.3	21.4
103.0	13.1	13.6	13.9	14.7	15.2	16.1	17.2	17.8	18.8	19.3	20.2	12.4	13.5	14.7	17.7	19.5	21.6
103.5	13.3	13.8	14.1	14.8	15.3	16.3	17.3	17.9	19.0	19.5	20.4	12.5	13.6	14.9	17.9	19.7	21.8
104.0	13.4	13.9	14.2	15.0	15.5	16.4	17.5	18.1	19.2	19.7	20.6	12.6	13.8	15.0	18.1	19.9	22.0
104.5	13.5	14.0	14.3	15.1	15.6	16.6	17.7	18.3	19.4	19.9	20.8	12.8	13.9	15.2	18.2	20.1	22.3
105.0	13.6	14.2	14.5	15.3	15.8	16.8	17.9	18.5	19.6	20.1	21.0	12.9	14.0	15.3	18.4	20.3	22.5
105.5	13.8	14.3	14.6	15.4	15.9	16.9	18.1	18.7	19.8	20.3	21.2	13.0	14.2	15.5	18.6	20.5	22.7
106.0	13.9	14.5	14.8	15.6	16.1	17.1	18.2	18.9	20.0	20.5	21.4	13.1	14.3	15.6	18.8	20.8	23.0
106.5	14.1	14.6	14.9	15.7	16.3	17.3	18.4	19.1	20.2	20.7	21.7	13.3	14.5	15.8	19.0	21.0	23.2
107.0	14.2	14.7	15.1	15.9	16.4	17.5	18.6	19.3	20.5	21.0	21.9	13.4	14.6	15.9	19.2	21.2	23.5
107.5	14.3	14.9	15.2	16.1	16.6	17.7	18.8	19.5	20.7	21.2	22.1	13.5	14.7	16.1	19.4	21.4	23.7
108.0	14.5	15.0	15.4	16.2	16.8	17.8	19.0	19.7	20.9	21.4	22.4	13.7	14.9	16.3	19.6	21.7	24.0
108.5	14.6	15.2	15.5	16.4	16.9	18.0	19.2	19.9	21.1	21.6	22.6	13.8	15.0	16.4	19.8	21.9	24.3
109.0	14.8	15.4	15.7	16.6	17.1	18.2	19.4	20.1	21.4	21.9	22.9	13.9	15.2	16.6	20.0	22.1	24.5
109.5	14.9	15.5	15.8	16.7	17.3	18.4	19.6	20.3	21.6	22.1	23.1	14.1	15.4	16.8	20.3	22.4	24.8
110.0	15.1	15.7	16.0	16.9	17.5	18.6	19.8	20.6	21.8	22.4	23.4	14.2	15.5	17.0	20.5	22.6	25.1
110.5	15.2	15.8	16.2	17.1	17.7	18.8	20.1	20.8	22.1	22.6	23.7	14.4	15.7	17.1	20.7	22.9	25.4
111.0	15.4	16.0	16.3	17.3	17.8	19.0	20.3	21.0	22.3	22.8	23.9	14.5	15.8	17.3	20.9	23.1	25.7
111.5	15.5	16.2	16.5	17.4	18.0	19.2	20.5	21.2	22.6	23.1	24.2	14.7	16.0	17.5	21.2	23.4	26.0
112.0	15.7	16.3	16.7	17.6	18.2	19.4	20.7	21.5	22.8	23.4	24.5	14.8	16.2	17.7	21.4	23.6	26.2
112.5	15.9	16.5	16.8	17.8	18.4	19.6	20.9	21.7	23.1	23.6	24.7	15.0	16.3	17.9	21.6	23.9	26.5
113.0	16.0	16.7	17.0	18.0	18.6	19.8	21.2	21.9	23.3	23.9	25.0	15.1	16.5	18.0	21.8	24.2	26.8
113.5	16.2	16.8	17.2	18.2	18.8	20.0	21.4	22.2	23.6	24.1	25.3	15.3	16.7	18.2	22.1	24.4	27.1
114.0	16.3	17.0	17.4	18.4	19.0	20.2	21.6	22.4	23.8	24.4	25.6	15.4	16.8	18.4	22.3	24.7	27.4
114.5	16.5	17.2	17.5	18.5	19.2	20.5	21.8	22.6	24.1	24.7	25.8	15.6	17.0	18.6	22.6	25.0	27.8
115.0	16.7	17.3	17.7	18.7	19.4	20.7	22.1	22.9	24.3	24.9	26.1	15.7	17.2	18.8	22.8	25.2	28.1
115.5	16.8	17.5	17.9	18.9	19.6	20.9	22.3	23.1	24.6	25.2	26.4	15.9	17.3	19.0	23.0	25.5	28.4
116.0	17.0	17.7	18.1	19.1	19.8	21.1	22.5	23.4	24.9	25.5	26.7	16.0	17.5	19.2	23.3	25.8	28.7
116.5	17.2	17.9	18.3	19.3	20.0	21.3	22.8	23.6	25.1	25.7	27.0	16.2	17.7	19.4	23.5	26.1	29.0
117.0	17.3	18.0	18.4	19.5	20.2	21.5	23.0	23.8	25.4	26.0	27.3	16.3	17.8	19.6	23.8	26.3	29.3
117.5	17.5	18.2	18.6	19.7	20.4	21.7	23.2	24.1	25.6	26.3	27.5	16.5	18.0	19.8	24.0	26.6	29.6
118.0	17.7	18.4	18.8	19.9	20.6	22.0	23.5	24.3	25.9	26.5	27.8	16.6	18.2	19.9	24.2	26.9	29.9
118.5	17.8	18.6	19.0	20.1	20.8	22.2	23.7	24.6	26.2	26.8	28.1	16.8	18.4	20.1	24.5	27.2	30.3
119.0	18.0	18.7	19.1	20.3	21.0	22.4	23.9	24.8	26.4	27.1	28.4	16.9	18.5	20.3	24.7	27.4	30.6
119.5	18.2	18.9	19.3	20.5	21.2	22.6	24.2	25.1	26.7	27.4	28.7	17.1	18.7	20.5	25.0	27.7	30.9
120.0	18.3	19.1	19.5	20.6	21.4	22.8	24.4	25.3	27.0	27.6	29.0	17.3	18.9	20.7	25.2	28.0	31.2

Table 5.10: Head circumference (cm) by age *Z* (SD) scores in boys and girls aged 0–5 years

Age		Boys							Girls						
Year	Mo	–3SD	–2SD	–1SD	Median	+1SD	+2SD	+3SD	–3SD	–2SD	–1SD	Median	+1SD	+2SD	+3SD
	0	30.7	31.9	33.2	34.5	35.7	37.0	38.3	30.3	31.5	32.7	33.9	35.1	36.2	37.4
	1	33.8	34.9	36.1	37.3	38.4	39.6	40.8	33.0	34.2	35.4	36.5	37.7	38.9	40.1
	2	35.6	36.8	38.0	39.1	40.3	41.5	42.6	34.6	35.8	37.0	38.3	39.5	40.7	41.9
	3	37.0	38.1	39.3	40.5	41.7	42.9	44.1	35.8	37.1	38.3	39.5	40.8	42.0	43.3
	4	38.0	39.2	40.4	41.6	42.8	44.0	45.2	36.8	38.1	39.3	40.6	41.8	43.1	44.4
	5	38.9	40.1	41.4	42.6	43.8	45.0	46.2	37.6	38.9	40.2	41.5	42.7	44.0	45.3
	6	39.7	40.9	42.1	43.3	44.6	45.8	47.0	38.3	39.6	40.9	42.2	43.5	44.8	46.1
	7	40.3	41.5	42.7	44.0	45.2	46.4	47.7	38.9	40.2	41.5	42.8	44.1	45.5	46.8
	8	40.8	42.0	43.3	44.5	45.8	47.0	48.3	39.4	40.7	42.0	43.4	44.7	46.0	47.4
	9	41.2	42.5	43.7	45.0	46.3	47.5	48.8	39.8	41.2	42.5	43.8	45.2	46.5	47.8
	10	41.6	42.9	44.1	45.4	46.7	47.9	49.2	40.2	41.5	42.9	44.2	45.6	46.9	48.3
	11	41.9	43.2	44.5	45.8	47.0	48.3	49.6	40.5	41.9	43.2	44.6	45.9	47.3	48.6
1	0	42.2	43.5	44.8	46.1	47.4	48.6	49.9	40.8	42.2	43.5	44.9	46.3	47.6	49.0
	1	42.5	43.8	45.0	46.3	47.6	48.9	50.2	41.1	42.4	43.8	45.2	46.5	47.9	49.3
	2	42.7	44.0	45.3	46.6	47.9	49.2	50.5	41.3	42.7	44.1	45.4	46.8	48.2	49.5
	3	42.9	44.2	45.5	46.8	48.1	49.4	50.7	41.5	42.9	44.3	45.7	47.0	48.4	49.8
	4	43.1	44.4	45.7	47.0	48.3	49.6	51.0	41.7	43.1	44.5	45.9	47.2	48.6	50.0
	5	43.2	44.6	45.9	47.2	48.5	49.8	51.2	41.9	43.3	44.7	46.1	47.4	48.8	50.2
	6	43.4	44.7	46.0	47.4	48.7	50.0	51.4	42.1	43.5	44.9	46.2	47.6	49.0	50.4
	7	43.5	44.9	46.2	47.5	48.9	50.2	51.5	42.3	43.6	45.0	46.4	47.8	49.2	50.6
	8	43.7	45.0	46.4	47.7	49.0	50.4	51.7	42.4	43.8	45.2	46.6	48.0	49.4	50.7
	9	43.8	45.2	46.5	47.8	49.2	50.5	51.9	42.6	44.0	45.3	46.7	48.1	49.5	50.9
	10	43.9	45.3	46.6	48.0	49.3	50.7	52.0	42.7	44.1	45.5	46.9	48.3	49.7	51.1
	11	44.1	45.4	46.8	48.1	49.5	50.8	52.2	42.9	44.3	45.6	47.0	48.4	49.8	51.2
2	0	44.2	45.5	46.9	48.3	49.6	51.0	52.3	43.0	44.4	45.8	47.2	48.6	50.0	51.4
	1	44.3	45.6	47.0	48.4	49.7	51.1	52.5	43.1	44.5	45.9	47.3	48.7	50.1	51.5
	2	44.4	45.8	47.1	48.5	49.9	51.2	52.6	43.3	44.7	46.1	47.5	48.9	50.3	51.7
	3	44.5	45.9	47.2	48.6	50.0	51.4	52.7	43.4	44.8	46.2	47.6	49.0	50.4	51.8
	4	44.6	46.0	47.3	48.7	50.1	51.5	52.9	43.5	44.9	46.3	47.7	49.1	50.5	51.9
	5	44.7	46.1	47.4	48.8	50.2	51.6	53.0	43.6	45.0	46.4	47.8	49.2	50.6	52.0
	6	44.8	46.1	47.5	48.9	50.3	51.7	53.1	43.7	45.1	46.5	47.9	49.3	50.7	52.2
	7	44.8	46.2	47.6	49.0	50.4	51.8	53.2	43.8	45.2	46.6	48.0	49.4	50.9	52.3
	8	44.9	46.3	47.7	49.1	50.5	51.9	53.3	43.9	45.3	46.7	48.1	49.6	51.0	52.4
	9	45.0	46.4	47.8	49.2	50.6	52.0	53.4	44.0	45.4	46.8	48.2	49.7	51.1	52.5
	10	45.1	46.5	47.9	49.3	50.7	52.1	53.5	44.1	45.5	46.9	48.3	49.7	51.2	52.6
	11	45.1	46.6	48.0	49.4	50.8	52.2	53.6	44.2	45.6	47.0	48.4	49.8	51.2	52.7
3	0	45.2	46.6	48.0	49.5	50.9	52.3	53.7	44.3	45.7	47.1	48.5	49.9	51.3	52.7
	1	45.3	46.7	48.1	49.5	51.0	52.4	53.8	44.4	45.8	47.2	48.6	50.0	51.4	52.8
	2	45.3	46.8	48.2	49.6	51.0	52.5	53.9	44.4	45.8	47.3	48.7	50.1	51.5	52.9
	3	45.4	46.8	48.2	49.7	51.1	52.5	54.0	44.5	45.9	47.3	48.7	50.2	51.6	53.0
	4	45.4	46.9	48.3	49.7	51.2	52.6	54.1	44.6	46.0	47.4	48.8	50.2	51.7	53.1
	5	45.5	46.9	48.4	49.8	51.3	52.7	54.1	44.6	46.1	47.5	48.9	50.3	51.7	53.1
	6	45.5	47.0	48.4	49.9	51.3	52.8	54.2	44.7	46.1	47.5	49.0	50.4	51.8	53.2
	7	45.6	47.0	48.5	49.9	51.4	52.8	54.3	44.8	46.2	47.6	49.0	50.4	51.9	53.3
	8	45.6	47.1	48.5	50.0	51.4	52.9	54.3	44.8	46.3	47.7	49.1	50.5	51.9	53.3
	9	45.7	47.1	48.6	50.1	51.5	53.0	54.4	44.9	46.3	47.7	49.2	50.6	52.0	53.4
	10	45.7	47.2	48.7	50.1	51.6	53.0	54.5	45.0	46.4	47.8	49.2	50.6	52.1	53.5
	11	45.8	47.2	48.7	50.2	51.6	53.1	54.5	45.0	46.4	47.9	49.3	50.7	52.1	53.5
4	0	45.8	47.3	48.7	50.2	51.7	53.1	54.6	45.1	46.5	47.9	49.3	50.8	52.2	53.6
	1	45.9	47.3	48.8	50.3	51.7	53.2	54.7	45.1	46.5	48.0	49.4	50.8	52.2	53.6
	2	45.9	47.4	48.8	50.3	51.8	53.2	54.7	45.2	46.6	48.0	49.4	50.9	52.3	53.7
	3	45.9	47.4	48.9	50.4	51.8	53.3	54.8	45.2	46.7	48.1	49.5	50.9	52.3	53.8
	4	46.0	47.5	48.9	50.4	51.9	53.4	54.8	45.3	46.7	48.1	49.5	51.0	52.4	53.8
	5	46.0	47.5	49.0	50.4	51.9	53.4	54.9	45.3	46.8	48.2	49.6	51.0	52.4	53.9
	6	46.1	47.5	49.0	50.5	52.0	53.5	54.9	45.4	46.8	48.2	49.6	51.1	52.5	53.9
	7	46.1	47.6	49.1	50.5	52.0	53.5	55.0	45.4	46.9	48.3	49.7	51.1	52.5	54.0
	8	46.1	47.6	49.1	50.6	52.1	53.5	55.0	45.5	46.9	48.3	49.7	51.2	52.6	54.0
	9	46.2	47.6	49.1	50.6	52.1	53.6	55.1	45.5	46.9	48.4	49.8	51.2	52.6	54.1
	10	46.2	47.7	49.2	50.7	52.1	53.6	55.1	45.6	47.0	48.4	49.8	51.3	52.7	54.1
	11	46.2	47.7	49.2	50.7	52.2	53.7	55.2	45.6	47.0	48.5	49.9	51.3	52.7	54.1
5	60	46.3	47.7	49.2	50.7	52.2	53.7	55.2	45.7	47.1	48.5	49.9	51.3	52.8	54.2

Table 5.11: Body mass index (kg/m²) for boys 0–5 years (WHO Standards)

Age		Percentiles					Z (SD) scores					
Year	Month	5th	15th	50th	85th	95th	–3Z	–2Z	–1Z	+1Z	+2Z	+3Z
	0	11.5	12.2	13.4	14.8	15.8	10.2	11.1	12.2	14.8	16.3	18.1
	1	12.8	13.6	14.9	16.4	17.3	11.3	12.4	13.6	16.3	17.8	19.4
	2	14.1	14.9	16.3	17.8	18.8	12.5	13.7	15.0	17.8	19.4	21.1
	3	14.7	15.5	16.9	18.5	19.4	13.1	14.3	15.5	18.4	20.0	21.8
	4	15.0	15.7	17.2	18.7	19.7	13.4	14.5	15.8	18.7	20.3	22.1
	5	15.1	15.9	17.3	18.9	19.8	13.5	14.7	15.9	18.8	20.5	22.3
	6	15.2	15.9	17.3	18.9	19.9	13.6	14.7	16.0	18.8	20.5	22.3
	7	15.2	15.9	17.3	18.9	19.9	13.7	14.8	16.0	18.8	20.5	22.3
	8	15.1	15.9	17.3	18.8	19.8	13.6	14.7	15.9	18.7	20.4	22.2
	9	15.1	15.8	17.2	18.7	19.7	13.6	14.7	15.8	18.6	20.3	22.1
	10	15.0	15.7	17.0	18.6	19.5	13.5	14.6	15.7	18.5	20.1	22.0
	11	14.9	15.6	16.9	18.4	19.4	13.4	14.5	15.6	18.4	20.0	21.8
1	0	14.8	15.5	16.8	18.3	19.2	13.4	14.4	15.5	18.2	19.8	21.6
1	1	14.7	15.4	16.7	18.1	19.1	13.3	14.3	15.4	18.1	19.7	21.5
1	2	14.6	15.3	16.6	18.0	18.9	13.2	14.2	15.3	18.0	19.5	21.3
1	3	14.5	15.2	16.4	17.9	18.8	13.1	14.1	15.2	17.8	19.4	21.2
1	4	14.4	15.1	16.3	17.8	18.7	13.1	14.0	15.1	17.7	19.3	21.0
1	5	14.3	15.0	16.2	17.6	18.6	13.0	13.9	15.0	17.6	19.1	20.9
1	6	14.2	14.9	16.1	17.5	18.5	12.9	13.9	14.9	17.5	19.0	20.8
1	7	14.2	14.8	16.1	17.4	18.4	12.9	13.8	14.9	17.4	18.9	20.7
1	8	14.1	14.8	16.0	17.4	18.3	12.8	13.7	14.8	17.3	18.8	20.6
1	9	14.1	14.7	15.9	17.3	18.2	12.8	13.7	14.7	17.2	18.7	20.5
1	10	14.0	14.6	15.8	17.2	18.1	12.7	13.6	14.7	17.2	18.7	20.4
1	11	14.0	14.6	15.8	17.1	18.0	12.7	13.6	14.6	17.1	18.6	20.3
2	0	13.9	14.5	15.7	17.1	18.0	12.7	13.6	14.6	17.0	18.5	20.3
2	1	14.1	14.8	16.0	17.4	18.3	12.8	13.8	14.8	17.3	18.8	20.5
2	2	14.1	14.7	15.9	17.3	18.2	12.8	13.7	14.8	17.3	18.8	20.5
2	3	14.0	14.7	15.9	17.3	18.2	12.7	13.7	14.7	17.2	18.7	20.4
2	4	14.0	14.7	15.9	17.2	18.1	12.7	13.6	14.7	17.2	18.7	20.4
2	5	14.0	14.6	15.8	17.2	18.1	12.7	13.6	14.7	17.1	18.6	20.3
2	6	13.9	14.6	15.8	17.2	18.0	12.6	13.6	14.6	17.1	18.6	20.2
2	7	13.9	14.5	15.8	17.1	18.0	12.6	13.5	14.6	17.1	18.5	20.2
2	8	13.9	14.5	15.7	17.1	18.0	12.5	13.5	14.6	17.0	18.5	20.1
2	9	13.8	14.5	15.7	17.0	17.9	12.5	13.5	14.5	17.0	18.5	20.1
2	10	13.8	14.4	15.7	17.0	17.9	12.5	13.4	14.5	17.0	18.4	20.0
2	11	13.8	14.4	15.6	17.0	17.9	12.4	13.4	14.5	16.9	18.4	20.0
3	0	13.7	14.4	15.6	17.0	17.8	12.4	13.4	14.4	16.9	18.4	20.0
3	1	13.7	14.4	15.6	16.9	17.8	12.4	13.3	14.4	16.9	18.3	19.9
3	2	13.7	14.3	15.5	16.9	17.8	12.3	13.3	14.4	16.8	18.3	19.9
3	3	13.6	14.3	15.5	16.9	17.7	12.3	13.3	14.3	16.8	18.3	19.9
3	4	13.6	14.3	15.5	16.8	17.7	12.3	13.2	14.3	16.8	18.2	19.9
3	5	13.6	14.2	15.5	16.8	17.7	12.2	13.2	14.3	16.8	18.2	19.9
3	6	13.6	14.2	15.4	16.8	17.7	12.2	13.2	14.3	16.8	18.2	19.8
3	7	13.5	14.2	15.4	16.8	17.7	12.2	13.2	14.2	16.7	18.2	19.8
3	8	13.5	14.2	15.4	16.8	17.7	12.2	13.1	14.2	16.7	18.2	19.8
3	9	13.5	14.2	15.4	16.8	17.6	12.2	13.1	14.2	16.7	18.2	19.8
3	10	13.5	14.1	15.4	16.7	17.6	12.1	13.1	14.2	16.7	18.2	19.8
3	11	13.5	14.1	15.3	16.7	17.6	12.1	13.1	14.2	16.7	18.2	19.9
4	0	13.4	14.1	15.3	16.7	17.6	12.1	13.1	14.1	16.7	18.2	19.9
4	1	13.4	14.1	15.3	16.7	17.6	12.1	13.0	14.1	16.7	18.2	19.9
4	2	13.4	14.1	15.3	16.7	17.6	12.1	13.0	14.1	16.7	18.2	19.9
4	3	13.4	14.0	15.3	16.7	17.6	12.1	13.0	14.1	16.6	18.2	19.9
4	4	13.4	14.0	15.3	16.7	17.6	12.0	13.0	14.1	16.6	18.2	19.9
4	5	13.3	14.0	15.3	16.7	17.6	12.0	13.0	14.1	16.6	18.2	20.0
4	6	13.3	14.0	15.3	16.7	17.6	12.0	13.0	14.0	16.6	18.2	20.0
4	7	13.3	14.0	15.2	16.7	17.6	12.0	13.0	14.0	16.6	18.2	20.0
4	8	13.3	14.0	15.2	16.7	17.6	12.0	12.9	14.0	16.6	18.2	20.1
4	9	13.3	14.0	15.2	16.7	17.6	12.0	12.9	14.0	16.6	18.2	20.1
4	10	13.3	13.9	15.2	16.7	17.6	12.0	12.9	14.0	16.6	18.3	20.2
4	11	13.3	13.9	15.2	16.7	17.7	12.0	12.9	14.0	16.6	18.3	20.2
5	0	13.3	13.9	15.2	16.7	17.7	12.0	12.9	14.0	16.6	18.3	20.3

Table 5.12: Body mass index (kg/m²) for girls 0–5 years (WHO Standards)

Age		Percentiles					Z (SD) scores					
Year	Month	5th	15th	50th	85th	95th	–3Z	–2Z	–1Z	+1Z	+2Z	+3Z
	0	11.5	12.1	13.3	14.7	15.8	10.2	11.1	12.2	14.8	16.3	18.1
	1	12.4	13.2	14.6	16.1	17.3	11.3	12.4	13.6	16.3	17.8	19.4
	2	13.5	14.3	15.8	17.4	18.8	12.5	13.7	15.0	17.8	19.4	21.1
	3	14.0	14.9	16.4	18.0	19.4	13.1	14.3	15.5	18.4	20.0	21.8
	4	14.3	15.2	16.7	18.3	19.7	13.4	14.5	15.8	18.7	20.3	22.1
	5	14.5	15.3	16.8	18.5	19.8	13.5	14.7	15.9	18.8	20.5	22.3
	6	14.6	15.4	16.9	18.6	19.9	13.6	14.7	16.0	18.8	20.5	22.3
	7	14.6	15.4	16.9	18.6	19.9	13.7	14.8	16.0	18.8	20.5	22.3
	8	14.6	15.4	16.8	18.5	19.8	13.6	14.7	15.9	18.7	20.4	22.2
	9	14.5	15.3	16.7	18.4	19.7	13.6	14.7	15.8	18.6	20.3	22.1
	10	14.4	15.2	16.6	18.2	19.5	13.5	14.6	15.7	18.5	20.1	22.0
	11	14.3	15.1	16.5	18.1	19.4	13.4	14.5	15.6	18.4	20.0	21.8
1	0	14.2	15.0	16.4	17.9	19.2	13.4	14.4	15.5	18.2	19.8	21.6
1	1	14.1	14.8	16.2	17.8	19.1	13.3	14.3	15.4	18.1	19.7	21.5
1	2	14.0	14.7	16.1	17.7	18.9	13.2	14.2	15.3	18.0	19.5	21.3
1	3	13.9	14.6	16.0	17.5	18.8	13.1	14.1	15.2	17.8	19.4	21.2
1	4	13.8	14.6	15.9	17.4	18.7	13.1	14.0	15.1	17.7	19.3	21.0
1	5	13.8	14.5	15.8	17.3	18.6	13.0	13.9	15.0	17.6	19.1	20.9
1	6	13.7	14.4	15.7	17.2	18.5	12.9	13.9	14.9	17.5	19.0	20.8
1	7	13.6	14.3	15.7	17.2	18.4	12.9	13.8	14.9	17.4	18.9	20.7
1	8	13.6	14.3	15.6	17.1	18.3	12.8	13.7	14.8	17.3	18.8	20.6
1	9	13.6	14.2	15.5	17.0	18.2	12.8	13.7	14.7	17.2	18.7	20.5
1	10	13.5	14.2	15.5	17.0	18.1	12.7	13.6	14.7	17.2	18.7	20.4
1	11	13.5	14.2	15.4	16.9	18.0	12.7	13.6	14.6	17.1	18.6	20.3
2	0	13.5	14.1	15.4	16.9	18.0	12.7	13.6	14.6	17.0	18.5	20.3
2	1	13.7	14.4	15.7	17.1	18.1	12.4	13.3	14.4	17.1	18.7	20.6
2	2	13.7	14.4	15.6	17.1	18.1	12.3	13.3	14.4	17.0	18.7	20.6
2	3	13.7	14.3	15.6	17.1	18.0	12.3	13.3	14.4	17.0	18.6	20.5
2	4	13.6	14.3	15.6	17.0	18.0	12.3	13.3	14.3	17.0	18.6	20.5
2	5	13.6	14.3	15.6	17.0	18.0	12.3	13.2	14.3	17.0	18.6	20.4
2	6	13.6	14.3	15.5	17.0	17.9	12.3	13.2	14.3	16.9	18.5	20.4
2	7	13.6	14.2	15.5	17.0	17.9	12.2	13.2	14.3	16.9	18.5	20.4
2	8	13.5	14.2	15.5	16.9	17.9	12.2	13.2	14.3	16.9	18.5	20.4
2	9	13.5	14.2	15.5	16.9	17.9	12.2	13.1	14.2	16.9	18.5	20.3
2	10	13.5	14.2	15.4	16.9	17.9	12.2	13.1	14.2	16.8	18.5	20.3
2	11	13.5	14.1	15.4	16.9	17.8	12.1	13.1	14.2	16.8	18.4	20.3
3	0	13.5	14.1	15.4	16.9	17.8	12.1	13.1	14.2	16.8	18.4	20.3
3	1	13.4	14.1	15.4	16.8	17.8	12.1	13.1	14.1	16.8	18.4	20.3
3	2	13.4	14.1	15.4	16.8	17.8	12.1	13.0	14.1	16.8	18.4	20.3
3	3	13.4	14.1	15.3	16.8	17.8	12.0	13.0	14.1	16.8	18.4	20.3
3	4	13.4	14.0	15.3	16.8	17.8	12.0	13.0	14.1	16.8	18.4	20.3
3	5	13.3	14.0	15.3	16.8	17.8	12.0	13.0	14.1	16.8	18.4	20.4
3	6	13.3	14.0	15.3	16.8	17.8	12.0	12.9	14.0	16.8	18.4	20.4
3	7	13.3	14.0	15.3	16.8	17.8	11.9	12.9	14.0	16.8	18.4	20.4
3	8	13.3	14.0	15.3	16.8	17.8	11.9	12.9	14.0	16.8	18.5	20.4
3	9	13.3	14.0	15.3	16.8	17.8	11.9	12.9	14.0	16.8	18.5	20.5
3	10	13.2	13.9	15.3	16.8	17.8	11.9	12.9	14.0	16.8	18.5	20.5
3	11	13.2	13.9	15.3	16.8	17.9	11.8	12.8	14.0	16.8	18.5	20.5
4	0	13.2	13.9	15.3	16.8	17.9	11.8	12.8	14.0	16.8	18.5	20.6
4	1	13.2	13.9	15.3	16.8	17.9	11.8	12.8	13.9	16.8	18.5	20.6
4	2	13.2	13.9	15.3	16.8	17.9	11.8	12.8	13.9	16.8	18.6	20.7
4	3	13.2	13.9	15.3	16.8	17.9	11.8	12.8	13.9	16.8	18.6	20.7
4	4	13.1	13.9	15.2	16.9	17.9	11.7	12.8	13.9	16.8	18.6	20.7
4	5	13.1	13.9	15.3	16.9	17.9	11.7	12.7	13.9	16.8	18.6	20.8
4	6	13.1	13.9	15.3	16.9	18.0	11.7	12.7	13.9	16.8	18.7	20.8
4	7	13.1	13.9	15.3	16.9	18.0	11.7	12.7	13.9	16.8	18.7	20.9
4	8	13.1	13.8	15.3	16.9	18.0	11.7	12.7	13.9	16.8	18.7	20.9
4	9	13.1	13.8	15.3	16.9	18.0	11.7	12.7	13.9	16.9	18.7	21.0
4	10	13.1	13.8	15.3	16.9	18.0	11.7	12.7	13.9	16.9	18.8	21.0
4	11	13.1	13.8	15.3	16.9	18.1	11.6	12.7	13.9	16.9	18.8	21.0
5	0	13.1	13.8	15.3	17.0	18.1	11.6	12.7	13.9	16.9	18.8	21.1

Table 5.13: Weight (kg) centiles and standard deviation for boys (5–18 years): IAP Growth Charts 2015

Age (y)	Percentiles							
	3	10	25	50	75	90	97	SD
5.0	13.2	14.3	15.6	17.1	19.0	21.3	24.2	3.2
5.5	13.8	15.0	16.5	18.2	20.3	22.9	26.1	2.9
6.0	14.5	15.8	17.4	19.3	21.7	24.6	28.3	3.6
6.5	15.3	16.8	18.6	20.7	23.3	26.6	30.8	3.8
7.0	16.0	17.6	19.6	21.9	24.9	28.6	33.4	4.2
7.5	16.7	18.5	20.7	23.3	26.6	30.8	36.2	4.9
8.0	17.5	19.5	21.9	24.8	28.5	33.2	39.4	5.7
8.5	18.3	20.5	23.2	26.4	30.5	35.7	42.6	6.5
9.0	19.1	21.5	24.3	27.9	32.3	38.0	45.5	6.3
9.5	19.9	22.4	25.6	29.4	34.3	40.5	48.6	7.0
10.0	20.7	23.5	26.9	31.1	36.3	43.0	51.8	7.9
10.5	21.6	24.6	28.3	32.8	38.5	45.8	55.2	8.3
11.0	22.6	25.9	29.8	34.7	40.9	48.7	58.7	8.9
11.5	23.8	27.3	31.6	36.9	43.5	51.8	62.5	9.3
12.0	24.9	28.7	33.3	39.0	46.0	54.8	66.1	10.0
12.5	26.1	30.2	35.1	41.2	48.6	57.8	69.5	10.6
13.0	27.5	31.8	37.0	43.3	51.1	60.7	72.6	11.3
13.5	29.0	33.6	39.1	45.7	53.8	63.6	75.6	11.4
14.0	30.7	35.5	41.3	48.2	56.4	66.3	78.3	12.1
15.0	34.5	39.8	45.9	53.1	61.6	71.5	83.1	12.1
16.0	37.5	43.1	49.5	56.8	65.2	74.8	85.8	12.2
17.0	39.8	45.6	52.1	59.5	67.8	77.1	87.5	12.3
18.0	41.8	47.7	54.3	61.6	69.7	78.6	88.4	11.3

Table 5.14: Weight (kg) centiles and standard deviations for girls (5–18 years): IAP Growth Charts 2015

Age (y)	Percentiles							
	3	10	25	50	75	90	97	SD
5.0	12.3	13.4	14.8	16.4	18.5	21.3	25.0	2.5
5.5	13.0	14.3	15.7	17.6	19.9	22.9	27.0	3.5
6.0	13.7	15.1	16.7	18.7	21.3	24.6	29.1	3.4
6.5	14.4	15.9	17.7	19.9	22.7	26.3	31.2	4.1
7.0	15.1	16.8	18.7	21.2	24.2	28.2	33.4	4.4
7.5	15.9	17.7	19.9	22.5	25.9	30.1	35.7	4.8
8.0	16.7	18.7	21.1	24.0	27.6	32.2	38.1	5.2
8.5	17.5	19.7	22.3	25.5	29.5	34.4	40.7	6.4
9.0	18.5	20.9	23.7	27.2	31.5	36.7	43.4	6.4
9.5	19.5	22.1	25.3	29.0	33.6	39.3	46.3	6.9
10.0	20.7	23.5	26.9	31.0	36.0	42.0	49.4	7.7
10.5	22.0	25.1	28.8	33.2	38.4	44.8	52.6	8.3
11.0	23.3	26.7	30.7	35.4	41.0	47.7	55.9	8.5
11.5	24.8	28.4	32.6	37.6	43.6	50.6	59.1	9.1
12.0	26.2	30.0	34.5	39.8	46.0	53.4	62.1	9.0
12.5	27.6	31.6	36.3	41.8	48.2	55.8	64.8	9.7
13.0	28.9	33.1	37.9	43.6	50.2	57.9	67.1	9.4
13.5	30.2	34.4	39.4	45.1	51.8	59.7	69.0	9.8
14.0	31.3	35.6	40.6	46.4	53.2	61.1	70.4	9.6
15.0	33.1	37.5	42.5	48.4	55.1	62.9	72.1	9.6
16.0	34.7	39.1	44.0	49.7	56.3	64.0	72.8	8.7
17.0	36.2	40.5	45.3	50.9	57.3	64.7	73.3	8.8
18.0	37.6	41.8	46.6	52.0	58.2	65.3	73.5	10.2

Source: IAP Growth Charts Committee. Indian Pediatrics 2015;52:47–55.

Table 5.15: Height (cm) centiles and standard deviation for boys (5–18 years): IAP Growth Charts 2015

Age (y)	Percentiles							
	3	10	25	50	75	90	97	SD
5.0	99.0	102.3	105.6	108.9	112.4	115.9	119.4	5.7
5.5	101.6	105.0	108.4	111.9	115.4	119.0	122.7	5.3
6.0	104.2	107.7	111.2	114.8	118.5	122.2	126.0	5.6
6.5	106.8	110.4	114.0	117.8	121.6	125.4	129.3	5.5
7.0	109.3	113.0	116.8	120.7	124.6	128.6	132.6	5.9
7.5	111.8	115.7	119.6	123.5	127.6	131.7	135.9	5.7
8.0	114.3	118.2	122.3	126.4	130.5	134.8	139.1	6.3
8.5	116.7	120.8	124.9	129.1	133.4	137.8	142.2	6.1
9.0	119.0	123.2	127.5	131.8	136.3	140.7	145.3	6.4
9.5	121.3	125.6	130.0	134.5	139.1	143.7	148.3	6.4
10.0	123.6	128.1	132.6	137.2	141.9	146.6	151.4	6.8
10.5	125.9	130.5	135.2	139.9	144.7	149.5	154.4	6.5
11.0	128.2	133.0	137.8	142.7	147.6	152.5	157.5	7.6
11.5	130.7	135.6	140.6	145.5	150.5	155.6	160.6	7.3
12.0	133.2	138.3	143.3	148.4	153.5	158.6	163.7	8.1
12.5	135.7	141.0	146.2	151.4	156.5	161.7	166.8	7.9
13.0	138.3	143.7	149.0	154.3	159.5	164.7	169.9	9.0
13.5	140.9	146.4	151.8	157.2	162.4	167.6	172.7	8.4
14.0	143.4	149.0	154.5	159.9	165.1	170.3	175.4	9.0
15.0	148.0	153.7	159.2	164.5	169.7	174.8	179.7	7.9
16.0	151.8	157.4	162.9	168.1	173.1	178.0	182.7	7.2
17.0	155.0	160.6	165.9	171.0	175.8	180.4	184.8	6.9
18.0	158.1	163.6	168.7	173.6	178.2	182.5	186.7	6.9

Table 5.16: Height (cm) centiles and standard deviations for girls (5–18 years): IAP Growth Charts 2015

Age (y)	Percentiles							
	3	10	25	50	75	90	97	SD
5.0	97.2	100.5	103.9	107.5	111.3	115.2	119.3	5.4
5.5	99.8	103.2	106.8	110.5	114.4	118.3	122.5	5.7
6.0	102.3	106.0	109.7	113.5	117.4	121.5	125.6	5.8
6.5	104.9	108.7	112.5	116.5	120.5	124.6	128.7	5.5
7.0	107.4	111.4	115.4	119.4	123.5	127.7	131.9	6.1
7.5	110.0	114.1	118.2	122.4	126.6	130.8	135.0	6.0
8.0	112.6	116.8	121.1	125.4	129.6	133.9	138.1	6.2
8.5	115.2	119.6	124.0	128.4	132.7	137.0	141.3	6.8
9.0	117.8	122.4	126.9	131.4	135.8	140.2	144.5	6.9
9.5	120.5	125.2	129.9	134.4	138.9	143.3	147.6	6.6
10.0	123.3	128.1	132.8	137.4	142.0	146.4	150.8	7.8
10.5	126.1	130.9	135.7	140.4	145.0	149.5	153.9	7.3
11.0	128.8	133.7	138.6	143.3	147.9	152.4	156.8	7.9
11.5	131.5	136.4	141.2	145.9	150.6	155.1	159.6	7.1
12.0	134.0	138.9	143.7	148.4	153.0	157.5	162.0	7.0
12.5	136.3	141.1	145.8	150.5	155.1	159.6	164.1	6.7
13.0	138.2	142.9	147.6	152.2	156.8	161.3	165.9	6.9
13.5	139.9	144.5	149.1	153.6	158.2	162.7	167.2	6.0
14.0	141.3	145.8	150.2	154.7	159.2	163.7	168.2	6.6
15.0	143.3	147.5	151.8	156.1	160.5	165.0	169.5	6.6
16.0	144.7	148.6	152.7	156.9	161.2	165.6	170.1	6.1
17.0	145.7	149.5	153.4	157.4	161.6	165.9	170.4	6.5
18.0	146.6	150.2	153.9	157.8	161.9	166.1	170.6	6.6

Source: IAP Growth Charts Committee. Indian Pediatrics 2015;52:47–55

Table 5.17: Extended Indian Academy of Pediatrics (IAP) Body Mass Index (BMI) Chart Percentiles for Boys Aged 5–18 Years

Age (y)	3rd	10th	25th	50th	Overweight (23 adult equivalent)	Obesity (27 adult equivalent)	Class 2 obesity (≥120% to <140% of 27 adult equivalent)	Class 3 obesity (≥140% of 27 adult equivalent)
5	12.1	12.8	13.6	14.7	15.7	18.3	21.9	25.6
5.5	12.2	12.9	13.7	14.8	15.8	18.4	22.1	25.8
6	12.2	12.9	13.7	14.9	16.0	18.6	22.3	26.1
6.5	12.3	13.0	13.8	15.0	16.1	18.9	22.6	26.4
7	12.3	13.1	13.9	15.1	16.3	19.1	23.0	26.8
7.5	12.4	13.2	14.1	15.3	16.5	19.5	23.3	27.2
8	12.5	13.3	14.2	15.5	16.7	19.8	23.8	27.8
8.5	12.6	13.4	14.4	15.7	17.0	20.2	24.3	28.3
9	12.7	13.5	14.5	15.9	17.3	20.7	24.8	29.0
9.5	12.8	13.7	14.7	16.2	17.6	21.2	25.4	29.7
10	12.9	13.8	14.9	16.4	18.0	21.7	26.1	30.4
10.5	13.0	14.0	15.1	16.7	18.3	22.3	26.7	31.2
11	13.1	14.1	15.4	17.0	18.7	22.8	27.4	32.0
11.5	13.2	14.3	15.6	17.3	19.1	23.4	28.1	32.8
12	13.3	14.5	15.8	17.7	19.5	24.0	28.7	33.5
12.5	13.5	14.6	16.0	17.9	19.8	24.5	29.4	34.2
13	13.6	14.8	16.3	18.2	20.2	24.9	29.9	34.9
13.5	13.7	14.9	16.5	18.5	20.5	25.3	30.4	35.5
14	13.8	15.1	16.7	18.7	20.8	25.7	30.8	36.0
14.5	14.0	15.3	16.9	19.0	21.1	26.0	31.3	36.5
15	14.2	15.5	17.2	19.3	21.4	26.4	31.7	36.9
15.5	14.4	15.8	17.4	19.6	21.7	26.7	32.0	37.4
16	14.6	16.0	17.7	19.9	22.0	27.0	32.4	37.8
16.5	14.9	16.3	18.0	20.2	22.4	27.3	32.7	38.2
17	15.1	16.6	18.3	20.5	22.6	27.5	33.0	38.5
17.5	15.4	16.8	18.6	20.8	22.9	27.8	33.3	38.9
18	15.6	17.1	18.9	21.1	23.2	28.0	33.6	39.2

Source: Indian Pediatr 2023;60:1013–31

Table 5.18: Extended Indian Academy of Pediatrics (IAP) Body Mass Index (BMI) Chart Percentiles for Girls Aged 5–18 Years

Age (y)	3rd	10th	25th	50th	Overweight (23 adult equivalent)	Obesity (27 adult equivalent)	Class 2 obesity (≥120% to <140% of 27 adult equivalent)	Class 3 obesity (≥140% of 27 adult equivalent)
5	11.9	12.5	13.3	14.3	15.5	18.0	21.6	25.2
5.5	11.9	12.6	13.4	14.4	15.7	18.3	22.0	25.6
6	12.0	12.7	13.5	14.5	15.9	18.6	22.3	26.1
6.5	12.1	12.8	13.6	14.7	16.1	18.9	22.7	26.5
7	12.1	12.8	13.7	14.9	16.4	19.3	23.1	27.0
7.5	12.2	12.9	13.9	15.1	16.6	19.7	23.6	27.5
8	12.3	13.1	14.0	15.3	16.9	20.1	24.1	28.1
8.5	12.3	13.2	14.2	15.6	17.2	20.5	24.6	28.7
9	12.4	13.3	14.4	15.8	17.6	21.0	25.1	29.3
9.5	12.5	13.5	14.6	16.1	18.0	21.4	25.7	30.0
10	12.7	13.7	14.9	16.5	18.4	21.9	26.3	30.7
10.5	12.8	13.9	15.2	16.8	18.8	22.5	27.0	31.5
11	13.0	14.1	15.5	17.2	19.3	23.0	27.6	32.2
11.5	13.2	14.4	15.8	17.6	19.8	23.6	28.3	33.0
12	13.4	14.7	16.1	18.0	20.2	24.1	29.0	33.8
12.5	13.7	15.0	16.5	18.4	20.7	24.7	29.6	34.6
13	13.9	15.2	16.8	18.8	21.1	25.2	30.2	35.2
13.5	14.1	15.5	17.1	19.1	21.5	25.6	30.7	35.8
14	14.3	15.7	17.3	19.4	21.8	25.9	31.1	36.3
14.5	14.5	16.0	17.6	19.7	22.0	26.2	31.4	36.6
15	14.7	16.1	17.8	19.9	22.3	26.3	31.6	36.8
15.5	14.9	16.3	18.0	20.1	22.4	26.4	31.7	37.0
16	15.0	16.5	18.2	20.3	22.6	26.5	31.8	37.1
16.5	15.2	16.7	18.4	20.4	22.8	26.6	31.9	37.3
17	15.4	16.9	18.6	20.6	22.9	26.7	32.0	37.3
17.5	15.5	17.1	18.7	20.8	23.1	26.7	32.1	37.4
18	15.7	17.3	18.9	21.0	23.2	26.8	32.2	37.5

Source: Indian Pediatr 2023;60:1013–31

Chapter

6

Developmental Assessment

Monica Juneja Piyush Gupta

Structure

Development denotes maturation of functions or acquisition of new skills and is intimately related to maturation and myelination of central nervous system.

6.1 IMPORTANCE OF DEVELOPMENTAL ASSESSMENT

Developmental assessment is an essential component of comprehensive evaluation of any child. A thorough knowledge of normal development and acceptable variations is essential to identify early patterns that are pathological and may indicate developmental disability. This would help in instituting early effective intervention strategies.

A thorough developmental assessment becomes especially important in the following situations:

1. Follow-up of high-risk babies.
2. Early diagnosis of vision and hearing impairment.
3. Children with sucking or swallowing problems in the newborn period, delay in any field of development and/or any behavioral problems.
4. During follow-up of children with conditions that may cause brain damage, e.g. meningitis, status epilepticus, and metabolic disorders.
5. If the parents have any concerns regarding their child's development; there is a family history of developmental delay or neurological illness; or before adopting a child for excluding developmental disabilities.

Developmental assessment includes a detailed history with emphasis on pregnancy, delivery, neonatal period, and course of development. Special emphasis has to be laid on the following in the child:

- Ascertain the status of hearing, vision, and motor control.
- Note all the milestones and the time of their appearance till date.

In this chapter, we introduce you to the principles and procedures for assessing development of a child. The steps required for developmental assessment are outlined in **Key Box 1**.

Laws of Development

1. *Development is a continuous process from conception to maturity and is commensurate with maturation of neurological function*. For example, at birth, a child is not able to turn around, sit, reach for objects voluntarily, laugh, or interact using language. In due course of time, the child acquires all these functions.

Key Box 1

Steps in Assessment of Development

1. Obtain history of development.
2. Identify the tools needed for developmental assessment (depending on the age of the child).
3. Perform developmental assessment including that of vision and hearing.
4. Calculate the developmental quotient (DQ).
5. Interpret, whether the development in a given child is normal or abnormal.
6. If development is abnormal, classify as *developmental delay or developmental regression.*
7. If there is a developmental delay, categorize whether it is *global or dissociative* **(Fig. 6.1)**.

2. *Normal development requires an anatomically and functionally normal central nervous system and pathways.* A child with a morphologically abnormal CNS (e.g. anencephaly, meningomyelocele) or damaged neurons and pathways (e.g. following hypoxic or ischemic insult) is unlikely to have a normal development.

   Abnormal development may result from intrauterine and perinatal insults (perinatal asphyxia, bilirubin encephalopathy, etc.) or any insult to the brain during early childhood period (meningitis, CNS hemorrhage, etc.).
3. *Infant development occurs in an orderly and predictable sequence* that is intrinsically determined, i.e. from cephalic to caudal (head to toe) and proximal to distal. For example, head control develops before the child learns to sit and stand. A child can do much with his hands before he can walk. Upper extremities become increasingly accurate in reaching, grasping, and transferring (proximal development) before achievement of pincer grasp (distal development).
4. *Even though the sequence of development is predictable and same, the rate of development varies from child to child.* For example, a child has to learn to sit before he/she can stand; but the age of attainment of sitting and standing varies between children.
5. *Responses to stimuli change from generalized mass activity involving the whole body, as seen in newborn, to discrete voluntary actions that are under cortical control.* This allows the child to move from non-specific and symmetrical responses when attending to a stimulus (e.g. vocalization, kicking with both arms and legs) to voluntary, asymmetrical, precise responses towards the stimulus (e.g. grasping or use of specific word).
6. *Certain primitive reflexes have to be lost before voluntary functions are acquired.*
   - For example, grasp reflex has to be lost before the infant can learn to reach for objects and grasp them voluntarily.

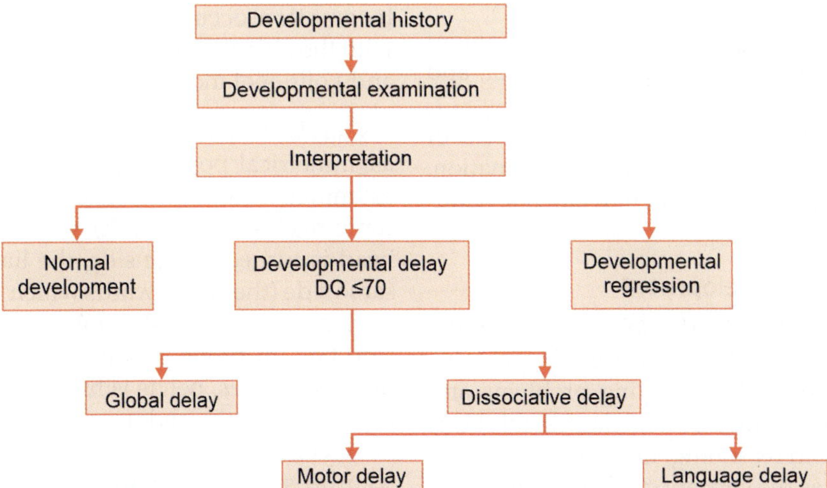

Fig. 6.1: Process of developmental assessment. Developmental delay (late achievement of certain functions) should be differentiated from developmental regression (loss of already acquired functions).

- Similarly, asymmetrical tonic neck reflex has to disappear before the infant learns to roll from back to front, bring the hands to midline, or reach for objects.
- Infant can gain progressive stability in a seated position only after disappearance of Moro reflex as this reflex interferes with head control and sitting equilibrium.

Persistence of primitive reflexes beyond the age at which they should disappear indicates and predicts abnormal development.

In the following sections, we will briefly review normal development, before proceeding to discussion on how to take a developmental history and conduct a developmental examination.

6.2 NORMAL DEVELOPMENT

Children accomplish maturation of different biological functions (level of development or **milestone**) at an anticipated age, with a margin of a few months on either side. For example, walking on her own is a major motor milestone in the life of a child. This is usually achieved at 12–13 months, but can vary from 10 to 15 months in different children.

Development is usually assessed in terms of achieving the milestones in the following domains:

1. Motor Development

Motor development depends on the maturation of muscular, skeletal, and nervous systems. It can be further classified into Gross Motor and Fine Motor domains.

- *Gross motor*—pertains to development of locomotion, general body control, and specific motor skills.
- *Fine motor*—pertains to development of finer body movements and coordination, i.e. grasping, fine hand movements, hand-eye coordination.

2. Cognitive Development

Cognition refers to the intellect or mental abilities of a child. This domain pertains to skills required for solving problems and learning new things through logical thinking, memory, and reasoning. In young children, it manifests as the concept of 'cause and effect', 'object permanence' and 'functional use of objects'.

3. Language Development

Development of the ability to communicate including comprehension (receptive language) and expression of language (expressive language).

4. Personal–Social Development

Child's personal reaction to other persons and his adjustment to domestic life, social groups, and community conventions.

5. Adaptive Development

Adaptive development refers to the ability of a child to use the information and skills acquired in the other domains in day-to-day functioning. As adaptive skills develop, the child's participation in personal care and daily routine increases. Also, his/her ability to adapt to a new environment or situation becomes better.

These major fields of child's development do not really belong to separate compartments. The child always reacts as an individual. Our categorical classification is simply for convenience and to facilitate observations and diagnostic analysis.

Tables 6.1 and **6.2** provide details of various milestones in all the developmental domains at various ages.

A. Motor Development

1. Gross Motor Development (Key Box 2)

As already discussed, development of locomotion occurs in an orderly sequence with the ultimate goal of gaining independent and volitional movements.

0–4 weeks: In first few weeks of life, flexed and asymmetrical postures predominate, due to asymmetric tonic neck reflex. In asymmetric tonic neck reflex (ATNR) when the baby's head is turned to one side, the limbs on the same side (the side towards which the head is turned) extend while the limbs on the opposite side flex. In prone position also, because of flexed postures, pelvis is high and knees are drawn under the abdomen. Because of poor neck control, there is no lifting of head in 'ventral suspension'; and there is complete head lag, when the baby is pulled to sitting position.

Table 6.1: Developmental milestones from birth to 6 months

Age	Supine	Pulled to sit	Gross motor				Fine motor	Adaptive/cognitive	Personal–social	Language
			Held sitting	Held standing	Prone	Ventral suspension				
4 weeks	ATNR at rest Arms and legs semiflexed	Complete head lag	Back rounded	Flops at hips and knees, walking reflex	Pelvis high, knees under abdomen	Head held up momentarily, elbows flexed, hips partially extended, knees flexed	Hands pre-dominantly closed, grasp reflex	Regards dangling object in line of vision (3 feet) in midline, follows 45° from midline on either side	Intent regard of mother's face	Quiets on hearing bell
6 weeks	ATNR intermittently	Considerable head lag	Intermittently holds head up	Head sags forward	Pelvis high, knees no longer under abdomen	Head held momentarily in plane of body	Hands often open	When supine, looks at objects in midline, follows it up to 90°	Smiles at mother in response to overtures	
8 weeks	Intermittent ATNR	Less head lag	Head held up but recurrently bobs forward, back less rounded	Holds head up, more than momentarily	Head mostly midline, lifts chin off couch ~45°	Head maintained in same plane as body	Hands frequently open, only slight grasp reflex	Fixation, convergence and focusing, follows moving person and dangling toy		Vocalizes when talked to
12 weeks	No more ATNR	Only slight head lag	Head mostly held up but still bobs forward	Partial weight bearing	Pelvis flat, head and shoulder off couch ~45–90°, weight borne on forearms	Head held up beyond plane of body	No grasp reflex, hands come together in midline while playing, brings hands to mouth, holds rattle transiently if placed in hand	Hand regard, binocular vision, promptly looks at object in midline, follows dangling toy from side-to-side ~180°, discriminates between colors	Recognizes mother	Turns head to sound, squeals with pleasure
16 weeks	Head in midline	Only slight head lag in beginning	Head held up but wobbles if swayed		Head and chest off the couch, plane of face ~90° to couch, limb stretched out		Tries to reach but overshoots objects. Plays with rattle, if placed in hand but cannot pick it up, if dropped	Immediately regards dangling objects, excited on seeing food, toys and shows pleasure by massive response	Smiles spontaneously at pleasurable sight/sound	Laughs aloud

Contd...

Table 6.1: Developmental milestones from birth to 6 months (*Contd...*)

Age	Supine	Pulled to sit	Gross motor				Fine motor	Adaptive/cognitive	Personal–social	Language
			Held sitting	Held standing	Prone	Ventral suspension				
20 weeks	Feet to mouth	No head lag	Back straight, no head wobble	Bears most of weight	Weight on forearms, rolls prone to supine		Voluntary grasp with accurate reaching, recovers rattle, if dropped **Cubes**—bidextrous approach	Mouthing no more hand regard	Smiles at mirror image	Razzing *Ah-goo*
24 weeks	Lifts head off the couch when about to be pulled up, rolls supine to prone		Sits supported in high chair (supported sitting)	Bears full weight on legs	Bears weight on hands, chest and upper abdomen off the couch		**Cubes**—unidextrous approach, ulnar palmar grasp, transfers cube from hand-to-hand, drops one cube when another offered, lifts cup by handle	Looks for dropped toy	Smiles and vocalizes at mirror images, stranger anxiety (beginning), drinks from cup when held to lips Imitates cough, displeasure at removal of toy, feeds self-finger foods Starts enjoying peek-a-boo	Mono-syllables—*ma, da, na*

Table 6.2: Developmental milestones from 6 months to 5 years

Age	Gross motor	Fine motor	Adaptive/cognitive	Personal–social	Language
28 weeks	Spontaneously lifts head off couch. Sitting with support (using own hands for support). Bears weight on one hand	**Cubes**–radial palmar grasp retains first cube when second offered	Explores different aspects of toys. Finds partially hidden objects. Observes cube in each hand	Imitates simple acts, e.g. tongue protrusion	Responds to name
32 weeks	Sits momentarily without support. Creeping/ commando crawling	Scissor grasp	Reaches persistently for toys out of reach	Engages in gaze monitoring, i.e. child follows adult's glance with own eyes	Imitates sound already in repertoire. Combines syllables—*da-da, ba-ba*
36 weeks	Sits steadily. Leans forwards and recovers balance. Pulls self to stand. Stands holding on to furniture.	**Cubes**–compares 2 cubes by bringing together **Pellet**–pincer grasp		Separation anxiety. Follows finger point	*Dada, mama* inappropriately
40 weeks	Crawling Pulls self to sitting position Cruises around furniture using 2 hands, walks with two hands held	Index finger approach **Cubes**–releases cubes	Responds to no	Waves bye-bye. Plays pat-a-cake. Pulls clothes to attract attention. Repeats performance laughed at	Responds to simple words. Uses *mama, dada* appropriately
48 weeks	Pivots while sitting. Cruises around furniture using one hand. Walks with one hand-held. Stands alone for a few seconds	Throws objects. Stirs with spoon	Releases toy to examiner. Finds toy under cup. Looks at picture in book. Gives toys to adult, for repeat demonstration	Cooperates with dressing	Imitates sound of dog, cow. Shakes head for no One word with meaning other than *mama, dada*
1 year	Stands well. Independent 2–3 steps	Casting **Pencil**–imitates scribbling **Cubes**–tower of 2 cubes	Mouthing and drooling stopped. Puts objects in and out of container	Proto imperative pointing	Speaks 2–3 words with meaning. Follows one step command with gesture
15 months	Gets into standing position without support. Stoops to pick up toys. Kneels without support. Creeps upstairs. Climbs on furniture	**Pencil**–spontaneous scribbling **Cubes**–builds 3 cubes tower **Pellet**–releases pellet into bottle	**Simple formboard**–inserts round block **Book**–turns pages 2–3 at a time **Body parts**–points to one	**Feeding**–manages cup well Uses spoon with spilling **Sphincter control**–indicates wet pants protodeclarative pointing starts (pointing at objects to express interest) Shows empathy, hugs adult in reciprocation	Speaks 3–5 words with meaning, follows one step command without gesture, e.g. getting objects from another room, Jargoning

Contd...

6

Developmental Assessment

Table 6.2: Developmental milestones from 6 months to 5 years (*Contd...*)

Age	Gross motor	Fine motor	Adaptive/cognitive	Personal–social	Language
18 months	Walks pulling toys Walks backward Runs stiffly Walks upstairs One hand-held Creeps downstairs Seats self on chair Throws ball without falling	**Pencil**–imitates vertical stroke **Cubes**–tower of 4 cubes	**Formboard**–inserts circle after it has been turned (usually with trial and error) **Book**–turns pages singly **Picture cards**–points to 1–2 objects Names one common object **Body parts**–points to 2–3, points to self and familiar people when named	**Feeding**–manages spoon well without rotation **Dressing**–takes off socks/unzips **Play**–domestic mimicry **Sphincter control**–dry by day with an occasional accident Begins to show shame when does something wrong	Understands mine Uses 10–25 words
24 months	Runs well, walks upstairs and downstairs holding rail both feet on each step. Kicks ball without falling Throws overhead	**Pencil**–imitates horizontal and circular stroke **Cubes**–tower of 6 cubes, imitates train of cubes without adding chimney Turns door knobs Unscrews lids	**Formboard**–places square (20 months) Completes at 2 years **Picture cards**–points to 5, names 3 **Body parts**–points to 4–6 objects, matches objects to pictures, shows use of familiar object	**Feeding**–sucks through a straw **Dressing**–pulls off pants, takes off clothes without button **Play**–parallel play **Sphincter control**–dry at night, if lifted out in evening	Begins to understand her/him/mine Follows 2-step command Says 2-word sentences Refers to self with name Uses 50+ words
30 months	Jumps on both feet Walks on tiptoes when asked	**Cubes**–tower of 8 cubes, imitates train and adds chimney Strings large beads awkwardly	**Formboard**–replaces all 3 shapes after it has been rotated (no trial and error) **Picture cards**–points to seven and names 5 pictures. Points to small details in pictures **Colors**–names 1, matches shapes and colors **Digit span**–repeats 2, one of three trials	**Dressing**–pulls pants up with assistance **Sphincter control**–attends to toilet need without help except for washing Washes hands Brushes teeth with assistance	Starts using pronouns, Echolalia and jargoning disappear, Follows two prepositions, Understands actions words: playing . . . coming . . .
3 years	Synchronous gait Stands on one foot for 3 seconds Walks upstairs alternating feet Pedals tricycle Catches ball with stiff arm	**Pencil**–copies circle **Cubes**–tower of 9–10 cubes, imitates bridge **Scissors**–cuts with scissors awkwardly Strings small beads well	**Goodenough test**–draws 2–3 parts person **Incomplete man**–adds 1–2 parts **Body parts**–Points to body parts based on function **Picture cards**–names 8–10 pictures, **Colors**–names 2 colors **Digit span**–repeats 3, one of three trials Understands long/short, big/small, more/less Knows gender and age	**Dressing**–dresses, undresses fully, if helped with buttons **Play**–joins in play Begins to take turns Starts to share Imaginative play Pours liquid from one container to other, tries to help with household tasks	Three-word sentences, uses pronouns correctly, uses plurals

Contd...

Table 6.2: Developmental milestones from 6 months to 5 years (*Contd...*)

Age	Gross motor	Fine motor	Adaptive/cognitive	Personal–social	Language
4 years	Balances on one foot for 4–8 seconds Goes downstairs alternating feet Hops on one foot 2–3 times Catches bounced ball (4.5 years)	**Pencil**–copies cross **Cubes**–imitates gate **Scissors**–cuts circle	**Goodenough test**–draws a 4–6 part person **Incomplete man**–adds 3 parts **Colors**–names 5–6 **Digit span**–repeats 3 Three of three trials **Number concept**–till 4 Reads several common signs/store names on the road Right–left discrimination	**Feeding**–uses fork Dressing–buttons **Play**–group play, has a preferred friend **Sphincter control**—goes to toilet alone Washes after bowel movement Brushes teeth alone	4-word sentences, understands adjectives: long, thin, follows 3-step command, Tells stories, Labels happiness, sadness, fear and anger in self, 100% intelligibility
5 years	Skips Running broad jump (2–3 feet) Jumps backward	**Pencil**–copies square (4.5 years) and triangle **Cubes**–copies gate (4.5 years)	**Goodenough test**–draws 8–10 parts person **Incomplete man**–adds 6–7 parts **Colors**–names 10 colors **Digit span**–repeats 4, two of three trials **Number concept**–till 10 Rote counting till 10 Identifies coins Names letters/numerals out of order Compares 2 weight	Independent dressing Bathes independently Has group of friends	5–8-word sentence knows telephone number responds to "why" questions Retells story with clear beginning, middle and end

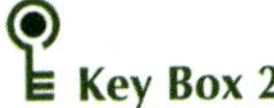

Key Box 2

Gross Motor Developmental Milestones

5 months	Head control is complete
6 months	Rolls prone to supine
7 months	Rolls supine to prone, sits without support for a few minutes
8 months	Creeping/commando crawling, sits without support
9–10 months	Crawls, sits up from supine
10–11 months	Pivots, cruises
12 months	Walks with one hand held
13 months	Walks without support
18 months	Runs stiffly, walks backwards
2 years	Walks upstairs with 2 feet per step, runs well, comes downstairs (two feet per step)
2½ years	Jumps on both feet
3 years	Walks upstairs with feet on alternating steps, rides a tricycle
4 years	Comes downstairs (alternating steps), hops/skips on one foot 2–3 times
5 years	Skips with both feet, jumps backwards

Gradually, the extensor muscles gain strength, head control develops, primitive reflexes disappear, and symmetric posture begins to predominate. Therefore, if the same infant is examined at 4 weeks, chin is lifted up momentarily and there is some intermittent partial extension of hips and knees in prone position.

1–6 months

- By 8 weeks, head is mostly in the midline and chin is lifted off the couch intermittently (so that the plane of face is at an angle of 45° to the couch) in prone position. In the position of ventral suspension, baby maintains the head in the plane of rest of the body.
- By 12 weeks, there is no more asymmetrical tonic neck reflex attitude in supine position. In prone position, pelvis is flat, legs are fully extended, chin and shoulders are lifted off the couch with weight borne on forearms. Developing head control is seen in ventral suspension as well whereby head is lifted

6

Developmental Assessment

and maintained well beyond the plane of the body.

- By 20 weeks, the head control is complete so that when held sitting, there is no head wobble even if the infant is swayed.
- By 9 months infant can stand holding on to furniture. Around 11 months the child starts to cruise, i.e. walk holding on to furniture.

This evolution in gross motor development (in supine position, in position of ventral suspension, by placing the infant in prone position, by pulling him to sitting position and holding him in standing position) is described in detail in section on developmental assessment.

6 months–1 year: Gross motor development proceeds from sitting to standing and achievement of ambulation. Initially, infant moves with abdomen on the ground (creeping/commando crawling; 8 months). Thereafter, he crawls (on hands and knees with abdomen off the ground; 9 months). Though the terms creeping and crawling are used synonymously in English literature, term crawling is used in general sense, when the baby moves with abdomen off the ground. So, we have retained the above terminology.

Later, infant stands and walks (with support, followed by without support). By 9 months infant can stand holding on to furniture. Around 11 months the child starts to cruise, i.e. walk holding on to furniture.

1–3 years: There is further refinement in balance, co-ordination, speed and strength.

Initially when the toddler learns to walk, he walks with a wide based gait with arms abducted and slightly elevated with steps of unequal length and direction.

Movements gradually smoothen, base narrows, arm swing evolves, and adult pattern of walking is achieved by 3 years of age.

3–6 years: Milestones evolve in the form of progress in the length of time, number of repetitions, or the distance, each task can be performed successfully.

2. *Fine Motor Development* (Key Box 3)

Fine motor skills are related to the use of upper limbs for exploring the environment. They are necessary for the child to perform self-help tasks, to play, and for progress in cognitive development (via exploration of objects).

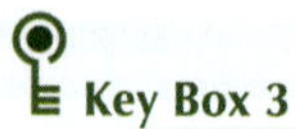

Key Box 3

Fine Motor Developmental Milestones

Age	Milestone
3 months	Opens hand spontaneously, holds objects when given in hand
4 months	Tries to reach for objects, overshooting
5 months	Reaches objects; bidextrous approach, ulnar palmar grasp, voluntary release (clumsily)
6 months	Unidextrous approach, transfers objects from hand-to-hand
7 months	Radial palmar grasp
8 months	Finger-thumb scissors grasp
9–10 months	Mature grasp, voluntary release (mature)
10–11 months	Pincer grasp
12 months	Tower of 2 cubes, casting, imitates scribbling
15 months	Tower of 3 cubes, scribbles, releases pellet into bottle
18 months	Tower of 4 cubes, imitates vertical stroke
2 years	Tower of 6 cubes, imitates horizontal stroke and circle, imitates train no chimney, turns door knobs
2½ years	Tower of 8 cubes, imitates train, adds chimney
3 years	Tower of 9–10 cubes, copies circle, imitates bridge
4 years	Copies cross, imitates gate
4½ years	Copies square, triangle, and gate

In initial few months, upper extremities are used for balance and mobility, e.g. rolling, sitting with support, pulling up to stand, and crawling. But as the gross motor development proceeds and infant becomes stable in upright position, hands are available for more purposeful exploration of objects. Thus, in the first year of life, there is a close association between gross and fine motor development that evolves into a similar relationship between fine motor and adaptive/cognitive domain.

In the second year of life, infant learns to use objects as tools for functional play.

0–3 months: In first few weeks of life, hands of baby are predominantly closed with a strong grasp reflex. Gradually, grasp reflex becomes weak and disappears by 12 weeks of life. So, in first 3 months of life, infants grasp the objects with eyes, i.e. look at objects as if they would like to grasp it and by 12 weeks will hold the object when given in hand.

3–6 months: Gradually, hands come together in midline while playing and baby tries to reach for objects clumsily, overshooting the mark (16 weeks). Thereafter, he is able to approach objects voluntarily, initially using the entire palm towards the ulnar side (ulnar palmar grasp) and with a bidextrous approach towards the objects (using both hands, 5 months) followed by unidextrous approach (6 months).

At the same time, infants learn to release objects voluntarily. Voluntary release is seen as the infant learns to transfer objects from one hand to the other, first using the mouth as an intermediate stage (5 months) and then directly hand-to-hand (6 months).

6–12 months: Grasp matures progressively from ulnar grasp (5 months: Cube grasped in the palm of hand on the ulnar side) to radial grasp (7 months: Cube held against the thenar eminence at the base of thumb) to finger-thumb scissors grasp (8 months: Index finger with the help of ring and little finger presses cube against the base of thumb), and finally to mature grasp (9–10 months: Cube held between distal volar pads of thumb and fingertips).

At 6 months, if baby is given one cube after the other, he drops the first one but by 7 months, he retains the first cube when second is offered. By 7 months, the child compares the cubes by bringing them together. Pincer grasp, i.e. picking up a crumble between index finger and thumb, comes at about 10 months. Voluntary release which is awkward at first (with all fingers extended) also becomes more accurate so that by 10 months of age as the infant starts to learn concept of object permanence, he enjoys releasing a cube into a container/dropping things on to the floor. By this time, intrinsic muscle control has developed considerably to allow the isolation of the index finger; and infant uses index finger approach to pry and palpate the objects and poke their fingers into small holes for exploration. By 12 months of age, most infants enjoy putting things into containers and dumping them out repeatedly.

After 1 year: As the infant moves into second year of life, mastery of skills of grasp and release achieved in first year of life allows him to use objects as tools and fine motor development becomes more closely associated with adaptive/cognitive development. The infant knows both what he wants to do and how he wants to do that. By 15 months of age, further accuracy of voluntary release enables him to stack 3–4 blocks and release small objects into containers. He starts to adjust objects after grasping to use them properly, e.g. picking up a crayon and adjusting it to scribble spontaneously (18 months of age) and adjusting a spoon to use it consistently for eating (20 months of age). Further refinements continue to occur allowing the toddler to draw, explore, problem-solve, create, and perform self-help tasks.

B. Cognitive Development

Cognitive development along with adaptive skills are the foundations of intelligence. Intelligence is defined as the ability to learn or deal with new situations **(Key Box 4)**.

In initial few weeks of life, infant explores the environment visually. Initially, he follows faces and then objects. After gaining better control of arms and hands, he starts batting at and then reaching for objects. At first, objects are brought to the mouth for oral exploration. Later, the infant visually examines an object held in one hand while manipulating it with the other. With maturation of vision, infant can focus on small objects by about 5 months of age.

By 1 year, this ability to focus on small objects combined with newly developed pincer grasp and index finger isolation allows the child to explore the objects by poking and the infant becomes successful in discovering how they work (e.g. fingering the clapper of the bell). Mouthing becomes less appealing.

As cognitive abilities continue to progress, infant learns to shift attention between two objects, compare, make choices, discard or combine objects. With maturation of concept of causality and object permanence, infant

Key Box 4

Adaptive/Cognitive Developmental Milestones

4 weeks	Follows red ring by 45°
6 weeks	Follows up to 90°
8 weeks	Follows moving person
3 months	Hand regard, follows to 180°
4 months	Excited on seeing food, toys; shows pleasure by massive response
5 months	Mouthing, no hand regards
6 months	Looks for dropped toy
7 months	Observes cubes in each hand, finds partially hidden objects
8 months	Reaches for toys out of reach
10 months	Responds to 'No'
11 months	Looks at picture in book, finds toys, under the cup
1 year	Mouthing and drooling stops, puts objects in and out of container
15 months	Turns 2–3 pages at a time
1½ years	Turns 1 page at a time, names one common object
2 years	Points at 4–6 body parts, sorts objects
2½ years	Names 1 color, matches shape/colors
3 years	Names 2 colors, knows gender and age
4 years	Names 5–6 colors, right–left discrimination
5 years	Counts till 10, names 10 colors, identifies coins

learns how his actions produce certain effects, how to repeat these actions to get the same effects and later how to vary the action to produce a novel effect. He looks for dropped objects and later for hidden objects. *Thus, the child moves on from 'learning to manipulate' to 'manipulate to learn'.*

C. Language Development (Key Box 5)

Language refers to the expression of thoughts and ideas. It includes both receptive and expressive languages.

- *Receptive language* is ability to understand what is being said.
- *Expressive language* refers to the ability to make thoughts, ideas known to others through speech, gestures, and facial expressions.

Key Box 5

Language Developmental Milestones

4 weeks	Quieting on sound of bell
2–3 months	Turns head to sound, begins vocalization
4 months	Laughs aloud, says *Ah-goo*
6–7 months	Monosyllables
8–9 months	Bisyllables
9–10 months	Imitates sounds, responds to No
10–11 months	First word with meaning
1 year	2–3 words with meaning
1½ years	Vocabulary of 10 words
2 years	Says 2 words sentence, uses 50+ words
3 years	3 words sentences
4 years	4 words sentences, tells stories
5 years	5–8 words sentences, knows telephone number.

Receptive Language

Infant shows receptive language skills at birth. He shows preference for voices.

- At 4 weeks, infant is heedful of sound and quietens on sound of bell and by 12 weeks starts turning head to sound.
- Afterwards, receptive language ability is shown by response to name (7 months), response to 'No' (10 months), and obeying of simple order (Give it to me).
- By 12–15 months, he can point to familiar objects and body parts.

Thereafter, growing receptive ability is shown by ever increasing understanding of words, following simple and then complex instructions, and understanding most of what is being said.

Expressive Language

Initial expressive language consists of musical-like vowel sounds (cooing). At about 3 months, the infant begins vocalizing immediately upon hearing an adult speak and talks a great deal when spoken to; he holds long conversations with his mother by 12–16 weeks (to and fro vocalization). By 16 weeks, he laughs aloud, squeals with pleasure and begins to say *ng, Ah-goo*. By 20 weeks, he enjoys razzing (i.e. blowing between partially closed lips) and imitates coughing and tongue protrusion. This is followed by monosyllables (*ba/da/ga*; 6–7 months) and bisyllables (8–9 months).

By this time, he vocalizes with many high and low pitched tones and vocalizes cough to attract attention. At 9–10 months, he starts imitating sounds.

First meaningful word, i.e. use of mono-/bi-syllables with a specific meaning for the child (e.g. saying mama only for referring to mother is a meaningful word which otherwise is a bisyllable), is spoken by 10–11 months.

After 1 year of age: By 12–13 months, he is saying 2–3 words with meaning and starts pointing at objects to communicate a request. Jargoning, speaking in an unintelligible language of his own, with modulations and phrasing, but only an occasional intelligible word, starts between 15 and 18 months.

There is an exponential gain in language 18 months onwards. An 18-month-old toddler boasts of a vocabulary of 10 different words. He repeats things said to him 21 months onwards and begins to join words other than in imitation by 21–24 months. Jargoning usually disappears. He starts using pronouns in order of mine, me, you and I in that order, though he is much more prone to call himself by his name rather than using I. He talks incessantly.

A 3-year-old is constantly asking questions, many of which seem meaningless and answers to these he already knows.

Questioning is at its peak at 4 years. Why and how frequently appear in questions and now he tells tall stories.

At 5, speech is much more mature. Language is now essentially complete in structure and form. He uses all types of sentences including complex sentences with hypothetical and conditional clauses.

Clarity of speech: Assessment of clarity of speech is also an important component of language assessment. While assessing speech clarity, it should be assessed whether the child is speaking as distinctly as expected of his age. Ability to pronounce words improves with age so that by 2 years of age, at least 50% of the speech is understandable to a stranger. At 3 years of age, 75% is understandable and by 4 to 5 years of age, speech is completely understandable to strangers. Lisping should disappear at 4 years of age. Slight stuttering may be present at 2–3 years of age, but if it is severe and persistent, referral to speech therapist is warranted.

D. Personal–Social Development (Key Box 6)

0–3 months

- A 4-week-old infant fixates on a face that bends over into his line of vision. This brief intent regard is the chief token of his social interest at this age. Infants soothe down when picked in lap and if snugly and warmly wrapped.
- By 6 weeks, infant begins to smile in response to overtures (social smile).
- By 3 months, infant shows considerable interest in the surroundings, engages in to and fro vocalization, watches movement of people in the room and may refuse to be left alone. He starts recognizing his mother and other familiar attendants and turns head to sound.

6 months–1 year: At 6 months, he smiles and then vocalizes at his mirror image. While lying

Key Box 6

Personal–Social Developmental Milestones

4 weeks	Fixates on a face for a brief moment
6 weeks	Starts smiling at mother
3 months	Recognizes mother, takes considerable interest in surroundings
5–6 months	Smiles/vocalizes at mirror image
6–7 months	Enjoys Peak-a-boo, responds to name
7–8 months	Imitates simple acts, gaze monitoring
8–9 months	Stranger anxiety
10 months	Waves bye-bye, plays pat-a-cake
11 months	Cooperates with dressing
1 year	Helps to dress
15 months	Uses spoon with spilling
1½ years	Takes off socks, dry by day
2 years	Sucks through a straw, pulls off pants, dry at night
2½ years	Washes hands, brushes teeth
3 years	Dress, undresses fully, if helped with buttons
4 years	Uses fork, goes to toilet alone
5 years	Independent dressing and bathing

down, he stretches his arms out on seeing that his mother is going to lift him up. He shows displeasure at removal of toy, starts imitating simple actions such as tongue protrusion and coughing and even tries to establish contact by coughing. A month later, he starts enjoying peek-a-boo, responds to his name, and starts differentiating unfamiliar and familiar people *(stranger anxiety)*. Between 10 and 12 months, he responds to words, e.g. 'Where is Papa' and repeats performances laughed at.

By 1 year, he helps to dress, begins to anticipate movement in nursery rhymes, starts showing interest in books, takes vocal and other means to elicit attention, and displays considerable perceptiveness of emotions of others.

Joint attention (process whereby an infant and caregiver share an experience) is the quintessential social milestone that develops towards the end of the first year after birth. The earliest demonstration of joint attention occurs around 8 months of age, when an infant follows a caregiver's gaze and looks in the same direction. By 10 months, he starts imitating pat-a-cake and bye bye.

After 1 year: Between 12 and 14 months, children begin to point to request something (*proto-imperative pointing*), and they usually integrate this pointing with eye contact directed between the object of interest and the caregiver, sometimes accompanied by a verbal utterance. This is followed by *proto-declarative pointing* by 16 months of age, characterized by the child pointing at something merely to indicate interest, usually accompanied by eye contact directed between the object and the caregiver. By 18 months, he brings objects or toys to his caregivers to show them or to share the experience.

Play skills: Play skills also follow a specific developmental course.

- By 18 months, child engages in *simple pretend play*, e.g. pretending to talk on a toy phone, pretending mother in domestic duties, e.g. dusting, cleaning, wiping (*domestic mimicry*).
- Two-year-old engages in *parallel play* (plays next to another child, but not with him, frequently looking at and imitating his actions) as he has not yet mastered the skill of cooperation.
- After his second birthday, the child begins to play with others of his own age. As a thumb rule, a child can play effectively only in groups of children in the same number as his age in years. Thus, a 2-year-old can play well only with one other child.
- By 30 months, the child uses *complex pretend play*, such as using generic items to represent other objects. A block may be used as a table in one scenario and a phone in another. By age of 3 years, a child is able to initiate a cooperative play with one or two peers, taking turns and having joint goals.
- 4-year-olds are able to play effectively with up to three other kids, become interested in tricking others, and concerned about being tricked themselves.
- By age 5, children have learned many adult social skills, their imaginative play is increasingly more complex, and they love to dress up and act out their fantasies.

E. Adaptive Development

Adaptive development includes self care skills (such as feeding, dressing, drinking independently, bathing and toilet training); assuming responsibility for oneself (putting away toys, avoiding dangers) and adapting to different environments or situations on a daily basis. This entails appropriate utilization of usual skills acquired in cognitive, communication, socio-personal and fine motor domains. Thus evaluation of adaptive domain, entails assessment of these skills in the child's daily repertoire.

6.3 HISTORY OF DEVELOPMENT

A. Timing of Developmental Assessment

Developmental surveillance, i.e. observing emergence of abilities in a child over a period of time, should be part of every well child visit (e.g. during routine immunization). During these visits, the pediatrician should monitor the development of child and be watchful for *Developmental Red Flags*. 'Developmental Red Flags' in each of the developmental domains are listed in **Table 6.3**. If any of these Red Flags is discovered, a thorough developmental screening is warranted and child should be referred for detailed evaluation **(Fig. 6.2)**.

Table 6.3: Red flag signs suggestive of developmental delay

Age	Red flag
Motor development	
1–2 months	Early rolling
3 months	Persistent fisting
4 months	Lack of steady head control while sitting
9 months	Inability to sit
18 months	Inability to walk independently
Prior to 18 months	Hand dominance
Any age	Scissoring, frog-leg posture, W sitting, bunny hopping
Adaptive/cognitive development	
2 months	Lack of fixation
4 months	Lack of visual tracking
6 months	Failure to turn to sound or voice
Language development	
6 months	Failure to turn to sound or voice
9 months	Lack of babbling consonant sounds
18 months	Does not use single words such as *mama, papa, dada*
24 months	Lack of words and two-word meaningful sentences; inability to follow simple commands
36 months	Failure to speak in three-word sentences
Personal–social development	
6 months	Lack of smiles or other joyful expressions
9 months	Lack of reciprocal (back-and-forth sharing of) vocalizations, smiles, or other facial expressions
12 months	Failure to respond to name when called, absence of babbling, lack of reciprocal gestures (showing, reaching, waving)
15 months	Lack of proto-imperative pointing (point to desired objects)
18 months	Lack of proto-declarative pointing (point to show interest) or showing gestures
24 months	Lack of simple pretend play
Any age	Loss of previously acquired babbling, speech, or social skills

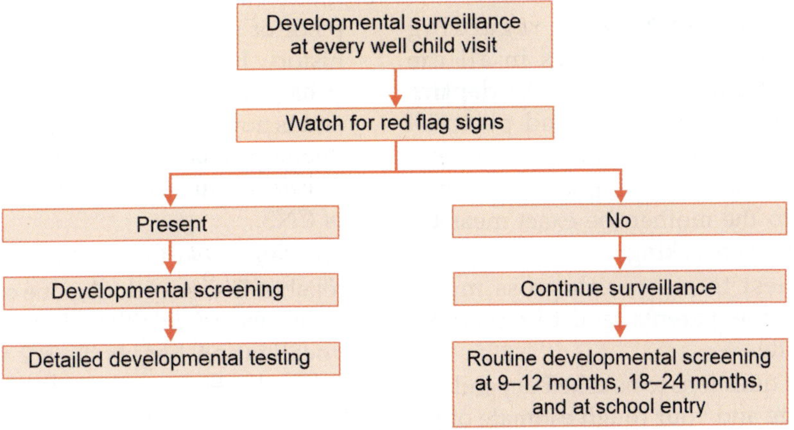

Fig. 6.2: Plan of developmental surveillance.

Indian Academy of Pediatrics (IAP) emphasizes the need for continuous developmental surveillance and recent guidelines recommend routine developmental surveillance during every immunization visit till 2 years of age. General developmental screening using standardized screening tools should be done for all children at 9–12 months, 18–24 months and at school entry, and additionally at 4–6 months and annually (till 5 years) for those with risk factors. Autism specific screening is recommended at 18 and 24 months using standardised autism screening tools.

Rashtriya Bal Swasthya Karyakaram, launched by Government of India in 2013, aims at screening for developmental delay including disabilities in children between 0–18 years. Screening tools cum reference cards and pictorial job aids have been developed for developmental screening under the program.

B. Developmental History

History is a vital part of the developmental diagnosis. It must include not only history regarding achievement of milestones (developmental history), but also all factors which may affect development, whether prenatal/perinatal/postnatal, especially in cases with abnormal development and these factors should be mentioned under appropriate headings. It is important to note that for assessment of language and social developmental domains, it is essential to take a detailed history as these domains are difficult to assess by observation alone in a clinician's office.

i. History of Milestones

1. Take a detailed history regarding achievement of milestones in all the domains, i.e. motor (*gross/fine*), adaptive and cognitive, language, and personal social, as described previously.
2. Questions should be simple and precise. Explain to the mother the exact meaning of what you are asking.
3. It is easiest to start with gross motor milestones as parents tend to remember them easily.
4. Choice of questions to be asked depends on child's age and your rough estimate of his mental age.

For example, in an average appearing 15-month-old child, asks the following questions:

> *Motor:* Can the child walk unsupported? Does the child try to feed himself with a spoon?
>
> *Adaptive and cognitive:* Does he scribble spontaneously? Does he watch pictures in a picture book?
>
> *Language:* Can the child say 2–3 words with meaning?
>
> *Personal–social:* Does the child indicate desire by pointing at objects?

If the child has acquired these functions, the development can be considered as normal. State as follows: *The development of this 15-month-old child matches the chronological age, in all 4 spheres of development.*

5. If the child has not acquired these functions, ask for a function that the child would have achieved by an earlier age. For example, if the child is not walking unsupported till now, ask whether he can walk with support. If yes, what kind of support is required, i.e. walking supported with one hand held or both hands held? If the child can walk with one hand held, his developmental age in gross motor domain corresponds to the chronological age of a child between 9 and 12 months. Record this as follows: *The development of this 15-month-old child in the gross motor domain corresponds to a chronological age of between 9 and 12 months.* Similarly, try to find the developmental age in each domain of development separately.
6. *Assess the rate of development:* This is a vital piece of information to be obtained from history. It will tell you whether the child (i) has been a slow starter, or (ii) had an illness and is now catching up; or (iii) had normal development followed by regression of development as in degenerative disorders of CNS.
7. History given by the mother is usually reliable. In case of doubt, one can check one milestone against the other. For example, vocalization begins 1 or 2 weeks after babies begin to smile. You can also check the mother's version against your own observation.

ii. History of Risk Factors Responsible for Developmental Delay (Key Box 7)

If developmental delay is expected, it is important to find the etiology for the same.

1. Inquire about *genetic, prenatal and perinatal factors* that may affect development, e.g. maternal age and diseases, smoking, drug intake, irradiation, birth asphyxia, bilirubin encephalopathy, infection, prematurity and present the relevant information in the antenatal, birth and postnatal history.
2. History must include *environmental factors* which may have a bearing on development. Overprotection, rejection, neglect, or abuse may all adversely affect development. Any relevant information should be presented in the family history.
3. Ask *history of relevant illness*, e.g. malnutrition, meningitis, encephalitis that may affect development and mention the same in past history.
4. *Prematurity:* History of prematurity is very important because, if baby is born premature, allowance must be made for prematurity till 2 years of age. For example, if a baby is born 2 months premature and is assessed at 4 months of age, he must be compared with an average 2-month-old baby and not with a 4-month-old.

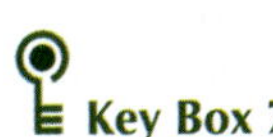

Key Box 7

Identify the Following Risk Factors in Developmental History

1. Prenatal maternal factors
   a. Acute or chronic illness (e.g. human immunodeficiency virus infection)
   b. Use of drugs or alcohol
   c. Toxemia, previous miscarriage or stillbirth
2. Perinatal factors
   a. Obstetrical complications
   b. Prematurity, low birth weight
   c. Multiple gestation
3. Neonatal factors
   a. Neurologic events (seizures or intraventricular hemorrhage)
   b. Sepsis or meningitis
   c. Severe hyperbilirubinemia
   d. Hypoxia due to respiratory compromise
4. Postnatal factors
   a. Seizures
   b. Sepsis or meningitis
   c. Recurrent otitis media
   d. Poor feeding, poor growth
   e. Exposure to lead or other toxins
5. Factors in the family history
   a. Developmental delay
   b. Deafness, blindness
   c. Chromosomal abnormalities
6. Factors in the social history
   a. History of abuse or neglect
   b. Limited social or financial support
   c. Teenage parent
   d. Single parent
   e. Mentally retarded parent
   f. Stressful life events (e.g. divorce, death or unemployment of parent)

6.4 DEVELOPMENTAL EXAMINATION

From the history, you can roughly assess the developmental age.

Example: Suppose a child is 1-year-old but he has achieved only those milestones, which he should have attained at the age of 6 months; then his development age will be taken as 6 months.

To confirm the developmental age, one needs to perform developmental examination.

A. Prerequisites for Developmental Examination

- The child should be in a happy and playful mood.
- The playtime of the child should coincide with the time of assessment.
- Child should not be hungry, thirsty, sleepy, or wet.
- Keep irrelevant toys and objects out of the sight in which you are assessing the child.
- Mother should be present. But she should not disturb or help the child during assessment.
- Watch the child as closely as possible, during free play.
- Establish rapport with the child otherwise he may not cooperate during examination.
- Perform developmental examination before doing the physical check-up as the child may cry during the later.
- Carry out the tests as quickly as possible, otherwise the child may loose interest and not cooperate.

B. Test for Hearing and Vision

Test for hearing and vision, before you begin with the proper developmental assessment. A visual or auditory handicap may affect the development as well as interpretation of developmental assessment.

An otherwise normal but deaf child is likely to be slow in development in the spheres of language acquisition and social domain.

Similarly, a child with a visual handicap may be delayed in adaptive and personal social domains.

1. Hearing Assessment

First of all, ask the parents whether the child responds to sound. The response could be an ocular movement (blink), a motor activity (startle), or behavioral change (crying or quietening).

It is important to note that deaf babies can gurgle, coo, vocalize, and say syllables (*dadada, bababa*), but language development does not progress further. More importantly, children who are hearing impaired, but not deaf; babble, laugh, startle to sound and show some, though delayed, language development. Thus, *normal early language development does not exclude hearing impairment and observation alone can miss hearing impaired children*. So, refer the child for detailed hearing evaluation on slightest suspicion of hearing impairment.

Hearing can be assessed by:

a. Observing the response to sound (in young infants 0–3 months);
b. By assessing sound localization (3–9 months); and
c. Later by assessing response to name, by asking the child to point at familiar objects and by giving him simple instructions to follow.

- In *first 3 months*, infants respond to sound by quieting (if crying), crying (if quiet), startle reflex, or blink. At 3 months, baby turns head to the side from which the sound is heard. Observe response to sound of crumpling a paper at ½ meter distance from the child's ear. A bell can also be used.
- *Between 4 and 6 months*, infants (i) turn head to sound (sound localization); (ii) imitate sound in their own speech repertoire; (iii) reciprocally vocalize with adults; (iv) notice toys that make sound; and (v) pay attention to music.

Sound localization is assessed by using a noisemaker, e.g. a small bell. Sound is produced behind the child to avoid giving visual stimulus and at a distance of about 18 inches from ear. Initially, the baby is able to localize sound only horizontally, but from 5 to 6 months, babies turn head not only to the side, but also look down, if the sound is made below the ears. At 6 months, he would turn head to the side, and then upwards, if the sound is made above the ear.

- *Between 7 months and 1 year*, infant turns head directly towards the sound and responds to his name. By the end of first year, his ability to localize sound is as good as that of an adult.
- *After 1 year of age*, hearing can also be assessed by assessing response of the child to various commands given by the examiner, provided that the examiner takes care not to give gestural/visual cues. For example, point to a picture of a cat and ask: What is it? *Cover your mouth while speaking, to avoid lip reading*.

For other details of hearing assessment, *see Chapter 13*. Clinical pointers to presence of a hearing defect are outlined in **Key Box 8**.

2. Vision Assessment

Defect of vision should be suspected, if mother or examiner notices absence of visual fixation or presence of nystagmus.

- Visual fixation can be tested in infants as young as 4 weeks by using a dangling object that does not produce sound (e.g. red ring on a string). A 4-week-old infant regards the dangling object when it is brought into his

Key Box 8

Pointers to Hearing Problem

1. Does not respond to sound or voice.
2. Does not begin to speak by 2 years of age.
3. Does not follow simple instructions.
4. Does not respond in the classroom.
5. Abnormal facial features.
6. History of birth asphyxia, or neonatal seizures neonatal jaundice.
7. Had meningitis/encephalitis.

line of vision (at a distance of ~ 8–10 inches to 3 feet from eyes) in midline and follows it less than 90°.

- A 6-week-old infant fixates on objects held in midline and follows it as it moves from midline to side and side to midline (90°).
- A 12-week-old infant promptly looks at objects in midline and follows it from one side to other (180°).
- A formal objective measurement of visual acuity can be done by 2.5 to 3 years of age by using picture charts.
- Objective measurement of refraction can be done at any age using a retinoscope by ophthalmologist.

It is important to note that hand regard (seen in normal infants between 12 and 24 weeks of age) is a developmental phenomenon and is not related to vision.

Snellen chart can only be used after 3 years of life. Details of vision testing at different ages are summarized in *Chapter* 12. Clinical pointers to presence of a visual defect are outlined in **Key Box 9**.

C. Tools for Developmental Assessment

You will need the following tools for developmental assessment of children till 5 years of age (Fig. 6.3):

- A red ring
- A small bell
- Pellets of 8 mm size (made of cardboard, wool, paper or plastic)
- 10 cubes of 1 inch each
- A pen and paper
- A picture book of common objects (scrap-book)

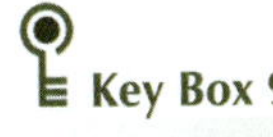

Pointers to Visual Handicap

1. Does not turn head to a light source or any object.
2. Mother complains of squint or that the pupils may look grey.
3. Slow in using hands or moving around.
4. Eyes are red, swollen and watering.
5. Eyes look dull, wrinkled.
6. Difficulty in seeing at night.
7. Child is slow in school, difficulty in reading.

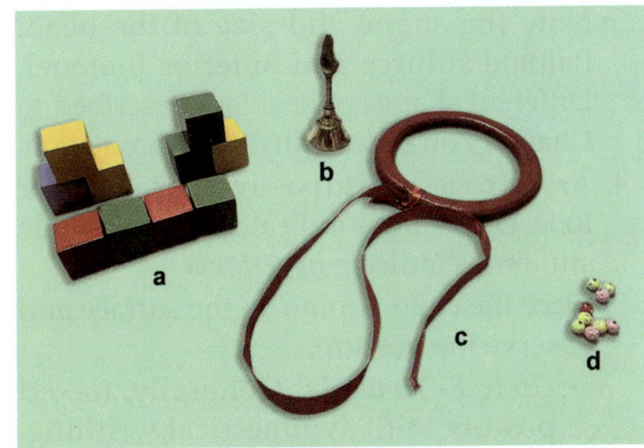

Fig. 6.3: Tools needed for development assessment: (a) cubes, (b) small bell, (c) red ring, and (d) pellets (8 mm size).

- Cards with circle, cross, square, triangle drawn on them
- Simple form board
- Colored and uncolored geometric forms
- Goddard's form board (for children >3 years of age)

General Tips for Developmental Examination

1. Perform developmental assessment prior to the physical examination.
2. Observe the child closely, throughout examination.
3. Look out for an abnormal movement (tremor, chorea, convulsion, etc.), or spasticity (tightening of body).
4. Note down what all the child babbles (for speech and language functions).
5. Record the child's interest, concentration and alertness.
6. Observe not only whether the child performs a certain task, but also see the rapidity with which the task is performed.
7. Undress the child last.
8. Do not stick to a rigid order of examination.

6.5 PROCESS OF ASSESSMENT

A. Between 1 and 3 Months

1. Observe the baby in the mother's lap; observe for any obvious abnormality such as fisting, tightness of body, etc.
2. Notice, if the child watches the mother, smiles or produces sound. The child starts smiling at the mother from 6 to 8 weeks onwards in response to visual/verbal contact.

3. Note the shape and size of the head. Palpate sutures and anterior fontanel. Different shapes of head are described in **Chapter 7** on general physical examination.
4. Assess resistance to passive movement for tone. Loose limbs indicate *hypotonia* while stiff limbs indicate *hypertonia*.
5. Place the child supine on the surface and observe the posture:
   - *Up to 8–10 weeks:* Generally, flexed posture with symmetrical writhing. Arms and legs extend on the same side, to which the baby's head is turned and extend on the opposite side (asymmetric tonic neck reflex) **(Fig. 6.4)**.
   - *12 weeks:* No more appearance of asymmetric tonic neck reflex.
6. Observe the hands:
   - *4 weeks:* Closed hands, presence of grasp reflex.
   - *8 weeks:* Opens hands frequently, slight grasp reflex.
   - *12 weeks:* Hands loosely open, may hold a rattle for a minute, if placed in hand. No grasp reflex.
7. Pull the child from supine position. Observe head lag and back:
   - *4 weeks:* Complete head lag, back completely rounded **(Fig. 6.5a)**.
   - *8 weeks:* Able to hold up head momentarily, less rounding of back **(Fig. 6.5b)**.
   - *12 weeks:* Head held up most of the time.

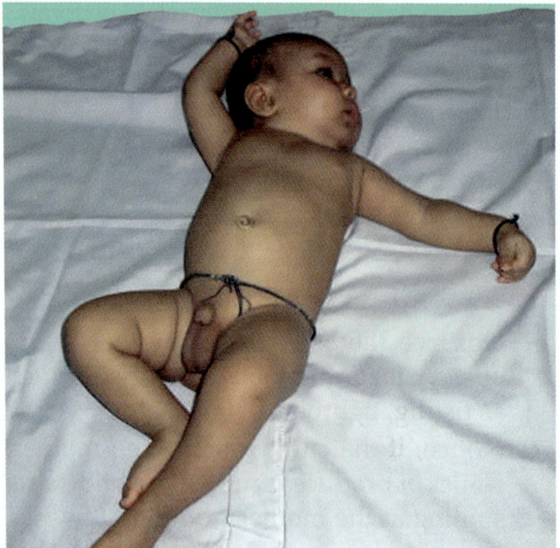

Fig. 6.4: Asymmetric tonic neck reflex.

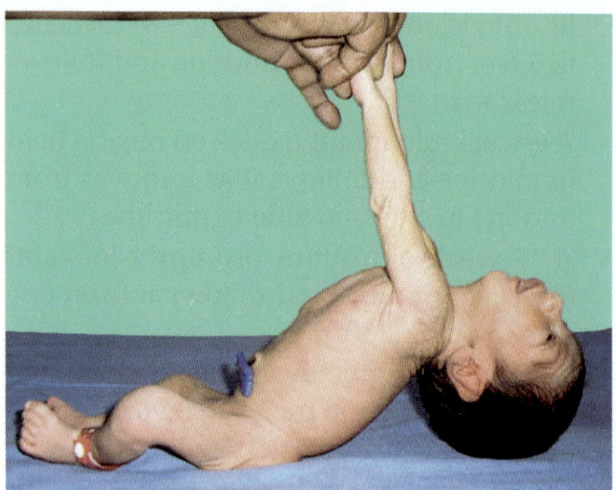

Fig. 6.5a: Pull from supine. Complete head lag, back completely rounded at 4 weeks.

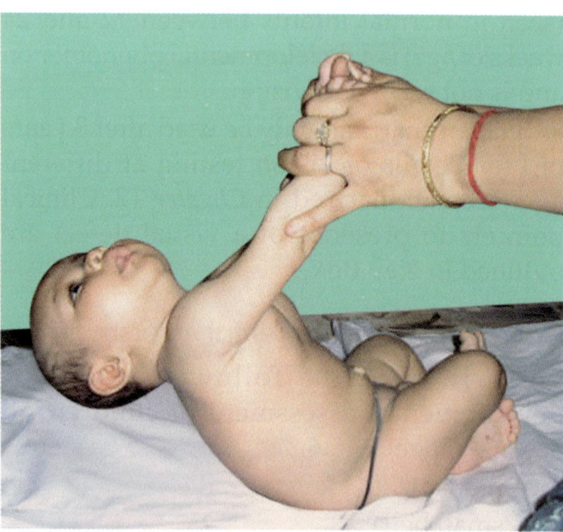

Fig. 6.5b: Pull from supine. Able to hold up head momentarily at 8 weeks; back is less rounded.

8. Hold the child in standing position:
   - Child should have some flexion at hips and knees and able to place sole on the surface **(Fig. 6.6)**.
   - In a hypotonic child, the arms and legs hang loosely; while in a spastic child, the two legs may cross each other in a scissoring position.
9. Hold the child in ventral suspension as shown in **Fig. 6.7** by placing the child prone in air with hand under the abdomen. Watch for position of limbs and head control:
   - *0–2 weeks:* Curled up on ventral suspension. Note flexion of elbows, knees with some extension at hips **(Fig. 6.7a)**.

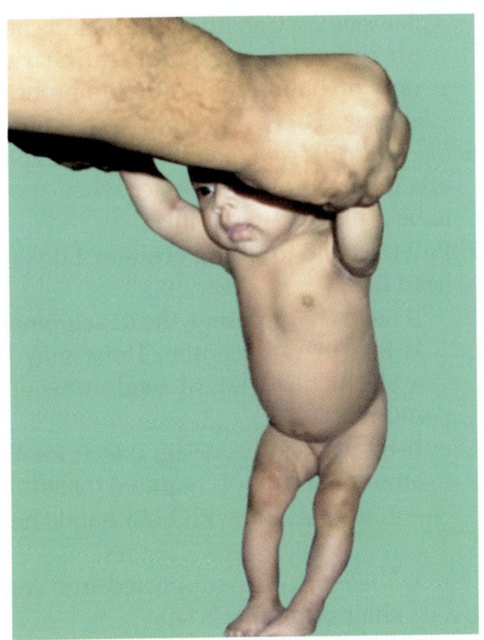

Fig. 6.6: Child less than 12-week-old is able to place sole on surface while held in stand position. No weight bearing.

- *4 weeks:* The child holds up the head momentarily. There is some flexion at the knees and hip. Back is rounded **(Fig. 6.7b)**.
- *6 weeks:* Head held momentarily in plane of body.
- *8 weeks:* Maintains head in the same plane as rest of the body **(Fig. 6.7c)**.
- *12 weeks:* The child holds the head up and above the plane of the body for considerable period of time.

10. Keep the child prone on an even surface. Observe the posture; specially chin, pelvis, and thighs **(Fig. 6.8)**:
    - *0–2 weeks:* The pelvis is high and the knees are drawn under the abdomen. Back is rounded, head remains on one side **(Fig. 6.8a)**.
    - *6 weeks:* Knees are not under abdomen. Hips extended. Chin raised from the couch intermittently.
    - *8 weeks:* Head mostly in midline. Lifts chin off the couch up to 45°C **(Fig. 6.8b)**.
    - *12 weeks:* Child can lift the chin as well as the shoulders off the surface or couch, up to 90°, bearing weight on the forearms. Pelvis is flat on the surface **(Fig. 6.8c)**.

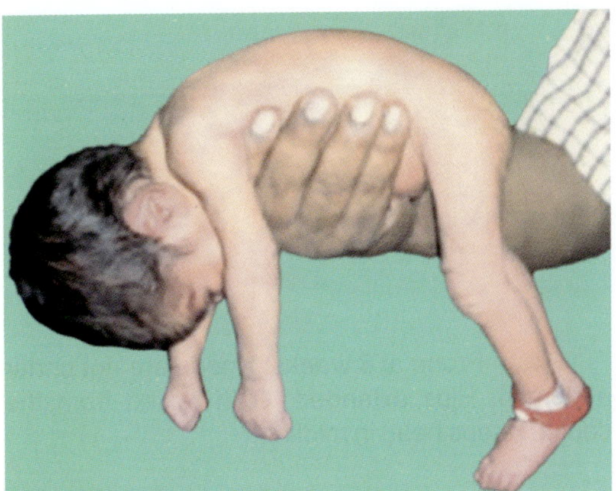

Fig. 6.7a: Ventral suspension at 0–2 weeks. Child curled up; flexion of elbows and knees with some extension at hips.

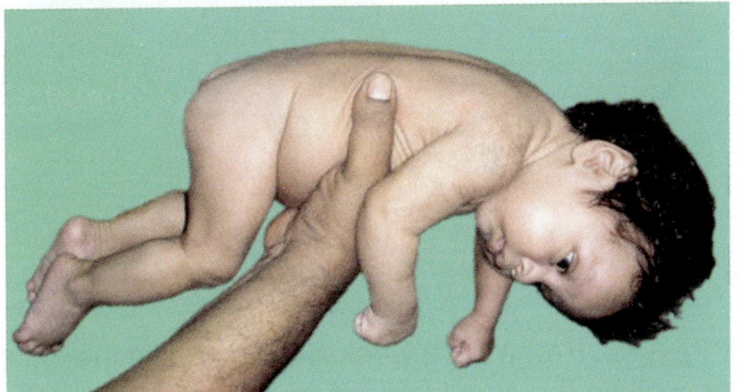

Fig. 6.7b: Ventral suspension at 4 weeks. Child holds up the head momentarily. There is some flexion at the knees and hip. Back is rounded.

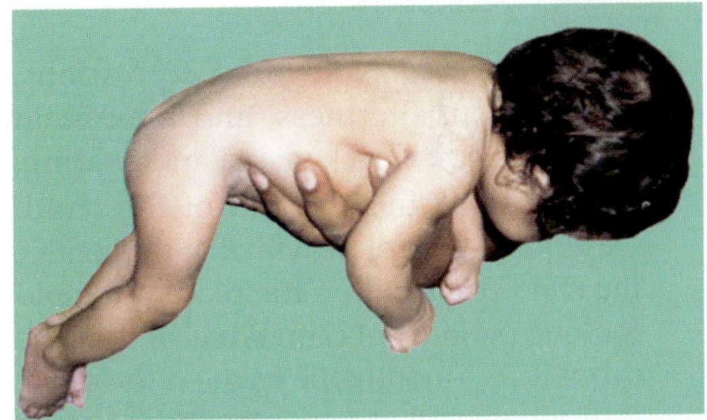

Fig. 6.7c: Ventral suspension at 8 weeks. Head is maintained in the same plane as rest of the body.

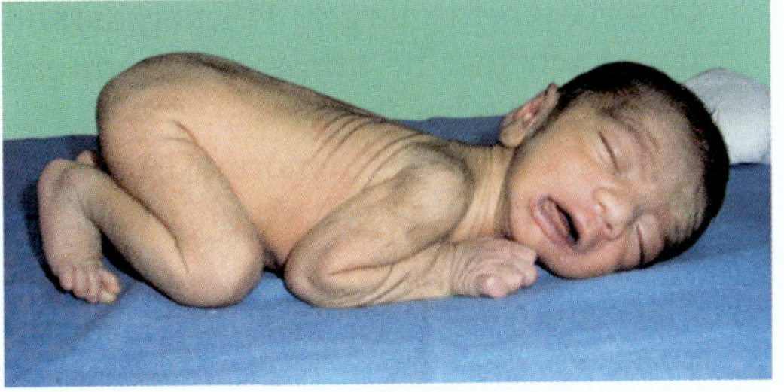

Fig. 6.8a: Prone at 0–2 weeks: The pelvis is high and the knees are drawn under the abdomen. Back is rounded, head remains on one side.

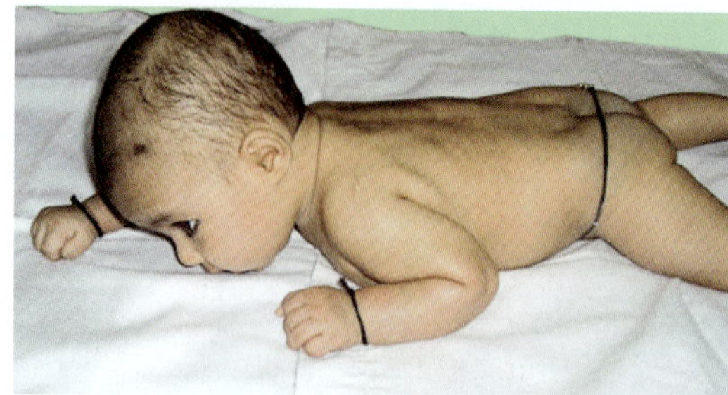

Fig. 6.8b: Prone at 8 weeks: Knees are not under abdomen. Hips extended. Chin raised from the couch. Keeps head in midline.

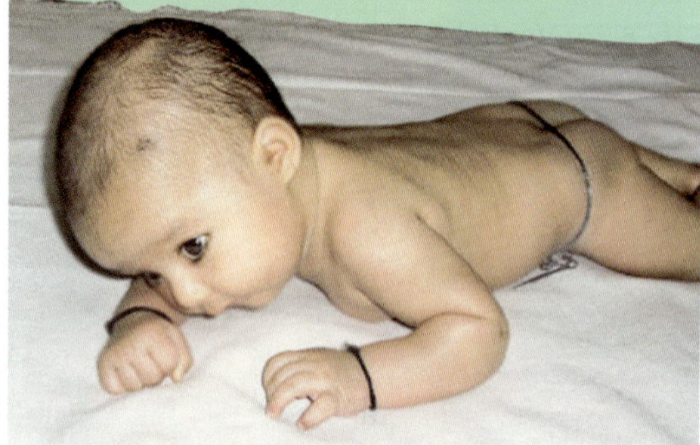

Fig. 6.8c: Prone at 12 weeks: Child can lift the chin as well as the shoulders off the surface or couch, up to 90°, bearing weight on the fore-arms. Pelvis is flat on the surface.

B. Between 4 and 6 Months

1. *Observe the child:* Note facial expressions, vocalization, altertness, and interest in surroundings. Check vision and hearing.
2. Place a rattle in the hand of the child. Observe, how he plays with it? At 4 months, the child plays with rattle placed in hand for long period; but cannot pick it up, if he drops it. At 5 months, he recovers the rattle, if dropped; and at 6 months, he looks for the dropped rattle.
3. Place a 1 inch cube in front of the child. Observe whether he gets it (5 months) and if yes, whether he transfers it from one hand to the other (6 months).
4. Watch for hand regard (normal between 3 and 5 months of age). It should disappear by 5 months of age.
5. Place the child in prone position and observe:
   - *4–5 months:* Can lift the head and chest off the surface, bearing weight on forearms (Fig. 6.9).
   - *5–6 months:* Can lift the head and chest off the surface with weight bearing only on hands, may roll from prone to supine.
6. *Place the child supine and observe:* The child lifts the head off the surface when about to be pulled up (6 months).
7. Pull the child to sitting position. Look for head lag:
   - If head lag is present, the development is less than 5 months. There may be a slight head lag at beginning of 4 months.
   - If there is no head lag, watch for the amount of support required for sitting:
     - *4 months:* Sits with both hands held (Fig. 6.10a).
     - *5 months:* Sits supported in a high chair or mother's lap.
     - *6 months:* Sits with his own hands on surface for support (Fig. 6.10b).
8. Hold the child in standing position. By 5–6 months, the child is able to bear most of the weight on legs.
9. *Show a mirror:* Smiles at mirror image by 6 months.
10. Observe the speech
    - *4 months:* Laughs aloud.
    - *5 months:* Speaks *Ah-goo*.

C. Between 6 and 12 Months

1. Observe the child's interest, alertness, and quality of vocalization/language as he sits or moves around. Does he differentiate

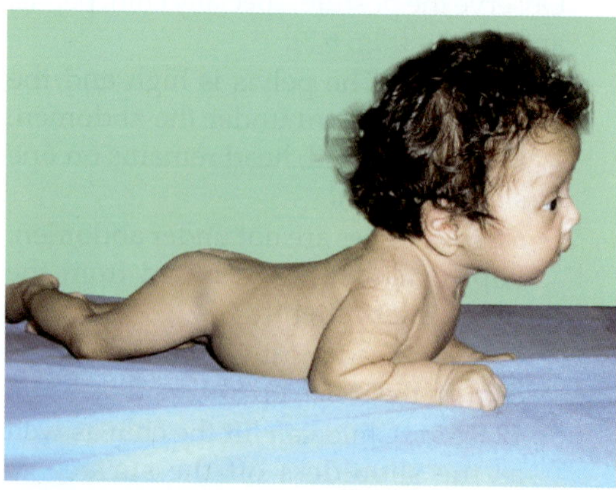

Fig. 6.9: Prone: A 4–5 months old child can lift the head and chest off the surface, bearing weight on forearms.

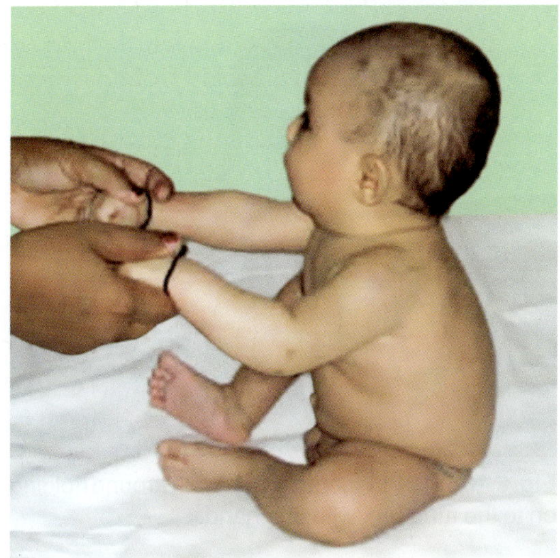

Fig. 6.10a: Pull the child to sitting position. Sits with both hands held at 4 months.

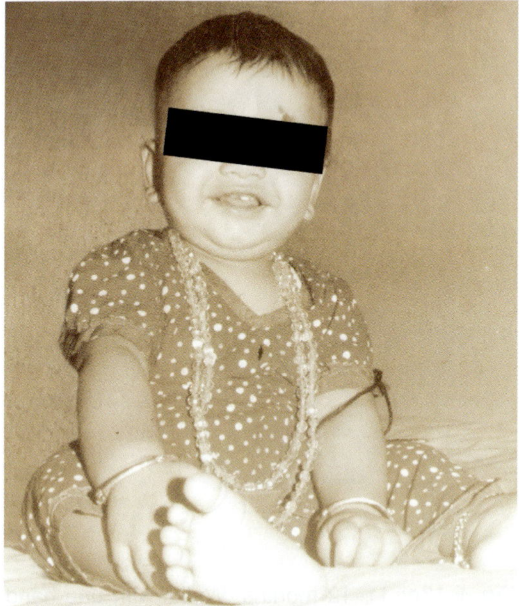

Fig. 6.10b: Pull the child to sitting position. Sits with hands on surface for support.

between family and strangers? Also, notice interaction with mother, e.g. in peek-a-boo and pat-a-cake games.

2. *Offer a cube:* With the child sitting in the mother's lap, place a cube on the table in front of the child. Observe, how the child approaches the cube and also observe what the child does with it:
   - *6 months:* Approaches cube with fingers and holds cube with the palm on the ulnar side (Fig. 6.11a). *Unidextrous approach.*
   - *7 months:* Radial palmar grasp of cube.
   - *8 months:* Scissor grasp (using all 4 fingers against the thumb).
   - *9–12 months:* Approaches cube by index finger and holds cube steady with index finger and thumb (Fig. 6.11b). This is mature grasp.
3. As soon as the child takes one cube, offer the second cube:
   - *5 months:* Drops first cube when second is offered.
   - *6 months:* Retains the first cube in hand, and takes the second cube also. Transfers from one hand to another.
   - *9 months:* Compares two cubes by bringing them together.
4. Offer a pellet. Watch the approach and the grasp:
   - *7–9 months:* Approaches with all the fingers/hand (rakes). Not able to pick it up.
   - *9–12 months:* Able to pick up the pellet between tip of thumb and forefinger (Fig. 6.12).

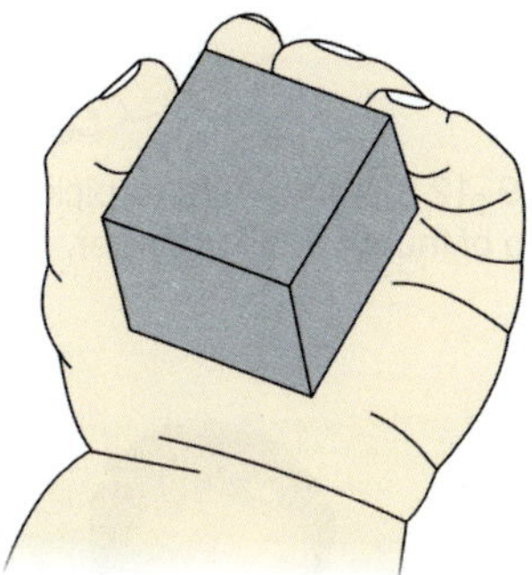

Fig. 6.11a: 6 months: Approaches cube with fingers and holds cube with the palm.

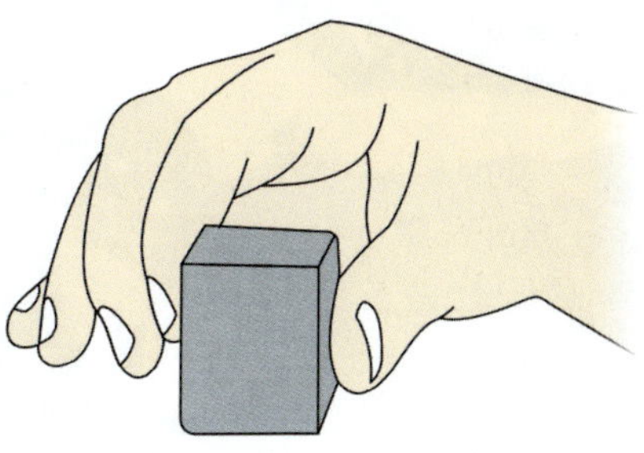

Fig. 6.11b: 9–12 months: Holds cube steady with index finger and thumb.

5. Place the child in the sitting posture and observe:
   - *7 months:* Can sit unsupported, momentarily.
   - *8 months:* Can sit steadily on floor without support.
   - *10 months:* Sits steadily without risk of imbalancing. Can pivot around to pick a toy from back/side.
6. Place in the prone position and observe for creeping (9–10 months).
7. Pull to the stand position, offer support of a table and observe. If the child can stand holding on to furniture and whether he can pull himself to standing position. Also watch, if he can walk around holding on to furniture.
   - *9–10 months:* Stands holding on to furniture, pulls to stand (Fig. 6.13a).

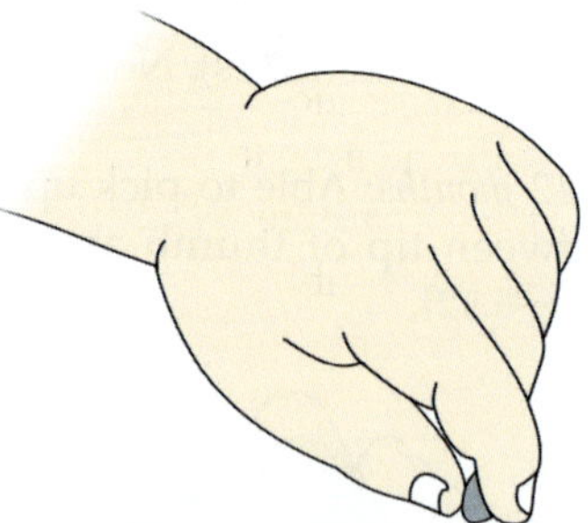

Fig. 6.12: 9–12 months: Able to pick up the pellet between tip of thumb and forefinger.

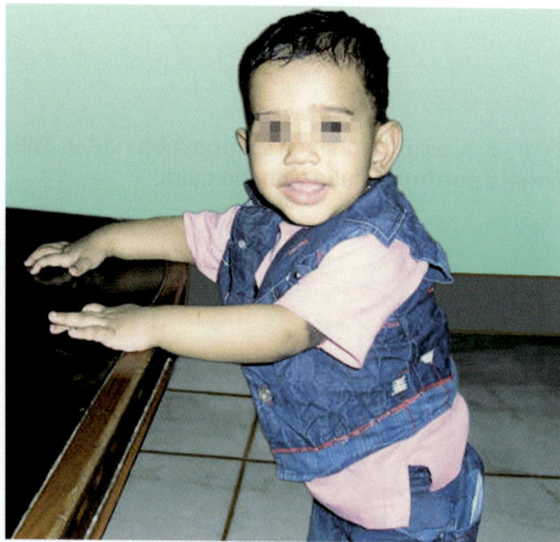

Fig. 6.13a: 8 months: Stands holding on to objects, with both hands.

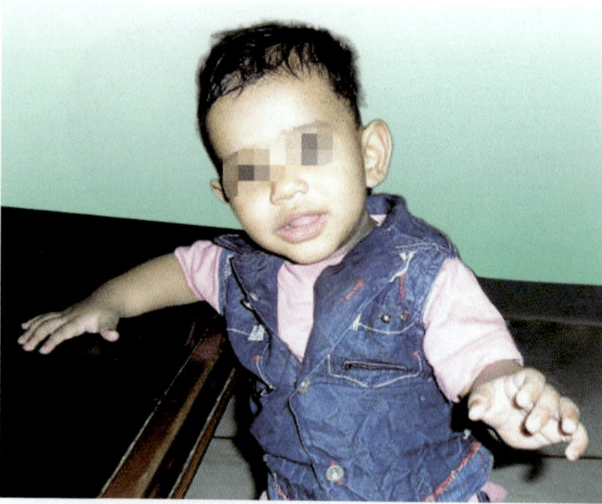

Fig. 6.13b: 10–11 months: Can walk around holding on to the furniture, with one hand.

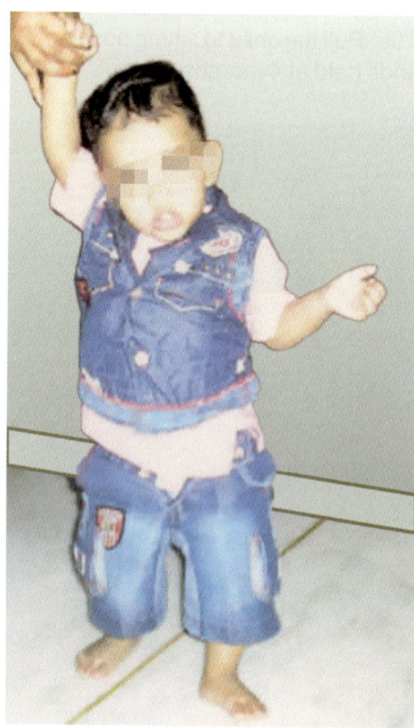

Fig. 6.13c: 11–12 months: Walks with one hand held.

   - *10–11 months:* Can walk around holding onto the furniture (Figs 6.13b and 6.13c).
   - *12–13 months:* Stands independently, takes a few independent steps.

D. Between 1 and 2 Years

1. If child comes walking into the room, watch his gait and assess its maturity. Observe his interest in toys or pictures hanging in the room. Does he point at things to ask for them or show something interesting to parents?

2. *Offer 10 cubes:* Show him how to build a tower and then let him do the same. This process is known as imitating. See how many cubes he can utilize in building a tower **(Fig. 6.14)**.
   - *15 months:* Tower of 2 cubes.
   - *18 months:* Tower of 3–4 cubes.
   - *2 years:* Tower of 6–7 cubes.

   Warning signs: The child should not take the cube to his mouth after the age of 15 months. Similarly, he should not be throwing cubes on the floor, one after another, after 18 months.
3. *Train and chimney:* Demonstrate, how to make a train of 9 cubes and place the 10th one on top of the first one (chimney). Ask him to do the same. A 2-year-old child can make the train, but fails to put the chimney **(Fig. 6.15)**.
4. *Picture identification and naming:* Show picture cards or book, and ask to identify them in the following format "where is the cat"? At a later age, you may ask "what is that"? This is known as picture naming and more difficult **(Fig. 6.16)**.
   - 18 months: Identifies 1 object and names 1 object.
   - 2 years: Identifies 5 objects; can name 3 objects.
5. *Give a picture book:* See, how many pages of a book, he can turn at one time.

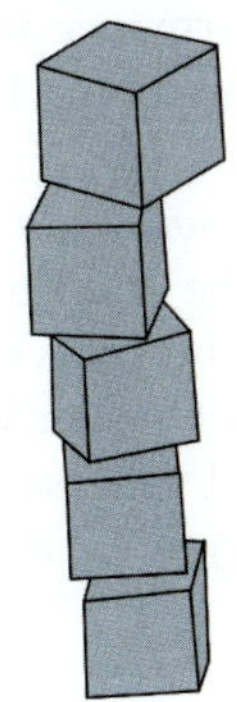

Fig. 6.14: Tower of cubes.

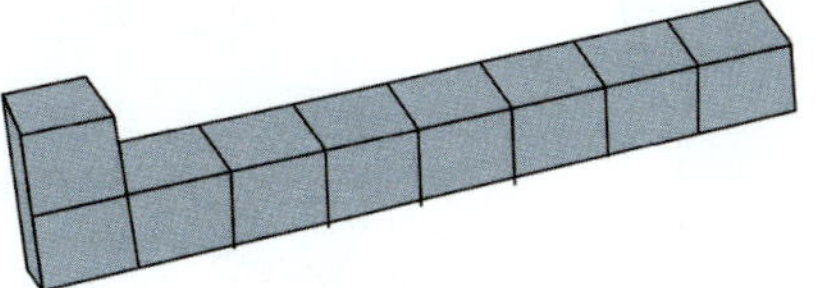

Fig. 6.15: Train with a chimney.

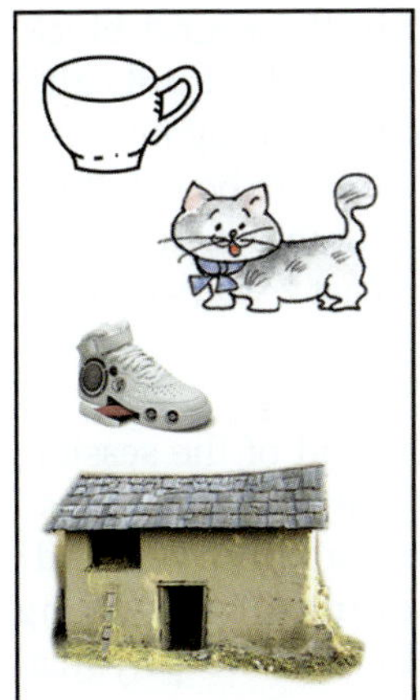

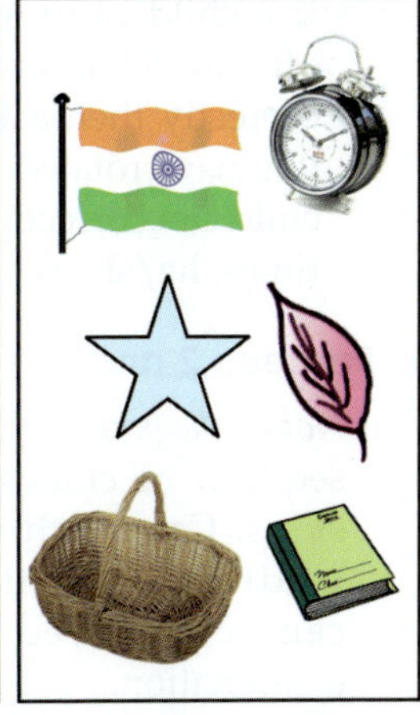

Fig. 6.16: Common pictures for identification.

   - *15 months:* Turns 2–3 pages at a time.
   - *18 months:* Turns 1 page at a time.
6. *Offer pen and paper and notice any spontaneous scribbling.* Ask to imitate (by showing how to do it by drawing in his/her sight) the drawing of a vertical stroke (|), horizontal stroke (—), and a circle. Interpret as follows:
   - *12 months:* Imitates scribbling.
   - *15 months:* Scribbles haphazardly.
   - *18 months:* Imitates vertical stroke.
   - *2 years:* Can imitate horizontal stroke and a circle.
7. *Offer simple form board:* First, offer only the round block **(Fig. 6.17)**.
   - If the child puts the round block in the correct slot without error, rotate the form board by 180 , take out the inserted block and ask the child to do it again. The child can do this by 15 months.

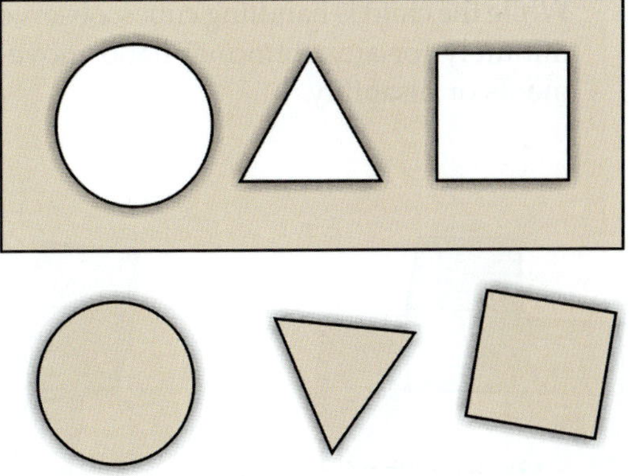

Fig. 6.17: Simple form board.

- If a child can put in the round block, offer all 3 blocks. If the child puts all 3 correctly then ask to do it again, after you have rotated the Form board. If the child can correctly put in the blocks 2–3 times, he/she is at least 2 years of age.

E. Between 2 and 5 Years

1. *Notice the gait*. At the end of the session, see how he climbs stairs, jumps/hops/skips. Can he throw a ball overhead? Undressing/buttoning-unbuttoning can be observed before the physical examination.
2. *Offer 10 cubes*
   - Usually, a child in this age group spontaneously begins to build a tower. Notice how many cubes he utilizes in making the tower.
   - Ask the child to imitate/copy (depending on expected maturity level) a train, bridge, gate and steps, one by one (Figs 6.18 to 6.20). (Note: **Imitation** means building the model while the child is watching and then asking him to build the same; while Copying means building the model out of sight of child, shielding with a paper, and then showing him the final model and asking him to build the same.)
     - *2½ years:* Tower of eight cubes; imitates train with chimney.
     - *3 years:* Tower of 9–10 cubes, imitates bridge.
     - *3½ years:* Copies bridge.
     - *4 years:* Imitates gate.
     - *5 years:* Copies gate.
     - *6 years:* May copy steps.

   While the child is handling cubes, observe minutely for any abnormal hand movements or disability.
3. *Give a pencil and paper:* Ask to imitate vertical and horizontal stroke, circle, cross, square, triangle, and diamond, in that order. If the child is able to imitate a task, ask to copy the same.
   - *2 years:* Imitates horizontal/circular stroke.
   - *3 years:* Copies circle and horizontal stroke. Imitates cross.
   - *4 years:* Copies cross.
   - *4½ years:* Copies square.
   - *5 years:* Copies triangle.
   - *6 years:* Copies diamond.
4. *Show the picture cards and ask to identify or name* the objects
   - *2½ years:* Identifies seven objects; names up to 5.
   - *3 years:* Names 8–10 objects.
5. Offer simple form board and observe the ability of the child to insert the blocks and the accuracy with which he does that.
6. If the child is successful with simple form board, he should be tried with the colored geometric forms followed by uncolored geometric forms. In each case, he is asked where the shapes fit, being given different forms one after the other. He is not told about his mistakes and is given another chance with those he has placed incorrectly.
7. After developmental age (DA) of 3½ years, time his performance in Goddard Form board, the score being based on the best of 3 trials.
8. *Goodenough draw-a-man test:* After DA of 3 years, ask the child to draw a man as completely as he knows. Child is given 1 point for each of the body parts added. For each 4 points, 1 year is added to the basal age which is 3 years. The test has 51 items,

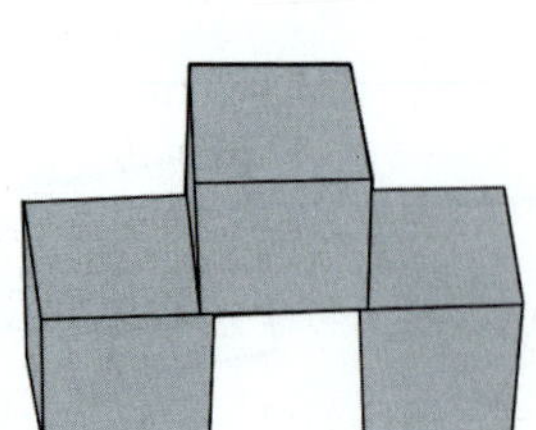

Fig. 6.18: Bridge of cubes.

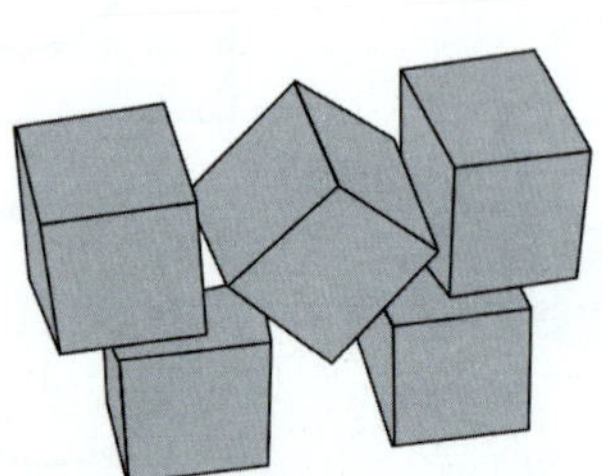

Fig. 6.19: Gate of cubes.

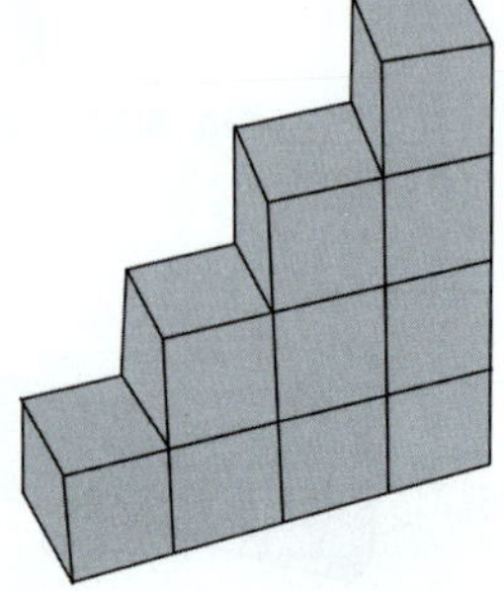

Fig. 6.20: Steps of cubes.

details of which can be found in textbooks. This test can be used for developmental assessment *between 3 and 10 years of age.*

9. *Gessel 'Incomplete Man' test:* In this test, picture of a man which is halfway complete is given to the child. The picture consists of a small circle for a head and below it a larger incomplete circle re-presenting the trunk with one stick arm and one stick leg protruding. The head has one ear, half hair, a mouth and a nose but is missing eyes, one ear, half hair, one arm and one leg and various connecting elements. Child is asked to complete the man. Depending on how many and in what way the child adds the parts, DA is deciphered.
10. *Digit repetition:* Child is asked to repeat digits, e.g. six, five, seven. Initially he is given 2 digits. If he can repeat them, ask him to repeat three and then four digits followed by five. In each case, he is given 3 trials with different numbers.
11. Ask the child to identify colors in pictures.

F. Perform Relevant Physical Examination

Key Box 10 provides a list of risk factors that you need to look for. If present, they place the child at a higher risk of having abnormal development. Note that you have to take anthropometric measurements; look for major and minor congenital anomalies; examine carefully the skin, eye, ear, extremities in detail; and conduct a thorough neurological examination. Also look for the presence of hepatosplenomegaly. A few warning signs of developmental delay are listed in **Key Box 11**.

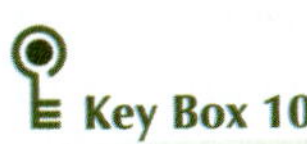

Key Box 10

Identifiable Risk Factors for Developmental Delay on Physical Examination

1. Abnormal growth (e.g. height or weight less than 3rd percentile or head circumference less than–3 SD or >2 SD).
2. Major congenital anomalies (e.g. spina bifida or midline defects).
3. Minor congenital anomalies (e.g. hypertelorism, hirsutism, or micrognathia).
4. Neurocutaneous skin lesions (e.g. neurofibromatosis or *cafe au lait* spots).
5. Abnormal optical findings (e.g. esotropia, exotropia, cataracts, or poor visual tracking).
6. Abnormal findings in ears (e.g. unusual shape or placement or recurrent acute or serous otitis media).
7. Visceral abnormalities (e.g. hepatosplenomegaly).
8. Skeletal abnormalities (e.g. brittle bones or dwarfism).
9. Neurologic abnormalities (e.g. lack of alertness, abnormal reflexes, hypertonia or hypotonia, or asymmetric findings).

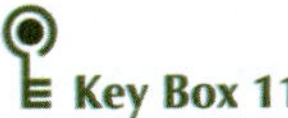

Key Box 11

Warning Signs of Delay in Development

1. Shrill/high pitched cry
2. Excessive sleepiness/irritability
3. Frog-legged positioning/opisthotonus
4. Tremors/convulsions
5. Small/large head size for age
6. Poor eye following/poor response to sound
7. Asymmetrical/increased/absent/persistent neonatal reflexes
8. Hypotonia/hypertonia/dystonia
9. Delayed developmental milestones

6.6 INTERPRETATION OF DEVELOPMENTAL ASSESSMENT

A. Development Quotient (DQ)

On the basis of his performance in developmental tests, child is assigned a developmental age (DA) that may or may not match with chronological age (CA).

Example: A child is 2-year-old. He has not attained the milestones expected at his age. After assessment, it is found that he has attained only those milestones which should have been attained by 1 year of age. Thus, CA of child is 2 years but his DA is 1 year.
Based on the DA and CA, DQ is calculated as follows:

$$DQ = DA/CA \times 100.$$

DQ is calculated separately for each developmental domain. Ideally, CA should be equal to DA and DQ should, therefore, be 100. *A child having DQ ≤70 is considered to be developmentally delayed.*

B. Developmental Delay and Developmental Regression

Developmental delay is said to be present, if the child does not achieve the developmental milestones at the age by which it is expected to be achieved with adequate consideration for the broad variation among normal children.

Developmental regression refers to loss of milestones that were achieved previously. Regression of milestones is characteristic of neurodegenerative disorders. It is important to note that there may be some temporary loss of milestones with acute severe illnesses which should recover in 3–4 weeks with recovery in general wellbeing. This should not be considered indicative of neuroregression.

C. Global Developmental Delay and Dissociative Delay

Development in one field usually parallels development in other fields.

Global developmental delay (GDD) is said to be present, if there is significant delay (two standard deviations or more below the mean) in 2 or more fields (out of—gross and fine motor, speech and language, cognition, socio-personal and activities of daily living) of development. The recent Indian Academy of Pediatrics (IAP) guidelines recommend to exclude children with delay in two or more domains in whom the delay can be explained primarily by (a) isolated motor delay or (b) severe uncorrected visual/ hearing impairment.

The term global developmental delay is usually used for younger children (i.e. typically less than 5 years of age), whereas the term *intellectual disability* is usually applied to older children when IQ testing is more valid. Cerebral palsy and other neuromotor, visual, and hearing impairment may co-exist with GDD. However, not all children with GDD are destined to develop intellectual disability.

In ***dissociative delay***, there is delay in one particular field with otherwise normal development in other domains; or delay is more pronounced in one domain as compared to others.

Sometimes, development in one field may not necessarily parallel that in other fields. When the rate of attainment of development skills varies significantly between two or more domains, it is termed '*Developmental dissociation*'. For example, a child with myopathy will have motor delay, but development in other fields will usually be normal.

D. Developmental Screening

Developmental screening is the process of using validated and standardized tools (that are norm referenced and standardized for target population) to assess development of a child. These tools provide objective information about the child's development and also inform the practitioner and the parents regarding the next important milestone to watch out for. Screening tools are really helpful as informal evaluation of development has been shown to be unreliable in early timely detection of developmental delay which can be missed if not specifically looked for. IAP recommends developmental screening of all children at 9–12 months, 18–24 months, and at school entry. For high risk infants, additionally, developmental screening should also be done at 4–6 months and yearly till 5 years of age.

An ideal screening test should be brief, with good psychometric properties (sensitivity and specificity >70–80%), available in local language and consist of items that have been culturally adapted and validated on local population. From an Indian perspective, such a screening test does not exist. Commonly used screening tests are listed below:

- ***Denver development screening test (DDST):*** This is a very popular international screening test for use in children up to 6 years of age. However, it is no longer recommended due to poor sensitivity and specificity.
- ***Bayley infant neurodevelopment screen (BINS):*** This is another international, interviewer administered screening test that screens children between 3 and 24 months of age and has acceptable psychometric properties.
- ***Ages and stages questionnaire (ASQ-3):*** This is a parent reported questionnaire to screen children between 3 and 66 months with acceptable psychometric properties and has been shown to have acceptable standards in a study done in India (after translation and substitution of a few items).
- ***Parent's evaluation of developmental status (PEDS):*** This is another parent reported developmental assessment tool to screen children up to 8 years of age, takes

only 2–10 minutes to administer and has been found reliable in some developing countries (Indian data lacking).

- *Developmental profile III (DP III):* This is also a parent reported tool (for children between 0 and 9 years of age) that has been used in numerous studies in India though has not been validated.

Developmental tools designed for use in community surveys of Indian population include Phatak's Baroda Developmental Screening Test (0–30 months) and Trivandrum Development Screening Chart (0–24 months) and ICMR Psychosocial Developmental Screening Test (0–6 years). However, drawbacks of these tests are less than optimal psychometric properties and lack of re-validation studies since initial formulation of these tests (more than two decades ago).

Rashtriya Bal Swasthya Karyakram (RBSK), a screening tool has recently been developed by the Government of India to screen children from 0–6 years for defects, deficiencies, diseases, and developmental delays. It takes 10–15 minutes to administer. The developmental screening section contains items which screens children for vision impairment, hearing impairment, developmental delay in different domains (gross motor, fine motor, cognitive, speech and language) as well as for neuromotor impairment and autism. The Mother and Child Protection (MCP) card is another tool being used in India for developmental screening (2–36 months).

E. Development Diagnostic Tests

As intelligence cannot be reliably assessed in young children, following development based tests are used for them:

Bayley Scale of Infant Development (BSID IV)

BSID has been extensively used worldwide to assess development of infants and toddlers between 1 and 42 months of age. The latest edition (BSID IV) evaluates children along 5 scales—cognitive, language, motor, social, emotional, and adaptive behavior.

Developmental Assessment Scale (DAS II) for Indian Infants

DAS II is Indian adaptation of Bayley Scale of Infant Development. It is the most widely accepted, effective and comprehensive tool for confirmation of developmental delay in Indian infants and toddlers (0–30 months). It consists of a motor scale (assesses gross motor and fine motor skills) and a mental scale (assesses cognitive and personal social development) and allows calculation of mental age and motor age and corresponding DQ. Composite DQ is calculated as average of Mental and Motor DQ.

F. Intelligence Tests

Various tests are available for testing the intelligence in an older child. These tests assess the problem-solving abilities of a child for his age and measure intelligence quotient (IQ). Some common tests used to measure intelligence include:

- Stanford Binet Intelligence Test
- Weschler Intelligence Scale for Children (WISC)
- Goodenough draw-a-man test
- Leiter International Performance Scale
- Wechsler preschool and primary scale of intelligence—revised
- Malin's Intelligence Scale for Indian Children (MISIC)—Indian adaptation of WISC
- Binet-Kulshreshtra—Hindi adaptation of Stanford Binet Intelligence Test.

G. Adaptive Scales

These scales assess adaptive behavior dysfunction, which is one of the essential criteria for the diagnosis of intellectual disability. The results are expressed as social quotient (SQ). Intellectual disability is usually diagnosed when SQ is ≤ 70. Vineland Adaptive Behavior Sclae (VABS) is the most commonly used scale for this purpose.

Intellectual disability (formerly called mental retardation) is characterized by a triad of (i) sub-average intelligence (intelligence quotient (IQ) ≤70); (ii) impairment of adaptive behavior; and (iii) onset before 18 years of age. Children less than 5 years with subnormal intelligence are labeled as having global developmental delay. Intellectual disability is classified on the basis of intelligence quotient (IQ) as mild: IQ 50–55 to 70; moderate: IQ 35–40 to 50–55; severe: I Q 20–25 to 35–40; and profound: IQ <20–25.

Chapter

7

General Physical Examination

❍ Pooja Dewan ❍ Piyush Gupta

Structure

In this chapter, we will discuss the pre-requisites for examination, tools needed, and proper positioning and preparation for examination. We will also discuss the first impression of the patient along with identification of dysmorphism, evaluation of vitals, signs of vitamin deficiency, and the general markers of disease. The general survey will be completed with a summarization of head to toe examination.

7.1 PREPARING FOR EXAMINATION

Though history-taking in clinical practice is the process which is needed to determine the sequence of events leading to the illness; yet a keen and systematic examination often holds the key to the patient's diagnosis. Any assessment in a child would be incomplete unless there are elements of *"observation, listening, and play"* in it.

Examination Room

Physical examination is mostly carried out in the outpatient setting which is often unfamiliar for the child causing undue anxiety. It is, therefore, important to make the environment pleasant, and the atmosphere friendly. The examination room must be warm, well-lit, and comfortable. Avoid putting curtains of yellow or blue color in the examination room as they may interfere with the assessment of jaundice and cyanosis in the child.

Equipment/Examination Kit

Before beginning examination, you need to equip yourself with certain tools needed during examination. These include a stethoscope, torch light, non-metallic inch-tape, weighing machine, spatula, sphygmomanometer, clinical thermometer, and developmental assessment tools including a red ring (6.5 cm diameter) and blocks (2.5 cm cubes, red).

Position of the Child

The child needs to be properly positioned so as to allow maximum access for examination. Older children are usually cooperative and allow examination in different positions:

- Children between 3 months and 1 year may be allowed to be seated in the mother's lap during examination.
- Between the age of 1 and 3 years, child may be examined in standing position or in mother's lap.
- Up to the age of 3 months and in children older than 3 years, examination can be performed on examination table (Fig. 7.1).

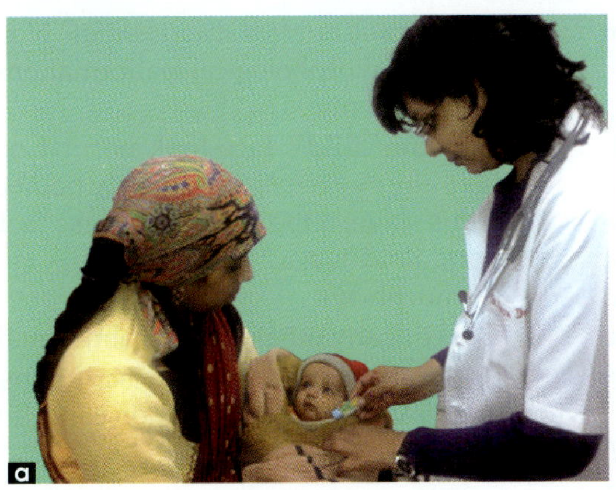

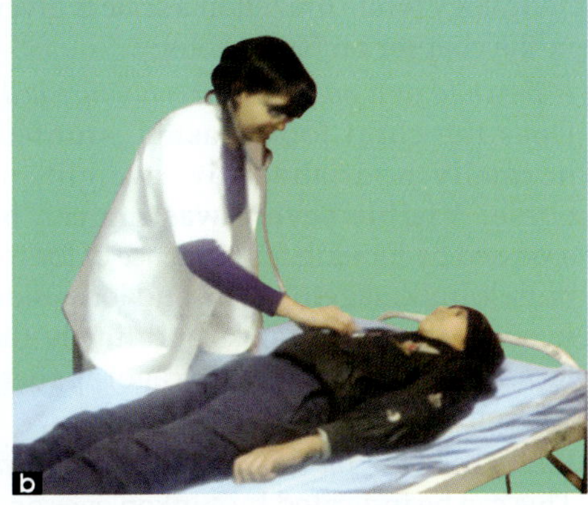

Fig. 7.1: Relative positions of the pediatrician and the child in (a) a younger child; (b) an older child.

7.2 THE FIRST IMPRESSION

Though a systematic approach to examination is imperative; an initial impression of the child can often clinch the diagnosis. The typical facies of a child having Down syndrome; posturing of a patient of tubercular meningitis; and the characteristic swelling of the body of a child with nephrotic syndrome are often sufficient to diagnose the clinical condition.

The opening sentence in the initial assessment should indicate whether the child *looks well or not*? If not, what are the obvious abnormalities. A child may be described as being comatose, having marked respiratory distress, cyanosed, having generalized swelling of the body, malnourished, or having a particular posture. Obvious jaundice, marked pallor, or overt bleeding may also be mentioned at this stage.

Note the Obvious Findings

1. *Is the child alert or apathetic?* Always assess the *level of consciousness* of the child (drowsy, delirious, stuporous, comatose). You may use the modified Glasgow Coma Scale (GCS) for children and the Brazelton's neurological assessment scale for neonates. GCS is detailed in chapter on

Tips for Examination

- Ensure that your hands are washed and warmed before examining the child.
- Have plenty of patience and observe keenly.
- Do not impose yourself on the child. Allow some time for interaction to build a rapport before you start examining the child.
- Avoid wearing a white apron, which may make the child wary of you.
- You should observe the child as discreetly as possible.
- At the same time, you may use a suitable toy or engage in conversation (ask about his school, friends, interests) to distract him.
- You can keep handy toys like a rattle, blocks (these may even be used to assess the child's fine motor development), soft ball, soft toys, paper, and pencil. You can also strap a toy on to your stethoscope to distract the child while auscultating.
- Make frequent eye contact with the child.
- If a child is to be undressed in order to examine him/her, you should undress him/her keeping his/her modesty into consideration. Also, you can ask the mother to undress her child to prevent undue anxiety on part of the child.
- If a child cries or is uncomfortable during examination, you must wait and spend more time to befriend him and win his confidence.
- Any painful examination or threatening maneuver, like per rectal examination or auscultation should be performed at the end of clinical examination. Perform rectal or vaginal examination only when specifically indicated.
- Obtain **Consent** from the parents of all children and **Assent** from the child (if >7 years old).

neurology while Brazelton's scale is given in the chapter on Neonatology.

2. *Is the child well nourished or malnourished?* Does the child look wasted, stunted, normally nourished, overweight, or obese? **Visible severe wasting** can be assessed by looking for evidence of loss of muscle bulk, sagging skin, and loose skin in arms, thighs, buttocks and finally the face. Bony skeleton (the rib cage) appears so prominent! **(Key Box 1)**.
3. *Assess whether the child looks dehydrated.* This can be indicated by sunken eyes and dry wrinkled skin.
4. *Does the child's age match his physical growth?* Is the child *precocious* or is the *growth delayed*?
5. Assess the child's posture (opisthotonus, decerebrate, decorticate, ambulatory), mobility, gait (wide-based, limping), and demenaour (restless, breathless, comfortable).
6. *Is the child having a respiratory problem* like respiratory distress or cyanosis?
7. *Is the child's color normal* or too pale/icteric/cyanosed?
8. *Are there any external abnormalities?* Notice any gross morphological malformations at this stage only.
9. Does the child's face look normal or is there any *dysmorphism*? You may point out at this stage, if the child has coarse facies, mongoloid facies, or any obvious facial dysmorphism.
10. Point out any other obvious abnormality.

Key Box 1 provides model descriptions of first impression for three common conditions in children.

7.3 VITAL PARAMETERS

An accurate assessment of vitals is important for diagnosis of the patient. This includes assessment of temperature, pulse rate, respiratory rate, blood pressure, and pulse oximetry **(Key Box 2)**.

A. Temperature

Normal Range of Body Temperature

Normal body temperature is 37°C or 98.6°F and ranges between 36.6° (97.9°F) and 37.2°C (99°F). The diurnal variation in temperature is usually 1°F (0.6°C). The temperature in the

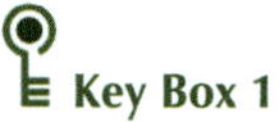
Key Box 1

The First Impression

Nephrotic syndrome

The child is alert and appears puffy. He has generalized edema with periorbital swelling. The abdomen also appears grossly distended and shiny.

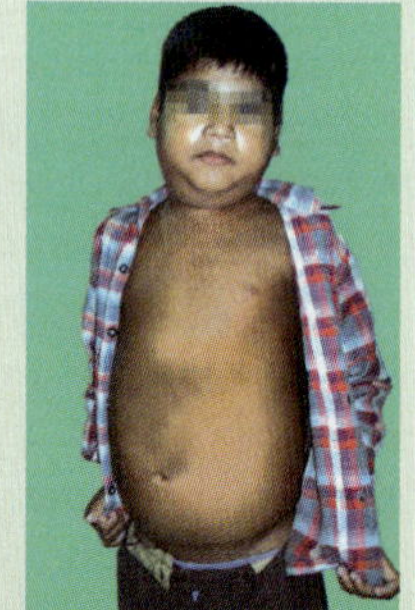

Severe malnutrition (*visible severe wasting*)

The child is conscious but listless, and markedly emaciated. There is noticeable loss of subcutaneous fat. Buccal pad of fat is absent and cheeks are sunken.

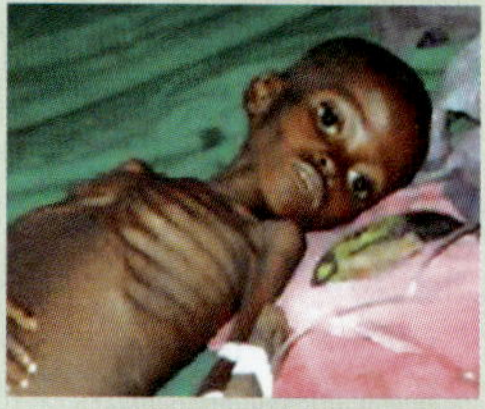

Tubercular meningitis

The child is comatose. He is lying in a decerebrate posture. The child is having central respiration.

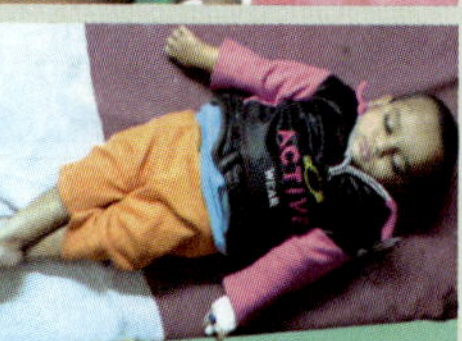

Key Box 2

Vital Parameters

1. Temperature
2. Arterial pulse
3. Respiration
4. Blood pressure
5. Capillary refill time
6. Hydration
7. Oxygen saturation

evening is usually higher. In neonates, the normal temperature is 36.5° to 37.5°C.

A neonate whose temperature is between 36° and 36.5°C is said to be in *cold stress* while one whose temperature is below 36°C is said to be having *hypothermia* and needs active rewarming and immediate management.

> A child whose rectal temperature is above 38°C/100.4°F is *febrile*. Rectal temperatures in excess of 41.5°C/107°F are suggestive of *hyperpyrexia (American College of Emergency Physicians)*.

Patterns of Fever

- ***Continuous fever:*** Daily fluctuations in the temperature do not exceed 2°C and temperature never touches the baseline (normal) temperature.
- ***Remittent fever:*** Daily fluctuations exceed 2°C and never touch the baseline.
- ***Intermittent fever:*** Temperature touches the baseline in between the febrile phases. *Quotidian fever* if it occurs daily (juvenile rheumatoid arthritis); *tertian fever* occurs every alternate day (*Plasmodium vivax* malaria), and *quartan fever* occurs every third day (*Plasmodium malariae* malaria).
- ***Relapsing fever:*** When afebrile phase in between febrile periods lasts more than 24 hours, the fever is said to be relapsing. *Pel-Ebstein* type of fever, seen in Hodgkin disease, is a type of relapsing fever where febrile period of a few days is followed by afebrile period of a few days to be followed again by a febrile period.
- ***Hyperpyrexia*** is seen in heat stroke, pontine hemorrhage, septicemia, malaria, and malignant hyperthermia.

Where and How to Measure Temperature?

The oral cavity or the axillae are the preferred sites to measure temperature. The other sites which may be used for measuring the temperature are forehead, rectum or tympanic membrane (ear canal). The rectal temperature is more than the oral temperature by 0.5°C while the axillary temperature is 1°C below the rectal temperature.

A glass mercury thermometer is no longer used because they can break and allow mercury to vaporize and be inhaled. We may use the following instruments to measure the temperature:

1. ***Digital thermometers:*** Rely on electronic heat sensors to measure the temperature. They may be placed in the mouth under the tongue (per oral), rectally, or in the axilla (or armpit) **(Fig. 7.2a)**.
2. ***Digital ear (tympanic membrane) thermometers:*** These thermometers rely on an infrared scanner to measure the temperature inside the ear canal. These should be used only in children older than 6 months **(Fig. 7.2b)**.
3. ***Temporal artery thermometers:*** These rely on an infrared scanner to measure the temperature of the temporal artery in the forehead **(Fig. 7.2c)**.

Digital thermometers: Wipe the area extending about 2 inches from the tip of the thermometer

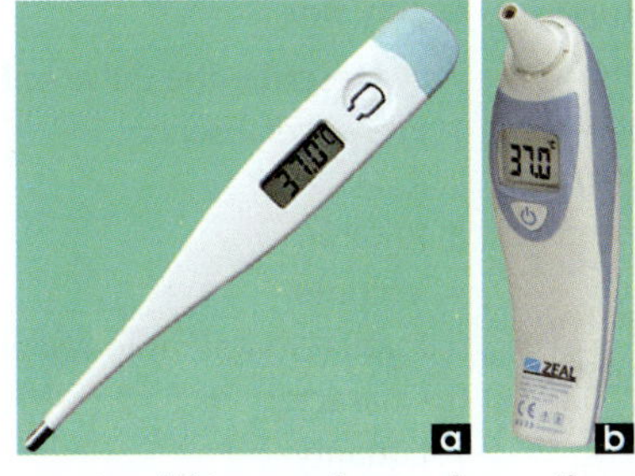

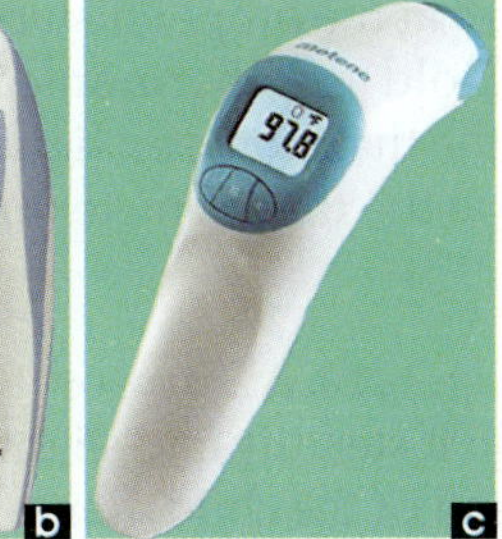

Fig. 7.2: (a) Digital thermometer; (b) tympanic membrane thermometer; and (c) temporal artery thermometer.

with 70% isopropyl alcohol before and after each use. Make sure you use separate digital thermometers for oral and rectal use. Label each thermometer, and do not use the same thermometer in both places.

Rectal temperature: Turn on the digital thermometer and lubricate the tip of the thermometer with petroleum jelly. Make the baby lie supine or sideways, and after lifting his or her thighs, insert the lubricated thermometer about 1/2 to 1 inch into the rectum. Do not attempt to force the rectal thermometer if you encounter any resistance. Hold the thermometer in place until you hear the beep and now remove the device and read the temperature.

Oral temperature: Turn on the digital thermometer. Place the tip of the thermometer under the child's tongue toward the back of the mouth and ask the child to keep his or her lips closed. Remove the thermometer when it signals that it is done and read the number. If the child has been eating or drinking, wait 15 minutes to take the temperature by mouth.

Axillary temperature: Place the tip under the child's axilla, taking care to direct the tip of the thermometer towards the apex of the axilla. Make sure the underarm is dry and there is no material between the chest and arm. Point the thermometer upward and place the tip well into the patient's underarm. Fold patient's arm over chest to hold the thermometer in place. Make sure that the tip of the thermometer touches the skin and not the clothing. Hold the thermometer in place until you hear the beep signal indicating the reading is finished. Remove the thermometer and note the reading.

Ear temperature: Turn on the thermometer. Gently place the thermometer in child's ear. Insert the thermometer at the proper distance into the ear canal. Hold the thermometer tightly in place until the thermometer signals that it is done. Remove the thermometer and note the reading.

Temporal artery temperature: Turn on the thermometer and hold it steadily and slightly away from the forehead of the child. Remove the thermometer and note the reading.

B. Arterial Pulse

Radial pulse is the most common to be assessed for its ease of access. Femoral pulse is felt especially in neonates or in children with circulatory collapse or shock. Other pulses to be assessed are brachial, carotid, popliteal, posterior tibial, and dorsalis pedis.

Key Box 3 outlines the pulse characteristics that need to be noted.

The vessel wall is usually not appreciable in children.

Presence of Peripheral Pulsations

The patient should be examined in a warm room as a cool environment may lead to peripheral vasoconstriction and reduce the peripheral pulse. The radial pulse is assessed using the index, middle, and ring fingers with the arm in slight pronation and the wrist slightly flexed. If the radial pulse is feeble or absent, check the pulsations in a bigger vessel, i.e. carotid or femoral artery. The femoral pulses may be diminished in coarctation of the aorta or hypoplastic left heart syndrome. Pulses are weak/absent in Takayasu arteritis.

Pulse Rate

Before counting the pulse rate, ensure that the child is relaxed and comfortable. Assess the pulse rate for a complete minute. In an emergency situation (as during neonatal resuscitation), count the pulse for 6 seconds and then multiply by a factor of 10 to get the pulse rate in beats per minute. The normal rates for various age groups are given in **Key Box 4**. In conditions like excessive crying, thyrotoxicosis, and fever, there may be tachycardia.

Key Box 3

Describe the Pulse in Following Terms

1. Presence/absence
2. Rate
3. Rhythm
4. Volume
5. Radiofemoral/radio-radial delay
6. Character
7. Equality

Key Box 4

Normal Pulse Rate

Preterm neonate	120–160 bpm
Term neonate	100–140 bpm
1 month to 1 year	100–120 bpm
1 to 5 years	90–110 bpm
5 to 10 years	80–100 bpm

Rhythm

Assess the rhythm of the pulse. Classify it as *regular* or *irregular*. The pulse may only vary with respiration (*sinus tachycardia:* heart rate increases with inspiration, *sinus bradycardia*: heart rate decreases with expiration).

If the pulse is irregular, look for any specific pattern of abnormality. In atrial fibrillation, the pulse is *irregularly irregular*. Sometimes few beats may be missed or ectopic beats (extrasystoles) may be present. A *regularly irregular* pulse is felt in heart block and atrial flutter.

Volume

The volume of the pulse is best assessed in the carotid artery. The volume of the pulse depends upon the pulse pressure. Low volume pulse is observed in shock, aortic stenosis, cardiomyopathy, and vasculitis (Takayasu arteritis). High volume pulse is present in aortic regurgitation, mitral regurgitation, patent ductus arteriosus, hypertension, cor pulmonale, arteriovenous fistula, thyrotoxicosis, beriberi, anemia, and high-grade fever.

Radiofemoral Delay

Feel the radial and femoral pulses simultaneously. The beats should be felt together, unless there is coarctation of aorta.

Character

The pulse may be described to have a specific character. These are diagrammatically shown in Fig. 7.3. The common characters of pulse are as follows:

Anacrotic pulse: Slow rising, twice beating pulse (both the anacrotic and tidal waves are felt during systole), seen in aortic stenosis.

Pulsus bisferiens: Rapid rising, twice beating pulse (tidal wave followed by a small wave, felt during systole), seen in idiopathic

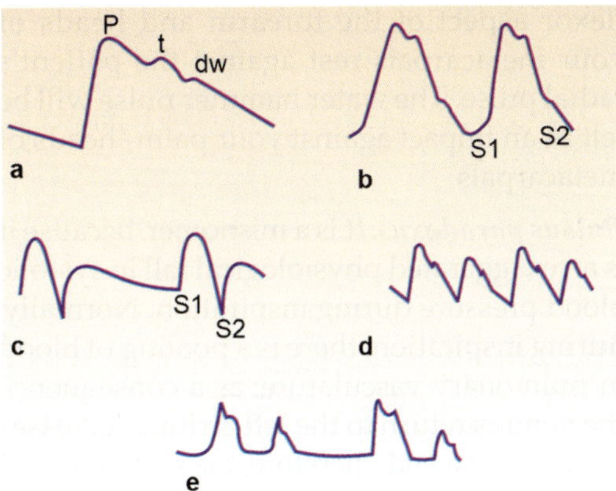

Fig. 7.3: Diagrammatic representation of the different types of pulses—(a) normal; (b) bisferiens; (c) dicrotic; (d) alternans; (e) bigeminus.

hypertrophic subaortic stenosis, severe aortic regurgitation, and mild aortic stenosis.

Dicrotic pulse: Twice beating pulse where the tidal wave is felt during systole and the second dicrotic wave is felt during diastole, seen in conditions with low cardiac output—like myocarditis, cardiac tamponade, and cardiomyopathy.

Pulsus parvus et tardus: Slow rising pulse, low volume pulse, anacrotic wave is not felt, present in aortic stenosis where the left ventricle takes much longer to push blood through the stenosed valve.

Pulsus alternans: Strong beat is followed by a weak beat, felt in left ventricular failure, myocarditis.

Pulsus bigeminy: Coupling of beats in pairs followed by a pause (a strong beat followed by a weak beat and then a pause followed again by a strong beat), present in AV block, sinoatrial block with ventricular escape, and digoxin toxicity. The reason is a premature ventricular contraction. It differs from pulsus alternans where this compensatory pause is absent.

Water hammer pulse or collapsing pulse: A sharp rise and steep fall of pulse volume felt in high output states like aortic regurgitation, mitral regurgitation, patent ductus arteriosus, chronic severe anemia, thyrotoxicosis, beriberi, etc. It is elicited in the radial or brachial pulse. Make the child recline or lie supine. Raise the arm vertically holding the muscular part of the forearm such that your palm covers the flexor aspect of the forearm and heads of your metacarpals rest against the patient's radial pulse. The water hammer pulse will be felt as an impact against your palm/heads of metacarpals.

Pulsus paradoxus: It is a misnomer, because it is an exaggerated physiological fall in systolic blood pressure during inspiration. Normally, during inspiration, there is a pooling of blood in pulmonary vasculature; as a consequence the venous return to the left atrium decreases in inspiration and, therefore, the systolic blood pressure is lower by up to 10 mmHg. When the fall in systolic blood pressure is more than 10 mmHg, the pulse is called pulsus paradoxus. The causes of pulsus paradoxus are given in **Key Box 5**.

In extreme cases, the peripheral pulse may even disappear though heart sounds are audible, hence the paradox.

Method to demonstrate pulsus paradoxus

- Ask the child to breathe normally and apply the cuff of the sphygmomanometer on his arm and inflate the cuff. Now, ask the child to hold his respiration in expiration and while allowing the mercury level to fall, auscultate for the Korotkoff sounds.
- Repeat the process in inspiration.
- The difference in the pressures in both the phases should not be more than 10 mmHg. Suspect cardiac tamponade, if this difference exceeds 20 mmHg.

Equality of Pulses

Radial, brachial, femoral and dorsalis pedis pulses should be felt on both the sides. If the pulse volume in upper limbs is felt unequal on both sides, a preductal coarctation of aorta should be suspected. If the pulse between upper and lower limbs is felt unequal (radio-femoral delay), a coarctation of aorta anywhere beyond the left subclavian artery should be suspected.

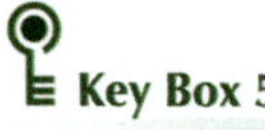
Key Box 5

Causes of Pulsus Paradoxus

1. Severe bronchial asthma
2. Pericardial effusion
3. Constrictive pericarditis
4. Severe congestive heart failure
5. Superior vena cava obstruction
6. Emphysema

C. Respiration

While assessing the respiration, comment on the parameters listed in **Key Box 6**.

Respiratory Rate

The respiratory rate coupled with color of the skin gives you an indication of the adequacy of ventilation and perfusion. The respiratory rate should be counted for complete 60 seconds when the child is at rest or sleeping. The physiological respiratory rates vary with the age of the child. The normal respiratory rates are given in **Key Box 7**. *Tachypnea* refers to fast respiration as per cut-offs defined by WHO **(Key Box 8)**.

Depth of Respiration

The normal sequence of respiratory events is inspiration–expiration–pause. The respiration may be *shallow* in narcotic poisonings and cervical cord compression; while it may be *rapid and deep* in metabolic acidosis (severe

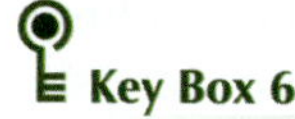
Key Box 6

Respiratory Parameters

1. Respiratory rate
2. Depth of respiration
3. Type of respiration
4. Rhythm
5. Work of breathing
6. Adventitious sounds (heard with naked ears)

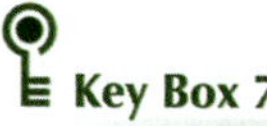
Key Box 7

Normal Respiratory Rates

• Preterm neonates	40–60 breaths per minute
• Term neonates	30–50 breaths per minute
• 1 month to 1 year	20–40 breaths per minute
• 1 to 5 years	20–30 breaths per minute
• 5 to 10 years	15–20 breaths per minute

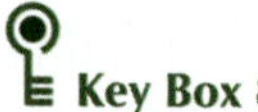
Key Box 8

Cut-off for Tachypnea

• 0–2 months	RR >60/min
• 2 months to 1 year	RR >50/min
• >1 year	RR >40/min

dehydration, diabetic ketoacidosis, salicylate poisoning and acute renal failure).

Kussmaul respiration refers to deep breathing (increase in tidal volume) seen in children with metabolic acidosis.

Type

The respiration is usually abdominal or abdominothoracic in infants; and thoracic in older children. In normal inspiration, the thorax and abdomen move out; the converse occurs in expiration. *Paradoxical respiration* occurs in diaphragmatic paralysis when the movement of abdomen is inwards in inspiration. In unilateral diaphragm paralysis, there is decreased movement of the diaphragm on the affected side.

Rhythm

Periodic breathing occurs normally in neonates when there are alternate periods of rapid respirations followed by apnea, which is not longer than 20 seconds and is not associated with bradycardia or cyanosis.

Cheyne-Stokes breathing is exactly similar to periodic breathing (period of apnea), but occurs in older children with cerebral edema or cardiac failure.

Pearls of Wisdom

Historical Pearls

Kussmaul Respiration: Reported by Adolf Kussmaul in 1874 in an adult with diabetic ketoacidosis as follows: *"A Peculiar Type of Dyspnea: In this type of dyspnea there is not the least suggestion as is so common in all other types that the passage of air to or from the lung has to combat obstruction in its path; to the contrary it passes in and out with the greatest of ease. The thorax expands noticeably in all directions without a pulling-in of the lower end of the sternum or intercostals spaces… and this complete inspiration is followed by a likewise complete expiration… Yet everything is indicative of extreme air hunger, such as the discomfort of angusty of which the patient complains, the extreme activity of the respiratory muscles, and the loud noise that the powerful inspirations and more so the expirations make… A true stridor, however, never exists… To the contrary, the noise of expiration often becomes a groan even when the patient lies unconscious in deep coma… The marked contrast between the extreme general weakness of the patient and the powerful respiratory movements is a striking peculiarity of this picture."*

Cheyne-Stokes Respiration: Reported by John Cheyne in 1818 in a patient of stroke with heart failure, as follows: *"The only peculiarity in the last period of his illness… was in the state of the respiration: For several days, his breathing was irregular; it would entirely cease for a quarter of a minute, then it would become perceptible, though very low, then by degrees it became heaving and quick, and then it would gradually cease again: This revolution in the state of his breathing occupied about a minute, during which there were about thirty acts of respiration."*

Reported by William Stoke in 1854 in heart failure as follows: *"It consists in the occurrence of a series of inspirations, increasing to a maximum, and then declining in force and length, until a state of apparent apnea is established. In this condition, the patient may remain for such a length of time as to [appear] dead, when a low inspiration… marks the commencement of a new ascending and then descending series of inspirations…The decline in the length and force of respirations is as regular and remarkable as their progressive increase. It is not entirely specific for congestive heart failure as he suggested. Less commonly, it can be a sign of stroke (apoplexy), toxic encephalopathies, traumatic encephalopathies, high-altitude pulmonary edema, and sleep apnea."*

Biot Respiration: Reported by Camille Biot, an intern from France, in 1876 described this pattern in a 16-year-old-patient with tuberculous meningitis as follows: *"Peculiarly, this breathing pattern lacks the crescendo-decrescendo cycles attributed to Cheyne-Stokes breathing and is completely irregular with varying periods of apnea. The breathing pattern is irregular and rapid, with rhythmical pauses lasting 10–30 seconds, but sometimes with alternating periods of apnea and tachypnea.This irregularity of the respiratory movements is not periodic, sometimes slow, sometimes rapid, sometimes superficial, sometimes deep, but without any constant relation of succession between the two types, with pauses following irregular intervals, preceded and often followed by a sigh more or less prolonged."*

Biot breathing occurs in conditions of raised intracranial pressure; it is characterized by apnea followed by 4–5 normal breaths.

Work of Breathing

The use of accessory muscles of respiration is visible by nasal flaring, recession of intercostal muscles, subcostal recession, supraclavicular and tracheal tug. *Tracheal tug* is the inward movement of trachea during inspiration.

Trail sign is the undue prominence of the clavicular head of sternomastoid on the side to which the trachea is deviated.

Adventitious Sounds

Listen for any obvious adventitious sounds during respiration, audible without a stethoscope **(Table 7.1)**. Observe whether they occur during expiration, inspiration, or in both the phases of respiration. Respiratory adventitious sounds usually are indicative of obstruction to the airway.

Different respiratory sounds include the following: *Snoring, rattling, grunting, groan, stridor, and wheeze*. These sounds differ in their pitch and intensity, depending on their site of origin.

- Sounds produced by obstruction near to oropharynx are more intense, but low pitched (e.g. snore).
- Sounds produced by obstruction in the terminal airways are high pitched (like blowing a whistle, e.g. wheeze), but less intense.

D. Blood Pressure

The proper technique for taking a blood pressure reading in children is the same as for measuring blood pressure in adults. As for all individuals, proper measuring technique is essential for obtaining accurate readings. Most devices for measuring blood pressure are dependent on one common feature, namely occluding the artery of an extremity (arm, wrist, finger or leg) with an inflatable cuff to measure blood pressure either oscillometrically, or by detection of Korotkoff sounds.

Prerequisites for Measuring Blood Pressure

1. *Appropriate cuff size:* The inflatable bladder should cover the circumference of the arm without overlapping. It should not exceed two-thirds the distance between axilla and cubital fossa. A cuff size of 2.5 to 4 cm wide is usually adequate for the neonate, 4–6 cm wide for an infant, 7.5–9 cm wide for young children, and 10 cm wide for older children and adolescents. The bladder length is approximately twice that of its width.

2. *Subject preparation:* A number of factors related to the subject can cause significant deviations in measured blood pressure. These include room temperature, exercise, alcohol or nicotine consumption, positioning of the arm, muscle tension, bladder distension, talking, and background noise. These need to be minimized.

- The child should be instructed to relax as much as possible and not to talk during the measurement procedure; ideally, *5 minutes should elapse before the first reading is taken*.
- Ask the child/parent to *remove all clothing from the area where the cuff is to be placed*.
- The child should be *comfortably seated*, with the legs uncrossed, and the back and arm supported, such that *the middle of the cuff on the upper arm is at the level of the right atrium* (the mid-point of the sternum) **(Fig. 7.4)**. Measurements with the patient lying on the examining table do not fulfil these criteria. BP should preferably be measured while the patient is seated in a chair.

Table 7.1: Respiratory sounds

Sound	Cause	Character
Snoring	Oropharyngeal obstruction	Inspiratory, low pitched, irregular
Grunting	Expiration against a partially closed glottis	Expiratory, occurs in hyaline membrane disease
Rattling	Secretions in airways	Inspiratory, may be felt by placing hands over the chest
Stridor	Obstruction in larynx/trachea	Inspiratory, sometimes an expiratory component
Wheeze	Lower airway obstruction	Whistling sound, predominantly expiratory

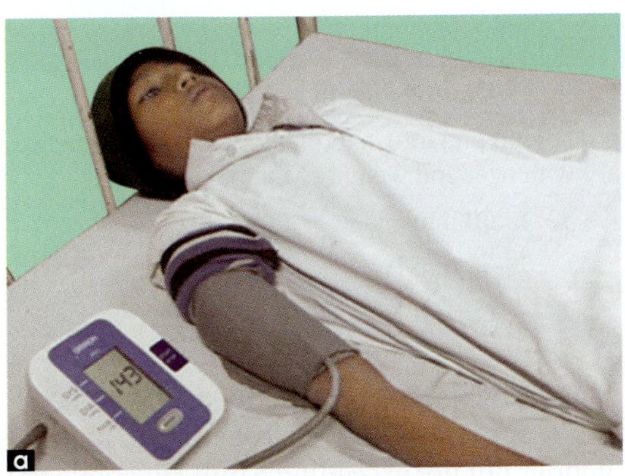

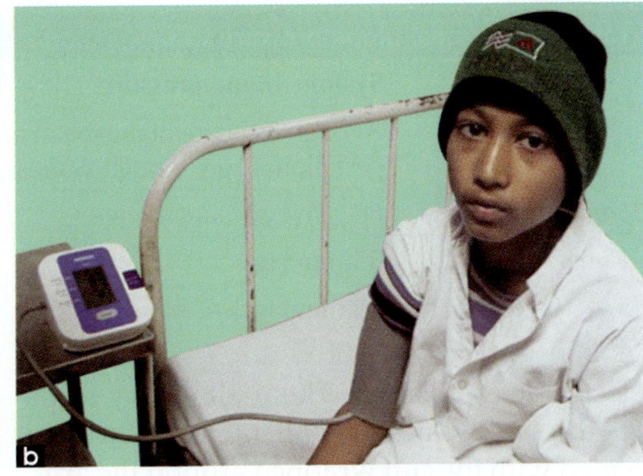

Fig. 7.4: Measurement of blood pressure in a child, in supine or sitting position; the manometer should be at the level of the heart.

- At the initial visit, blood pressure should be measured in both arms.

3. Remove observer related bias

- *Repetition:* Record at least 2 separate readings taken at least 2 minutes apart.
- *Consistency:* Blood pressure readings should be taken by the same person whenever possible. On a single visit to the doctor's office, the same person should obtain both readings for that day.
- *Instrument used:* The cuff should be wide enough to cover two-thirds the length of the upper arm.

Techniques of Blood Pressure Measurement

1. Auscultatory method

- Deflate the bladder of the cuff, and place it around the upper arm, so it fits snugly, but not too tightly. If you are right handed, you should hold the bulb/pump in your left hand to inflate the cuff. Hold it in the palm, so your fingers can easily reach the valve at the top to open/close the outlet to the air bladder wrapped around the child's arm.
- Put the head of the stethoscope just under the edge of the cuff, a little above the crease of the person's elbow. Hold it there firmly with the thumb, or with a few fingers of your right hand. Put the earpieces of the stethoscope in your ears.
- Inflate the cuff with brisk squeezes of the bulb, while palpating the radial artery pulsations. Watch the pressure gauge as you do it. Inflate till a pressure 20–30 mmHg above the level when the pulsations of radial artery had disappeared. For most kids, you should not need to go over 150 (the markings indicate "pressure" in mmHg or mercury).
- Now, slightly open the valve on the air pump (held in your left hand, as above). It is important that you do not let the air out too suddenly. Likewise, your friend will be quite irritated with you, if you let it out too slowly.
- Now, pay attention very carefully to what you hear through the stethoscope as the needle on the pressure gauge falls. You will be listening for a slight "blrrpp" or a something that sounds like "prrpshh". The first time you hear this sound, called Korotkoff sounds, note the reading on the pressure gauge. This value represents the *systolic blood pressure*.
- The sounds should continue, and become louder in intensity. Note the pressure reading when you hear the sound for the last time. This value represents the *diastolic blood pressure*.
- Afterwards, open the air valve completely to release any remaining pressure.

2. Palpatory method: Palpate the arterial pulse while the mercury column in the sphygmomanometer is allowed to fall. Note the level when the artery pulsations return, this indicates the systolic blood pressure.

3. Automated (digital) sphygmomanometer: The digital blood pressure monitor has an LCD screen to show the accurate reading and comes with self-inflating cuff, that is, the cuff inflates once it is secured and the device is turned on. It is based on oscillometric measurements and

Table 7.2: Normal blood pressure values

	Systolic blood pressure	Diastolic blood pressure
Neonates	A rough estimate of the mean arterial blood pressure in term neonates is equal to the gestational age, though values vary with age, and weight of the baby.	
1 month to 1 year	80 mm Hg	50 mm Hg
1 year to 5 years	85 mm Hg	55 mm Hg
5 to 10 years	95 mm Hg	60 mm Hg

electronic calculation. The preliminary steps are the same. Once the patient is comfortably seated with the cuff wrapped around the arm, press the power button to turn on the digital sphygmomanometer so that the cuff starts to inflate. Once the cuff reaches full pressure, it will begin to deflate at 2 to 5 mmHg per second. The final readings on the screen will depict the blood pressure (systolic, mean and diastolic blood pressure) and heart rate.

7

4. Flush method: This method is more useful in infants and younger children, and used to measure the systolic blood pressure. Wrap the cuff around the upper limb, limb is then raised vertically, and held above the head till the palm becomes pale. Now, inflate the cuff above the expected systolic blood pressure, while the arm is maintained in vertical position. Now, bring the arm down alongside the body and the cuff is deflated, till the palm becomes pink again; the level on the manometer at this point indicates the systolic blood pressure.

5. Other methods: *Doppler* is a non-invasive method to record blood pressure in neonates and infants. Alternatively, in critical settings, invasive arterial recording can also be taken.

Normal Values

These are summarized in **Table 7.2**. A rough guide to estimation of average (50th centile) systolic and diastolic blood pressures in children older than 1 year is as follows:

Systolic blood pressure = 90 + (age in years × 2)
Diastolic blood pressure = 55 + (age in years × 2)

Generally, boys have higher blood pressure values than girls of comparable age. The lower normal limit for systolic blood pressure, i.e. 5th centile is [70 + (age in years × 2)]. A child whose blood pressure exceeds the 95th centile for age and sex is said to have hypertension.

Stage 1 hypertension is defined as systolic BP (and/or diastolic BP) >95th centile for age and gender but not exceeding 5 mm Hg above the 99th centile. Average systolic or diastolic blood pressure > 99th centile plus 5 mm Hg suggests stage 2 hypertension.

E. Capillary Filling Time (CFT)

This test is performed at bedside to assess the peripheral perfusion of tissues.

Press with your thumb against a bony prominence (sternum or forehead) for 5 seconds to allow the skin to be blanched, and note the time taken for the skin to regain its color.

You can also blanch the finger pulp or nail-beds, but ensure that hands are warm.

The skin regains its usual pink color within 3 seconds, if the perfusion is good.

A CFT more than 3 seconds is considered prolonged and indicates poor perfusion and shock.

CFT is prolonged in severe dehydration, and shock.

F. Assessment of Hydration

Any child presenting with a history of diarrhea should be evaluated for dehydration. The following clinical signs are used to assess the hydration:

- *Child's general condition/sensorium:* Assess if the child is alert, lethargic or restless/irritable or drowsy. Offer water to drink. Note whether the child accepts readily (thirsty) or refuses drink.
- *Observe the eyes and note whether sunken.*
- *Elasticity of skin/skin turgor:* Pinch the skin over the abdomen midway between the umbilicus and side, and release it. The skin goes back either very slowly (longer than 2 seconds); slowly (skin stays up even for a brief instant); or immediately.

Table 7.3: Assessment of dehydration

	No dehydration	Some dehydration	Severe dehydration
Sensorium#	Alert, well	Irritable, restless	Lethargic, unconscious
Eyes#	Normal	Sunken	Very sunken
Tears	Present	Absent/present	Absent
Oral mucosa and tongue	Moist	Dry	Very dry
Skin pinch#	Goes back immediately	Goes back slowly*	Goes back very slowly**
Thirst	Normal, not thirsty	Drinks eagerly	Not able to drink
Urine output	Normal	Decreased	Very decreased/absent

#According to IMNCI, at least 2 of the following signs should be present to classify as some or severe dehydration.

Skin pinch: Check the elasticity of the skin using the 'skin pinch test'. Locate the area on the child's abdomen between the umbilicus and the side of the abdomen; then pinch the skin between the thumb and index finger. Pick up all the layers of the skin for one second, and then release it and observe the return of the skinfold. This test is not useful in malnourished and obese children and in infants.

*When released, the skinfold stays up briefly.

**When released, the skinfold stays up longer than 2 seconds.

The oral mucosa may be otherwise dry in a child who is a mouth-breather, and may be wet in a dehydrated child who has just vomited or if he has been drinking fluids.

In a marasmic child, the skin may go back slowly even if the child is not dehydrated. The reverse may occur in an edematous or obese child.

Classifying Severity of Dehydration

A child with *severe dehydration* would have the following clinical markers of dehydration: Lethargic/unconscious, sunken eyes, not able to drink or drinking poorly, skin pinch goes back very slowly.

A child with *some dehydration* would have the following clinical markers of dehydration: Restless/irritable, sunken eyes, drinks eagerly, thirsty, skin pinch goes back slowly.

Classify dehydration as *No, Some* or *Severe* **(Table 7.3)**.

G. Oxygen Saturation

It is a useful bedside tool to assess hypoxemia in a patient. It measures the percentage saturation of hemoglobin bound with oxygen in blood.

Method

An oxygen saturation probe is attached to a pulse oximeter applied across a capillary rich area, like pulp of finger/toe or ear lobule. A red and infrared rich light source allows light to pass through tissue and depending upon the concentration of the oxygenated hemoglobin, some of the light is absorbed and what comes out at the receiving end of the probe is analyzed by a microprocessor. Values are expressed as percentage of oxygen saturation of hemoglobin. A saturation of less than 90% in under-five children indicates hypoxemia.

Advantages and Disadvantages

The main advantages of pulse oximetry are that it is non-invasive, reproducible, requires minimal training, and is useful especially in infants and young children. However, its accuracy is less when there is severe desaturation (<70%), hemoglobinopathies, hypotension, hypothermia, or carbon monoxide poisoning. Also it needs maintenance and when used alone may not identify sick children needing hospitalization.

7.4 GENERAL MARKERS OF DISEASE

Now, we will discuss a few general markers of disease which should be assessed in every child **(Key Box 9)**. As far as possible, these signs should be looked for in natural daylight.

A. Pallor

Pallor is the paleness of skin or mucous membranes, which is usually due to diminished number of circulating red cells resulting in anemia and may also be a manifestation of shock.

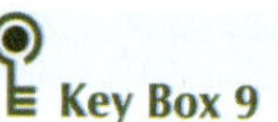

Key Box 9

General Markers of Disease

1. Pallor
2. Icterus
3. Cyanosis
4. Clubbing
5. Lymphadenopathy
6. Edema
7. Jugular venous pressure

Where to Look?

Look for pallor at the following sites:

i. Lower palpebral conjunctiva (upper palpebral conjunctiva may be scarred due to trachoma making assessment difficult);
ii. Dorsum of the tongue;
iii. Oral mucosa;
iv. Palmar or plantar creases;
v. Skin (Fig. 7.5); and nails.

Grading of Pallor

Clinically, pallor may be graded as moderate and severe. In *severe* pallor, the palmar creases become faint and pale. In *moderate* pallor, there is paleness of the mucosae, but pink hue of the palmar creases is maintained.

Tips to Aid Assessment

Look for the coexistence of other signs, which may help to aid in diagnosis of the etiology or complications of anemia.

i. Tachycardia (congestive heart failure)
ii. Edema (CHF, nephritic syndrome)
iii. Pulse volume (low in shock)
iv. Nail changes (koilonychia, platynychia in iron deficiency anemia, splinter hemorrhages in associated thrombocytopenia)
v. Skin changes (hyperpigmentation in megaloblastic anemia, petechiae in malignancies, aplastic anemia)
vi. Lymphadenopathy and hepatosplenomegaly (infection, hemolysis, or infiltration)
vii. In the presence of jaundice, sometimes it may be difficult to distinguish pallor from icterus.

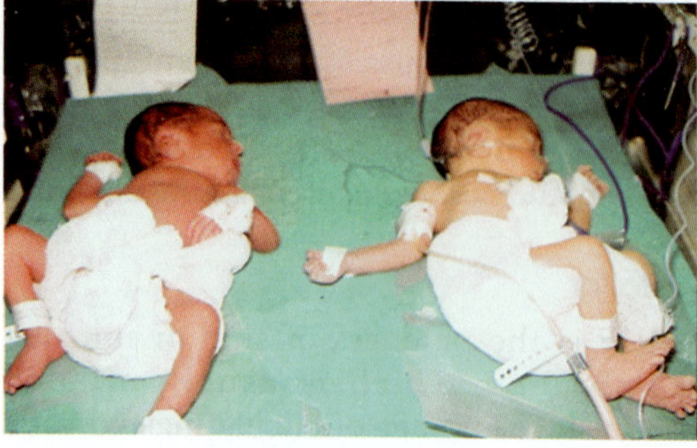

Fig. 7.5: The baby on the left appears pink compared to the baby on the right who is pale.

B. Icterus

Icterus is the yellowish discoloration of skin and mucosal membranes seen in children with jaundice. Usually, jaundice becomes apparent clinically as icterus at serum bilirubin levels exceeding 2 mg/dL in older children and at more than 5 mg/dL in neonates.

Where to Look?

Icterus is, usually, observed at the following sites:

i. Sclera (Fig. 7.6)
ii. Palate
iii. Under surface of tongue
iv. Tip of nose
v. Palms and soles (in neonates)

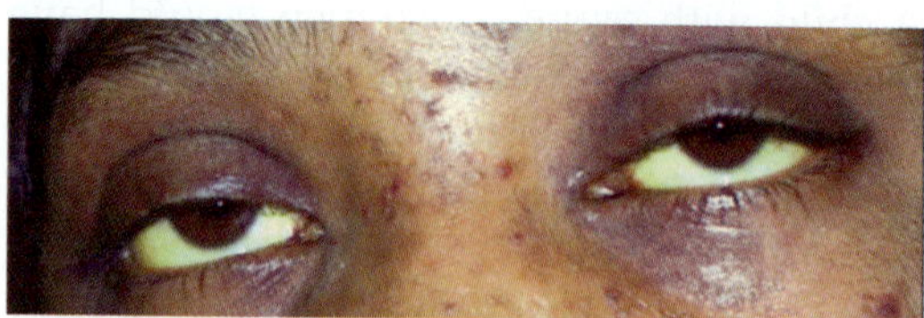

Fig. 7.6: Icteric sclerae.

Assessment in a neonate: Press the skin against a bony surface for 5 seconds to blanch the skin and observe the skin color. You can even provide a rough estimate of the level of bilirubin by seeing the extent of jaundiced discoloration of skin **(Key Box 10)**.

Look at the type of yellow discoloration as it may even provide a clue to the etiology.

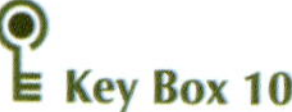

Key Box 10

Evaluation of Extent of Hyperbilirubinemia in Newborn

Face and neck	4–6 mg/dL
Upper trunk	6–9 mg/dL
Lower trunk and thighs	9–12 mg/dL
Legs	12–15 mg/dL
Palms and soles	>15 mg/dL

7

Clinical Methods in Pediatrics

A lemon yellow tint indicates underlying hemolysis, while a dark yellow or an orange tint indicates obstructive jaundice.

C. Cyanosis

Cyanosis refers to the bluish discoloration of skin and mucous membranes due to the presence of reduced hemoglobin in the blood (Fig. 7.7). Cyanosis becomes apparent when the reduced hemoglobin level exceeds 5 mg/dL. However, in severely anemic children, cyanosis may not be apparent even in the presence of hypoxemia. Usually, cyanosis is associated with oxygen saturation (SpO_2) below 85%. **Key Box 11** enlists the important causes of cyanosis.

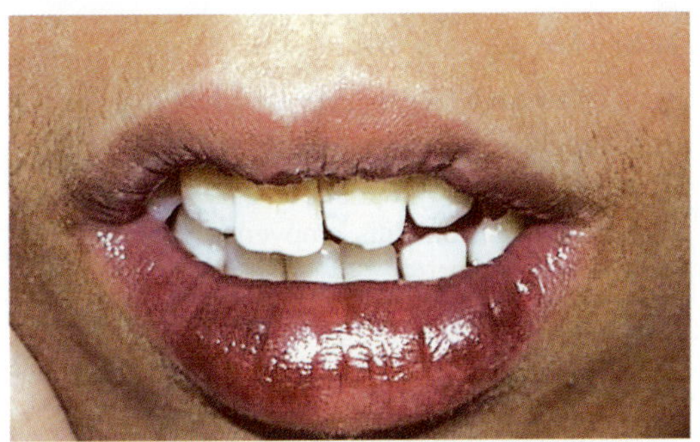

Fig. 7.7: Central cyanosis in a child.

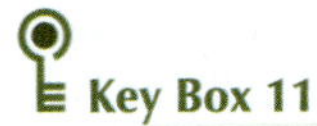

Key Box 11

Causes of Cyanosis

A. Central cyanosis

1. *Impaired pulmonary function:* Alveolar hypoventilation, ventilation-perfusion mismatch, impaired oxygen diffusion
2. *Cardiac shunts:* Cyanotic congenital heart diseases (TOF, TGA with VSD, TAPVR, tricuspid atresia, etc.), pulmonary AV fistulas, multiple small intrapulmonary shunts
3. *Hemoglobin abnormalities:* Methemoglobinemia, sulfhemoglobinemia, carboxyhemoglobinemia

B. Peripheral cyanosis: Cold exposure, congestive heart failure, arterial obstruction (Raynaud phenomenon, emboli), venous obstruction (thrombophlebitis)

Classification

Depending upon the distribution of cyanosis, it is classified as:

- *Central:* Cyanosis of mucosae and extremities.
- *Peripheral:* Cyanosis in extremities but not the mucosae.
- *Differential:* In the first variety, the hands are blue but feet are pink (coarctation of aorta with transposition of great vessels). Alternatively, the hands are pink, but the feet are blue (patent ductus arteriosus with shunt reversal due to pulmonary hypertension).

D. Clubbing

It is a condition affecting the fingers and toes in which proliferation of distal soft tissues, especially the nail beds, results in thickening and widening of the extremities of the digits. The nails are abnormally curved, the nail beds excessively compressible, and skin over them becomes red and shiny. It occurs due to the opening up of anastomotic channels in the nail-bed due to anoxic stimuli.

Clubbing is usually painless (except hypertrophic pulmonary arthropathy) and a slow process indicating a chronic hypoxic or toxic stimulus for hypervascularity and opening of arteriovenous anastomosis.

How to Assess Presence of Clubbing?

1. *Nailfold angle:* In normal fingers, the nail extends from the base (the profile angle) at about 160°, but in clubbed fingers this angle approaches 180°.

2. *Phalangeal depth ratio:* In normal fingers, the distal phalangeal depth (DPD) should be smaller than the interphalangeal depth (IPD); this relationship is reversed in the finger with clubbing. Since calipers may not be readily available, physicians may estimate the phalangeal depth ratio. Clubbing is considered present, if the DPD/IPD ratio is greater than 1.0.

3. *Schamroth sign:* The *Schamroth sign* describes the "window" that is created when the dorsal surfaces of the terminal phalanges on opposing fingers are placed together. A normal finger shows a diamond-shaped window, while the clubbed finger will have no space visible between the opposing nails (Fig. 7.8).

Figure 7.9 shows clubbing of fingers.

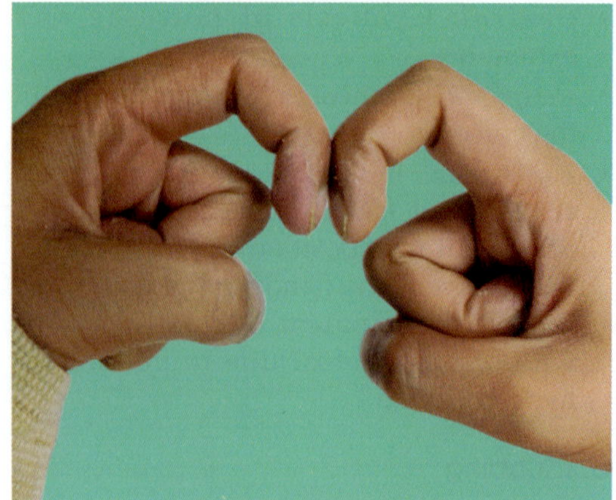

Fig. 7.8: Schamroth sign (Grade II clubbing).

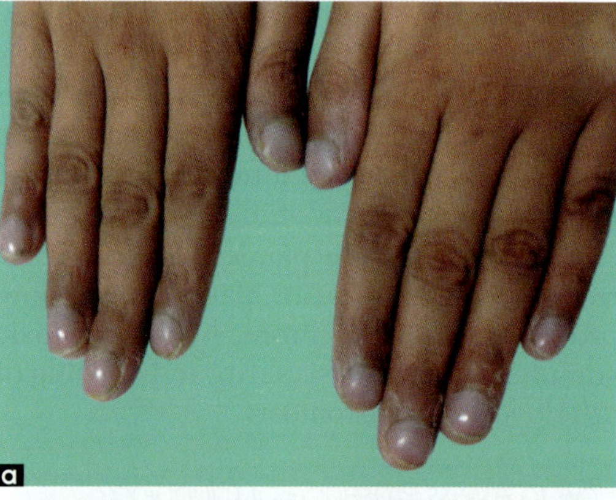

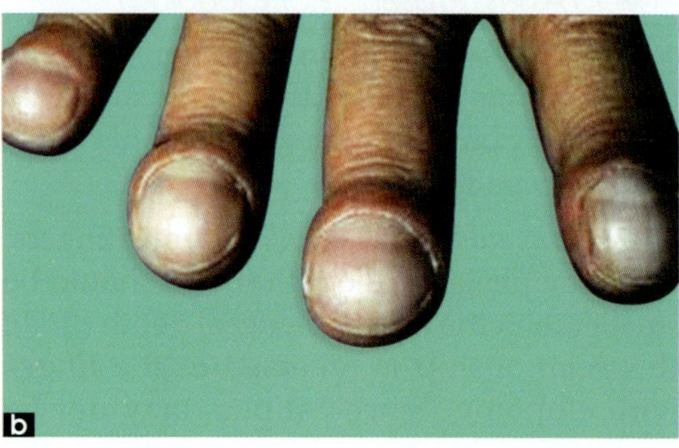

Fig. 7.9 Clubbed nails. (a) Grade III (top); (b) grade IV.

Grades of clubbing

Grade I: Softening of the nailbed (fluctuation of nailbed).

Grade II: Obliteration of the angle between nail base and adjoining skin (nailfold) (*Schamroth sign*).

Grade III: Swelling of subcutaneous tissues over the base of nail making the overlying skin shiny, and increased curvature of nail (*parrot beak or drumstick appearance*).

Grade IV: Swelling of fingers in all dimensions associated with hypertrophic pulmonary arthropathy (pain and swelling of wrist and hands with radiographic evidence of new subperiosteal bone formation).

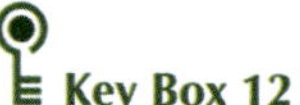

Key Box 12

Diseases Associated with Clubbing

A. Symmetrical Clubbing

1. *Respiratory diseases:* Bronchiectasis, chronic bronchitis, empyema, tuberculosis, cystic fibrosis
2. *Liver diseases:* Biliary cirrhosis, chronic active hepatitis
3. *Cyanotic:* Congenital heart diseases and infective endocarditis
4. *Others:* Celiac disease, thyrotoxicosis, Hodgkin lymphoma, familial

B. Asymmetrical Clubbing

1. *Unilateral:* Anomalous aortic arch, aortic or subclavian artery aneurysm, pulmonary hypertension with patent ductus arteriosus, brachial arteriovenous aneurysm or fistula, recurrent shoulder dislocation, superior sulcus (Pancoast) tumor
2. *Unidigital:* Median nerve injury, sarcoidosis
3. *Clubbing of toes without fingers:* Coarctation of aorta

Key Box 12 lists the important causes of clubbing.

E. Lymphadenopathy

1. Cervical Lymph Nodes

Lymph nodes of the neck: Stand behind the child, and flex the neck of the child slightly. Alternatively, neck can also be flexed from the front with the head tilted to the side being examined. The superficial cervical lymph nodes must be examined from above downwards: Submental, submandibular, tonsillar, cervical (upper, middle, lower), posterior auricular and occipital.

- Systematically palpate with the pads of your index and middle fingers for the various cervical lymph nodes in the sequence indicated in **Key Box 13**.
- *Deep cervical lymph nodes* should be palpated, one side at a time. Gently bend the child's head forward and roll your fingers over the deeper muscles along the carotid arteries.

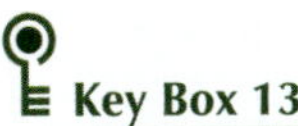

Key Box 13

Feel for the Following Cervical Lymph Nodes, in this Sequence

1. *Pre-auricular:* In front of the ear
2. *Post-auricular:* Behind the ear
3. *Occipital:* At the base of the skull
4. *Tonsillar:* At the angle of the jaw
5. *Submandibular:* Under the jaw on the side
6. *Submental:* Under the jaw in the midline
7. *Superficial (anterior) cervical:* Over and in front of the sternomastoid muscle
8. *Posterior cervical:* Along the anterior margin of trapezius
9. *Deep cervical:* Feel behind the sternomastoid with your thumb and finger
10. *Supraclavicular:* In the angle of the sternomastoid and the clavicle

- To feel *scalene nodes*, roll your fingers gently behind the clavicles. Instruct the child (older) to cough or to bear down like he is having a bowel movement. Occasionally, an enlarged lymph node may pop up.

Figure 7.10 is a line diagram depicting the location of the cervical glands. **Figures 7.11 to 7.13** show the palpation of submental, submandibular, and supraclavicular groups of cervical nodes, respectively.

2. Axillary Lymph Nodes

- Axillary nodes should be examined by inserting the fingers in the axillae with the patient's arm slightly abducted.
- The apical, anterior, posterior, medial, and lateral groups are examined.

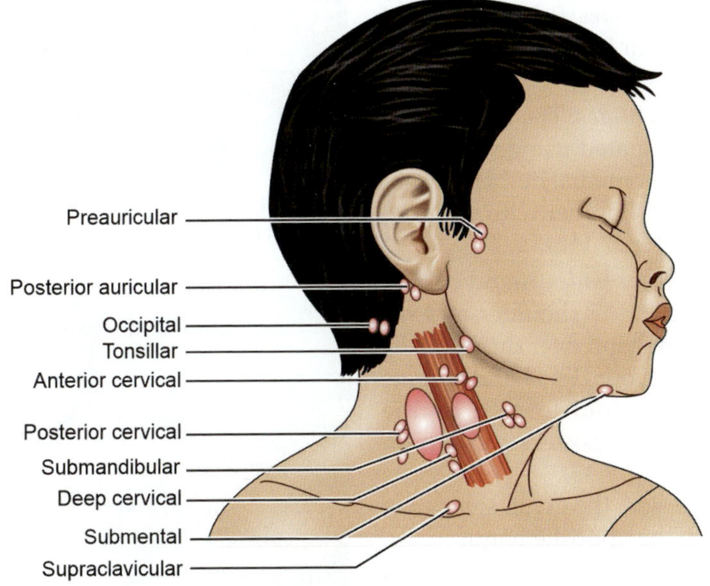

Fig. 7.10: Location of different cervical glands.

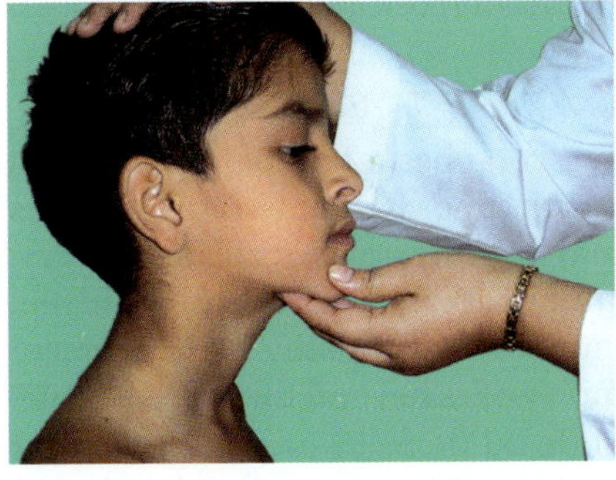

Fig. 7.11 Palpation of submental lymph node.

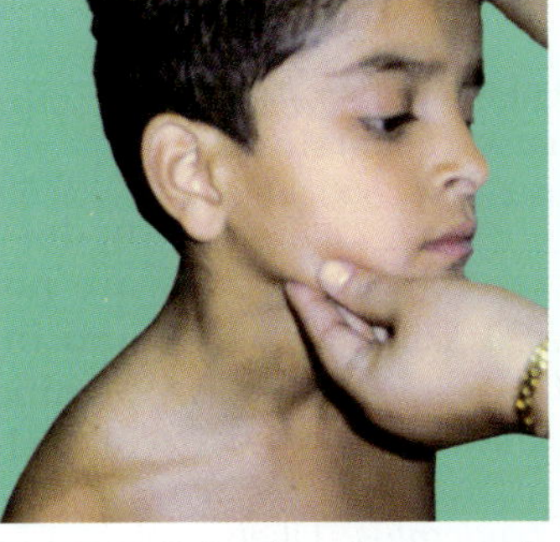

Fig. 7.12 Palpation of submandibular lymph nodes.

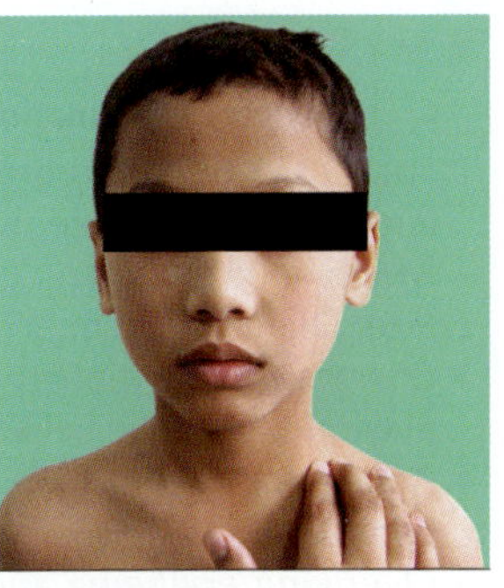

Fig. 7.13 Palpation of the supraclavicular lymph node.

- You can examine the apical, anterior, medial, and lateral group of axillary lymph nodes while standing in front of the child, while the posterior group of axillary lymph nodes is examined while standing behind the child.

Right anterior axillary nodes: These should be palpated by your left hand (palmar surface). Abduct the child's arm slightly, flex the elbow, and passively place the forearm on your right palm. Now, use your left hand to palpate the pectoralis major forming the anterior axillary fold, and the lymph nodes on its posterior surface.

Right apical axillary nodes: In the same position by depressing the child's shoulder with your right hand, palpate the right apical group by insinuating your fingers of left hand, deeper into the axilla.

Right medial axillary nodes: Palpate the right medial group with your left hand against the upper lateral chest wall (Fig. 7.14a).

Right lateral axillary nodes: The right lateral axillary nodes are palpated using your right hand against the upper medial humerus, after abducting the child's shoulder with your left hand on the elbow (Fig. 7.14b).

Right posterior axillary nodes: Stand behind the child, abduct the child's shoulder, and ask to place his/her right hand over the opposite shoulder. Now, using your right hand palpate the posterior axillary fold formed by the latissimus dorsi and the posterior group on its anterior surface (Fig. 7.15).

For the opposite side, the given steps may be performed with the opposite hand.

Describe the lymph node in terms of the parameters outlined in **Key Box 14**.

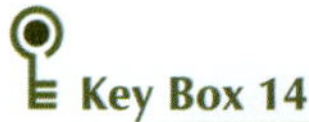

Physical Examination of the Node

1. *Location:* Local, regional or generalized (enlargement of more than 2 non-contiguous lymph node groups).
2. *Size:* Diameter in cm.
3. *Character:* Firm, rubbery, etc. is subjective and may or may not be helpful.
4. *Adherence to underlying structures:* Fixed or non-fixed.
5. *Overlying erythema and tenderness:* Likely infectious or non-infectious.

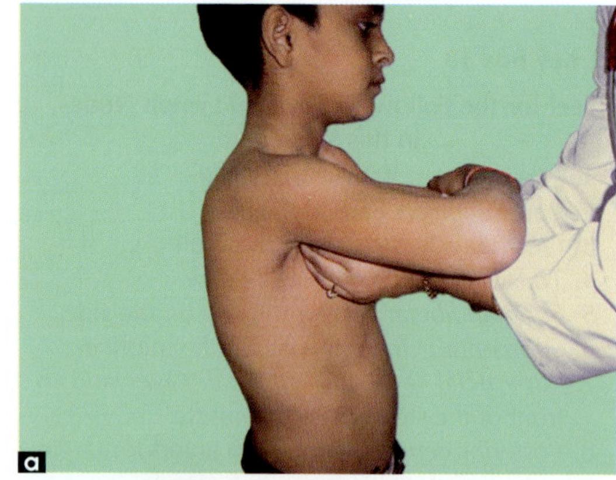

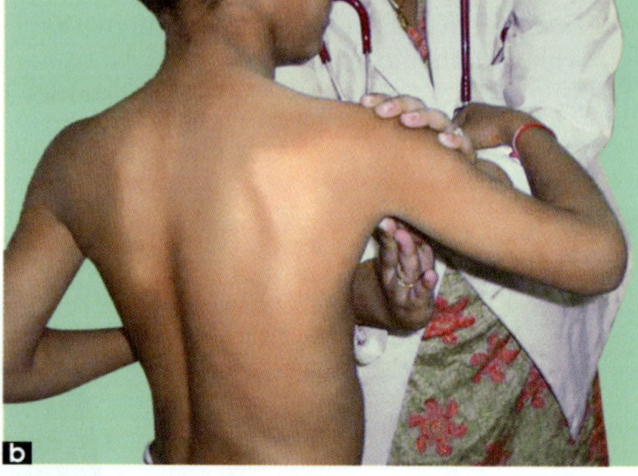

Fig. 7.14: (a) Palpation of medial; (b) lateral axillary group of lymph nodes.

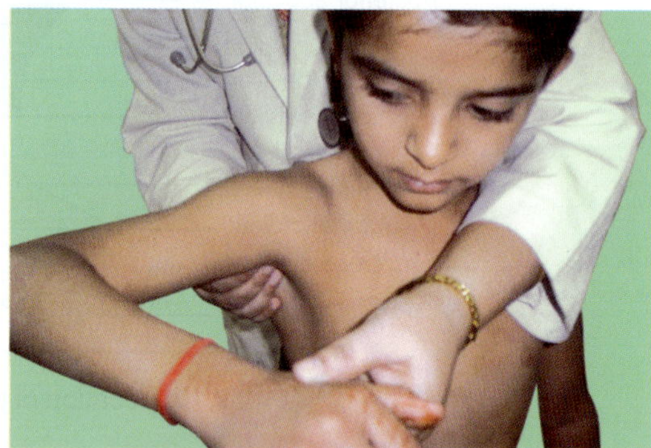

Fig. 7.15 Palpation of posterior axillary lymph nodes.

3. What is Significant Lymphadenopathy?

Almost everyone has a few palpable lymph nodes at any time. Palpable lymph nodes are normal in anterior cervical, axillary, and inguinal regions in healthy children. Significant lymphadenopathy is enlargement of the lymph nodes beyond this normal state.

Any node >1.0 cm in greatest diameter can be significant, but certain nodes should be considered enlarged at different sizes (i.e. epitrochlear nodes >0.5 cm, inguinal nodes >1.5 cm, submandibular nodes >1.5 cm). The presence of even shotty (<0.5 cm) supraclavicular or epitrochlear nodes is reason for concern and further evaluation.

Examination of lymphadenopathy is complicated by age. A 1.5 cm inguinal or a 2 cm anterior cervical node in a 7-year-old child might be of little concern, but in a 2-month-old infant would be an indication for further evaluation.

Nodes that are matted together, firm, and non-tender increase the risk of malignancy.

Lymphadenitis is suggested by erythema, tenderness, warmth, and fluctuance.

Localized or regional lymphadenopathy is more likely to be infectious while generalized lymphadenopathy is more suggestive of a malignancy or inflammatory or immune disorders. Detailed etiology of lymphadenopathy is given in **Key Box 15**. Figure 7.16 shows a child with marked inguinal lymphadenopathy.

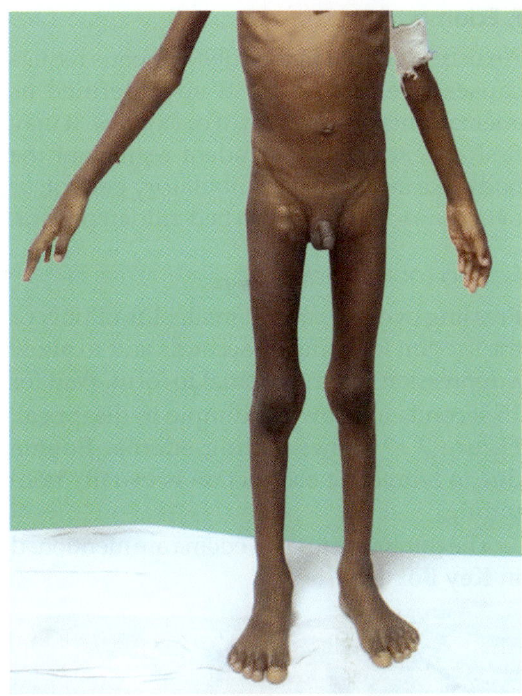

Fig. 7.16: Inguinal lymphadenopathy.

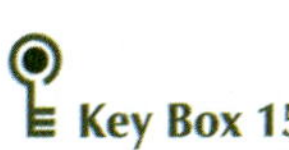

Key Box 15

Etiology of Lymphadenopathy

A. Generalized lymphadenopathy (enlargement of >2 contiguous lymph node groups)

Viral: Common upper respiratory infections, infectious mononucleosis, CMV, acquired immunodeficiency syndrome, rubella, varicella, measles

Bacterial: Septicemia, typhoid fever, tuberculosis, syphilis, plague

Protozoal: Toxoplasmosis

Fungal: Coccidioidomycosis

Autoimmune disorders and hypersensitivity states: Juvenile rheumatoid arthritis, systemic lupus erythematosus, serum sickness

Drug reactions: Phenytoin, allopurinol

Storage diseases: Gaucher disease, Niemann-Pick disease

Neoplastic and proliferative disorders: Acute leukemias, lymphomas (Hodgkin, non-Hodgkin), neuroblastoma, histiocytoses

B. Regional lymphadenopathy

Cervical: Viral upper respiratory infection, infectious mononucleosis, rubella, cat scratch disease, streptococcal pharyngitis, acute bacterial lymphadenitis, toxoplasmosis, tuberculosis/atypical mycobacterial infection, acute leukemia, lymphoma, neuroblastoma, rhabdomyosarcoma, Kawasaki disease

Submaxillary and submental: Oral and dental infections

Occipital: Pediculosis capitis, tinea capitis, secondary to local skin infection, rubella, roseola

Pre-auricular: Local skin infection, chronic ophthalmic infection, cat scratch disease

Mediastinal: Acute lymphoblastic leukemia, lymphoma, sarcoidosis, cystic fibrosis, tuberculosis, histoplasmosis, coccidioidomycosis

Supraclavicular: Lymphoma, tuberculosis, histoplasmosis, coccidioidomycosis

Axillary: Local infection, cat scratch disease, brucellosis, reactions to immunization, lymphoma

Abdominal: Acute mesenteric adenitis, lymphoma

Inguinal: Local infection, diaper dermatitis, insect bites, syphilis, lymphogranuloma venereum

F. Edema

An excess of fluid in the subcutaneous tissues causes swelling of the tissues defined as edema. It may be *generalized* or *localized*. It may first appear in the dependent regions of the body like the feet in an ambulatory patient; or over the sacral region in a bed-ridden patient.

How to Look for Edema?

Pressing over the medial malleolus of tibia or the sacrum for about 30 seconds and to allow a depression (pitting edema) to form. Wait for 15 seconds to allow the dimple to disappear. **Figure 7.17** shows pitting edema. Edema due to lymphatic obstruction is usually non-pitting.

The common causes of edema are mentioned in **Key Box 16**.

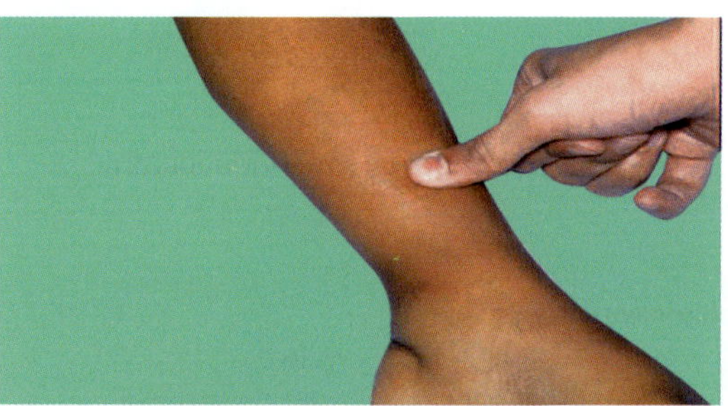

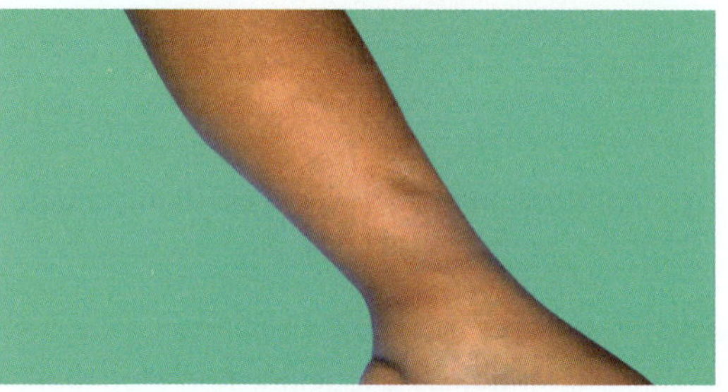

Fig. 7.17: Pitting pedal edema.

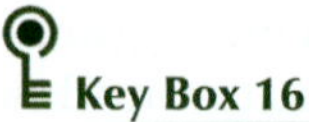

Key Box 16

Common Causes of Edema

A. Generalized edema

1. Nephrotic syndrome
2. Congestive heart failure
3. Kwashiorkor
4. Hepatic failure

B. Localized edema

1. Angioneurotic edema
2. Urticaria
3. Cellulitis
4. Trauma
5. Filariasis
6. Congenital (Milroy disease is congenital edema usually confined to the legs)

G. Jugular Venous Pressure (JVP)

The pressure in the internal jugular vein reflects the pressure of the right atrium, however, the external jugular vein is more readily visible and, therefore, JVP is usually estimated by examining the external jugular vein. This is more so in smaller children who have shorter necks. Ideally, JVP should be measured in internal jugular vein.

How to Measure JVP?

- Incline the child's back at 45° sitting on the bed. Allow him to rest his back against your arm or a backrest **(Fig. 7.18)**.
- The neck muscles must be relaxed; so it is also important to support the neck.
- The upper level of pulsations in the external jugular vein is seen using a torch beam directed tangentially across the neck.

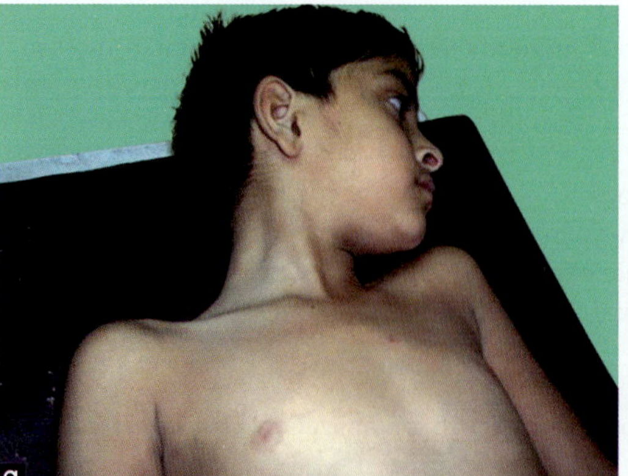

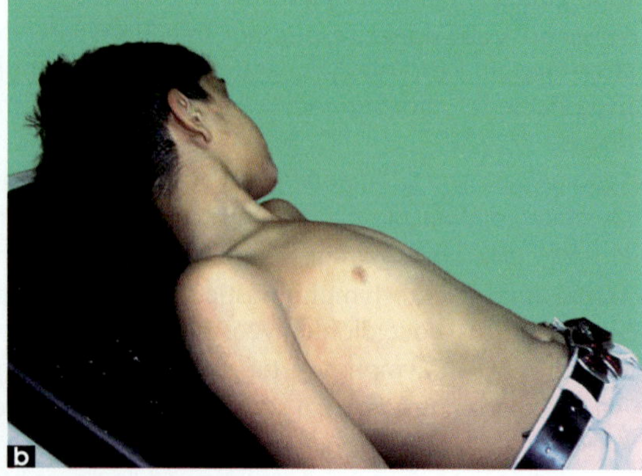

Fig. 7.18: (a) Look for the two heads of sterno-scleidomastoid; (b) position of patient for assessing JVP.

- Do not mistake the carotid pulsations for venous pulsations. The venous pulsations have a predominant inward motion and the upper level falls with inspiration as opposed to arterial pulsations which have a predominant outward motion.
- Measure the top of the pulsations from the sternal angle. The sternal angle is at a distance of 5 cm from the center of the right atrium in any position of the body.
- In a normal child, the distance of the upper level of pulsations from the sternal angle does not exceed 2 cm when reclining at 45°. Therefore, in a healthy child reclining at 45°, the mean level will be invisible and when reclining at 90°, this level should not be more than the level of the clavicle.
- Causes of raised JVP are summarized in **Key Box 17**.

Jugular Venous Pulse

- The normal jugular venous pulse consists of three positive waves *a*, *c*, and *v* and two negative waves x and y. **Figure 7.19** shows a line diagram of the jugular venous pulse.
- The *a* wave occurs due to right atrial contraction.

Key Box 17

Causes of Raised Jugular Venous Pressure

1. Right ventricular failure
2. Cardiac tamponade
3. Tricuspid stenosis
4. Superior vena cava obstruction
5. Hyperkinetic circulatory state
6. Increased blood volume
7. Lung diseases, e.g. asthma, emphysema

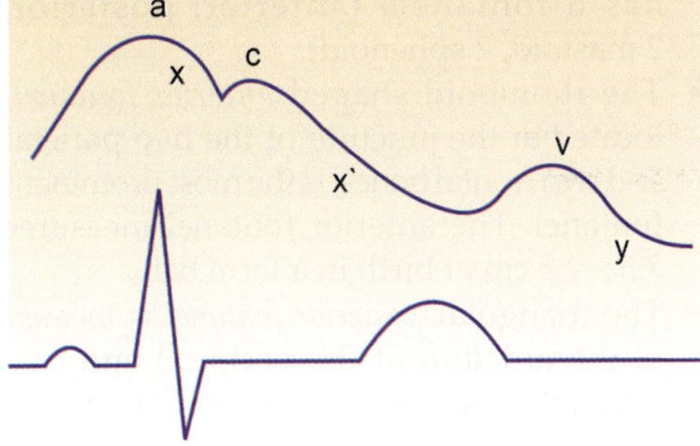

Fig. 7.19: Waveforms of jugular venous pulse.

- The *c* wave occurs due to impact of the carotid artery adjacent to the jugular vein and retrograde transmission of a positive wave in the right atrium produced by the right ventricular systole and the bulging of the tricuspid valve into the right atrium.
- The *x* wave is produced by the downward displacement of the tricuspid valve during ventricular systole and due to continued atrial relaxation.
- The *v* wave is produced because of right atrial filling with the tricuspid valve closed during ventricular systole.
- The *y* wave is produced by the opening of the tricuspid valve and subsequent rapid inflow of blood from the right atrium into the right ventricle leading to a sudden fall in right atrial pressure.
- The ascending limb of *y* wave is due to continuous diastolic inflow of blood into the great veins, right atrium and ventricle which are all in free communication during diastole.

Hepatojugular reflux

When pressure is applied over the liver by pressing firmly below the right costal margin for 30 seconds, the venous pressure gets exaggerated initially due to increased venous return. Later the myocardium accommodates the extra venous return and the level falls. However, in early cardiac failure, there is a positive hepatojugular reflux.

7.5 HEAD-TO-TOE EXAMINATION

Complete general examination should be done stepwise starting from head to the toes **(Key Box 18)** and must always include all the four basic techniques, *viz.* inspection, palpation, percussion, and auscultation.

A. Cranium

1. Size and Shape

- Observe whether the shape of the skull looks normal or not. **Key Box 19** describes different abnormal shapes of skull.
- Also look for and palpate for any swelling over the scalp. In a newborn baby, look for a soft fluctuant swelling on the scalp which may either be a caput succedaneum (crosses the suture lines) or a cephalhematoma (does not cross suture lines).

Key Box 18

The 10 Components of Head to Toe Examination

1. Cranium
2. Face
3. Eyes
4. Ears
5. Nose
6. Mouth and oral cavity
7. Neck
8. Hands, feet, and limbs
9. Skin and nails
10. Genitalia

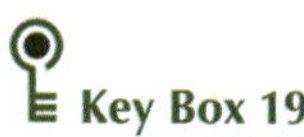

Key Box 19

Abnormal Shapes of the Skull

1. *Brachycephaly:* Anterior–posterior flattened skull (square and short) due to premature closure of coronal suture, e.g. Down syndrome.
2. *Scaphocephaly/dolichocephaly:* Anteroposteriorly elongated skull due to premature fusion of sagittal suture. The parietal eminences are usually absent.
3. *Trigonocephaly:* Pointed skull due to closure of metopic suture.
4. *Plagiocephaly:* Skewing of skull due to premature unilateral fusion of coronal or lambdoid suture or it may be a flattened occiput which is postural in infancy.
5. *Oxycephaly/acrocephaly/turricephaly:* Elongation of the skull like a tower due to premature closure of multiple sutures.

- Record the head circumference (*see* anthropometric examination) and compare with the normal value expected for the child's age and sex from the growth standards. Look for any abnormally large head (>2 SD for age, macrocephaly) **(Fig. 7.20)**, or abnormally small head (<–3 SD for age, microcephaly) **(Fig. 7.21)**. **Figure 7.22** depicts the various abnormal skull shapes.

2. Sutures

Palpate the sutures. Are the sutures closed prematurely (*craniosynostosis*) or are they widely separated (may occur in vitamin D deficiency, hydrocephalus, achondroplasia, prematurity, osteogenesis imperfecta, raised intracranial tension, congenital hypothyroidism)?

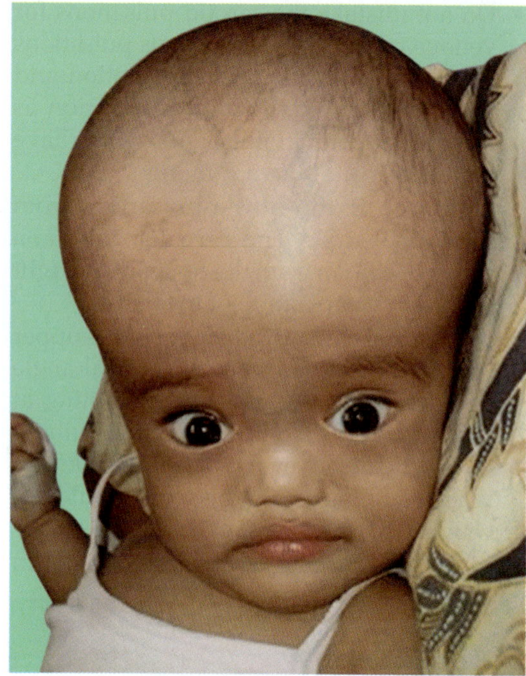

Fig. 7.20: A child with macrocephaly.

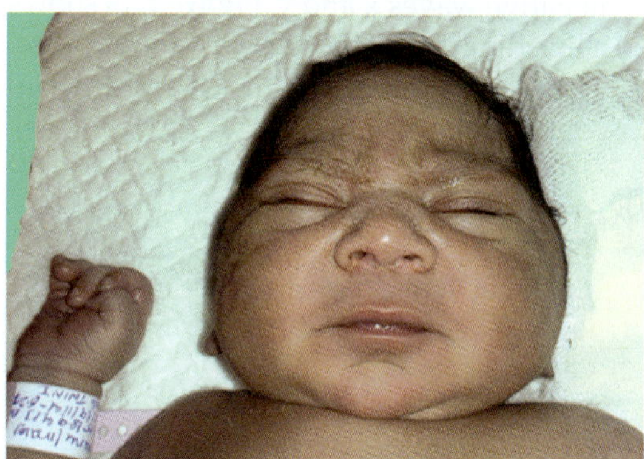

Fig. 7.21: A child with microcephaly.

3. Fontanels

- Palpate the fontanels. A neonate normally has 6 fontanels (anterior, posterior, 2 mastoid, 2 sphenoid).
- The rhomboid-shaped *anterior fontanel*, located at the juncture of the two parietal and two frontal bones, is the most prominent fontanel. The anterior fontanel measures 2.5 × 2.5 cm at birth in a term baby.
- The triangular *posterior fontanel* is located at the junction of the occipital and two parietal bones. The posterior fontanel at birth usually is the size of tip of the little finger (0.5 cm).

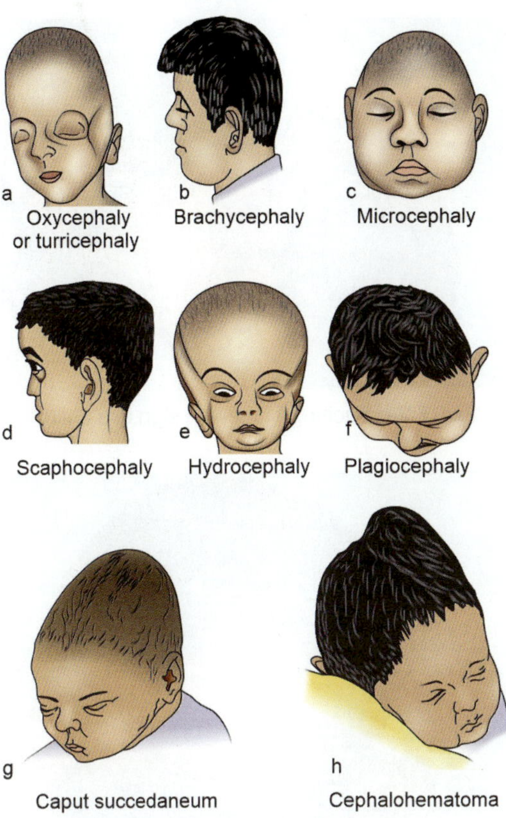

Fig. 7.22: Abnormal skull shapes.

- Sometimes, a *third fontanel* between the anterior and posterior fontanels is seen. It is associated with congenital hypothyroidism and Down syndrome.
- Usually, the anterior fontanel closes between 9 and 24 months of age while the posterior fontanel closes by six weeks of age.
- Delayed closure may be suggestive of malnutrition, rickets, raised intracranial tension, achondroplasia, or hypothyroidism.
- Also measure the size of the anterior fontanel, obtained by measuring the lines joining the mid-points of opposite sides. Another method is to measure it in length and breadth **(Fig. 7.23)**.
- Palpate to decide, if the fontanel is bulging (raised ICT) or depressed (depressed). Ensure that the child is not crying during examination and that his head is held upright.
- A bulging fotanel in a crying child does not necessarily indicate raised intracranial tension. Also feel, if the fontanel is pulsatile or not (normal pulsations are masked by the raised ICT). Scalp veins also become prominent in children with hydrocephalus.
- Note any associated dysmorphism.

4. Craniotabes

This refers to a reduction in the rigidity of the cranial bones. Presence of craniotabes is indicated by softened or parchment like skull bones which may get indented like a ping pong ball when pressed away from the lines. Craniotabes is a characteristic of rickets; it is also normally present in skull of premature babies. Also look for "bossing of skull bones". Frontal bossing is present in rickets, Hurler syndrome, and thalassemia.

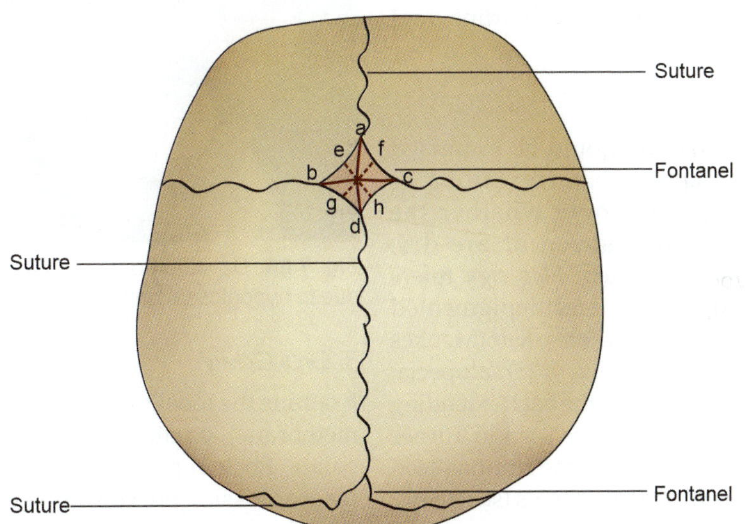

Fig. 7.23: The anterior fontanel can be measured as (ad × bc) or (eh × gf).

5. Transillumination

This should be attempted, if subdural effusion, hydrocephalus, porencephaly, or hydrancephaly is suspected. Illuminate with a torch light with a rubber foam cuff or cold light source over the frontal and occipital areas in a dark room. When transillumination exceeds 2.5 cm in the frontal area and 1 cm in the occipital area it is considered abnormal.

6. Crack-pot Sign (Macewen Sign)

This should be elicited only in children, whose fontanels have closed. A positive sign indicates raised intracranial tension.

Method: Raise the head above the bed **(Fig. 7.24)**. Tap lightly on one side of the parietal eminence, and listen to the reverberating sound on the opposite parietal eminence; you may also use a stethoscope to listen for the quality of the sound. A characteristic sound as if coming from a cracked pot indicates raised intracranial tension.

7. Cranial Bruits

These should be auscultated for over the vertex, occipital or temporal regions.

B. Face

1. Facies

First of all, look for any characteristic facies **(Key Box 20)**, especially when dealing with dysmorphic syndromes. Observe symmetry of the face, and record malformations of the mouth, eyes, ears, nose, teeth, hairline, and forehead, if present.

2. Hair

Character of scalp hair should be examined first: Whether dense or sparse; strong or easily pluckable. Also note whether the hair have the normal sheen or are dry, lustureless, hypopigmented. *Flag sign* refers to alternately pigmented and depigmented hair in malnutrition. Notice *kinky hair* (Menkes disease), white forelock **(Fig. 7.25)**, alopecia, low hairline (low hairline in the back extending up to spine of C4 vertebrae as seen in Turner syndrome or low hairline in the front as seen in hypothyroidism), and eyebrows (*synophrys*, i.e. the two eyebrows meet in midline or sparse eyebrows).

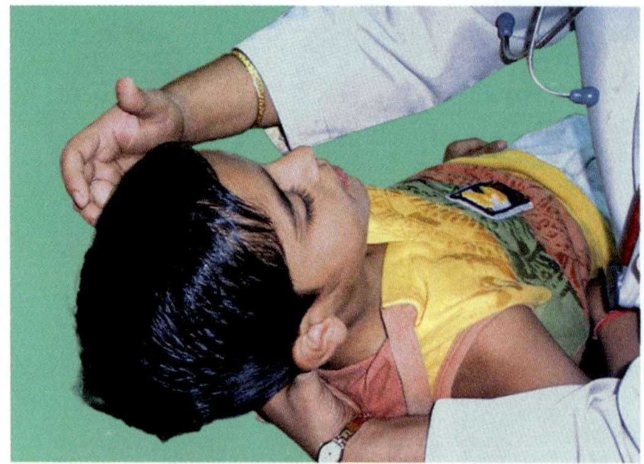

Fig. 7.24: Eliciting Macewen sign in a child.

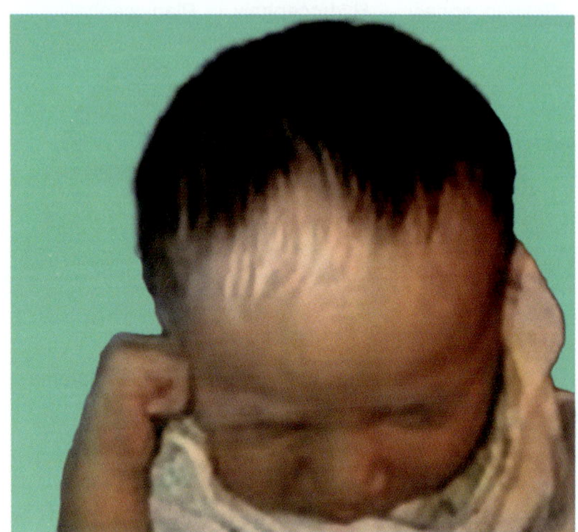

Fig. 7.25: White forelock.

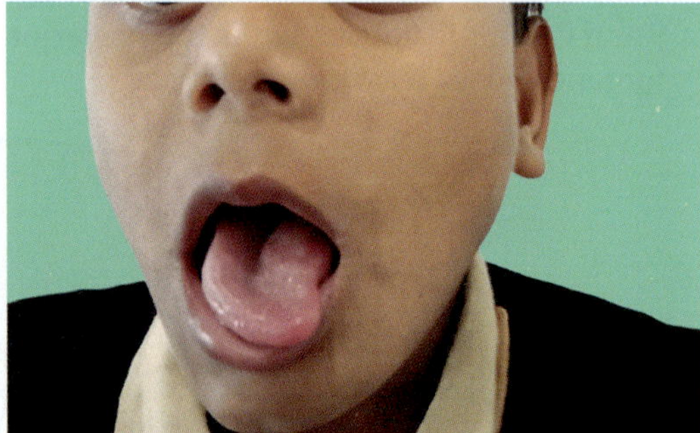

Fig. 7.26: Deviation of tongue to left with atrophy due to hypoglossal nerve palsy.

3. Oral Cavity

Examine the tonsils (hypertrophy, congestion, membrane), palate (cleft palate, high-arched palate, Ebstein pearls), tongue [glossoptosis, macroglossia, microglossia, tongue-tie or any deviation suggestive of hypoglossal nerve palsy **(Fig. 7.26)**], mouth (retrognathia,

Key Box 20

Description of Some Characteristic Facies

- *Mongoloid/Down facies:* Upward slant of eyes, epicanthic folds, hypertelorism, flattened nasal bridge, protuberant tongue.

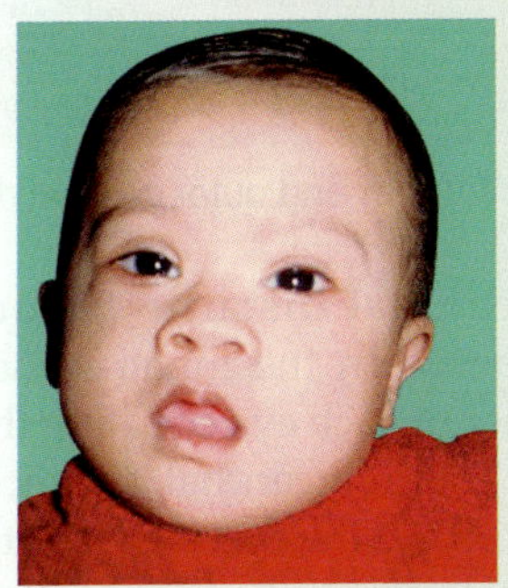

Down syndrome

- *Elfin facies:* Upturned nose, broad upper lip, small mandible, prominent maxilla, short stature.

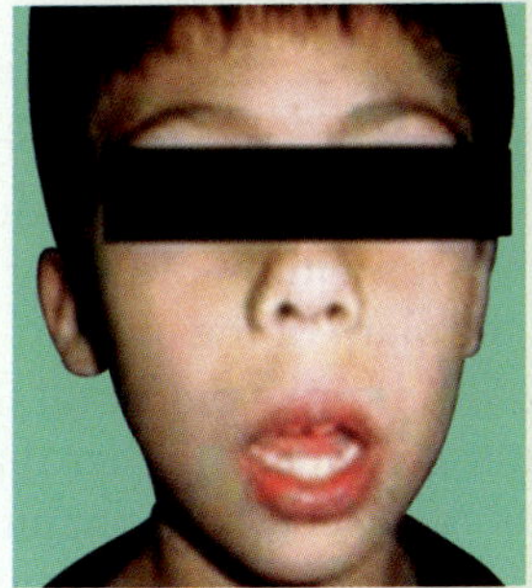

William syndrome

- *Moon/steroid/cushingoid facies:* Rounded face, chubby and puffy look, double chin, hirsutism.

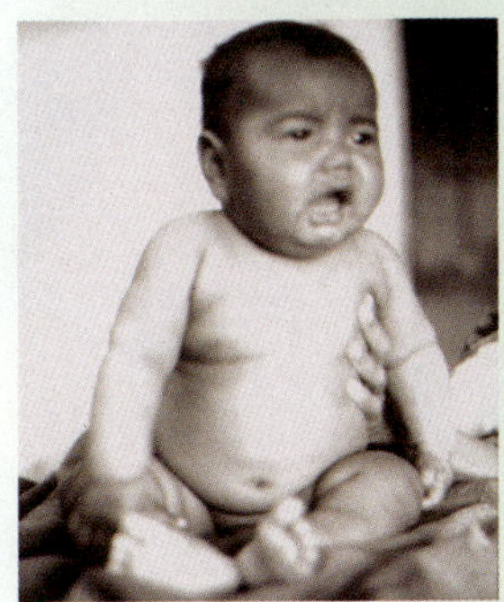

Cushing syndrome

- *Hemolytic facies:* Pallor, malar prominence, frontal bossing, depressed nasal bridge.

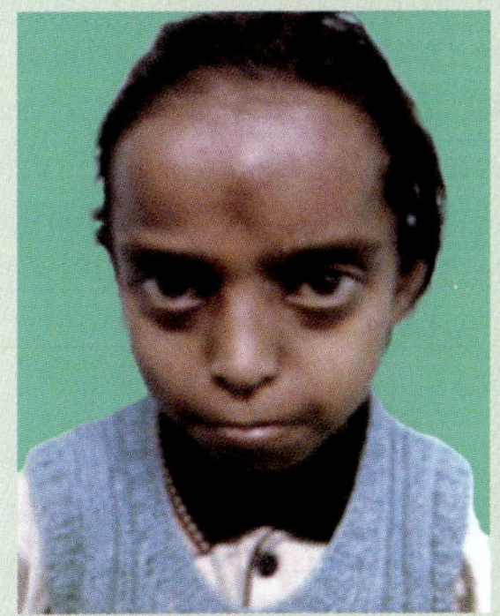

Thalassemia

- *Risus sardonicus:* Due to spasm of the platysma muscle, the corners of the mouth move downwards and outwards, the lip is stretched across the incisor teeth.

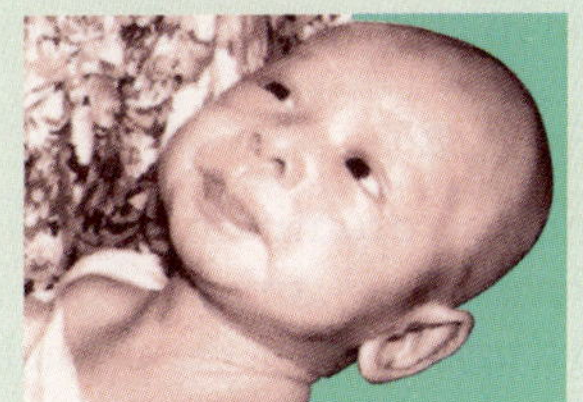

Tetanus

- *Coarse facies:* Dry skin, thick tongue, thickened facial outlines

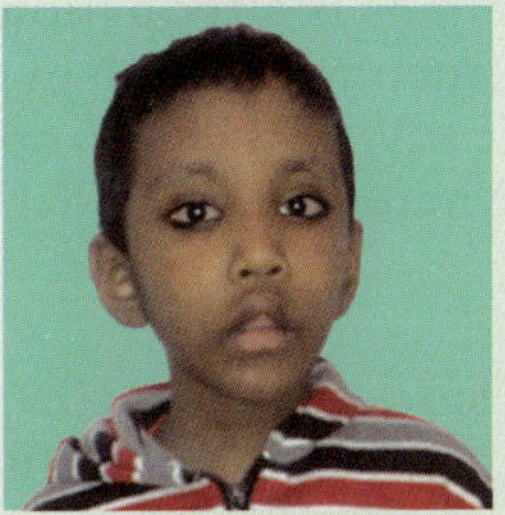

Hypothyroidism, mucopolysaccharidosis

- *Potter facies:* Suborbital creases, depressed nasal tip, low set ears, retrognathia, associated with positional deformities of limbs, like clubfeet.

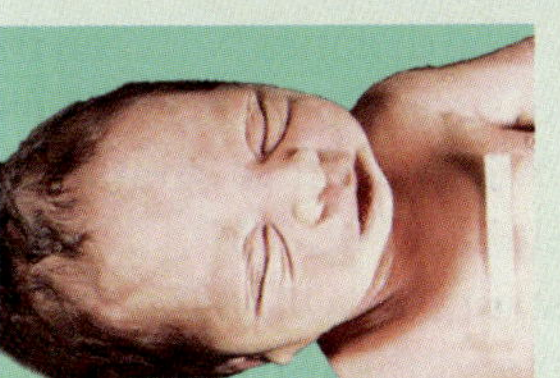

Renal agenesis

micrognathia, prominent lips), and teeth (hypodontia, anodontia).

4. Forehead

See the shape of the forehead. A pointed forehead is suggestive of trigonocephaly and midline brain defects. Vertical height of the forehead is increased in hydrocephalus, Crouzon syndrome, and Apert syndrome. A narrow forehead due to a low frontal hairline is present in Hurler syndrome and Cornelia de Lange syndrome.

C. Eyes

Observe for any obvious anatomical, congenital, or acquired defect in the eye. Test the functions of the extraocular muscles, visual acuity (in children older than 7 years) and color vision, and light reflex (direct and consensual). Lastly, examine the fundus. A brief scheme of external ocular examination is provided below. For details of ocular examination in children, *see* Chapter 12.

1. Size of Eyeballs

Eyeballs may be prominent (*exophthalmos*), sunken (*enophthalmos*), small (*microphthalmos*), or enlarged (*buphthalmos*). Exophthalmos may be seen in thyrotoxicosis, Crouzon syndrome, neuroblastoma, or neurofibromatosis, while enophthalmos is seen in Horner syndrome, or phthisis bulbi (post-traumatic). Microphthalmos is a reduction in size of all ocular structures as seen in congenital infections (CMV, rubella, toxoplasmosis), Goldenhar syndrome or CHARGE syndrome.

2. Placement

Are the eyes too closely placed (hypotelorism) or too widely spaced (hypertelorism)? *Hypertelorism* may be seen in Down syndrome, cretinism, thalassemia, Turner syndrome, Noonan syndrome and Rubinstein-Taybi syndrome. *Hypotelorism* is seen in arhinencephaly, cyclopia, trisomy 13 and holoprosencephaly. The distance between the two eyes may be measured in terms of inner canthal distance, mid-pupillary distance, or outer canthal distance (Fig. 7.27).

The distance between the inner corner of the left eye and the inner corner of the right eye, is called *intercanthal distance*. Normally, the intercanthal distance is equal to the distance between the inner corner and the outer corner of each eye equaling the width of the eye. If the intercanthal distance is bigger than the width of the eye, it may be telecanthus or hypertelorism. If the intercanthal distance is increased, but the interpupillary distance is normal, it indicates *telecanthus*; but if both are increased, it indicates *hypertelorism* (Fig. 7.28).

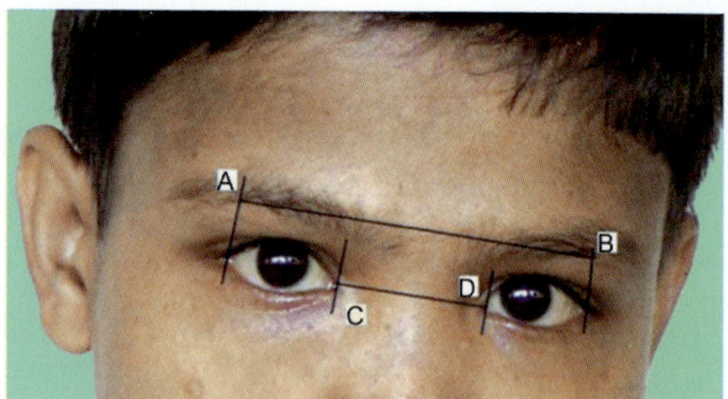

Fig. 7.27: Inner and outer canthal distance.

3. Slant and Palpebral Fissure Length

Is the palpebral fissure length too short (fetal alcohol syndrome, William syndrome)? Look for any obvious squint, ptosis, or nystagmus. Examine the slant of the eyes.

- ***Mongoloid slant:*** A palpebral slant wherein the outer canthus is higher than the inner canthus is called the mongoloid/upward slant; it is seen in Down syndrome, Prader-Willi syndrome, ectodermal dysplasia,

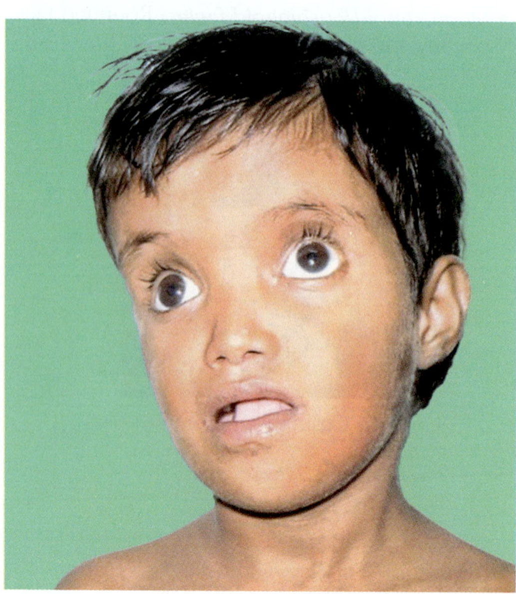
Fig. 7.28: Hypertelorism.

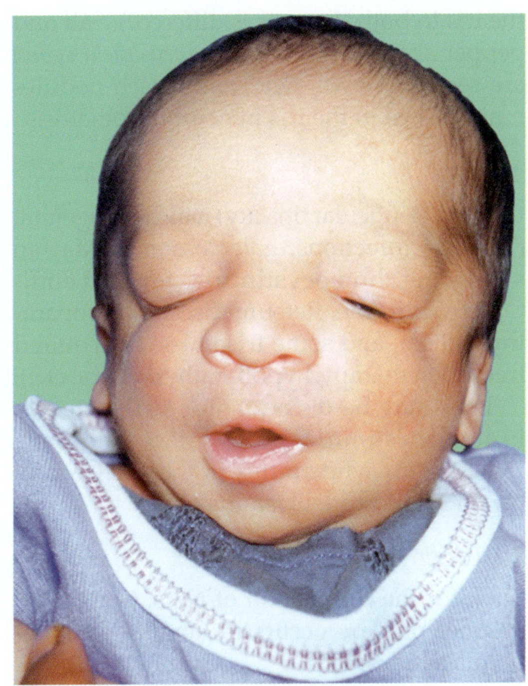

Fig. 7.29: Antimongoloid slant.

Aarskog syndrome, and Zellweger syndrome. This slant is normal in certain races (Mongols, hence the name mongoloid slant).

- ***Antimongoloid slant:*** If the inner canthus is higher than the outer canthus, the slant is downward slant (antimongoloid slant) seen in Treacher Collins syndrome (Fig. 7.29), 10p deletion syndrome, Turner syndrome, Apert syndrome, Noonan syndrome, Smith-Lemli-Opitz syndrome, and cri-du-chat syndrome.

4. Epicanthic Folds

Epicanthic folds are folds of skin which project from the upper lid over the medial epicanthus (Fig. 7.30). Epicanthic folds are seen in Down syndrome, Turner syndrome, Noonan syndrome, Smith-Lemli-Opitz syndrome, cri-du-chat syndrome and Cornelia de Lange syndrome. Epicanthic folds are normally seen in some newborns till 1–3 months of age, and may be seen normally in Chinese.

5. Eyelids

Look for colobomas (developmental defects) of the eyelids (seen in Goldenhar syndrome, Treacher Collins syndrome). Lid edema can be seen in pertussis, measles, acute nephritis, conjunctivitis, and infectious mononucleosis. Drooping of eyelids (ptosis) can be congenital or acquired, or may be unilateral or bilateral. Ptosis is seen in Horner syndrome, oculomotor palsy, botulism, myasthenia gravis, Mobius syndrome, or Noonan syndrome.

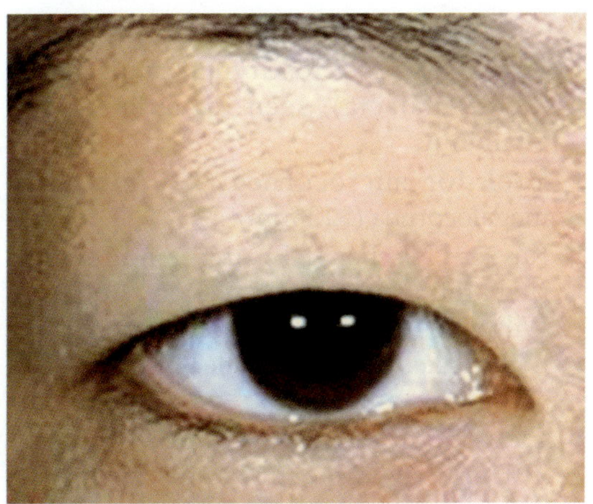

Fig. 7.30: Epicanthic folds.

6. Eyelashes and Eyebrows

- Long and curly eyelashes are seen in Cornelia de Lange syndrome, and malnourished children.
- Scanty or absent eyelashes occur in children with Treacher Collins syndrome, Hallermann-Streiff syndrome, cartilage hair hypoplasia, and premature babies.
- Eyebrows are sparse in premature babies and in children of Hallermann-Streiff syndrome. Eyebrows may meet in midline (synophrys) in patients with Cornelia de Lange syndrome and Waardenburg syndrome.
- Hypopigmentation of eyelashes and eyebrows occurs in children with albinism.

7. Conjunctiva

- Examine the conjunctiva for any dryness (vitamin A deficiency), scarring (seen in trachoma), vascularization (riboflavin deficiency), or hemorrhages (vitamin C deficiency, whooping cough).
- Epibulbar dermoids are seen in Goldenhar syndrome.
- Look for any pinguecula (Gaucher disease) or pterygium (exposure to sun or dust).

8. Cornea

- Assess the cornea for dryness or ulceration (keratomalacia), seen in deficiency of vitamin A.
- Look for microcornea (<10 mm) and megalocornea (>13 mm).
- Kayser-Fleischer (KF) ring is a brownish ring around the cornea seen in patients of Wilson disease. Often KF ring is not visible to the naked eye and can be appreciated on slit-lamp examination.
- Clouding of cornea **(Fig. 7.31)** can occur in Hurler syndrome, Morquio syndrome, Scheie syndrome, GM1 gangliosidosis, tyrosinosis, Mareoteaux-Lamy syndrome, and congenital syphilis (interstitial keratitis).

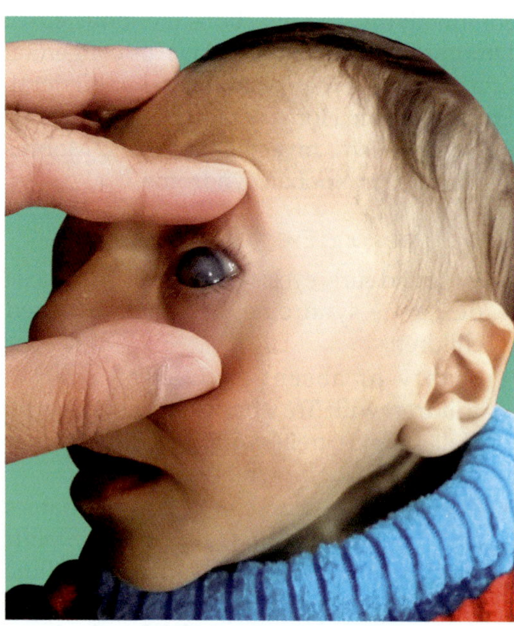

Fig. 7.31: Corneal clouding

9. Sclera

Icterus should be looked for in the sclera. Blue sclera can be seen in Ehlers-Danlos syndrome, Marfan syndrome, osteogenesis imperfecta, and congenital glaucoma.

10. Pupils

Assess the pupil size, symmetry, and reaction of the pupil to light.

11. Iris

Look for absent iris (aniridia), seen in Wilms tumor and heterochromia iridis (the color of the iris in both the eyes is different). Salt and pepper speckling of the iris (*brushfield spots*) are seen in Down syndrome. Lisch nodules may be seen in the iris in neurofibromatosis.

12. Lens

Cataract (lenticular opacity) may be congenital (TORCH infections, galactossemia, Marfan syndrome, homocystinuria, Smith-Lemli-Opitz syndrome, Refsum disease, hypoparathyroidism, and some trisomies) or acquired (radiation therapy, hypoparathyroidism, etc.).

Lens may be dislocated or subluxated as in homocystinuria and Marfan syndrome. Evaluate for white reflex in the eye (seen in cataract and retinoblastoma).

13. Lacrimal Glands and Tears

Look for the production of tears. Congenital absence of tears occurs in familial dysautonomia syndrome.

14. Vision

Visual acuity should be tested in children older than 7 years using a Snellen chart. Color vision can be tested using Ischihara chart. Children older than 5 years can be asked to identify common colors. Assess for diplopia (uniocular/binocular).

15. Fundoscopy

An ophthalmoscope can be used to examine the fundus after dilating the pupils with a topical mydriatic like atropine eye ointment or tropicamide eyedrops. *Remember to assess the pupil size and papillary reaction before instilling mydriatic agent into the eyes*. Look for the optic disk margins and depth of the optic disk. Papilledema is seen in conditions with raised intracranial tension. Look for any retinal hemorrhages, optic atrophy, cherry-red spots, choroids tubercles, and chorioretinitis. Both eyes should be tested separately.

D. Ears

The ears should be evaluated for their external structure and hearing.

1. Placement: Whether Low-set?

If a horizontal line is drawn joining both the medial canthi and extended outwards, then the helix usually lies above this line. If the helix

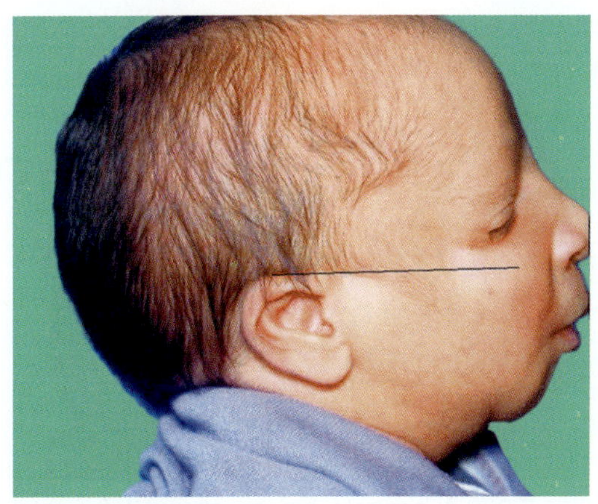

Fig. 7.32: Low-set ears and retrognathia in a baby with Treacher Collins syndrome.

lies below this line, the ears are said to be "low set." *Low-set ears* **(Fig. 7.32)** are often associated with other congenital abnormalities. Low-set ears are seen in Down syndrome, Noonan syndrome, Turner syndrome, Apert syndrome, other trisomy syndromes, DiGeorge syndrome and fetal hydantoin syndrome.

2. External Ear Abnormalities

- External ear may be small and dysplastic (microtia) or absent (anotia).
- ***Microtia* (Fig. 7.33)** is commonly seen in patients of Goldenhar syndrome and Treacher Collins syndrome.
- ***Preauricular tags*** or pits are often seen due to maldevelopment of the first branchial arch **(Fig. 7.34)**.
- ***Darwinian tubercle*** is a small thickening seen on the posterior aspect of the helix.
- Large bat-like ears are seen in Fragile X syndrome.

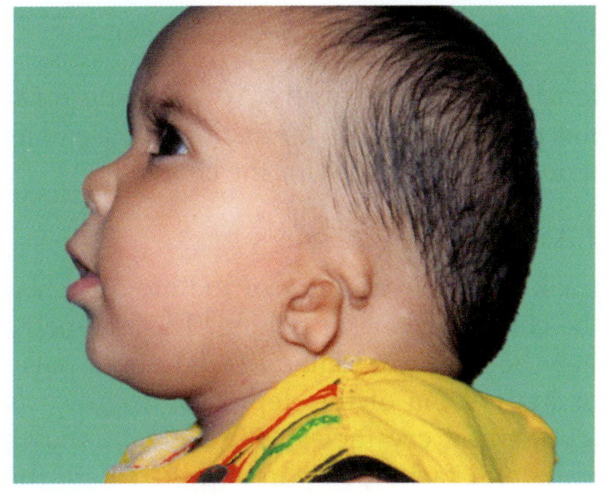

Fig. 7.33: Microtia.

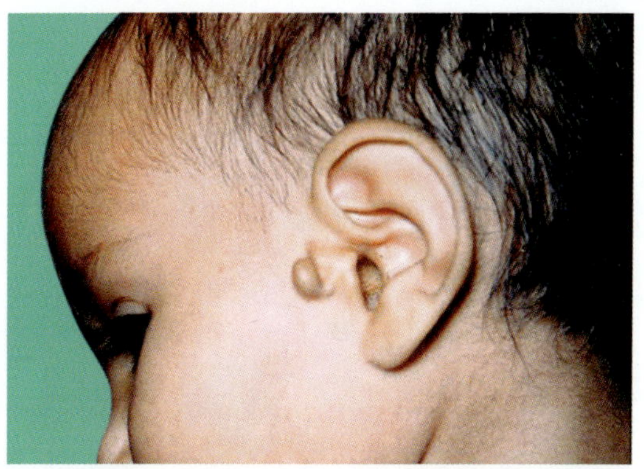

Fig. 7.34: Preauricular tag.

3. Otoscopic Examination

Otoscopy is indicated to diagnose wax, foreign body, and abnormalities of the tympanic membrane. Details are provided in Chapter 12.

Method: The pinna is pulled horizontally in infants, and upwards and backwards in older children while holding the handle of the otoscope between the thumb and the index finger.

Abnormalities

- The cone of light which extends from the tip of the handle of the malleus downwards and forwards may be obliterated in ear infections, while the handle of the malleus may become more prominent in retraction of the tympanic membranes.
- Observe the tympanic membrane for color (dusky), tension (bulging, retracted), or perforation.

E. Nose

1. Size and Shape

The nasal length from the root of the nose to the highest concavity at the tip of the base of the nose in a vertical axis ranges from 20 to 32 mm at birth in term neonates. The nasal width approximates the distance between the medial margins of the irides.

- The nose may be small (trisomy 18, Down syndrome, Apert syndrome) or large (Seckel dwarf, 13q deletion).
- Beaking of the nose is seen in Apert syndrome **(Fig. 7.35)**, progeria, pyknodysostosis, and Rubinstein-Taybi syndrome.
- Rudimentary nose is seen in holoprosencephaly. The nose tip may often be upturned.

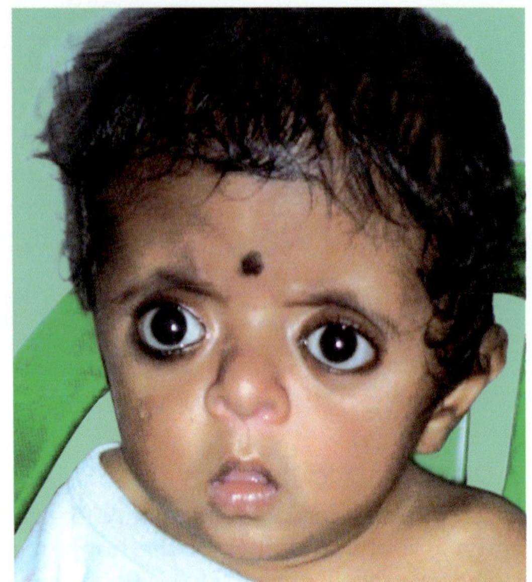

Fig. 7.35: Beaking of the nose (Apert syndrome).

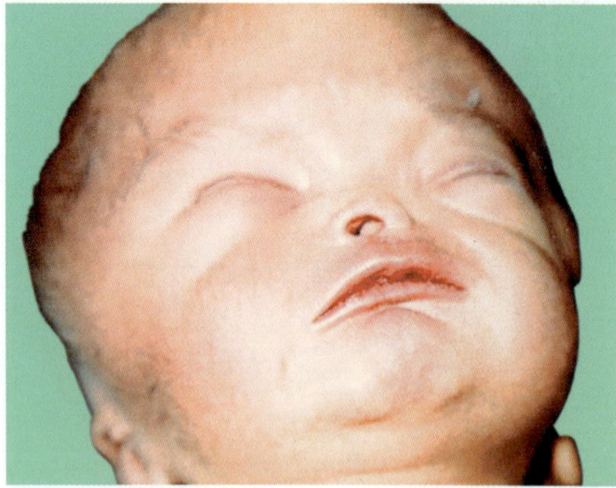

Fig. 7.36: A neonate having absent left nostril, bilateral anophthalmia, and hydrocephalus.

2. Nasal Bridge

The nasal bridge is depressed in syphilis, Down syndrome, Hurler syndrome, chondrodystrophy, congenital hypothyroidism, and hemolytic anemia.

3. Alae Nasi

The alae nasi may be hypoplastic as in infant of diabetic mother.

4. Nares

- Exclude choanal atresia by passing a nasogastric tube through each nostril one by one.
- In bilateral choanal atresia, usually a newborn baby becomes blue unless he is crying.
- Sometimes there may be absence of one of the nostrils (Fig. 7.36).

5. Nasal Cavity

Look for the presence of any foreign body, purulent discharge, nasal crusts (Fig. 7.37) or polyps using a nasal speculum. The presence of a deviated nasal septum is a common finding.

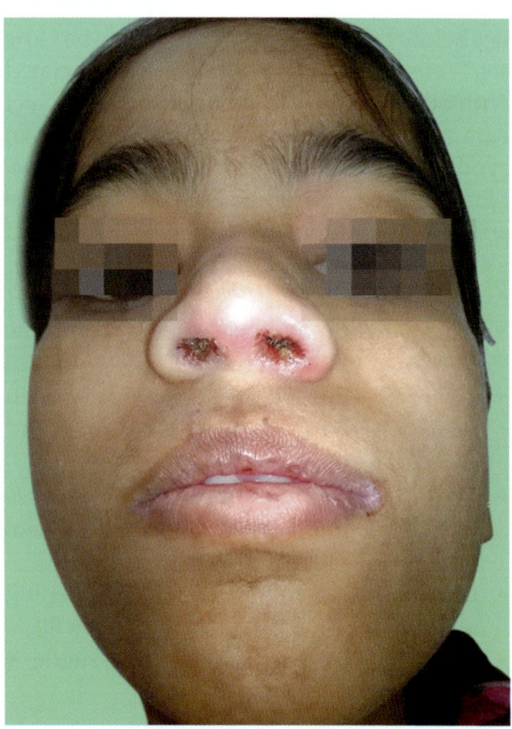

Fig. 7.37: Crusted nasal discharge.

F. Mouth and Oral Cavity

Examination of the mouth and oral cavity includes examination of the lips, philtrum, buccal mucosa, gums, palate, tongue, teeth, tonsils, and oropharynx. You may perform this part of general examination in the end as it may be unpleasant for the child.

1. Mouth

Look for the symmetry of the mouth when the child is crying or talking. The symmetry may be lost in unilateral facial nerve palsy or hypoplasia of the depressor anguli oris (congenital cry facies). Figure 7.38 shows unilateral facial palsy in a child where the mouth is drawn to the normal side while

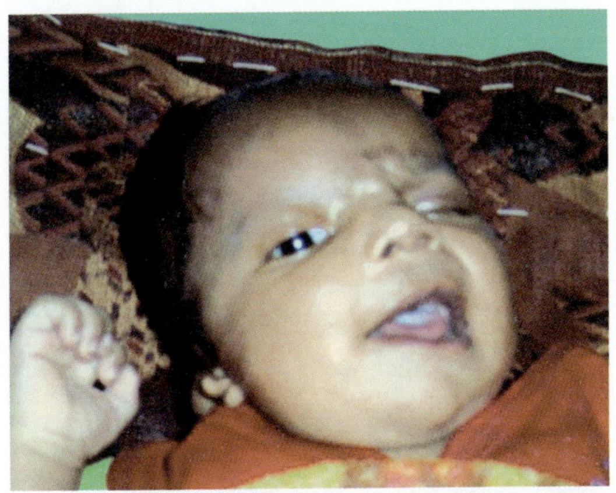

Fig. 7.38: A child with right-sided facial nerve palsy.

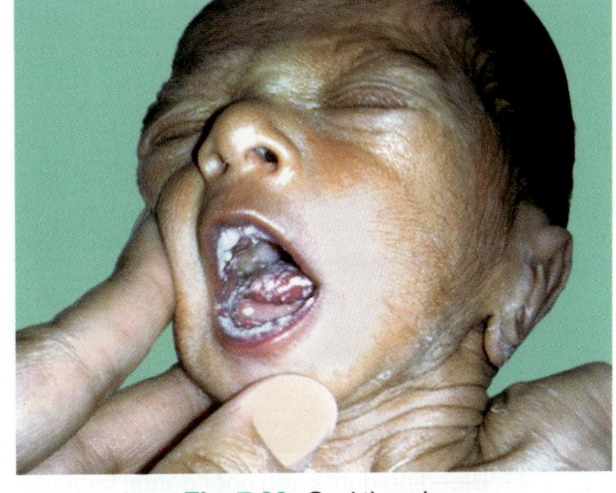

Fig. 7.39: Oral thrush.

crying and there is inability to close the eye on the affected side.

2. Lips

- The lips may show edema (*angioneurotic edema*), pallor, cyanosis, or signs of vitamin deficiency or infection.
- Cleft lip may occur unilaterally or bilaterally with or without cleft palate.
- Dryness, scaling, and cracking of lips (*cheilitis*) is seen in acute febrile illness or seasonal chapped lips.
- *Angular stomatitis* is seen in ariboflavinosis.
- In congenital syphilis, moist lesions radiate from the corners of the mouth (*rhagades*).
- In candidiasis and streptococcal infection, fissuring and scaling of angles of the mouth can occur (*perleche*).

3. Philtrum

The philtrum may be short (orofacial digital syndrome, DiGeorge syndrome) or long (femoral hypoplasia, fetal alcohol syndrome, fetal hydantoin syndrome, Smith-Lemli-Opitz syndrome, and Hurler syndrome).

4. Buccal Mucosa

- Assess for hydration, color, ulceration, and inflammation.
- White curd-like plaques which are difficult to scrape off may be deposited on the oral mucosa in candidiasis or thrush **(Fig. 7.39)**.
- Greyish white spots surrounded by reddish hue may be seen in the oral cavity opposite the lower molar teeth in measles (*Koplik spots*).

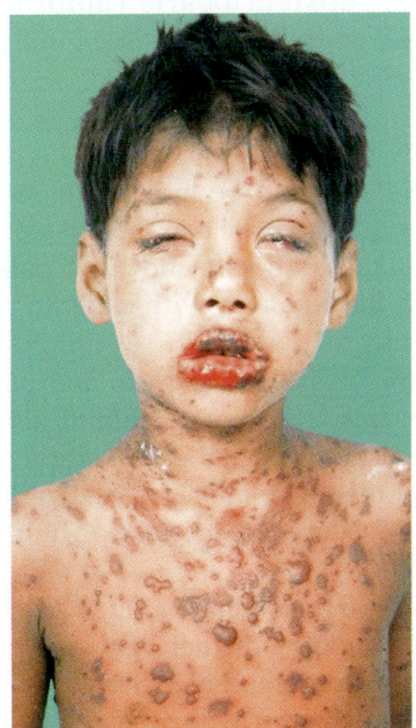

Fig. 7.40: A child with Stevens-Johnson syndrome with extensive bullous lesions over the skin and oral mucosae.

- Oral mucosa may be erythematous in Kawasaki disease.
- Also look for petechiae or bullae in the oral cavity. **Figure 7.40** shows a child with Stevens-Johnson syndrome with extensive involvement of oral mucosae, conjunctiva, and skin.

5. Gums

The gums may be hypertrophied (phenytoin therapy, acute monocytic leukemia, mouth breathers, poor oral hygiene, epulis, scurvy) or may show ulceration **(Fig. 7.41)** or bleeding

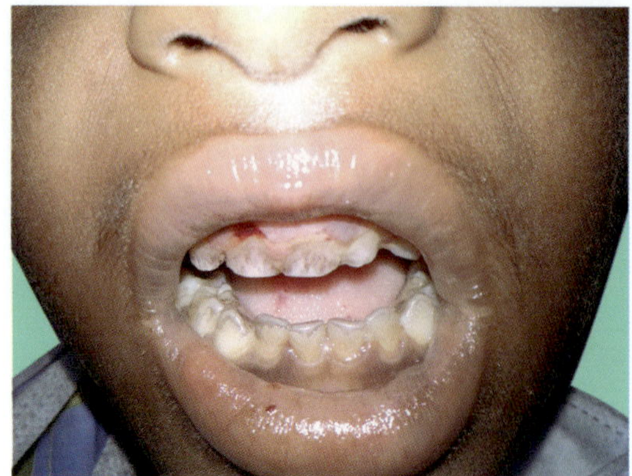

Fig. 7.41: Bleeding gums and poor dental hygiene.

(scurvy). Epstein pearls (Bohn nodule) (Fig. 7.42) or epulis may be seen in the gums of a newborn baby.

6. Palate

The palate should be looked for structural defects which may be confined to soft palate, hard palate, both soft and hard palates, or soft and hard palates with clefts in alveolar processes.

- Figure 7.43 shows cleft lip and palate. In a neonate, cleft palate should always be looked for by digital examination in order to not miss out small clefts. An older child may be examined after asking him to open his mouth.
- A high-arched palate (Fig. 7.44) may be seen in mouth breathers, Down syndrome, Marfan syndrome, Ehlers-Danlos syndrome, and in neonates who received prolonged ventilation.

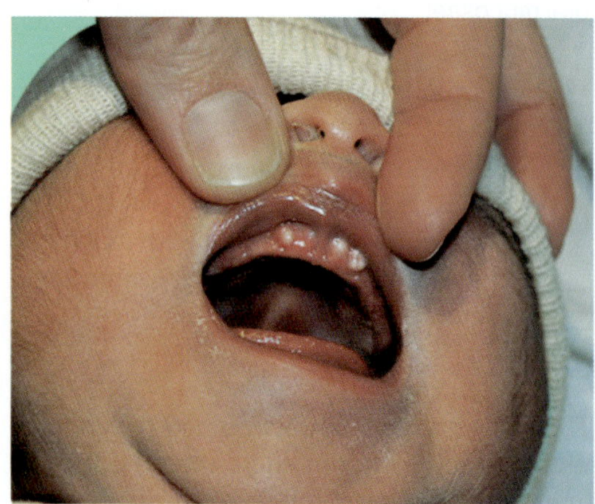

Fig. 7.42: Bohn nodule on the gums.

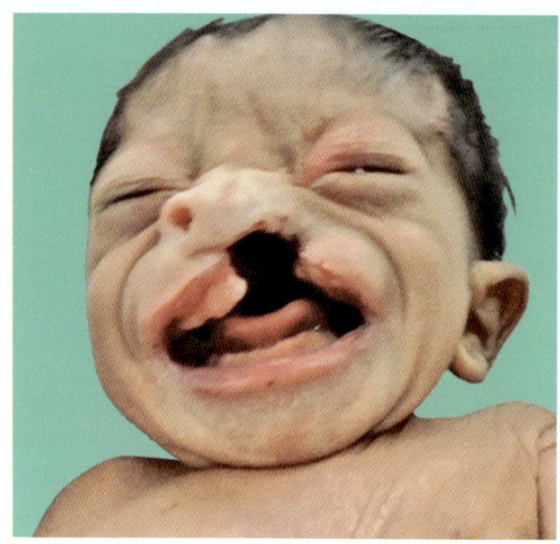

Fig. 7.43: Cleft lip and palate in an infant.

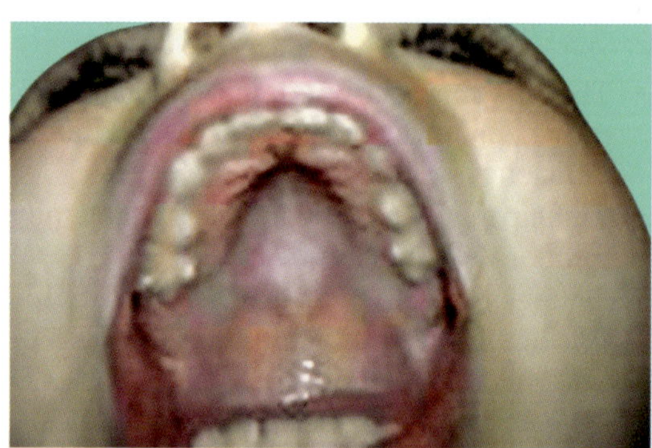

Fig. 7.44: High-arched palate.

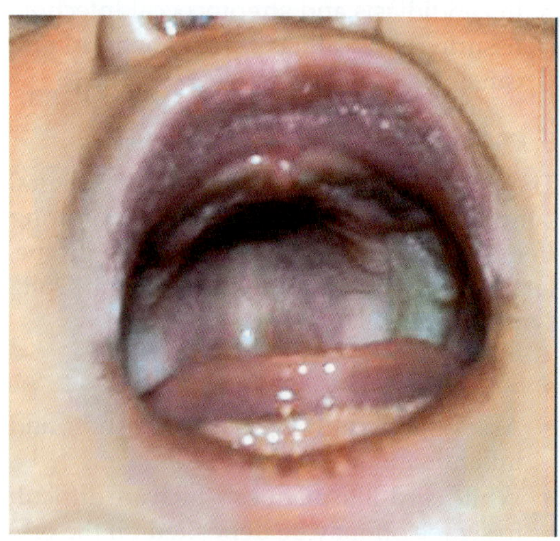

Fig. 7.45: Epstein pearl on palate in midline.

- Epstein pearls (benign epithelial swellings) are seen on palate in the midline in neonates (Fig. 7.45).

7. Tongue

Look for color (pallor, cyanosis, strawberry red), fissures, ulceration, presence of follicles (bald tongue in iron deficiency anemia) and its symmetry and movement of the tongue.

- Tongue is large (macroglossia) in certain conditions like congenital hypothyroidism, mucopolysaccharidosis, Pompe disease, amyloidosis, Beckwith-Wiedemann syndrome, Down syndrome, hemangioma, lymphangioma, neurofibromatosis, angioneurotic edema, and Angelman syndrome.
- A small tongue is seen in lesions of hypoglossal and facial nerves.
- A tongue tie (*ankyloglossia*) is unusual.
- Fasciculations may be seen in the tongue in Werdnig-Hoffman disease.

8. Mandible and Chin

- Look for a small mandible (*micrognathia*) or a receding chin (*retrognathia*) (*see* **Fig. 7.32**).
- Retrognathia is often seen to occur in association with cleft palate.
- A *lockjaw* may occur in tetanus, strychnine poisoning, rhabdomyosarcoma of the jaw, encephalitis, arthritis of temporomandibular joint, and infantile Gaucher disease.

9. Teeth

Count the number of teeth: Deciduous or primary teeth appear from 6 to 24 months age while secondary or permanent teeth usually start appearing from the age of 6 years.

Deciduous teeth are usually white in color and have a smooth edge. In contrast, permanent teeth are ivory-white in color with a serrated edge. In children, often mixed dentition is seen.

Color/staining of teeth

- Black/brown staining of teeth occurs in children receiving oral iron preparations (**Fig. 7.46**), having caries, fluorosis, osteogenesis imperfecta, and hypophosphatemic rickets.
- Yellow staining of teeth is seen in children receiving tetracycline.
- Children with porphyria may have reddish brown or pink teeth.

Look for dental caries: Assess the shape of the teeth. Peg-like incisors are seen in congenital syphilis. Mulberry molars have irregularly formed crowded cusps on a small occlusal surface.

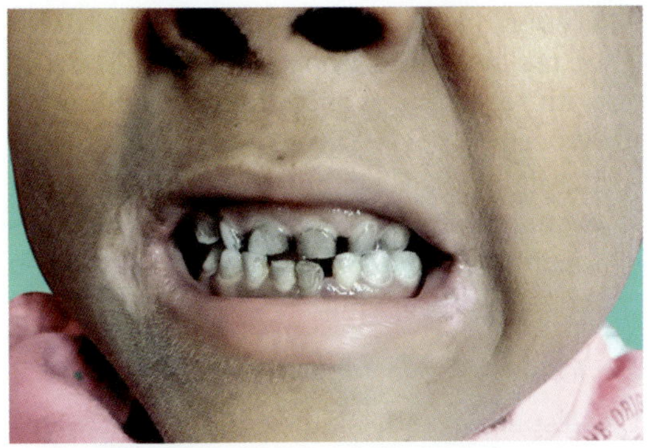

Fig. 7.46: Brownish-black staining of teeth.

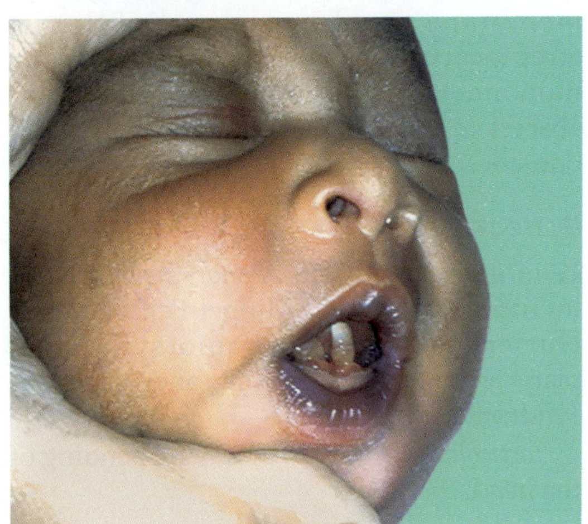

Fig. 7.47: Natal teeth.

Natal teeth: Sometimes a newborn may have teeth at birth (**Fig. 7.47**).

10. Pharynx

Ask the child to open the mouth and protrude his tongue. Use a spatula to depress the tongue to get a clearer view of the pharynx. A good lighting is essential for which you may use a head mirror or torch light.

- Examine the pharynx for congestion or any bulge in the posterior pharyngeal wall (retropharyngeal and parapharyngeal abscess).
- Redness of the epiglottis and pharyngeal congestion occur in epiglottitis.
- Check if the uvula is central or deviated to one side (in palatal palsy, uvula is drawn towards the normal side).
- Look for the gag reflex.

- Hyperplasia of the lymphoid follicles of the posterior pharyngeal wall occurs with recurrent pharyngitis and adenoidal hypertrophy.
- If epiglottitis is suspected, do not attempt examination of the pharynx unless facilities for intubation and mechanical ventilation are available at hand.

11. Tonsils

Use a spatula, and ask the child to say "aah". Examine the tonsillar size, color, and surface (presence of a membrane). A gray or yellow membrane may be seen in diphtheria, streptococcal pharyngitis, and infectious mononucleosis. In case of a peritonsillar abscess (quinsy), tonsil may be displaced to one side.

G. Neck

Length and position: A *short neck* is seen in Turner syndrome, Klippel-Feil anomaly, Hurler syndrome, Morquio syndrome, platybasia, Sprengel deformity and Goldenhar syndrome.

Torticollis may lead to the lateral bending of the head.

Stiffness or neck rigidity may occur in meningitis, tetanus, caries of spine, retropharyngeal abscess, Arnold-Chiari malformation, and acute poliomyelitis.

Look for any swelling in the neck, e.g. cystic hygroma, cervical lymph nodes, thyroid swelling, thyroglossal cyst or fistula, branchial cyst, sternomastoid tumor. **Figure 7.48** shows a large transilluminant neck swelling (cystic hygroma).

Observe *prominence of neck veins* or presence of *visible pulsations* in the neck (dancing carotids).

H. Hands, Feet, and Limbs

1. Handedness

Handedness usually develops by 3 years of age. In case of early development of handedness, look for evidence of other neurological abnormalities.

2. Size and Shape

Abnormalities of size and shape of hands and fingers are shown in **Key Box 21**. Observe the foot for eversion, equinus, adduction, plantar, or dorsal flexion deformities.

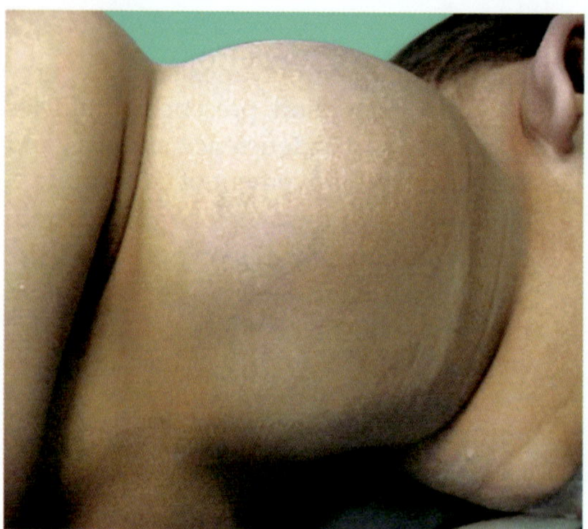

Fig. 7.48: Cystic hygroma.

Assess for the presence of a *rocker-bottom foot* (abnormal vertical position of the talus and calcaneus) or club foot (congenital talipes equinovarus). At birth, the foot length is very close to the femoral length. Refer to the section on dysmorphism.

3. Color

Observe the color of palms and soles. Palmar or plantar erythema may be seen in hand-foot and mouth disease, sympathetic dystrophy, high output failure, or liver failure; bluish hue may be seen in cyanosis or Raynaud phenomenon while yellowish appearance is seen in jaundiced patients.

4. Rash

Palms and soles may have macules (erythema multiforme, SLE), papules (scabies), vesicles (scabies, herpes simplex, staphylococcal scalded skin syndrome, burns, congenital syphilis), nodules [(Osler nodes in bacterial endocarditis: tender red nodules over finger pulps **(Fig. 7.49)**], or purpura [(meningococcemia, Henoch-Schönlein purpura, Rocky-mountain spotted fever **(Fig. 7.50)**].

5. Nails

Look for clubbing, *koilonychia* (spoon-shaped nails in iron deficiency anemia) **(Fig. 7.51)**, *splinter hemorrhages* (infective endocarditis, **Fig. 7.52**), pitting and discoloration of the nails (**Fig. 7.53**, chromonychia) and infection (*paronychia*), and dystrophy of nails.

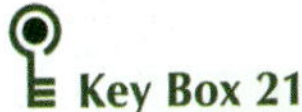

Key Box 21

Abnormalities of Hands and Fingers

Small hands: Achondroplasia, Down syndrome, Cornelia de Lange syndrome, Prader-Willi syndrome

Large hands: Soto syndrome

Arachnodactyly (unduly long fingers): Marfan syndrome, homocystinuria

Polydactyly: Trisomy 13, Laurence-Moon-Biedl syndrome

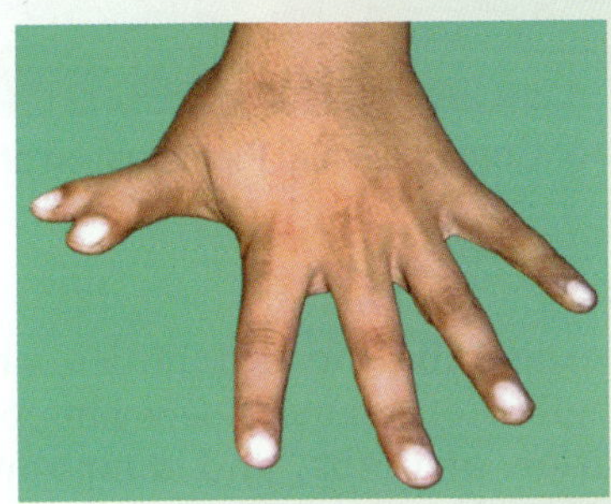

Polydactyly

Syndactyly: Apert syndrome, Carpenter syndrome, Smith-Lemli-Opitz syndrome

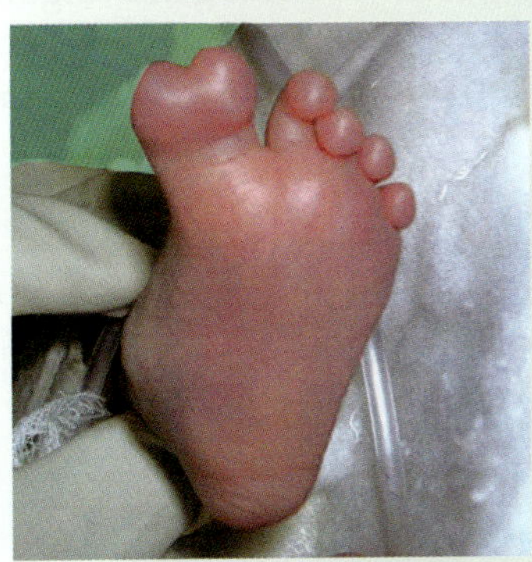

Syndactyly

Camptodactyly (flexion deformity of fifth finger): Down syndrome

Hitchiker thumb: Diastrophic dwarfism

Distally placed thumb: Trisomy 18

Proximally placed thumb: Trisomy 22, Cornelia de Lange syndrome, distrophic dwarfism

Clinodactyly (short fifth middle pharynx): Down syndrome, Silver-Russell syndrome

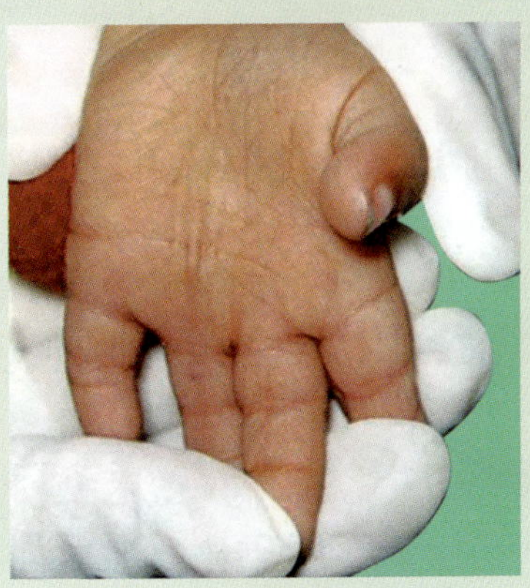

Clinodactyly

Macrodactyly: Mafucci syndrome, neurofibromatosis

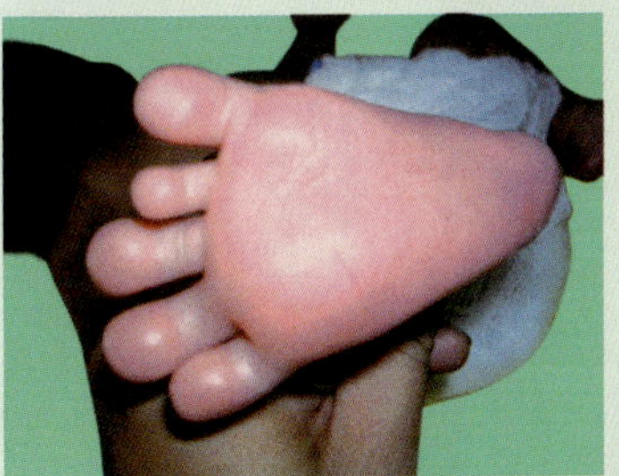

Macrodactyly of the lateral three toes

Ectrodactyly: Split hand and foot syndrome (Lobster foot/hand)

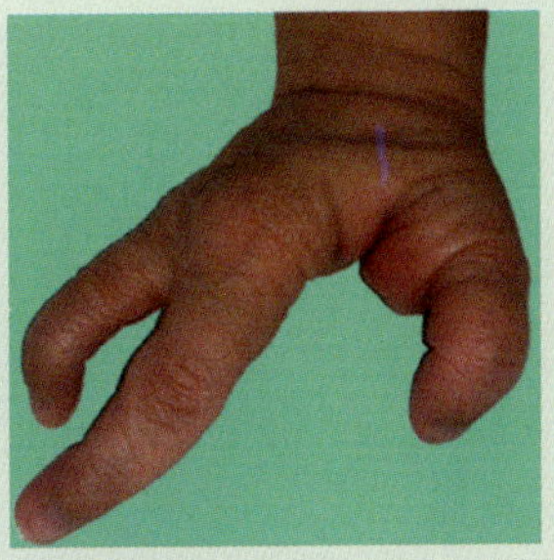

Ectrodactyly

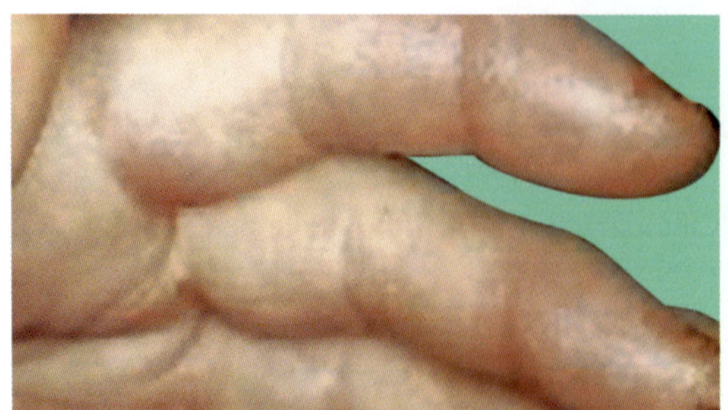

Fig. 7.49: Osler nodes.

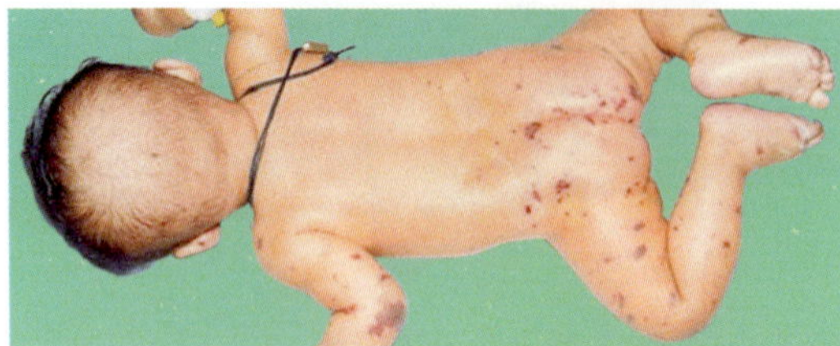

Fig. 7.50: Petechial rash in meningococcemia.

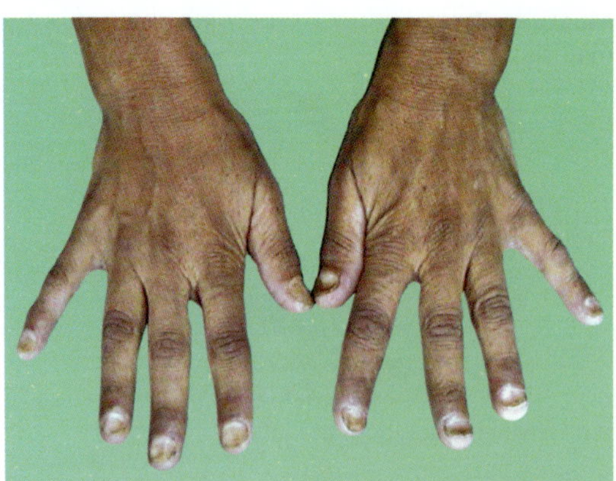

Fig. 7.51: Koilonychia.

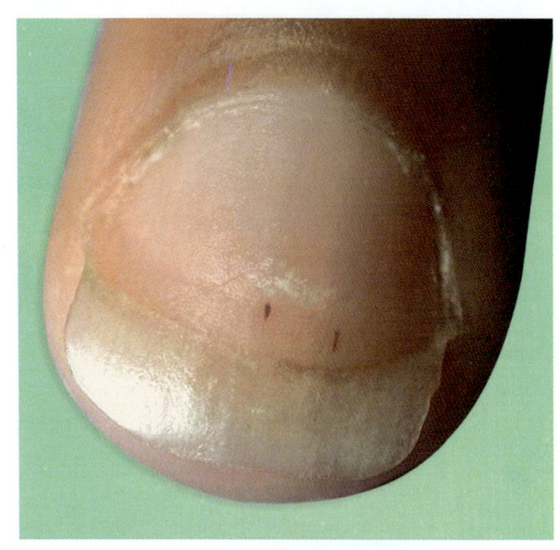

Fig. 7.52: Splinter hemorrhages.

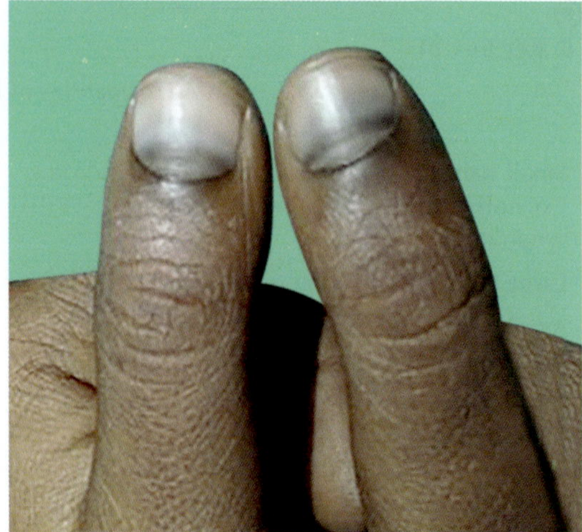

Fig. 7.53: Chromonychia: Pigmentation of nails.

6. Bones and Joints

When examining the extremities, observe their length, proportions, movements, posture or position of limbs, and their range of movement. Look for any joint swelling, tenderness, and erythema. Look for evidence of rickets in the form of wrist widening and double malleoli. Look for genu valgum/genu varum (Fig. 7.54). Look for tenderness of limbs, which may be seen in scurvy or syphilis.

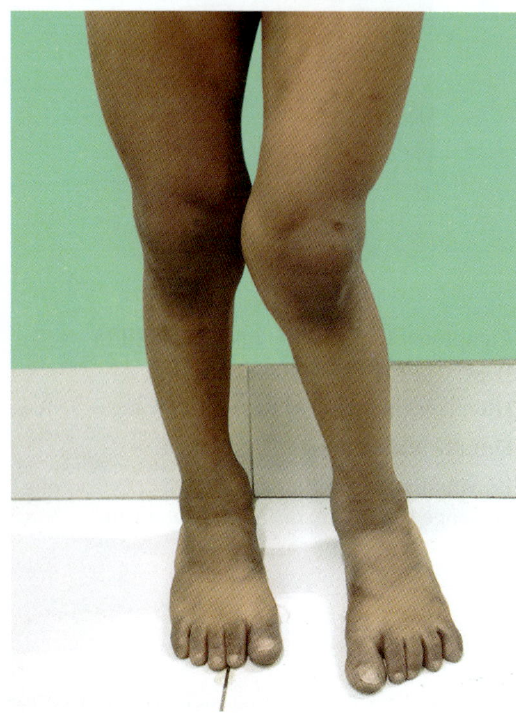

Fig. 7.54: Genu valgum deformity (knock knees).

7. Involuntary Movements

Look for tremors (essential tremor, Wilson disease, anxiety, thyrotoxicosis, and hepatic failure: Asterixis). Chorea (rheumatic chorea, SLE, Huntington disease), ballismus, and tetanic spasms (carpopedal spasm may occur with hypocalcemic or hypomagnesemic tetany) should be looked for, besides seizures.

8. Dermatoglyphics

Look for *simian crease* (Down syndrome) which is a single transverse palmar crease or for the *Kennedy crease* which is a plantar crease between the great toe and the second toe (abnormal dermatoglyphics are discussed in the section on dysmorphology).

Limb length/ proportions: Look for any obvious shortening or increased length of limbs. Shortening may involve the entire limb (*micromelia*), proximal limb (*rhizomelia*), middle segment (*mesomelia*), or the distal limb segment (*acromelia*). The height, upper segment (US), lower segment (LS) and the US to LS ratio should be measured (as detailed in Chapter on anthropometry). The arm span should also be measured.

I. Skin

Examine the skin for its color, texture, turgor, pigmentation, scars, rash, hemorrhages, vesicles, pustules, subcutaneous nodules, striae, telangiectasia, hirsutism, nevi, xanthoma, and dermographism. Terms used to describe the morphology of skin changes are highlighted in **Key Box 22**. Detailed examination of skin is discussed in Chapter 14.

Examination

Skin is examined mainly by inspection; palpation is required only in a few instances.

- The *texture of skin* can be assessed by rubbing a hand over the skin. The skin may be dry, scaly, and coarse in deficiency of vitamins A and E and essential fatty acids; and congenital hypothyroidism.
- The *skin turgor* should be assessed by pinching the skinfold midway between the umbilicus and flanks making sure that all the layers of skin are pinched and then observing the return of the pinch. Failure of the skinfold to go back in <3 seconds suggests dehydration.

Key Box 22

Terms Used to Describe Important Skin Lesions

1. **Macule:** Non-palpable area of altered color
2. **Papule:** Elevated lesions up to 5 mm in diameter
3. **Nodule:** Palpable, solid lesion more than 5 mm in diameter
4. **Plaque:** Palpable discoid lesion more than 2 cm in diameter
5. **Vescicle:** Fluid-filled blister less than 5 mm in diameter
6. **Bulla:** Fluid-filled blister more than 5 mm in diameter
7. **Pustule:** Blister containing pus
8. **Petechiae:** Subdermal bleed which is less than 3 mm in diameter
9. **Purpura:** Subdermal bleed 3–6 mm in diameter
10. **Ecchymosis:** Subdermal bleed more than or equal to 6 mm in diameter

- Look for any *rash*. Note its character, distribution, symmetry, involvement of palms and soles, and blanching, etc.
- Look for neurocutaneous stigmata, like café au lait spots (brownish macular lesions) **(Fig. 7.55)** or any melanocytic nevi **(Fig. 7.56)**, or an hemangioma **(Fig. 7.57)**.

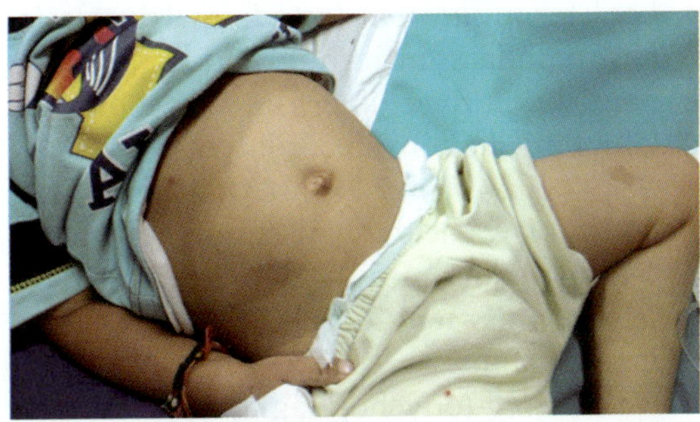

Fig. 7.55: Café au lait spot on abdomen and thigh.

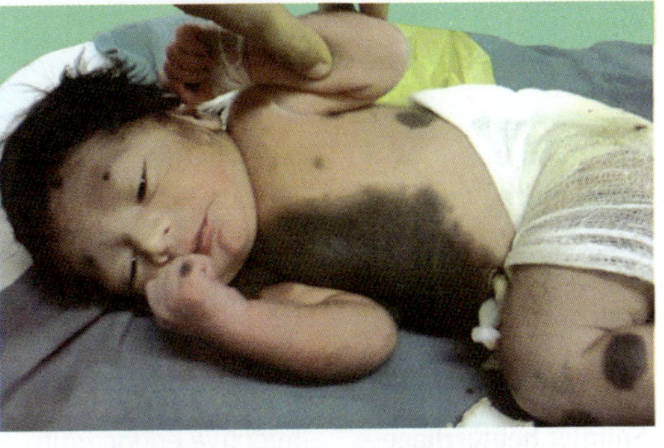

Fig. 7.56: Giant melanocytic nevus.

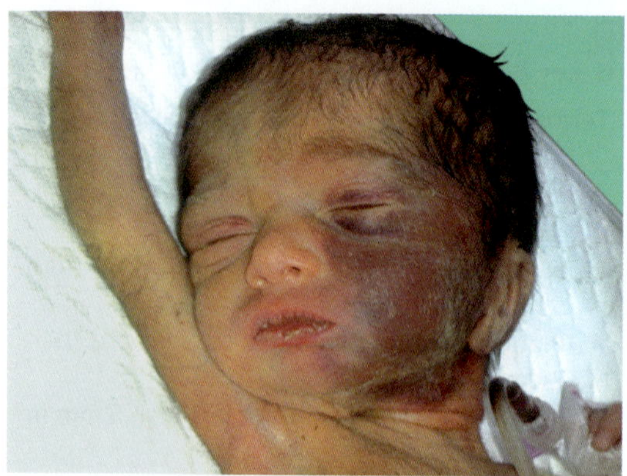

Fig. 7.57: Hemifacial staining in an infant with Sturge-Weber syndrome.

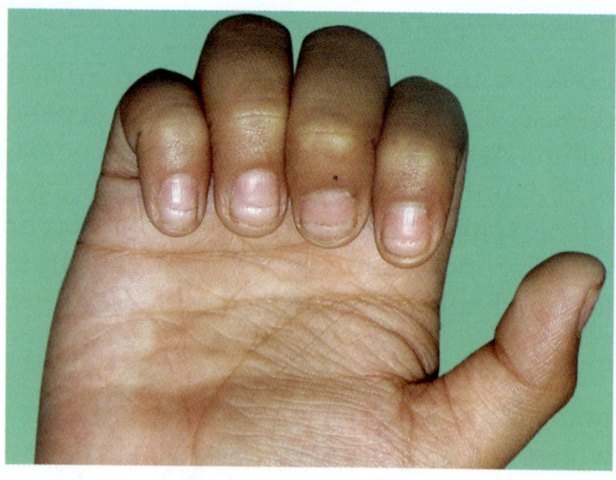

Fig. 7.58: Beau lines.

- Look for spider nevi (small capillary lesions distributed over the upper trunk and back) and palmar erythema (for hepatic failure).

J. Nails

Nail changes may be primary where the disease is affecting the nail or secondary to a systemic disease.

- *Hypertrophy* of the nails may be congenital, such as in *Mal de Meleda*, or acquired, when the nail becomes deformed with claw-like appearance as in trauma or failure to cut nails regularly, leprosy, and peripheral vascular disease.
- Look for any *atrophy* (ectodermal dysplasia, nail-patella syndrome) or dystrophy of nails. Look for *changes in shape* of nails (clubbing, koilonychia, platynychia).
- *Beau's lines* (Fig. 7.58) are transverse lines and furrows at the nail lanula, which are seen in trauma, measles, and drug reactions.
- *Pitted nails* may occur in psoriasis and lichen planus.
- *Nail biting* (onychophagia) is a common habit in children, biting and clipping of the tip of the nails by teeth. All fingernails are often bitten, but occasionally, one or more are spared. The nail is often bitten right back to the point of separation from the nail.
- *Color:* The nails may be discolored in several disorders **(Key Box 23)**.

K. Genitalia

This is a very important part of examination in every child and often missed. Older child may feel hesitant to allow for examination of genitals, so it is important to explain the procedure along with its significance to them before starting this examination. Adolescent girls should be examined in the presence of a female attendant.

Boys

Look for the presence of testes in scrotum (undescended, retractile testes) and size of testes (large testes in fragile X syndrome, germinoma), rugosity of scrotum, bifid scrotum, urethra (hypospadias, epispadias), penile length, hydrocele, hernia, and epididymo-orchitis in boys.

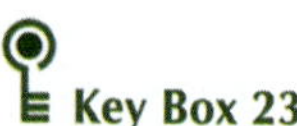

Key Box 23

Color Change of Nails

Black	Addison disease, Cushing disease, melanoma, pigmented nevus
Blue/Azure	Hepatolenticular discoloration
Brown	Drug reaction (antimalarial, phenolphthalein, potassium permanganate soaks, mercury compounds), post-inflammatory
Half and half moons	Chronic renal failure (Fig. 7.59)
Yellow	Syphilis
Green	*Pseudomonas aeruginosa* infections
Splinter hemorrhage	Infective endocarditis, scurvy, trauma, dermatomyositis

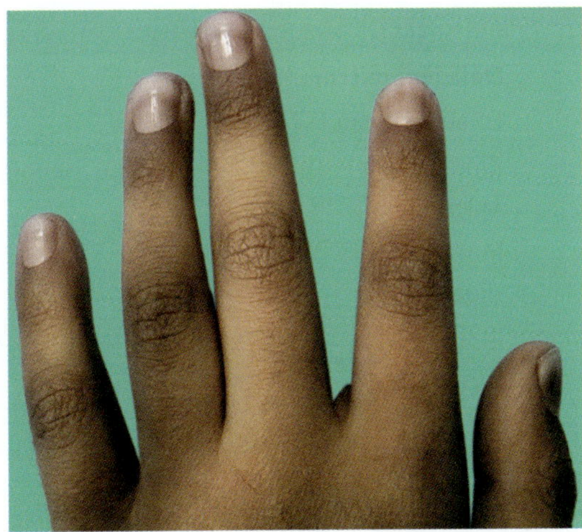

Fig. 7.59: Half moon nails.

Girls

Examine the breasts (size, shape, galactorrhea, premature thelarche), and see the distribution of pubic and axillary hair. Sexual maturity may be *delayed* as in hypothyroidism, hypopituitarism, Turner syndrome, or may be *precocious* as in polycystic ovarian disease, McCune-Albright syndrome, teratoma, hydrocephalus, and CNS tumors. Sexual maturity must be graded as per the Tanner pubertal staging described in Chapter 5.

7.6 PERIPHERAL SIGNS OF MICRONUTRIENT DEFICIENCY

You must look for evidence of nutritional deficiency during examination. You may examine either from head to toe, or look specifically for signs of deficiency of each nutrient. Certain features are almost diagnostic of a particular micronutrient deficiency **(Key Box 24)**. **Table 7.4** summarizes the peripheral changes characteristic of various micronutrient deficiencies.

1. Vitamin A Deficiency

Vitamin A deficiency is characterized by night blindness and xerophthalmia. WHO classifies eye changes of vitamin D deficiency as follows:

- X1A Conjunctival xerosis
- X1B Bitot spots **(Fig. 7.60)**
- X2 Corneal xerosis
- X3A Corneal ulceration less than two-thirds of cornea
- X3B Keratomalacia (corneal ulceration more than two-thirds of cornea), **(Fig. 7.61)**
- XS Corneal scarring
- XF Xerophthalmic fundus

Key Box 24

Diagnostic Signs of Micronutrient Deficiency

Finding	Description	Deficiency
Hyperpigmented knuckles	Dark bilateral brown-black coloration over the knuckles of fingers of hands	Folate, Vitamin B_{12}
Angular stomatitis	Superficial erosions or fissures at the angles of the mouth	Vitamin B_2 (riboflavin)
Cheilosis	Dry scaling and fissuring of the vermillion surfaces of the lips	Vitamin B_2 (riboflavin)
Blepharitis	Inflammation of the eyelids	Vitamin B_2
Bitot spots	Chalky white spots on the temporal side of corneo-scleral junction	Vitamin A
Harrison sulcus	Deep groove along the spaces where the diaphragm is inserted into the inner aspects of the rib	Vitamin D
Rachitic rosary	Prominence of costochondral junction due to flaring of anterior ends of ribs	Vitamin D
Scorbutic rosary	Angulation of costochondral junctions due to posterior dislocation of the sternum	Vitamin C
Phrynoderma	Toad-like skin due to follicular hyperkeratosis	Essential fatty acids, vitamin A, vitamin E

Table 7.4: Peripheral changes characteristic of micronutrient deficiencies

Body part	Sign	Deficient micronutrient
Hand nails	Hyperpigmentation	Folate, vitamin B_{12}
	White spots and ridges	Zinc
	Brittle nails	Magnesium
	Koilonychia, platynychia	Iron
	Splinter hemorrhages	Vitamin C
Skin	Stretch marks	Zinc
	Follicular hyperkeratosis	Vitamin A
	Spontaneous hemorrhages	Vitamin C or vitamin K
	Dry scaly skin with hair follicles plugged with coiled distorted hairs and a red halo	Vitamin C
Mouth	Pale fissured and bald tongue	Iron
	Sore burning tongue and lips and peeling of lips	Vitamin B_2
	Painful sore tongue with smooth appearance	Folic acid
Gums	Bleeding gums	Vitamin C
Face	Greasy red scaly skin of face and sides of nose	Vitamin B_6
	Seborrheic dermatitis around nose and acne like forehead rash	Vitamin B_2
Eyes	Xerophthalmia	Vitamin A
	Cataracts	Chromium
	Blue eyes and blond hair	Zinc, magnesium
	Circumcorneal vascularization	Vitamin B_6, essential fatty acid, vitamin B_2
	Blue eyes and premature gray hair	Vitamin B_{12}
Throat	Thyroid swelling	Iodine
Heart	Irregular beat, high blood pressure, cardiomegaly	Magnesium, vitamin B_1 and CoQ10
Legs	Tender calf muscles	Magnesium
	Hypotonia and hyporeflexia	Potassium
	Paresthesia and tetanic spasms	Calcium, magnesium
	Double malleoli, bow legs	Vitamin D

2. Vitamin B Deficiency

Vitamin B_1: Dry beriberi: Irritability, fatigue, emotional disturbances, difficulty in walking or standing, edema, tender calf muscle, hyporeflexia; *Wet beriberi:* Congestive heart failure.

Vitamin B_2: Sore throat and tongue, watering of eyes, glossitis (strawberry, glazed tongue, Fig. 7.62), cheilosis (Fig. 7.63), nasolabial dysbacea, circumcorneal vascularization, and keratinization, photophobia, hyperesthesia, altered pain and temperature sensation.

Niacin: Dermatitis (pigmented scaly cracked skin on exposed area of body, casal necklace, pellagrous glove, pellagrous foot), dementia.

Pyridoxine: Pallor, hyperaccusis, convulsions.

Vitamin B_{12}: Pallor, icterus, jaundice, loss of position and proprioception.

3. Vitamin C Deficiency

Bleeding tendency, ecchymosis, mucosal bleeds (Fig. 7.64), pallor, gum swelling, tenderness of muscles, bone pains, pseudoparalysis,

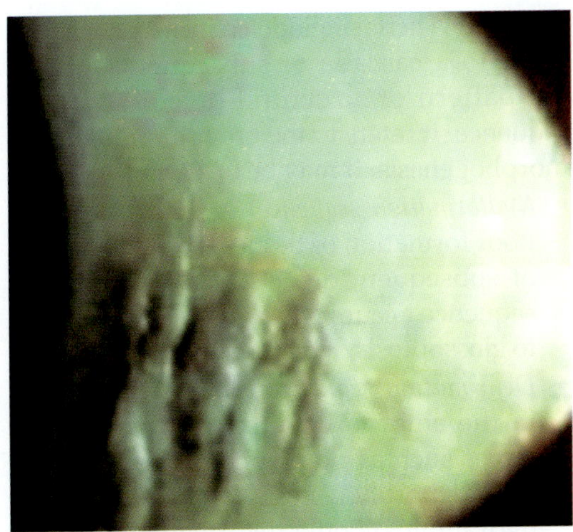

Fig. 7.60: Bitot spots, chalky white patch at corneo-scleral junction.

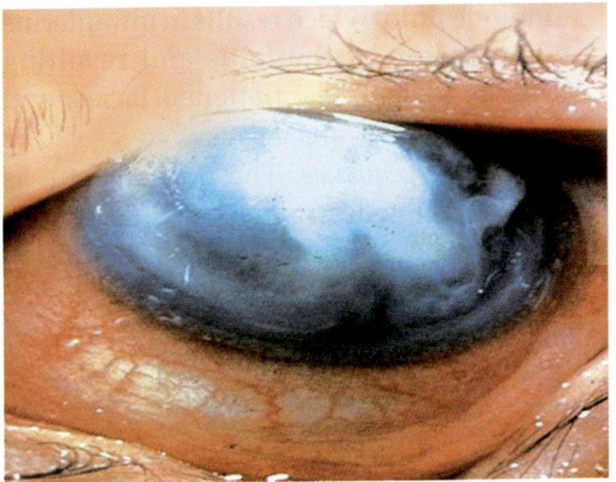

Fig. 7.61: Keratomalacia.

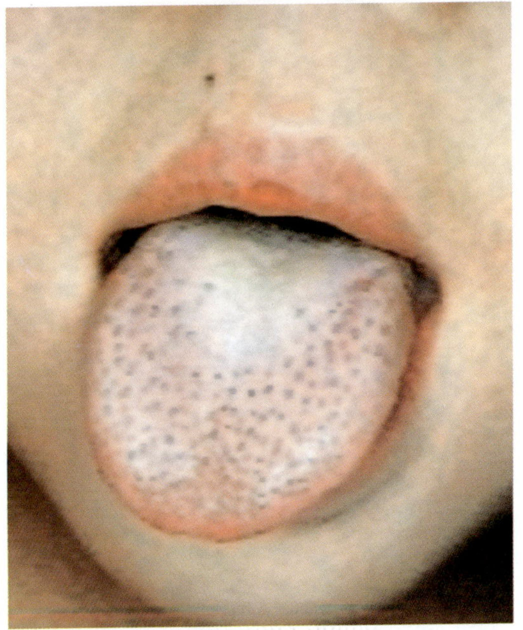

Fig. 7.62: Strawberry tongue.

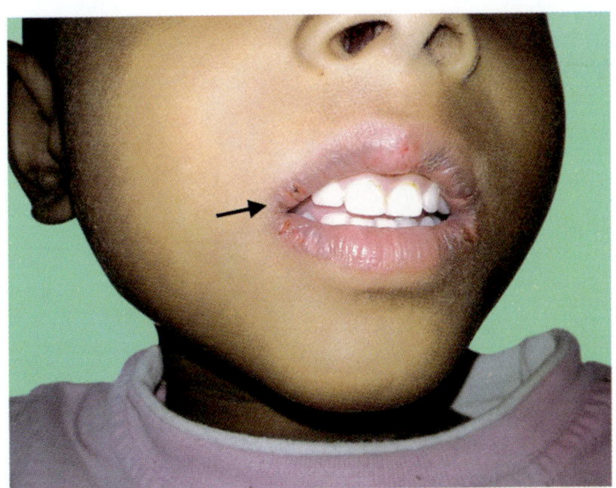

Fig. 7.63: Cheilosis

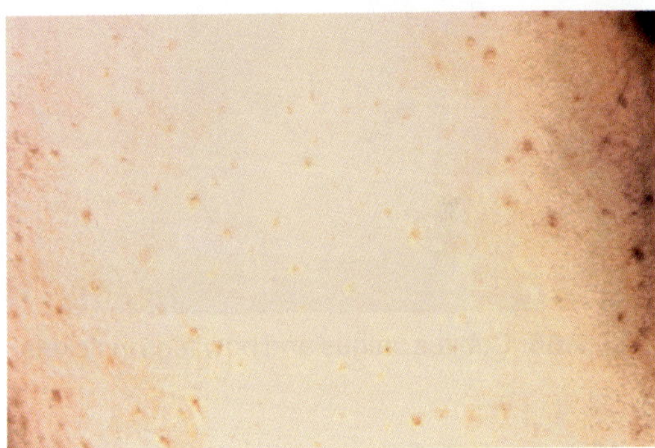

Fig. 7.64: Skin hemorrhages seen in scurvy.

scorbutic rosary, hyperkeratosis, conjunctival and subperiosteal hemorrhages.

4. Vitamin D Deficiency

Frontal and parietal bossing, craniotabes, rachitic rosary, pigeon chest, harrison sulcus, wrist widening **(Fig. 7.65)**, double malleoli, bow legs **(Fig. 7.66)**, visceroptosis, hypotonia, short stature, tetanic spasms, and seizure.

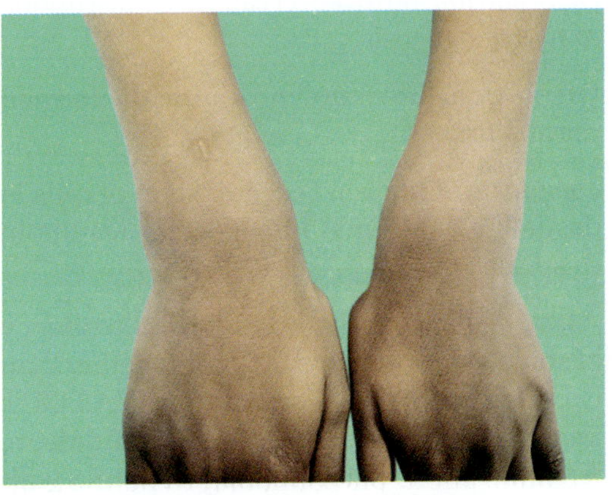

Fig. 7.65: Widening of wrists.

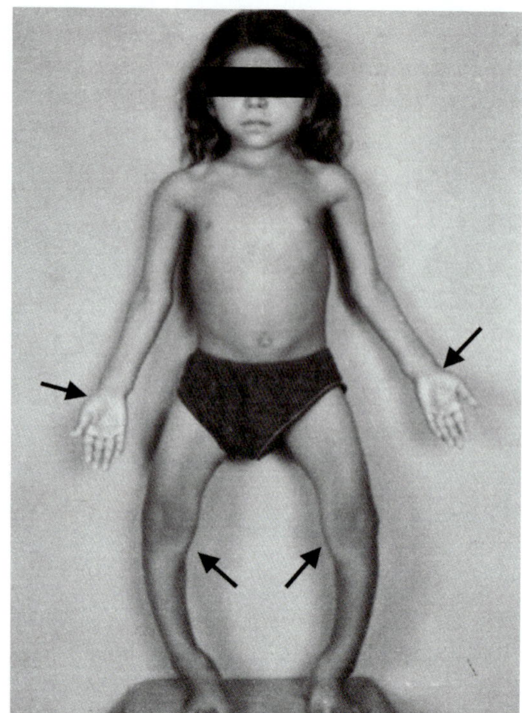

Fig. 7.66: Cubitus valgus and bow legs in rickets.

5. Vitamin E Deficiency

Phrynoderma (rough and scaly skin), ataxia, visual disturbances, pallor.

7.7 LOOKING FOR DYSMORPHISM AND CONGENITAL ABNORMALITIES

Dysmorphism refers to abnormal morphology; it can result from any of the mechanisms given below:

Malformation: Birth defect arising because of poor formation of tissues.

Deformation: Birth defect caused by disruption of morphogenesis.

Disruption: Breakdown of already formed normal tissues.

Dysplasia: Abnormal organization of cells in tissue, i.e. abnormal histogenesis results in dysplasia.

Association: It is the non-random tendency of some malformations to occur together than expected by chance. For example, **VATER** is an acronym that includes **V**ertebral defects, **A**nal atresia, **T**racheoesophageal fistula with **E**sophageal atresia, and **R**enal dysplasia.

Sequence: When a single defect in morphogenesis leads to a cascade of subsequent defects, the pattern of structural defects is called sequence. It refers to the order of problems in morphogenesis. It may be of 4 types:

- *Malformation sequence:* A single localized poor formation of tissue leading to a chain of subsequent defects, e.g. Pierre Robin sequence occurs when micrognathia leads to glossoptosis, which results in cleft palate.
- *Deformation sequence:* There is no defect in the embryo or fetus, but mechanical forces such as uterine constraint result in altered morphogenesis. For example, oligohydramnios/Potter deformation sequence due to chronic leakage of amniotic fluid or renal agenesis; leading to decreased amniotic fluid; which results in intrauterine compression of the fetus and resulting limb abnormalities, flattened facies, and pulmonary hypoplasia.
- *Disruption sequence:* The normal fetus is subjected to a destructive problem and its consequences. Amniotic band disruption sequence is characterized by varied clinical manifestations ranging from partial amputations to major craniofacial and limb-body wall defects, as a consequence of early amnion rupture, and vascular disruption events (Fig. 7.67).

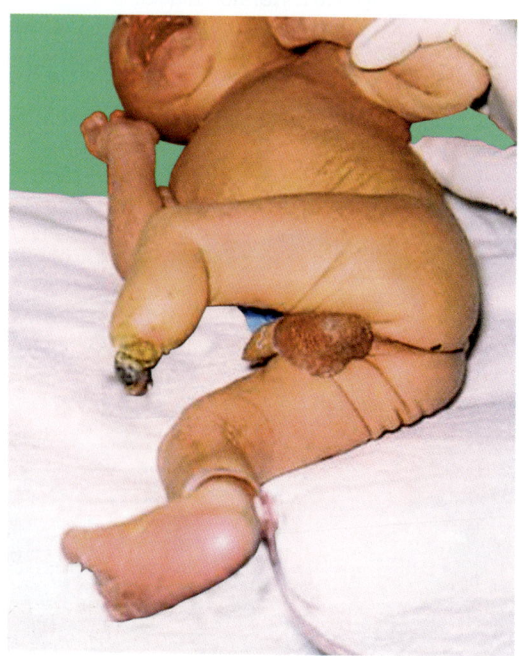

Fig. 7.67: Amniotic band sequence.

- *Dysplasia sequence:* The primary defect is a lack of normal organization of cells into tissues. Neurocutaneous melanosis sequence is due to lack of migration of melanoblastic precursors from the neural crest which results in melanocytic hamartomas of the skin in conjunction with similar changes in the pia and arachnoid.

Syndromes: When multiple structural defects occur together that cannot be explained on the basis of a single initiating defect and its consequences, but are due to multiple defects in one or more tissues, the recurrent patterns of maldevelopment are called *malformation syndromes*. For example, William syndrome is characterized by *Elfin facies* (broad upper lip, small mandible, prominent maxilla, upturned nose), cocktail party chatter, supravalvular aortic stenosis, peripheral pulmonary stenosis, and hypercalcemia.

Common terms used to describe dysmorphology are defined in Table 7.5.

Table 7.5: Common terms used to describe dysmorphology

Dysmorphic feature	Definition	Associated conditions
Acromelia	Dwarfism associated with shortened distal fragment of limb	Acromesomelic dysplasia
Anotia	Complete absence of the auricle or pinna, and narrowing or lack of external auditory meatus	Oculo-auriculo-vertebral spectrum, Treacher Collins syndrome
Anti-mongoloid slant	Nasal corners of the palpebral fissure are higher than the temporal corners, as opposed to the typical mongoloid slant	Treacher Collins syndrome, cri-du-chat syndrome
Arachnodactyly	Spider like or long fingers or toes	Marfan syndrome, Stickler syndrome,
Brachydactyly	Short fingers or toes	Down syndrome, Rubinstein-Taybi syndrome
Camptodactyly	Flexion deformity at the proximal interphalangeal joint, usually involves the little finger	Trisomy 13 (Patau syndrome), Trisomy 18 (Edward syndrome)
Carrying angle	Angle subtended by the forearm on the humerus	Cubitus valgus in Turner syndrome
Clinodactyly	Incurving of little finger; radial in direction, and is most often associated with a short middle phalanx which is shorter on its radial than ulnar side.	Down syndrome, Carpenter syndrome, Miller-Dieker syndrome
Clubfoot (congenital talipes equinovarus, CTEV)	A foot deformity in which the foot is twisted inward with the toes pointing down.	Sporadic, often associated with spinal deformities, such as spina bifida or other neuromuscular diseases
Cryptophthalmos	Complete failure of development of the eyelid folds with continuity of the skin from the forehead to the cheek.	Fraser syndrome
Cubitus valgus	Valgus deformity at the elbow due to an increased carrying angle at the elbow, so it deviates away from the midline of the body when extended.	Apert syndrome, Cornelia de Lange syndrome, Noonan syndrome, Turner syndrome

Contd...

Table 7.5: Common terms used to describe dysmorphology (*Contd...*)

Dysmorphic feature	Definition	Associated conditions
Cubitus varus (Gunstock deformity)	Varus deformity of the elbow in which it deviates towards the midline of the body when extended	Supracondylar fracture of humerus
Ectrodactyly (split hand/split foot malformation)	Deficiency or absence of one or more central digits of the hand or foot	Tibial aplasia-ectrodactyly syndrome, ectrodactyly-ectodermal dysplasia-clefting syndrome
Epicanthic fold	A skinfold covering the medial epicanthus of the eye	Down syndrome, cri-du-chat syndrome, Treacher Collins syndrome
Epispadias	Congenital absence of the upper wall of the urethra, occurring in both sexes, but more often in the male, with the urethral opening somewhere on the dorsum of the penis	Exstrophy-epispadias complex
Hypertelorism (wide set eyes)	Increased distance between the eyes manifests as increased distance between inner and outer canthi. The interpupillary distance is increased (telecanthus). Canthal index (inner canthal distance/outer canthal distance × 100) is higher than 42	Edward syndrome (Trisomy 18), craniofrontonasal dysplasia, Noonan syndrome, neurofibromatosis, Apert syndrome, Crouzon syndrome, mucopolysaccharide metabolism disorders, Coffin-Lowry syndrome
Hypospadias	Opening of the urethra is on the underside of the penis	Sporadic, Prader-Willi syndrome, Aniridia-Wilms tumor association, Beckwith-Wiedemann syndrome
Hypotelorism	Reduced distance between the medial walls of the orbits with reduced inner and outer intercanthal distances. Canthal index is lower than 38 in hypotelorism	Holoprosencephaly, trigonocephaly
Low-set ears	When the helix meets the cranium at a level below that of a horizontal plane passing through the inner canthi	Down syndrome, Noonan syndrome, Smith-Lemli-Opitz syndrome, Treacher Collins syndrome
Mesomelia	Shortening of middle fragment of limb	Mesomelia-synostoses syndrome, Ellis-van Creveld syndrome
Micropenis	A normally structured penis that is below the normal size range for age. A stretched penile length (SPL) of less than 1.9 centimeters (0.75 inches) in a newborn is usually considered micropenis. SPL that is more than 2.5 standard deviations below the average size for age is also regarded as micropenis	Prader-Willi syndrome
Microtia	Congenital deformity where the pinna (external ear) is underdeveloped	Hemifacial microsomia, Goldenhar syndrome, Treacher Collins syndrome
Mongoloid slant	A palpebral slant wherein the outer canthus is higher than the inner canthus	Down syndrome, Noonan syndrome
Phocomelia	Absence of limb	Thalidomide syndrome

Contd...

Table 7.5: Common terms used to describe dysmorphology (*Contd...*)

Dysmorphic feature	Definition	Associated conditions
Pre-axial polydactyly	Extra finger on the side of the great toe or thumb	Holt-Oram syndrome, Greig cephalo-polysyndactyly syndrome, Fanconi anemia
Post-axial polydactyly	Extra finger on the side of the little finger/little toe	Ellis-van Creveld syndrome, Greig cephalopolysyndactyly syndrome
Rhizomelia	Shortening of the proximal limb resulting in dwarfism	Achondroplasia
Sirenomelia	A congenital defect resulting in fusion of both lower legs presenting as mermaid's tail	Mermaid syndrome
Syndactyly	Fusion of fingers (cutaneous or osseous)	Apert syndrome
Synophyrs	Fusion of the eyebrows in the midline	Cornelia de Lange syndrome, Waardenburg syndrome, Sanfilippo syndrome
Telecanthus	The distance between the inner canthi is increased, but the interpupillary distance is normal	Associated with encephaloceles, meningoencephaloceles, and frontonasal dysplasia
Wide spaced nipples	Distance between the nipples > ¼ of the chest circumference	Turner syndrome, Noonan syndrome

Key Box 25 provides a summary of the check-list for examination of a dysmorphic child.

Dermatoglyphics

Dermatoglyphics refers to the dermal ridge patterns, which can be seen on the palm, soles, fingers, and toes of an individual.

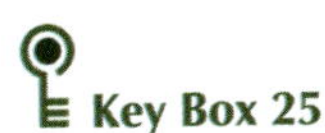

Key Box 25

Summary of the Checklist for Examination of a Dysmorphic Child

Head
- Does the head look normal in shape and size?
- Is there microcephaly/macrocephaly? Are the sutures closed?
- Measure the occipitofrontal circumference.

Eyes
- Are the eyes spaced normally?
- Is there hypotelorism/hypertelorism? Is there microphthalmia/buphthalmos?
- Look at the palpebral fissures, epicanthic folds, synophrys, coloboma, ptosis, corneal clouding, blue sclera, heterochromia iridae and shallow or prominent orbits.

Ears
- Are the ears low-set?
- Look at ear shape (microtia/anotia), size (small/large or bat-like), auricular tags or pits.

Face
Look for mandibular/maxillary hypoplasia, hypertrophied gums, cleft lip or palate, prominent lips, pallor, cyanosis, macroglossia, teeth caries and pigmentation.

Hands
Look for simian crease, brachydactyly, clinodactyly, polydactyly, syndactyly, arachnodactyly, broad thumbs, absent or hypoplastic radii.

Skin
Look for alopecia, hirsutism, café au lait spots, hypo-/hyperpigmentation, neurofibromas.

Genitalia
Look for cryptorchidism, hypospadias, micropenis.

Fingertip Patterns

The various patterns seen on fingertips include: Whorls, loops (ulnar, radial), and arches (Fig. 7.68). Some characteristic patterns seen in certain dysmorphic syndromes are as follows: Ulnar loops on most fingers in Down syndrome, mostly arches seen in trisomy 18, and mostly whorls seen in fingertips in congenital rubella syndrome. In Klinefelter syndrome, these patterns are markedly reduced.

Flexion Creases

Three flexion creases are usually present in each palm.

- *Simian crease* (Fig. 7.69) is a single transverse mid-palmar crease which occurs when the two distal palmar creases are fused (characteristically seen in Down syndrome). It is seen in 4% of normal individuals.
- *Sydney crease* occurs when the proximal crease runs through the entire palm while the distal crease is normally present.

Tri-radii

The ridges in the palms meet at certain points which are called tri-radii. The tri-radii in each palm are called *a*, *b*, *c*, *d* and *t*. The angle formed at tri-radii *t* by joining *a*, *t* and *d* is called ATD angle which is usually about 40°. In Down syndrome, Turner syndrome, and congenital rubella syndrome, the ATD angle is obtuse as the proximal tri-radius is shifted distally (Fig. 7.70).

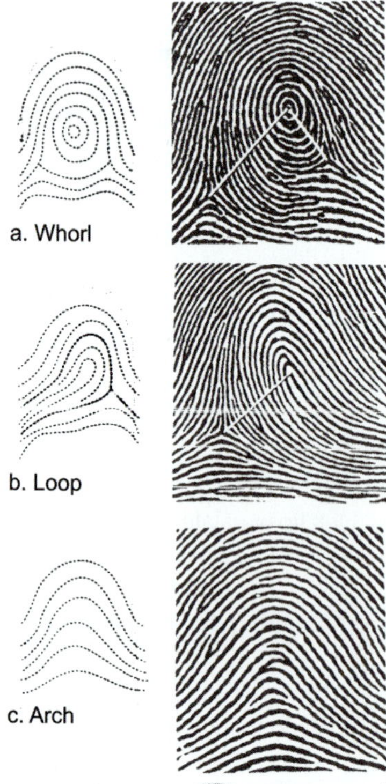

Fig. 7.68: Dermal ridge patterns.

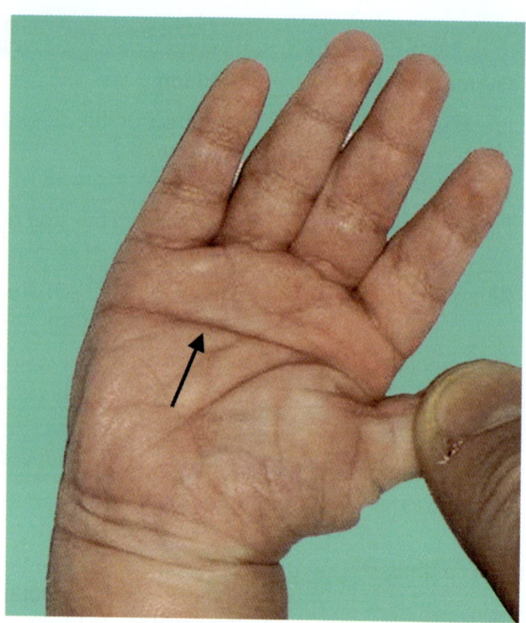

Fig. 7.69: Simian crease in Down syndrome.

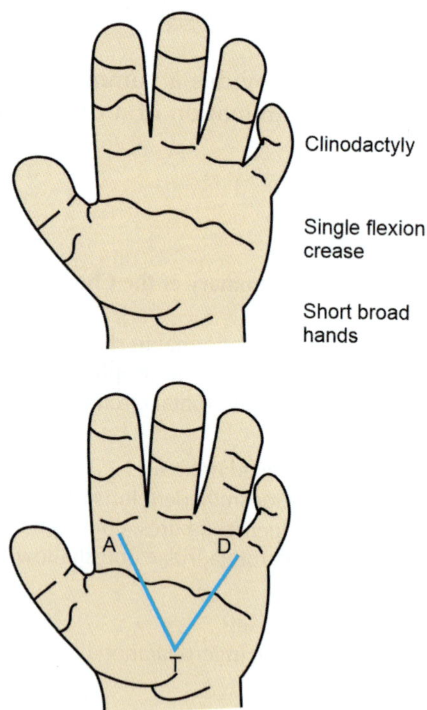

Fig. 7.70: ATD angle in Down syndrome.

Common Dysmorphic Syndromes

1. Syndromes Associated with Chromosomal Abnormalities

Down syndrome/Trisomy 21: It is the commonest chromosomal disorder caused by the presence of all or part of a third copy of chromosome 21. Children with Down syndrome may have some or all of the following physical characteristics—hypotonia, poor Moro reflex, hyperflexibility of joints, excess skin on the back of neck, flat facial profile, downward slanted palpebral fissures (mongoloid slant), epicanthic folds on the inner corner of the eyes, Brushfield spots/ white-speckled spots on the iris, cataract, keratoconus, strabismus, refractive errors, anomalous auricles, clinodactyly, flat occiput, protruding tongue, macroglossia, small and broad hands, characteristic dermatoglyphics [simian crease (*see* Fig. 7.69), more ulnar loops, absence of whorls on ball of foot, obtuse ATD angle (Fig. 7.70), flat and broad feet with deep plantar crease), increased gap between the great toe and second toe, i.e. sandle gap (Fig. 7.71)], short stature, joint laxity including atlantoaxial dislocation, pelvic bone dysplasia, protuberant abdomen, Hirschsprung disease, pyloric stenosis, duodenal atresia, biliary atresia, hypothyroidism, and predisposition to Alzheimer disease. There is an increased tendency to have associated cardiac defects, like endocardial cushion defect, ventricular septal defects, and ASD.

Patau syndrome/trisomy 13: Features include holoprosencephaly, microcephaly, microphthalmia, abnormal helices with low-set ears, cleft palate and lip, simian crease, hyperconvex and narrow fingernails, overlapping of fingers over the thumb, polydactyly, rocker-bottom feet, cutis aplasia, calvarial and scalp defects (Fig. 7.72), coloboma and cataracts in eyes, cryptorchidism, congenital heart defects (VSD, ASD, PDA), kidney defects, meningomyelocele, and single umbilical artery. Majority of children with Patau syndrome die within the first year of life.

Edward syndrome/Trisomy 18: It is characterized by slow growth before birth (intrauterine growth retardation) and a low birth weight. Congenital heart disease (VSD, ASD, PDA), small and abnormally-shaped head, a small jaw and mouth, clenched fists with overlapping fingers, low arch dermal ridge patterning in fingertips, single umbilical artery, prominent occiput, hypertonicity, low-set ears, short palpebral fissures, micrognathia, small pelvis, limited hip abduction, cryptorchidism, and hypoplastic supraorbital ridges are seen.

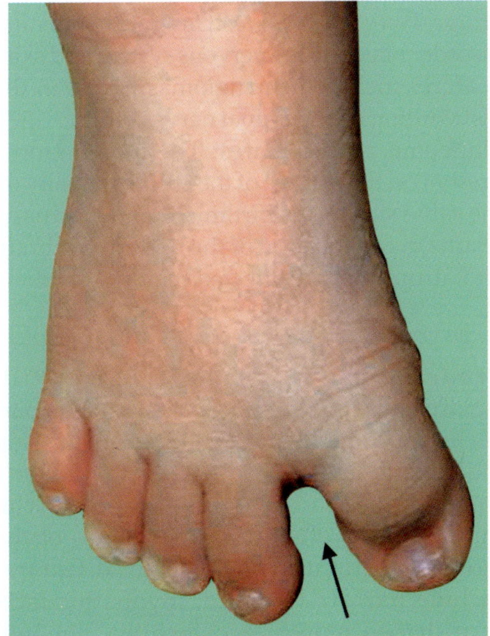

Fig. 7.71: Sandle gap seen in Down syndrome.

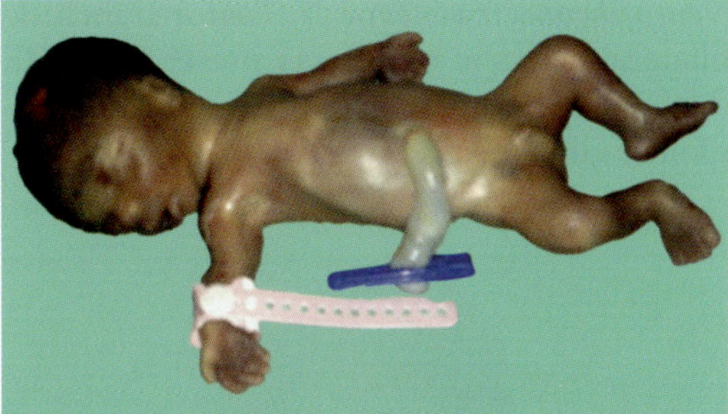

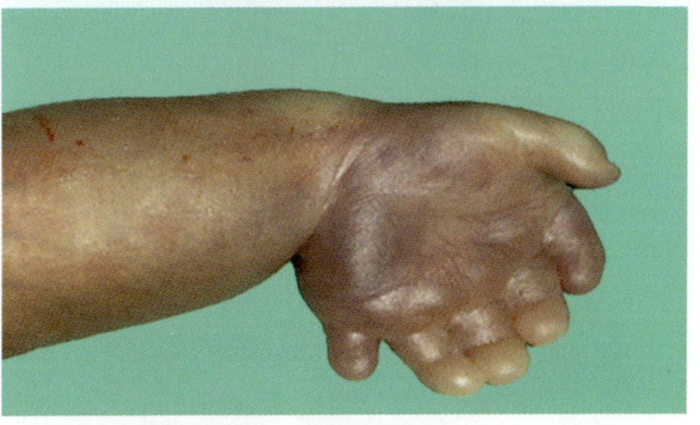

Fig. 7.72: Stillborn neonate with Patau syndrome showing scalp defects and polydactyly.

Due to the presence of several life-threatening medical problems, many individuals with trisomy 18 die before birth or within their first month.

Cri-du-chat Syndrome (5p deletion syndrome): It is characterized by abnormalities of the larynx and the nervous system as consequence of which infants have a cry resembling the meoing of kitten. Other features include microcephaly, antimongoloid slant, hypertelorism, global developmental delay, hypotonia, simian crease, round face, and epicanthic folds.

2. Syndromes Associated with Neurocutaneous Stigmata

Neurofibromatosis (von Recklinghausen disease): It is a genetically-inherited disorder characterized by abnormal growth of nerve tissues which form benign tumors. The disorder affects all neural crest cells (Schwann cells, melanocytes, and endoneurial fibroblasts).

Neurofibromatosis type I: Features include café au lait spots (≥6 in number, >5 mm size in prepubertal children and >15 mm size in postpubertal individuals), ≥2 neurofibromas (Fig. 7.73), axillary/inguinal freckling, Lisch nodules (hamartomas of iris), tibial bowing, kyphoscoliosis, macrocephaly, and short stature.

Neurofibromatosis type II: Features include bilateral acoustic neuromas presenting with deafness and tinnitus. Neurofibroma, meningioma, glioma, and schwannomas are seen.

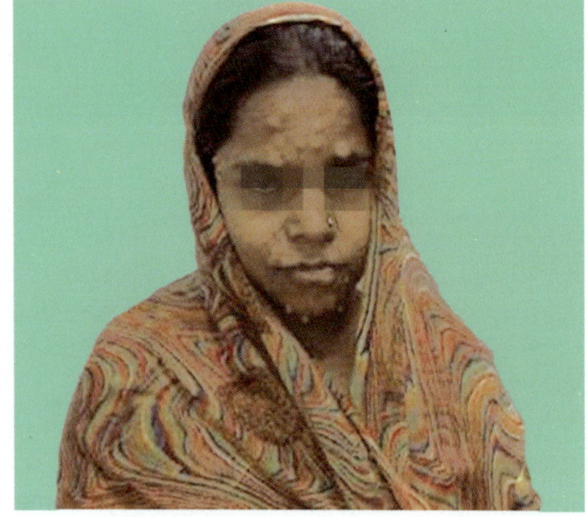

Fig. 7.73: Neurofibroma.

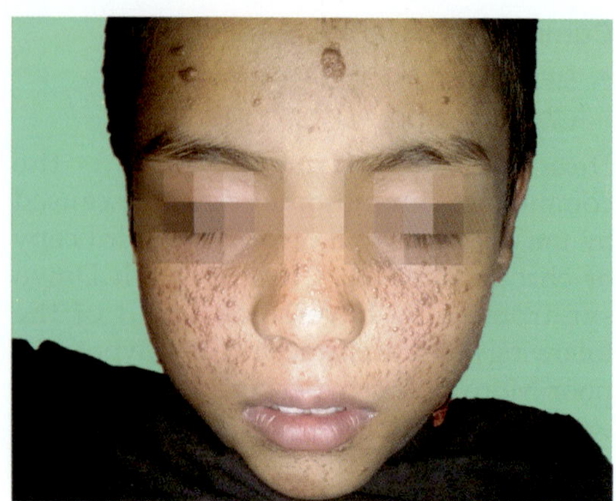

Fig. 7.74: Adenoma sebaceum (fibrous angioma of face).

Tuberous sclerosis: It is a group of two genetic disorders that affect the skin, brain/nervous system, kidneys, and heart, and cause tumors to grow. Features include hypopigmented macules (ash leaf spots or confetti appearance), adenoma sebaceum (fibrous angiomas along nasolabial folds and spreading to cheeks) (Fig. 7.74), periungual fibroma, shagreen patch (raised patches of skin with an orange-peel texture over sacral region), café au lait spots, tuberous hamartomas, malignant glioma, hydrocephalus, renal angiomyolipoma, polycystic kidneys, cardiac rhabdomyomas, and cystic hamartomatous nodules in lungs. Myoclonic seizures occur in childhood.

Sturge-Weber syndrome: It is a rare congenital disorder affecting the nervous system and skin. Features include hemangiomas of face in the distribution of trigeminal nerve (*see* Fig. 7.57), glaucoma, and seizures. The hemangioma present on the surface of the brain is usually on the same side as the birthmark and gradually results in calcification of the underlying brain and atrophy of the affected region.

3. Syndromes Associated with Short Stature

Prader-Willi syndrome: Prader-Willi syndrome is caused by a gene missing on part of chromosome 15; most children are missing the genetic material on part of the father's chromosome while the rest of children with this condition often have two copies of the mother's chromosome 15. Clinical features include narrow forehead, myopathic face, carp-shaped mouth, micrognathia, almond-shaped eyes, strabismus, small hands and feet, short stature, hypotonia in infancy, cryptorchidism in male neonates, mental retardation, gross obesity, and hypogonadism.

Turner syndrome (45 XO, gonadal dysgenesis): It is a chromosomal disorder in which all or part of one of the X chromosomes is absent. It is seen in phenotypic females who may present with shield chest, cubitus valgus, webbed neck, low posterior hairline, high-arched palate, short fourth metacarpal, hyperconvex nails, ovarian dysgenesis, hypogonadism, lymphedema of hands and feet, short stature, and cardiac defects (coarctation of aorta, bicuspid aortic valve).

Achondroplasia: It is an autosomal dominant disorder affecting the bone growth that causes the most common type of dwarfism. Features include prominent forehead, midfacial hypoplasia, short limbs (Fig. 7.75), disproportionately large head-to-body size difference, broad hands with short metacarpals, phalanges with trident configuration, thoracolumbar kyphosis, and spinal stenosis.

A trident hand (Fig. 7.76) is a description where the hands are short with stubby fingers, with a separation/gap between the middle and ring fingers.

Russell-Silver syndrome: It is a disorder present at birth characterized by slow growth before (intrauterine growth retardation) and after birth. Many children with Russell-Silver syndrome have a small, triangular face with distinctive facial features including a prominent forehead, a narrow chin, a small jaw, and down-turned corners of the mouth. Other features of this disorder can include clinodactyly, asymmetric or uneven growth of some parts of the body, one side of the body also will appear to be larger than the other, clinodactyly, café au lait spots, blue sclerae in infancy, with an increased risk of delayed development and learning disabilities.

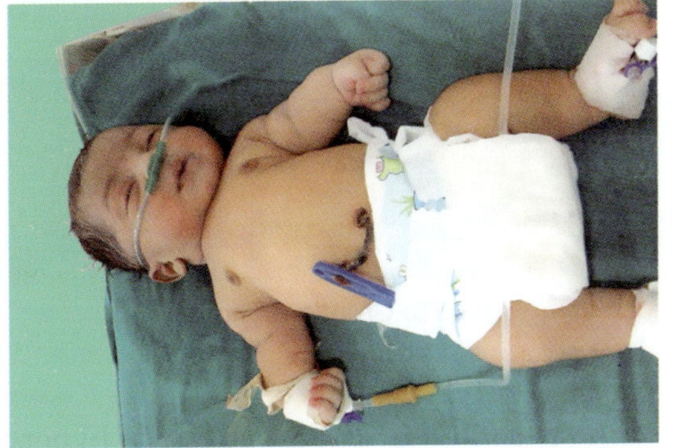

Fig. 7.75: Achondroplasia.

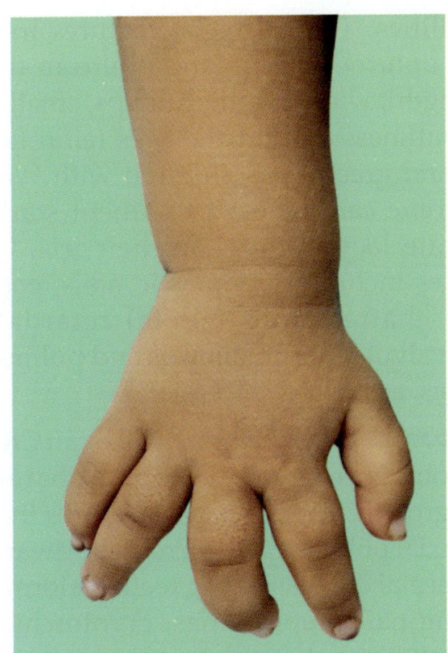

Fig. 7.76: Trident hand.

Fetal alcohol syndrome: It is a pattern of mental and physical defects (smooth philtrum, thin upper lip, small palpebral fissures, small nose, growth retardation, maxillary hypoplasia) that can develop in a fetus in association with high levels of alcohol consumption during pregnancy.

4. Syndromes Associated with Cardiovascular Disease

Noonan syndrome: It is an autosomal dominant disorder associated with defects in several genes. It is often referred to as Turner-like syndrome which may affect males and females. The spectrum of dysmorphic features includes hypertelorism, antimongoloid slant (downward slanting), epicanthic folds, micrognathia, high- arched palate, bilateral ptosis, low posterior hairline, webbed and short-appearing neck, short stature, shield chest, cubitus valgus, pectus excavatum or carinatum, kyphosis, scoliosis, small penis and cryptorchidism in males, delayed menarche in females.

William syndrome: This genetic condition is present at birth and is characterized by medical problems, including cardiovascular disease, developmental delays, and learning disabilities. Typical facial features include small upturned nose, long philtrum (upper lip length), wide mouth, full lips, small chin, and puffiness around the eyes (elfin facies). Blue and green-eyed children with William syndrome can have a prominent starburst or white lacy pattern on their iris. Other features include hypoplastic nails, cocktail party chatter, mild mental retardation, supravalvular aortic stenosis and pulmonary stenosis, and hypercalcemia.

Ellis-van creveld syndrome: Ellis-van Creveld syndrome is a rare genetic disorder that affects bone growth. The abnormal features include post-axial polydactyly, micromelic dwarfism, ectodermal dysplasia (peg teeth, deformed or missing nails), epispadias, cryptorchidism, and cleft lip or cleft palate.

Holt-oram syndrome: It is a genetic disorder that affects bones in the upper limbs and may also cause cardiac problems (atrial or ventricular septum defects). Bone abnormalities include polydactyly, a hypoplastic thumb or a thumb that looks like a finger, partial or complete absence of bones in the forearm, an underdeveloped bone of the upper arm, and abnormalities that affect the collar bone and shoulder blades. Its presentation resembles the teratogenic effects of thalidomide.

5. Syndromes Associated with Craniosynostoses

Apert syndrome (acrocephalosyndactyly): It is a rare autosomal dominant disorder characterized by craniosynostosis, craniofacial anomalies (brachycephaly with large forehead, proptosis, midfacial hypoplasia) and severe symmetrical syndactyly (mitten hands, Fig. 7.77) of the hands and feet.

Carpenter syndrome (acrocephalopoly-syndactyly): It is an autosomal recessive disorder characterized by acrocephaly (tower-shaped skull), obesity, flat nasal bridge, preaxial/polydactyly of feet, partial syndactyly of hands and feet and reduced height.

Crouzon syndrome (branchial arch syndrome): It affects the first branchial (or pharyngeal) arch and features include maxillary hypoplasia, proptosis, hypertelorism, low-set ears, parrot-nose and dental anomalies, like hypodontia and crowding of teeth (Fig. 7.78).

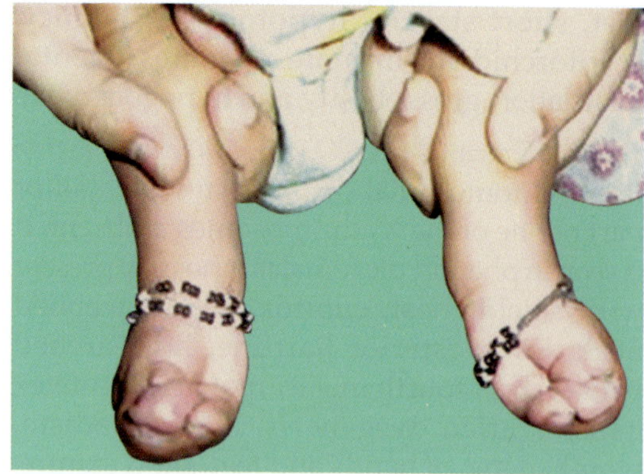

Fig. 7.77: Mitten hands in Apert syndrome.

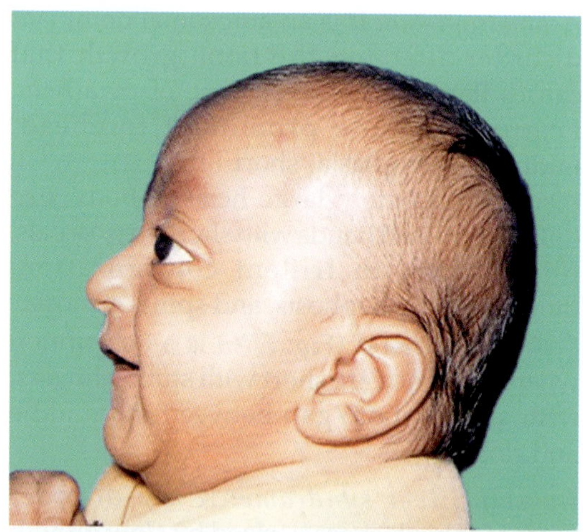

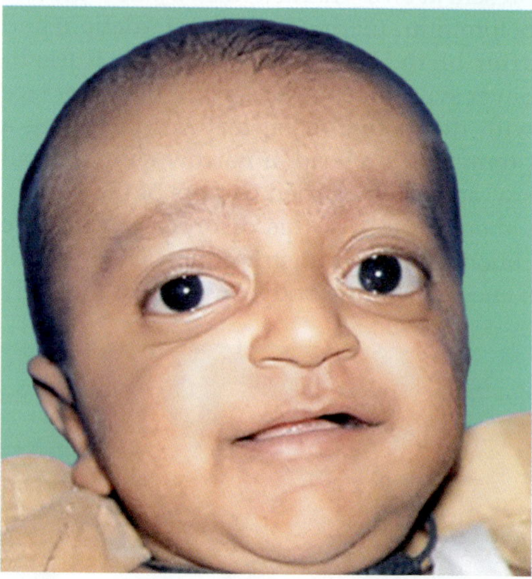

Fig. 7.78: Crouzon syndrome.

6. Other Syndromes

Marfan syndrome: Arachnodactyly, hyper-extensibility, lens subluxation, aortic dilatation.

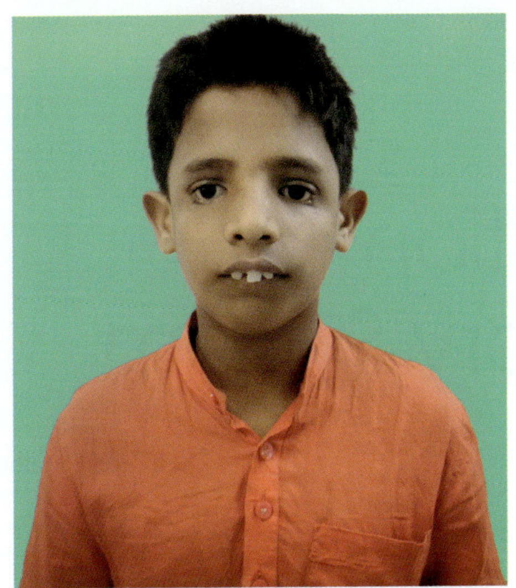

Fig. 7.79: Antimongoloid slant in Treacher Collins syndrome.

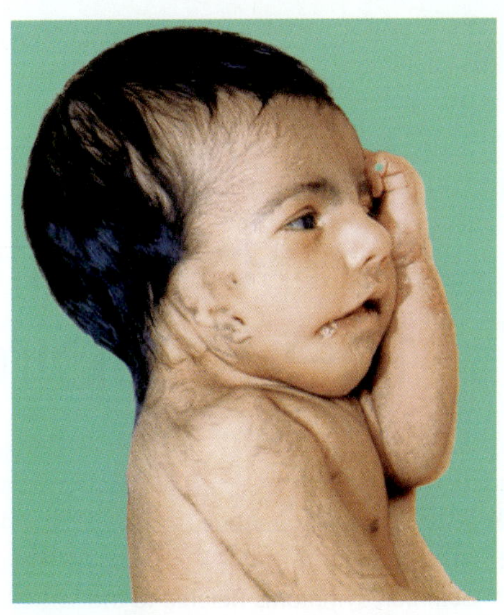

Fig. 7.80: Goldenhar syndrome showing facial cleft, and preauricular pit.

Ehlers-Danlos syndrome: Hyperextensibility of joints and skin, poor wound healing, and thin scar.

Treacher Collins syndrome: Malar hypoplasia, anti-mongoloid slant of palpebral fissure (Fig. 7.79), coloboma of lower eyelids, malformed external ears, micrognathia.

Beckwith-Wiedemann syndrome: Exomphalos, macroglossia, nevus flammeus over forehead, hemihypertrophy, creases/clefts in ear lobes.

Goldenhar syndrome (Oculo-auriculovertebral syndrome): Facial asymmetry, lateral cleft-like extention of corner of mouth, ear abnormalities (preauricular tags, microtia), spina bifida, dermoids of eye (Fig. 7.80).

Rubinstein-Taybi syndrome (Broad thumb hallux syndrome): Microcephaly, hypoplastic maxilla with narrow palate, low-set ears, anti-mongoloid slant, beaked nose, hypertrichosis, broad toes and thumbs, mental retardation, short stature, cryptorchidism.

Cornelia de Lange syndrome: Hirsutism, synophrys, long curly eyelashes, long philtrum, thin downturned upper lip.

Chapter 8

Examination of the Respiratory System

Joseph L Mathew

Structure

8.1 INTRODUCTION

The examination of the respiratory system involves a systematic evaluation of the entire respiratory tree starting from the nose through the upper airways and the lungs. Therefore, it is not synonymous with examination of the chest alone. In addition, there are often findings in other systems that are related to respiratory system pathology. Therefore, a comprehensive respiratory system examination, necessitates (at times) evaluation of other systems also.

Detailed examination of the respiratory system requires considerable skill on the part of the examiner, cooperation of the child, and facilities in terms of a quiet, thermally comfortable area, where this can be done conveniently. Infants and young children are usually apprehensive of any examination, and this is heightened if an attempt is made to expose the chest. Therefore, examiners must be very sensitive. Such children may be best examined in the lap of the caregiver.

8.2 COMMON SYMPTOMS RELATED TO THE RESPIRATORY SYSTEM

1. Cough

Cough is probably the most frequent presenting symptom in children. On the one hand, cough is a symptom that can appear innocuous to the family but represents serious underlying disease. On the other hand, it could be a trivial clinical problem, but very disturbing for the child and family. There are a few clinical pointers that suggest that the cough is not trivial. These are discussed in greater detail below.

Whatever the type of cough, it must be stressed that cough is an essential, normal protective response that occurs several times during the day, in healthy children. In fact, the absence of cough (or inability to cough) would be a more serious problem than its mere presence. **Table 8.1** shows a partial list of conditions that cause chronic cough in children. Approach to a child with cough is shown schematically in **Key Box 1**.

A. History: Ask the Following

1. What is the duration?

Cough is categorized as 'acute' when it is present for less than 3–4 weeks and 'chronic' beyond that, although some prefer 8 weeks to apply this label. The algorithm of the National Tuberculosis Elimination Programme (NTEP) Guidelines (and endorsed by the Indian Academy of Pediatrics) for the management of childhood tuberculosis (TB) considers cough

Table 8.1: Causes of chronic cough in children (partial list)
Young infant
• Viral infection
• Congenital anomalies of upper and lower airways
• Gastroesophageal reflux disease (GERD)
• Interstitial lung disease
Older infant and toddler
• Infections
• GERD
• Asthma
• Cystic fibrosis
School age and older child
• Asthma
• Upper airway allergy
• Postnasal drip
• Viral infections
• Tuberculosis
• Irritative cough
• Psychogenic cough

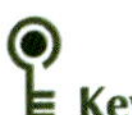
Key Box 1

Evaluation of a Child with Cough

Ask

1. What is the duration?
2. How did it begin?
3. What is the nature?
4. Is there noisy breathing?
5. Is there diurnal variation?
6. What aggravates and relieves the cough?
7. Family history, living conditions and environmental details.

Look for

1. Assessment of growth
2. Digital clubbing
3. Peripheral signs of congestive cardiac failure
4. Superficial lymphadenopathy
5. Patency of nares and nasopharynx
6. Mucosa of the pharyngeal wall and larynx
7. Tonsils and ear canals
8. Signs of allergic rhinitis, such as 'allergic rub' and 'allergic shine'
9. Skin lesions suggestive of atopic dermatitis or eczema
10. Detailed chest examination

of greater than 2 weeks duration significant enough to trigger a search for TB.

Acute cough, generally suggests a disease of shorter duration, while chronic cough points towards a long-standing problem. However, there are some caveats. Acute cough can represent exacerbations of long-standing lung disease. Likewise, post-infectious (viral) cough can persist for several weeks following an acute viral upper respiratory infection.

2. What event(s) occurred at the onset?

- A sudden bout of cough in an otherwise healthy older infant or child may suggest an acute event such as aspiration of a foreign body, even if there is no history of choking.
- Parents often do not recollect the event/incident that led to aspiration of a foreign body in young infants. Sometimes, there is a suggestive history that the cough began while consuming nuts, or other edible items. However, often these are not witnessed. In some instances, it is worth asking whether any small parts of toys or other objects (such as pens) are missing/lost. It is also helpful to inquire whether an older sibling (especially toddler age group) could have fed the infant anything on any occasion; this history has sometimes been rewarding in identifying foreign body aspiration.
- Current cough that started with an upper respiratory infection (described loosely as 'common cold' or 'viral' episode) could indicate a post-viral cough. It can last for several weeks, but the usual history is that there is improvement over time.
- Presence of cough from birth or early infancy is observed in congenital developmental anomalies of the airways (usually upper airways) such as tracheoesophageal fistula, tracheomalacia, etc. The usual history in such infants is that the onset of cough was associated with feeding. The timing of the cough in relation to feeding can be instructive. Cough occurring before or during swallowing suggests aspiration due to neuromuscular incoordination affecting the normal protective reflexes that operate during swallowing (especially if the cough is associated with a gurgling sound characteristic of pooling of feed). Cough occurring immediately after swallowing suggests communication between the esophagus and airway, as seen in H-type

tracheoesophageal fistulae. Cough that occurs several minutes after feeding may reflect high-grade gastroesophageal reflux and aspiration into the airway.

- Wet-sounding cough and tachypnea, from the neonatal period should alert to a possibility of primary ciliary dyskinesia (PCD).

3. What is the nature?

Cough is generally categorized as dry or wet. Dry cough usually results from airway irritation, whereas wet cough represents underlying airway secretions. The former is more common and often does not point towards a specific condition. The presence of dry cough helps to rule out suppurative lung disease. The cough in persistent asthma is usually 'dry'.

If there is a history of wet cough with expectoration, the nature of the expectorated material is important. Frank sputum, especially if it is foul-smelling (or rarely streaked with blood) may indicate suppurative lung disease. A history of foul-smelling breath (halitosis) may also indicate underling bronchiectasis.

Although, it would be useful to elicit a description of specific sounds produced by cough in certain conditions, this is often not easy. Nevertheless, 'barking cough' is often heard in laryngotracheobronchitis (croup). In tracheomalacia, there is a harsh crowing sound (stridor) and the paroxysmal cough (often with a whoop) is characteristic in pertussis.

Post-tussive vomiting, often regarded as a hallmark of pertussis, is non-specific and can occur with any forceful cough, especially in young children.

4. Is there associated noisy breathing?

This is important because additional sounds can point towards airway pathology, and it is possible to differentiate between intra-thoracic and extra-thoracic airway problems.

It is more difficult to reach a specific diagnosis when parents describe chest sounds as 'noisy', 'rattly' (khar-khar) or 'congested'.

Intrathoracic airway (lower airway) obstruction produces wheezing, which is better appreciable during expiration, while extrathoracic (upper airway) obstruction causes stridor, better heard during inspiration. Stridor is low-pitched while wheeze is a high-pitched sound. These can be differentiated even by an untrained observer. It is important to remember that parents may not understand "wheeze" in the same way as physicians do. Asking about a "whistling" sound may not be helpful. In such situations, producing a wheezing type of sound, helps parents to better understand the information being sought.

It is sometimes helpful to ask parents whether they perceive that the noisy breathing originates from the nose, throat, or chest. Rarely, an astute parent describes this well, giving a vital clue to the site of pathology in the airway.

5. Is there diurnal variation?

- Night-time cough is often (mis) labeled as asthma, but this should be considered only if it occurs after the child has gone to sleep, particularly in the early hours of the morning.
- Night cough at the onset of sleep (when the child is lying down) is more likely to be related to GER than asthma.
- Sometimes children cough at night in the absence of any pathology.
- Cough during the first few minutes after waking may suggest more serious conditions, such as suppurative lung disease, particularly if it is productive.
- Cough present during the daytime but absent at night suggests a habit rather than disease. The characteristic hallmark of habit cough is its absence when there are no witnesses, and the dramatic, distressing nature when witnessed.

6. What aggravates or relieves the cough?

Cough worsened by exposure to dust, aero-allergens, or smoke (from burning solid fuel, or pollution, or exposure to tobacco smoking) suggests increased airway reactivity, and can point towards asthma. Strenuous physical activity also exacerbates cough in such children; although the so-called "exercise-induced asthma" wherein symptoms of asthma are provoked only by physical activity, is not frequently encountered in children. The provocation of cough by social circumstances, such as the presence of people, stress, or an unfamiliar environment, suggests a habit cough. Relief of cough within minutes of inhaling a bronchodilator is very likely to be related to asthma; although some children with post-viral cough also report relief with bronchodilators.

Cough that is exacerbated with particular postures may point towards the presence of suppurative lung conditions. In addition, cough from extrapulmonary problems, such as congestive heart failure or where the gastrointestinal tract communicates with the airway, may also vary with posture.

7. *Presence of atopy*

In children with long-standing cough (especially if it is episodic), the presence of atopic manifestations is helpful to confirm airway allergy. Usually this includes symptoms of allergic rhinitis (frequent runny nose, multiple bouts of sneezing, often in the morning), allergic conjunctivitis (redness and/or watering from the eyes), or atopic dermatitis (itchy lesions in the flexures, face, etc.).

8. *Family and environmental history*

The traditional query seeking a family history of tuberculosis should be expanded to ask less specific questions about any (similar or other) long-standing respiratory symptom(s) in any household contacts (including those who work part-time or participate in childcare). Asking about current or previous history of any family member taking anti-tuberculosis therapy, can be helpful. The reason is that many caregivers are reluctant to disclose history of tuberculosis or its therapy. Family history should also explore allergic tendency (upper airway, lower airway, or skin) in any family member, and exposure of the child to passive smoking within the family. Family history should also include the presence of atopy (as described above) or asthma in any family member, or treatment being taken for these conditions.

It is also worth inquiring whether the child attends a creche or day-care center; cross-infections are common in these settings.

The importance of exposure to tobacco smoke (from cigarettes, *biris*, *hookahs*, etc.) is very well-known. Parents are often reluctant to admit the presence of a smoker in the family, and hence often state that the smoking individual indulges the habit outside the house.

An assessment of living conditions with reference to allergen exposure, industrial fumes, smoke from burning of biomass fuel, exposure to dampness, and presence of molds can strengthen a diagnosis suggestive of reactive airways. In recent years, children have been reported to be sensitive to the smoke/odour produced by the burning of incense sticks (*agarbatti*), mosquito repellent coils, other insect repellent liquids, and even deodorant sprays. It is also useful to inquire about the presence of pets and domestic animals within the living areas. History of storage of large quantities of grain in rural families may be associated with allergic airways.

B. Examination: Look for the Following

1. *General physical examination*

In addition to the 'generic' features looked for in general physical examination (pallor, icterus, cyanosis, etc. that have been described in preceding chapters), particular attention should be paid to (i) the nutritional status; (ii) digital clubbing (including its grade); (iii) peripheral signs of congestive cardiac failure; and (iv) superficial lymphadenopathy.

When assessing the nutritional status, calculating the Z-scores is helpful to quantify the problem, and also when a child with chronic conditions is serially followed-up over time. Signs of fat-soluble vitamin (A, D, E, K) deficiency are often observed in children with cystic fibrosis. Other micronutrient deficiency signs are sometimes present in those with long-standing malnutrition.

Certain respiratory conditions may be associated with characteristic general physical examination signs. For example, some children with cystic fibrosis have a fine salt-crusting on the skin. The phenomenon of 'aquagenic wrinkling' (akin to washerwoman hands) when the hands are dipped in water is often considered a marker of cystic fibrosis. Skin lesions suggestive of atopic dermatitis or eczema can assist in confirming a suspicion of asthmatic airways.

Tracheo-esophgeal fistula may be a component of the VACTERL syndrome; therefore, it is worth searching for anorectal anomalies, vertebral defects, and limb anomalies. Similarly, some cardiac conditions associated with left-to-right shunting may have associated limb anomalies (such as polydactyly, syndactyly, etc.). Pulmonary Langerhans cell histiocytosis (LCH) may have a characteristic seborrheic dermatitis, and bony defects (although these are better seen on an X-ray). Needless to mention, pulmonary involvement in systemic diseases, such as storage disorders, metabolic syndromes, hepatic/renal conditions would show up some of the characteristic general examination findings.

2. Upper airway

Examine the patency of the nares, mucosa of the pharyngeal wall, tonsils, and ear canals. Ensure that there is no nasal polyp. Follow it with a detailed evaluation including the tympanic membrane with an otoscope, nasopharynx, and larynx by indirect laryngoscopy (if possible). Signs of allergic rhinitis, such as 'allergic rub', and 'allergic shine,' can be helpful, if they are obvious.

Some respiratory conditions with cough have characteristic upper airway findings; for example the condition referred to (formerly) as Wegener's granulomatosis is associated with nasal septal perforation. Similarly, there may be nasal polyps in cystic fibrosis.

3. Chest

Inspection

- Inspect the chest for the shape and symmetry to confirm whether the lung condition causing cough is localized (to one side) or generalized.
- An obvious barrel-shaped chest suggests diffuse air-trapping as seen in chronic untreated asthma.
- Flattening suggests volume loss due to collapse or malformed lungs or lobes. Similarly, shoulder drooping and flattening of the scapula suggest loss of lung volume.
- Unilateral hyperinflation could point towards obstruction of an airway or pleural collections.
- A precordial bulge suggests cardiac hypertrophy and may point to an underlying heart disease, as the cause of cough.

Palpation: Palpation in respiratory system examination is oriented towards identifying the position of the mediastinum. The position of the trachea is examined, followed by localizing the cardiac apex. Shifts towards a particular side depend on the underlying lung or pleural condition.

Percussion: Percussion is useful to confirm air-trapping or the presence of fluid in the pleural space. Characteristic impressions of 'dull' or 'stony dull' recognized with considerable practice, point to specific underlying conditions.

Auscultation: Auscultation of breath sounds will usually give an accurate estimate of the pathological process producing cough, although not necessarily a clinical diagnosis.

For example, coarse crackles can suggest bronchiectasis of any cause; *fine velcro crackles* could point to interstitial lung disease, wheeze suggests narrowing of smaller airways which could be diffuse in asthma or localized in obstructions of particular airways. *Absence of breath sounds* may suggest complete collapse, obstruction of a main bronchus, or presence of pleural collections.

2. Noisy Breathing

These include snoring, stridor, wheezing, and other noisy respirations. Most parents are unable to characterize these noises properly, except for snoring. A general history should thus be asked.

A. History: Ask the Following

1. What is the nature of the noise?

Most often parents describe a 'rattly' (*khar-khar*) sound that occurs with coughing or even at rest. This occurs concomitantly with what is described as a 'cold', 'viral infection' or 'sore throat'. These terms are better described in the vernacular and may convey a more precise meaning. Asking for other symptoms along with the noisy breathing can point towards a diagnosis. Thus, the presence of dry cough, running nose, sore throat, change in voice, difficulty in feeding in younger children, and low-grade fever (singly or in combination) may point towards upper airway infection/inflammation.

High-grade fever, productive cough (or otherwise), and sick appearance usually point towards lower respiratory infection. Here also, the rattly noise may be similar, but parents tend to use more evocative terms, such as 'chest congestion', 'chest blockade' and even 'pneumonia'.

Snoring: Snoring is a sound that is easy for most parents to relate to, and they are usually able to accurately describe this. Snoring points to obstruction of nasopharyngeal airway by enlarged adenoids and often occurs concomitantly with mouth-breathing, upper respiratory tract inflammation, and disturbed sleep.

Snoring is increasingly recognized as a manifestation of 'sleep disordered breathing' which comprises a spectrum of clinical conditions ranging from benign snoring (with no functional consequences) at one end, to obstructive sleep apnea at the other (which has serious consequences). In children with snoring, it is helpful to ask for history of recent (excessive) weight gain, and the presence of any obvious stress factors that could be responsible.

Stridor: Stridor is described as a harsh sound originating from critical narrowing of the extrathoracic airways (larynx, upper trachea, main bronchus).

Stridor is the hardest 'noisy sound' to describe. Here again, it is easier if the physician creates a harsh, crowing sound by breathing in forcefully. Stridor rarely presents in a chronic fashion; hence, most parents will be aware of this unusual symptom. However, chronic stridor can be encountered in laryngomalacia where parents present a history of noisy breathing starting in the neonatal period but the baby might look quite well during the visit to the physician.

Wheezing: Wheezing is almost never accurately described by parents and, hence, it may be easier to elicit this, if the physician artificially creates a high-pitched sound by breathing out forcefully.

Although, wheezing is described as a musical whistling sound in Western textbooks, asking for a "whistle-like sound" as opposed to "whistling sound" confuses most parents. Here too, descriptions of the sound in the local vernacular can be more helpful than strict textbook descriptions.

Grunting: Grunting is a low pitch, expiratory sound generated by breathing against the closed glottis in an effort to increase airway pressure and prevent collapse of small sized lower airways and alveoli. This is not a sign of airway disroder, but indicates lung paranchymal disease in infants.

2. What are the associated symptoms?

An evaluation of associated symptoms is most helpful in pointing towards a specific condition.

- Ask for the usual symptoms of upper respiratory tract inflammation/infection, especially adenotonsillitis and lower respiratory infection.
- Remember to inquire about earache, tugging at the ear, and unexplained crying because these point towards otitis media; which is often missed in the evaluation.

3. Where does the noise appear to originate?

This is a tricky question for most parents, but an extremely useful one from the physician's point of view. This is because, if the origin of the noise could be pin-pointed to the nose, throat, or chest; subsequent evaluation and diagnosis become much easier. Most parents (and indeed many physicians) are unable to appreciate the site of origin of the noise, but it is relatively simple to request parents to place an ear at the nose, in front of the throat, and over the chest serially to determine the site. Of course, the physician could do the same thing with gratifying results, when the child is present.

4. Is there diurnal variation?

As mentioned for cough, presence of noisy breathing during sleep (loosely described as 'at night' by many parents) points towards bronchoconstriction and is often due to asthma. This suspicion is strengthened, if the noise can be categorized as 'wheezing' and occurs as recurrent episodes with intervening periods of well-being. Airway obstruction due to other causes usually does not present with the latter two features.

5. What aggravates and relieves the noise?

As described for cough, the same set of queries should be directed here as well. Relief with a bronchodilator is a very important point, and this is often described as 'relief by nebulization' since many physicians use this route to deliver bronchodilator therapy.

B. Examination: Look for the Following

1. ***Height:*** Chronicity of the condition will often affect height; this should not be missed during examination.
2. ***Weight:*** Some overweight children have symptoms and signs of reactive airway disease. Likewise, children with asthma often have excessive weight gain, for various reasons.
3. ***Upper airway:*** Perform a thorough upper airway examination including ear canals and tympanic membrane. Although detailed examination of the larynx may be difficult without specialized instruments, attempt this and seek the assistance of a specialist, if necessary.
4. ***Chest:*** During chest examination, look for the following:
   i. Signs of air-trapping in asthma;
   ii. Localization of findings, if unilateral airway obstruction by foreign body aspiration is suspected;
   iii. Features of consolidation in pneumonia; and
   iv. Coarse crackles in bronchiectasis due to any cause.

3. Difficulty in Breathing

This is a very vague term but encompasses a wide range of abnormalities in the rate, pattern, or effort of respiration. Therefore, its value for the physician is great, but unfortunately most parents are unable to characterize their description of breathing difficulty. Some of the following may be helpful in such situations.

A. What to Ask for?

1. What is the nature of the difficulty?

Ask two questions:

a. Is the child breathing faster than usual? (for tachypnea)
b. Is the child breathing harder than normal? (for dyspnea)

Both indicate increased work of breathing that can occur in a variety of conditions ranging from airway problems, parenchymal disease, other thoracic abnormalities including pleural, extrapulmonary conditions, and even extrathoracic pathology.

2. What are the associated symptoms?

Quickly ask for the usual symptoms of upper airway problems, lower airway conditions (wheezing, noisy breathing), parenchymal pathology (cough, productivity, retractions, chest pain), pleural disease (pain while breathing), and extrapulmonary disease (trauma, muscle pull, cardiovascular symptoms). Retractions (ribcage being drawn in) are useful to ask for, but need evocative descriptions to establish its presence.

3. Is there alteration in activity?

Ask this to assess the extent of severity. Enquire about inability to feed, interrupted sleep, altered behavior, inability to play and participate in usual activities, and inability to speak. To gauge the severity of hypoxia—ask for cyanosis, altered sensorium, and convulsions.

4. What makes it better and worse?

Postural changes, deep breathing, coughing, movement, and medication can all affect respiratory distress variably. Therefore, it may be prudent to try and elicit this, although the difficulty in terms of accuracy and specificity has to be acknowledged.

8.3 RELEVANT ANATOMY AND SURFACE LANDMARKS

The respiratory system includes the entire respiratory tract starting from the nose through the nasopharynx, oropharynx, and larynx; via the glottis into the trachea, bronchi, and their several divisions till termination into the alveoli.

Besides this air conducting system, it also includes the blood supply (arterioles, capillaries, and venules) coming in contact with the conducting system; extrapulmonary structures, such as pleura, muscles involved in respiration (diaphragm, intercostal muscles, accessory muscles), and thoracic bony structures particularly the ribs and musculoskeletal framework. Some experts prefer to include the components of cellular respiration also; this gives an idea of all possible pathology in the process of respiration.

Perhaps, it is equally important for the clinician to learn the demarcation of anatomical structures on the surface that is examined, as it is to remember the actual anatomical detail.

Since this has relevance to clinical examination and interpretation of findings, it will be dealt within some detail.

1. Trachea

The trachea can be traced from the cricoid cartilage to the sternal angle anteriorly. Posteriorly, it can be marked up to the spinous process of the fourth thoracic vertebra. Thereafter, the trachea divides into the two major bronchi. Thus, the trachea has both an intra-, and extrathoracic component. It should be remembered that the trachea may be normally slightly curved towards the right.

2. Angle of Louis

Another important surface landmark is the angle of Louis. This refers to the angle between the body of the sternum and the manubrium. The second rib articulates to the manubrium at this site. Therefore, when the ribs are counted anteriorly, one starts with the second rib and not the first. Therefore, the space that is palpable immediately inferior to this rib is the second intercostal space.

The angle of Louis also marks the site where the trachea divides into the two bronchi. The mediastinum is also divided into superior and inferior at this level.

3. Thoracic Areas

The thorax is arbitrarily divided into various spaces drawing artificial lines, using the ribs and intercostal spaces as landmarks. Anteriorly, the ribs are counted downwards starting from the second rib as mentioned above. Posteriorly, this may be more cumbersome, but it is useful to remember that the inferior angle of scapula lies in line with the seventh rib.

The arbitrary 'spaces' on the thorax are defined as follows:

i. *Infraclavicular* (space below clavicle): This can again be subdivided into *mammary* and *inframammary*.
ii. *Supraclavicular* (space above clavicle)
iii. *Interscapular* (space between the scapulae)
iv. *Suprascapular* (space above scapula)
v. *Infrascapular* (space below scapula).

4. Thoracic Lines

The following lines represent important landmarks on the thorax:

i. *Mid-sternal line* (vertical line passing through the middle of sternum). Posteriorly, this line is expected to pass through the center of the spinous processes;
ii. *Parasternal line* (vertical line along the lateral edge of sternum). Posteriorly, this line is the paravertebral line;
iii. *Mid-clavicular line* (vertical line passing through the mid-point between acromian process and mid-sternal line);
iv. *Anterior axillary line* (vertical line along the anterior axillary fold);
v. *Mid-axillary line* (vertical line at the mid-point between anterior and posterior axillary lines); and
vi. *Posterior axillary line* (vertical line along the posterior axillary fold).

Figures 8.1 and 8.2 show the important imaginary lines and spaces on the chest.

5. Lungs

The *right lung* corresponds to a line starting about 1 inch above the clavicle in the mid-clavicular line, it touches the parasternal line at the angle of Louis, passes vertically

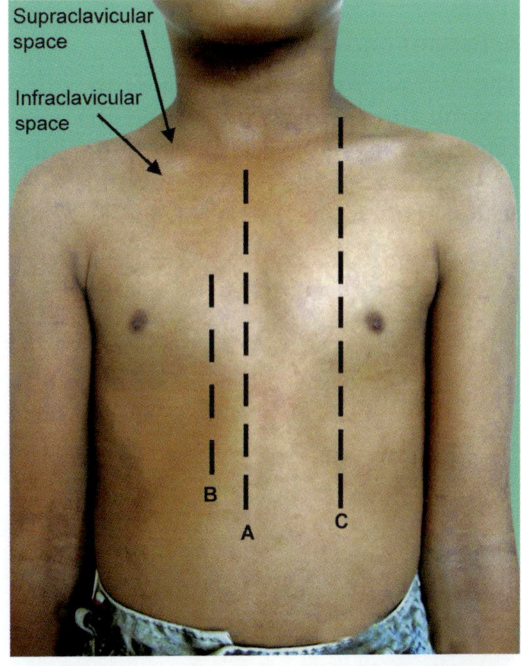

Fig. 8.1: Imaginary lines on the thorax that are useful in surface anatomy. Line A represents mid-sternal line, B is the parasternal line and C is the mid-clavicular line. Note that the mid-clavicular line does not necessarily pass through the nipples.

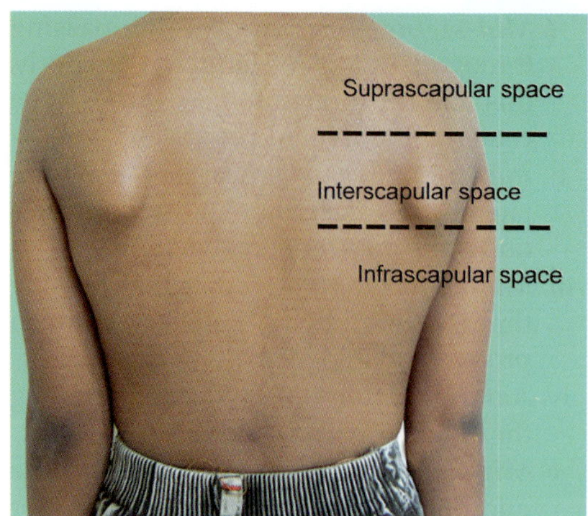

Fig. 8.2: The spaces when examined posteriorly. Note the arms of the child by the side of the body, in symmetry on both sides.

downwards through the right parasternal line, onwards to the sixth rib in the mid-clavicular line, eighth rib in the mid-axillary line, the tenth rib posteriorly, and then the vertebral line (Fig. 8.3).

The *left lung line* starts at the angle of Louis, follows the outer margin of heart to the sixth rib in the mid-clavicular line and follows the same course as the right lung subsequently.

6. Fissures and Lobes

The *oblique fissure* corresponds to a line passing through the sixth rib in the mid-clavicular line and the fifth rib in the mid-axillary line; along the medial margin of scapula (when the arms are held above the head) till the third spinous process. The surface marking on both sides is similar.

The *transverse fissure*, on the right side, is drawn by joining a line from the fifth rib in the mid-axillary line to the fourth rib anteriorly.

Delineating the fissure lines helps to identify the lobes of the lungs for examination purposes. Thus, most of the lower lobe is in the back, most of the upper lobe is in the front, and the entire middle lobe lies anteriorly.

Physicians often talk in terms of regions and zones of the lung. Strictly speaking, this is incorrect because regions are simple descriptive terms that do not conform to specific pulmonary anatomy. Thus, mammary region simply means the area over the breast, and nothing more is conveyed. Likewise, zones (upper, middle and lower) are defined on chest radiographs for describing the site of pathology, and these also do not conform to lung anatomy.

8.4 GENERAL EXAMINATION RELEVANT TO THE RESPIRATORY SYSTEM

1. Central Cyanosis

Cyanosis refers to bluish color of the skin and mucous membranes that occurs due to excessive concentrations of reduced hemoglobin in the capillary blood (Figs 8.4 and 8.5). It is classically described as *central* or *peripheral*. From the standpoint of the respiratory system, central cyanosis is of greater importance.

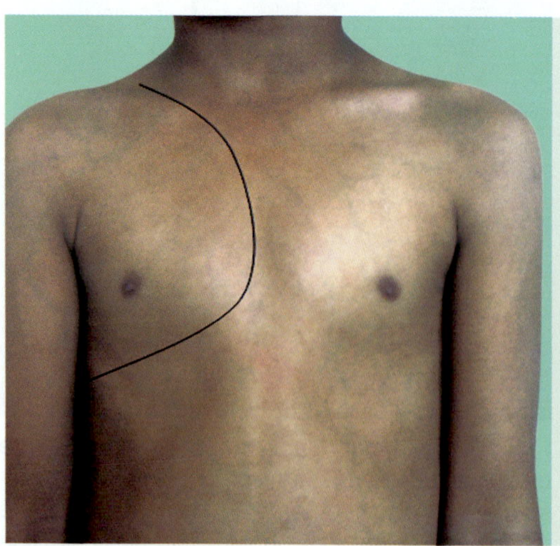

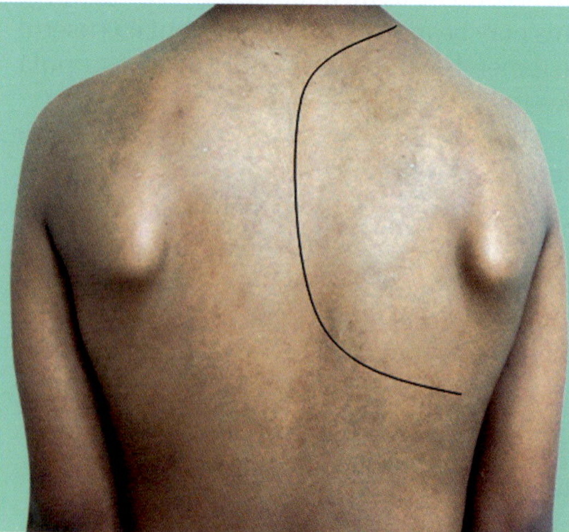

Fig. 8.3: Surface marking of the right lung.

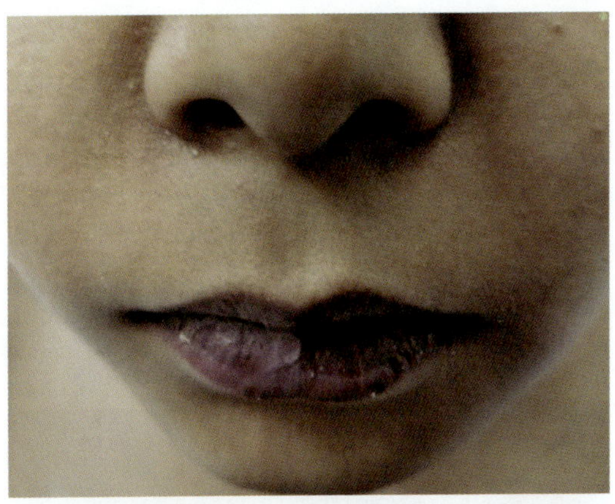

Fig. 8.4: Cyanosis manifesting as dusky lips.

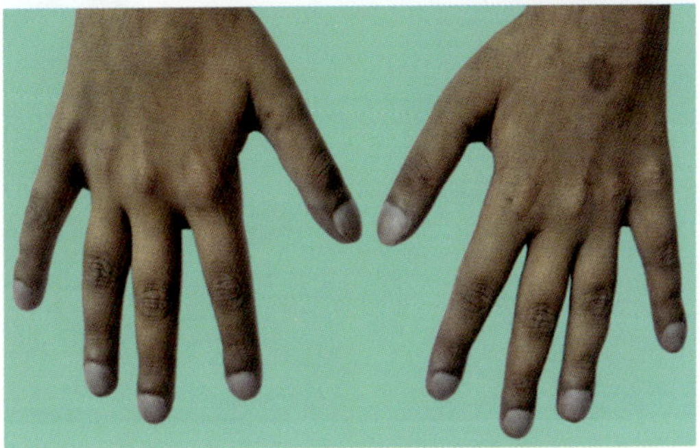

Fig. 8.5: Peripheral cyanosis.

- Look for central cyanosis in the tongue and mucous membranes under good illumination, preferably daylight or white light from fluorescent lamps.
- The presence of central cyanosis represents reduced hemoglobin concentration greater than 5 g/dL in capillary blood.
- Look for differential cyanosis. This is a somewhat rare phenomenon wherein the digits of the lower limbs are cyanosed, while those of the upper limbs are not. It is seen in children with patent ductus arteriosus with pulmonary hypertension, wherein blood with low oxygen, enters the aorta distal to the left subclavian artery.
- Central cyanosis can occur through any of the following mechanisms:
  - i. Alveolar hypoventilation;
  - ii. Diffusion impairment;
  - iii. Right-to-left shunting;
  - iv. Mismatch of ventilation and perfusion; and
  - v. Inadequate oxygen transport by hemoglobin due to abnormal hemoglobin (as in methemoglobinemia).

2. Clubbing

Clubbing is produced by the enlargement of the connective tissue in the terminal phalanges of fingers and toes. Clubbing is conveniently graded from Grade 1–4. *See* Chapter 7 for details.

Mechanism

The exact mechanisms, that result in clubbing, have still not been fully elucidated. It is, generally accepted that endothelial growth factors released during sustained hypoxia and consequent vasodilatation, contribute to changes that result in clubbing.

Clubbing not only indicates chronic hypoxia, but also can reflect its progression or resolution with time. It is still not clear how much time it takes and what degree of hypoxia is required to manifest with clubbing.

Generally, it is believed that clubbing is uncommon in the first few months of life. However, acquired causes can result in clubbing within a period of few weeks. In this case, clubbing will resolve, if effective treatment is instituted before connective tissue changes become fixed. Figure 8.6 shows a

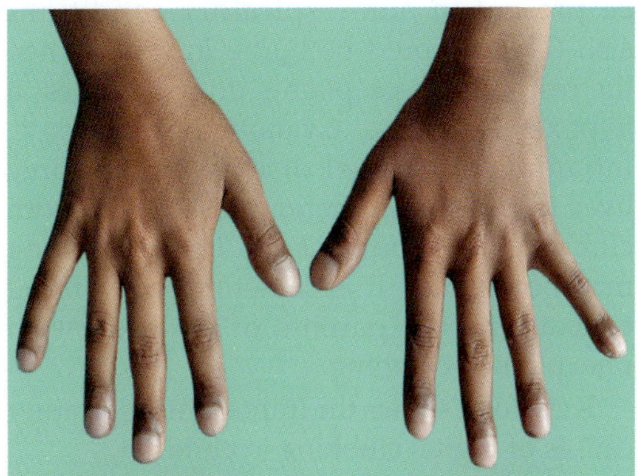

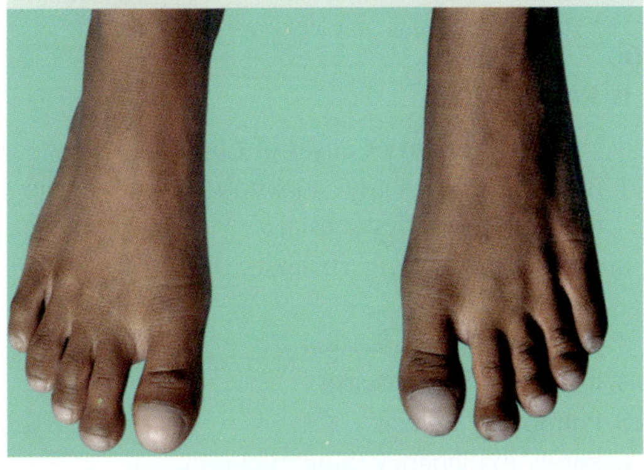

Fig. 8.6: Pandigital clubbing.

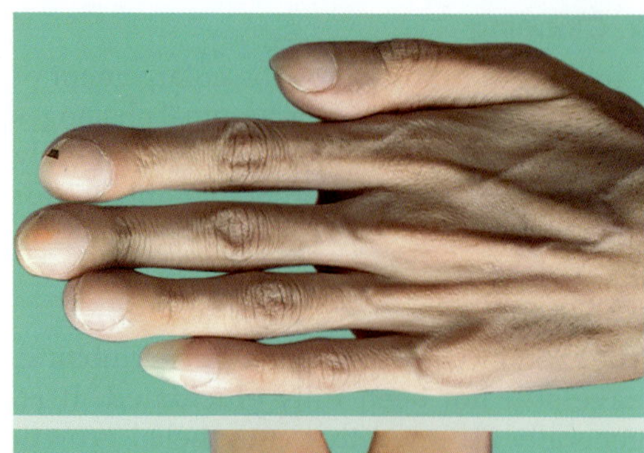

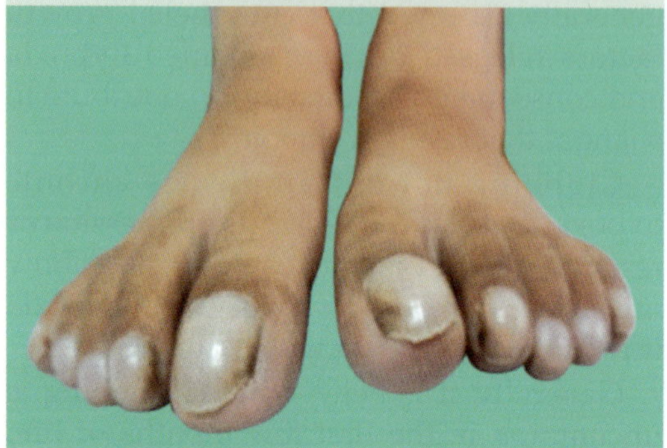

Fig. 8.7: Grade IV Pandigital clubbing.

child with pandigital clubbing, and Fig. 8.7 depicts advanced clubbing.

It is important to note that clubbing can be present in non-respiratory conditions also. These should be borne in mind when the respiratory complaints do not suggest a hypoxemic process. Cyanotic heart disease, inflammatory bowel disease and chronic liver disease are sometimes associated with clubbing. Last but not the least, clubbing may be familial. It is sometimes rewarding to examine the parents of children with unexplained clubbing.

Key Box 2 shows the important respiratory causes of digital clubbing in children.

Key Box 2

Respiratory Causes of Clubbing

1. Bronchiectasis of any cause (tuberculosis, cystic fibrosis, ciliary dyskinesia)
2. *Suppurative lung disease:* Lung abscess, empyema
3. Pulmonary hypertension
4. Interstitial lung disease
5. Pulmonary fibrosis
6. Rarely malignancy (lung, pleura)

3. Examination of Regional Lymph Nodes

The lymph nodes of greater importance while examining the respiratory system are the superficial cervical group, supra- and infraclavicular, and axillary lymph nodes. These are sometimes easy to identify even on routine inspection (Fig. 8.8).

Note the size, shape, firmness (consistency), and mobility of the lymph nodes.

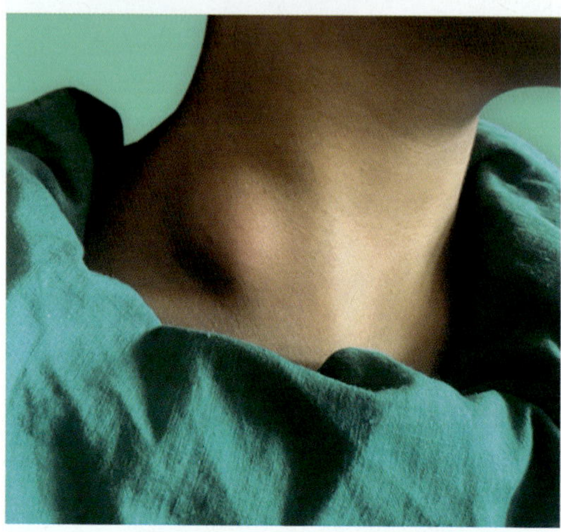

Fig. 8.8: A single enlarged (and inflamed) cervical lymph node.

Significant lymphadenopathy: In adults, lymphadenopathy is described as 'significant' when it is greater than 1.0 cm in diameter (>1.5 cm for inguinal nodes). This is apparently applicable to children as well.

Most lymph nodes are round in shape and generally firm in consistency. A rubbery feel, matting of nodes, presence of scars and sinuses over the nodes, and tenderness are also hallmark of significant lymphadenopathy.

Cervical Lymph Nodes

The cervical nodes are grouped into a horizontal chain that includes pre-auricular, post-auricular, and suboccipital nodes and a vertical part that can be felt along the sternocleido-mastoid muscle anteriorly and posteriorly. The jugulodigastric node is part of the deep cervical group and is often enlarged and painful in acute tonsillitis.

After warming the hands, place the tips of the fingers on the neck of the child from the front or behind and gently feel for enlarged nodes (Figs 8.9 and 8.10).

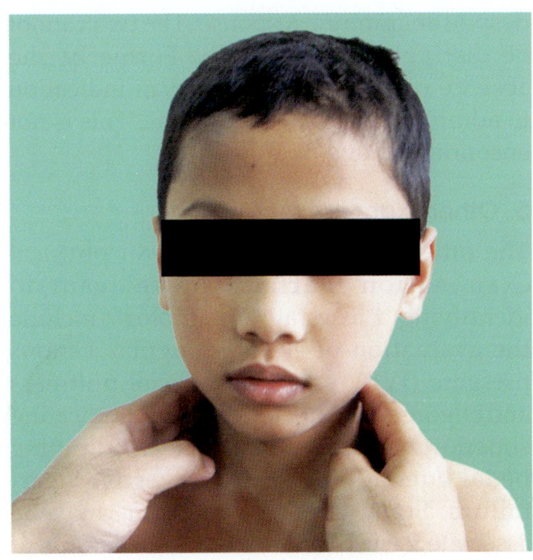

Fig. 8.9: Palpation of the superficial cervical nodes from front.

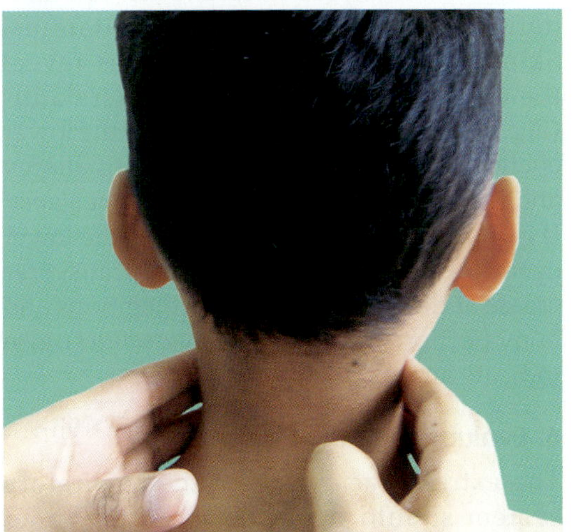

Fig. 8.10: Palpation of the superficial cervical nodes from behind.

The other superficial nodes in the neck include the submandibular and submental nodes that are palpated in a similar manner **(Figs 8.11 and 8.12)**. Use the pulp of the fingers and avoid poking with the fingertips.

Supraclavicular Nodes

Place the fingertips above the clavicle and apply gentle but firm pressure in small circular movements **(Fig. 8.13)**.

Infraclavicular Nodes

The same action as above is performed with fingertips placed below the clavicle.

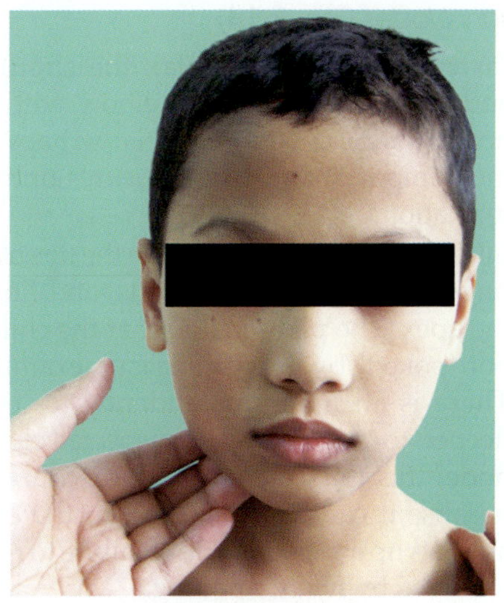

Fig. 8.11: Palpation of the submandibular lymph nodes.

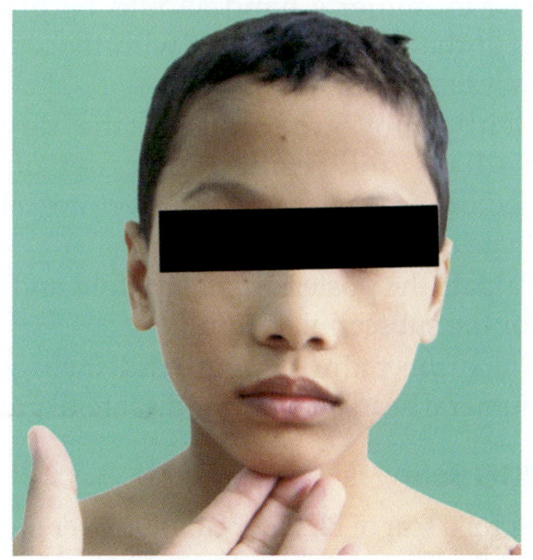

Fig. 8.12: Palpation of the submental lymph node.

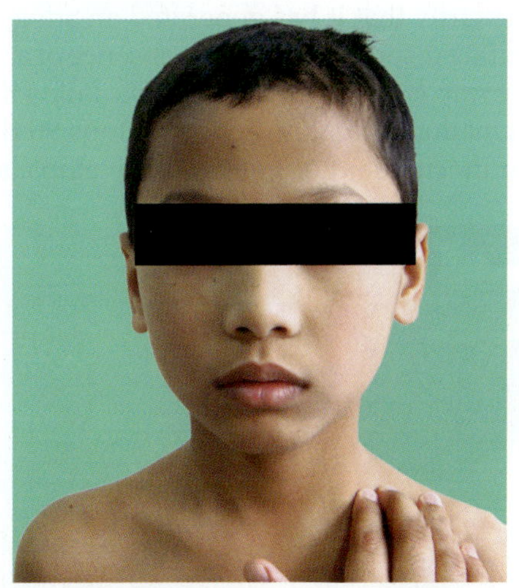

Fig. 8.13: Palpation of the supraclavicular lymph node.

Axillary Nodes **(Fig. 8.14)**

- Instruct the child to relax the shoulder and support the arm and elbow with the non-examining hand. This is perhaps the most important step and ensures optimal relaxation.
- Introduce the pads rather than the tips of the fingers into the axillary walls, and finally the apex. The pads ensure that the child is not 'poked' by an enthusiastic examiner. There is an inherent tendency to 'push deeper' to try and locate a suspected elusive node; this must be strongly discouraged because it causes discomfort to the child and sets up a vicious cycle of failure to relax, followed by further poking.
- With gentle but firm circular motions, feel the central group in the apex of the axilla. The examiner's hand should be placed with the palm in contact with the side of the chest.
- Gently move the pads of the fingers medially and inside the border of the pectoral muscle and the pectoral node chain.
- Palpate the posterior axillary fold and feel for the subscapular group.
- Place the palm of the hand facing the humeral head and feel for the lateral group.

4. BCG Scar

Look for a scar of BCG vaccination over the left shoulder. The presence of a scar only suggests that the vaccine has been administered, but not necessarily that it has generated an adequate immune response. Likewise, absence of a scar can mean either of two things, *viz.* failed BCG vaccination (when no scar develops 90 days after inoculation) or failure to develop a scar despite an immune response. The two cannot be distinguished clinically. Formerly, the absence of a scar was taken as an indication to administer BCG a second time. This is not encouraged now.

5. Other Examination Findings

The other components of general physical examination that may be relevant to identifying a respiratory pathology include the evaluation of elevated jugular venous pressure (JVP), presence of facial puffiness and engorgement of the neck veins (indicating superior mediastinal syndrome), and pitting pedal edema indicating congestive heart failure. Some clinical conditions may be associated with abnormal facies. Features of general and specific nutritional deficiencies provide clues to underlying conditions. Children with cystic fibrosis often manifest deficiencies of the fat-soluble vitamins. Skin examination may sometimes reveal the characteristic rash of atopic dermatitis (Fig. 8.15). A bluish discoloration of the lower eyelid may be seen in children with allergy and is sometimes referred to as '*allergic shiner*' (Fig. 8.16). A fold of skin just below the lower eyelid called *Dennie lines*; and a transverse crease at the junction of the cartilaginous and bony portion of the nose (*allergic salutes*), also indicate airway allergy.

6. Evaluation of the Upper Airway

The extrathoracic parts of the respiratory system should never be forgotten in an eagerness to examine the chest. Simple inspection often provides clues towards a diagnosis, and may reveal the existence of co-morbid conditions.

Fig. 8.14: Examination of axillary lymph nodes.

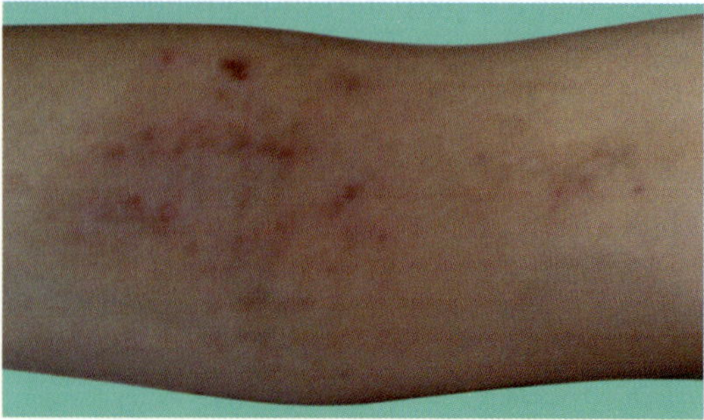

Fig. 8.15: Characteristic rash of atopic dermatitis in the cubital fossa.

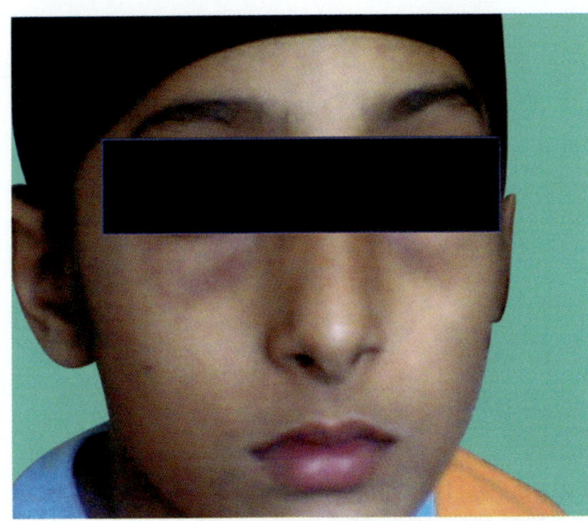

Fig. 8.16: Allergic shiner.

Nose

- Examine the nose and confirm bilateral patency by occluding each side while feeling and listening for airflow through the other nostril. This can also be done more safely using a metal surface to observe misting.
- In infants with early-onset respiratory distress, confirmation of the airway patency may require the insertion of a thin catheter through both the nostrils in addition to clinical examination. It is also instructive to note that there are cases of narrowed airways that allow a thin catheter to pass through, but not a slightly wider one.
- Lift the tip of the nose with a finger to view the nasal passage, and observe the color of the mucosa, presence of polyps, and secretions. The presence of polyps in a child can be a pointer towards cystic fibrosis.
- Examine the maxillary and frontal paranasal sinuses for tenderness in older children since this often provides a clue to chronic sinusitis.

Oral Cavity

Inspect the oropharynx either by requesting the child to open the mouth wide and say 'ah' with the tongue thrust out as much as possible. This is relatively easy for cooperative toddlers and older children, if the examiner demonstrates how it is to be done. It then obviates the need for using a tongue depressor. However, it can be tricky in infants and young children. In such situations, it is best done later in the examination sequence.

Examine the posterior pharyngeal wall, tonsillar pillars, and tonsils with particular attention to presence of follicles or pus. Examination of the adenoids requires indirect laryngoscopy.

Ears

Examine the ear canals for presence of wax, discharge, and any abnormalities on the walls. Gently pull the pinna outwards, upwards and backwards to view the tympanic membrane (Fig. 8.17).

In acute otitis media, the membrane appears inflamed and bulges outwards. The 'cone of light' appears obliterated. An otoscope aids in confirming the findings.

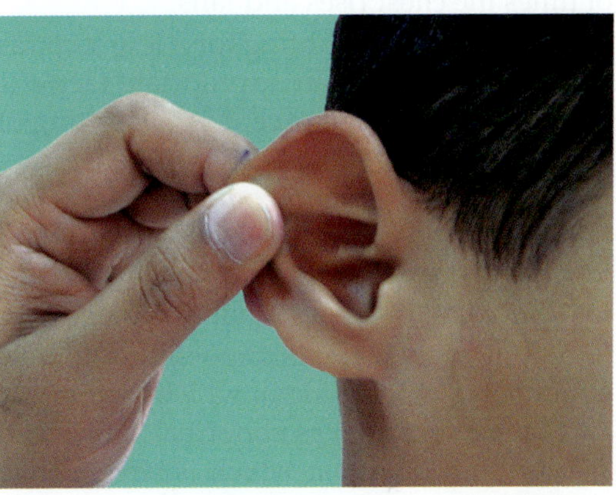

Fig. 8.17: Retracting the pinna posteriorly and superiorly facilitates inspection of the external auditory meatus and tympanic membrane without the need for an otoscope.

8.5 EXAMINATION OF THE CHEST

Traditionally, chest examination (as for other systems) proceeds in the order of inspection, palpation, percussion, and auscultation. However, in children, the sequence of these steps may be altered depending on the comfort of the child and feasibility of examination.

A. Inspection

Inspection of the chest must be done with the entire chest completely exposed (from the neck to the waist) with adequate light being present. This necessitates unclothing the child (including garments that can be rolled upwards easily) and can be quite distressing both for the child and parents.

A useful tip is to ask the parents to do it slowly and calmly so that the child is comfortable and not disturbed by vigorous actions geared to save time. Generally, it is easier if the parent rather than the examiner performs this. The practice of rolling up one or more layers of clothing to uncover part of the chest must be strongly discouraged. Figures 8.18 to 8.23 show the correct method of inspecting the chest, and some of the common errors to be avoided. Inspection should focus on the aspects highlighted in **Key Box 3**.

1. Respiratory Rate

Count the respiratory rate for a full minute: The ideal recommended practice is to count the rate for a full minute, by noting the number of times the chest rises and falls.

The practice of counting for a few seconds and multiplying by an appropriate factor is strongly condemned; except in the setting of cardiorespiratory resuscitation. There is not much point in trying to count the rate when the child is crying or agitated; it would be ideal, if a sleeping respiratory rate could be obtained, but this is often not feasible.

Strictly speaking, it is impossible to define a number on either side of which respiratory rate can be regarded as abnormal. Abnormal rate is defined as that which is beyond two standard deviations of the mean respiratory rate for that age. In general, rate greater than 60/min in infants less than 2 months, more than 50/min between 2 months and 1 year; and beyond 40 per minute between 1 and 5 years of age is considered as *tachypnea*.

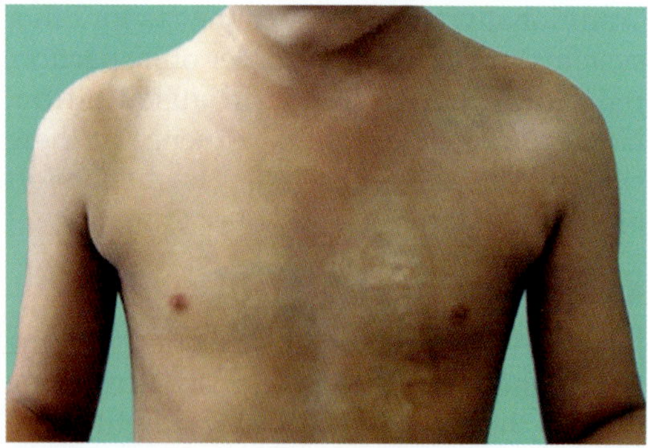

Fig. 8.18: Inspection in the sitting posture. Observe that the chest is completely exposed. Also note the emphasis on bilateral symmetry in the child's posture.

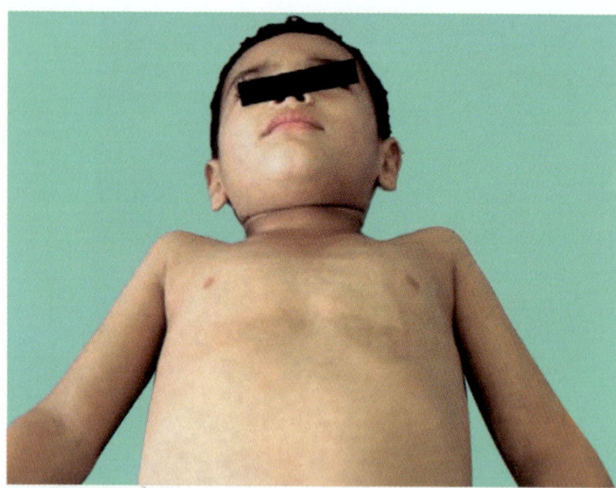

Fig. 8.19: The chest should be inspected from the foot (or head) end in the lying position. Again note the child's posture with emphasis on bilateral symmetry.

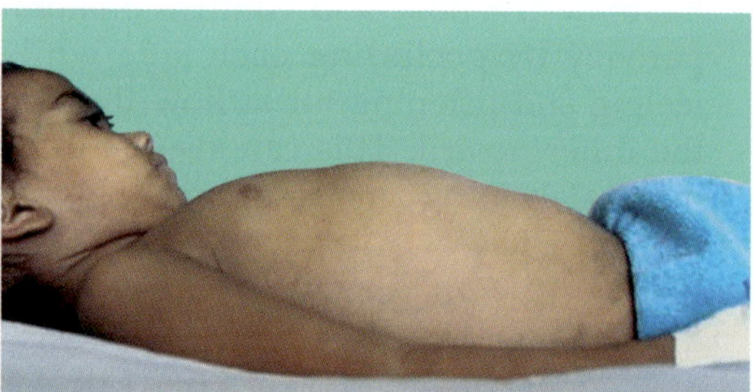

Fig. 8.20: It is important to inspect the chest from the side also. Here, the chest appears to bulge, an effect created by the bed that is sagging in the center rather than a true bulge.

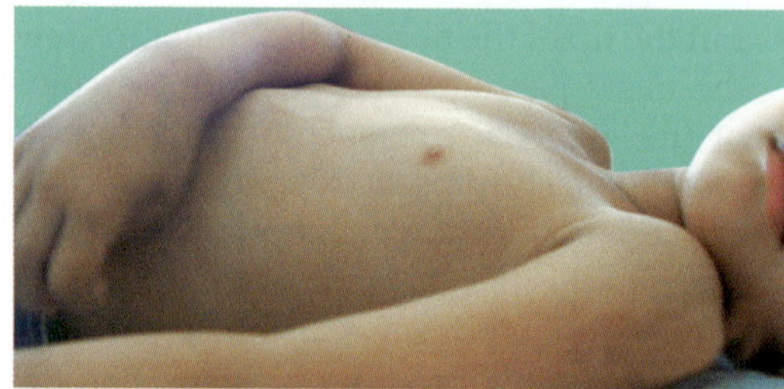

Fig. 8.21: Note the apparent 'bulge' on the right side of the chest. This is because of incorrect position of the child.

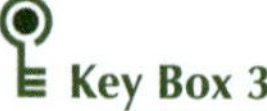

Key Box 3

Inspection of the Chest

1. Respiratory rate
2. Breathing pattern
3. Effort of breathing
4. Chest shape
5. Chest symmetry

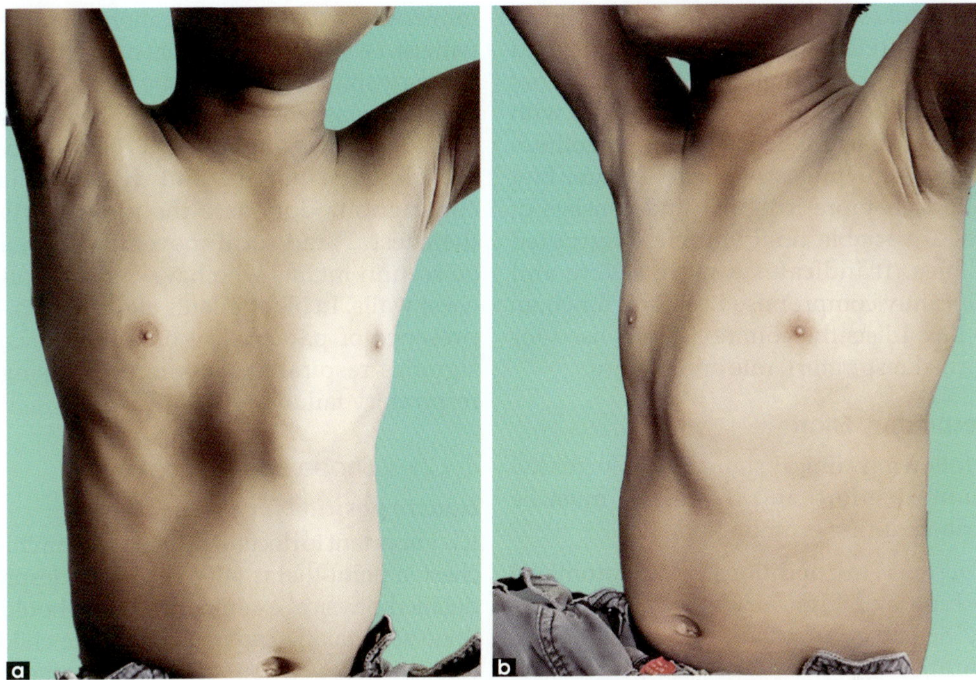

Fig. 8.22: Holding the arms above the head can accentuate some of the chest deformities.

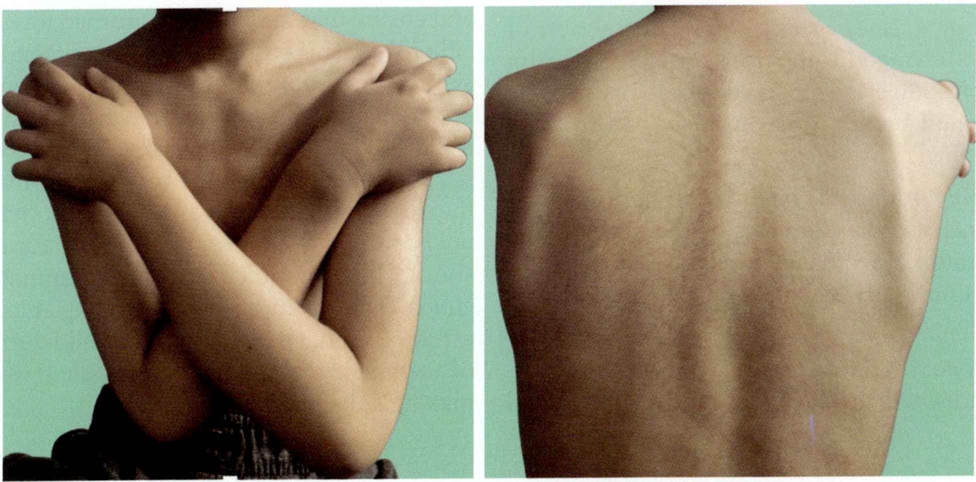

Fig. 8.23: Folding the arms in front can widen the area available for examination posteriorly.

However, it should be remembered that this is a rough guide for health-care workers in the field and is designed for screening purposes, rather than management. Some clinicians use a cut-off of 30 per minute for children between 5–12 years of age.

2. Respiratory Rhythm

Periodic breathing: Most children have a regular breathing rhythm, but infants, especially younger ones and premature babies may have brief pauses during respiration. Normally, these are short and less than 5–6 seconds in duration. When there are 3 or more such pauses that are separated by intervals shorter than 20 seconds, it is referred to as periodic breathing. It is very rare for these pauses to be associated with bradycardia and cyanosis; in which case they are of greater concern?

Cheyne-stokes breathing and biot breathing: The former refers to cycles of increasing and decreasing tidal volumes separated by brief episodes of apnea. It is seen in children with increased intracranial tension and sometimes in those with congestive heart failure. Biot breathing is more irregular and consists of cycles at variable tidal volume interrupted by apnea. It indicates a more severe and significantly compromised cerebral function. **Key Box 4** lists the common terms used for abnormal respiratory rate and pattern.

3. Respiratory Effort

The following clinical signs reflect increased respiratory effort; and if present, must be described during examination.

Retractions: In conditions of compromised breathing and high airway resistance, the more negative intrapleural pressure during inspiration 'pulls' the pliable portions of the chest wall inwards; this manifests as intercostal, subcostal, supraclavicular, and suprasternal retractions.

Use of accessory muscles: Contraction of the sternocleidomastoid muscles during inspiration is the most seen accessory muscle. In small babies, this can also lead to head bobbing.

Flaring of the alae nasi: Nasal flaring serves to increase the diameter of the airway and, therefore, decreases airway resistance in the upper airways and also the total airway resistance.

Paradoxical movement: In normal circumstances, both the chest wall and abdominal wall move outward during inspiration. The reverse pattern, i.e. inward movement of the chest wall during inspiration is called *paradoxical breathing*. This happens when the thoracic cage loses its stability. For example, when the intercostal muscles are inactive and diaphragmatic contractions dominate the movements of the chest. Paradoxical movements can also be seen in infants who have very compliant chest walls. In older infants and children, the presence of paradoxical breathing usually signifies respiratory fatigue progressing to respiratory failure.

4. Chest Shape and Symmetry

How to position for examination?

It is important to document the shape of a child's chest, a point that is often neglected despite a detailed physical examination. This should be done after taking care to position the child in the 'anatomic position'. The key is that the child (if standing) must be absolutely erect with arms hanging loosely by the sides and feet together. Take care to make the child's head face forward and ensure that the neck is not turned towards either side. This ensures that the chest remains symmetric on both sides so that impressions of apparent asymmetry are not created. Likewise, if the child is examined supine, take care that he/she is lying flat on the back with arms by the sides and facing upwards. The neck should not be turned to either side, and both scapulae should be in contact with the examination couch. These simple precautions enable the astute examiner to quickly detect mild degrees of asymmetry which can be valuable towards making a diagnosis.

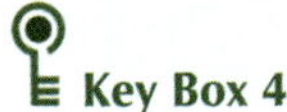

Terminology for Abnormal Patterns of Respiration

Term	Description
Tachypnea	Abnormally high (fast) respiratory rate
Bradypnea	Abnormally low (slow) respiratory rate
Hyperpnea	Abnormally deep respiration
Hypopnea	Abnormally shallow respiration
Dyspnea	Difficult breathing
Orthopnea	Breathing difficulty in the recumbent position
Platypnea	Breathing difficulty in the upright position
Periodic breathing	Respiratory pauses that occur in groups of three or more and separated by less than 20 seconds of respiration
Cheyne-Stokes breathing	Cycles of increasing and decreasing tidal volume with pauses in between
Biot breathing	Irregular cycles of breathing at variable tidal volume and apneic pauses

How to inspect?

Whether the child is standing or lying supine, you should try and inspect the chest from the front at first; then examine from the sides. This will enable the determination of asymmetry that is often not apparent when viewed from the front.

In the supine position, it is a wise idea to bend down so that your eye is level with the child's chest; this should always be followed by inspection from the foot-end. It enables the child to have an idea of what the examiner is doing and the view is not obscured by the face. Ensure that the child does not turn his head to follow you when you change your position.

Figures 8.24 to 8.27 show the importance of inspecting the chest from all possible angles. **Figures 8.28 to 8.30** highlight the challenges with incorrect positioning when examining for chest wall symmetry.

What to look for?

Normally, the chest is symmetric on both sides; this pattern can be altered in certain conditions. When one side appears less prominent, determine whether this is a spurious impression due to curvature of the spine or the child's position; or whether there is volume loss on that side. Alternatively, there could be hyperinflation/increased volume of thoracic contents on the contralateral side.

Estimating the anteroposterior 'diameter' of the chest in comparison to the side-to-side measurement has value in objectively determining hyperinflated states. The thoracic index which is the ratio of anteroposterior to transverse diameter; measured at the level of the nipples, can sometimes help to confirm this. The normal ratio is less than 1.0. Severe hyperinflation in chronic obstructive lung disease results in the chest resembling a barrel.

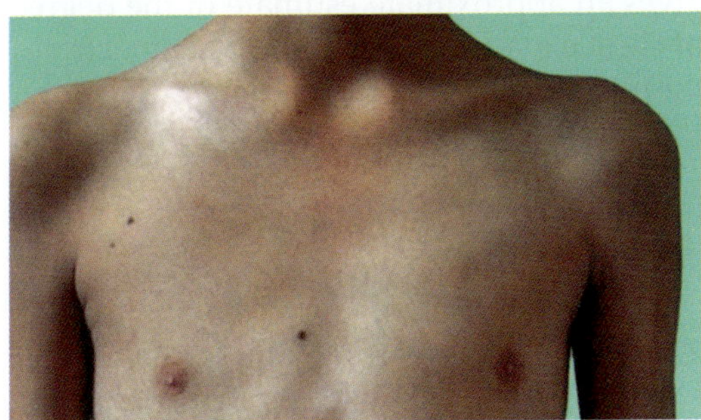

Fig. 8.24: Inspecting the exposed chest from the front does not reveal gross asymmetry.

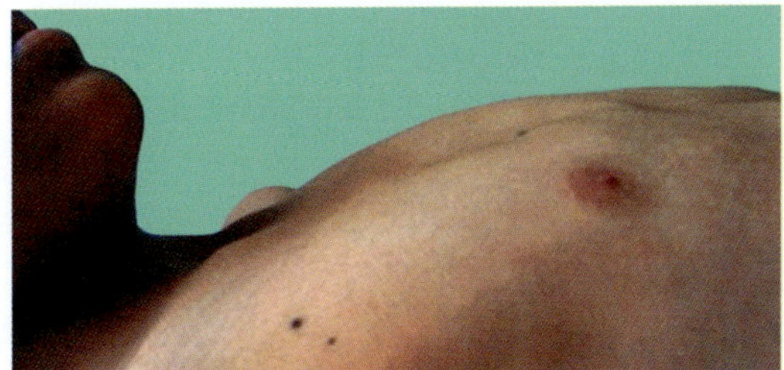

Fig. 8.25: The same child when examined from the side shows flattening on the right side.

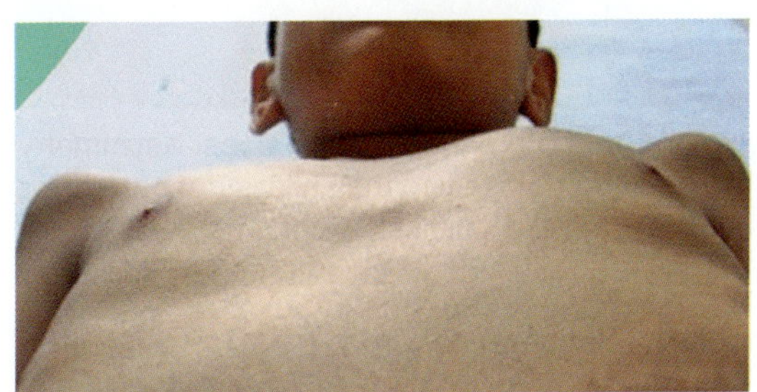

Fig. 8.26: This is even more clear when the child is examined from the foot-end.

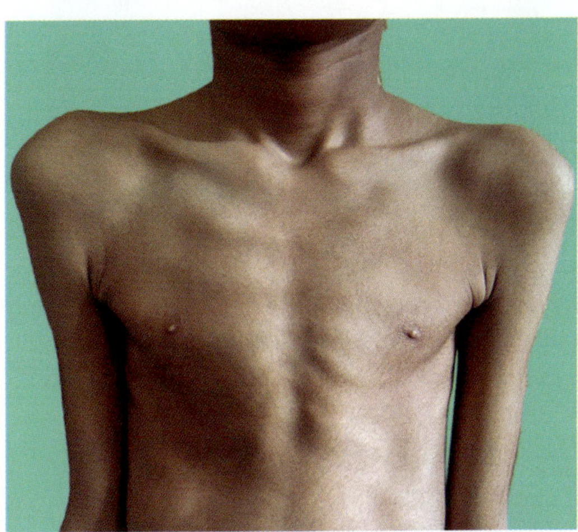

Fig. 8.27: With correct positioning, chest wall asymmetry can be easily appreciated.

Harrison sulcus refers to a deep 'groove' along the spaces where the diaphragm is inserted into the inner aspect of the ribs. This was regarded as a classical sign of rickets, but is not seen very frequently these days except in children with severe lung disease **(Fig. 8.31)**.

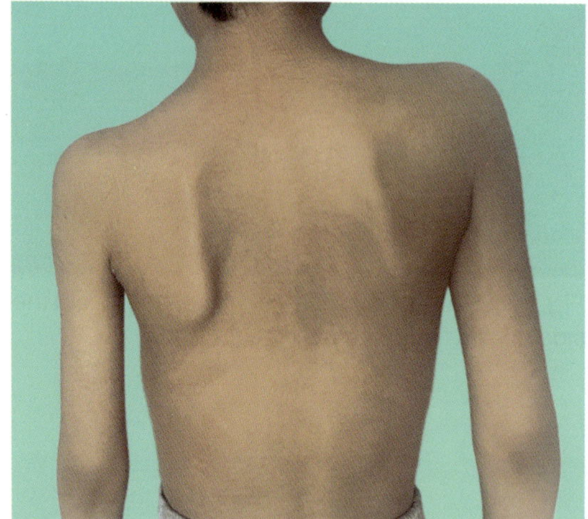

Fig. 8.28: There appears to be chest asymmetry on inspection. However, the child is not positioned correctly, making it difficult to confirm.

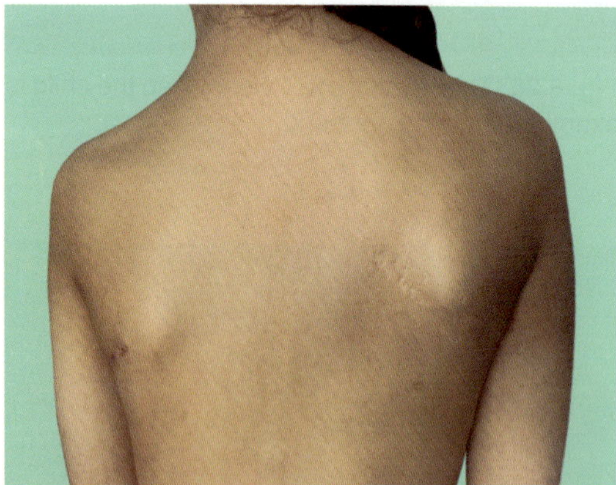

Fig. 8.29: This child also appears to have an asymmetric chest but the incorrect positioning makes it difficult to be certain.

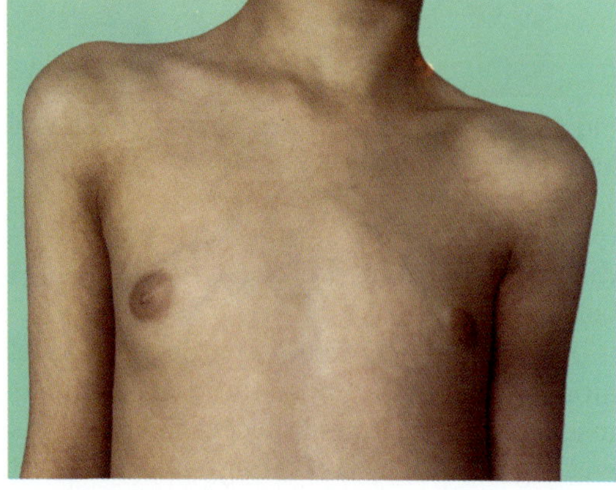

Fig. 8.30: An apparent left-sided volume loss due to incorrect positioning.

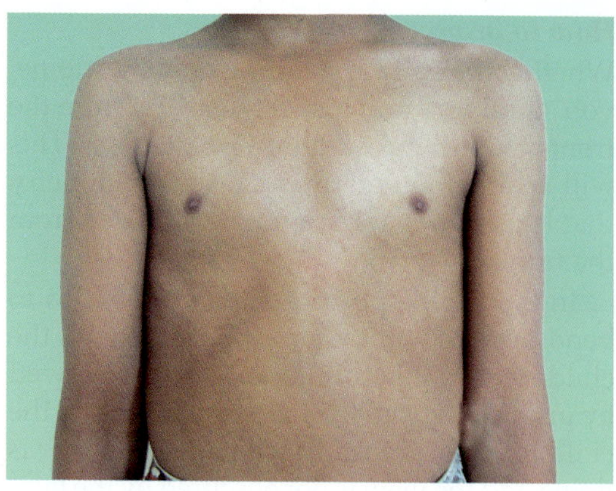

Fig. 8.31: Harrison sulcus.

5. Chest Movements

Inspection should also focus on the symmetry of chest movements with respiration. Clinical conditions that affect one side of the thorax including lungs, pleura, chest wall, or diaphragm can cause asymmetric breathing movements. Injury can cause the chest to be 'splinted' with localized decrease in movements.

B. Palpation

Palpation follows chest inspection and is essential to confirm and better define abnormalities that have already been picked up during inspection. Although often repeated, warm hands are must when examining children. **Key Box 5** highlights the points to be looked for during palpation.

1. Chest Expansion

Determine the degree and symmetry of chest expansion by placing the palms on either side of the thorax at the level of the nipples and gently apposing the thumbs in the midline. The thumbs separate during inspiration and this gives an approximate estimate of the degree of chest expansion. Figure 8.32 demonstrates the method when the child is lying supine, and Figures 8.33 to 8.35 demonstrate the method

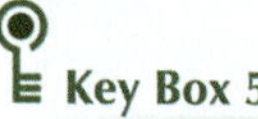

Key Box 5

Palpation of the Chest

1. *Chest expansion:* Measure and symmetry of expansion
2. Tracheal position
3. Tactile fremitus

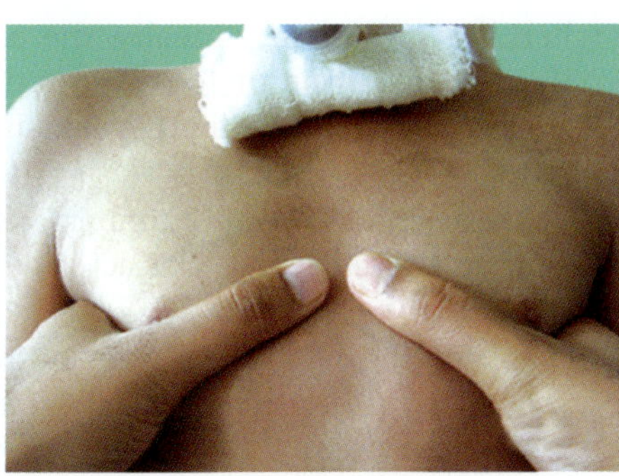

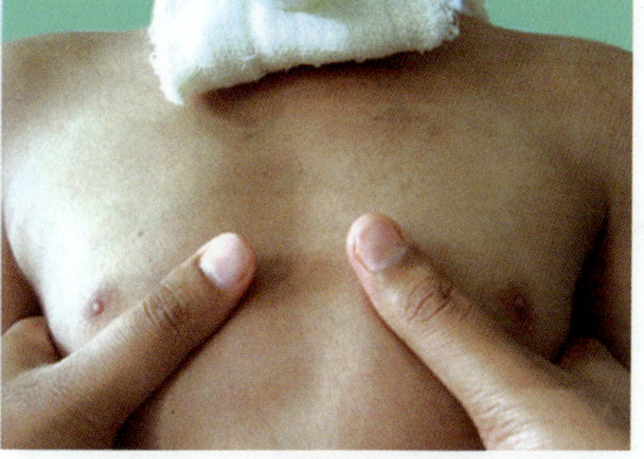

Fig. 8.32: Assessing chest expansion by palpation.

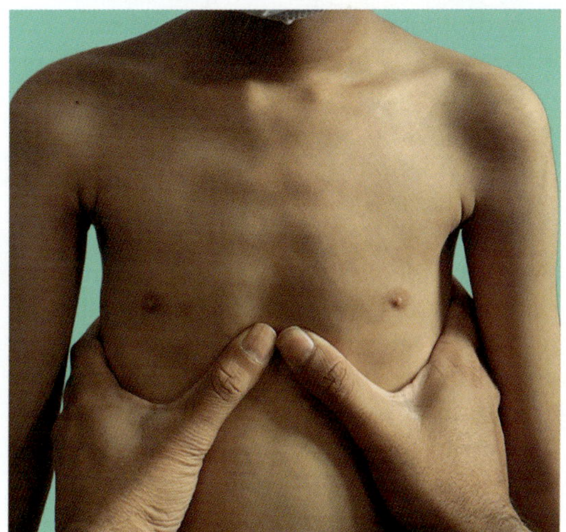

Fig. 8.33: Chest expansion being assessed during palpation.

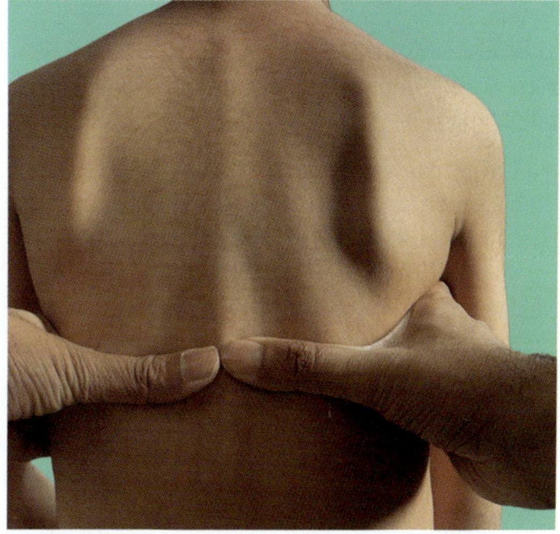

Fig. 8.35: It is helpful to assess chest expansion at multiple sites.

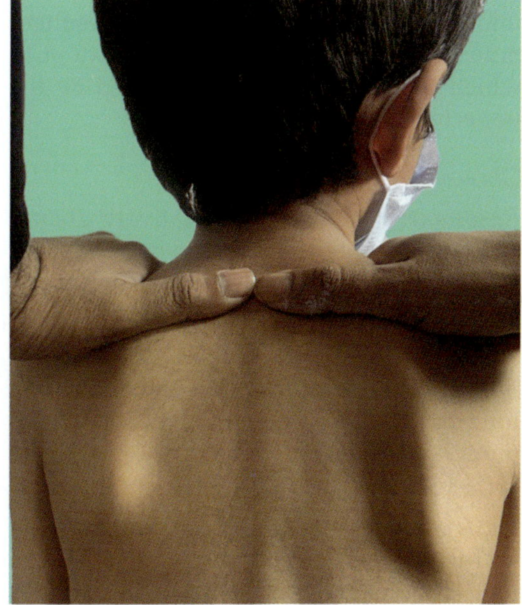

Fig. 8.34: Chest expansion being assessed posteriorly.

when the child is sitting up. It is important to assess expansion anteriorly and posteriorly. For greater accuracy, use a tape measure to quantify the chest expansion.

The normal chest expansion is 3–5 cm in older children and less in younger children and infants.

2. Tracheal Position

The trachea is normally central in position, however, a slight deviation towards the right is not uncommon. The child should be in such a position that no deviation due to posture occurs.

- Determine the position of the trachea by placing the second and fourth fingers on the two sternal attachments of the sternocleidomastoid muscles. Then, gently pass the third finger over the trachea to assess its relationship to the two fixed landmarks (Fig. 8.36).

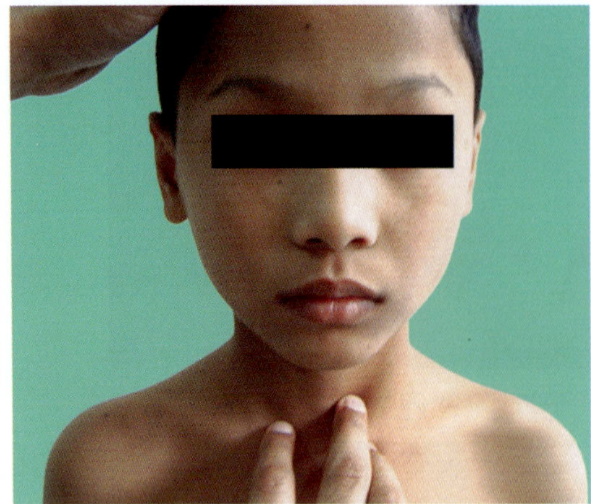

Fig. 8.36: Determining the tracheal position on palpation.

- The practice of 'holding' the trachea between the thumb on one side and the last three fingers; and then trying to assess its position with the index finger should be discouraged. However, in young babies, the trachea may be easier to palpate with a single finger over the suprasternal notch.
- Tracheal position may be shifted markedly in three sets of conditions **(Key Box 6)**:
  - i. Abnormalities in thoracic structure;
  - ii. Loss of thoracic volume creating a 'pull effect'; and
  - iii. Increased volume creating a 'push' to the opposite side.

3. *Tactile Vocal Fremitus*

Tactile fremitus is usually only practiced in older children. However, it can also be assessed to some extent in younger babies, when they are crying. Ideally, the aim is to palpate vibrations of low-frequency that are set up when the patient speaks in a low-pitched voice.

- Ask the child to count numbers, since it is difficult to elicit the 'classic' ninety-nine, repeatedly.
- Feel for the vibrations with both hands placed on either side of the chest to assess asymmetry, if any.
- Tactile fremitus is decreased when air or fluid in the pleura (pneumothorax, hydrothorax) impairs transmission.
- Atelectasis and collapse also decrease fremitus.
- The tactile fremitus appears increased in consolidation of a lobe or lung.

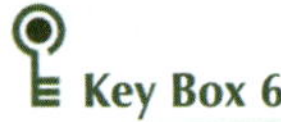

Key Box 6

Deviations of Trachea

1. Deviations of trachea due to scoliosis and kyphoscoliosis usually occur towards the concave side.
2. The trachea is *'pulled'* when the ipsilateral lung has undergone atelectasis, collapse, or in situations where the lung has been partially or totally removed. Congenital anomalies, such as pulmonary aplasia and agenesis, also create this effect.
3. Tracheal *'push'* occurs in pneumothorax and pleural effusion. Rarely, the trachea may be 'shifted' posteriorly due to pressure by masses in the mediastinum.

C. Percussion

The principle behind chest percussion is the same as in the musical instruments that come under the category of percussion, *viz.* to set a membrane into vibration and generate a sound. In musical instruments, such as the drum, *tabla*, etc., the impulse generates vibrations that persist without being damped and the sound is heard as a resonant note. The pitch is altered by the degree to which the membrane is stretched; and the amplitude varies with the force of the impulse.

In the chest, striking the surface causes the underlying tissues to vibrate and the resultant note is altered depending on the extent to which the vibrations are dampened by the underlying structures.

Character of Notes

Resonant: When there is relatively greater amount of air in the lungs as in hyperinflated states, the sound is heard as more *resonant* and persists longer than usual.

Hyper-resonant: When there is excess air between the chest wall surface and underlying lung tissue as in a pneumothorax, the note perceived as *hyper-resonant* as might be expected.

Dull: When there is fluid or a relatively solid structure, such as a consolidated lung intervening, the note is *dull* as well as shortened in duration. An incomplete dull note is sometimes also referred to as impaired.

Stony dull: In children with pleural effusion, percussion over fluid creates greater damping of the vibrations and the sound of the note is described as *stony* dullness (as if one is percussing on a stone).

How to Percuss?

Chest percussion is an art learned with experience; astute examiners rely heavily on this even when examining young babies. Inexperienced examiners tend to percuss repeatedly in order to elicit a note that they can describe; *this is usually neither desirable nor necessary.*

- Place the hand on the child's chest so that the middle finger is resting along an intercostal space. The other fingers of the hand must not come into contact with the chest wall; this is achieved by lifting them slightly.
- Tap the middle phalanx bringing the index or middle finger of the other hand straight downwards **(Figs 8.37 to 8.39)**. This action requires movement only at the wrist joint; and not the finger or shoulder joints. Lift the tapping (plexor) finger immediately off the pleximeter finger and listen carefully for the note that is produced. While percussing the posterior areas, the hands of child should be folded across so that right hand touches the left shoulder and the left hand touches the right shoulder. This draws the scapulae outwards allowing a larger area of the lung to be percusssed.
- All areas of the chest should be percussed and each compared with the contralateral side, immediately.

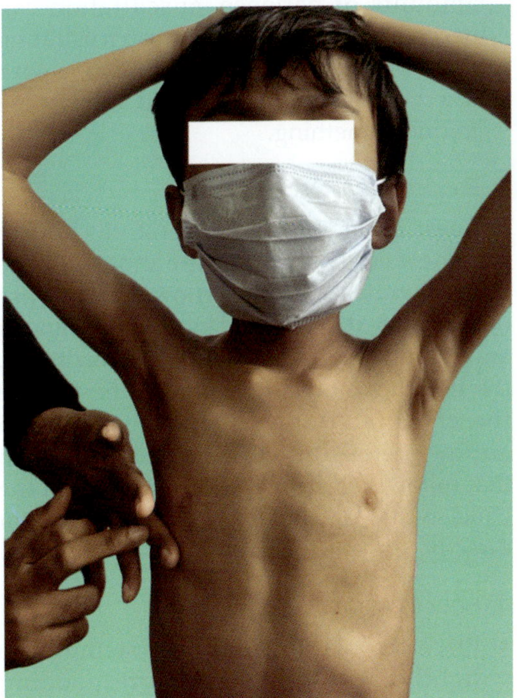

Fig. 8.37: The correct method of chest percussion. Note the examiner's left hand; where only one finger is in contact with the chest along an intercostal space. The plexor finger strikes the pleximeter finger vertically with movement at the wrist joint. It is often helpful to request a cooperative child to place the hands above the head.

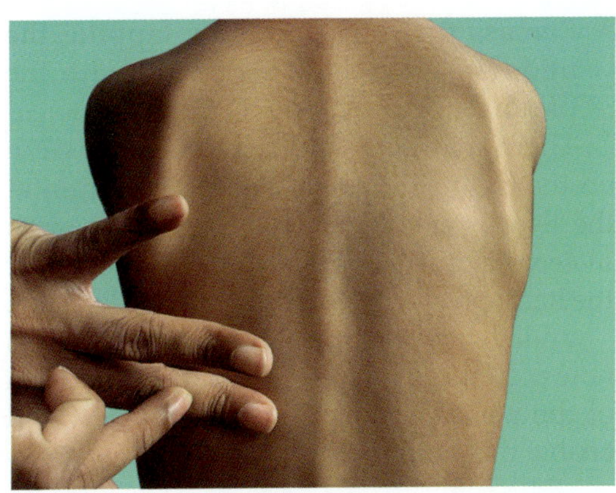

Fig. 8.38: Percussion also should be performed at multiple sites. While percussing the posterior areas, the hands of child should be folded across so that right hand touches the left shoulder and the left hand touches the right shoulder. This draws the scapulae outwards allowing a larger area of the lung to be percussed.

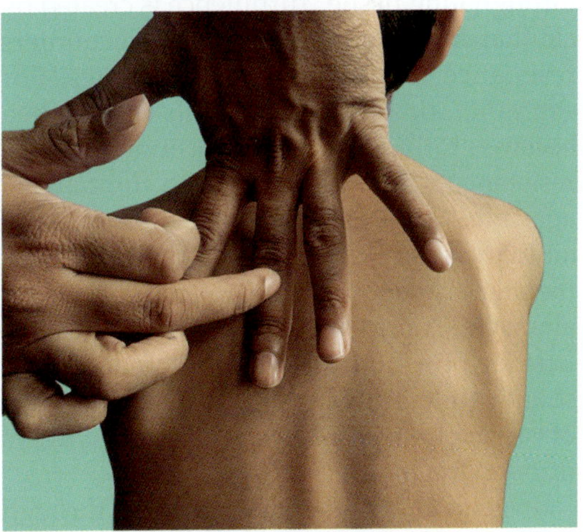

Fig. 8.39: An alternate method to percuss the chest when it is not possible to place the finger along an intercostal space.

- Percuss the lung apices by tapping the middle of the clavicle directly with the plexor finger.

  There will be a dull note on percussion on the right side when the upper margin of the liver is encountered at the fifth or sixth intercostal space; likewise, percussion over the heart produces a dull note on the left side.

  Initially, it may appear difficult to describe a note accurately, but practice and appreciation of the percussion note in normal chest will enable this with time.

D. Auscultation

1. Physiology of the Breath Sounds

Breath sounds are generated in the large airways. Their quality keeps on altering as airflow becomes turbulent during passage through the airways and later transmission through lung tissue. Turbulence is created by air that flows within tubes and encounters resistance that alters flow dynamics. For example, air passing through the trachea becomes turbulent when it encounters a high resistance at the glottis due to the narrow aperture. This resistance causes the velocity of air to increase. When air is 'distributed' from the single channel (trachea) to multiple smaller airspaces, considerable sound energy is lost. Besides flow and turbulence, the quality of sound is altered by its frequency since sounds of varying frequencies take different pathways through the lung.

In general, lower frequencies pass through the lung and are directed towards the chest wall. On the other hand, high frequency sound passes preferentially through the airways before being directed through the parenchyma and then the chest wall. The importance of this is that, sounds need not be exactly symmetrical on both sides even in normal persons.

2. The Stethoscope: Tool for Auscultation

A reasonably good stethoscope is an essential tool for every pediatrician, and it is all that is needed for auscultation. While it is difficult to choose (or recommend) between the various models available, a few basic principles must be borne in mind.

- The stethoscope should be of sufficient length to make examination comfortable for the child and physician.
- The rubber tubes must be supple and easily flexible, but not stretch.
- The earpieces should not be cracked or torn.
- The parts of the instrument encountering the child's exposed chest must be warm.
- ***Bell or diaphragm:*** It is feasible to examine children using either the diaphragm or the bell; this is a matter of personal choice. However, in small babies, the diaphragm may be larger than the intercostal space and not fit snugly, in such cases, the bell may be preferable.
- ***Digital stethoscope:*** These days, digital stethoscopes are available that allow recording of the sounds for storage, transmission, etc.
- ***Your skill:*** The successful interpretation of auscultation does not depend on the set of earpieces alone, but also on what lies between the earpieces; in other words, the auditory perception and interpretative skill of the examiner. With a fair amount of time, good degree of practice and infinite amounts of patience, auscultation can become a joy for you rather than frustrating attempt at pressing the stethoscope over the chest of a struggling child and hoping to find something.

3. Prepare for Auscultation

Request an older and cooperative child to breathe deeply through the mouth, since this generates a good airflow. You should demonstrate it to the child by doing it yourself and asking the child to simulate. In an infant, the breath sounds are evaluated best while the child is crying, since the maximum airflow occurs during prolonged inspiration that follows a robust cry. Turn the face of the child so that he/she does not breathe on you directly.

4. How to Auscultate?

- Place the diaphragm of the stethoscope lightly, but firmly over corresponding parts of the chest on both sides; so that all lobes are covered sequentially. Listen to the breath sounds.
- Auscultate all areas in a systematic manner: Supraclavicular, mammary, inframammary, axillary, infra-axillary, interscapular, and infrascapular of both sides.

- Describe what is heard in terms of the location, intensity, pitch, and timing.
- Location should be described according to the lobar anatomy rather than the chest surface anatomy.

Intensity refers to the amplitude of the sound (how 'loud' or how 'soft' it is heard); this must not be confused with 'harsh' which reflects the pitch and the amplitude together.

An important point to remember is—we are trying to assess breath sounds, and hence this should be described as such—the practice of mentioning air entry when one means breath sounds is both irritating and incorrect. Air entry is not assessed by auscultation except perhaps in an intubated patient when the physician is checking tube position by listening to air entering through the airway. Likewise, in patients who are being ventilated, auscultation does not strictly pick up breath sounds, though these can still be described as such.

5. Breath Sounds

Vesicular breathing: Inspiration is immediately followed by expiration; there is no gap between the two phases. These are generated by turbulence of airflow and, therefore, are heard when flow is maximal, therefore, they are audible throughout inspiration and the early part of expiration. Vesicular breath sounds are heard over normal lungs.

Bronchial breathing: Inspiratory and expiratory phases are equal, and there is a gap in between the two phases of respiration. The term '*bronchovesicular*' is used to describe breath sounds that are difficult to categorize into either. This is not to be encouraged.

- Bronchial breathing is heard when sound generated in the central airways is transmitted unchanged through the lung substance. This happens in consolidation because the alveoli that are normally filled with air and dampen sound transmission are now relatively solid and conduct the sound straight to the chest wall.
- Bronchial breathing can also be heard just above the air–fluid interface in a pleural effusion.
- Rarely, it can be heard over a collapsed portion of the lung, if there is a patent airway overlying the collapse.
- Older texts referred to tubular, cavernous, and amphoric qualities of bronchial breath sounds, but these are not used in current practice.

6. Additional Sounds

Pitch and timing are used to categorize abnormal breath sounds into two broad groups: '*Musical*' sounds over a relatively long duration are called wheeze (*rhonchi*) as opposed to 'non-musical', discontinuous sounds of shorter duration that are called crackles (*crepitations*).

Wheeze: Wheeze is produced by oscillations within narrowed airways.

a. When a large airway is narrowed or obstructed, the wheeze has a single frequency/pitch, and this is described as monophonic.
b. Narrowing of multiple smaller airways over a wide area of the lung creates sounds with varying frequencies and is referred to as polyphonic wheezing.

Wheezing sound is heard more often during the expiratory phase, since it is produced by limitation of flow. However, when airway obstruction is severe enough to limit airflow even during the active inspiratory phase, wheezing can be heard during inspiration also.

Crackles: These are produced when air passes through an air–fluid interface or secretions. It can also be produced by the 'popping effect' during sudden opening or closure of airways. Crackles are sub-categorized as fine and coarse.

a. ***Coarse crackles*** are more commonly heard in children than fine crackles. These usually occur during inspiration in pneumonia.
b. ***Fine crackles*** during late inspiration are heard in restrictive lung diseases, especially interstitial lung disease where the sound is described as 'velcro crackles'.

It is good practice to describe breath sounds with reference to these terms rather than a host of other terms that may not convey the same meaning. For example, the word rhonchi is used interchangeably with wheeze. Some examiners interpret it as a low-pitched wheeze while others use it to describe any sound that is heard in a child with airway obstruction including sounds produced by secretions in the chest. 'Crepitations' is a term that is used to describe crackles; however, the current classification of breath sounds does not encourage this terminology. Likewise, older texts mention 'rales', a term that encompasses both wheezes and crackles depending on how the term is described further.

7. Vocal Resonance

Vocal resonance refers to the sounds heard over the chest (with the help of a stethoscope or ear pressed to the chest wall) when the patient generates sound from the larynx. When these sounds pass through the airways and lungs, the higher frequency components get filtered off. However, when there is consolidation, the relatively solid lung does not filter off these frequencies, and sounds produced at the larynx are transmitted with good clarity to the examiner. *Egophony* or *aegophony* refers to nasal or bleating quality of speech transmitted through consolidation with patent bronchus. *Bronchophony* is the voice of the bronchus where spoken voice is heard loud (near the earpiece of stethoscope) but not very clear. *Pectoriloquy* is the voice of the chest where the spoken voice is heard loud and clear. In *whispering pectoriloquy*, the whispered sound is also heard clearly (not otherwise heard over normal lung tissue).

8. Pleural Rub

Pleural rub is a sound that can be auscultated in pleural disease. It is a creaky sound that is produced by rubbing of the visceral and parietal layers when the pleura is inflamed. Therefore, a typical rub will be audible during both phases of respiration.

8.6 PHYSICAL FINDINGS IN COMMON RESPIRATORY CONDITIONS

1. Lobar Pneumonia (Consolidation)

Consolidation is a pathological term that implies a heavy lung where air is replaced by more solid material. Radiologists use it liberally to describe alveolar opacification due to any cause. For a physician, consolidation is often synonymous with lobar pneumonia although this is not always the case.

- ***Inspection*** of the chest shows normal shape and symmetry; however, an astute examiner may detect diminished movement on the affected side.
- ***Palpation*** reveals a central tracheal position and reduced chest expansion. Tactile fremitus may be increased and the percussion note is impaired.
- ***Auscultation:*** Bronchial breath sounds are audible over the affected area with bronchophony and whispering pectoriloquy. These findings usually occur when a lobe is 'consolidated'. In pneumonia, these findings may not be heard until the disease process has reached this stage. Earlier in the course, fine crackles are the more usual findings. Likewise, coarse crackles can be heard when pneumonia is 'resolving'.

Characteristics of consolidation are summarized in **Key Box 7**.

2. Collapse

Physical examination findings in 'collapse' depend on whether an entire lung is involved or a single lobe only is collapsed. The former results is gross asymmetry of the chest on inspection with 'flattening' on the affected side; therefore, the shoulder droops down and the scapula of the affected side appears to be lower than the contralateral side. The trachea deviates towards the affected side. Movements of the chest in the affected side are diminished and the cardiac apex is shifted towards the side of the lesion. The percussion note is impaired and auscultation reveals diminished breath sounds and decreased vocal resonance.

These findings are much more subtle, if only a lobe is collapsed. In such cases, it may be difficult to appreciate the diminished movements and expansion, as also the decreased vocal resonance. When a lobar

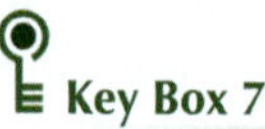

Consolidation: Chest Findings

1. Intercostal retractions
2. Trachea central
3. Increased vocal fremitus over affected area
4. Dull/impaired note on percussion
5. Diminished breath sounds
6. Bronchial breathing
7. Crackles (localized in lobar pneumonia, scattered in bronchopneumonia)
8. Wheeze in younger children

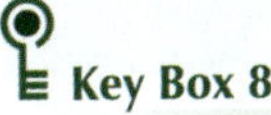
Key Box 8

Collapse/Fibrosis: Chest Findings

1. Diminished movement and expansion
2. Tracheal shift to ipsilateral side
3. Mediastinal (cardiac apex) shift to ipsilateral side
4. Impaired note on percussion
5. Diminished breath sounds on affected area

collapse involves the upper lobe, direct transmission of sound from the trachea can result in the perception of bronchial breathing, increased vocal resonance, and even whispering pectoriloquy.

Characteristics of collapse are summarized in **Key Box 8**.

3. Pleural Effusion

Depending upon the volume of fluid that accumulates in the pleural space, the signs in a pleural effusion can vary. Large collections are associated with an apparent 'bulging' of the affected side of the chest on inspection with reduced movements. The trachea is shifted towards the opposite side as also the cardiac apex. Vocal fremitus is reduced, percussion note has a characteristic stony dullness, and breath sounds are absent or markedly reduced. It is possible sometimes to appreciate bronchial breathing at the site of the air–fluid level. In the early stages of an effusion, a pleural rub may be audible.

Characteristics of pleural effusion are summarized in **Key Box 9**.

4. Pneumothorax

Pneumothorax is associated with features of 'volume excess' on the affected side as in a pleural effusion; hence there is tracheal and mediastinal shift to the contralateral side, decreased movements and expansion, reduced vocal fremitus, but a normal or hyper-resonant percussion note. Breath sounds and vocal resonance are decreased.

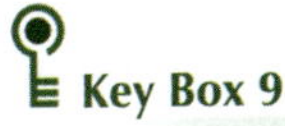
Key Box 9

Pleural Effusion: Chest Findings

1. Respiratory distress
2. Diminished movement and expansion in localized area
3. Tracheal shift to contralateral side
4. Mediastinal (cardiac apex) shift to contralateral side
5. Stony dullness on percussion
6. Diminished breath sounds on affected area

5. Chronic Air-trapping

When there is chronic air-trapping as in long-standing asthma, the chest appears hyper-inflated throughout; the bulging results in a barrel-shaped chest. The expansion may be normal or reduced, with trachea being central. Tactile fremitus remains normal, percussion note may show increased (resonant) note with reduction or obliteration of the cardiac and hepatic dullness. Breath sounds are usually vesicular with polyphonic wheezes all over the chest. Characteristics of acute asthma are summarized in **Key Box 10**.

6. Foreign Body Aspiration

A foreign body can sometimes be a tricky issue in children; the examination findings

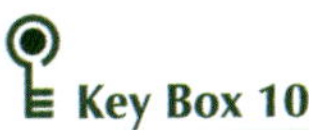
Key Box 10

Acute Asthma Episode

Typical history

1. Wheezing, history of similar episodes in past
2. May be preceded by upper respiratory infection
3. History of exposure to trigger may be present
4. Cough, breathing difficulty, inability to feed
5. Difficulty in speaking
6. Relief with bronchodilator

Physical examination

1. Sensorium may be normal to altered depending on severity
2. Tachycardia, tachypnea, pulsus paradoxus (in severe episodes)
3. Signs of upper respiratory tract infection may be present
4. Signs of respiratory distress
5. Cyanosis in severe cases
6. Skin lesions suggesting atopic dermatitis/eczema

Chest examination

1. Hyperinflation in uncontrolled asthma
2. Prolonged expiration
3. Bilateral rhonchi
4. Silent chest in very severe cases

Table 8.2: Typical findings in upper respiratory tract afflictions

Criteria	Upper respiratory tract infection	Laryngotracheo-bronchitis (croup)	Upper airway obstruction
History	Acute onset, fever, running nose, cough, no breathing difficulty, sore throat, change in voice, swallowing difficulty, decreased feeding, suggestive family history	Preceded by symptoms of upper respiratory infection, brassy/barking cough, audible stridor, inability to feed/drink, occasionally drooling, symptoms worse on supine	1. High-grade fever, toxic appearance, pain on one side of throat, characteristic 'hot potato' voice suggest peritonsillar abscess 2. Triad of acute fever, dysphagia and drooling suggest epiglottitis 3. Choking episode followed by respiratory distress suggest aspiration of foreign body 4. Fever, respiratory distress and toxic appearance point towards bacterial tracheitis
Examination	Fever, inflamed pharynx/ tonsils/ tympanic membrane, nasal discharge, regional superficial lymphadenopathy, occasionally rash associated with a viral infection	Behavior may range from irritable to lethargic, audible stridor, signs of respiratory distress (suprasternal indrawing, nasal flaring)	Features of upper airway obstruction as in croup with added signs as described above
Chest examination	Usually normal chest, sometimes wheeze and/ or crackles	Usually normal, wheeze may be present	Usually normal, wheeze may be present

vary depending upon the stage at which the child presents.

In an acute setting, the usual history of choking followed by respiratory distress associated with features of air-trapping on one side, contralateral tracheal shift, diminished breath sounds, and impaired vocal resonance all suggest obstruction of a large bronchus. These findings are much more subtle and difficult to appreciate, if the foreign body had slipped more distally to obstruct a segmental airway.

In long-standing cases, referred to as 'forgotten foreign body', there is collapse with secondary infection and bronchiectasis of the affected segments/lobes/lung. In such cases, loss of volume with coarse crackles in the affected area is easily appreciable.

7. Diseases of the Upper Airway

Three sets of conditions need to be differentiated in an upper airway affliction:

i. Upper respiratory tract infection;
ii. Laryngotracheobronchitis; and
iii. Upper airway obstruction.

Their characteristics and differentiating features are outlined in **Table 8.2**, based on the history, general physical examination, and examination of the respiratory system.

8.7 INVESTIGATIONS RELATED TO THE RESPIRATORY SYSTEM

The purpose of this section is to highlight some commonly used investigative modalities in children with respiratory system problems and not to provide a detailed guide to the methodology, interpretation, and accuracy of the tests.

A. Microbiology of Airway Secretions

Microbiologic analysis of respiratory specimens can yield important information at relatively low cost; if properly collected, processed and analyzed. In most cases, the aim is to obtain material from the lower airway to establish the etiology of infectious processes. However, interpretation of microbiologic results in children is often hampered by 'contamination' of many samples with upper airway secretions that are colonized with a variety of organisms, some of which are potentially pathogenic.

1. Upper Airway Samples

Throat swab: It is relatively easy to obtain a throat swab specimen in a cooperative child. With the mouth wide open, a sterile swab is inserted and 'swabbed' over the pharynx and tonsils. It is then transferred to a sterile container or ideally, plated directly on to culture medium. A variety of bacteria colonize the throat in children and adults; all of these are not pathogenic. Therefore, mere isolation of organisms may not point towards pathology.

Nasopharyngeal aspirate (NPA): A nasopharyngeal aspirate (NPA) works in the same way as a throat swab. However, the technique is different. A thin sterile catheter is introduced through the nostril to a fixed length that corresponds to the distance between angle of the mouth to the tragus of the pinna. About 1 mL of normal saline is instilled and secretions are aspirated into a mucus trap. This can be analyzed for antigens of organisms or plated for culture.

2. Lower Airway Secretions

Sputum: Sputum expectorated by coughing is perhaps the easiest and best method of obtaining lower airway samples that are minimally contaminated with material from the upper airway. However, most young children do not expectorate properly and sputum often yields a mixture of upper airway organisms. Therefore, many laboratories confirm the quality of sputum by measuring the number of epithelial cells relative to neutrophils. It is a good practice to send sputum for detailed examination in terms of cytology, Gram staining, and bacterial culture. Specific investigations, such as staining for acid-fast bacilli and mycobacterial culture, staining for fungal hyphae and fungal culture, analysis for hemosiderin, etc., should be considered as per the need.

Expectoration of sputum can be 'induced' in children who are unable to do so naturally. This is done by pre-medication with a bronchodilator (such as salbutamol) followed by inhalation of saline for 10–15 minutes. The yield of induced samples can be enhanced by active chest physiotherapy using percussion of the chest. For very young children and infants, this can be done using a silicon airway mask. Lower airway samples can be better collected in these children using nasopharyngeal aspiration following induction and physiotherapy.

Gastric lavage: Early morning gastric lavage is yet another method that is helpful to collect lower airway samples. The principle is that children swallow secretions that can be obtained from the stomach. It is a good method to detect the presence of acid-fast bacilli that are otherwise difficult to obtain in children. A gastric lavage must be distinguished from a gastric aspirate. The latter involves placing a catheter in the stomach and aspirating the contents, early in the morning, prior to the child's waking up. This is an important precaution because an awake child starts swallowing and this propels the swallowed contents distally, reducing the yield of organisms. Therefore, the nasogastric catheter be placed the previous night so that the effect of swallowing or crying during the placement does not hamper the collection of secretions. The following morning, the stomach contents are aspirated prior to the child's waking up till 10 mL is collected. The stomach is then washed by instilling 30 mL normal saline and the contents aspirated again. The two aspirates are sent in the same container for microbiologic processing.

B. Invasive Procedures

1. Lung Puncture

Direct puncture of lung parenchyma can be used for obtaining specimens in cases of consolidation wherein the lung tissue is relatively solid. This is done by inserting a needle attached to a syringe containing sterile saline; through an intercostal space over consolidated tissue. Within the span of a single breath, the needle is advanced, the saline is instilled and aspirated, and the needle is withdrawn.

2. Bronchoscopy

Fiberoptic bronchoscopy with bronchoalveolar lavage (BAL) has greatly enhanced the examination of the lower airway and collection of specimens for analysis. BAL is done by wedging the bronchoscope into a segmental bronchus under direct vision. Sterile normal saline is instilled and aspirated by suction; this procedure washes the distal airway and results in significant yield of specimens for cytologic and microbiologic analysis.

3. Thoracocentesis

Thoracocentesis or pleural tap enables collection of fluid from the pleural cavity for diagnostic and (rarely) therapeutic purposes. A needle attached to a syringe is inserted through the intercostal space in the posterior axillary line at a site determined by chest percussion. Fluid aspirated is analyzed in terms of cytology (type and number of cells), biochemistry (protein, sugar, glucose, pH, LDH, etc.) and microbiology (Gram staining, bacterial culture, mycobacterial culture, fungal culture, etc.).

C. Imaging Modalities

1. Radiography

A conventional radiograph of the chest is perhaps the most frequently used investigation in children. It is used justifiably in many cases primarily to assess lesions in lung parenchyma. It also serves well for evaluation of the other parts of the upper and lower respiratory systems.

Proper position of the child is essential to get a good radiographic record; ideally the child should be placed in an 'anatomical position' with arms by the side, chest in contact with the radiographic plate and timed to the mid-inspiratory position. Thus, the erect posture with a posteroanterior (PA) imaging is the standard modality. Obviously, this is impossible to achieve in most children; but every effort must be made to ensure a position as close to this as feasible, even in young infants where simple things like turning of the head to one side can give impression of gross abnormality. The anteroposterior (supine) (AP) radiograph is often used in babies, and children confined to bed. Interpretation of such films differs from the posteroanterior (PA) films.

Radiographs should be checked for exposure and quality prior to interpreting them. In a properly exposed chest radiograph, spinous processes to the level of the third or fourth thoracic vertebra are clearly visible. Over exposed films appear 'more black' and will show spines below this level also.

It is good practice to interpret radiographs covering all parts starting from outwards to inwards. The examiner should observe and comment upon the ribcage and bony structures, soft tissue that lies within, pleural space abnormalities, pulmonary parenchyma, trachea and airway, cardiac, mediastinal and vascular shadows, and presence of any objects, such as feeding tubes, catheters, central venous lines, etc. In children, most chest radiographs also cover a small portion of the abdomen wherein gross pathology is sometimes visible.

Chest radiography can yield more information when special views are taken for specific purposes. Lateral views are particularly useful to determine pleural contents and the differentiation of parenchymal lesions from others in the vicinity. The decubitus film that is hardly ever ordered can easily differentiate pleural fluid opacity from parenchymal opacity. Incidentally, it is the recommended mode to calculate the thickness of pleural fluid for the purpose of intervention, a point that is missed by most clinicians.

Conventional radiographs of the respiratory system also include the Water's view for evaluation of the paranasal sinuses and a lateral film to evaluate the soft tissues of the neck for airway obstruction.

More specialized radiographic evaluations of the respiratory system include fluoroscopy which enables visualization of the airway and respiratory movements. It was used fairly frequently for observing diaphragmatic movements. These days, it is used more often as a contrast study to assess diverse pathology, such as swallowing dysfunction, gastroesophageal reflux, and aspiration into the airway.

Figures 8.40 to 8.50 depict some common chest radiography findings in children.

However, it is emphasized that the habit of some physicians to order radiological studies without a proper clinical examination, is strongly discouraged. In most situations, physical examination can reveal the findings identified in chest radiographs. A few case summaries provided ahead highlight this.

2. Ultrasonography (USG)

Ultrasonography has become a preferred investigative tool in many conditions because it is non-invasive in nature and free from radiation. It has an emerging role in evaluation of the respiratory system. Hitherto, its main use in children is to assess the approximate volume and consistency of fluid in the pleural space. These days, chest ultrasonography has been used in suspected pneumonia also. It can sometimes be used to resolve the nature of an opacity on conventional radiographs. As for abdominal masses, the contents and consistency of solid lesions in the thorax can also be delineated by ultrasonography, but this is rarely required in children.

Invasive procedures (such as placement of central venous catheters, intercostal drainage tubes, etc.) are generally done under point-of-care ultrasonographic guidance in many hospitals.

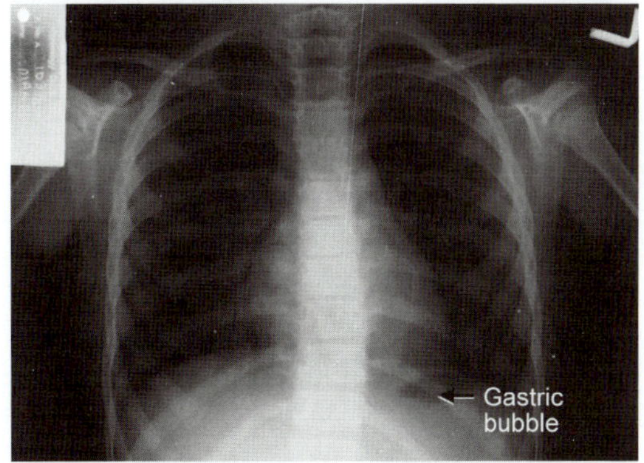

Fig. 8.40: Normal chest radiograph. Note the appropriate exposure suggested by the clearly visible intervertebral spaces till T_4. Bilateral symmetry of clavicles, scapulae, and upper limbs suggests good centering (no undue rotation). This is a postero-anterior (PA) view suggested by the clearer anterior structures (heart and anterior part of ribs) and less visible posterior structures (scapulae). The gastric bubble suggests that the radiograph has been taken in the erect position.

3. Computed Tomography

The computed tomography (CT) scan has overtaken most other radiological investigative tools, judging by the number and frequency with which these are ordered. It is fast becoming a highly misused modality, with serious consequences in terms of radiation hazards, cost, and ethics. It should be remembered that the CT scan works on the principle of taking 'slices' of the body (chest) at fixed intervals; therefore, it is excellent to pick up diffuse lesions as in interstitial disease or localized lesions that occupy considerable space, such as lobar consolidation, abscess,

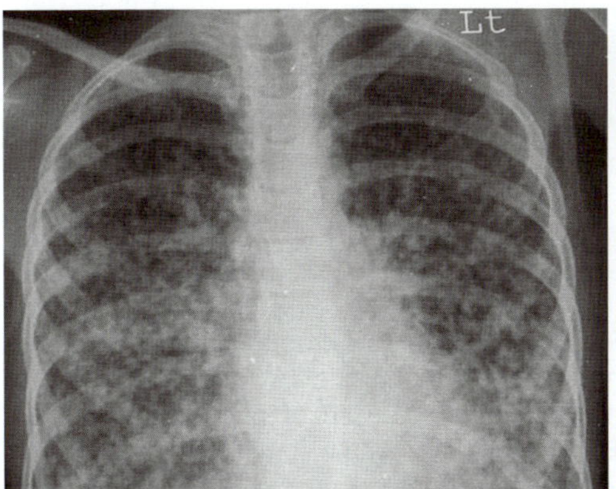

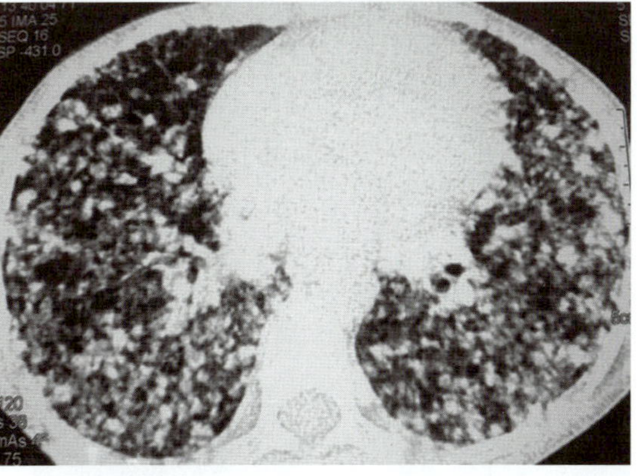

Fig. 8.41: Miliary shadows. This pattern is characteristic of miliary tuberculosis. However, it can also be seen with pulmonary metastasis from thyroid carcinoma, as in this child.

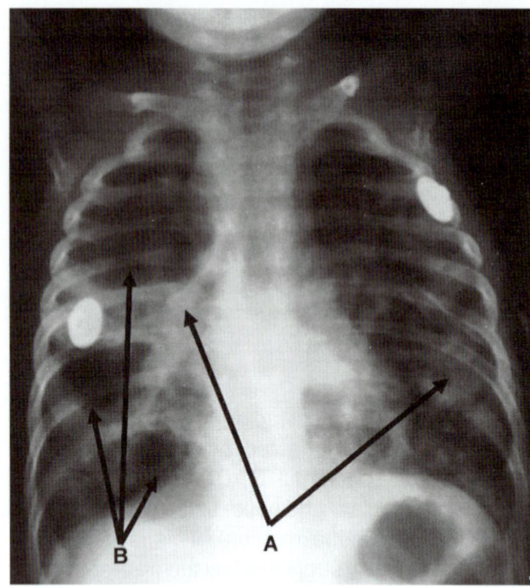

Fig. 8.42: Necrotizing pneumonia. Note the bilateral consolidation (A) and multiple pneumatoceles (B). This pattern is characteristic of staphylococcal lung disease.

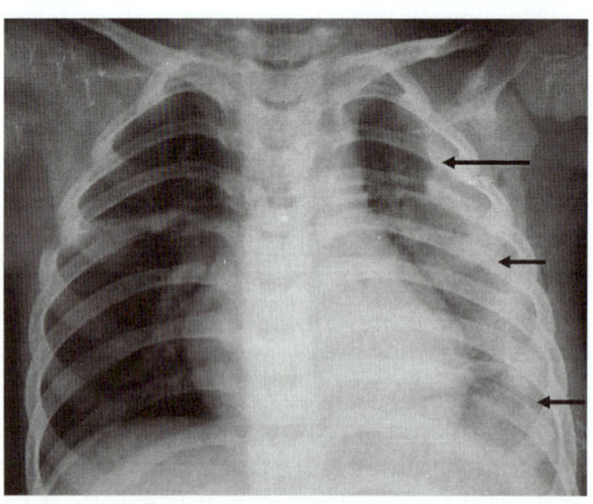

Fig. 8.43: Pleural effusion. Observe the clear demarcation between the lung margin and pleural fluid (arrows). An intercostal drainage tube is just visible. The classical 'fluid level' is seen only with 'thin' effusions on an erect radiograph. It is not visible here.

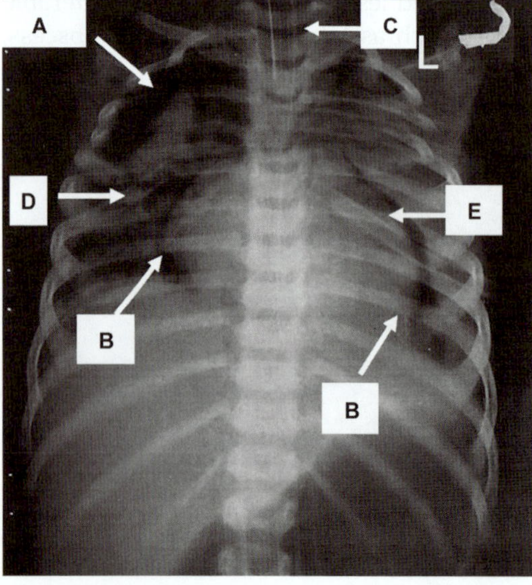

Fig. 8.44: Air-leak syndrome. Note the pneumothorax on the right side (A) and silhouetting of the heart characteristic of pneumomediastinum (B). These are probably complications of manual ventilation suggested by the endotracheal tube *in situ* (C). Intercostal (D) and mediastinal (E) drainage tubes are visible.

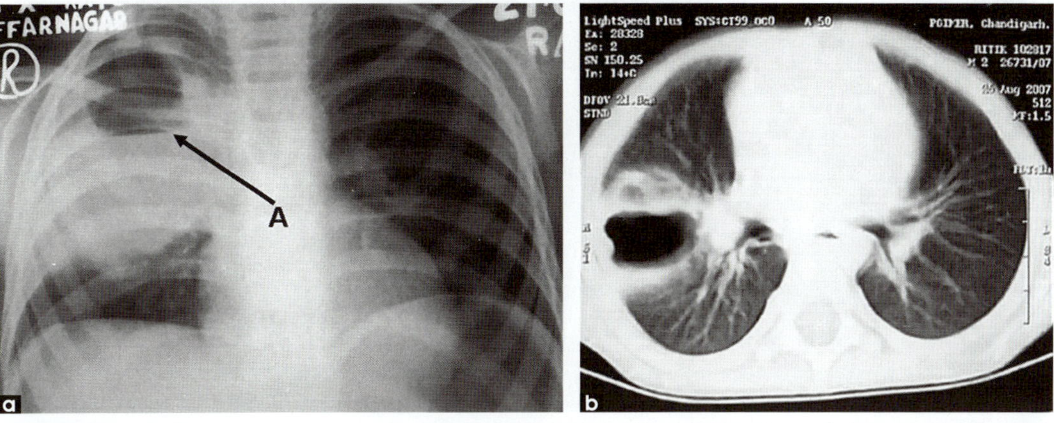

Fig. 8.45: Lung abscess. (a) Note the rounded lesion with an air–fluid level A; (b) CT scan of the same patient.

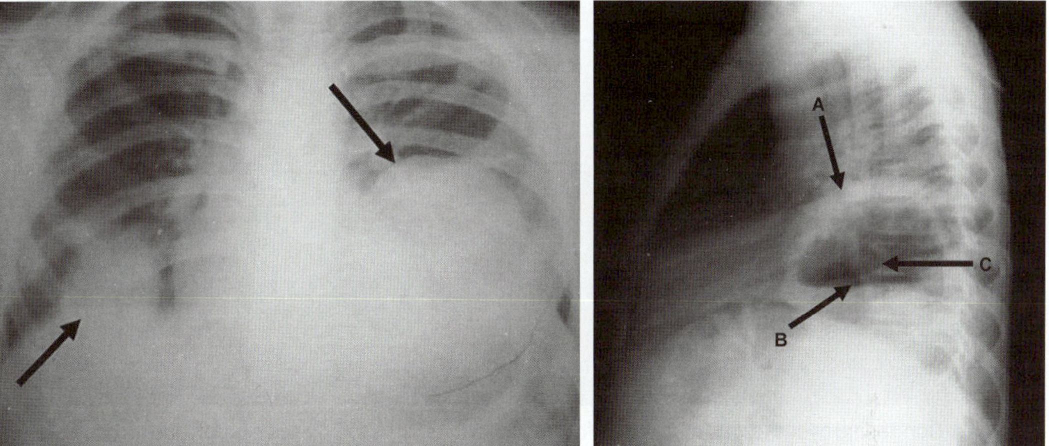

Fig. 8.46: Bilateral hydatid cysts. Observe the two well-defined round solid-appearing lesions in both lungs. The lateral radiograph shows a well-defined cystic lesion with (A) thick wall, (B) air–fluid level and (C) lack of homogeneous internal opacification.

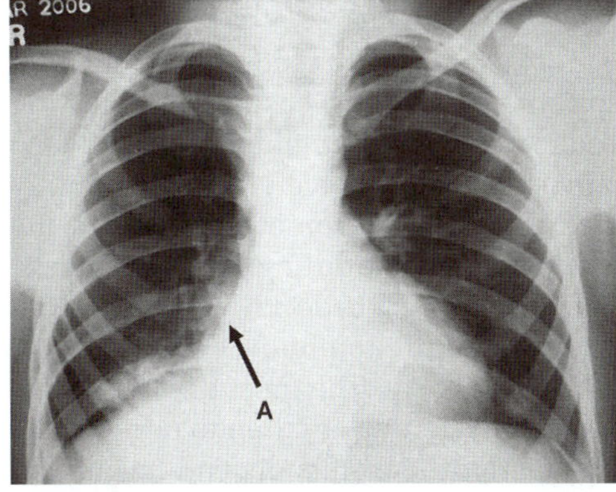

Fig. 8.47: Foreign body obstructing segmental bronchus. Note the segmental collapse (A).

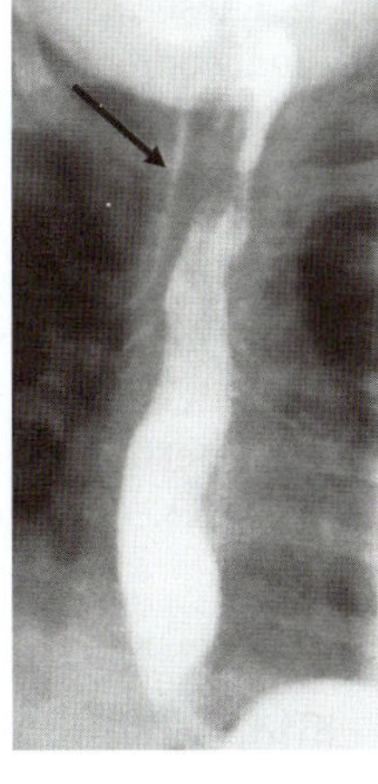

Fig. 8.48: Contrast esophagogram. This test was performed to detect gastroesophageal reflux, which was absent. The esophageal contour, gastroesophageal junction, and gastric filling are normal. Note the aspiration of a small quantity of contrast into the airway (arrow). This is why water-soluble contrast is preferred to barium in young children.

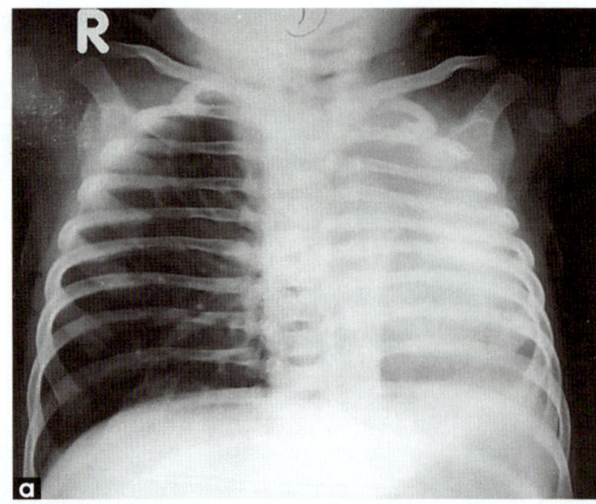

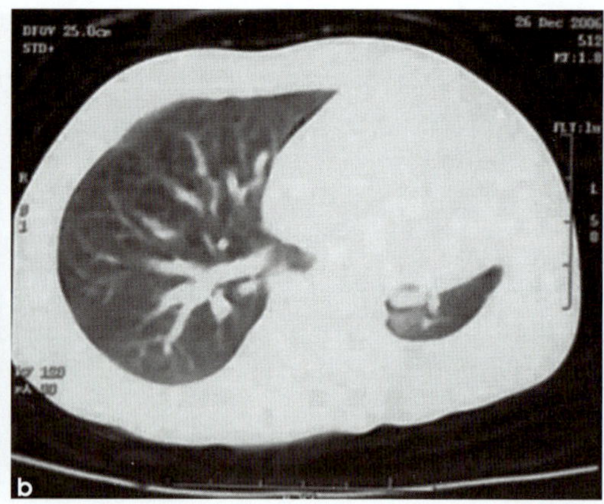

Fig. 8.49: Hypoplastic lung. (a) Chest radiograph: Note the absence of aeration and vascular shadows on the left side. Note also the ipsilateral mediastinal shift, relative 'crowding' of ribs and curvature of spine with concavity towards the left side; (b) CT scan of the same patient.

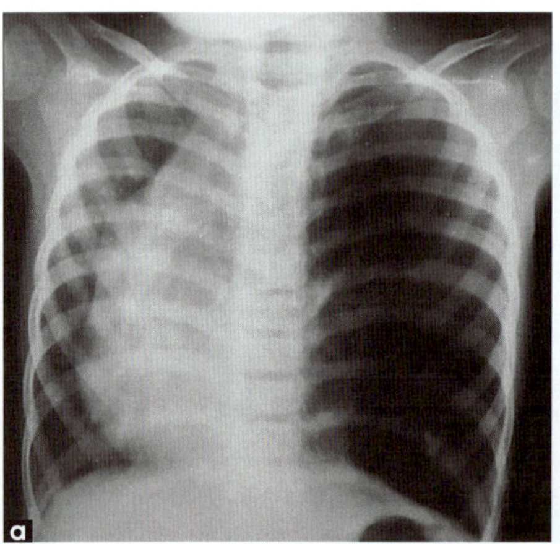

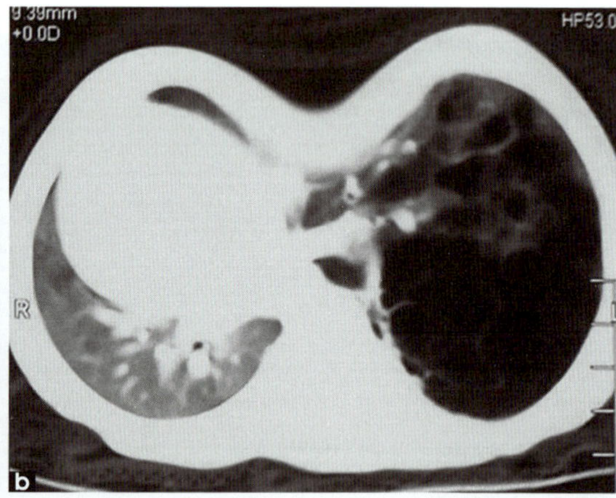

Fig. 8.50: Congenital cystic adenomatoid malformation (CCAM-II). (a) The radiograph shows contralateral mediastinal shift due to hyperlucent cysts; (b) CT scan shows multiple cyst-like lesions, prominence of the ipsilateral chest and a pectus excavatum.

etc. However, it has the potential to miss small millimeter size lesions within the parenchyma.

CT imaging has been considerably augmented by contrast enhancement, high resolution scans, and spiral CT. These also permit evaluation of the mediastinal contents and vasculature. CT scans must be ordered judiciously, and this is currently best left to the expert.

More advanced imaging modalities, such as magnetic resonance imaging (MRI), positron emission tomography (PET), and SPECT-CT, are neither routinely feasible nor perhaps required in children with chest diseases.

D. Lung Function Tests

Lung function tests have variable benefit in making a diagnosis in children with respiratory conditions; however, they are more useful in serial monitoring and follow-up of these children.

1. Spirometry

The most used lung function test in children is spirometry which measures flow during forced respiration. The child must take a deep breath and exhale as forcefully and as rapidly as possible. The spirometer measures the volume and flow rate during these maneuvers. Spirometry can help to decide whether airway obstruction is predominantly in the larger or smaller airways. The great difficulty with spirometry is getting children to perform the test properly; the results depend heavily on the motivation and capability of the child to perform the test. Therefore, the test is often

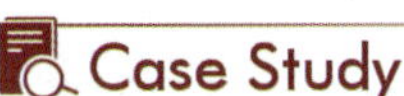

Case Study

CASE VIGNETTE 1

A 10-year-old girl underwent a left sided pneumonectomy. She presented with an episode of fever, cough, and rapid breathing. Chest examination revealed drooping of the left shoulder and tracheal deviation towards the left side. The position of the left nipple was slightly lower than the right nipple. The cardiac apex was palpable in the left fifth intercostal space approximately 3 cm lateral to the mid-clavicular line. There was a dull note on percussion over the left lung fields. Additionally, breath sounds were absent in the same area.

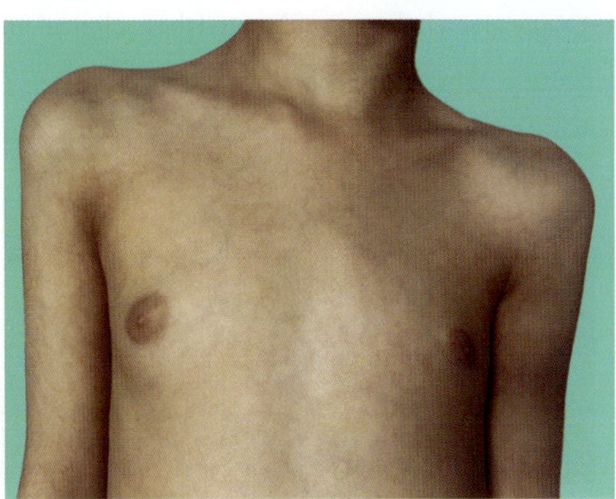

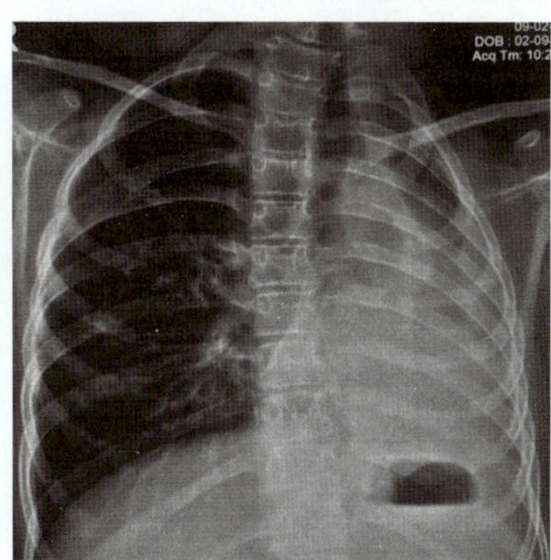

What do these findings suggest?

Volume loss on the left side that is likely long-standing in duration. The photograph showing drooping of the left shoulder, and the left nipple at a level lower than the right.

What does the chest X-ray show?

It shows trachea-mediastinal shift towards the left with relative hyperinflation of the right lung.

CASE VIGNETTE 2

A 2-year-old infant with pulmonary Langerhans cell histiocytosis (LCH) presented with sudden-onset respiratory distress, characterized by rapid breathing and subcostal retractions. On examination, she had a rightward shift of the trachea and a bulging of the left chest wall. Palpation revealed decreased vocal fremitus and decreased chest expansion on the left side. Percussion over the left intercostal, axillary, infrascapular, and interscapular areas revealed hyper-resonance, while auscultation in the same area revealed diminished breath sounds and decreased vocal resonance.

What do these findings suggest?

Left-sided pneumothorax.

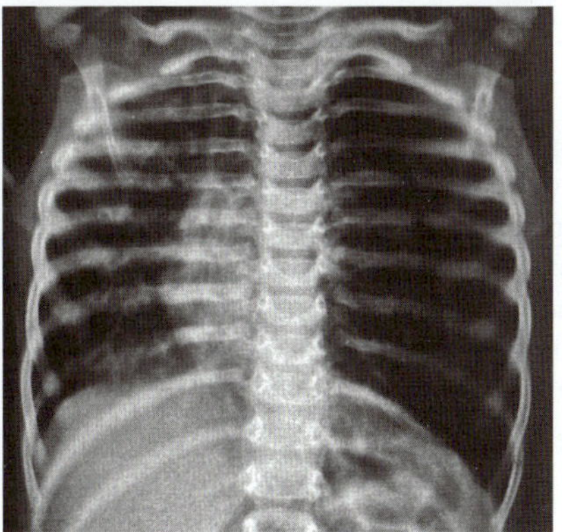

What does the chest X-ray show?

Chest X-ray shows left sided massive pneumothorax, with tracheal and mediastinal shift to the contralateral side, and a flattened dome of the diaphragm.

CASE VIGNETTE 3

A 4-year-old girl with cystic fibrosis presented with a 2-day fever, rapid breathing, and increased cough. On examination, there was right shoulder drooping, tracheal deviation towards the right, and flattening of the right side of the chest as compared to the left (shown below). Percussion revealed dullness over the right infra-axillary and infrascapular areas, with decreased vocal resonance and diminished breath sounds in the same area.

What do these findings suggest?

Clinical examination findings suggest volume loss on the right side. There could be a right-sided lung collapse, most likely secondary to mucus plugging. The chest X-ray given below corroborated these clinical findings.

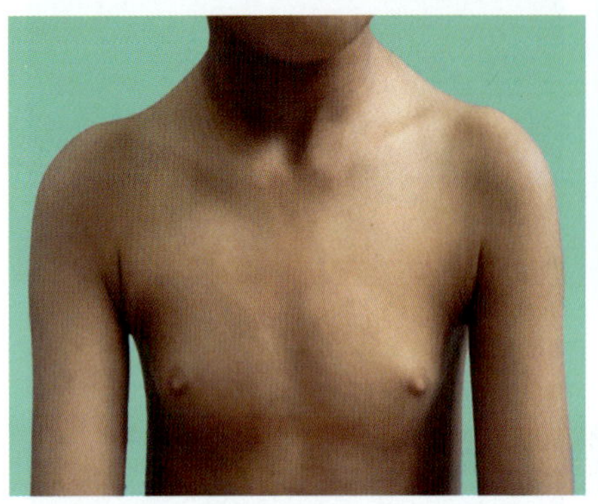

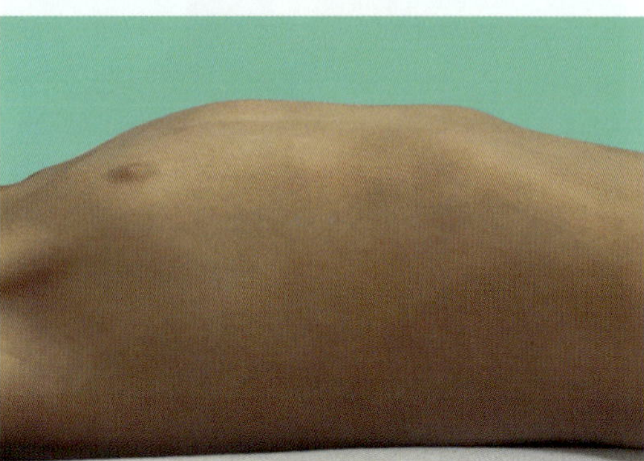

What does the chest X-ray show?

Tracheal deviation towards the right, along with mediastinal shift; and segmental collapse in the right lower lobe.

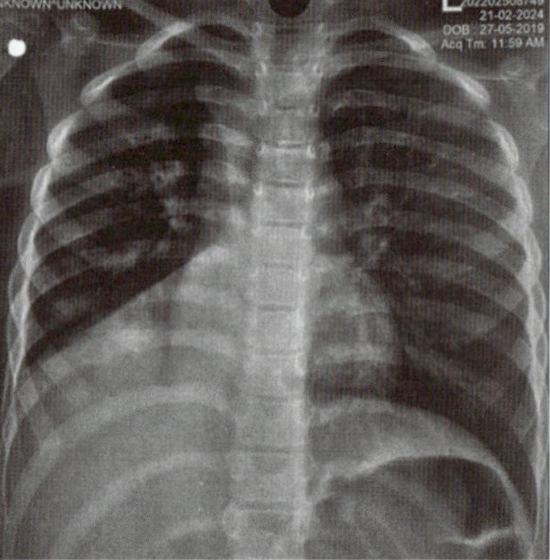

CASE VIGNETTE 4

An 8-year-old boy presented with intermittent fever over a period of 10 months. It was associated with intermittent pain in the upper chest (on both sides) increasing with deep breaths. ON clinical examination, the trachea was centrally placed, chest expansion was symmetrical, the apex beat was positioned normally, but there was a stony dull note in the infra-axillary and infra-scapular areas on both sides. Breath sounds were diminished in these areas.

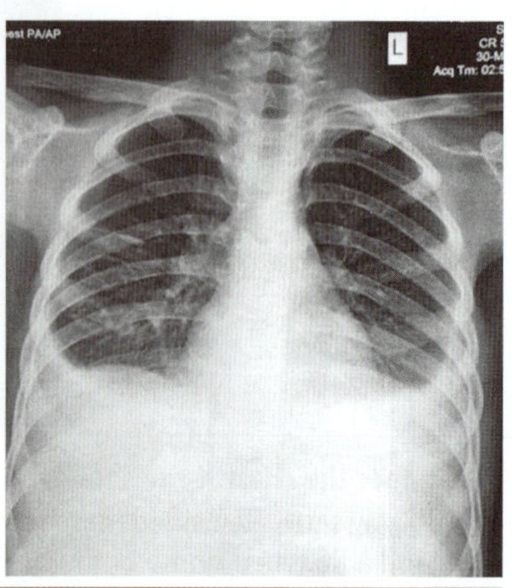

What do these findings suggest?

Bilateral pleural effusion.

What does the chest X-ray show?

The chest X-ray shows bilateral pleural effusion, which explains the absence of mediastinal shift.

CASE VIGNETTE 5

A 10-year-old boy developed fever, followed by cough after 5 days. He gradually developed left-sided chest pain and difficulty in breathing. At a private clinic, a chest X-ray was done without clinical examination. It suggested pleural effusion, hence an intercostal drainage tube was inserted. When he was examined at a referral hospital after 10 days, the chest tube was *in situ*, the trachea was centrally placed, cardiac apex did not appear to be shifted, and there was drooping of the left shoulder with flattening of the left side of the chest. Percussion revealed a stony dull note on the entire left side, bronchial breath sounds in the left infraclavicular area and diminished breath sounds on the entire left side.

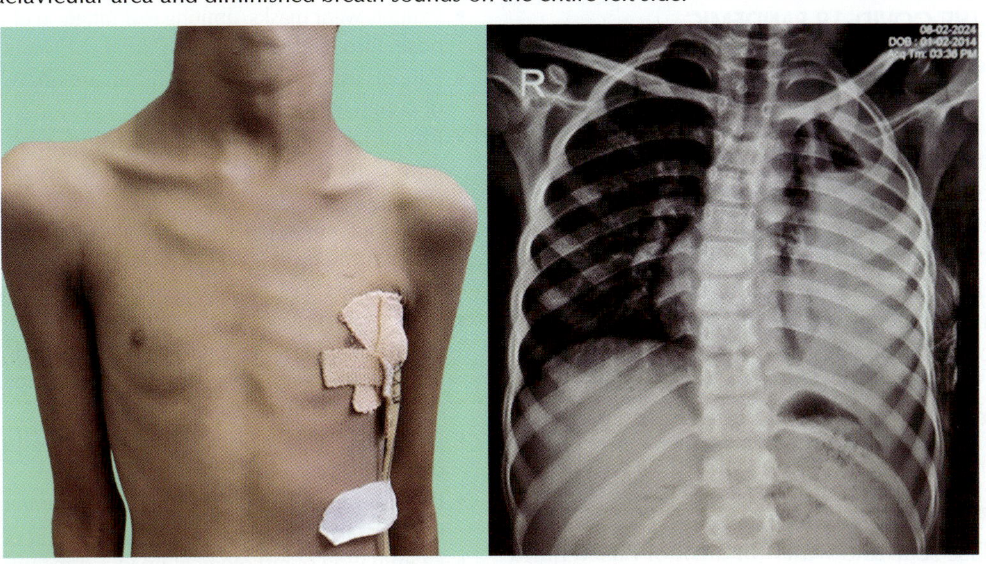

What do these findings suggest?

The clinical findings suggest left lung with consolidation with parapneumonic effusion (or empyema). The features of volume loss can be explained by associated collapse of the ipsilateral lung.

What does the chest X-ray show?

The chest X-ray matches the clinical findings. It additionally shows crowding of the ribs confirming volume loss. The chest tube is difficult to identify.

---

unreliable in young children, especially below 5 to 6 years of age.

2. Peak Expiratory Flow Rate (PEFR)

A simpler tool that is less expensive and easy to perform is the measurement of peak expiratory flow rate using a peak flow meter. This is a handy device into which the child blows as hard as possible. A sliding marker directly gives the peak expiratory flow; this is compared against norms based on height or against the personal best recording of the child himself. Peak flow monitoring is useful to follow-up children with obstructive airways especially asthma.

3. Forced Oscillation Technique

This technique measures the mechanical properties of the respiratory system. In this, sound waves of different frquencies are superimposed on tidal breathing. The machine analyses the flow and pressure pattern of distortion of returned oscillation waves providing resistance (R) and reactance (X). R is the measure of frictional forces applied by the airway on sound waves and X is measure of elsaticity (compliance) of airways. As it can be performed during tidal breathing, it requires minimal coppertion of the child, hence it can be performed in children as young as 3–6 yeard old, who cannot perform spirometry. However, large variability in parameters among the population and lack of normative data are major limitations in applying this technique widely.

4. Plethysmography

Measurement of lung volumes is a useful lung function test that is not widely available in our country. This requires complex equipment that measures dilution of a gas or direct measurement of volumes by whole body plethysmography. Lung volume measurement helps to quantify restrictive lung disease and also air trapping in obstructive conditions.

8.8 SPECIAL CONSIDERATIONS RELATED TO THE COVID-19 PANDEMIC

The current COVID-19 pandemic poses several challenges to successful examination of the respiratory system in children. Some of these are listed in **Key Box 11**. To overcome these challenges, it is important that physicians, policymakers (or hospital administrators), parents and patients (i.e. children) work together to ensure a safe examination procedure for all concerned. This necessitates basic education, implementation of standard guidelines, and following standard precautions. Some of the elements are highlighted below.

Hand Hygiene

- Use soap and water (or alcohol-based hand sanitizer solution).
- Ensure all steps are followed diligently.
- Avoid taking shortcuts in the interest of saving time.
- Educate parents and families about appropriate hand hygiene.

Respiratory Hygiene/Cough Etiquette

- Request parents to cover their and their child's mouth and nose during coughing or sneezing.
- If a handkerchief or tissue paper is/are used, it should be handled and/or disposed appropriately.
- Clean hands after coughing/sneezing.

Personal Protective Equipment

- Use a facemask.
- Ensure that the patient and family members are also using face masks.
- Use (non-sterile) gloves during examination procedures that may result in contact with airway secretions.
- Consider additional protection layers (such as a gown) especially when handling a crying infant.

Key Box 11

Challenges in Respiratory System Examination during the COVID-19 Pandemic

- Risk of droplet transmission during normal breathing in those with suspected infection.
- Generation of aerosol during crying.
- Patients wear masks, limiting examination of the nose, throat, etc.
- Patients especially young children are unaware of cough etiquette.
- Physicians may need to examine a child from behind a transparent screen (rather than directly).
- Direct examination is somewhat cumbersome through multiple layers of personal protective equipment (PPE).
- Remote respiratory system evaluation through tele-health platforms of Information Technology (IT) systems (using video-conferencing or social media apps) can be prone to errors.
- Donning full PPE (in COVID or SARI wards) precludes auscultation altogether.
- Post-examination sanitization of the room/area is necessary.
- Examination of radiological images transmitted through low fidelity apps (notably on social media) can mask as well as unduly emphasize findings.
- Special precautions are required for (otherwise) routine aids to respiratory examination, such as peak flow measurement, spirometry, collection of respiratory specimens for microbiologic analysis, etc.
- Safe disposal of biomedical waste at the point-of-care.

- Aerosol generating procedures should be undertaken only with full PPE including N-95 respirator, hazmat suit, eye protection and splash guard.

Safe Handling of Biomedical Waste

- Follow institutional guidelines for cleaning and sterilization of reusable equipment, devices, accessories.
- Dispose non-reusable items in appropriate bins, using the recommended disinfection solutions.
- Ensure disinfection of the room/area where physical examination is performed.
- For details of donning/doffing of masks, gloves, and PPE, refer to Chapter 18.

Chapter

9

Evaluation of the Cardiovascular System

❍ S Srinivasan ❍ Photographs by Arul Raj

Structure

"We were never tired of visiting and examining and auscultating, and of examining and auscultating again and again."

Peter Mere Latham (1789–1875)

9.1 APPROACHING A CHILD WITH POSSIBLE CARDIOVASCULAR DISORDER

Clinical evaluation of a possible cardiovascular disorder in adult medicine has always laid emphasis on systematic and sequential approach (e.g. eliciting history of illness, performing inspection, palpation, percussion and auscultation, considering the diagnostic possibilities and arriving at the most probable diagnosis). Such an approach has been recommended so that no essential physical findings—positive and negative—get missed or omitted.

In neonates and small children, especially those who are apprehensive, uncooperative or extremely sick, it is common sense that such an approach is not always possible.

- Follow a flexible approach as permitted by the child.
- Gain the child's confidence by developing your own style of diplomatic, tactful, and patient approach.
- Realize beyond doubt that a good history followed by careful inspection of the child will be the most rewarding experience in arriving at a diagnosis.
- General instructions are listed in **Key Box 1**.

Main Objectives of Evaluation of a Child with Symptoms Suggestive of a Cardiac Problem

1. Assess the child quickly for any life-threatening emergency. Defer detailed history taking and physical examination till the child gets stabilized and is out of danger, in the following situations: Severe state of breathlessness, cyanotic spell, shock state, pallor with lethargy, and heart failure. Quickly assess, resuscitate, and stabilize.
2. Obtain and record the chronological evolution of all symptoms of presenting illness and relevant illness in the past and other related details.
3. Perform a thorough physical examination of the child, anthropometry, presence of any external dysmorphic features, malformations and anomalies, microcephaly, cataracts, epicanthus, ear, lip,

Key Box 1

General Important and Useful Instructions

- Do not address the child under discussion as a case.
- Do not refer the index child as an *"interesting case."* What is interesting academically to you is often an agonizing experience for the child and parents.
- Do not make inappropriate comments or discuss the findings, diagnosis, prognosis, or offer your opinion regarding the child's condition in the presence of the child and parents.
- Do not laugh or crack jokes with fellow students at the child's bedside.
- Give due regards to the personal feelings, emotions, dignity, and privacy of the child and parents.
- Avoid placing hands or stethoscopes of many at the same time over the chest or abdomen to appreciate the demonstrated findings.
- Be polite while talking to parents and empathize with their concerns and anxieties.
- Do not be rough in handling the child.
- Do not disturb a sleeping child to elicit findings. In cardiac cases, findings can be more easily obtained when a child sleeps than in one who is awake, crying, and apprehensive.
- Do not examine the older children or the adolescent in the absence of their parents or chaperone.

palatal anomalies, short neck with webbing, clinodactyly, arachnodactyly, xanthomas, neurocutaneous lesions, e.g. neurofibromas, hemangiomas, cobble stone appearance of skin, etc. suggestive of primary etiology as mentioned in Point no 4.

Relevant organ system suggested by the symptoms must be examined in a systematic manner so as not to miss any vital diagnostic clinical sign or clue.

4. Analyze and synthesize the data collected by history taking and positive and negative clinical findings to postulate the most plausible, sensible and acceptable working diagnosis of the cardiovascular problem the child has , its etiology (congenital—genetic/ chromosomal or acquired—infective, nutritional, postinfective/autoimmune , endocrinal, traumatic, etc.), type, severity, associated complications, its impact on growth and development, functional limitation and its social, psychological and financial impact on the family.
5. Arrive at a diagnostic possibility, consider the alternate diagnostic possibilities, and chalk out appropriate cost-effective and rational plan of investigative work up and treatment options. Communicate patiently and effectively to the parents about the condition, management, follow-up plan, and preventive measures.
6. Demonstrate the proficiency and competency level in the acquisition of essential clinical skills in performing cardiac examination in children, cognitive skills in discussing differential diagnosis, and in counseling skills **(Table 9.1)**.
7. Take care to minimize the physical and mental discomfort to the child and parents.

9.2 HISTORY-TAKING

History-taking for clinical evaluation of a child with cardiac problem is as valuable as a road map navigator to a car driver trying to reach a destination in a new, untraveled, unfamiliar territory. A carefully elicited history and proper clinical examination still retain their relevance in arriving at an accurate diagnosis in more than 60% of childhood cardiac conditions.

A. Clinical Evaluation of a Child presumed to have a Cardiac Condition

Step 1

Observe the child right from the moment of entry into the chamber for medical consultation.

Step 2

Assess rapidly the child's airway, breathing and circulation status for presence of life-threatening cardiocirculatory and respiratory emergencies: Cardiogenic shock states, cyanotic spells, acute left ventricular failure with pulmonary edema, life-threatening tachy- or bradyarrhythmias **(Key Box 2)**. Stabilize the child before proceeding further.

Step 3

Elicit and record (a) symptoms—their evolution and analysis; and (b) details of relevant events and illness, admissions, medications,

Table 9.1: Four areas of skills and competencies expected of a clinician

The learner must be able to demonstrate comprehensive understanding and performance in the following areas:

Expected skills	Areas of performance
Cognitive	• Theoretical aspects • Analytical and interpretative capabilities in arriving at a reasonably good diagnosis • Management: Plan of investigations, treatment and preventive aspects, e.g. medical, surgical, etc.
Clinical	• History eliciting skills • Skills in: Observation, palpation, percussion, and auscultation
Attitudinal	• Approach to the child (flexible) • Manner of performance of examination (gentleness and ease in handling the child; caring, kind and friendly attitude) • Respecting the privacy and sentiments of the child and parents • Follow hand hygiene during examination
Communication	• Case presentation • History-taking • Case discussion • Differential diagnoses • Plan of management • Parental counseling

surgeries, records of previous investigations, antenatal period, birth details, growth and development, and immunizations received.

Step 4

Perform general physical examination for:

- General appearance and well-being, posture (decubitus-squatting), comfort level, activity, behavior
- *Vital parameters:* Respiratory rate, pattern of breathing, pulse, heart rate and rhythm, capillary refilling time, jugular venous pulse (JVP), blood pressure recording in both upper and lower limbs
- *Stature and build:* Weight, height, BMI, upper/lower segment ratio, arm span *vs* height
- Dysmorphic features of chromosomal or genetic syndromes, other minor and major external malformations
- Anemia, cyanosis, dependent pitting limb or sacral edema, puffiness of eyelids, clubbing of fingers and toes, oral cavity, teeth and pharynx, skin and joints

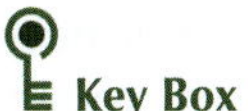

Key Box 2

Life-threatening Cardiac Emergencies in Newborn

Neonates with weak pulses, shock-like states in the absence of sepsis, lethargy, inactivity, pale ashen or cyanosed appearance

Consider: Ductus-dependent lesions with reduced blood flow to:

a. *Pulmonary circulation:* Transposition of great arteries with intact ventricular septum; pulmonary atresia (PA); and tricuspid atresia (TA)
b. *Systemic circulation:* Hypoplastic left heart syndrome (HLHS), aortic atresia or critical aortic stenosis (AS); interrupted aortic arch syndrome; and coarctation of aorta

Step 5

- Examine the cardiovascular system
- *Inspect:* Chest and precordium
- *Palpate:* Peripheries, pulse, blood pressure, precordium, liver, spleen
- *Percuss:* Specific areas
- *Auscultate "prescribed areas" over the precordium.* Heart sounds, other sounds (clicks, rub), murmurs, and over the chest for abnormal lung auscultatory findings and other areas outside the chest, whenever necessary.

Step 6

Analyze and discuss the collected data to offer a comprehensive diagnosis, discuss differential diagnosis; offer investigative and treatment plan.

B. Symptoms of Cardiovascular Disorders in Neonates and Infants

Enquire for presence of the following symptoms that often indicate a cardiac condition in neonates and infants. Their postulated pathophysiology is described below:

- *Interrupted feeding and 'suck-rest-suck cycle' during breastfeeding:* Respiratory muscle fatigue because of increased work load and reduced blood flow to these muscles, equivalent to exertional dyspnea in older children.
- *Fast breathing (tachypnea):* Stimulation of pulmonary interstitial J receptor.
- *Shortness of breath (breathing difficulty/ dyspnea):* Increased work of breathing due to lung congestion causing decrease in lung compliance.
- *Sudden collapse:* Shock secondary to obstructed or compromised blood supply.
- *Excessive forehead sweating:* Increased adrenergic output to support increased cardiac output.
- *Recurrent lower respiratory tract infection:* Lung congestion, airways compression by bronchial vessel and pulmonary vessel, dilation due to increased blood flow and resultant stasis of secretion—predisposing to infection.
- *Bluishness of oral cavity, tongue (cyanosis):* Increased deoxygenated hemoglobin.
- *Bluish spells on crying:* Increased chemoreceptor sensitivity, physical activity, and cry-induced infundibular spasm.
- *Failure to thrive:* Increased calorie demand and decreased intake.
- *Restlessness, lethargy, irritability, sleep disturbances:* Decreased perfusion to the CNS.
- *Inactivity, easy fatigability, decreased activity:* Decreased perfusion to the various organs and/or perfusion of blood with decreased oxygen saturation.
- *Abnormal precordial activity, feeling of abnormal pulsations and thrill by mother while giving bath:* Increased sympathetic drive and compensatory increase of heart rate, hyperdynamic circulation.
- *Swelling of eyelids and feet, abdominal distension, hepatomegaly, and ascites:* Renal salt and water retention, CCF, increase in venous hydrostatic pressure and increased fluid transudate across capillaries.
- *Precordial bulge* and chest wall deformity in severe and chronic cardiac problem.
- *Decreased urination:* Decreased effective renal blood flow, salt and water conservation.
- *Delayed gross motor development:* Recurrent hospitalization, decreased CNS stimulation, and limited calorie supply.
- *Rash:* Kawasaki disease, congenital systemic lupus erythematosus, infective endocarditis, myocarditis.
- *Dysmorphic facies or extracardiac anomalies:* Many of these are genetic or chromosomal disorders/syndromes with associated congenital heart defects.

C. Symptoms in Older Children

The common symptoms reported by parents in children beyond 2 years of age are as follows: Shortness of breath with physical activity while engaged in peer-related games and motor activities, like climbing stairs or going up a slope, easy fatigability and excessive tiredness, not showing interest in outdoor games, recurrent lower respiratory infections, bluishness, squatting, palpitation, chest pain, fainting episodes, failure to gain weight or sudden weight gain with decreased urination with swelling of feet, pain in calf muscles on walking (intermittent claudication), shortness of breath and cough on lying down, cough with hemoptysis, prolonged fever, and rarely sudden paralytic attacks secondary to embolic phenomena. Common symptoms are discussed below.

1. Breathing Difficulty

(*Dyspnea, shortness of breath, getting out of breath*) **(Key Box 3)**.

Breathing difficulty or shortness of breath is uncomfortable breathing experienced and expressed by older children. They express this difficulty in breathing in many ways, such as getting out of breath with fast and labored breathing or feeling short of breath or getting

Key Box 3

History of Breathing Difficulty

Ask for

- Type of onset? (sudden in few seconds or minutes, gradual over days)
- Nature or rapidity of progression (Rapid/Slow)?
- Severity (Grading)?
- Duration?
- Frequency?
- Precipitating events? Triggers?
- Aggravating and relieving factors?
- Associated symptoms (chest pain, cough, palpitation, sweating, anxiety, fear, swelling of feet, puffiness of eyelids, decreased urination, sleep disturbances)?

suffocated. In infants and young children, the same is perceived and reported by their parents. Dyspnea indicates difficult breathing which may be associated with working of accessory respiratory muscles.

Episodes of dyspnea are not unusual with more than the usual levels of physical activities and in exhaustive exertion, e.g. climbing high hills and mountains. But if it occurs at usual levels of physical activities and in exhaustive exertion or in the absence of respiratory problems, like bronchiolitis, asthma, or anemia, this suggests the possibility of an underlying cardiac disorder.

This suspicion is strengthened when the child is afebrile and has associated forehead sweating, even at rest. The cause of cardiac dyspnea is related to the decreased filling or emptying ability of the affected heart, resulting in elevation of pulmonary arterial and venous pressures and congestion of lungs.

Rapid breathing with chest indrawing in an otherwise happy, smiling, and active infant strongly suggests an underlying cardiac cause.

2. Suck-stop Cycles in Neonates

It presents as frequent pauses (stops) during breastfeeding; necessitated by increasing, rapid, labored breathing while the neonate sucks at the breast. This is the only vital exercise needing efforts by neonates and young infants.

3. Dyspnea

After 1 year of age, when children become mobile, breathing difficulty is brought about by motor exertions (such as active sitting, crawling, and walking).

4. Orthopnea

The child experiences increasing difficulty in breathing on lying down in a recumbent position. The child gets greatly relieved in the sitting position, more on bending forwards while sitting. This is also associated with cough while lying down.

5. Paroxysmal Nocturnal Dyspnea (PND)

PND refers to episodes of sudden onset of severe breathing difficulty associated with apprehensive feelings of suffocation or choking sensation and air hunger at nights in a sleeping child. The paroxysm results in sudden awakening. On awakening and after sitting up, the child gets some relief which is often transient. The rapid, shallow respiration when accompanied by cyanosis or bouts of wet cough with frothy sputum and streaks of blood indicates grave prognosis.

PND occurs in conditions where there is increased left atrial pressure and pulmonary venous hypertension, e.g. mitral stenosis, acute pulmonary edema, and hypertensive left ventricular failure.

The basic mechanisms involved are left ventricular dysfunction, fall in PaO_2 and a rise in left atrial pressure during sleep in recumbent position. It is often a medical emergency necessitating immediate hospitalization for appropriate control of left ventricular failure.

6. Palpitations

Palpitation is a subjective symptom of one's own awareness of heartbeats and hence is not a common complaint in young children below 5 years **(Key Box 4)**. Sometimes in younger children, an intelligent mother will note rapid, obvious precordial activity and bring to the notice of the physician.

It is likely to indicate cardiac problems (heart blocks, arrhythmias, volume overload states secondary to regurgitant lesions, large left to right shunts, or mitral stenosis) or non-cardiac problems, such as anxiety states,

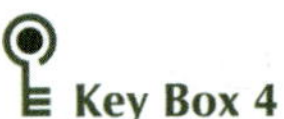

Key Box 4

History for Palpitation

1. When? – At rest or on exertion
2. How sudden?
3. How long? – Duration
4. How often? – Frequency
5. How severe? – Functional limitation of child's activities like school absenteeism; inability to play games? What precipitates?
6. What aggravates and what relieves? – Physical activity, emotional disturbances, drugs, etc.
7. What are other associated cardiac symptoms?

severe anemia, thyrotoxicosis, or other high cardiac output states.

Palpitation assumes greater significance when associated with breathlessness, chest pain, giddiness, or syncope. Palpitation at rest or with minimal activity needs immediate evaluation.

7. Cyanosis (Bluishness of body, nails, mouth and tongue) and Cyanotic Spells

- *Ask parents:* Have they noticed bluish discoloration of body or in any other body part, like skin, tongue, lips, oral mucosa, conjunctiva, or nails?
- Probe further by asking the following questions, if they had noticed bluish discoloration:
  a. *Time of onset:* Since when? From birth **(Key Box 5)**, from day 1 of life, or later in the neonatal period, infancy, or later childhood.
  b. *Sites of bluishness:* Where are all noticeable? Generalized—whole body, tongue, nails; and toes; or Localized to a few areas—upper or lower part of the body.
  c. *Severity:* Markedly bluish and hence easily noticed by all in the family; Moderate—seen only on careful observation by parents, and minimal—seen only after being informed earlier by the treating pediatrician.
  d. *Episodes of severe or intense bluish spells* with breathlessness (cyanotic spells), its frequency, precipitating, aggravating and relieving factors of such episodes, hospitalizations for the same, and treatment details.
  e. *History of cyanotic spells,* along with episodes of *squatting* indicates a lesion with decreased pulmonary blood flow, such as tetralogy of Fallot (TOF).
  f. *History suggestive of heart failure and recurrent respiratory infections* suggests a cyanotic heart disease with increased pulmonary blood flow, e.g. TGA.

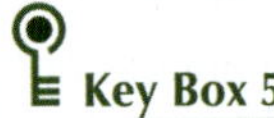

Key Box 5

Cyanosis from Birth and Persisting till now

- Transposition of great arteries (TGA)
- Tricuspid atresia
- Pulmonary atresia
- Severe pulmonary stenosis with interatrial defect

**Obstructive type of infradiaphragmatic total anomalous pulmonary venous drainage presents with severe cyanosis soon after birth with marked respiratory distress resembling hyaline membrane diseases or Group B streptococcal pneumonia.*

8. Squatting

Squatting is the posture assumed for symptomatic relief from exertional breathlessness. This posture is suggestive of a cyanotic heart disease with decreased pulmonary blood flow **(Key Box 6)**. Usually, there is an underlying large ventricular septal defect, with associated pulmonary obstructive lesion and a delicate right to left shunting. Tetralogy of Fallot is the most common example.

Mechanism of relief: Squatting promptly relieves the increasing breathlessness by improving the oxygen saturation.

9. Chest Pain

Chest pain of cardiac origin is relatively a rare symptom in children. Though chest pain in children and adolescents does not have the

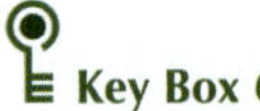

Key Box 6

Conditions in which Squatting causes Relief

1. Tetralogy of Fallot
2. Tricuspid atresia
3. Double outlet right ventricle with pulmonary stenosis
4. Single ventricle with pulmonary stenosis
5. Transposition of great arteries with pulmonary stenosis
6. Common atrioventricular canal with pulmonary stenosis

Two-phase response to squatting		
Phases	**Hemodynamic response**	**Mechanism of relief**
Initial first 15 seconds after squatting	Transient sudden phase of decreased venous return	Initial trapping of highly unsaturated blood in the lower extremity
Continued squatting beyond 2 minutes	• Steady increase in the venous return • Sustained increase in the pulmonary blood flow following decreased right to left shunt during the entire squatting period • Greater diversion of the blood flow more into the pulmonary artery and less into the over-riding aorta	• Increase in the systemic vascular resistance • Increase in the left ventricular pressure and the aortic afterload

same connotation as that experienced by the adults, the possibility of a cardiac cause cannot be totally ignored **(Key Box 7)**.

Enquire (from parents or directly from the child, if he/she is old enough to describe) and record the following:

a. ***Location, severity, and type of pain:*** Heaviness or pressure on the left side of the chest or squeezing pain strongly suggests ischemic pain; sharp, stabbing retrosternal pain points towards pericarditis.
b. ***Radiation:*** Pain radiating towards neck, throat, jaw, arm and shoulder suggests ischemic cardiac pain. Pain that radiates to left arm and/or shoulder suggests pericarditis. Pain radiating to the back or scapula suggests aortic dissection.
c. ***Timing, onset, and duration:*** Chest pain of aortic dissection or pulmonary embolism is acute in onset, whereas ischemic chest pain is more often gradual in onset.
d. ***Aggravating and relieving factors:*** The likelihood that the chest pain is of cardiac origin increases, if it is aggravated or precipitated by exertion.

Key Box 7

Common Causes of Chest Pain in Children

1. Unknown causes	25–45%
2. *Musculoskeletal* (Myalgia, osteochondritis)	30–40%
3. *Pleuropulmonary* (Pleuritis, pneumonia, severe asthma)	10–15%
4. *Gastrointestinal* (Gastroesophageal reflux, esophagitis, gastritis)	5–10%
5. *Psychological anxiety* and *stress*	3–5%
6. *Cardiac conditions*	1–3%

e. ***Associated cardiac symptoms:*** Fever, cough, vomiting, dysphagia, headache, palpitation, light headedness, syncope, exertional dyspnea, sweating, scanty micturition, and edema increase the possibility of a cardiac cause.

Cardiac causes of chest pain in children

1. Pericarditis
2. Severe aortic stenosis
3. Moderate-to-severe aortic regurgitation
4. Anomalous origin of left coronary artery from pulmonary artery (ALCAPA)
5. Kawasaki disease with coronary artery vasculitis
6. Autoimmune vasculitis states as in polyarteritis nodosa
7. Prolonged tachyarrhythmias (shortened diastolic interval decreases the coronary blood flow)
8. Hypertrophic obstructive cardiomyopathy (HOCM)
9. Mitral valve prolapse and dissecting aneurysm—Marfan syndrome
10. *Metabolic conditions:* Familial hypercholesterolemia, familial triglyceridemia, mucopolysaccharidosis, and homocystinuria.

10. Syncope

Syncope (dizzy spells) refers to sudden and near or transient loss of consciousness. Before reaching adolescence, between 15% and 50% of children experience at least one episode of syncope.

Most of the causes of syncope are benign, e.g. vasovagal attacks, prolonged standing,

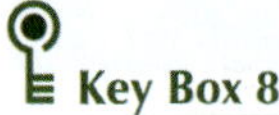

Key Box 8

Cardiac Causes of Syncope in Children

1. Severe aortic stenosis
2. Severe pulmonary stenosis
3. Coarctation of aorta
4. Dissecting aortic aneurysm
5. Mitral valve prolapse
6. Some types of heart blocks and tachyarrhythmias
7. Sick sinus syndrome and prolonged QT syndrome

postural changes, brief hypoglycemic episodes, and severe cough. Syncope associated with visual loss, scintillating scotomas, nausea, and vomiting may suggest other non-cardiac causes.

Syncopal episodes in association with other common cardiac symptoms of low cardiac output, such as dizziness, blurring of vision, easy fatigability, scanty micturition, and cold extremities, suggest a possible cardiac etiology **(Key Box 8)**. Syncope indicates severe forms of obstructive lesions in the outflow tracts of the great vessels. It may also point to the presence of cardiac arrhythmias.

D. Symptoms Suggestive of Associated Complications

1. Symptoms of Heart Failure

Sudden or insidious onset of increasing breathlessness, orthopnea, easy fatigability, decreased exercise tolerance, disturbing cough on lying down, wheeze, feeding difficulties, sleep disturbances with breathlessness or cough, brow sweating even in cold climate, eyelid and facial puffiness, dependent edema, decreased urine output, cold extremities, abdominal distension, and right quadrant pain indicates heart failure.

Remember: Pedal edema is uncommon and a late feature of heart failure in neonates and infants.

2. Symptoms of Bacterial Endocarditis

These include fever, skin rashes, hematuria, sudden onset of pallor, reddish streaks or spots in the nail beds, painful fingertips, and history suggestive of embolic phenomena.

3. Symptoms of Central Nervous System Complications

Symptoms of central nervous system complications (cerebrovascular thromboembolic accidents, intracranial abscess) include: Headache, vomiting, convulsions, syncope, altered sensorium, and limb weakness or paralysis.

E. Other Aspects in History

1. History of Abnormal Facies/ Congenital Malformations

Enquire tactfully from the mother without upsetting her whether she or her family members had noticed in her child anything special/odd in the facial and body features in comparison to her other children.

Parents may also bring children for check up to rule out the presence of a congenital heart disease, as they had previous children or other family members who had similar illness.

Many chromosomal disorders, other genetic, metabolic conditions and isolated malformations are associated with congenital heart diseases. Some common conditions are listed in the next section.

2. Growth and Development History

Both congenital and acquired heart diseases of moderate severity cause growth impairment and developmental delay. Many chromosomal and other genetic syndromes, maternal infections, metabolic disturbances, drug intake in first trimester are all associated with gross physical growth and developmental retardation.

3. Nutritional History

Nutritional intake, digestion, absorption, and assimilation are all affected to a variable extent. Nutritional deficiencies and excesses in mothers during pregnancy may result in cardiac malformations. Deficient intakes of vitamins, minerals, trace elements, and electrolytes may present with cardiac dysfunction.

4. Functional Status

Record the impact of the cardiac problem on the normal daily activities, educational school attendance, and sport activities.

- History of acute or chronic infections in various trimesters—fever, rashes, maternal rubella, and mumps.
- Other maternal illness—metabolic disorders, like diabetes mellitus, phenylketonuria, and other, e.g. systemic lupus erythematosus **(Table 9.2)**.
- Drugs—phenytoin, lithium, other anticonvulsants, herbal and native medicines **(Table 9.3)**.
- Substance abuse—alcohol.
- Exposure to irradiation, toxins, and environmental pollutants.

Table 9.2: Maternal metabolic conditions and associated cardiac conditions in the child

Metabolic conditions in the mother	Clinical features in the child	Cardiac association
Diabetes mellitus	Congenital malformations of CVS, CNS, and skeletal system; macrosomia, birth injuries, hypoglycemia, hypocalcemia, polycythemia, hyperbilirubinemia, caudal regression syndrome, respiratory distress syndrome	Hypertrophic obstructive cardiomyopathy, d-transposition of great arteries, double outlet RV, tetralogy of Fallot, truncus arteriosus
Phenylketonuria	Low birth weight, mental retardation, microcephaly, congenital heart defects	Coarctation of aorta, hypoplastic left heart syndrome
SLE	IUGR, thrombocytopenia, severe hydrops	Congenital heart block

Table 9.3: Maternal medications and cardiac malformations

Drugs	Congenital heart disease	Other clinical features
Valproate	Ventricular septal defect, coarctation of aorta, tetralogy of Fallot (TOF), hypoplastic left heart syndrome, valve defects	Trigonocephaly, medial eyebrow deficiency, epicanthal folds, infraorbital groove, anteverted nares, flat nasal bridge, cleft lip and palate, neural tube defects (spina bifida, meningomyelocele).
Hydantoin	Pulmonic or aortic stenosis, coarctation of aorta, patent ductus arteriosus	Dysmorphic facies; microcephaly, epicanthal folds, motor delay, cleft lip and palate, hypoplastic nails and distal phalanges, mental retardation
Carbamazepine	d-Transposition of great arteries, atrial septal defect	Neural tube defects (spina bifida)
Primidone	Ventricular septal defect (VSD)	Neonatal hemorrhage; short stature, poor somatic development
Diazepoxides	Transposition of great arteries (TGA)	Hypotonia, respiratory depression
Lithium	Ebstein anomaly, tricuspid atresia, atrial septal defect	Hypotonia, limb anomalies
Trimethadione	Transposition of great arteries, tetralogy of Fallot, hypoplastic left heart syndrome	Ear malformation, hypoplastic midface, unusual eyebrow configuration
Sex hormones	VSD, TGA, TOF	Virilization of female fetus
Clomiphene	TOF	Microcephaly, harelip and cleft palate, undescended testes, polydactyly, conjoined twins, omphalocele, spina bifida occulta
Alcohol	VSD, TOF	*Fetal alcohol syndrome* microcephaly, epicanthal folds, small palpebral fissures, microphthalmia, ptosis, flat nose, smooth philtrum, thin upper lip, maxillary–midface–hypoplasia, cleft lip and palate, deafness, under-developed pinna, camptodactyly, clinodactyly, motor delay

6. Family History

Record the presence of any of the following in family members: Rheumatic fever, sudden unexplained deaths, SIDS, structural or congenital cardiac abnormalities in siblings, genetic, dysmorphogenic or inherited metabolic syndromes in the family.

The estimated recurrence risk of congenital heart disease is 2–6% when a previous sibling is affected, nearly 30% with 2 siblings affected, and 3%, if one of the parents is affected.

7. Treatment History

Document treatment, investigations, and intervention details during the neonatal period, early and late infancy. Note the following:

- Medications prescribed as drops, syrup, tablets, injections—name, dose, frequency, duration of drug treatment, compliance with recommended treatment, their effect in the control and relief of symptoms.
- Minor or major cardiac or non-cardiac surgical interventions or catheter procedures.
- Details of admissions—indications and hospital management details.
- Treatment for recurrent acute lower respiratory infections, rheumatic fever or carditis, recommended prophylactic treatment; if any.

9.3 PHYSICAL EXAMINATION

- Instruct the mother to uncover the chest of the infants and young children before her entry to your chamber. This step is extremely important as the child starts crying as soon as the mother removes the dress in front of the examiner.
- Keep a confident, reassuring, cheerful look when child enters your chamber.
- Do not touch the child at once.
- Initiate dialogue with parents or the mother in a very friendly manner.
- Do not stare at the child but glance periodically with an engaging smile.
- Hand over a colorful toy, block, or a picture book as a distraction or even the stethoscope to the child so that he gets familiarized with it.
- Make gentle and friendly gestures by touching his hands at the wrist or touching the dorsum of the feet on both sides over the dorsalis pedis, with him/her seated in the mother's lap. Note the warmth of the peripheries and the ease with which the arterial pulsations of radials and dorsalis pedis are felt. Also note whether pallor, cyanosis, or clubbing is present.

Few important findings related to cardiovascular system in general physical examination are shown in Fig. 9.1.

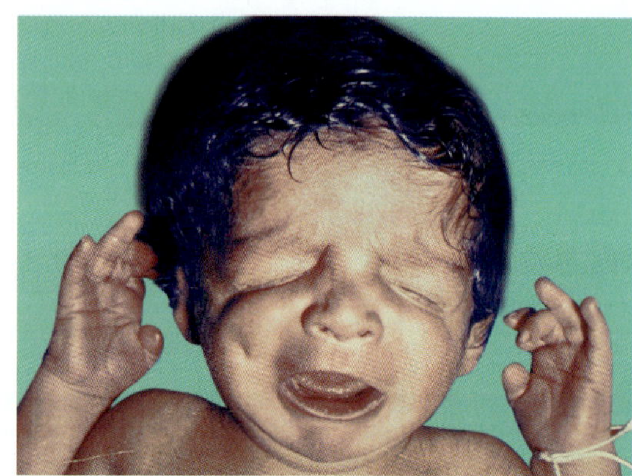

Fig. 9.1a: Antimongoloid slant.

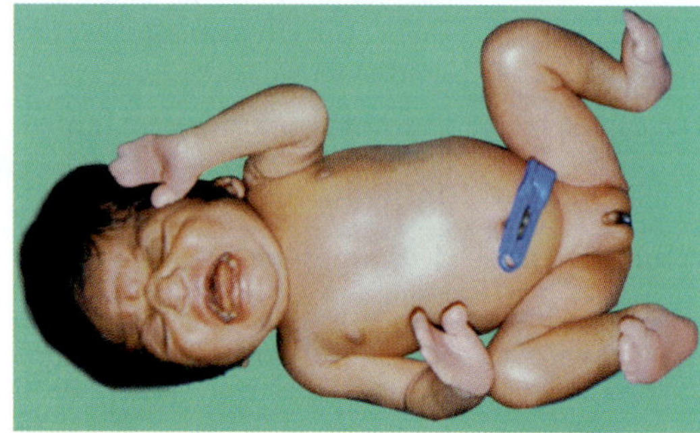

Fig. 9.1b: Tower skull, broad forehead, low set ears, depressed nasal bridge, cleft palate, and syndactyly of fingers and toes.

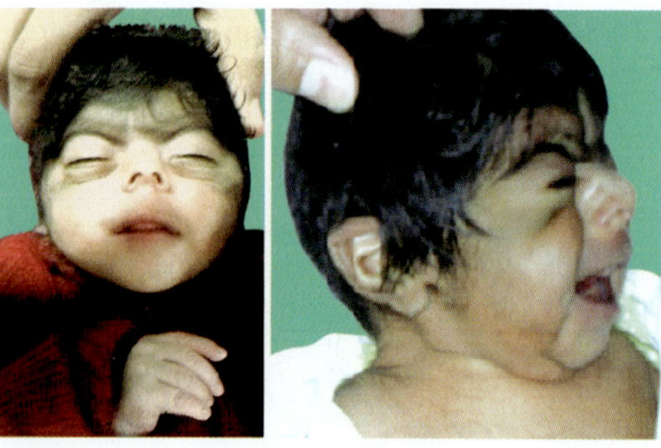

Fig. 9.1c: Synophrys in Cornelia de Lange syndrome.

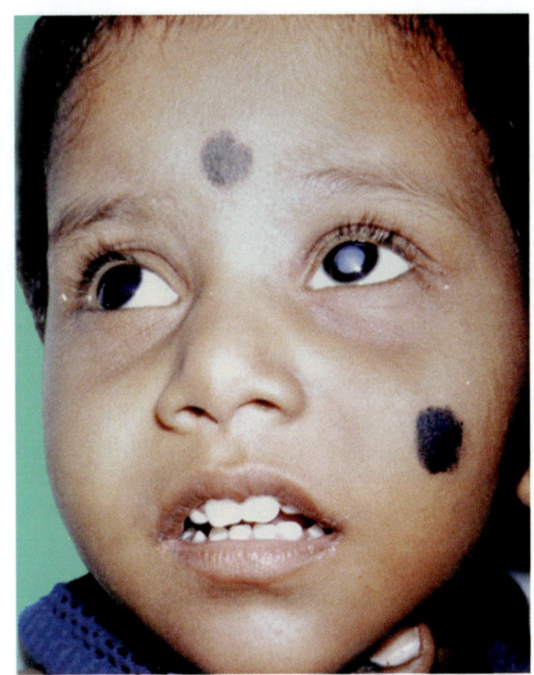

Fig. 9.1d: Unilateral cataract of lens in the left eye-association with congenital rubella syndrome, DiGeorge syndrome, and myotonic dystrophy.

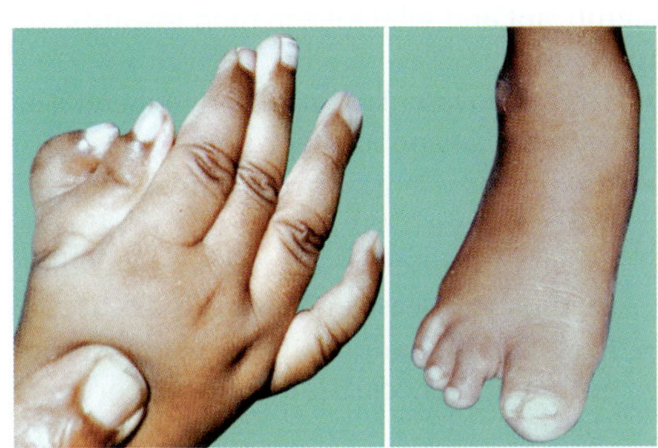

Fig. 9.1e: Preaxial polydactyly of fingers and toes.

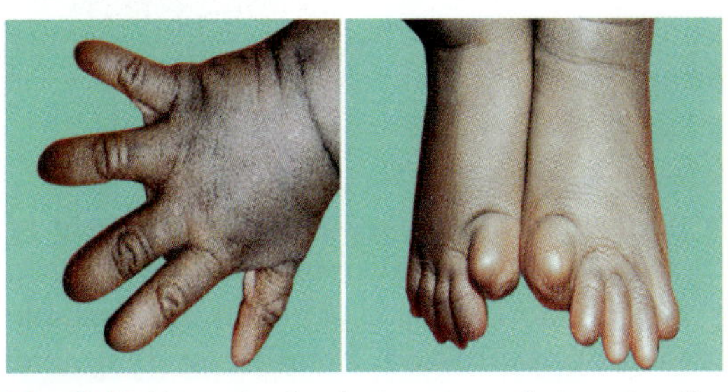

Fig. 9.1f: Hypoplastic phalanges and absent nails.

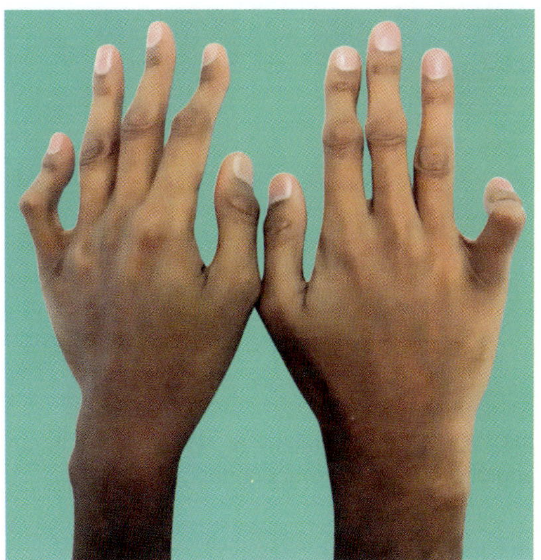

Fig. 9.1g: Arachnodactyly in Marfan syndrome.

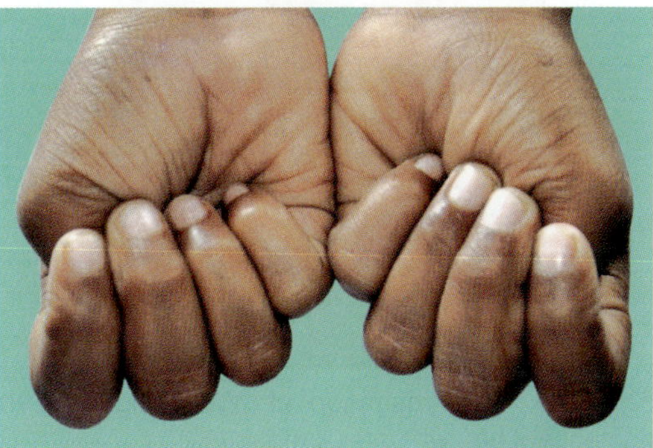

Fig. 9.1h: Demonstration of "Thumb Sign" in a normal child. Thumbs are well inside the clenched fingers.

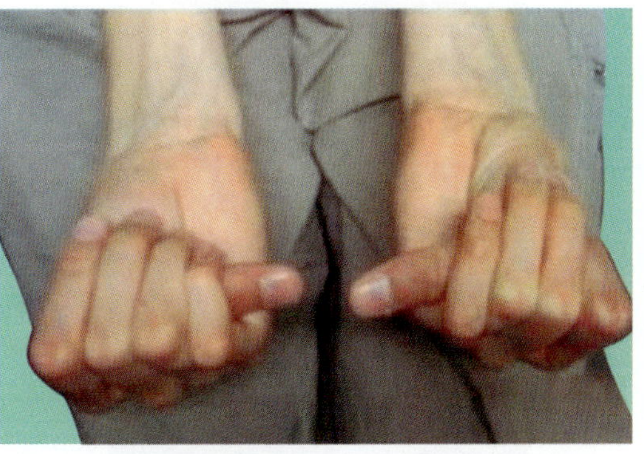

Fig. 9.1i: Demonstration of "Thumb Sign" in arachnodactyly in Marfan syndrome. Thumbs are projecting well outside the flexed fingers.

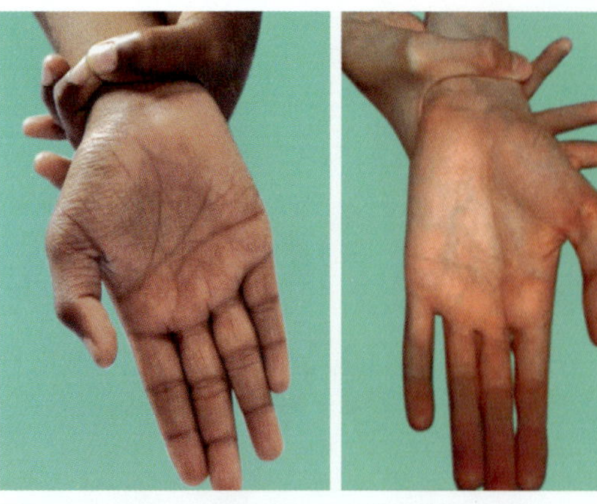

Fig. 9.1j: Demonstration of "Wrist Sign" in an adolescent boy with arachnodactyly.

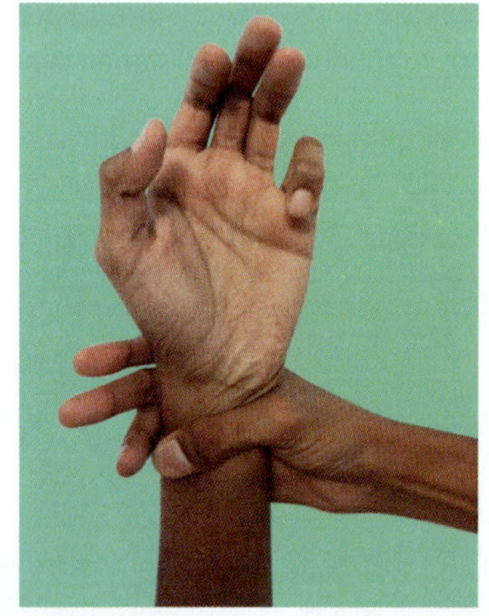

Fig. 9.1k: Demonstration of "Wrist Sign" in an adolescent boy with arachnodactyly.

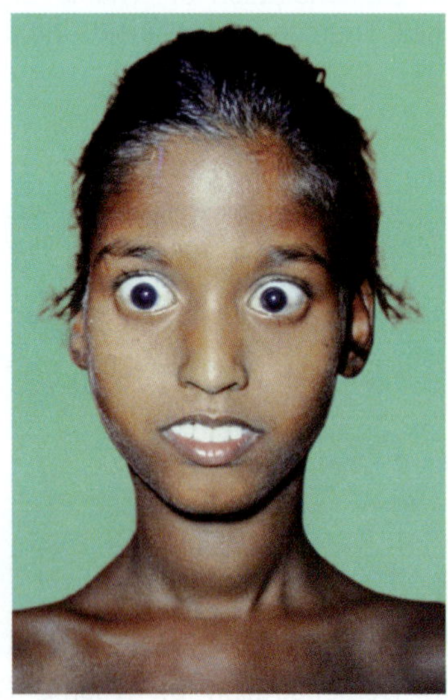

Fig. 9.1l: Bilateral exophthalmos and thyroid swelling—hyperthyroidism.

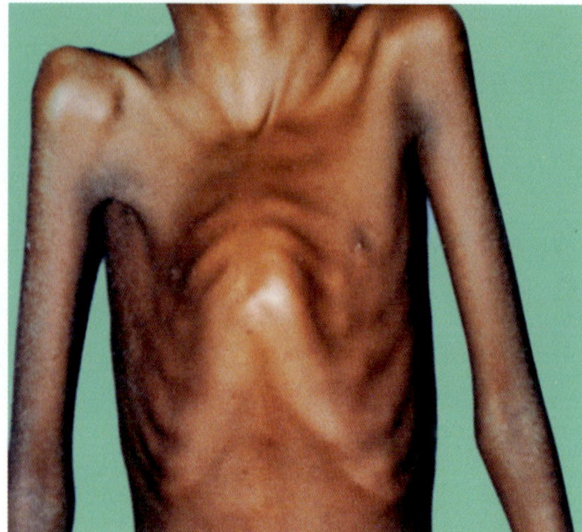

Fig. 9.1m: " Pigeon chest ": Pectus carinatum.

> "There is no more difficult art to acquire than the art of observation, and for some men it is quite as difficult to record an observation in brief and plain language."
>
> —William Osler

Inspect

Inspection when done properly gives significant and vital information towards the following:

- The cardiovascular diagnosis (congenital or acquired, cyanotic or acyanotic);
- Its etiology, e.g. chromosomal or dysmorphogenic syndromes, infective cause (intrauterine—congenital rubella), rheumatic disease or Kawasaki disease;
- Presence of complications, like bacterial endocarditis, cardiac failure, cerebral abscess;
- Presence of precipitating cause, like anemia, infections, or thyrotoxicosis; and
- The overall cardiac status.

Inspection starts the moment the child is brought for consultation or the moment you reach the bed where the child is already admitted.

Observe and Record

- ***General appearance (look) and state of well-being:*** Healthy or unwell, ill, very sick, toxic, pale, cyanosed or bluish, comfortable or not, distressed, breathless, dyspneic, tachypneic, orthopneic.

- ***Posture and position:*** In which position the child is comfortable or becomes uncomfortable or distressed.
- ***Sensorium, general activity, interactive level and behavior***
  - Apprehensive, excessively sleepy or drowsy
  - Active, alert and playful or tired, inactive
- ***Build:*** Tall (Marfan syndrome, homocystinuria) or short (Turner syndrome, Noonan syndrome)
- ***Dysmorphic facial features:*** Single or a combination of abnormal external physical anomalies in the body from head to foot.

Look at the following:

- ***Head and face:*** Eyes (puffiness/edema of eyelids), oral cavity, lips, tongue, palate (for cyanosis, glossitis, petechiae, enanthems), mucous membranes of eyes, mouth and oral cavity for congestion, teeth (for caries), tonsils, pharynx (sore throat and tonsillitis in streptococcal infection leading to rheumatic fever and carditis).
- ***Neck:*** Short or, long, webbing, hairline, pulsations, thyroid swelling.
- ***Extremities:*** Arms, legs, hands and fingers, upper arms and forearms, feet and toes.
- ***Nails:*** Color—pink, pale or cyanosed; clubbing of fingers and cyanosis of the nail bed; splinter bleeding spots.
- ***Palms:*** Erythema, Janeway lesions, rashes, desquamation (skin peeling in Kawasaki disease; and myocarditis following hand-foot-mouth disease), Osler nodes.
- ***Skin:*** Look for rashes, desquamation, subcutaneous nodules, erythema marginatum, photosensitivity, angiokeratomas, neurofibromas and xanthoma tuberosum over extensor surfaces of elbows, knees, ankles, and gluteal regions and xanthelasma near the inner canthi. Observe any laxity of skin (Down syndrome, Ehlers-Danlos syndrome, and pseudoxanthoma elasticum), subcutaneous nodules, and rashes.
- ***Bones and joints:*** Spine, sternum, joints, skeletal deformities: swelling, effusion. Possible clues for rheumatic fever, vasculitidis, cardiomyopathies. Swelling of the large and small/joints.

Key Box 9 enlists signs of infective endocarditis in general physical examination.

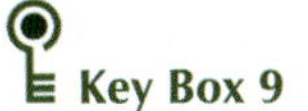

Signs of Infective Endocarditis in General Physical Examination

- Elevated body temperature
- Pallor and clubbing
- Palmar erythema
- *Janeway lesions:* Non-tender nodular lesions over the palms of hands and soles
- *Osler nodes:* Painful, tender, erythematous nodules or swellings at the palmar surface of pads of fingers and toes
- Splinter hemorrhages in the nails
- Roth spots Oval, flame-shaped hemorrhages in the fundus
- Splenomegaly
- Neurological deficit (variable) in presence of cerebral embolic phenomenon

A. Dysmorphic Features

Perform careful clinical evaluation of cardiovascular system in any child with following abnormal body physical features:

- ***Skull abnormalities:*** Microcephaly, macrocephaly, brachycephaly, oxycephaly, and plagiocephaly are associated with specific congenital heart diseases.
- ***Face:*** *Coarse facies* indicates conditions like Hurler syndrome, or Hunter syndrome that may be associated with cardiac disorders.
  - *Absence of depressor anguli oris* is associated with VSD, TOF, and ASD.
  - *Elfin facies* is characteristic of William syndrome. Also look for facial hypoplasia and abnormal grooves or clefts in the face.
- ***Eyes***
  - *Hypertelorism:* Noonan-Ullrich syndrome (pulmonary stenosis), Turner syndrome (coarctation of aorta), Klippel-Feil syndrome (ventricular septal defect), William syndrome (supravalvular aortic stenosis, pulmonary stenosis), Hurler syndrome (valvular regurgitation), and Leopard syndrome (pulmonary stenosis, hypertrophic obstructive cardiomyopathy)
  - *Epicanthus:* Down syndrome, Turner syndrome, William syndrome, fetal hydantoin syndrome

- *Mongoloid slant:* Down syndrome, Alagille syndrome
- *Anti-mongoloid slant* (outward and downward slanting of palpebral fissure) Cri-du-chat syndrome, Apert syndrome, Treacher Collins syndrome
- *Lens:* Cataract in congenital rubella syndrome, DiGeorge syndrome, and congenital myotonic dystrophy. Dislocation of lens in Marfan syndrome (anteriorly) and homocystinuria (posteriorly)
- *Eyebrows:* Synophrys (Cornelia de Lange syndrome), absent eyebrows (fetal alcohol syndrome)

- ***Ears:*** Low set, microtia, ear lobe crease, deafness, and pre-auricular sinus
- ***Nose:*** Broad, upturned, flat, or beaked
- ***Philtrum, mouth, tongue***
  - *Absent philtrum:* Thin upper lip in fetal alcohol syndrome
  - *Macroglossia:* Cretinism, Hurler syndrome, acromegaly, and Pompe disease
  - *Pseudomacroglossia:* Down syndrome
- ***Palate***
  - *High-arched palate:* Look for Marfan syndrome, Turner syndrome, Noonan syndrome, pseudoxanthoma elasticum, and Friedreich ataxia
  - *Cleft palate:* Velocardiofacial syndrome, fetal hydantoin syndrome, fetal alcohol syndrome, trisomy 13
  - *Bifid uvula:* Look for septal defects—ASD, VSD
- ***Neck***
  - *Short neck:* Ratio of height to the distance between external occipital protuberance and C7 processes (*Bird's index*): <12.8 is normal; >13.6 indicates short neck (platybasia, Klippel-Feil syndrome, Morquio syndrome)
  - *Webbed neck:* Turner syndrome, Noonan syndrome, trisomies
- ***Low hair line:*** Turner syndrome, Noonan syndrome
- ***Forearm, hand, and feet:*** Look for anomalies of extremities (forelimb or distal limb anomalies), phocomelia, camptomelia, and pes cavus
- ***Fingers and toes:*** Preaxial or postaxial polydactyly, syndactyly, clinodactyly, arachnodactyly, brachydactyly, hammer toe–cardiac conditions with its associated syndromes are given in **Table 9.4**.
- ***Chest deformities***
  - *Pectus excavatum (funnel chest):* Congenital deformity of lower sternum with posterior depression and consequent bowing of anterior ribs. You need to look for Marfan syndrome (aortic root anomalies—AR, AS, dissecting aneurysm)
  - *Pectus carinatum (pigeon chest):* Anterior elevation of sternum, reverse of pectus excavatum is also seen in Marfan syndrome. Also, look for ASD or VSD.
  - *Harrison sulcus:* Bilateral transverse grooving on either side of xiphisternum due to the traction exerted by costal diaphragmatic attachment on the softened ribs. Most common underlying cardiac cause is a left to right shunt, mostly VSD.
  - *Thoracic kyphoscoliosis* (abnormal lateral and anteroposterior curvature of thoracic spine) seen in Marfan syndrome, Morquio syndrome, other mucopolysaccharidosis, myopathies and other metabolic disorders due to underlying-mitral valve prolapse, MR, or TR.
  - *Straight back syndrome:* Look for mitral valve prolapse.
  - *Shield, broad chest with wide-spaced nipples:* Turner syndrome, Noonan syndrome. Look for coarctation of aorta and pulmonic stenosis.
  - *Absence of costosternal portion of pectoralis major* and pectoralis minor with 2–6 ribs is a feature of Poland syndrome which may have dextrocardia and ASD.
- ***Bones, joints and muscles:*** Cubitus valgus, muscle weakness, hypo- or hypertonia, myotonia, vertebral bone anomalies, absence of muscles.

Table 9.4 provides a list of abnormal features, their association with a cardiac disorder, and the final clinical syndromic diagnosis.

Table 9.4: Congenital cardiac diseases in genetic disorders

Disorder	Congenital heart defect	Other clinical features
Trisomy 21 (Down syndrome)	Endocardial cushion defects, VSD, TOF, PDA	Typical facies with brachycephaly, mongoloid slant, epicanthic folds, simian crease, clinodactyly, brachydactyly, hypotonia, delayed milestones
Trisomy 18 (Edwards syndrome)	VSD, DORV (95%)	Low birth weight, microcephaly, micrognathia, closed fist with overlapping fingers, rocker bottom feet
Trisomy 13 (Patau syndrome)	VSD (80–90%)	LBW, central facial anomalies, low-set ears, polydactyly, visceral and genital anomalies
Turner syndrome	Coarctation of aorta	Short female, webbing of neck, broad chest with widely placed nipple, congenital lymphedema, gonadal dysgenesis
Trisomy 9	DORV, VSD, PDA	Mental retardation, wide fontanel, short sternum, upslanting palpebral fissure, rocker bottom foot
10 q deletion	TOF	Growth retardation, craniofacial anomaly, urogenital anomalies, neuropsychiatric problems
Apert syndrome	TOF, VSD, common atrium	Craniosynostosis, low-set ears, downslanting palpebral fissure, exophthalmos, crowded teeth, syndactyly, mental retardation, megalencephaly
Carpenter syndrome	PDA, VSD, PS, TGA	Brachycephaly with variable craniosynostosis, midfacial hypoplasia, polydactyly, syndactyly, mitten hands
De Lange syndrome	VSD, TOF, PDA, DORV	Short stature, microcephaly, synophrys, underdeveloped orbital arches, micromelia
Goldenhar syndrome	TOF, VSD, ASD	Facial asymmetry, microtia, ear tag, cleft lip/palate, epibulbar dermoid
DiGeorge (CATCH 22) syndrome	VSD, Truncus arteriosus, TOF, DORV, interrupted aortic arch	Hypertelorism, retrognathia or micrognathia, long face, high and broad nasal bridge, cleft soft palate, bifid vula, small teeth, asymmetric crying face, downturned mouth, narrow palpebral fissures, downslanting eyes, hypoplasia/absence of thymus, and parathyroid, hypocalcemia, deficient cell-mediated immunity, FTT, GER
Klippel–Feil syndrome	ASD, Cor Triatriatum	Short webbed neck, decreased cervical range of movements, low hairline, short (middle and distal) limbs, postaxial polydactyly, nail dysplasia, teeth anomalies, synkinesia
CHARGE syndrome	Right-sided heart lesions, pulmonary artery branch stenosis, conotruncal lesions: TOF, DORV, VSD, ASD, PDA, TOF, ECD	Coloboma, choanal atresia, mental retardation, genitourinary anomalies, ear anomalies, genital hypoplasia
VACTERL syndrome	TOF, VSD	Vertebral anomalies, anal atresia, congenital heart syndrome defects, tracheoesophageal fistula, renal dysplasia, limb anomalies
TAR syndrome	ASD, VSD, TOF, conduction defects	Thrombocytopenia, absent or hypoplastic radius, normal thumb

Contd...

Table 9.4: Congenital cardiac diseases in genetic disorders (*Contd...*)

Disorder	Congenital heart defect	Other clinical features
Lawrence-Moon-Biedl syndrome	Cardiomyopathies: Hypertrophic or dilated, PDA,TGA, PS	Retinitis pigmentosa, obesity, polydactyly, hypogonadism
Silver–Rusell syndrome	TOF, VSD	Pre- and postnatal growth delay, triangular facies, bilateral fifth finger clinodactyly
Marfan syndrome	Aortic aneurysm, AR and/or MR	Arachnodactyly, tall stature, increased arm span, hyper-extensibility, subluxation of lens
Crouzon syndrome	PDA, ECD, coarctation of aorta, TGA, PS	Craniosynostosis, low-set ears, downslanting palpebral fissure, hypertelorism, maxillary hypoplasia, exophthalmos, crowded teeth, syndactyly, mental retardation
Noonan syndrome	PS, ASD, hypertrophic cardiomyopathy	Features resembling Turner syndrome, seen in boys
William syndrome	AS (supravalvular), PS, aortic and mitral valve anomalies	Typical facial dysmorphic features, periorbital fullness, Elfin facies, upturned nose, prominent upper lip, open wide mouth, short stature, hypercalcemia, hypothyroidism
Alagille syndrome	Pulmonary valve, artery or branch stenosis, TOF in <15% of cases	Typical facial dysmorphic features, hepatic disease, renal anomalies, butterfly vertebra, neurovascular anomalies
Holt-Oram syndrome	ASD (ostium secundum), first degree A-V block	Upper limb radial and thumb anomalies (absent, distally displaced, duplicated, triphalangeal), carpal and metacarpal anomalies, especially of the fourth or phocomelia with rudimentary limbs, hypoplastic radius, short deformed forearm with limited supination, sloping shoulders
Rubinstein-Taybi syndrome	ASD, TOF, VSD, PDA in 33% cases	Macrocephaly, downward slanted eyes, drooping eyelid, coloboma, cataract, low-set ears, broad thumbs and big toes, short stature

B. Cyanosis

- Look for presence of cyanosis at the following sites: Lips, tongue, oral mucous membrane, soft palate, underside of the tongue, conjunctival membrane, ear lobes, nose, nails of fingers and toes.
- Once bluishness is noted in all the above areas and not only in the peripheries, perform the following steps to differentiate central cyanosis from peripheral cyanosis.
- Feel for warmth of the hands by gently taking the child's hands as you are looking for cyanosis in the nails.
- Look for associated clubbing of fingers and toes.
- When the peripheries are warm to touch and not cold and cyanosis is associated with clubbing of fingers, the diagnosis is likely to be central cyanosis.
- Warm the extremities to improve the circulation in the extremities and see whether the bluishness becomes less or disappears **(Key Box 10)**.

Exposure to cold is the most frequent cause of acrocyanosis, leading to blue hands and feet in neonates and circumoral cyanosis in older children.

1. Central Cyanosis

Central cyanosis is visible only when the circulating reduced hemoglobin or deoxyhemoglobin in capillaries is more than 4 (3–5) g/dL. The absolute quantity of reduced hemoglobin determines the visibility of cyanosis rather than the relative quantity. Central cyanosis is easily noticeable in fair-skinned children with normal hemoglobin levels when arterial oxygen saturation is less than 85%. In dark-skinned children, central

Key Box 10

Steps to differentiate central cyanosis from peripheral cyanosis

Examination steps	**Central cyanosis**	**Peripheral cyanosis**
Observe		
Site of bluishness/cyanosis	Lips, tongue (tip, underside), palatal and conjunctival mucosa, nails	Only in the peripheries: Tip of nose, pinna of the ears, tips of fingers and toes
Touch and feel		
Peripheries of all limbs for local warmth	Warm on touching	Cold extremities, ears
Perform		
Capillary filling time	Normal, less than 3 seconds	Prolonged, ≥3 seconds
Look		
Clubbing of fingers and toes	Often present, especially in cardiac origin of central cyanosis	Absent
Perform following measures to improve peripheral circulation and observe for decrease or disappearance of the bluishness:		
a. Warm the extremities	No change	Decrease or disappear
b. Resuscitate with fluids to improve the peripheral circulation	No change	Decreases
c. Administer 100% oxygen for 10 minutes	Improvement seen only in pulmonary causes of central cyanosis	Decreases

cyanosis may not be easily discernible until the oxygen saturation is 75% and less.

Children with marked polycythemia appear cyanotic at higher levels of arterial oxygen saturation (<92%) than children with normal hematocrit levels (<85%). In children with significant anemia, cyanosis will not appear at 85% arterial oxygen saturation levels, but only at lower levels of arterial oxygen saturation (<65%). For example, a child with a hemoglobin level of 18 g/dL and visible cyanosis at a desaturated hemoglobin level of 3 g/dL will have arterial oxygen saturation of 83%, whereas a cyanosed child with a hemoglobin level of 9 g/dL and 3 g/dL of desaturated hemoglobin will have an arterial oxygen saturation of 67%.

Cardiac conditions cause central cyanosis by structural abnormalities which divert portions of the systemic venous return (desaturated blood) away from the lungs. Two categories of cardiac anomalies cause central cyanosis: Conditions with obstruction to pulmonary blood flow and an intracardiac septal defect (e.g. tetralogy of Fallot), or conditions in which the systemic venous and pulmonary venous returns are mixed in a common chamber before being ejected (e.g. single ventricle).

Cyanosis resulting from acute pulmonary edema in left ventricular failure may be strikingly improved by oxygen administration, whereas cyanosis occurring with structural cardiovascular anomalies shows little change with this maneuver.

Central cyanosis may rarely be due to the presence of abnormal hemoglobin derivatives, like methemoglobinemia.

2. Steps to Correlate the Presence of Central Cyanosis with a Cardiac Cause

1. Confirm central cyanosis **(Fig. 9.2)** by differentiating from peripheral cyanosis (refer to cyanosis in history).
2. Analyze the history which gives adequate weightage in differentiating cardiac causes of central cyanosis from respiratory causes and abnormal hemoglobin derivatives.
   - History of acute fever, cough, breathlessness, pleuritic type of chest pain, and acute episode of wheeze in a child with asthma points to a respiratory cause.

Acute pulmonary causes of central cyanosis include severe pneumonia, acute tension pneumothorax, acute severe asthma, ARDS and other causes of acute respiratory failure. In these conditions, areas of the lungs, though not ventilated, are perfused, and blood flowing through that portion of the lung is unoxygenated. Thus, desaturated blood returns to the left atrium and mixes with fully saturated blood from the ventilated portions of the lungs.

- History of drug intake, well water, or some toxic substances before the onset of cyanosis indicates methemoglobinemia, which is a dysfunctional hemoglobin disorder. It results in central cyanosis because these abnormal hemoglobin molecules are unable to bind normal quantities of oxygen.

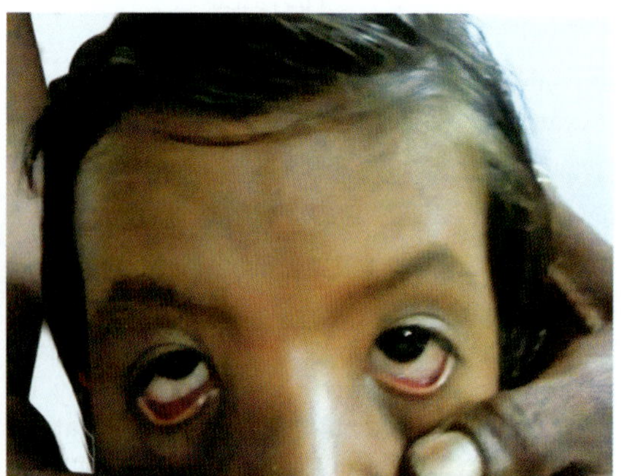

Fig. 9.2a: Central cyanosis in the palpebral conjunctiva.

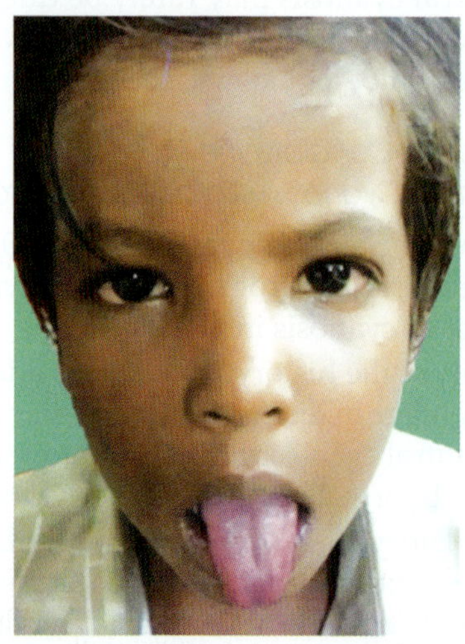

Fig. 9.2b: Central cyanosis seen in the tongue.

3. Look for clubbing of fingers and toes. Clubbing is more often associated with cardiac causes of central cyanosis.

   In acute respiratory conditions causing cyanosis, clubbing of fingers is not seen. But in chronic suppurative lung diseases, e.g. bronchiectasis or cystic fibrosis, clubbing of fingers may be seen. But in these two conditions, the history and physical examination will easily distinguish them from cardiac conditions.
4. Look for the presence of *differential cyanosis* in all limbs:

- Note the type of differential cyanosis:
  - *Cyanosis absent in the upper part of the body and right hand; and present in lower limbs*
    Seen in patent ductus arteriosus with severe pulmonary arterial hypertension and reversal of shunt—Eisenmenger syndrome. Face and fingers are pink, but toes are blue.
  - *Cyanosis more marked in the upper part of the body than in the lower limbs*
    This is known as reverse differential cyanosis and most commonly due to complete d-transposition of great arteries or Taussig-Bing anomaly with increased pulmonary vascular resistance and reversed flow through a PDA.

3. Pulse Oximetry

Pulse oximeter readings of oxygen saturation are obtained routinely in the screening for detection of cyanotic heart conditions. The screening is considered positive, if:

1. Any oxygen saturation measure is <90% (in the initial screen or in repeat screens);
2. Oxygen saturation is <95% in the right hand and foot on three different occasions done one hour apart; or
3. Presence of more than 3% absolute difference in oxygen saturation between the right hand and right foot on three occasions done one hour apart.

These children are subjected to a diagnostic echocardiographic evaluation.

4. Hyperoxia Test

This test was considered till recent times to be a gold standard for differentiating pulmonary disorders and abnormal hemoglobin disorders from cardiac causes of central cyanosis.

- Obtain arterial blood gas from the right radial artery when the infant is breathing room air (FiO_2 0.21).
- Administer 100% oxygen (FiO_2 1) to the infant for 10 to 15 minutes.
- Repeat arterial blood gas values after 100% oxygen administration.
- Observe increase in PaO_2 values.

Interpret the observed change

- *In congenital cyanotic heart diseases*, the PaO_2 will not change much and it will not go beyond 150 mmHg even after 100% oxygen administration.
- *In pulmonary conditions*, the PaO_2 increases beyond 150 mmHg after hyperoxia test, indicating that the cyanosis is not the result of a significant shunt.
- *Methemoglobinemia or other abnormal hemoglobin disorder* will be considered when the PaO_2 rises beyond 200 mmHg but still the pulse oximetry reading continues to remain low.

C. Clubbing

Clubbing refers to the soft, fluctuant swelling at the root of the nails resulting in a visible bulbous prominence of the distal portion of the terminal phalanges of fingers and toes. Clubbing of fingers and toes at its mildest form is noted when the normally seen angle at the skin–nail junction gets obliterated, and in its advanced condition, the digit assumes a drumstick appearance.

- Look for swelling at the root of the nails (Fig. 9.3).
- Elicit fluctuation in early stages of clubbing by applying gentle pressure by your right forefinger in the root of the nail bed of the child's forefinger or middle finger which is gently held by your thumbs. Appreciate the elicited fluctuation by your other forefinger.
- *Schamroth window sign:* Keep the dorsal sides of the distal phalanges of corresponding fingers of both the hands of the child touching so that the nails are touching opposed to each other. In case of normal nails, there is a small visible diamond-shaped or quadrangular space at the root of the nail base. In children with clubbing of fingers, no such space will be formed because of the swelling at the nail base (Fig. 9.4).

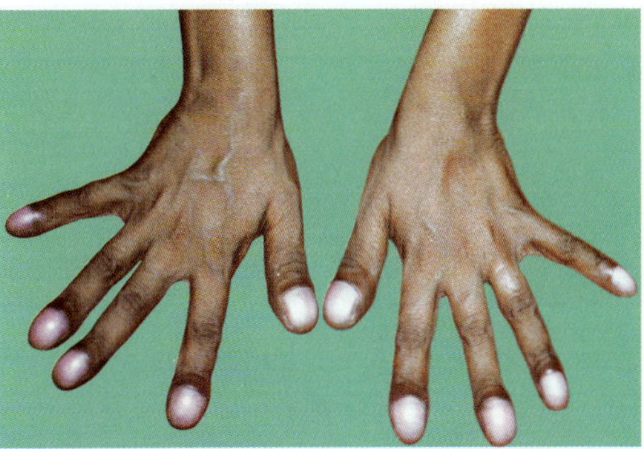

Fig. 9.3: Central cyanosis and clubbing seen in the fingers of both hands.

- *Lovibond angle criteria or Lovibond "profile sign":* Lovibond angle (normal angle: 160°) is created by the nail as it emerges from the proximal nailfold. According to the Lovibond angle criteria, an angle greater than 180° is indicative of true clubbing. The conditions that are mistaken for clubbing, such as normal nail curving or paronychia, have angle closer to 160° and never more than 180° (Fig. 9.5).
- *Curth modified profile angle:* Look at the angle between the back surface of the middle phalanx and that of the terminal phalanx. In clubbing of fingers, this angle decreases from 160° to less than 145°.
- *Rice and Rowl and interphalangeal depth ratio:* Estimate the ratio of distal phalangeal depth (DPD) diameter to interphalangeal depth (IPD) diameter of the middle finger; in normal children, it is less than 1. DPD: IPD ratio greater than 1.1 indicates presence of clubbing.

Grading of Clubbing

Grade I	Visible nail bed filling and swelling of root of the nail bed; fluctuation and softening of nail bed
Grade II	Obliteration of nail bed angle with increased Lovibond angle >180° and positive Schamroth sign
Grade III	Parrot beak or drumstick appearance with increased convexity of the nail-fold
Grade IV	Swelling of fingers at all phalangeal joints and wrists with hypertrophic pulmonary osteoarthropathic changes

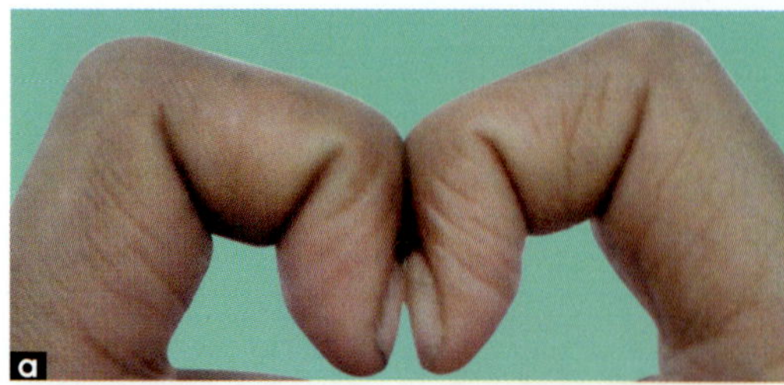

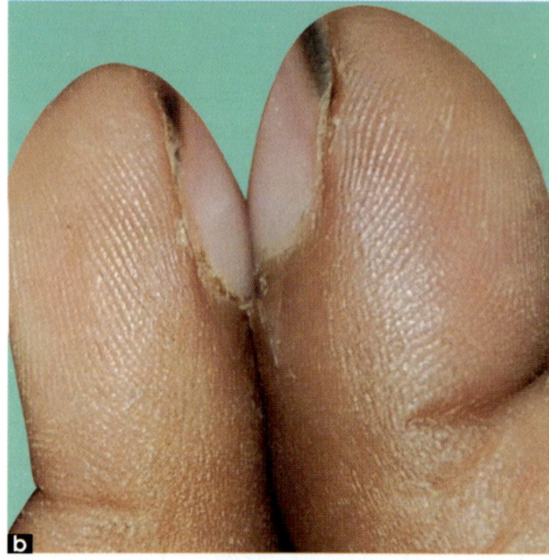

Fig. 9.4: Schamroth sign: (a) No clubbing showing quadrangular window in normal child; (b) obliteration of normal window indicating clubbing.

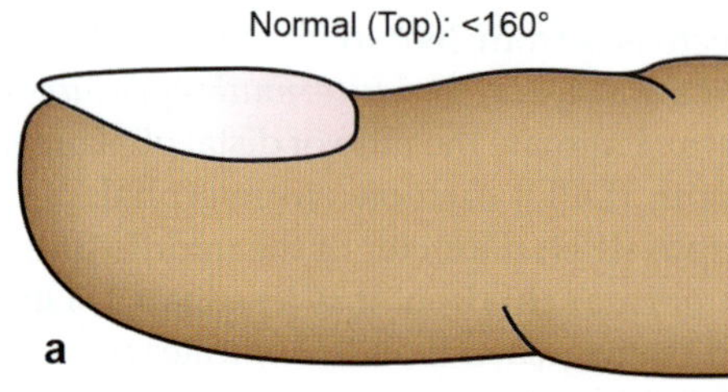

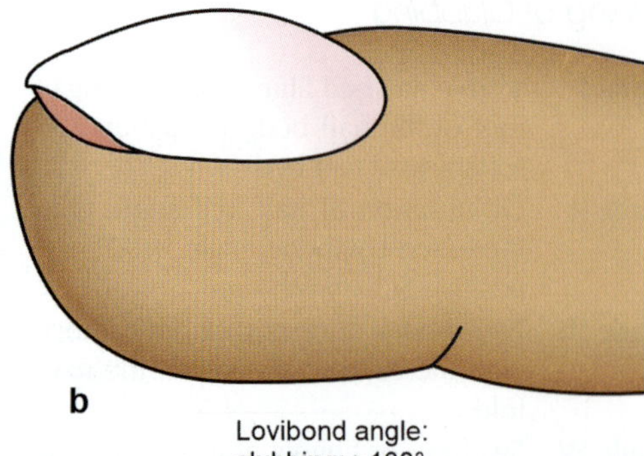

Fig. 9.5: Lovibond angle: (a) Normal (<160°); (b) in clubbing of fingers (>180°).

Etiopathogenesis of Clubbing

- ***Basic pathogenetic mechanisms:*** Vasodilatation of nail bed capillaries; small capillary arterio-venous anastomosis and fistula formation, connective tissue proliferation.
- ***Etiology dependent factors and stimuli***
  a. Hypoxia in cyanotic heart diseases;
  b. Increased levels of unoxidized ferritin escaping oxidative degradation in the lungs by shunt bypass;
  c. Chemical substances and factors, such as ATP and 5-HT;
  d. Prostaglandin E2 and other increased hormonal levels of estrogens, growth hormone, and parathormone;
  e. TNF, platelet-derived growth factor (PDGF), and hepatocyte growth factor;
  f. Neurogenic vasodilatory mechanism mediated by vagus nerve; and
  g. Genetic predisposition—genes identified in familial clubbing.

Causes of Clubbing

- ***Cardiac:*** Congenital cyanotic heart diseases, bacterial endocarditis
- ***Pulmonary:*** Suppurative lung diseases, e.g. bronchiectasis, lung abscess, empyema, interstitial lung diseases, and fibrocavitatory tuberculosis
- ***Intestinal and hepatic:*** Ulcerative colitis, Crohn regional ileitis, some malabsorption states, biliary cirrhosis
- ***Neoplasms:*** Mesotheliomas, other rare tumors
- ***Endocrinal:*** Thyrotoxicosis, myxedema
- ***Familial:*** Genes identified
- ***Idiopathic***
- ***Unilateral clubbing:*** Local AV malformations and aneurysms, trauma, sarcoidosis, gout, and occupational (in child laborers).

D. Jugular Venous Pressure (JVP)

Steps in the Assessment of JVP

- Request the parents to place their child supine in a reclining posture on an examination couch/cot. In infants and young children, request the mother to keep the child on her lap in a reclined position at 45° angle.

- Elevate the head and shoulders properly supported and place at an angle of 45° with the help of a backrest.
- Keep the neck slightly extended and turned a little to the left making sure that the neck muscle is not kept contracted.
- Take care to have an illuminating source to provide adequate lighting tangentially over the right supraclavicular area.
- Look carefully for any visible pulsations over the right supraclavicular region near the sternal edge.
- Identify the right carotid arterial pulse seen and felt medial to the sternocleidomastoid and lateral to the end of the hyoid bone as a single outward thrust with every S1 (no wavy pattern seen).
- Concentrate, focus, and train your eyes to discern and identify internal jugular venous pulsations seen in between the two heads of sternocleidomastoid muscle **(Fig. 9.6)** as subtle, repeatedly distending or filling, undulating waveforms with 3 elevations and 2 troughs for every single carotid arterial pulsation.
- Differentiate jugular venous pulsations from carotid arterial pulsations **(Table 9.5)**.
- Identify the "meniscus", the highest oscillation point of the JVP.
- Identify the angle of Lewis (mildly elevated junction felt at the junction of manubrium sterni with the body of sternum).
- Measure the elevation/vertical height in cm by keeping a scale or thin cardboard horizontally projected from the top most point of JVP to a measuring centimeter ruler or scale kept vertically at the Lewis angle of the sternum.

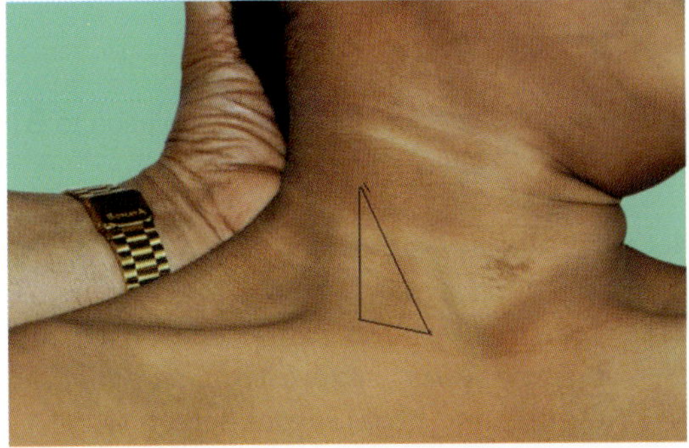

Fig. 9.6: Inspection for JVP: Look for wavy undulating pulsations of internal jugular vein between the two heads of sternomastoid (in the triangular area shown).

- Add this reading with 5 cm to get the central venous pressure (CVP); as the center of the right atrium is 5 cm below the angle of Lewis.
- Next, observe the waveforms—positive filling waves (3 elevations, e.g. "a, c and v waves" and 2 troughs, e.g. "x and y" waves) **(Fig. 9.7** and **Key Box 11)**.

Abnormal JVP and its Clinical Interpretation (Fig. 9.8)

1. ***'a' wave (atrial contraction) abnormalities***
   - *Cannon (very large) 'a' waves* occur when right atrium contracts against a closed tricuspid valve, e.g. in tricuspid atresia, AV dissociation, and complete heart block. Cannon waves can be regular, (junctional rhythm, isorhythmic AV dissociation) or irregular (complete heart block, classic AV dissociation, ventricular pacing, or ventricular ectopics).
   - *Giant (large)'a' waves* occur due to:
     - i. Forcible contraction of right atrium against obstruction at AV valve area: *tricuspid stenosis, right atrial myxoma.*
     - ii. Forcible contraction of right atrium against increased resistance offered by non-compliant right ventricle with increased end diastolic pressure: *severe pulmonary artery hypertension, moderate to severe pulmonary stenosis, acute pulmonary embolism.*
     - iii. Right ventricular endomyocardial fibrosis.
   - *Absent 'a' waves* occur when there is ineffective atrial contraction as in atrial fibrillation, or marked sinus tachycardia.

2. ***'v' wave (atrial filling wave) abnormalities:*** *Mechanism:* Rapid and excessive right atrial filling with good compliance.

Causes

- Tricuspid regurgitation (combined large "cv" wave without "x" descent in severe tricuspid regurgitation).
- Atrial septal defect with mitral regurgitation.
- Total anomalous pulmonary venous drainage with restrictive atrial septal defect.

Table 9.5: Differentiation of jugular venous pulsations from carotid arterial pulsations		
Differentiate by	**Jugular venous pulsations**	**Carotid artery pulse**
Location	Seen in the right supraclavicular triangle lateral to the top of the sternum between the two heads of the sternocleidomastoid muscle	Seen and felt internal—medial to this muscle and lateral to the hyoid bone
Upper meniscus	Seen	None
Palpation	Only seen, not palpable	Always easily palpable
Obliteration by finger pressure above the clavicle	Disappearance of visible pulsations	Cannot be obliterated
Undulations-elevations and troughs for every single heart beat	Yes	Single impulse with every heartbeat
Number of pulsations per systole	2 Pulsations per systole (x and y descents)	1 Pulsation per systole
Prominent waves	2 Descents (downslopes)—gradual upslope and a dramatic collapse	Upstroke—dramatic upstroke and a gentle collapse
Variation in the meniscus level with posture and respiration	Yes fall in level with inspiration	No variation
Effect on waves by right subcostal abdominal pressure	May become prominent	No effect

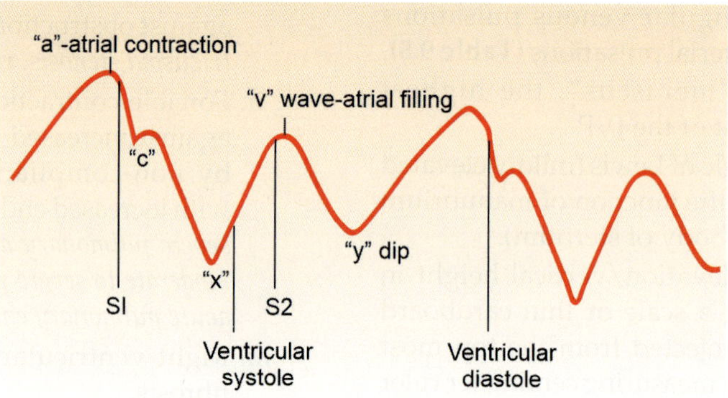

Fig. 9.7: Positive "a", "c", "v" and negative "x", "y" waves of Jugular venous pulsations in relation to S1 and S2.

3. *'x' descent abnormalities*
   - *Prominent descent:* Constrictive pericarditis, early pericardial effusion and sometimes in atrial septal defect; and conditions with large or cannon "a" waves
   - *Decreased or absent 'x' descent:* Early sign of moderate to severe tricuspid regurgitation (cv waves are seen)

4. *'y'descent abnormalities*
   - *Rapid and deep "y" descent (Friedreich sign):* Constrictive pericarditis, severe tricuspid regurgitation, severe right ventricular failure, and atrial septal defect
   - *Absent "y" descent:* Pericardial tamponade. Presence of rapid "y" descent (diastolic collapse) rules out the presence of cardiac tamponade.

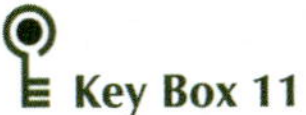
Key Box 11

Cardiac Events Causing the Waves of Jugular Venous Pulsations

JVP waves	Cardiac event causing the wave	Timing
"a" wave	Atrial contraction	Presystolic; occurs just before S1 and carotid pulse
"c" wave	Upward bulging motion of tricuspid valve into the right atrium during isovolumetric contraction of ventricle	Peak seen immediately after S1
"x" descent	Right atrial relaxation causing systolic descent (early and mid-ventricular)	"x" descent collapses before S2
"v" wave	Passive atrial filling in late systole with tricuspid valve closed	Starts in late systole, peaks immediately after S2 with subsequent y downslope during early diastole
"y" descent	Opening of the tricuspid valve with passive right ventricular filling in early diastole (diastolic descent)	After S2

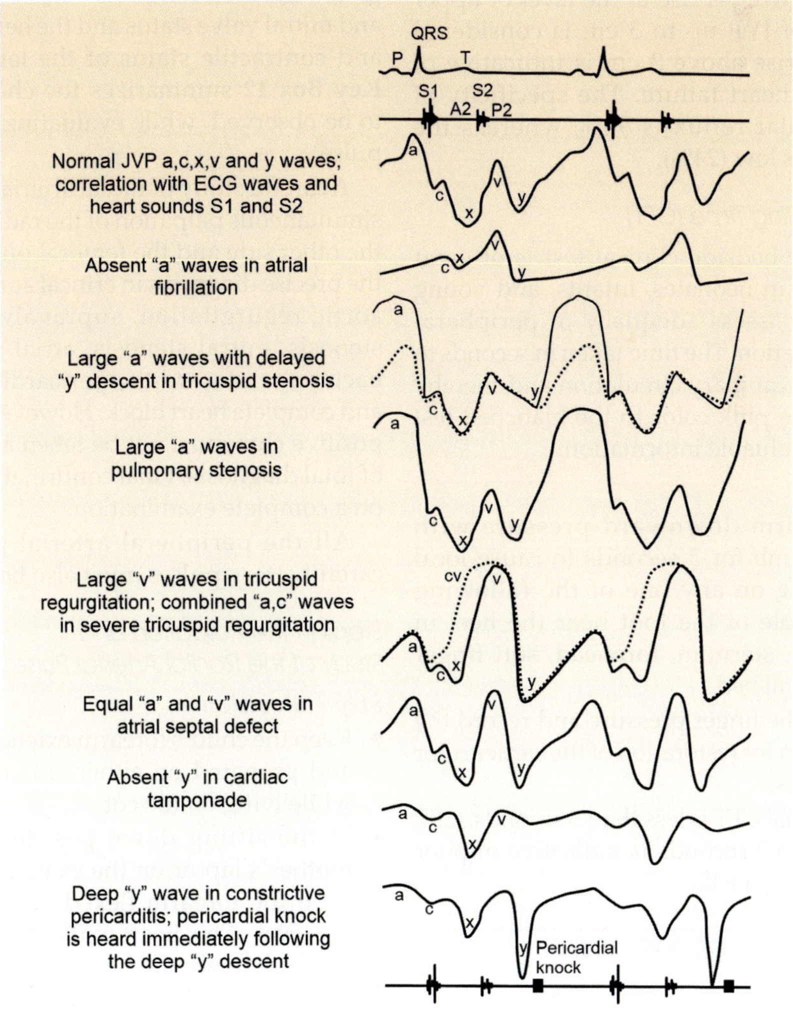

QRS
P
T
S1
S2
A2
P2
Normal JVP a,c,x,v and y waves; correlation with ECG waves and heart sounds S1 and S2
Absent "a" waves in atrial fibrillation
Large "a" waves with delayed "y" descent in tricuspid stenosis
Large "a" waves in pulmonary stenosis
Large "v" waves in tricuspid regurgitation; combined "a,c" waves in severe tricuspid regurgitation
Equal "a" and "v" waves in atrial septal defect
Absent "y" in cardiac tamponade
Deep "y" wave in constrictive pericarditis; pericardial knock is heard immediately following the deep "y" descent
Pericardial knock

Fig. 9.8: Normal and abnormal wave patterns of jugular venous pulsations.

Kussmaul Sign

During inspiration, the mean venous pressure and JVP fall as phasic flow of blood occurs in the superior vena cava (SVC) and the right ventricle accommodates this increased venous return. In constrictive pericarditis, cardiac tamponade, severe right heart failure, and restrictive cardiomyopathy, this phasic blood flow does not occur in the SVC during inspiration, the mean venous pressure rises and the JVP column rises. This is a sensitive (but not specific) sign for constrictive pericarditis.

Hepatojugular Reflux

Apply slight upward pressure with the four fingers of the right hand for 30 seconds in the right hypochondrium just below the lower edge of the liver. A rise in the level of upper meniscus of JVP up to 3 cm is considered normal. A rise above 3 cm is indicative of congestive heart failure. The specificity of hepatojugular reflux is 96%, whereas the sensitivity is low (24%).

Capillary Filling Time (CFT)

This simple bedside clinical test is of great importance in neonates, infants, and young children to assess adequacy of peripheral blood circulation. The time taken in seconds to re-establish capillary circulation and thereby restoring the pink color to the blanched test area gives valuable information.

Procedure

- Apply firm downward pressure with your thumb for 5 seconds to cause local blanching on any one of the following areas—sole of the foot near the heel in neonates, sternum, forehead, soft finger pad, or nail bed.
- Release the finger pressure and record the time taken for restoration of the earlier color in seconds.
- The normal CFT is less than 3 seconds. CFT more than 3 seconds is indicative of poor perfusion (shock).

9.4 PULSE AND BLOOD PRESSURE

Arterial Pulse

Arterial pulse is the transmitted and propagated wave of centripetal arterial blood flow from the aortic root into the peripheral arterial branches. It is felt as a palpable pulsatile impulse by the fingers at various sites where the arterial course is very near to the body surface.

This forward central and peripheral arterial flow is primarily determined by the intrinsic contractile ability of the ventricular musculature, its size and shape, and the rate at which it contracts and the intrinsic resistance of the blood vessels. The speed of this arterial pulse wave is ten times faster than that of the blood column.

Palpation of radial arterial pulses and interpretation of its characteristics is one of the most basic essential steps in the evaluation of adequacy of circulation and diagnosis of the cardiac condition. A careful clinical analysis of the characteristics of radial artery pulsations gives valuable information regarding the aortic and mitral valve status and the hemodynamic and contractile status of the left ventricle. **Key Box 12** summarizes the characteristics to be observed, while evaluating the arterial pulse.

A careful study of radial arterial pulse with simultaneous palpation of the radial artery on the other side and the femoral pulse can give the precise diagnosis in critical aortic stenosis, aortic regurgitation, supravalvular aortic stenosis, mitral stenosis, atrial fibrillation, bacterial endocarditis, pericardial effusion, and complete heart block. However, one single positive clue must not be taken as indicative of total diagnosis. Final confirmation is based on a complete examination.

All the peripheral arterial pulses and carotid artery pulses must also be palpated.

Steps in the Palpation and Study of the Radial Arterial Pulse

Step 1: Position

- Keep the child's forearm extended, relaxed and pronated on either side of the body while lying on the cot.
- In the sitting down position either on mother's lap or on the examination chair, keep the forearm flexed at the elbow at the level of his heart with wrist flexed and fingers extended.

Step 2: Hold the wrist

- Place the pads (most sensitive area at the end of finger) of your right index, middle

Key Box 12

Assessment of Arterial Pulse

1. Rate
2. Rhythm
3. Presence of pulse deficit
4. Volume and waveform characteristics
5. Symmetry
6. Arterial wall thickness

and ring fingers on the radial side of the wrist of the child, close to the proximal crease (**Fig. 9.9**).

- Evaluate both radial arteries at the same time (**Fig. 9.10**).

Step 3: Feel

Get the feel of the radial artery pulsations. Beginners must spend a few minutes practicing and appreciating the feel of the pulse, the speed and height of upstroke, contour or fullness of the pulse, and the downstroke velocity.

Step 4: Assess the following characteristics

- *Rate:* Count for a full minute and record the pulse rate per minute. The normal range of pulse rate in various age groups differs from an average of 124 per minute in neonates to 86 per minute in adolescents.

Age groups	Normal range of *resting pulse rate per minute*
Birth–4 weeks	
Preterm	120–160
Term	100–140
28 d–1year	100–120
1–5 years	90–110
6–12 years	80–100
Adolescents	60–90

- ***Rhythm* (Table 9.6):** Observe, whether pulse is regular or irregular? In infants and young children, you may appreciate a normal physiological variation in the pulse rate during inspiration and expiration, termed *sinus arrhythmia*—increase in pulse rate during inspiration and a slight decrease during expiration.
  a. If irregular, is it *regularly irregular* or *irregularly irregular*?
  b. Is there and how much is the *pulse deficit*? (difference between heart rate and pulse rate simultaneously calculated by two persons in the same minute).

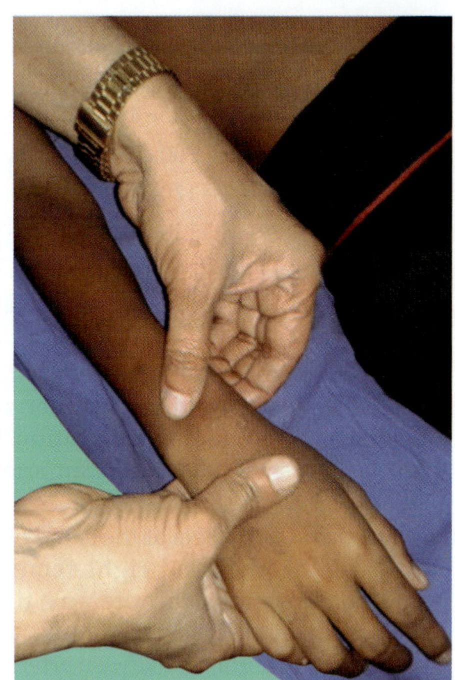

Fig. 9.9: Palpation of radial arterial pulse with three fingers with child's arm pronated.

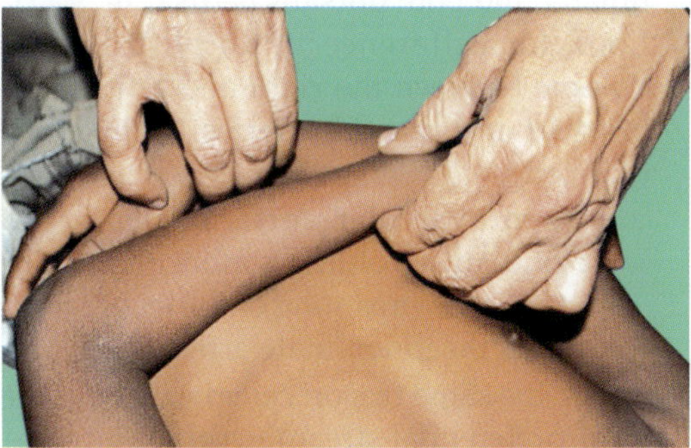

Fig. 9.10: Palpation of bilateral radial artery for inequality in volume and any radio-radial delay.

- ***Volume and waveform characteristics:*** Feel whether pulse volume is normal, low, or high. Notice both the upstroke (whether normal, slow rise, or rapid rise) and downstroke (whether normal, slow descent or sudden collapse of pulse). Also, look for alternating high and low volume peaks (**Key Boxes 13–16**).
- ***Symmetry***
  a. *Radio-radial delay:* Feel both radial arteries at the same time and record, if there is time delay between the right and left

Table 9.6: Pulse rate and rhythm in some common arrhythmias

Conditions	Rate per minute	Rhythm
Sinus tachycardia	More than the upper limit for age and sex	Regular
Atrial tachycardia	180–300	Regular
Atrial flutter	120–300	Regularly irregular
Atrial fibrillation	120–300	Irregularly irregular
Sinus bradycardia	Less than the lower limit for age and sex	Regular
Complete heart block	Very slow, often less than 50	Irregular

radial arteries. A delayed left radial arterial pulsation indicates either the presence of preductal coarctation or post-aneurysmal left subclavian artery stenosis.

b. *Radiofemoral delay:* Feel at the same time both right radial and right femoral arterial pulsations to note any time delay. A delay indicates the presence of coarctation of aorta or Takayasu arteritis.

- *Assess peripheral pulse* for palpability and pulsatality—carotids, axillary, and brachial arteries, femorals, popliteals, posterior tibialis, and both dorsalis pedis (Fig. 9.11). Look for difference in amplitude and volume between the right and left radial, brachial and carotid arteries (right more than left):
  a. In supravalvular aortic stenosis, the carotid pulse volume is more because of preferential streaming of the jet of blood toward the innominate artery.
  b. For the same reason called *Coanda effect* of preferential streaming of jet into the innominate artery, the right arm BP may exceed the left arm BP by 15 mm or more.
- *Arterial wall thickness:* Feel the condition of the vessel wall by gently pressing and rolling the radial artery with the index finger (one of the three fingers kept over the radial artery) over the underlying radial bone. This is important for certain conditions, like familial hyperlipidemia, hypercholestero-lemia, and progeria.

Pulsus Paradoxus

The term pulsus paradoxus is a misnomer, because it represents an exaggeration of a normal phenomenon—a marginal physiological decrease in systolic BP during inspiration, ranging from 5 to 10 mmHg. It can be apprecia-

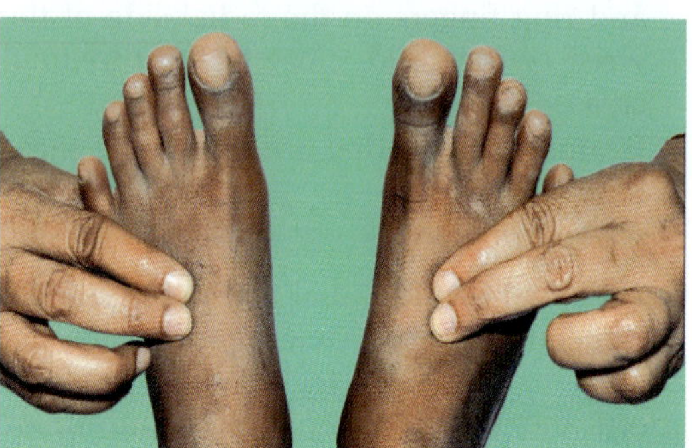

Fig. 9.11: Palpation of bilateral dorsalis pedis.

ted by experienced clinicians on feeling the arterial pulse in the absence of tachycardia. The mechanism of this normal physiological decrease in systolic BP during inspiration is summarized in Fig. 9.12. Common causes are listed in **Key Box 17**.

Definition

Pulsus paradoxus is present when the difference between the two readings (the first taken during expiration and the second during inspiration) is greater than 10 mmHg. Often, this difference is greater than 20 mmHg. The term paradoxus was given by Kussmaul who observed visible apical impulse in the near absence of peripheral arterial pulse during inspiration.

Physiology of Pericardial Effusion and Cardiac Tamponade

The raised intrapericardial pressure does not affect the augmented venous return to the right side of the heart during inspiration; neither it affects the increased pooling of blood in pulmonary vascular bed. But, the raised intrapericardial pressure results in an increase in the left atrial and left ventricular pressures which further lower the blood returning to the left heart chambers. This results in a

Key Box 13

Other Abnormal Arterial Pulse Waveforms

1. Pulsus Alternans

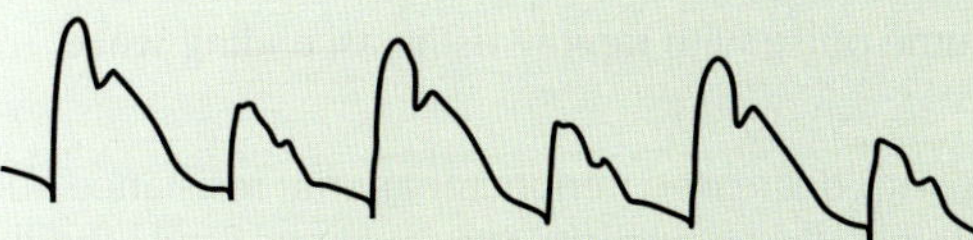

- Pulsus alternans occurs when you appreciate the occurrence of strong (high volume) pulse alternating with weak, low volume pulse in the presence of normal rhythm.
- *Interpretation:* Moderate-to-severe left ventricular failure (LVF), myocarditis.

2. Pulsus Bigeminus

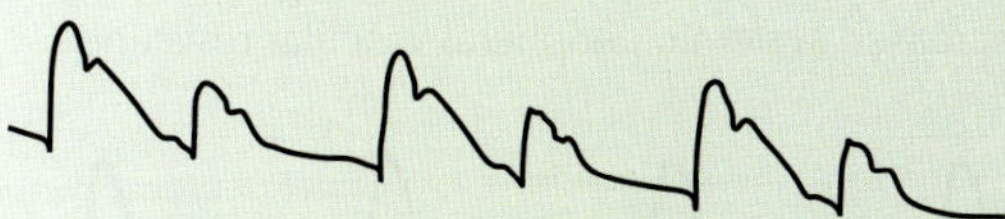

- Pulsus bigeminus refers to regular premature ventricular ectopics occurring alternately after every normal beat; the normal beat is stronger and the immediately following ectopic is weaker; hence this may be misinterpreted with pulsus alternans. There is a longer interval (compensatory pause) between the weaker ectopic and the next normal stronger beat.
- *Interpretation:* Ventricular arrhythmia, AV block, premature contractions, digoxin toxicity.
- The pulse is brisk and jerky with a sharp, tapping upstroke with normal volume and downstroke in hypertrophic cardiomyopathy.

3. Pulsus Trigemini

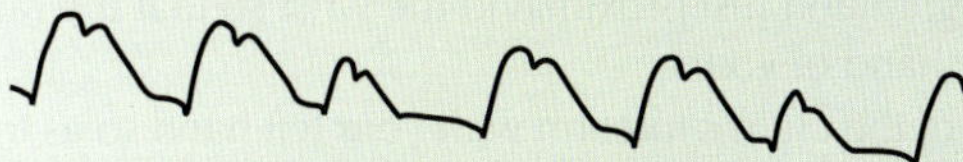

Coupling of three beats because of ectopic ventricular premature beat occurring regularly after two normal beats.

4. Bisferiens Pulse

- This normal or high volume pulse has two palpable impulses in the rapidly rising systolic upstroke, the latter second impulse occurring at the peak of the upstroke (tidal wave).
- It is better appreciated over the carotids than radials.
- *Interpretation* Severe aortic regurgitation (AR) or AR with aortic stenosis (AS) or hypertrophic obstructive cardiomyopathy (HOCM).

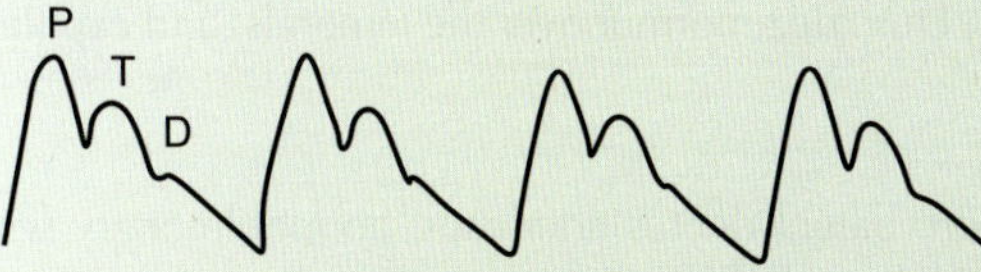

- Differentiate pulsus bisferiens from the other types of arterial pulse where two impulses are felt per beat, e.g. anacrotic pulse and dicrotic pulse.
  a. In *anacrotic pulse*, the pulse is a low volume pulse, the systolic upstroke is slow unlike the rapid stroke of bisferiens pulse. The third difference is the timing of the second impulse—in anacrotic pulse, it occurs in the anacrotic upstroke (percussion limb) much before the start of the tidal wave.
  b. In *dicrotic pulse*, the first palpable impulse is in the systolic upstroke and the second in the dicrotic limb in the diastolic period.

5. Sinus Arrhythmia

Marginal slowing of heart rate during expiration and a faster rate during inspiration is physiological and often noted in infants and young children.

Key Box 14

High Volume Arterial Pulse

1. Hyperkinetic (Bounding) Pulse

High amplitude, large volume pulse with rapidly rising ascending wave

Interpretation

- High cardiac output states with decreased peripheral arterial resistance and wide pulse pressure, e.g. anxiety, exercise, fever, anemia, thyrotoxicosis, arteriovenous fistula, beriberi
- Aortic regurgitation (AR), moderate MR, moderate sized VSD, PDA

2. Water Hammer/Collapsing Pulse

A large volume pulse with abrupt and rapid upstroke with an equally rapid downstroke due to the rapid and reverse diastolic run off into the left ventricle in aortic regurgitation (AR) and rapid run off to the peripheral vessels due to decreased systemic peripheral vascular resistance.

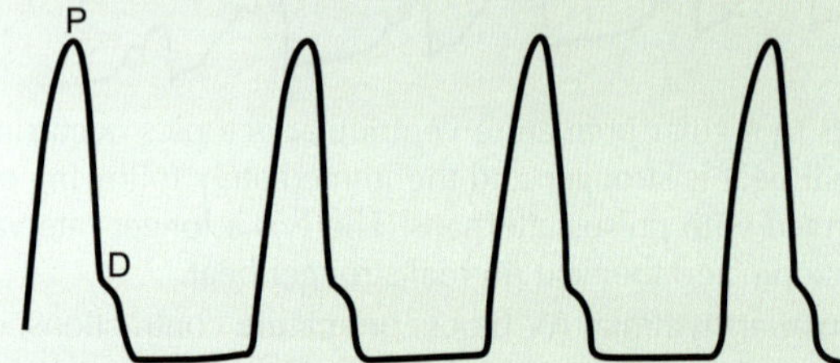

Method of elicitation of collapsing pulse

- Feel the radial pulse of the child with pad of fingers.
- Encircle the arm in your right hand just proximal to the wrist so that the radial pulse is still felt by the palmar surface of gripping hand of yours.
- Encircle the proximal part of the child's forearm with your left hand so as to feel the easily transmitted pulsations of the brachial artery over the brachioradialis muscle.
- Elevate suddenly yet gently the child's arm vertically above his/her shoulder.
- You will feel the thump of the water hammer (a famous Victorian era English toy) collapsing radial pulse on the palmar grip of your right hand and the transmitted impact of the brachial artery pulse across the brachioradialis on your left hand.

If you are almost sure about the collapsing pulse

- Record BP to note high normal systolic and low or very low diastolic BP readings with a pulse pressure of more than 60 mmHg.
- Elicit other peripheral signs of aortic regurgitation or other aortic diastolic run off conditions—pistol shot sounds over femorals, Duroziez murmur over the femorals, and capillary pulsations over the nail bed.

Interpretation

- *Causes:* Aortic regurgitation, patent ductus arteriosus, aortopulmonary window, rupture of sinus of Valsalva into the right ventricle and AV fistulas.
- Collapsing pulse in a cyanotic child suggests truncus arteriosus with truncal regurgitation, pulmonary atresia with aortopulmonary collaterals, and tetralogy of Fallot with collaterals or PDA.
- Also felt in hyperkinetic states, like anemia, fever, thyrotoxicosis, pregnancy, and beriberi.

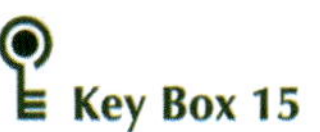

Key Box 15

Causes of Regular and Irregular Pulse Patterns

Regular, rapid pulse	*Irregularly irregular pulse*
• Sinus tachycardia	• Atrial fibrillation
• Supraventricular tachycardia (SVT), paroxysmal atrial tachycardia (PAT), junctional tachycardia (JT)	• Atrial tachycardia or atrial flutter with varying degrees of AV conduction blocks
• Atrial tachycardia or atrial flutter with fixed block	• Multifocal atrial and ventricular ectopics
• Ventricular tachycardia	• Multifocal ventricular tachycardia

Pulse deficit: Presence of a disparity of 10 or more between the auscultated heart rate and the palpated radial arterial pulse rate, both estimated at the same time for a full minute. Causes: Atrial fibrillation, frequent ventricular premature and weak contractions.

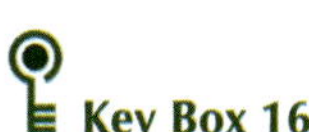

Key Box 16

Low Volume Arterial Pulses

1. *Hypokinetic pulse*
   - Weak, small volume pulse felt with difficulty
   - *Interpretation:* Low cardiac output and shock states, severe heart failure, myocarditis, severe left heart obstructive lesions, such as mitral and aortic stenosis, aortic outflow obstructions, like aortic arch syndromes and coarctation of aorta (especially in neonates and infants); and cardiac tamponade
2. *Pulsus tardus*
   - Slow rising pulse with a late peaking closer to the S2
   - *Interpretation:* Severe heart failure, also reported in fixed left ventricular obstructive lesions
3. *Pulsus parvus et tardus*
   - A low volume pulse with slow rise without the feel of anacrotic notch and the double systolic impulse described in anacrotic pulse
   - *Interpretation:* Severe aortic stenosis; severe low cardiac output states
4. *Anacrotic pulse*
   - Refers to a slow rising (ana = up and crotos = beat) percussion (upstroke) wave with late peaking, small volume (low amplitude) radial arterial pulse.
   - Feel and appreciate this slow upstroke with a notch in early or mid-upstroke resulting in two systolic impulses on radial artery—both the percussion (anacrotic) and tidal waves with every beat.
   - *Interpretation:* Diagnostic of aortic stenosis (AS) of moderate-to-severe degree. The anacrotic notch occurs during the early half of the ascent and earlier it is felt, severe is the AS. In severe mitral stenosis (MS), the notch is felt in the later half of the ascending limb.

greater, exaggerated fall in systolic BP during inspiration.

Recording of Pulsus Paradoxus

- Concentrate and appreciate any appreciable decrease in the volume of the pulse during inspiration **(Fig. 9.13)**. Make it a routine every time you feel the radial arterial pulse.
- Once you appreciate this decrease in volume during inspiration, confirm by using the BP apparatus.
- Inflate the cuff pressure rapidly above the systolic pressure and then deflate slowly.
- Record the appearance of first Korotkoff sound as the systolic pressure during expiration because the initial few sounds are heard irregularly only during expiration.
- Release slowly the cuff pressure further until the Korotkoff sounds are heard both in inspiration and expiration, at which point the sounds become regular and almost doubled. The difference between these two

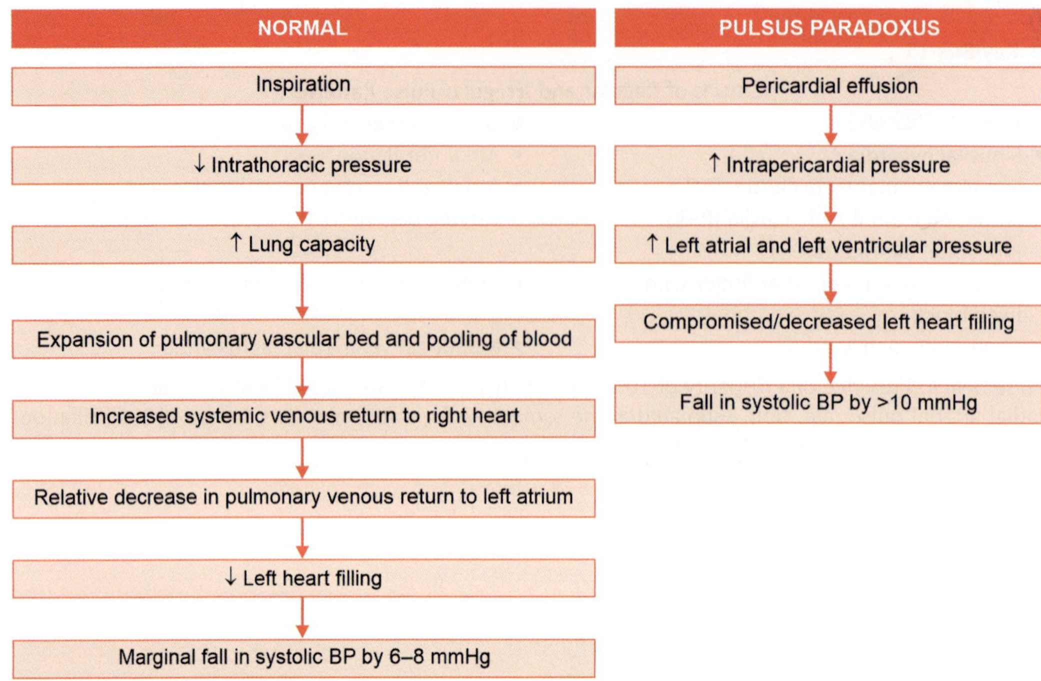

Fig. 9.12: Physiology of decrease in systolic BP in inspiration.

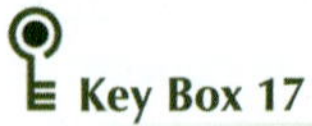

Key Box 17

Causes of Pulsus Paradoxus

1. *Cardiac:* Cardiac tamponade, pericardial effusion, constrictive pericarditis
2. *Pulmonary:* Acute severe asthma
3. Conditions that obstruct superior vena caval return to right atrium as in anterior and superior mediastinal tumors

points in BP gives the difference in systolic BP between expiration and inspiration.

- The systolic BP recordings are taken during regular breathing. In older children and adolescents with a normal respiratory rate of less than 32 per minute, the recording of systolic BP during expiration and inspiration is done without asking the child to hold the breath in the respective phases.
- But when the respiratory rate is faster, if it is difficult to record during inspiration, the child may be asked to hold the breath briefly during inspiration.

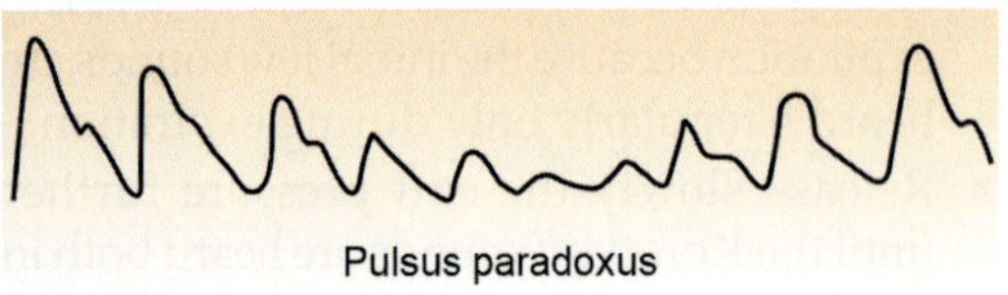

Fig. 9.13: Diagrammatic representation of pulsus paradoxus.

BLOOD PRESSURE

1. Recording with Sphygmomanometer

Select and keep in readiness: (a) *properly functioning BP recording* instrument—mercury column sphygmomanometer (getting replaced in many centers), aneroid or an automated device with a manual inflate mode; (b) appropriately sized blood pressure cuffs; and (c) a good stethoscope.

Cuff size: For brachial arterial pressure recording, choose the appropriate cuff size; the air bag inside the cuff should encircle three-fourths of the arm circumference and its width should be adequate to cover two-thirds of the length of the upper arm.

Age group	Width	Length
Neonate	3–4 cm	5–8 cm
Infant	5–6 cm	8–9 cm
Child	7–9 cm	13–18 cm
Adolescent	10–13 cm	24 cm
Large arm	16–18 cm	34–38 cm
Thigh	20 cm	42 cm

2. Preparation

Ensure the child is restive, quiet, calm and relaxed with help of parents and not involved in any motor activities. Get the child to be seated comfortably on the mother's lap. Be patient and allow adequate time for the anxious or crying child to settle down.

3. Tie the Cuff

- Expose the upper arm below the shoulder by removing excess clothing where the BP cuff will be applied.
- Place the right upper arm of the child on the table with the elbow flexed and forearm and palm facing upwards so that the center of the upper arm is in level with the child's heart.
- Wrap the appropriate sized cuff snugly around the child's arm 2 cm above the crease of the elbow. Ensure the bladder in the BP cuff encircles 75% of the arm circumference.

4. Methods of Recording

Palpatory Method for Recording Systolic BP

- Feel the radial artery pulse on the same side.
- Inflate the BP cuff by pumping the cuff bulb or bladder repeatedly so as to elevate the mercury column 30–40 mm above the level where no longer the radial pulse is felt.
- Deflate the BP cuff slowly to bring down the mercury column level by 2–3 mmHg per second as you continue to feel the radial arterial pulse for its reappearance.
- Record the systolic BP as shown in the mercury gauge level where you start feeling the re-emergence of radial arterial pulsations as you are deflating.

Auscultatory Method for Recording Systolic and Diastolic BP

- Feel the brachial artery pulsations over the anterior cubital fossa.
- Place the diaphragm of the stethoscope over the area where brachial artery pulsations are felt with both the earpieces plugged in your ears.
- Elevate the mercury column again by inflating the cuff to a level (20 mm in children and 30 mm in adults) above the recorded systolic BP by palpatory method.
- Deflate BP cuff pressure slowly as mentioned earlier as you continue listening to the first appearance of audible sound.

5. Record the Systolic BP

The gauge reading in mmHg where the first tapping sound is heard marks the systolic pressure. Note and record the value at which you start hearing the occurrence of first transmitted rhythmic sound (1st Korotkoff sound) of resumed onward blood flow beyond the cuffed brachial arterial segment.

6. Record the Diastolic BP

Continue listening as the stepwise deflation of cuff is carried on below the systolic BP reading. The sounds start fading in intensity and beyond a reading; you can no longer hear the sound. The diastolic pressure is that reading (5th Korotkoff sound) where the brachial arterial sound is no longer heard. In young children, the fourth Korotkoff sound is considered as indicative of diastolic pressure.

If the sounds disappear soon after the recording of systolic pressure, you have to elevate the arm above the heart level for 2–3 minutes and then inflate the cuff in the same elevated position. Before deflating the cuff, bring back the arm to be placed on the table as mentioned above.

7. Interpret the Findings

- Chart the systolic and diastolic BP of the child in numbers.
- Mention how and where BP was recorded: (i) the arm or leg; (ii) the position (seated, standing or lying down); (iii) cuff size used and the type of BP apparatus (mercury sphygmomanometer, or others).
- Plot both the readings on locally available standard BP percentile charts according to the age, sex, and the height of the child.
- Stage the BP—normotension, prehypertension, or established hypertension **(Key Box 18)**. Normal values are given in **Key Box 19**.

Important Tips

- Take a repeat reading later when the child is quiet and relaxed, if the first reading was obtained with the child anxious or crying.

- Do not label a child as hypertensive based on only one casual high reading. Take a second reading after 5–10 minutes in the same arm and later in the other arm.
- Consider the child as having hypertension only after obtaining a minimum of three abnormal high readings at different sittings.
- In cardiac cases, BP must also be similarly recorded in the lower limbs in the popliteal fossa with an appropriate cuff tied around the mid-thigh region (auscultate over the popliteal artery).

The American Heart Association (AHA) recommends taking a reading with both arms and averaging the readings. To check the pressure again for accuracy, wait about 5 minutes between readings. Typically, blood pressure is higher in the mornings and lower in the evenings. If the blood pressure reading is a concern or masked or white coat hypertension is suspected, a 24-hour blood pressure study may be required to assess the patient's overall blood pressure profile.

9.5 EXAMINATION OF THE PRECORDIUM

Precordium refers to the anterior chest wall area overlying the heart. The heart is normally positioned beneath the sternum and to the left of the sternum. Its apex is usually located just inside of the midclavicular line in the 5th left intercostal space.

- The ***right heart border*** lies within 1 cm lateral to the right border of the sternum. The right heart border is formed from above downwards by superior vena cava, right atrium, and inferior vena cava.
- The ***left heart border*** is formed from above downwards by arch and descending aorta, pulmonary artery, left atrial appendage, and the left ventricle.

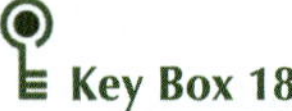

Key Box 18

Interpretation of Blood Pressure

- After recording the systolic and diastolic BP, obtain the expected (50th centile) height percentile for the child's age and sex.
- Plot the recorded systolic and diastolic BP under his/her height percentile against locally available BP percentile charts.
- If the recorded systolic and diastolic BP falls below 90th percentile for the child's height percentile, the child is said to have normal *blood pressure*.
- If the readings fall in between 90th and 95th percentile, the child is labeled as *pre-hypertensive*.
- Readings above 95th percentile indicate the child to have *hypertension*.

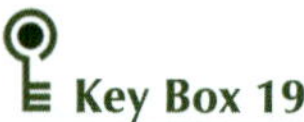

Key Box 19

Normal Blood Pressure

In the absence of a readily available nomogram, the following formula will be of use as a guide to decide whether the child is having BP within normal limits in children above one year of age:

1. Systolic BP (50th percentile)
   = 90 + [2 × age in years]
2. Systolic BP (5th percentile)
   = 70 + [2 × age in years]
   (lower limit of normal systolic)
3. Diastolic BP (50th percentile)
   = 55 + [2 × age in years]

In preterm and term neonates, the mean arterial blood pressure (MAP) must be equal to or more than the gestational age; it must not be less.

A. Inspection of Precordium

Look for symmetry and shape of the anterior chest wall, precordial chest deformities, pectus carinatum, pectus excavatum, Harrison sulcus, apical impulse, and pulsations in the left parasternal region, epigastric pulsations, and pulsations in the suprasternal region and the neck.

1. Precordium

In the absence of pleural or pulmonary conditions or pectus carinatum or other skeletal abnormalities, precordial bulge or asymmetry of the chest indicates the presence of a chronic cardiac condition like ventricular enlargement. Pulmonary hypertension with a large left to right shunt results in bulge of the upper sternum.

2. Apical Impulse

Note the location, and character of apical impulse, if visible. Diffuse apical impulse is highly suggestive of hyperdynamic conditions and if it is seen down and out, it indicates cardiac enlargement or cardiac displacement.

Also look for abnormal pulsations in the following areas: (i) left parasternal,

(ii) epigastric, (iii) suprasternal, (iv) localized pulsation in the pulmonary area—second left intercostal space; (v) both sides of the neck and also over the back of the chest, (vi) right parasternal and intercostal spaces in conditions of dextrocardia, dextroposition, or marked cardiac enlargement.

- The presence of abnormal pulsations noticed in any of the above areas is subsequently confirmed by palpation. The clinical significance of each of these is discussed in detail in the next section.

3. Venous Prominence

Prominent veins over specific regions in the neck or over precordium indicate superior vena caval obstruction.

B. Palpation (Key Box 20)

Palpation gives valuable information regarding the cardiac position or malposition, its size (normal or enlarged), status of ventricular chambers (dilated or hypertrophied), and the status of valves and major arteries.

The clinical objectives of palpation over the precordium are to localize, characterize, record, and interpret from the characteristics of: (i) Apical impulse (or point of maximal impulse); (ii) precordial pulsations over specified areas, (iii) heaves, and thrusts, (iv) palpable sounds; and (v) thrills.

Palpate routinely and systematically all the specified conventional areas of palpation over the precordium and adjacent areas starting from: (a) Apex, (b) mitral area, (c) aortic area, (d) pulmonary area, (e) tricuspid area, (f) left parasternal region, (g) right parasternal region, (h) suprasternal notch, (i) epigastric (subxiphoid) region, (j) right and left supraclavicular areas and (k) over carotid arteries **(Key Box 21)**.

Initial Preparatory Steps before Undertaking Palpation over the Precordium

- Conduct the examination of the child from the right side of the child.
- Keep talking to the mother in a friendly manner eliciting clinical details and take time to touch the child. This step is extremely important to get optimum cooperation from the child.

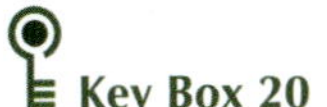

Key Box 20

Cardiac Palpation

1. Apex beat
2. Precordial pulsations
3. Heave and thrusts
4. Palpable heart sounds
5. Thrill

- Keep the child sitting either in the mother's lap or in a comfortable chair so that child's chest and precordium is in alignment with your elbow.
- Keep periodically looking at the child with a warm, smiling and friendly facial expression while you are engaged in taking the history of illness.
- Only sick children who cannot sit down must be asked to lie down. A feeling of anxiety, helplessness and vulnerability occurs as soon as you make the child lie down on an examination couch.

Tips for Improving Palpatory Skills

- Palpate as many normal children's precordium as possible during your clinical postings.
- Get to appreciate that normally the cardiac impulse is felt in the left side of the chest.
- Be aware of the fact that no pulsations or cardiac impulse will be felt over the right side of the chest as the heart is beneath the sternum and to the left of the sternal border.
- Ensure that the heart is placed normally on the left in its usual place and this is the first step and objective in palpation. For this, keep the palms of both hands on either side of the sternum to feel the cardiac impulse and pulsations. This simple step is rewarding in identifying dextrocardia wherein the apical impulse and pulsations are felt more easily on the right side of the chest than on the left side.

Steps in Performing Palpation

1. Take care not to place a cold hand over the chest wall.
2. Prewarm your palm of the hand after appropriate handwashing.
3. Encircle the anterolateral rib cage with your right hand so as to place the palm of

Key Box 21

Palpation of Precordium

Specified areas	*What is to be felt and recorded*
Apical	• To localize precisely the site and to identify the character • Normal or abnormal: Left side or right side; shifted outwards, downwards or outwards and downwards • Diffuse, tapping, hyperdynamic, heaving, thrusting, or non-localizable
Precordial	To identify the presence and localize the abnormal pulsations in the following areas: (i) Left parasternal areas, (ii) epigastric region, (iii) suprasternal notch, (iv) pulmonary area
Left parasternal • Mitral area • Aortic area • Pulmonary • Tricuspid • Carotids – Right and left supraclavicular – Upper or lower parasternal regions – Suprasternal notch	Lift or heave—present or absent; if present, grading of its severity (1, 2 or 3) • Thrills and their timing • Pulsations • Heaves/lifts • Sounds • Others } Systolic, diastolic, or continuous

your right hand over the precordial area so that the ulnar side of the hypothenar area is overlying the palpable apical impulse.

4. Feel for the outermost and lowermost area where the apical impulse is best felt by the palm.
5. Notice the presence of any thrill either in the left parasternal area or over the apex.
6. Localize precisely the apical impulse (apex beat) using the pad of your right index finger or right middle finger.
7. The next step is to find out the intercostal space in which this maximum impulse is felt.
8. Keep the index finger of the left hand over the sternal angle of Lewis as the landmark. Second left intercostal space is identified as the space just below and lateral to the sternal angle of Lewis. Each of the pads of tips of four fingers of the right hand is placed in the left intercostal spaces. The index finger is now moved to be placed finger over the 2nd space, the middle finger over the 3rd space, the ring, 4th finger over the 4th space, and the 5th (little finger) over the 5th space. The normal apical impulse is felt 1 cm inside the left midclavicular line, in 4th or 5th space **(Fig. 9.14)**.
9. Characterize the type of the apical impulse **(Fig. 9.15)**.
10. Interpret the clinical implication of your finding.

1. Apical Impulse

Apical impulse refers to the *outermost and lowermost definitive palpable outward thrust of cardiac impulse* in the lower precordium. Impulse is imparted by the anterior movement of left ventricular apex during early systolic contraction of the left ventricle. When the spirally arranged musculature contracts during the systole, the ensuing rotatory movement brings forward the left ventricular apical impulse towards the anterior chest wall. This is felt by the examining finger as a brief, light tap.

Location

- The site of normal apical impulse at different ages is as follows:

Birth till 1 year	3rd left intercostal space 0.5–1 cm lateral to the midclavicular line
1–4 years	4th left intercostal space mostly just lateral to the midclavicular line and occasionally in the 5th left intercostal space *(Contd...)*

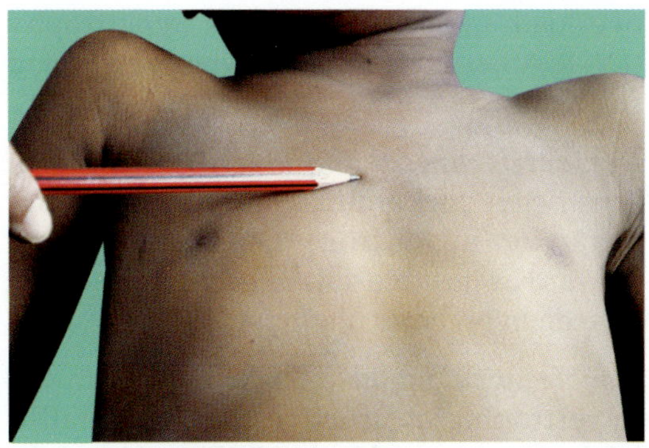
Fig. 9.14a: The most crucial step in CVS examination is identification of angle of Lewis and 2nd left intercostal space.

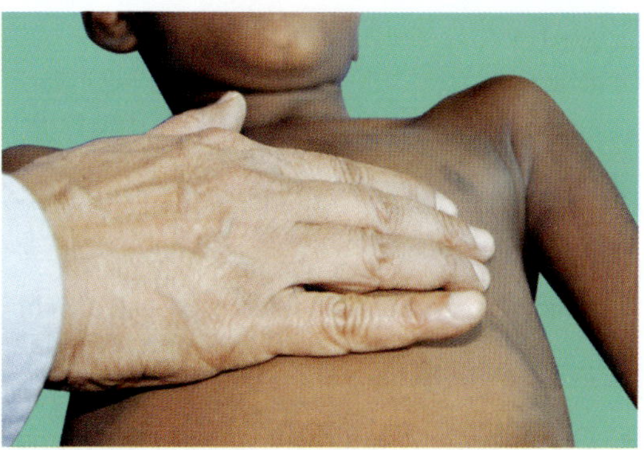
Fig. 9.14b: Palpation: Initial step to locate the position of heart.

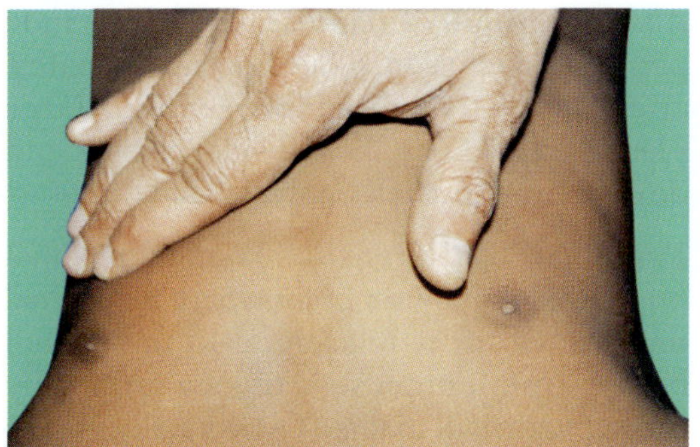
Fig. 9.14c: Palpation for precise localization of the apical impulse.

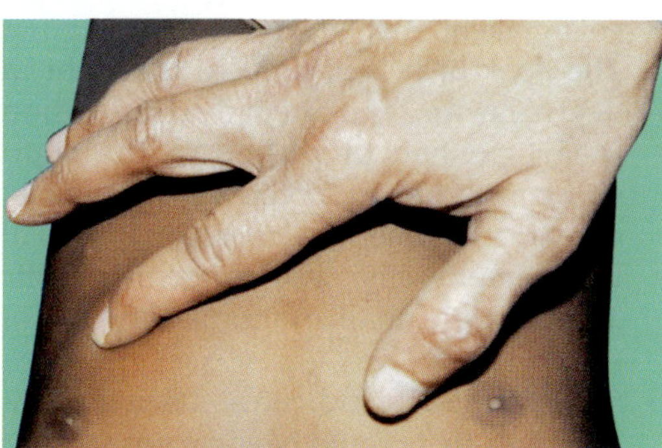
Fig 9.14d: Precise localization of apical impulse with pad of index finger.

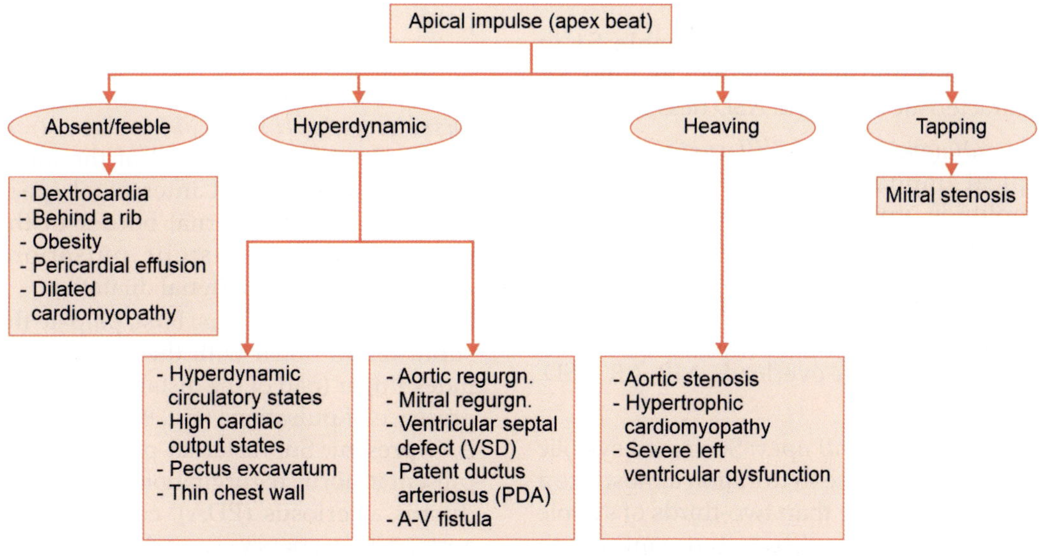

Fig. 9.15: Types of apical impulse and the possible causes.

(Contd...)	
4–8 years	4th (mostly) or 5th left intercostal space in the midclavicular line
8–12 years	4th or 5th left intercostal space 1 cm medial to the midclavicular line
Beyond 12 years	5th left intercostal space 1 cm medial to the midclavicular line

- Displacement laterally and/or inferiorly indicates cardiac enlargement.
- An apex that is displaced downwards and outwards suggests left ventricular enlargement or left ventricular hypertrophy.
- Lateral and/or outward displacement alone is characteristic of right ventricular enlargement.
- The apex beat is shifted to the right in dextrocardia. Acquired dextroposition (heart pushed or pulled to the right side) may be observed in congenital diaphragmatic hernia (left side); congenital lobar emphysema, and congenital cystic adenomatoid malformation (CCAM) of the lung.
- Shift to the left indicates cardiomegaly. However, there could be some non-cardiac causes of shift to left, such as abnormality of the spine (scoliosis), sternum (pectus excavatum), or lung (contralateral pneumothorax or pleural effusion; ipsilateral collapse of the lung).

Character of apical impulse

Tapping apical impulse: Palpable S1 in mitral area and heard by bell as loud S1. Characteristic of MS and ASD (less common).

Hyperdynamic (forceful/ill-sustained) apex: Apical impulse with rapid, brisk, large amplitude, upstroke, occupying more than one intercostal, exceeding 3 cm; ill-sustained with impact duration between one-third and half of systole. Suggests left ventricular dilatation. Seen in high cardiac output states, ventricular volume overloads, MR, AR, VSD, and PDA.

Heaving (sustained) apex: Sustained systolic thrust with increase in duration almost like a wave felt for more than two-thirds of systole with increased amplitude but confined to one intercostal space. Indicative of pressure overload and left ventricular hypertrophy (LVH), AS, systemic arterial hypertension, and coarctation of aorta.

Retractile apical impulse: Indicative of constrictive pericarditis where there is systolic retraction away from the chest wall and forward or positive diastolic thrust. Also may be seen in biventricular hypertrophy.

Double apical impulse: Suggests AS with AR, hypertrophic obstructive cardiomyopathy, left bundle branch block (LBBB) and in adults left ventricular aneurysm. In hypertrophic cardiomyopathy, the second apical impulse is due to diastolic filling of the enlarged ventricle. Triple or quadruple impulse may also be felt in HOCM.

Absence of apical impulse: Causes include peri-cardial effusion, dilated cardiomyopathy, apex under the rib, emphysema or large pleural effusion on the left side, obesity, and dextrocardia (not felt on the left side).

Point of maximal impulse: Point of maximal impulse is the lowest point where a maximal impulse or lift is felt lateral to the sternal border. Apical impulse is usually formed by the left ventricular apex. Occasionally, due to the rotational movement of the heart due to right ventricular dilatation or hypertrophy, the ventricular apex is no longer felt by the examiner's hand. In such instances, the lowermost and outermost impulse felt by the examiner is referred to as the point of maximal impulse.

2. Precordial Pulsations

- *Systolic pulsation in pulmonary area:* Palpate by placing the pad of the index finger in the 2nd left intercostal space just lateral to the sternal border in the pulmonary area. Systolic pulsations indicate pulmonary arterial dilatation.
- *Suprasternal pulsations:* First, palpate the suprasternal notch with the pad of your index finger (pad of the distal phalanx) for presence of pulsations **(Fig. 9.16a)**. Record it, if present. Suprasternal pulsations are present in aortic regurgitation (AR), patent ductus arteriosus (PDA), coarctation of aorta, aortic aneurysm, and poststenotic dilatation of pulmonary or aortic stenosis.

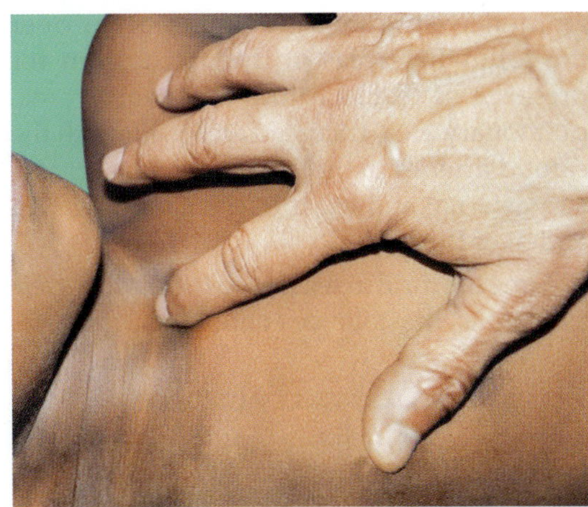

Fig. 9.16a: Palpation of suprasternal pulsations.

- *Epigastric pulsations* Next, palpate gently the epigastric (subxiphoid) region with the pads of two or three fingers of your right hand with a mild upward slant towards the substernum **(Fig. 9.16b)**. Epigastric pulsations are suggestive of right ventricular volume overload states, including atrial septal defect, tricuspid regurgitation, and moderate to large ventricular septal defect.
- *Parasternal pulsations:* Place the four fingers of the right hand over the left parasternal region in such a manner that index finger is over the 2nd left intercostal space, middle finger over the third space, the fourth in the fourth space, and the little finger in the fifth space. Feel for the presence of systolic pulsations; also feel for any forward thrust or heave beneath the same areas.

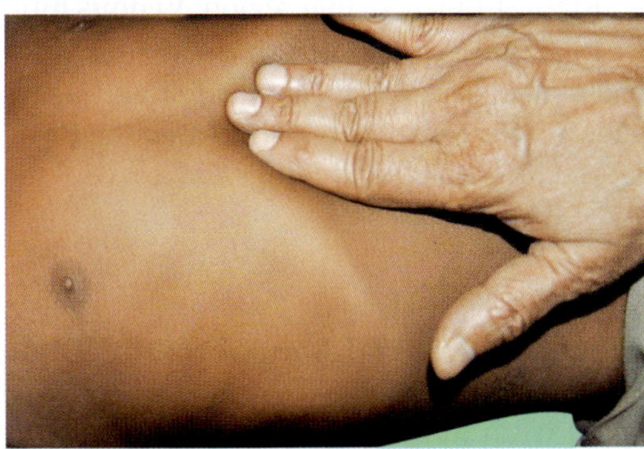

Fig. 9.16b: Palpation of epigastric pulsations indicative of right ventricular enlargement with three fingers.

a. Parasternal pulsations without lift may be felt in very thin children with muscle wasting.
b. Pulsations in the parasternal area without a perceptible or palpable left parasternal lift is characteristic of right ventricular volume overload conditions, like ASD, TR, moderate-to-large VSD without pulmonary arterial hypertension, besides hyperdynamic high output states.
c. Pulsations along the right sternal edge are characteristic of large right atrium as in Ebstein anomaly.

3. Parasternal Heave

How to elicit parasternal heave

- *Step 1:* Observe the left parasternal region over the precordium for the presence of visible pulsations in the intercostal spaces or forward lift or thrust/heave.
- *Step 2:* Place the finger pads (2nd—index, 3rd, 4th, and 5th—little finger) of your right hand in the 2nd, 3rd, 4th, and 5th left intercostal spaces over the precordium and feel these pulsations.
- *Step 3:* Place the ulnar border of your right hand and record any forward thrust or heave over the left parasternal region **(Fig. 9.17)**.
- *Step 4:* Try to obliterate by applying gentle downward pressure by your right hand ulnar/hypothenar eminence.
- *Step 5:* Grade the lift/heave into grade 1, 2 or 3.
- *Step 6:* Interpret the finding.

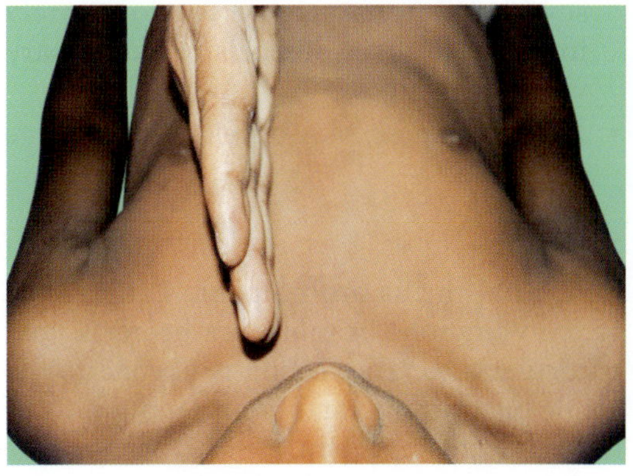

Fig. 9.17: Palpating with the ulnar border for parasternal pulsations and heave.

Grading of parasternal heave

Grade 1

- Noticeable left parasternal pulsatile impulse in the left intercostal spaces with mild upward lift—seen by placing a pencil or ballpoint pen over that area.
- Seen in right ventricular enlargement and left atrial enlargement (lesser possibility).

Grade 2

- Forward obvious forceful left parasternal lift obliterated by firm pressure by fingers or ulnar side of the palm.
- Caused by mild right ventricular hypertrophy.

Grade 3

- Outward forceful and sustained left parasternal lift not obliterated by firm pressure by ulnar side of the palm.
- Suggests significant right ventricular hypertrophy.

4. Other Palpable Sounds

- *Palpable first sound (S1) over the apex:* Mitral stenosis (felt as tapping apex).
- *Palpable second sound (S2) in pulmonary area:* Pulmonary hypertension.
- *Palpable third sound (S3):* Severe MR or dilated cardiomyopathy.
- *Palpable fourth sound (S4):* More often palpable in adults than in children in the following conditions: Hypertrophic cardiomyopathy, severe AS, acute MR, and longstanding hypertension.
- *Opening snap* in the early diastolic period may sometimes be felt in mitral stenosis.
- *Systolic ejection clicks:* May be palpable in severe pulmonary hypertension, rarely in valvular aortic stenosis or pulmonary valvular stenosis.
- *Pericardial knock:* May be felt in constrictive pericarditis.

5. Thrills

Precordial thrills are palpable equivalents of the vibrations of murmurs heard in that particular area. The feeling is likened to the gentle purring of a cat. The site and timing of murmurs are important.

Palpate (use the medial border of the palm of your right hand mainly the hypothenar eminence—the most sensitive area) over the following areas of the precordium for presence of thrills: Mitral area, aortic area, pulmonary area, tricuspid area, over both the carotid arteries in the supraclavicular region, suprasternal and left infraclavicular regions, and over the back.

Time the thrill in relation to the cardiac cycle as systolic, diastolic, or continuous.

Systolic Thrill: Diagnosis by Location

- Mitral region in the apical region and lateral to mitral area: **MR**
- Aortic area—2nd right intercostal space outside the right sternal border, suprasternal notch; and over both the carotids: **AS**. This murmur is better felt in the sitting position, with the child leaning forwards.
- Pulmonary area—2nd left intercostal space (LICS) just outside the sternal border: **PS**
- Anywhere in the left parasternal region from pulmonary to mitral area, but mostly in the lower left parasternal region: **VSD**
- Over the carotids: **AS**

Diastolic Thrill

- *Apex and internal to apex:* **MS**. The diastolic thrill in mitral stenosis is better felt with child lying in the left lateral position.
- *3rd LICS just lateral to the sternal border:* **AR**

Continuous Thrill

- 2nd LICS, left supraclavicular area: **PDA**
- 2nd LICS and down: **Rupture of sinus of Valsalva**
- Right supraclavicular region: **Venous hum**

Perform follow-up auscultation over the area where the thrill was felt and again identify the murmur which created the thrill. Correlate with other findings and arrive at the most likely diagnosis.

C. Percussion

There is a general opinion that cardiac percussion has a limited value. There may be some truth in this for neonates and infants. But in older children who are cooperative and non-apprehensive; percussion, when done properly, gives invaluable information.

Recommended Steps of Percussion

Step 1: Delineate the upper border of the liver

Start percussing downwards over each intercostal space from right infraclavicular area till you reach the area of dullness, usually felt in the 5th space **(Fig. 9.18a, b)**. The intercostal space with dullness marks the level of upper border of the liver.

This step will also help to recognize dextrocardia with or without situs inversus.

Step 2: Define the right heart border: Percuss inwards from right midclavicular line in each of the five upper intercostal spaces and proceed medially towards the right sternal border **(Fig. 9.18c)**. Direct the percussion parallel to the right heart border. The dullness of the right heart border does not usually extend beyond the right sternal border.

Step 3: Delineate the left heart border: Percuss inwards starting from the mid-axillary space in the 2nd, 3rd, 4th, and 5th left intercostal spaces from the resonant to the dull area **(Fig. 9.18d, e)**. The lower and outermost area of cardiac dullness on the left side corresponds to the apex of the heart.

Percussion Findings and Interpretations

1. Extension of dullness beyond the right sternal border indicates right atrial enlargement. Indicates atrial septal defect (moderate to large), pericardial effusion or pericardial cyst, dilated cardiomyopathy, Ebstein anomaly, or dextrocardia.
2. Dullness beyond the apical impulse on the left side indicates pericardial effusion.
3. Dullness >2.5 cm beyond left sternal border in the second left intercostal space

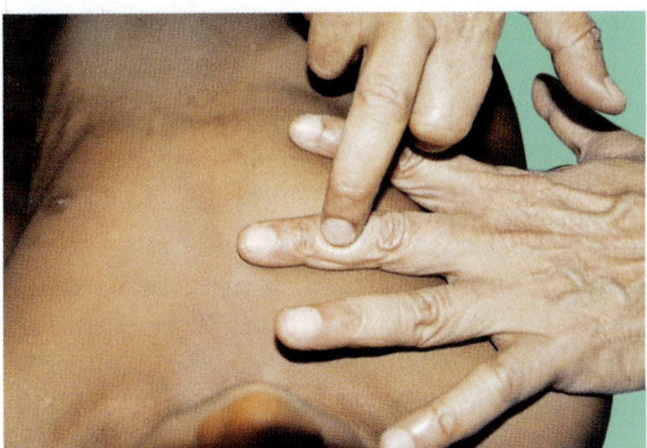

Fig. 9.18a: Percussion to locate the upper border of the liver. Percuss from second right intercostal space downwards to find out the area of upper border of liver dullness.

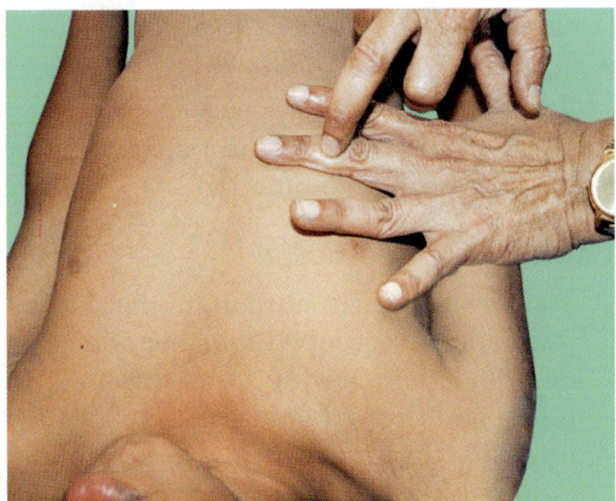

Fig. 9.18b: Percussion to locate the lower border of the liver.

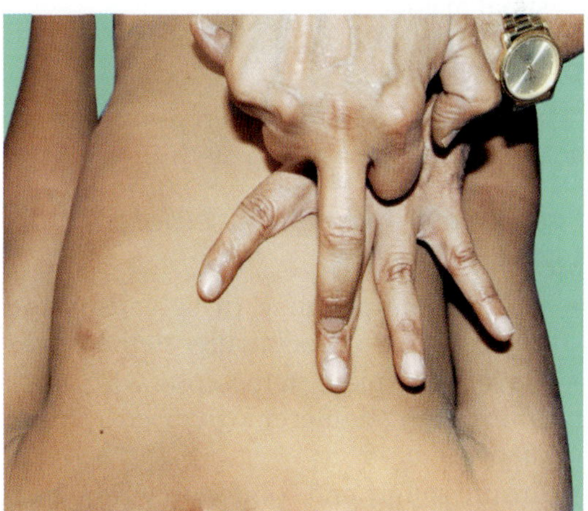

Fig. 9.18c: Percussion over the intercostal spaces from right midclavicular line towards the right sternal border to delineate the right heart border.

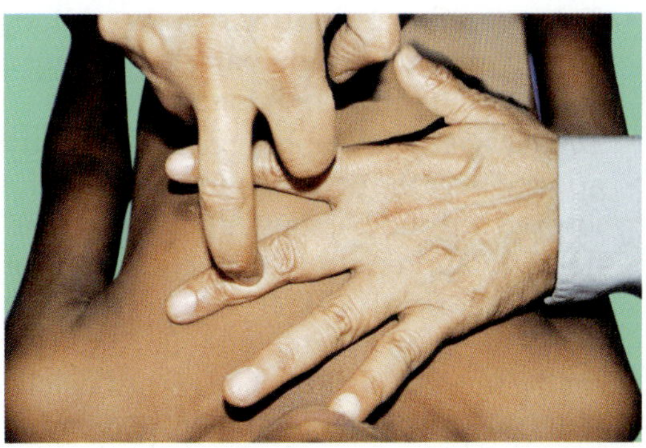

Fig. 9.18d: Percussion over the 2nd left intercostal space to find out dullness in pulmonary area for pericardial effusion and pulmonary artery dilatation.

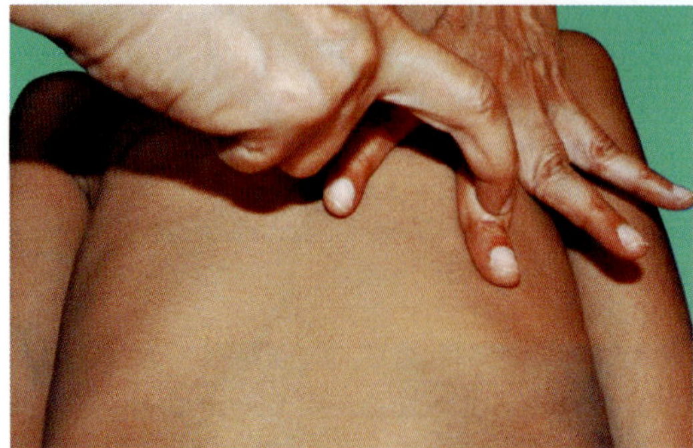

Fig. 9.18e: Percussion laterally away from the apical impulse to feel for extension of cardiac dullness.

indicates pulmonary arterial hypertension, idiopathic pulmonary artery dilatation, patent ductus arteriosus (PDA), left atrial enlargement, pericardial effusion **(Key Box 22)**, aortic aneurysm, or mediastinal mass.

Key Box 22

Percussion Signs in Pericardial Effusion

1. Rotch sign

Percussion dullness in the right cardiohepatic angle in the fifth intercostal space extending outwards beyond the right sternal border.

2. Ewart sign

In significantly large pericardial effusions, an area of dullness on percussion with bronchial breath sounds and increased tactile fremitus below the left scapular angle was described by Ewart in 1986. This occurs because of the compressive atelectatic effect on the left lower lobe segment by the massive pericardial fluid collection.

3. Shifting dullness in the Trendelenburg position

Wider band of dullness on percussion over the base of the heart due to the gravitational shifting of pericardial fluid towards the base. This must be done only in older children who are not anxious and not severely breathless.

D. Auscultation

"Cardiac auscultation should not become a lost art, or the stethoscope a medical relic."

Essentials for Meaningful Auscultation

Stethoscope

- Do not compromise in selection and possession of a good quality stethoscope.
- Have a two piece stethoscope with a bell (minimum diameter of 2.5 cm) and a diaphragm.
- Ensure snugly and comfortably fitting ear knobs.
- The angle of earpieces must be oriented forwards and directed towards the external auditory meati and canals.
- ***Tubings:*** Good quality, thick-walled, weather-proof, double-barreled tubings, 25–30 cm (10–12 inches) long.
- ***Diaphragm:*** The diaphragm when tightly applied over the precordium filters out the low pitched audible sounds (<150/Hz) and helps to appreciate selectively events of high frequencies (>300/Hz up to 1000/Hz) (e.g. S2, ejection and mid-systolic clicks and for the soft, but high-pitched early diastolic murmur of aortic regurgitation, pericardial friction rub).
- ***Bell:*** The bell must be applied lightly to listen to low frequency heart events between 35 Hz and 150 Hz (e.g. heart sounds S3 and S4 gallops, mid-diastolic rumble of mitral stenosis).

Auscultator: Auscultator should have a proper frame of mind (unbiased, undisturbed, tension free) and open ears. Attitude, concentration, focus, practice, training, keenness in learning, and practicing the art matter a lot.

Environment

- Quiet room with no noise from fans and air conditioners.
- Adequate lighting to detect even minimal degree of cyanosis.
- Child friendly, non-threatening examination setting.
- Toys and colorful picture books to distract the child.
- Appropriate presence of a chaperone or parents during examination.

Objectives of Auscultation

1. Train your ears to auscultate the normal heart sounds (grouped together and often described as lubb-dup, lubb-dup)—S1 in mitral and tricuspid areas, S2—its relative intensity and its splitting in aortic and pulmonary areas, its normal variation with respiration, physiological S3 in specific age groups, normal intensity of these sounds,

the normally silent systolic and the diastolic intervals without any murmurs, or other sounds.

2. To identify abnormal additional sounds and murmurs; to distinguish normal sounds and innocent murmurs from abnormal sounds; and to characterize pathological murmurs based on location, timing, pitch, and tonal qualities.

Areas for Auscultation **(Fig. 9.19)**

1. Apex—mitral area (MA)
2. Aortic area (AA) and second aortic area—2nd right intercostal space near right sternal border and 3rd left intercostal space near left sternal border
3. Tricuspid area (TA) at the lateral end of the left sternal border opposite 4th and 5th left intercostal spaces, internal to the apical impulse
4. Pulmonary area (PA)—2nd left intercostal near the left sternal border
5. Left and right infraclavicular regions
6. Left anterior axillary line and over both axillae
7. Over both carotid arteries on either side of neck
8. Over both interscapular regions (for pulmonary/aortic collateral murmurs)
9. Over femorals, brachials, popliteals (especially while taking lower limb BP, pistol shot sounds, and Duroziez murmur in aortic regurgitation, peripheral AV malformations)
10. Cranium, fontanelle, and both lumbar regions (renal areas).

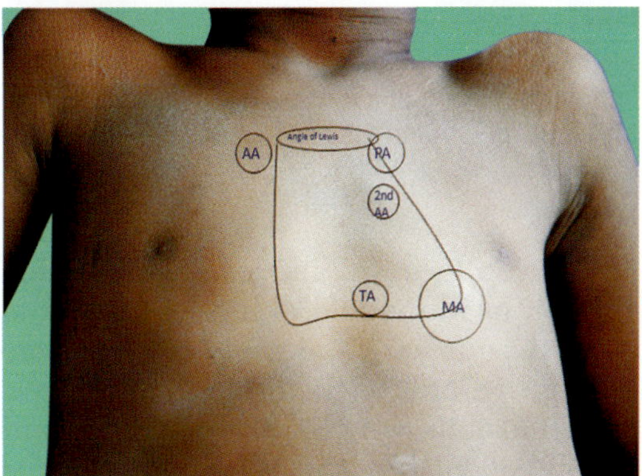

Fig. 9.19: Areas of auscultation.

Steps in Cardiac Auscultation **(Fig. 9.20)**

1. Sequence

- Start auscultation from apical region (mitral area) either in sitting position or in supine position. The child may be slightly turned to the left side.
- From the apex, move your stethoscope internally inch by inch (*inching* technique) and at every stop auscultate in a similar manner.
- Then proceed to tricuspid area, then upwards along the left parasternal margin to pulmonary area.
- Proceed next across the sternum to the aortic area in the 2nd right intercostal space and finally over both carotid arteries on either side of the neck.
- Timing of cardiac events is done in relation to carotid artery impulse or apical impulse by simultaneous palpation.

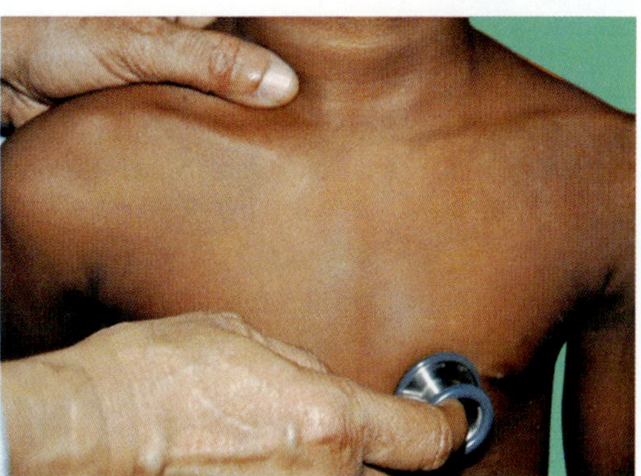

Fig. 9.20a: Auscultation: Identification of S1 by timing it with carotid arterial pulse.

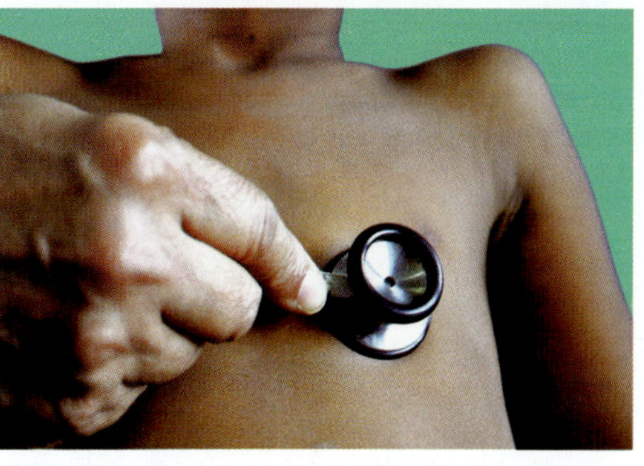

Fig. 9.20b: Auscultation over the mitral area where the apical impulse has been localized.

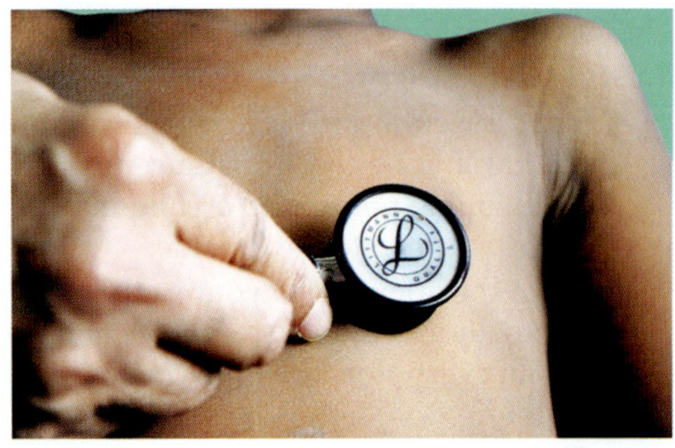

Fig. 9.20c: Auscultation over the mitral area for low-pitched heart sounds and mid-diastolic murmur of mitral stenosis.

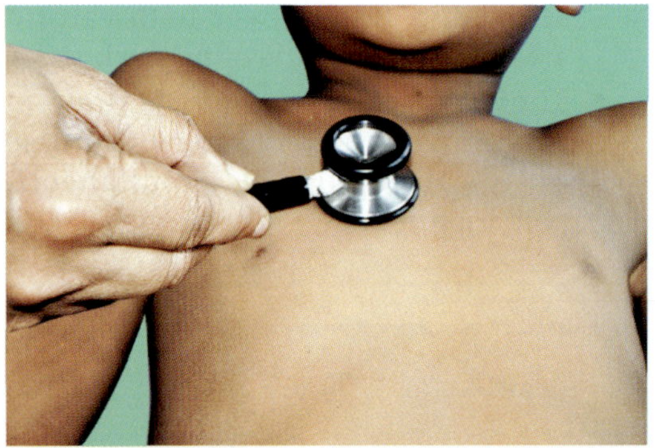

Fig. 9.20d: Auscultation over aortic area in the right second intercostal space just lateral to the sternal border.

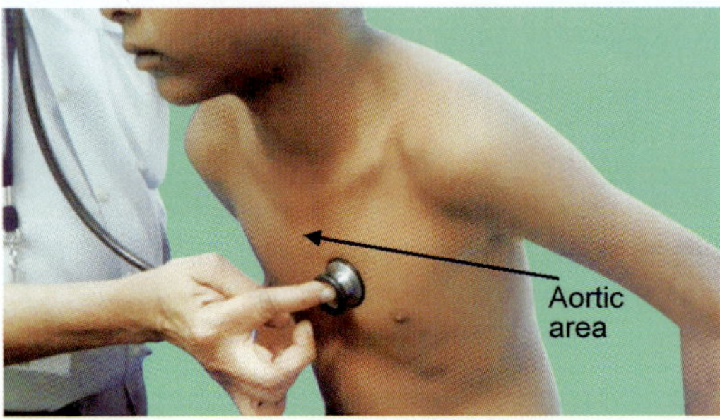

Fig. 9.20e: Auscultation over the 2nd aortic area (3rd left intercostal space just lateral to right sternal border) for high-pitched early diastolic murmur of AR.

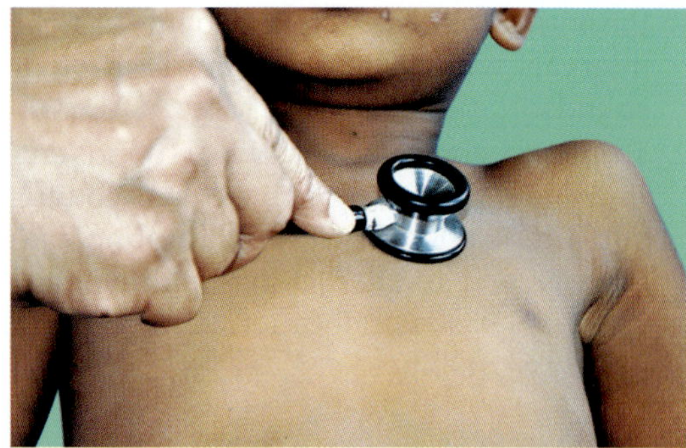

Fig. 9.20f: Auscultation of the pulmonary area over the left 2nd intercostal space just lateral to the left sternal border for pulmonary component of S2, character of splitting, and murmurs.

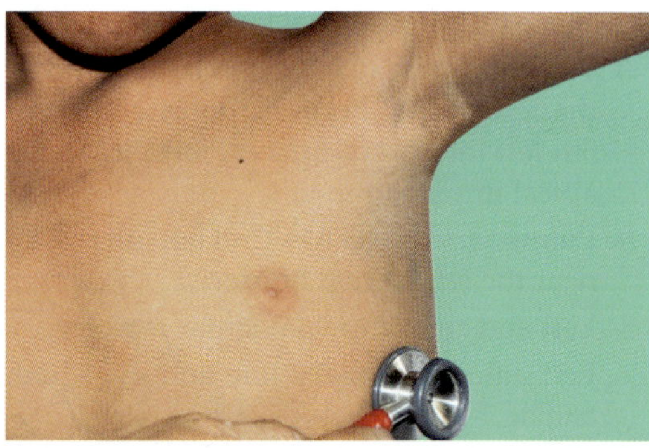

Fig. 9.20g: Auscultation away from the apical area towards the axilla for conduction of pansystolic murmur of mitral regurgitation.

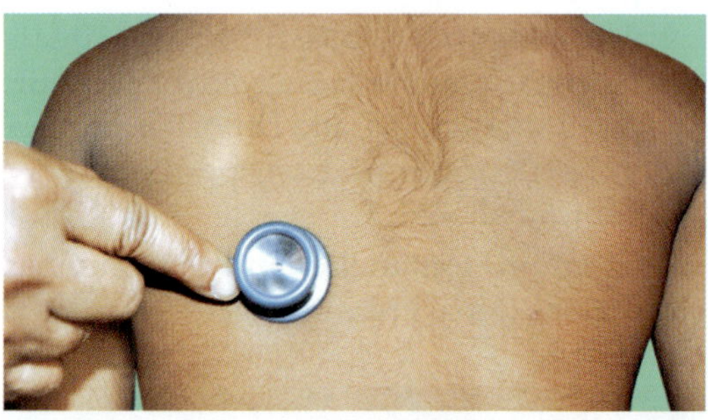

Fig. 9.20h: Auscultation over the upper back on the left side for conduction of pansystolic murmurs of MR, VSD or continuous murmurs of collaterals.

2. As beginners, first focus your attention and identify the first heart sound (S1) by auscultating in the mitral area over the apex and simultaneously palpating the carotid pulse. With practice, identifying S1 becomes a habit, when no longer one has to time it with the carotid pulse.
3. Develop focussed and selective listening habit of individual events—concentrate with your ears and mind only on one event, i.e. only on S1, then only the systolic period following S1, then only S2, and subsequently on the early, mid, and late diastolic period, and again on S1.

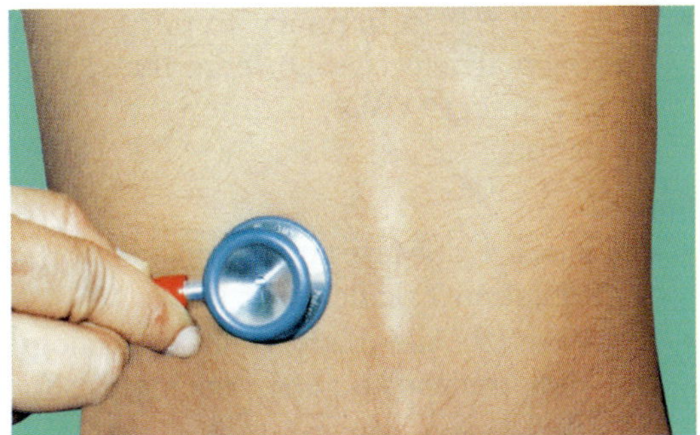
Fig. 9.20i: Auscultation over the back for bruit or murmur—coarctation of aorta and renal artery stenosis.

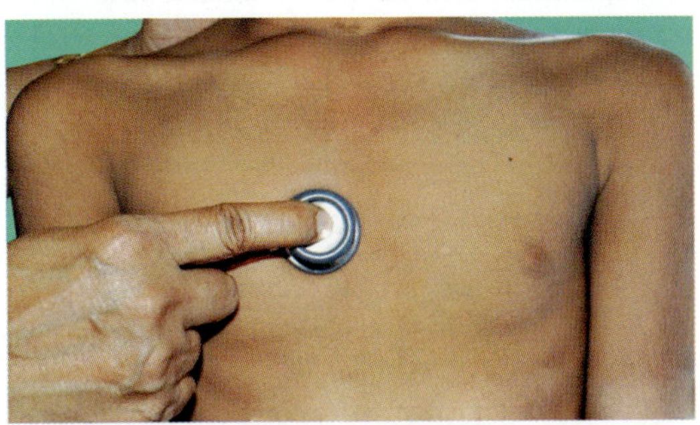
Fig. 9.20j: Auscultation over the 3rd and 4th right parasternal regions for heart sounds and murmurs in cases of right heart enlargement, dextrocardia, and pericardial effusion.

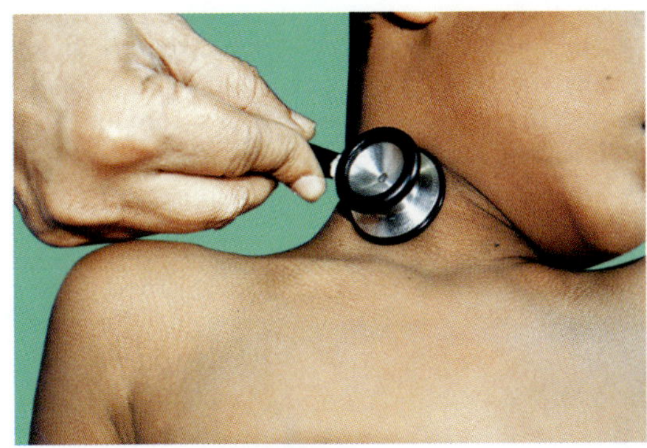
Fig. 9.20k: Auscultation over carotid artery for systolic bruit in aortic stenosis.

4. After you are confident about the identity of S1, assess and document its intensity—normal/loud/soft or quiet.
5. Listen to detect the presence and character of any additional sound and/or systolic murmur immediately after S1 and before S2.
6. In pulmonary and aortic areas, identify the intensity and splitting characteristics

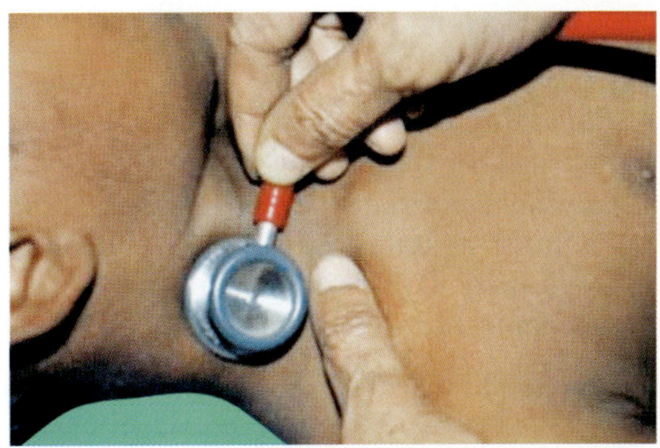
Fig. 9.20l: Auscultation over the neck after finger pressure at the base of the neck for obliteration of venous hum.

(normal, wide, fixed, or paradoxical) of both aortic and pulmonary components of S2.

7. After S2, listen for opening snap, S3, S4, and diastolic murmurs (early, mid, and late diastolic murmurs with or without presystolic accentuation).

9.6 HEART SOUNDS

A. First Heart Sound (S1)

- S1, produced by closure of tricuspid and mitral valves, is usually heard as a single sound as the interval between the earlier mitral valve closure and the later tricuspid valve closure is less than 20 to 30 msec which the human ear cannot discriminate.
- S1 signifies the onset of systolic interval.
- S1 is best heard over the apical impulse in the mitral area.

How to Identify S1

- Palpate simultaneously the external carotid arterial pulsation with index and middle fingers or thumb of your left hand while you are auscultating the apex (mitral area) with the bell of the stethoscope.
- Listen and focus only on the sound which is heard just before the carotid arterial pulsation. S1 (*lubb*) just precedes the carotid pulse and is louder at apex. It is lower pitched and longer than S2 (*dup*) which follows carotid pulse.
- Assess the characteristics of S1, once you are confident about S1 (low-pitched a longer bisyllabic sound—resembling conventionally the sound–"lubb").

Intensity of S1

Loud S1

- ***Physiological:*** Exercise, anxiety, certain high output states, sinus tachycardia.
- ***Cardiac conditions:*** Mitral stenosis, short PR interval states, like WPW syndrome, tricuspid stenosis, atrial myxoma, mechanical prosthetic valve.

Soft S1

- Muscular thick chest wall, obesity, emphysema.
- Long PR interval, acute rheumatic fever with prolonged PR interval, pericardial effusion, mitral regurgitation, tricuspid regurgitation, certain types of AV block, calcific mitral stenosis, myocarditis and LV dysfunction, cardiogenic shock, cardiomyopathy, proximal left bundle branch block (LBBB).

Variable intensity: Complete atrioventricular dissociation or complete heart block, (reason: short PR intervals with early ventricular systole even before atrial emptying); atrial fibrillation, multiple ventricular ectopics.

Splitting of S1

In the following 5 conditions, the splitting of S1 can be appreciated.

1. Ebstein anomaly
2. Right bundle branch block (RBBB)
3. Large atrial septal defect (ASD)
4. Premature ventricular ectopics
5. Severe pulmonary arterial hypertension

B. Second Heart Sound (S2)

Second heart sound is produced because of closure of semilunar valves of aorta and pulmonary artery. It has two components—the first component (A2) is by aortic valve closure and the second and later (P2) is caused by closure of the pulmonic valve. S2 signifies the end of systolic interval and beginning of the diastolic interval.

Record the intensity and split of S2.

Intensity of S2

Loud S2

- *Increased A2:* Systemic hypertension, aortic root dilatation, L-transposition of great arteries (L-TGA), tetralogy of Fallot (TOF).
- *Increased P2:* Pulmonary hypertension, atrial septal defect (ASD), large ventricular septal defect (VSD), pulmonary artery dilatation.

Soft S2

- *Decreased A2:* Severe aortic stenosis, aortic regurgitation, calcific aortic valve.
- *Decreased P2:* Pulmonary stenosis, tetralogy of Fallot, transposition of great arteries.

Splitting of S2 (Key Box 23)

Focus and appreciate the normal variable split of S2, i.e. almost single or closely split S2 in expiration and an easily discernible, well audible split during inspiration (Fig. 9.21). Reason for this respiratory variation in the splitting of S2 is explained in Fig. 9.22.

Key Box 23

Normal variable Splitting of Second Heart Sound (S2)

Expiration

- Both aortic and pulmonary components of S2 are very close to each other (less than 20–30 msec)
- Hence, this close splitting in expiration cannot be appreciated by human ears during auscultation.

Inspiration

- The aortic component of S2 occurs much earlier and the pulmonary component of S2 occurs later (the interval between the two components is more than 30 msec)
- The splitting of S2 is easily appreciated by everyone.

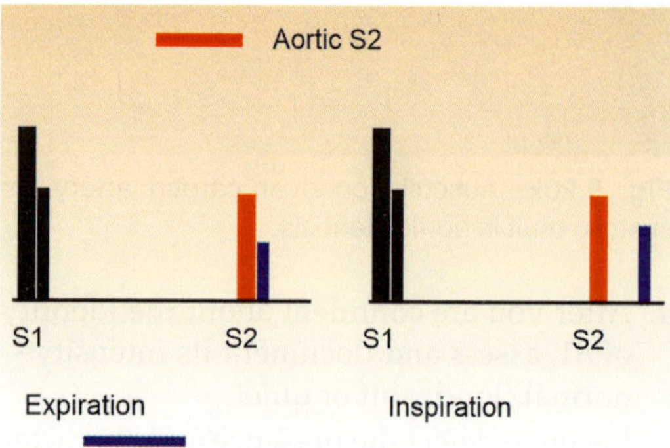

Fig. 9.21: Normal variation in splitting of S2 during expiration and inspiration—pulmonary component of S2 is better heard in inspiration because the splitting is wider.

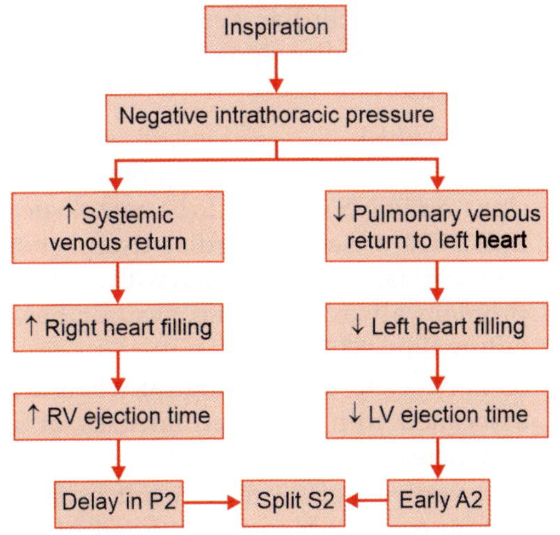

Fig. 9.22: Mechanism of splitting of second heart sound.

1. Wide, variable splitting of S2: Wide, variable splitting of S2 refers to audible aortic and pulmonary components of S2 both in inspiration and expiration. The three possibilities for the occurrence of such a wide, variable splitting are as follows:

a. *Early closure of aortic valve (A2):* Ventricular septal defect, mitral regurgitation
b. *Late closure of pulmonary valve (P2):* Pulmonary arterial hypertension, pulmonary stenosis, right bundle branch block, pulmonary embolism, left ventricular ectopic beat
c. *Increased hangout interval due to decreased impedance to pulmonary artery:* Atrial septal defect, pulmonary stenosis, total anomalous pulmonary venous connection, Ebstein anomaly, idiopathic dilatation of pulmonary artery.

2. Wide, Fixed Splitting of S2: Wide, fixed splitting occurs in ostium secundum-atrial septal defect (OS-ASD) and severe right ventricular failure **(Fig. 9.23)**.

Mechanism: In ASD, the second heart sound is widely split because of the delayed or wider *pulmonary hangout interval*. Pulmonary hangout interval refers to the time gap between the pulmonary arterial pressure curve and the right ventricular systolic pressure curve at the time of closure of semilunar valves of pulmonary and aortic arteries. The normal pulmonary hangout interval is 60–80 msec and the aortic hangout interval is 20 msec.

As in normal children, there is an increase in venous return to the right side of the heart during inspiration even in children with atrial septal defect. But during expiration, the pressure in the right atrium decreases as there is relatively less venous return. This decreased pressure in right atrium increases the left to right shunt blood flow into the right atrium from high pressured left atrium. This causes increased flow through the pulmonic valve, prolonged right ventricular ejection time and delayed closure of pulmonary valve.

But with the development of moderate to severe pulmonary arterial hypertension, the splitting of S2 is no longer wide and it becomes narrow, but it may still remain fixed.

3. Single S2: S2 is said to be single when no split is heard either in expiration or in inspiration. Causes are listed below:

a. *Absence of the aortic component of S2:* Severe aortic stenosis (valvar, supravalvar AS), hypoplastic left heart syndrome, aortic atresia, aortic regurgitation
b. *Absence of the pulmonary component of S2:* Pulmonary atresia, truncus arteriosus, absent pulmonary valves

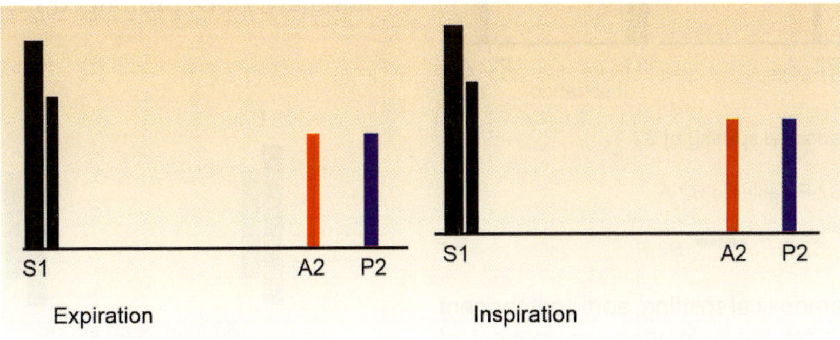

Fig. 9.23: Wide, fixed splitting of S2 in ostium secundum-atrial septal defect.

c. *Very soft or masked pulmonary component of S2-feeble S2-P:* Tetralogy of Fallot, transposition of great arteries, posteriorly placed pulmonary artery, severe pulmonary stenosis

d. *Synchronous aortic and pulmonary component of S2* severe pulmonary arterial hypertension, primary pulmonary arterial hypertension, Eisenmenger complex.

4. Paradoxical or reverse splitting of S2: Instead of the normal occurrence of aortic component before pulmonary component, in paradoxical splitting, pulmonary component of S2 is heard before the aortic component of S2 (split audible in expiration but not in inspiration) **(Fig. 9.24)**. This occurs in the following conditions:

1. Patent ductus arteriosus, and post-stenotic dilation of aortic stenosis.
2. *Aortic stenosis and hypertension:* Due to delayed closure of aortic valve, mechanical obstruction, or functional resistance to systolic emptying of left ventricle.
3. *Electrical conduction disturbances:* Proximal left bundle branch block and right ventricular ectopics.

C. Third Heart Sound (S3)

S3 is a low-pitched protodiastolic sound best heard with the bell, 120–200 msec after S2 (A2) during the rapid ventricular filling phase.

Physiological S3 is normally heard in infants, children, adolescents, and athletes.

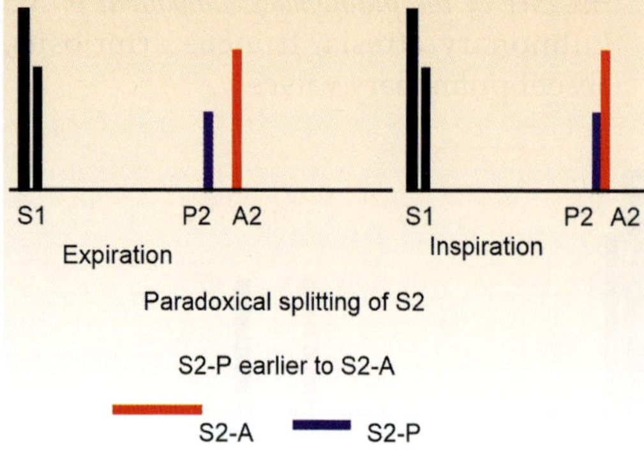

Fig. 9.24: In paradoxical splitting, aortic component of S2 occurs after the pulmonary component of S2, in expiration, the splitting is heard, whereas in inspiration, both components are close to each other that splitting cannot be appreciated.

If there are no cardiac symptoms and no other positive cardiac signs, S3 is likely to be physiological.

Pathological S3

- In children with cardiac symptoms and/or signs, audible S3 is likely to be pathological indicative of serious cardiac dysfunction and heart failure. S3 in a child with a cardiac problem always signifies systolic heart failure **(Fig. 9.25)**.
- S3 is likely to be pathological when it is associated with decreased intensity of S1 and increased intensity of S2.
- Left ventricular S3 may result because of volume or pressure overload of left ventricle. Other causes include constrictive pericarditis and pericardial effusion.
- Right ventricular S3 is heard best over the 3rd, 4th and 5th left parasternal intercostal spaces and epigastrium. It occurs due to overload of right ventricle (as in severe TR or ASD).

D. Fourth Heart Sound (S4)

S4 is a low frequency, presystolic sound, best heard with lightly applied bell over the mitral area. It occurs in the late diastolic period due to atrial contraction against ventricular non-compliance or left ventricular resistance to left atrial blood flow across mitral valve **(Fig. 9.26)**. It is an important sign of diastolic heart failure or active ischemia. Except in very old geriatric population, S4 is always pathological in all the other age groups. Causes are as follows:

- *Left atrial S4 gallop:* Aortic valvular stenosis, systemic arterial hypertension.
- *Right atrial S4 gallop:* Pulmonary arterial hypertension, pulmonary stenosis, Ebstein anomaly, ASD, prolonged PR interval.

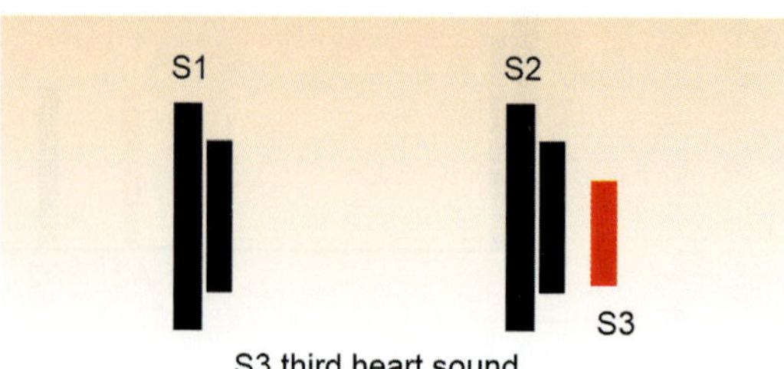

Fig. 9.25: Sudden appearance of third heart sound (S3) in a child with a cardiac problem always signifies systolic heart failure.

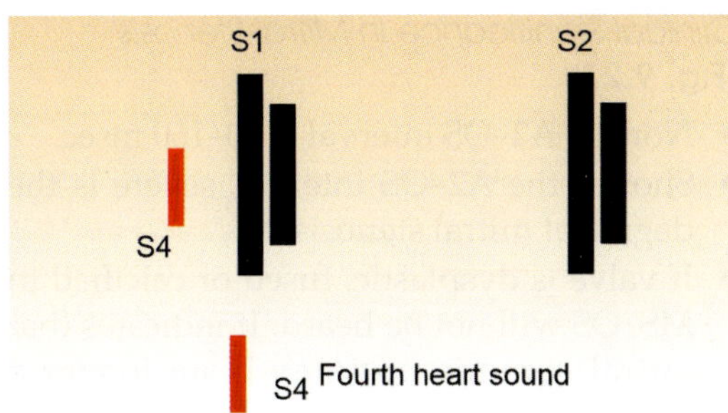

Fig. 9.26: Fourth heart sound (S4) occurs in the late diastolic period due to atrial contraction against ventricular non-compliance; it is almost always pathologic.

E. Gallop Rhythms

Presence of S3/S4 when associated with tachycardia and normally audible S1 and S2 will give on auscultation an impression of a triple or quadruple cadence likened to the galloping sound (canter) of a horse on the run. The significance is the same as mentioned earlier regarding presence of S3 and S4; but because of associated marked tachycardia, there is a greater probability of presence of underlying myocardial or valvular cardiac dysfunction.

Triple Rhythm

- S3 gallop/ventricular or protodiastolic gallop: S1, S2 and S3 heard in tachycardia
- S4 gallop/atrial or presystolic gallop: S1 + S2 + S4 (forceful atrial contraction sound)

Quadruple rhythm: All the four heart sounds are heard in presence of tachycardia.

Summation gallop: Marked tachycardia shortens the diastolic interval; and both S3 and S4 are heard together because of their closeness to each other.

F. Clicks

1. Vascular Clicks

Multiple systolic clicks (sharp, high frequency sounds) are heard in moderate or large sized patent ductus arteriosus which can be appreciated in spite of a loud, continuous murmur. The large left ventricular volume ejected into the aorta results in dilatation of ascending aorta and arch of arota, resulting in aortic ejection clicks.

2. Valvular Ejection Clicks (EC)

Systolic ejection clicks occur in early systole (prior to ventricular ejection) close to S1 as a result of abrupt halting of opening semilunar valves which are stenosed. Clicks can originate from aortic valve or pulmonary valve. Stenosis can be structural or functional.

Aortic Ejection Clicks **(Table 9.7)**

It is a sharp, high frequency, loud sound, best heard at apex during early systole. It is also heard well between the right upper sternal border and apex across the mid and left sternal area than in the aortic area. Conditions where aortic ejection clicks are heard include aortic stenosis (AS), bicuspid aortic valve and dilated aortic root as seen in tetralogy of Fallot (TOF), truncus arteriosus, and systemic arterial hypertension. In aortic stenosis, the ejection click is invariably followed by ejection systolic murmur. Greater the severity of aortic stenosis, closer is the occurrence of aortic ejection click to first heart sound.

Table 9.7: Aortic and pulmonary ejection clicks

Differentiating features	Aortic click	Pulmonary click
Maximally heard site	Aortic area and apex	Pulmonary area–2nd LICS
Conduction	Carotids	Localized
Variation with respiration	No variation	Phasic, louder in expiration
Arterial pulse	Low volume	Normal volume
Precordial palpation	Heaving LV apex Left parasternal heave	
Thrill	Aortic area and carotids Pulmonary area	
S2	Closer or paradoxical split	Wider splitting

Pulmonary Ejection Click **(Table 9.7)**

Pulmonary ejection click is less common than aortic click. It is best heard at the sternal edge of 2nd and 3rd LICS preceding an ejection systolic murmur. It decreases in intensity during inspiration. Conditions where pulmonary ejection clicks are heard include pulmonary valvular stenosis (PS), pulmonary arterial hypertension (PH), and pulmonary arterial root dilatation.

Remember

- Severe the pulmonary stenosis, shorter is the S1-EC interval.
- In PS, with increasing severity, EC occurs earlier, whereas in PH, with increasing severity, the click occurs later.
- In PH, there is no increase in intensity of the click during expiration which is noticed in PS.

Non-ejection Clicks

These include mid or late systolic clicks heard frequently in prolapse of mitral or tricuspid valve. These clicks are variable in intensity, better heard in a standing position, or during a Valsalva maneuver.

G. Opening Snap (OS)

Opening snap occurs due to the opening of pliable, non-calcific atrioventricular valves (mitral or tricuspid) across high pressure gradient generated between the respective atria and ventricles, as in mitral or tricuspid valve stenosis. It is heard immediately after S2 in the early diastolic period, just medial to the apex in mitral stenosis.

The opening snap is a high-pitched, fairly loud, snappy, sharp, clicking sound appreciated best by the diaphragm pressed firmly over the mitral or tricuspid area. Opening snap is heard till the valve leaflets or cusps (especially the anterior cusp of the mitral valve) remain mobile. The opening snap disappears once the leaflets calcify.

> Auscultate and focus total attention in the early diastolic period after second heart sound (S2) to hear for opening snap, whenever you hear loud S1 with rough, rumbling mid-diastolic murmur.

Clinical Significance in Mitral Stenosis **(Fig. 9.27)**

- Normal A2–OS interval is 40–160 msec.
- Shorter the A2–OS interval, severe is the degree of mitral stenosis.
- If valve is dysplastic, fused or calcified in MS, OS will not be heard. It indicates that mitral commissurotomy is no longer a reasonable surgical option. Mitral opening snap may also be heard in MR, large VSD, PDA, hypertrophic obstructive cardiomyopathy, and left atrial myxoma.
- Tricuspid opening snap may be heard in tricuspid stenosis, large ASD, and right atrial myxoma.

H. Pericardial Friction Rubs

1. Pericardial Rub

Pericardial friction rub is produced by friction of visceral and parietal layers of pericardium, often caused in children by inflammation of the pericardium. Pericardial friction rub has high specificity nearing 100% in the diagnosis of acute pericarditis, but has low sensitivity.

This intense high-pitched rubbing sound is superficially heard over the precordium; it has a to and fro grating, scratching or rasping, machine-like quality. It has classically three components, in nearly half of patients. The first

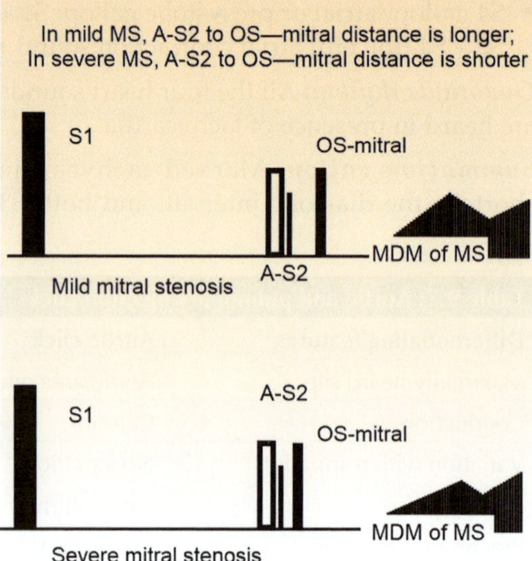

Fig. 9.27: Above: loud S1, wider distance between aortic S2 and OS of mitral stenosis (mild) within mid-diastolic murmur; below: closer aortic S2–OS in severe mitral stenosis.

component is heard throughout ventricular systole and the latter two components in the diastole—second in mid-diastole (rapid ventricular filling phase) and the third one in late diastole (presystolic atrial contraction period). The systolic component is more constantly heard.

Being high-pitched; these interrupted scratchy sounds are best heard with the diaphragm during inspiration in 2nd and 3rd left intercostal spaces and in end-expiration over the left lower sternal border when the child leans forward. The pericardial rub is differentiated from pleural rub by appreciating its presence even with breath held in expiration.

As it may be transient, repeated auscultation is essential. Once picked up by auscultation, other physical signs of pericardial effusion must be looked for.

2. Pericardial Knock

Pericardial knock is a high frequency sound heard throughout the precordium in constrictive pericarditis. It occurs in the early diastole—usually 90 to 120 msec after A2, but slightly earlier than the average S3. It occurs at the trough of the deep y wave of jugular venous pulse **(Fig. 9.28)**. This is caused by sudden cessation of the ventricular filling. It gets augmented in inspiration.

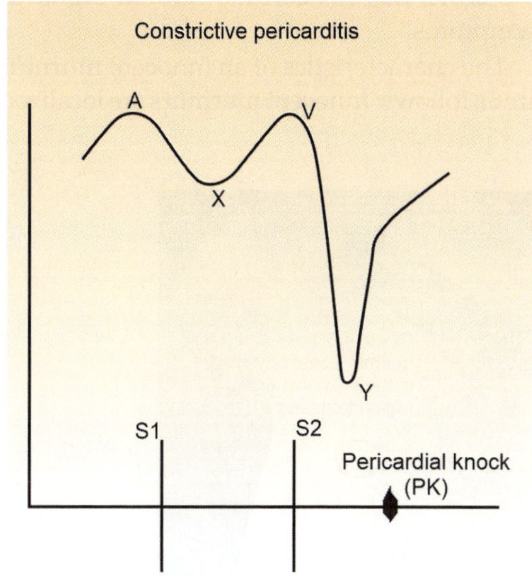

Fig. 9.28: Pericardial knock—in relation to 2nd heart sound and 'y' wave of JVP.

9.7 HEART MURMURS

Heart murmurs are audible sound energy waves in the range of 20 Hz and 2000 Hz transmitted to the precordial surface. They occur as a result of turbulent blood flow created by functional or structural hemodynamic alterations in the pattern of blood flow in the heart chambers (a) across the valves or the atrial or ventricular septum; or (b) in the vessels as in coarctation of aorta, renal artery stenosis, or pulmonary arteriovenous collaterals malformations.

Characteristics of Murmurs

1. ***Site of origin:*** Identify the region where the murmur is loudest and hence is best heard, (point of maximal intensity, e.g. mitral, aortic, pulmonary or tricuspid area)
2. ***Phase and timing:*** Time in relation to the cardiac cycle and heart sounds as systolic/diastolic/continuous/to and fro murmur, etc.
3. ***Duration (length):*** Short, long, pan, early, mid, or late.
4. ***Intensity-amplitude or loudness:*** Grading of murmur **(Key Boxes 24 and 25)**.
5. ***Frequency:*** Expressed as pitch of the murmur—high/medium/low.
6. ***Shape or configuration:*** Crescendo (progressively louder), decrescendo (progressively softer), diamond (increasing loudness with a peak and then decreasing), or plateau

Key Box 24

Grading of Systolic Murmurs (Levine, 1933)

Grade 1	Barely audible, faint; heard only by trained ears with intense concentration in a quiet room
Grade 2	Faint, but clearly audible immediately
Grade 3	Moderately loud without palpable thrill
Grade 4	Loud with a thrill (a palpable vibration on the chest wall)
Grade 5	Very loud, thrill present, and audible even with the edge or rim of the diaphragm of the stethoscope touching the chest wall area where thrill is felt
Grade 6	Very loud, heard with the stethoscope lifted off the chest wall by a few mm.

Key Box 25

Grading of Diastolic Murmurs

Grading	*Degree*
I	Very soft/faint murmur
II	Faint but heard easily without difficulty
III	Loud without a palpable thrill
IV	Loud with a thrill

(same intensity from the beginning to the end).

7. ***Conduction and radiation:*** Conduction is when a murmur is propagating with the same loudness in an outward direction from the area of origin. Radiation is when the murmur is progressively less intense along a direction from the site of origin **(Fig. 9.29)**.
8. ***Tonal quality:*** Presence of harmonics and overtones—blowing, rumbling, vibratory, musical, etc.
9. ***Dynamic variation:*** Alteration in murmur intensity with respiration, posture, exercise, and a few maneuvers.

Steps of Auscultation

Step 1: Listen for murmurs in all precordial areas with the help of either the diaphragm or bell of the stethoscope—mitral, aortic, tricuspid, pulmonary areas, all along left parasternal region inside of the midclavicular line from first to the lowermost intercostal spaces overlying the heart, over both the carotid arteries on either side of the neck, and in the left infra- and supraclavicular regions.

Key Box 26

Characteristics of Pathologic Murmurs

A murmur with the following characteristics is NEVER considered INNOCENT.

1. All pansystolic murmurs
2. All diastolic murmurs
3. Late systolic murmurs
4. *Loud murmurs:* 3/6–6/6 (very loud murmur with and without thrill)
5. Continuous murmurs (except venous hum and mammary soufflé)
6. Murmurs with abnormal cardiac findings

Step 2: Identify the site of origin and other characteristics of the murmurs as listed above.

Step 3: Decide the nature of murmur based on the above characteristics. Is the murmur: (a) Functional or Innocent; or (b) Organic (pathological) **(Key Box 26)**.

Step 4: Interpret the hemodynamic cause of murmur from its site of origin, timing, conduction and others.

Step 5: Evaluate the severity and sometimes the etiology of the heart problem by correlating the murmur with symptoms and other clinical signs.

A. Innocent Murmurs

A murmur heard in a child without structural heart disease is termed innocent murmur; the child has no cardiac related signs or symptoms.

The characteristics of an innocent murmur are as follows: Innocent murmurs are localized

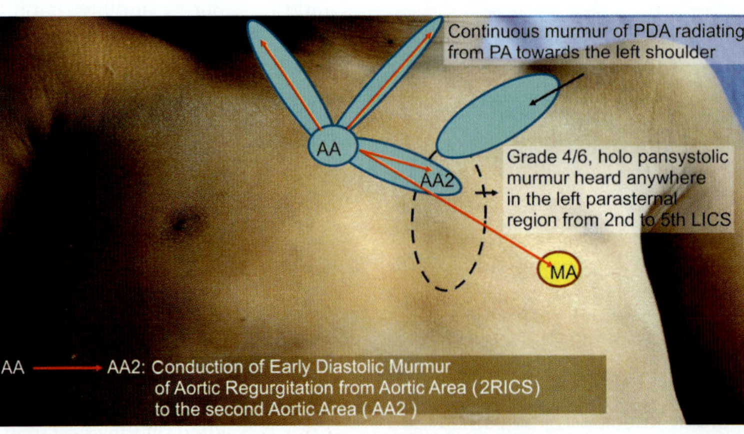

Fig. 9.29: Conduction and radiation characteristics of murmurs from the area of origin.

to specific area, short, often early or mid-systolic, grade 1/6 or 2/6 (not associated with thrill), and they vary in intensity with change in posture, decreasing in intensity when the child stands, sits up, or strains during a Valsalva maneuver.

A few common causes of innocent murmurs are discussed below.

1. Physiologic Pulmonary Branch Stenosis of the Neonates

Listen to this low pitched, grade 1 or 2 early to mid-systolic, ejection murmur in newborns and infants below 6 months of age.

It is due to the turbulence occurring at the bifurcation of the relatively narrower right and left pulmonary artery branches arising at comparatively sharp angles from the dilated main pulmonary trunk. The main pulmonary trunk is dilated because it receives the combined cardiac output from the high pressure right ventricle during the fetal period. The other reason for the turbulence is a physiologic drop in pressure from the main to the proximal branch pulmonary arteries.

This murmur disappears anywhere between 2–6 months after birth when these vessels grow larger in diameter. It is physiologic as there is no permanent narrowing or obstruction of branching pulmonary arteries.

2. Innocent Pulmonary Flow Murmurs

Theses murmurs are heard in many school age children, adolescents, and athletes (age group of 8 to 14 years). The murmur is ejection systolic, grade 2–3, and best heard at the left upper sternal border. It is better heard in expiration and in the supine position. Pulmonary flow murmurs are exaggerated in anterior chest wall deformities, like pectus excavatum, those with a straight back, or kyphoscoliosis and in children with high output states, like anemia.

3. Venous Hum

Venous hum is one of the commonest innocent murmurs in children below 5 years. It is a blowing, low-pitched, continuous murmur often associated with thrill. It is the turbulent vibration created by the venous drainage from the internal jugular and subclavian veins into the superior vena cava or by the angulation of internal jugular vein over the transverse process of the atlas. It may also be heard on the left supraclavicular area. Anemia exaggerates its intensity. It is not to be mistaken for the continuous murmur of PDA.

Differentiating venous hum from murmur of PDA

- Place the index finger to feel for any palpable thrill and hear by auscultation with the bell for presence of any murmur over the right lower part of the neck in the infraclavicular area and supraclavicular area, lateral to the insertion of sternocleidomastoid.
- Perform the following steps, if a murmur is present with or without a thrill:
  - i. Locate the site of murmur and identify where the murmur is loudest.
  - ii. Appreciate and record any change in the intensity of the murmur or disappearance of thrill and murmur with (a) change of posture—sitting and lying down position; (b) turning the head; and (c) Valsalva maneuver (in an older child).
  - iii. Apply light finger pressure just above the clavicle and try to appreciate the disappearance of thrill and murmur observed earlier.
  - iv. Auscultate and listen for presence of associated clicks along with the murmur.
  - v. Interpret as per **Key Box 27**.

4. Still's Murmur

It refers to a long crescendo-decrescendo mid-systolic murmur with a musical, vibratory quality heard in children between 3 and 6 years of age. The quality is likened to the strumming of guitar or buzzing of a bee. It is rare in infancy. As a low to mid frequency murmur, it is heard better by the bell over left mid-sternal and lower parasternal areas. The intensity of the murmur increases in the supine position and with exercise, fever, and other hyperkinetic states associated with increased heart rate. It is proposed to be caused by the vibrating chordae tendinae of mitral valve or by the vibrating false tendon of the left ventricle.

Key Box 27

Differentiating Venous Hum from Patent Ductus Arteriosus

Differentiating features	*Venous hum*	*Continuous murmur (PDA)*
1. Site where best heard	Right infraclavicular and supraclavicular areas	Pulmonary area and in the left infra- and supra-clavicular regions
a. Loudest part of the murmur	During diastole (maximum venous flow into the right atrium)	In systolic phase
2. Variation with:	Yes	No change
a. Posture	Present and better heard in sitting position; disappears or less distinct on lying down	
b. Head turning	May totally disappear, if not less intense	
c. Valsalva maneuver	Disappearance	
3. Application of light finger pressure just above the clavicle	Disappearance of thrill and the murmur	
4. Clicks	No	May be present

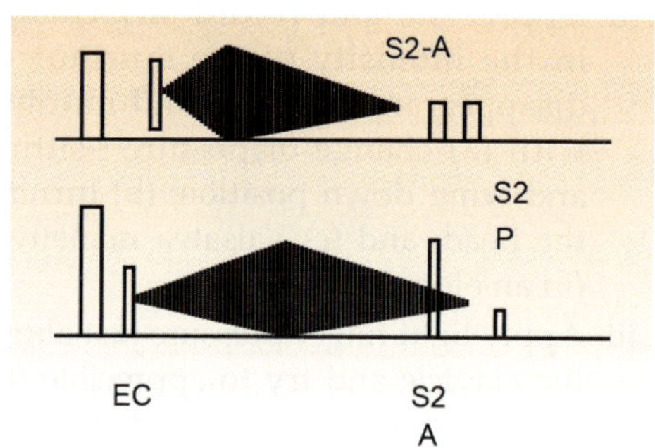

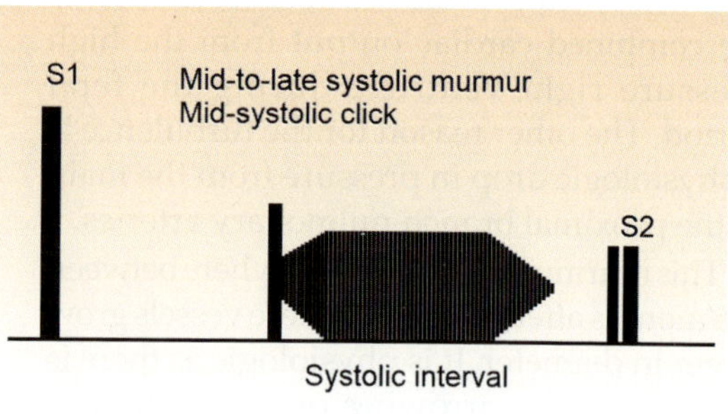

Fig. 9.30: Systolic murmurs.

B. Organic Murmurs

1. Organic Systolic Murmur (Fig. 9.30)

Pansystolic murmur

- Isointensity murmur from S1 to S2
- *Causes:* MR, TR, VSD

Ejection systolic murmur

- Crescendo-decrescendo diamond-shaped murmur
- *Causes:* Aortic stenosis (AS), pulmonic stenosis (PS), ASD, VSD

Mid/late systolic murmur

- Grade 2–3 loud mid/late systolic murmur following click
- *Cause:* Mitral valve prolapse (MVP)

2. Organic Diastolic Murmurs (Fig. 9.31)

- *Early diastolic murmur:* Aortic regurgitation (AR), pulmonary regurgitation (PR)
- *Mid-diastolic murmur:* Mitral stenosis (MS), tricuspid stenosis (TS), Carey-Coombs murmur (of mitral valvulitis), Austin-Flint

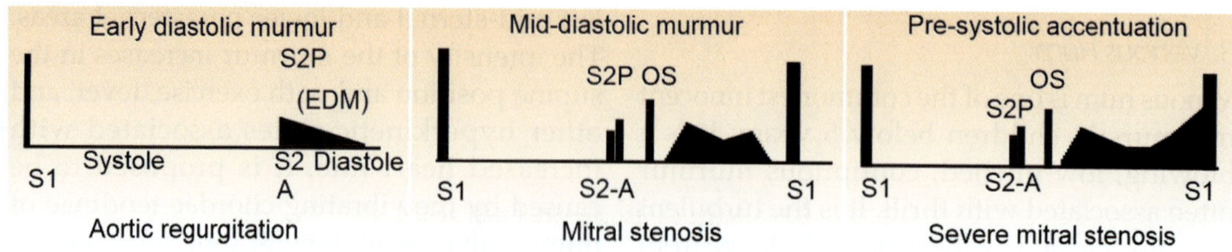

Fig. 9.31: Three types of diastolic murmurs and their causes.

murmur in AR, secondary flow murmurs heard in ASD, VSD, PDA, MR, and TR

- *Presystolic murmur:* Severe mitral stenosis.

3. Organic Continuous Murmurs (Fig. 9.32)

Acyanotic: Patent ductus arteriosus (PDA), aortopulmonary window, rupture of sinus of Valsalva, AV fistulas, peripheral pulmonary artery branch stenosis, and abnormal origin of left coronary artery from pulmonary artery (ALCAPA).

Cyanotic: Truncus arteriosus, pulmonary AV fistulas, and Blalock-Taussig shunt.

Secondary collaterals: Tetralogy of Fallot, aortic coarctation, aberrant left coronary artery with RCA collaterals.

4. Organic Murmurs (systolic-diastolic) Resembling Continuous Murmurs

When there are more than one cardiac lesion, one causing systolic murmur and the other producing diastolic murmur, combination of these two murmurs in presence of tachycardia may be mistaken for a continuous murmur. Only by practice, the examiner can differentiate this systole-diastolic murmur from a continuous murmur.

Combination of defects with systolic and diastolic murmurs that often get misinterpreted as continuous murmur, are as follows:

i. VSD (pansystolic murmur) + AR (early diastolic murmur)
ii. AR (early diastolic murmur) + AS (ejection systolic murmur)
iii. MR + AR
iv. MS + TR

C. Dynamic Auscultation

1. Respiration and Change in Intensity of Murmur

Increased inspiration

- All murmurs of right heart, i.e. murmurs of pulmonary stenosis, tricuspid regurgitation, pulmonary regurgitation and tricuspid stenosis intensify during inspiration.
- All heart sounds (S3, S4) of right ventricle accentuate during inspiration.

Increased expiration

- All murmurs from left heart events: Mitral stenosis and regurgitation; aortic stenosis and regurgitation increase in expiration.
- Pulmonary ejection click.
- Heart sounds—S3, S4 of left ventricle.

2. Posture and Change in Intensity of Murmur

Supine

- Increased still murmur, pulmonary flow murmur
- Decreased or total disappearance of venous hum

Standing

- *Increased:* Murmurs of mitral valve prolapse, hypertrophic obstructive cardiomyopathy
- *Decreased:* Pulmonary flow murmur, pulmonary stenosis, aortic stenosis murmur

Squatting

- *Increased:* Mitral regurgitation, aortic regurgitation, aortic stenosis, pulmonary stenosis
- *Decreased:* Mitral valve prolapse, hypertrophic obstructive cardiomyopathy

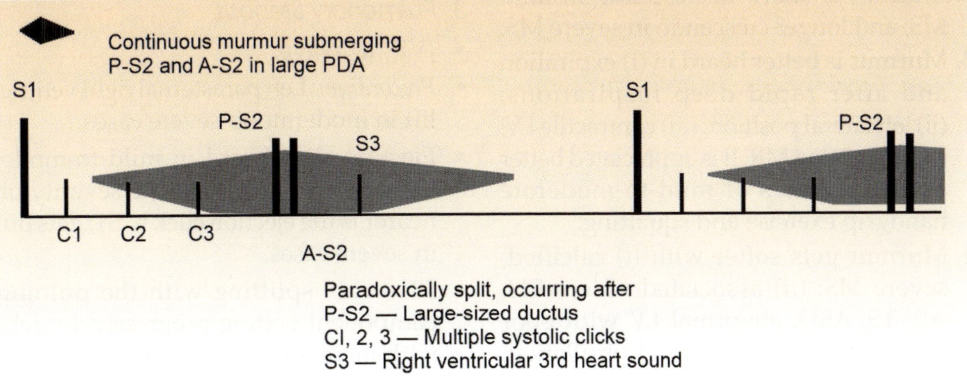

Fig. 9.32: Causes of continuous murmurs.

3. Other Maneuvers

- *Valsalva maneuver:* Increases the intensity of murmur of mitral valve prolapse and HOCM. Decreases the intensity in aortic stenosis and pulmonary stenosis.
- *Isometric exercise handgrip:* The maneuver increases the murmur intensity in mitral regurgitation, aortic regurgitation, and pulmonary stenosis. Decreases the intensity in MVP and HOCM.
- Application of finger pressure at the base of the neck. This maneuver decreases the intensity of venous hum.
- Application of pressure in the abdomen in neonates and children increases the intensity of murmur of VSD.

9.8 SPECIFIC VALVULAR LESIONS

A. Obstructive Lesions

1. Mitral Stenosis

- *Cause:* Often acquired and almost always secondary to rheumatic fever beyond 3 years of age
- *Symptoms:* Progressive dyspnea on exertion (exercise, stress and fever), orthopnea, paroxysmal nocturnal dyspnea, palpitation, fatigue
- *Pulse:* Low volume, pulsus parvus in severe or critical MS
- *Apex:* Tapping with diastolic thrill
- *Heart sound:* S1 loud, S2 normal; gets louder with increasing severity; opening snap heard in MS with non-calcified, mobile cusps.
- *Murmurs*
  1. Low-pitched mid-diastolic murmur often with a presystolic accentuation.
  2. Murmur is short, decrescendo in mild MS; and longer crescendo in severe MS.
  3. Murmur is better heard in (i) expiration and after rapid deep inspirations; (ii) left lateral position; (iii) contractile LV; (iv) associated MR. It is appreciated better after 3 minutes of mild-to-moderate handgrip exercise and squatting.
  4. Murmur gets softer with (i) calcified, severe MS; (ii) associated severe PH, AS, TS, ASD, abnormal LV with poor myocardial function, atrial fibrillation; (iii) large RV rotating the LV posteriorly; and (iv) obesity.
- Differential diagnosis Tricuspid stenosis, left atrial myxoma, cor triatriatum, flow diastolic murmurs of ASD, VSD, MR, and Austin-Flint murmur of AR.

2. Aortic Stenosis **(Table 9.8)**

- *Causes:* (a) Congenital in children below 12 years; (b) rheumatic between 12–18 years; and (c) idiopathic calcification.
- *Pulse:* Low volume (pulsus parvus et tardus or anacrotic slow rising pulse)
- *Apex:* Heaving, left ventricular
- *Thrill* over the aortic area, carotids, left ventricular heaving apical impulse
- *Heart sound:* S1—normal. Louder (especially in congenital) in mild-to-moderate valvular AS; soft in severe AS; S2—normal; paradoxical splitting in severe AS (splitting is wider in expiration and narrower in inspiration); aortic component may be absent in severe AS; S2—very soft and often inaudible in subaortic stenosis.
- *Murmurs:* Grade 3–6, harsh, mid-systolic ejection crescendo-decrescendo murmur best heard in the aortic area and second aortic area with radiation to the carotids. Severe the stenosis, longer the murmur and later the peaking.
- Early diastolic murmur is heard in 30–50% cases of subaortic stenosis.
- *Ejection click:* Heard best at the apex, 0.05 sec after S1, in AS with non-calcified, mobile cusps; EC is not heard in the discrete subaortic stenosis. S1-EC interval becomes progressively shorter with increasing severity.

3. Pulmonary Stenosis

- JVP "a" wave;
- *Precordium:* Left parasternal right ventricular lift in moderate-to-severe cases.
- Ejection click heard in mild-to-moderate valvar stenosis; greater the severity of PS, nearer is the ejection click to S1; gets buried in severe cases.
- S2—wide splitting with the pulmonary component getting progressively delayed with increasing severity; becomes fixed in the most severe forms due to fixed right ventricular output.

Table 9.8: Characteristics of aortic stenosis (AS)

	Valvular AS	Subvalvular AS	Supravalvular AS	HOCM
Etiology	Congenital uni- or bicuspid aortic valve; RHD (usually after 30 years)	Congenital discrete membrane or fibro-muscular ring	Congenital discrete or localized narrowing of ascending aorta; William syndrome	
Carotid pulse	Normal to anacrotic (pulsus et tardus)	Normal to anacrotic (pulsus et tardus)	Unequal; right-sided carotid and radial arteries stronger	Brisk, jerky, systolic rebound
Thrill (maximum)	2nd RICS	2nd RICS	1st RICS	4th LICS
Premature ventricular ectopics	Increased	Increased	Increased	Decreased
Paradoxic splitting of S2	Present in severe cases	No	No	Rather common
S4	AS (severe)	Uncommon	Uncommon	Uncommon
Ejection systolic click	Mostly present, except in calcified valve	Absent	Absent	
Early diastolic murmur of AR	Common in RHD and bicuspid AS with bacterial endocarditis	Sometimes	Rare	No
Dilated ascending aorta	Common	Rare	Rare	Rare

RICS: right intercostal space; LICS: left intercostal space

- Right-sided S4 is heard in severe cases with marked right ventricular hypertrophy with poor compliance.
- 3–6 Grade, harsh, mid-systolic ejection crescendo-decrescendo murmur; severe the stenosis, longer the murmur and later the peaking.

4. Tricuspid Stenosis

Extremely rare. Prominent "a" wave in JVP, and grade 2–3 audible mid-diastolic murmur in tricuspid area increasing in intensity with inspiration indicates presence of moderate to severe TS.

B. Regurgitant (Incompetent) Valvular Lesions of the Heart

1. Mitral Regurgitation

Etiology: Above 3 years often rheumatic in tropical countries; mitral valve prolapse, dilated annular ring secondary to marked left ventricular dilatation as occurs in myocarditis, dilated cardiomyopathies, severe anemia, beriberi, and connective tissue disorders.

Mild MR: Pulse, BP: normal; no cardiomegaly; apex: normal site; heart sounds: normal; no S3; grade 2–3 pansystolic murmur at the apex; no mid-diastolic murmur.

Moderate MR: High volume pulse; apex: may be shifted downwards and outwards and is hyperdynamic; heart sounds: widened S2 splitting; S3 present in many; murmur: grade 3–4 blowing, pansystolic murmur at the apex conducted towards axilla.

Severe MR: Pulse: normal or low; apex: moderate cardiac enlargement with apex shifted downwards and outwards; hyperdynamic; heart sounds: S1—soft; S2—widened; may be loud with development of pulmonary hypertension; murmurs: S3 and flow diastolic murmur heard in addition to grade 4–6 blowing, pansystolic murmur at the apex conducted towards axilla.

Mitral regurgitation in MVP: Mid-systolic click with late systolic murmur; gets louder with standing, during Valsalva maneuver, and during inspiration.

2. Tricuspid Regurgitation (TR)

- TR is most commonly secondary to pulmonary hypertension. Rheumatic heart disease is the second most common etiology.
- TR is often associated with MS, MR.
- Congenital TR is rare.
- Other causes include tricuspid valve prolapse, and Ebstein anomaly.

9 ***Characteristics:*** Prominent "v" wave, and obliteration of "x" descent in JVP; pansystolic murmur, intensity increasing during inspiration; prominent systolic pulsations of the liver.

3. Aortic Regurgitation

Etiology: Rheumatic after 5 years; endocarditis affecting bicuspid aortic valve, seen in connective tissue disorders—mucopolysaccharidosis, Marfan syndrome, rheumatoid arthritis, ankylosing spondylosis, and Reiter disease. Other causes include aortic dissection, and prolapse of right or non-coronary cusp of aortic valve in ventricular septal defect.

Mild AR: Pulse, BP: normal; no cardiomegaly; Apex: normal site; S1 and S2: normal; no peripheral signs of AR **(Key Box 28)**; high-pitched early diastolic murmur heard only in silent room with the child sitting and holding the breath in expiration. Often diagnosed by echocardiography.

Moderate AR: High volume pulse with wide pulse pressure (>50 mmHg and <80 mmHg); diastolic BP is <50 mmHg; peripheral signs of AR may be present ; apex: may be shifted downwards and outwards and is hyperdynamic; high-pitched early diastolic murmur heard easily with the diaphragm applied firmly in the aortic area.

Severe AR: Pulse: high volume, collapsing pulse; with very wide pulse pressure (>80 mmHg); systolic BP—elevated; diastolic BP is <40 mmHg and may be even 0 mmHg; peripheral signs of AR are present; apex: shifted downwards and outwards and is hyperdynamic; S1 and S2: soft; S3 and S4 in severe cases; soft, high pitched early diastolic murmur; short and soft mid-diastolic Austin-Flint murmur heard in mitral area (due to anterior mitral valve flutter caused by impingement of jet of diastolic backflow in rheumatic AR).

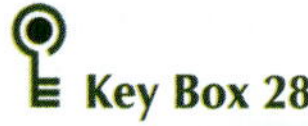

Key Box 28

Peripheral Signs of Aortic Regurgitation

- Water hammer, collapsing pulse
- *Hill sign:* Lower limb systolic BP—15 mmHg ≥Upper limb systolic BP
- *Pistol shot sounds* on auscultation over brachials and femorals, appreciated by the bell of the stethoscope
- *Duroziez murmur:* Diastolic murmur appreciated by the application of pressure distally by the edge of the diaphragm over the femoral artery; with proximal pressure application, a systolic murmur will be heard **(Fig. 9.33)**
- *Becker sign:* Retinal artery pulsations
- *Landolfi sign:* Rhythmic dilatation and contraction of pupils
- *Muller sign:* Visible uvular pulsations
- *Corrigan sign:* Dancing carotids
- *DeMusset sign:* Head nodding with each cardiac systole
- *Light house sign:* Flushing of face with each cardiac cycle
- Dancing brachialis
- *Quincke sign:* Nail bed pulsation
- *Rosenbach sign:* Liver pulsations
- *Gerhardt sign:* Splenic pulsations felt when enlarged

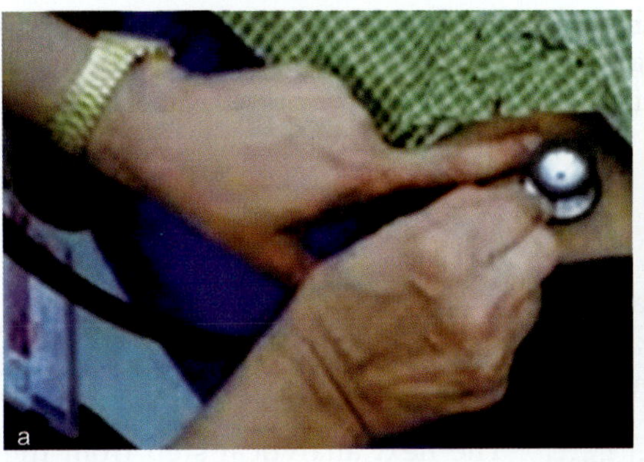

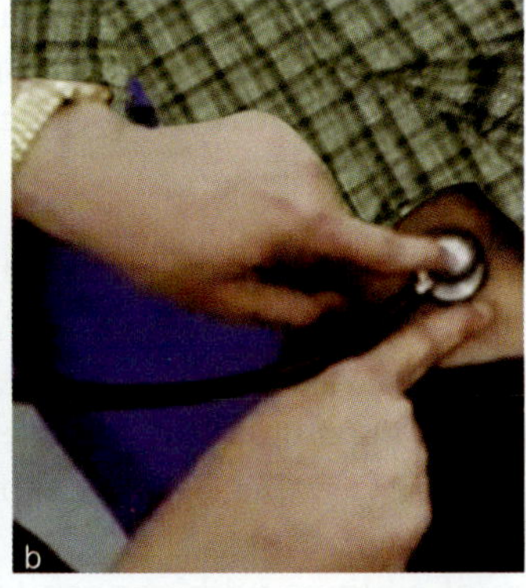

Fig. 9.33: Auscultation over right femoral artery for Duroziez murmur in aortic regurgitation: (a) after proximal finger pressure: systolic component; (b) after finger pressure distal to femoral artery: diastolic component.

4. Pulmonary Regurgitation

Usually, it is the result of severe pulmonary hypertension; rarely congenital due to absence of pulmonary valve or rheumatic fever and heart disease.

Auscultation: Ejection click with S2: Loud in pulmonary hypertension. No click and soft S2 in absent pulmonary valve; early diastolic murmur of Graham-Steele.

Examination of Other Systems

Upper and lower respiratory system: Perform routinely a thorough clinical examination of throat, pharynx, tonsils, teeth, oral cavity, ears, sinuses (Kartagener syndrome with dextrocardia, sinusitis and bronchiectasis), lungs, and pleural cavities (hydrothorax in cardiac failure, pleural rub).

Abdomen: Palpate liver for size, position—right side or left side; (mirror image dextrocardia with situs inversus totalis) and spleen—size, splenic rub.

Palpate for any abdominal mass (pheochromocytoma) and palpate for ascites.

Feel for aortic, external iliac, femoral and renal artery pulsations and listen for bruit.

Central nervous system: Look for evidence of arterial embolization due to bacterial endocarditis, thromboembolic phenomena, and cerebral abscesses in cyanotic congenital heart diseases; and bleeding secondary to anticoagulation therapy.

After history and physical examination, try to fit in the puzzle in the appropriate slot after careful consideration of evidence for and against each of the diagnostic possibilities.

9.9 CARDIAC DIAGNOSIS

Diagnostic questions that must be addressed following analysis of history and complete physical examination findings, are discussed as follows.

1. Does this Child have a Cardiac Problem?

Proper symptom analysis with clinical data collected by meticulous examination will leave no doubt in deciphering unequivocally the presence of a cardiac problem. Nada's criteria **(Key Box 29)** is an objective tool to guide to

Key Box 29

Nada's Criteria for Presence of Heart Disease

Major criteria	*Minor criteria*
1. Systolic murmur grade III or more	1. Systolic murmur less than grade III in intensity
2. Diastolic murmur	2. Abnormal second sound
3. Cyanosis	3. Abnormal ECG
4. Congestive heart failure	4. Abnormal chest X-ray
	5. Abnormal blood pressure

Presence of 1 major or 2 minor criteria suggests the presence of a heart disease.

probability of a heart disease, though presence of criteria laid by Nada is not mandatory for presence of a heart disease, specially in newborn infants.

2. Is the Identified Cardiac Problem Congenital or Acquired?

The following presentations indicate the presence of a congenital heart disease:

- Early onset of cardiac related symptoms from neonatal period or infancy.
- History of siblings with congenital heart diseases.
- Presence of dysmorphism or specific physical and morphological features of genetic, chromosomal syndromes, or single or multiple congenital malformations.
- Presence of cyanosis. Nearly all cyanotic heart diseases with a few rare exceptions are congenital heart diseases though the onset of cyanosis may occur even beyond the neonatal period.
- Presence of clinical features suggestive of either left to right shunts (VSD, ASD, PDA) or obstructive lesions (coarctation of aorta, AS, PS).
- History of adverse events like infections, drug intake, substance abuse, irradiation, other metabolic or autoimmune disorders in the early pregnancy, or abnormal fetal ultrasound findings during antenatal checkups.
- Presence of parasternal murmurs.

3. Whether the Congenital Heart Disease is Cyanotic or Acyanotic?

Confirm that cyanosis, if present, is of cardiac origin only. Detection of cyanosis and ascribing its etiology has been described earlier in this chapter. Obtain a hematocrit and oxygen saturation by pulse oximetry to corroborate the diagnosis. Cyanotic congenital heart diseases (CCHD) need earlier intervention than many of the congenital acyanotic heart diseases.

4. If the Heart Condition is Cyanotic, Assess Whether Pulmonary Blood Flow is Decreased or Increased?

The next analytical step from the history and clinical features is to decide whether the congenital cyanosis heart condition (CCHD) is associated with (a) decreased pulmonary blood flow; or (b) increased pulmonary blood flow. **Table 9.9** helps in categorization of congenital cyanotic heart disease according to pulmonary blood flow.

A list of cardiac disorders follows, based on the pulmonary blood flow:

CCHD with decreased pulmonary blood flow: TOF, tricuspid atresia, pulmonary atresia, Ebstein anomaly, single ventricle with PS, double outlet right ventricle (DORV) with PS, TGA with VSD with PS.

CCHD with increased pulmonary blood flow: TGA, TAPVC, hypoplastic left heart syndrome, Eisenmenger syndrome, single ventricle without PS, DORV without PS, TGA with VSD without PS.

ECG Diagnosis of CCHD

A. Decreased pulmonary blood flow

(Features of moderate to marked cyanosis, cyanotic spells, squatting)

- *Left ventricular hypertrophy:* Tricuspid atresia, pulmonary atresia with intact

Table 9.9: Cyanotic heart disease categorized according to pulmonary blood flow

Parameter	Pulmonary blood flow	
	Decreased	**Increased**
Intesity of cyanosis	Moderate-to-severe	Mild
Hypercyanotic spells	Present	Absent
Squatting	Present	Absent
Recurrent chest infection	Absent	Present
Congestive heart failure	Absent	Present
Cardiomegaly	No	Yes
Lung fields (on X-ray)	Oligemic	Plethoric

ventricular septum (hypoplastic right ventricle).

- *Right ventricular hypertrophy:* Tetralogy of Fallot (TOF) and other conditions with Fallot's hemodynamics due to the associated presence of pulmonary stenosis (PS), e.g. TGA + VSD + PS, single ventricle + PS, DORV+ VSD + PS, and endocardial cushion defect + PS; severe PS with ASD; pulmonary atresia with VSD.
- *Biventricular hypertrophy:* Persistent truncus with hypoplastic pulmonary arteries, single ventricle.

B. Increased pulmonary blood flow

(Features of heart failure, recurrent LRIs, and respiratory distress)

- *Left ventricular hypertrophy:* Tricuspid atresia associated with large VSD + TGA, double inlet left ventricle.
- *Right ventricular hypertrophy:* Transposition of great arteries (TGA), total anomalous pulmonary venous return (TAPVR)—unobstructed type, hypoplastic left heart syndrome.
- *Biventricular hypertrophy:* Persistent truncus arteriosus, transposition of great arteries (TGA) + ventricular septal defect (VSD), single ventricle without pulmonic stenosis (PS).

Figures 9.34 and 9.35 portray an algorithmic approach to diagnosis of congenital cyanotic heart disease.

5. If the Congenital Heart Condition is Acyanotic: Assess Whether it is a Shunt, Obstructive Lesion, or Others?

Acyanotic lesions are classified in **Fig. 9.36**.

Left to Right Shunt

Symptoms of "suck and stop" cycles during breastfeeding, sweating over the forehead, fast breathing, mother's perception of increased precordial activity, strange palpable feeling of "purring of a cat" over the chest while bathing, presentation at 4–6 weeks, associated with symptoms of feeding difficulty, failure to thrive, frequent respiratory infections, and rapid breathing, suggest the possibility of a left to right shunt.

If the history and physical examination suggest the possibility of a left to right shunt, find out the level of the shunt—atrial (ASD), ventricular (VSD), or at the level of great arteries (PDA). Most common is a VSD, followed by PDA. ASD (ostium secundum) is usually asymptomatic in the first decade of life in the majority of cases. Ostium primum ASD presents in a manner similar to VSD or PDA.

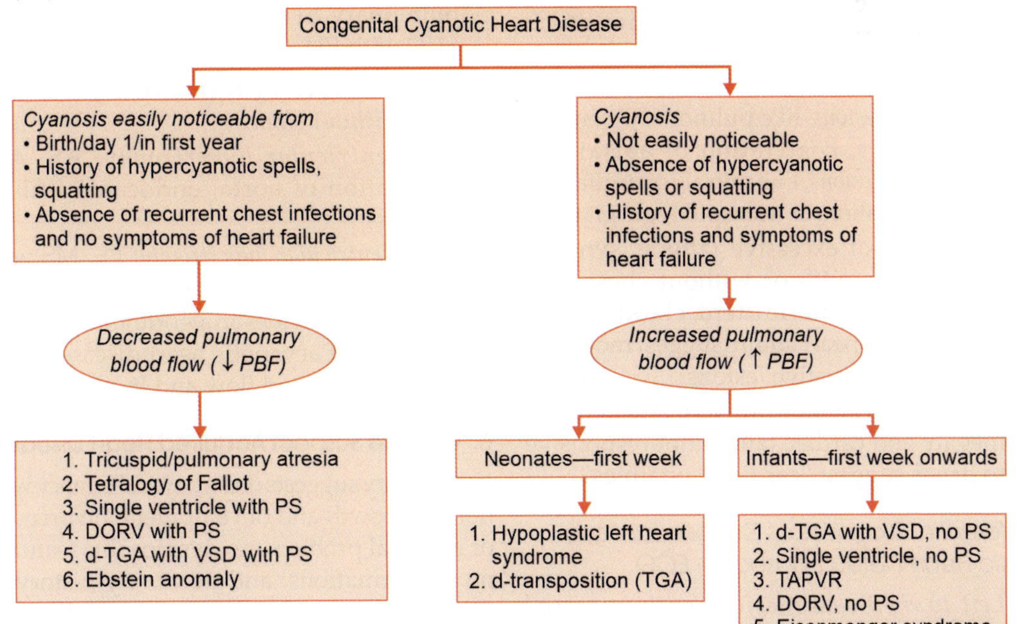

Fig. 9.34: Algorithmic analysis of history in a child with suspected congenital cyanotic heart disease. DORV: double outlet right ventricle. PS: pulmonary stenosis.

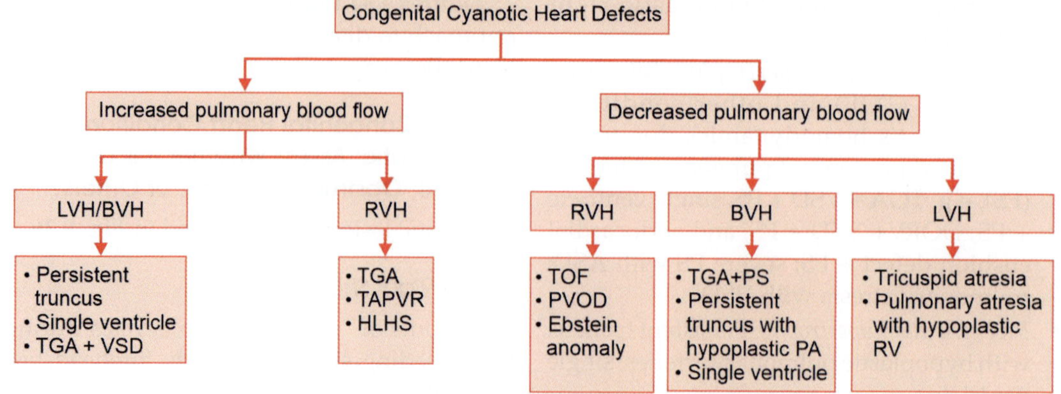

RVH: right ventricular hypertrophy; **LVH:** left ventricular hypertrophy; **BVH:** biventricular hypertrophy; **TGA:** transposition of great arteries; **VSD:** ventricular septal defect; **TAPVR:** total anomalous pulmonary venous return; **HLHS:** hypoplastic left heart syndrome; **TOF:** tetralogy of Fallot; **PVOD**: pulmonary vascular obstructive disease; **PS:** pulmonary stenosis; **PA:** pulmonary artery; **RV:** right ventricle

Fig. 9.35: Algorithmic approach to a "Child with congenital cyanotic heart disease".

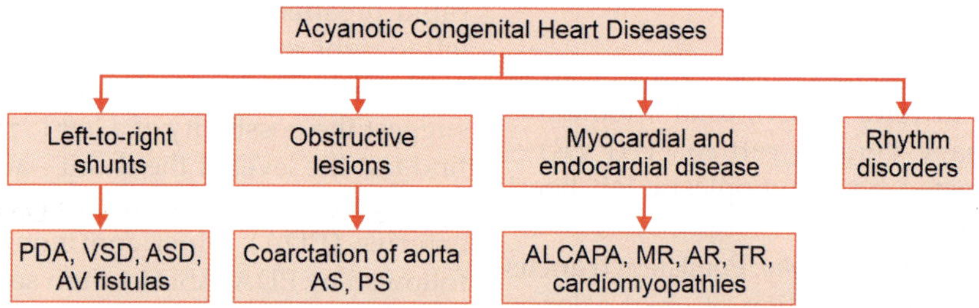

Fig. 9.36: Classification of acyanotic heart lesions.

Other Lesions

In the absence of findings suggestive of left to right shunts, the next set of acyanotic heart conditions to be considered are (a) *obstructive lesions*, like pulmonary stenosis, aortic stenosis, coarctation of aorta; and (b) *regurgitant lesions*, like mitral regurgitation, aortic regurgitation, or tricuspid regurgitation.

- Symptoms of excessive fatigue, syncope or dizziness with or without chest pain on exertion, intermittent claudication, symptoms of heart failure suggest moderate to severe obstructive lesions.
- Symptoms of failure to thrive, marked cardiomegaly and cardiac failure not responsive to drugs suggest "cardiomyopathies".

Differential Diagnosis of Congenital Acyanotic Heart Defects based on ECG

A. Left to right shunt lesions with increased pulmonary blood flow

- *Left ventricular hypertrophy:* PDA, VSD, ECD
- *Right ventricular hypertrophy:* ASD
- *Biventricular hypertrophy:* PDA with pulmonary hypertension, VSD with PH, ECD with PH

B. Obstructive/regurgitant/myocardial lesions without shunt

- *Left ventricular hypertrophy:* AS, AR, coarctation of aorta, endocardial fibroelastosis.
- *Right ventricular hypertrophy:* PS, MS with pulmonary hypertension.

Figure 9.37 provides an algorithmic approach to diagnosis of acyanotic heart disease, based on pulmonary blood flow and ECG findings.

6. When to Suspect Acquired Heart Disease?

If the history suggests onset beyond infancy with normal growth and development, no prenatal or neonatal problem, no dysmorphic features, no malformations, and no family history of congenital heart diseases in the siblings or parents, the possibility of an "acquired heart disease" must be entertained. History (e.g. rheumatic migratory joint pains, rashes,

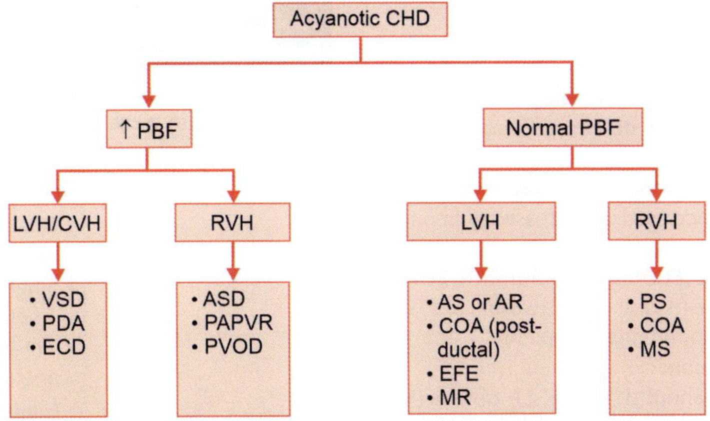

CHD: congenital heart disease; **PBF:** pulmonary blood flow; **RVH:** right ventricular hypertrophy; **LVH:** left ventricular hypertrophy; **CVH:** combined ventricular hypertrophy; **PDA:** patent ductus arteriosus; **VSD:** ventricular septal defect; **ECD:** endocardial cushion defect; **PAPVR:** partial anomalous pulmonary venous return; **ASD:** atrial septal defect; **AS:** aortic stenosis; **AR:** aortic regurgitation; **PVOD:** pulmonary vascular disease; **PS:** pulmonary stenosis; **COA:** coarctation of aorta; **MS:** mitral stenosis; **MR:** mitral regurgitation; **EFE:** endocardial fibroelastosis

Fig. 9.37: Algorithmic approach to a child with acyanotic congenital heart disease.

cervical lymph node, oromucosal lesions with fever, etc.) and certain specific physical findings and structural (valvular) lesions may strongly suggest acquired heart disease.

- Joint pains or joint swelling in the past or present, fever, subcutaneous nodules over the bony prominences, like ribs, back of head, sternum, and spine and over the muscle tendons near joints, abnormal involuntary jerky movements suggest rheumatic heart disease.
- If the child has fever for more than 5 days, diffuse rashes, non-purulent conjunctivitis, intense redness of the mouth, oral cavity, a few cervical lymph nodes and skin desquamation of skin over the palms, soles, lips and periungual zone must make you think of Kawasaki disease.
- Fever and rashes for a few days, sudden onset of breathlessness and inactivity, fatigue, symptoms of failure indicate a possible myocarditis.

7. Answer the Following Questions for Suspected Acquired Heart Diseases

i. Where is the anatomical lesion (*site of lesion*)? Valvular, myocardial, pericardial, vascular, or conduction tissue?
ii. What is the *nature of the pathophysiological lesion*? Stenosis, regurgitation, myocardial failure, pericardial effusion, etc.
iii. What is the *severity of lesion*?
iv. *What is the etiology*? Infective? Rheumatic or other autoimmune mediated inflammatory problem? Traumatic? Degenerative?
v. *What are the complications*? Cardiac failure, arrhythmias, bacterial endocarditis, respiratory infections, growth and developmental retardation. Remote secondary complications secondary to bacterial endocarditis like neuroparalysis, and embolic nephritis must also be mentioned in the diagnosis.
vi. *What is the functional limitation* imposed on the child's activities and behavior?

Final Clinical Step

Analyze the history and the physical examination findings and arrive at the most likely diagnosis. Present or record your diagnosis: The diagnosis must contain the 10 aspects outlined in **Key Box 30**.

9.10 PRENATAL DIAGNOSIS OF CARDIOVASCULAR DISORDER

Prenatal diagnosis is possible by ultrasound evaluation of the fetal heart during pregnancy. The objectives are 3-fold.

1. To provide accurate information regarding the cardiovascular status
2. To facilitate delivery of optimized antenatal care

Key Box 30

Complete Cardiac Diagnosis

1. **Nature of heart disease:** Congenital or acquired?
2. **If congenital:** Cyanotic or acyanotic?
3. **If cyanotic:** Increased or decreased pulmonary blood flow
4. **If acquired:** *Etiology:* Rheumatic fever, rheumatic heart disease, Kawasaki disease, infective, autoimmune, idiopathic
5. **Nature of lesion:**
   Congenital: Shunt (L-R or R-L), obstructive, myocardial, endocardial, conduction defect
   Acquired: Pericardial, endocardial, or myocardial
6. **Specific defect:**
   Congenital: VSD, coarctation, TOF, PS, endocardial fibroelastosis, etc.
   Acquired: MR, MS, AR, TR, pericardial effusion, myocarditis, cardiomyopathy, etc.
7. **Severity of lesion:** Mild/moderate/severe (for valvular defects) or small/moderate/large (for shunts)
8. **Complications, if any:** CHF, bacterial endocarditis, active carditis, cerebral abscess, pulmonary hypertension, arrhythmia.
9. **Functional limitations, if any:** Grade IV dyspnea, growth and developmental retardation.
10. Associated chromosomal or dysmorphogenetic syndrome (if any)?

3. To ensure the best possible outcomes for mother and fetus

Details, timings, and objective of ultrasound examinations for fetal heart defects are listed in the following **Table 9.10**.

9.11 NEONATAL SCREENING FOR CONGENITAL HEART DEFECT

Critical congenital heart disease (CHD) is defined as any cardiac lesion from which infants die or require early surgery or cardiac catheterization within the first 28 days of life for survival or to prevent organ damage. Early detection of a critical CHD by using sensitive pulse oximeter by trained hands before acute discharge of the neonate from the hospital plays significant role in reducing instances of cardiovascular shock leading to better cardiopulmonary and neurological outcomes. As most newborns are asymptomatic at birth, newborn screening for CHD helps in identifying some cases to allow prompt diagnosis and treatment and may prevent disability or fatal outcome.

Table 9.10: Ultrasound examination for fetal heart defects

Ultrasound evaluation	Timing in weeks	Objective
First	11–14	To confirm/identify/ determine: • Fetal viability by seeing heart beating • Single fetus/plurality → 1 Fetus • Chromosomal aneuploidies • Major structural anomalies
Second *Anomaly scan*	18–22/24	Situs of fetal heart, chambers, flow patterns of SVC, IVC into RA and pulmonary veins into LA, atrioventricular continuity, aortic mitral continuity, etc.
Third trimester	28–42	To evaluate fetal heart anomaly and function

Pulse Oximetry

It is an important and highly recommended neonatal screening test that is universally adapted and made mandatory in many nations across the globe before a neonate is discharged from the hospital. Ideally done 24 hours after birth with oximetry readings.

- Pulse oximetry readings must be taken using sensitive pulse oximeter from right hand (preductal) and either foot (post-ductal) with infant breathing room air.
- Pulse oximetry is interpreted as abnormal if oxygen saturation at room air measured less than 90% or difference between right hand and foot is more than 3%.

In a study from Delhi, the sensitivity, specificity, positive predictive value, negative predictive value and odds ratio (95% CI) of pulse oximetry were 95.2%, 52.4%, 9.5, 99.5 and 22, respectively. It was concluded that neonatal screening by pulse oximetry is an essential and valuable screening test to detect cyanotic congenital heart defects and for those needing early surgical intervention procedures for their survival.

Chapter 10

Examination of the Abdomen

○ Ruchi Rai ○ DK Singh

Structure

10.1 AIM AND SCHEME OF ABDOMINAL EXAMINATION

It is important to examine the abdomen in every child as it is very often secondarily involved even when the primary disease involves some other system. The abdomen is occupied by the gastrointestinal, genitourinary, and hepatobiliary systems. Therefore, examination of the abdomen is complex. The key to simplify the examination is to approach it in a systematic manner. The aim is to do a stepwise examination and decide which system is involved; which organ(s) is (are) affected; what is the nature of the disease; and what is the differential diagnosis.

The steps of examination remain the same as for other systems, i.e. inspection, palpation, percussion, and auscultation.

10.2 COMMON SYMPTOMS RELATED TO THE ABDOMEN

Symptoms that point towards an abdominal involvement should be assessed in detail to have an idea about the exact problem and a probable diagnosis. Many symptoms related to the abdomen may not be due to a localized disease, but arise due to extra-abdominal pathology. Symptoms in a child are what the parents perceive the problem to be, unless the child is old enough to tell about symptoms. The parents many times are wrong in interpreting their child's symptoms; they may sometimes totally miss a problem and sometimes exaggerate a simple problem. A child less than 3 years of age may not be able to complain about abdominal pain at all and the attendants may falsely interpret crying or any other problem due to abdominal pain. Even an older child may not be able to give a reliable history. A methodical examination will ultimately help you decide about the importance and the severity of each symptom and clinch the diagnosis. Some common symptoms related to the abdomen are discussed below.

1. Abdominal Pain

Pain in abdomen can be acute, chronic, or recurrent. A detailed history regarding the frequency, site, timing, severity, nature, relieving and aggravating factors, and associated symptoms is very important. Evaluation of chronic abdominal pain sometimes becomes a challenge, as the child with functional pain may appear as uncomfortable as the one with an organic cause. Features that help in differentiating between an organic and psychological cause of pain abdomen are listed in **Key Boxes 1 and 2**.

Key Box 1

Cause of Pain Abdomen: Psychologic or Organic

1. A periumbilical pain is usually non-organic.
2. The site of pain, if pointed by a finger, is more likely to be significant rather than when pointed vaguely by the whole hand.
3. Pain abdomen occurring typically before going to school or during examination may be more psychological than pathological.
4. Pain severe enough to interfere in the child's play or forcing the child to remain in bed or occurring at midnight when the child was sleeping is more likely to be significant.

Key Box 2

Pain Abdomen: Points to Remember

1. Pain abdomen may not be a symptom at all, even in advanced conditions, like chronic liver disease, hydronephrosis, malignancy, massive splenomegaly, chronic renal failure, etc.
2. Non-abdominal causes of pain abdomen should always be kept in mind while evaluating a patient. These include abdominal migraine, abdominal epilepsy, sickle cell crisis, lead poisoning, acute intermittent porphyria, diabetic ketoacidosis, and Henoch-Schönlein purpura.

Site of Pain

The site of pain can give a rough idea about organ of origin.

- ***Right hypochondrium:*** Liver is the main organ in this area. Stretching of the hepatic capsule or inflammation of liver gives rise to pain, e.g. acute hepatitis, amebic abscess, or congestive hepatomegaly as in congestive heart failure. Pain due to pleurisy or a pneumonic patch on the right side can also be referred to the right hypochondrium.
- ***Epigastrium:*** Gastritis is the most common cause of epigastric pain. Pancreatitis is not so common in children. Pain arising from liver and upper bowel is also felt at the epigastrium.
- ***Left hypochondrium:*** Pain may be due to splenic enlargement or infarct; or left sided pleurisy.
- ***Periumbilical:*** Pain arising from distal small bowel, cecum, appendicitis, or proximal colon is felt in the periumbilical area.
- ***Suprapubic region:*** May be due to cystitis, bladder calculus, distal large bowel, or pelvic organs.
- ***Backache:*** Renal pain causes pain in the back especially in the renal angle. Ureteric pain typically radiates from the loin to the groin along the course of the ureters.
- ***Lumbar region or flanks:*** Pain of renal origin is typically felt in the lumbar region.
- ***Right iliac fossa:*** In chronic appendicitis, pain is felt in the right iliac fossa at the McBurney's point (junction of lateral one-third and medial two-thirds of the right spino-umbilical line joining the right anterior superior iliac spine and umbilicus).

Common causes of acute abdominal pain are summarized in **Table 10.1**.

Shifting of Pain

This is characteristically seen in acute appendicitis. The pain is initially felt around umbilicus, but later shifts to the right iliac region with the onset of parietal peritonitis.

Table 10.1: Common causes of abdominal pain

	Acute pain	Recurrent abdominal pain	
Children (<2 yrs)	**Children (>2 yrs)**	**Children (<2 yrs)**	**Children (>2 yrs)**
Malrotation, volvulus	Appendicitis	Colic	Functional
Intussusception	Intestinal obstruction	Malabsorption	Inflammatory bowel syndrome
Gastroenteritis	Peritonitis	Milk allergy	
Urinary tract infection	Urinary tract infection	Rotational defects	Parasitic infection
Peritonitis	Hepatitis	Chronic constipation	Urolithiasis
Colic	Ureteric colic	Lactose intolerance	Peptic ulcer
Perforation	Perforation		Meckel diverticulum

Referred Pain

This is more important in surgical problems. The pain is said to be *referred* when it is felt at some other region having the same segmental innervations as the site of lesion. The pain arising from stomach, duodenum, and jejunum is referred to the epigastrium; that from the ileum and appendix is referred to the umbilicus; and that from the colon is referred to the hypogastrium. Any irritation to the under surface of the diaphragm may get referred to the corresponding shoulder. The diaphragm is supplied by the phrenic nerve (C3, 4, 5) and the cutaneous nerves from the same segments supply the skin over the shoulder.

In renal colic, the pain is referred from loin to groin and inner side of the thigh, i.e. the distribution of genitofemoral nerve (L1, 2). Irritation of the parietal pleura in pleurisy, hemothorax, or pneumothorax may get referred to the abdominal wall and mimic acute abdominal condition.

Character of Pain

- ***Colicky:*** Sharp intermittent griping pain suggests obstruction of a hollow organ (ureteric calculus or bowel obstruction).
- ***Burning:*** Pain in the epigastrium or retrosternal area due to gastritis or esophagitis.
- ***Throbbing:*** Pain due to inflammation (hepatitis or cholecystitis).

2. Vomiting

Differentiate between Vomiting and Regurgitation

Regurgitation of feeds is a normal phenomenon in infants. This is due to poor lower esophageal sphincter tone. As the tone improves with age, the regurgitation decreases and stops. Regurgitation can also be due to aerophagy, i.e. ingestion of air while feeding which is common in babies receiving bottle feeds.

Find out the Cause

Ask about the frequency, whether bilious or non-bilious, relationship to food, and associated symptoms.

- Vomiting can be due to *abdominal* or *extra-abdominal* reasons **(Table 10.2)**.
- Vomiting may be a *functional* problem.
- Vomiting may also occur, if the child is being forcefully fed.
- If the vomiting is succeeding bouts of cough, then it is just post-tussive vomiting.
- Vomiting is bilious, if there is obstruction below the second part of duodenum.
- Children with congenital hypertrophic pyloric stenosis typically present with persistent vomiting after each feed from the second or the third week of life and failure to thrive.
- Vomiting is frequent and profuse in acute intestinal obstruction.
- Vomiting which is projectile (involuntary forceful ejection of a large quantity) is generally due to raised intracranial pressure as in cases of hydrocephalus, septic meningitis, intracranial hemorrhage; or in high intestinal obstruction.
- Nausea is an early symptom of chronic appendicitis and hepatitis.
- Vomiting is a prominent symptom of hepatitis.

Table 10.2: Important causes of vomiting in children

Children (<2 yrs)	Children (>2 yrs)
Gastroenteritis	Gastroenteritis
Intestinal obstruction	Intestinal obstruction
Congenital pyloric stenosis	Acute appendicitis
Gastroesophageal reflux	Hepatitis
Hydrocephalus, CNS infections	Renal colic
Perforation, peritonitis	Perforation, peritonitis
Uremia, inborn errors of metabolism	CNS space occupying lesion
Systemic infection	Uremia
Volvulus, intussusception	Diabetic ketoacidosis
Overfeeding, faulty feeding	Psychogenic

Persistent vomiting is associated with weight loss or failure to gain weight. If the mother complains of persistent vomiting for quiet sometime, but you find that the child looks well, and is gaining adequate weight then most probably it is not pathological.

3. Constipation

Mere passage of infrequent stools is not constipation. What is more important is the consistency and the difficulty in passage of stools. Constipation is usually related to the fluid and fiber content of the child's diet, but may be pathological in many instances.

A normal child may pass stools every second or third day, but if the stools are soft, and there is no difficulty in passing stools, this is not constipation. Such a situation is common in exclusively breastfed babies. Infants on top feeds are constipated and may need intervention.

- Children with intestinal obstruction will present with acute constipation along with abdominal distention and vomiting.
- Children with Hirschsprung disease present with chronic constipation since birth, if they are not diagnosed in the neonatal period. In such a child, there is history of passage of first meconium after 24 hours of birth.
- Children with hypothyroidism will be chronically constipated but it will be associated with other features of hypothyroidism.
- *Absolute constipation*, i.e. arrest of both feces and flatus is seen in intestinal obstruction and peritonitis.
- Some neonates on exclusive breastfeeds may pass stools once in 4–5 days which are paste-like and soft. This is a normal phenomenon.

While you are examining a child with constipation, look for signs of intestinal obstruction, palpate for fecoliths and also assess the development of the child. Common causes of constipation are listed in **Table 10.3**.

Table 10.3: Common causes of constipation
Hirschsprung disease
Anorectal stenosis
Anal stricture
Volvulus
Lead toxicity
Cystic fibrosis
Hypothyroidism
Hypokalemia
Psychomotor retardation
Functional

4. Diarrhea

Ask about the frequency, consistency, color, associated blood and mucus, and vomiting. Differentiate between normal stools and diarrhea. Consistency and frequency of stools of a particular child should be assessed keeping in mind the normal routine of that child. Semi-formed stools 5–6/day, especially after feeds in infants should not be interpreted as diarrhea, if the child is otherwise healthy and gaining weight. A normal toddler may also pass 3–4 semi-formed stools in a day.

- Diarrhea in infants is usually viral in origin.
- Presence of loose stools that resemble rice-water and have a fishy odor is characteristic of cholera.
- Dysentery is characterized by loose motions associated with blood and/or mucus; the etiology is bacterial or amebic. There may be associated fever and constitutional symptoms.
- Presence of bulky, frothy, and sticky stools suggests malabsorption.
- Diarrhea can also be non-infective in origin.
- Newborn babies may pass loose stools after each feed due to gastrocolic reflex. This is not diarrhea.

Tenesmus is a feeling to pass stools even when the bowel is empty. It can be associated with abdominal cramps, pain, and straining. This is seen in inflammatory bowel diseases or motility disorders.

Common causes of diarrhea are listed in **Table 10.4**.

Persistent diarrhea: Diarrhea starting as an acute episode and lasting for more than 14 days is called persistent diarrhea. History of weight loss is important in such cases. While examining a case of diarrhea, look for anal excoriation, signs of dehydration, and signs of systemic involvement.

Table 10.4: Common causes of diarrhea

Infant	Child	Adolescent
Gastroenteritis	Gastroenteritis	Gastroenteritis
Systemic infection	Food poisoning	Food poisoning
Antibiotic associated	Antibiotic associated	Antibiotic associated
Lactase deficiency	Systemic infection	Hyperthyroidism
Cow's milk protein intolerance	Giardiasis	Irritable bowel syndrome
Celiac disease	Lactose intolerance	Inflammatory bowel disease Giardiasis

5. Abdominal Distention

The reasons for abdominal distention can be many, therefore, mere presence of distention may not lead you to any diagnosis **(Key Box 3)**. The distension may just be physiological as in infants after feeds; or in toddlers who generally have a protuberant abdomen. Ask relevant questions and perform a thorough examination to reach a conclusion.

Visceromegaly (hepatomegaly or splenomegaly), intra-abdominal lump (malignancy, Wilms tumor, neuroblastoma, cyst), gas (ileus or intestinal obstruction) and fluid (ascites) are the common causes of abdominal distention.

6. Urinary Complaints

- Burning micturition or crying during micturition is a symptom of urinary tract infection.
- Passing of urine as drops or in very small quantity after frequent and painful attempts at micturition is due to a *bladder stone impacted in the urethra.*

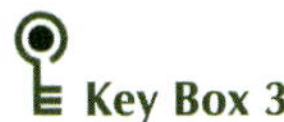
Key Box 3

Extra-abdominal Causes of Abdominal Distension

1. *Generalized hypotonia* as seen in rickets or in protein energy malnutrition. Due to hypotonia of abdominal muscles, the abdominal contents tend to bulge out especially when the child is standing.
2. *Hypokalemia* can lead to ileus causing abdominal distention.
3. *Respiratory distress* in severe bronchopneumonia, congestive cardiac failure, bronchial asthma, etc. may lead to abdominal distention due to ingestion of air while working hard to breathe.

- Poor urinary stream or passing of urine in drops since birth may be due to the presence of *posterior urethral valve.*
- Anuria in which the urinary output is minimal or nil (be careful to palpate for the urinary bladder to rule out retention of urine) can be due to shock, dehydration, acute renal failure, or acute tubular necrosis.
- *Strangury* refers to painful and frequent attempts at micturition, passing only a small quantity or only drops on straining each time is often seen in vesical calculus or cystitis. This is also associated with urgency.
- Young infants sometimes cry just before the act of micturition and stop crying as soon as they start passing urine. This is normal.

While examining a urinary case, you must palpate for renal and bladder lump, look for renal tenderness, and examine urethral meatus. Also look for edema or anasarca, signs of fluid overload, and do not forget to measure the blood pressure.

7. Jaundice

Jaundice occurs as a result of accumulation of bilirubin in the blood **(Key Box 4)**.

- *Conjugated hyperbilirubinemia* localizes the problem to liver or biliary tract.
- Red blood cell destruction (hemolysis) is yet another cause of jaundice, but this results in *unconjugated hyperbilirubinemia.*

Ask about the course of jaundice, whether it is waxing and waning or progressively deepening.

Conjugated hyperbilirubinemia is usually associated with passage of dark yellow- colored urine. Passage of clay-colored stools indicates an obstructive type of jaundice. Itching often accompanies obstructive jaundice; presence

Key Box 4

Jaundice: Points to Remember

1. Sometimes severe pallor is interpreted as jaundice by the caregivers. Ask specifically whether the child is getting pale (whiter) or icteric (yellowish).
2. Jaundice can also be unconjugated in nature and in that case it is due to hemolysis and the liver is not affected.

of scratch marks over the chest or abdomen gives a clue, even if jaundice is doubtful.

A previous history of jaundice is also important. Past history of blood transfusion is important in hepatitis B or C infection for knowing the source of infection. In a child with jaundice, obtain history suggestive of bleeding from any site and symptoms of deficiency of fat-soluble vitamins A, D, E and K. Palpate for the liver and if it is enlarged, note its characteristics. Also look for splenomegaly, edema or anasarca, and signs of liver cell failure. Assess the sensorium.

Children may pass dark-colored urine when they have fever or have poor intake due to concentrated in urine. Intake of drugs, like rifampicin or multivitamin preparations, may cause dark-colored urine.

Jaundice may be absent in some conditions involving liver, like Reye syndrome, amebic or pyogenic liver abscess, and hydatid disease.

8. GI Bleeding (Key Box 5)

Ask for history of blood in stool, urine, or vomitus. Hepatic involvement leads to coagulation disorder because of defective production of various coagulation factors, so a history of bleeding from any site should be asked for in patients of chronic liver disease. In many instances, you may not get a history of bleeding from the gastrointestinal tract, but if you suspect, then the stool can be examined for occult blood. The amount of bleeding can be assessed by the degree of anemia.

Melena

It is the presence of black tarry stools, and is indicative of bleeding proximal to the distal ileum. The blood gets denatured and the presence of this denatured blood leads to blackish stools. Swallowed blood due to bleeding in the oral cavity, nose, or upper respiratory tract also leads to melena.

Key Box 5

Common Causes of GI Bleeding

1. Dysentery
2. Cow's milk protein intolerance
3. Intussusception
4. Anal fissure
5. Colonic polyp
6. Esophageal varices
7. Inflammatory bowel disease
8. Coagulopathy
9. Hemorrhoids
10. Peptic ulcer

Hematemesis

- Presence of blood-stained vomitus is characteristic of esophageal varices of portal hypertension.
- It can also be a presenting complaint in severe gastritis or raised intracranial pressure.
- Children with bleeding or coagulation disorder may also present with hematemesis.
- Hematemesis (vomiting of blood) should not be confused with hemoptysis (coughing out of blood).

Bleeding Per Rectum

Fresh bleeding per rectum occurs due to hemorrhoids, anal fissure, fistula, or polyps. Another important cause of bleeding per rectum is varices at the anal canal secondary to portal hypertension. Features of intestinal obstruction along with passage of blood per rectum is suggestive of intussusception or enterocolitis.

Hematuria

Red color of the urine can be due to hematuria, hemoglobinuria, myoglobinuria, or porphyria **(Key Box 6)**. Hematuria is the most common of these. The bleeding may be fresh and red as in cystitis or a bladder stone; or it can be dark brown or cola-colored as in acute glomerulonephritis.

Common causes of hematuria in children include acute glomerulonephritis, calculi:

Key Box 6

Red Color Urine

1. Hematuria
2. Hemoglobinuria
3. Myoglobinuria
4. Porphyria
5. Drugs: Pyridium, rifampicin, desferoxamine
6. Food items: Beetroot, black berries

Ureteric or vesical; urinary tract infection, cystitis, renal vein thrombosis, DIC, thrombocytopenia, renal trauma, and Wilms' tumor.

9. Alteration in Appetite

Loss of appetite is typical of chronic illnesses, such as tuberculosis, chronic liver or renal disease, malabsorption, malignancy, or in acute conditions, like dysentery, colitis, diarrhea, and urinary tract infection. Loss of appetite is associated with loss of weight, if it persists for long.

- Beware of the constantly worrying mothers who are always dissatisfied with their child's appetite.
- See for the nutritional status of the child, and observe the weight gain over a period of time before coming to a conclusion.

Increased appetite can be due to worm infestation, recovery phase of hepatitis, or may be observed in a patient on steroids.

10. Scrotal Swelling

History of scrotal swelling is quite frequently encountered in boys.

Acute or Chronic

It can be *acute* or *chronic;* and painless or painful. Immediate attention and evaluation is mandatory in boys with acute and painful scrotal swelling to rule out testicular torsion or incarcerated inguinal hernia, which requires urgent surgical intervention. Hydrocele is the most common chronic swelling of the scrotum.

- Testicular torsion presents as an acute painful scrotal swelling.
- Epididymo-orchitis also presents in a similar way as torsion testis but needs to be urgently differentiated because of the need of urgent surgery in case of torsions.

Painful or Painless

Ascertain whether testicular swelling is *painful* (causes: testicular torsion, epididymitis, and incarcerated inguinal hernia) or *painless* (hydrocele, inguinal hernia, testicular tumor, and varicocele).

11. Other Points in History

- ***Menstrual history*** should be taken in adolescent girls.
- ***Family history:*** History of tuberculosis in the family is important in a child with suspected tubercular abdomen. History of unexplained death of one or both parents can suggest HIV infection.
- ***Drug history:*** History of intake of hepatotoxic drugs, like phenytoin, valproic acid, isoniazid, rifampicin, pyrazinamide, etc., should be asked for in children presenting with hepatitis. Rifampicin causes dark yellow to orange discoloration of urine which may be mistaken for jaundice.
- ***Blood transfusion:*** History of blood or blood component transfusion during the present illness can tell us about the course of the disease before child approached us. The child may not be severely pale or bleeding at the time of presentation, if he/she had a recent transfusion. A history of repeated transfusions in the past may point towards a chronic illness, like a congenital hemolytic anemia, chronic liver disease, or portal hypertension. A blood transfusion can be source of blood-borne infections, such as hepatitis B, hepatitis C, and HIV.
- ***Antenatal history:*** History suggestive of intrauterine infections in the mother during antenatal period is important in an infant with hepatosplenomegaly, mental retardation, and cataract suggesting a congenital rubella infection.
- History of ***umbilical catheterization*** or umbilical sepsis is important in patients suspected of having extra hepatic biliary atresia.
- ***Fever*** may be a prominent or the only symptom in patients of abdominal tuberculosis, malaria, kala azar, hepatic abscess or malignancies.

10.3 RELEVANT ANATOMY AND THE LANDMARKS

For convenience, we divide the abdomen into 9 regions. It becomes easier to describe the site of abnormality, and also helps in pointing the organ from which the problem originates depending upon which organ occupies that region.

- Draw four imaginary lines (2 vertical and 2 horizontal) to divide the abdomen into 9 regions (Fig. 10.1).
- *Vertical lines:* Two vertical lines are drawn passing through the tips of both the ninth costal cartilages above and midpoint between the pubis and the anterior superior iliac spine, below.
- *Horizontal lines:* One horizontal line is drawn between lowest points of both the costal margins (transpyloric). The other horizontal line passes through the upper borders of the iliac crests.
- The abdomen is thus divided into the following 9 regions (from above downwards):
    i. Right hypochondrium, epigastrium, and left hypochondrium;
    ii. Right lumbar, umbilical, and left lumbar; and
    iii. Right iliac, hypogastrium or suprapubic, and left iliac.
- Contents of various regions are shown in Key Box 7 (Fig. 10.2).

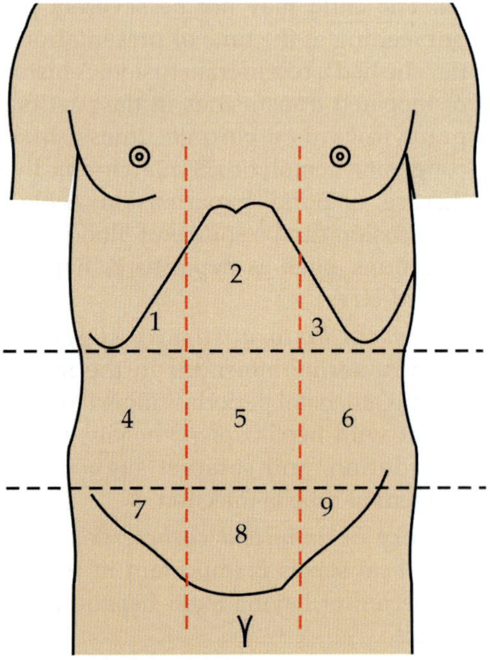

Fig. 10.1: Regions of the abdomen: 1,3: right and left hypochondrium; 2: epigastrium; 4,6: right and left lumbar; 5: umbilical; 7,9: right and left iliac; 8: hypogastrium or suprapubic.

Key Box 7

Contents of 9 Regions of Abdomen

1. *Right hypochondrium:* Liver, gallbladder and large colon
2. *Left hypochonvdrium:* Spleen, colon
3. *Epigastrium:* Stomach, pancreas, left lobe of liverv
4. *Right lumbar:* Right kidney, large colon
5. *Left lumbar:* Left kidney, large colon
6. *Umbilical:* Small intestine
7. *Right and left iliac:* Large bowel
8. *Suprapubic:* Urinary bladder

10.4 GENERAL EXAMINATION RELEVANT TO ABDOMINAL EXAMINATION

A. Vitals

1. Respiratory Rate

Respiratory rate should be counted carefully in all patients for full one minute when the patient is calm and at rest.

- Abdominal distention can be severe enough to cause respiratory compromise and lead to tachypnea or respiratory distress. Such massive distention can be due to massive ascites or massive gaseous distention secondary to large bowel obstruction. The distention pushes up both the diaphragms into the thorax compromising the lung volume.
- Abdominal distention can also be a consequence of respiratory distress or tachypnea, which leads to aerophagy thus causing gaseous distention.
- Increased respiratory rate can be due to fluid overload secondary to acute renal failure.
- Tachypnea will also be associated with fever seen in infective abdominal conditions.

2. Heart Rate

Count the heart rate in all the patients for one minute. It can be altered in the following:

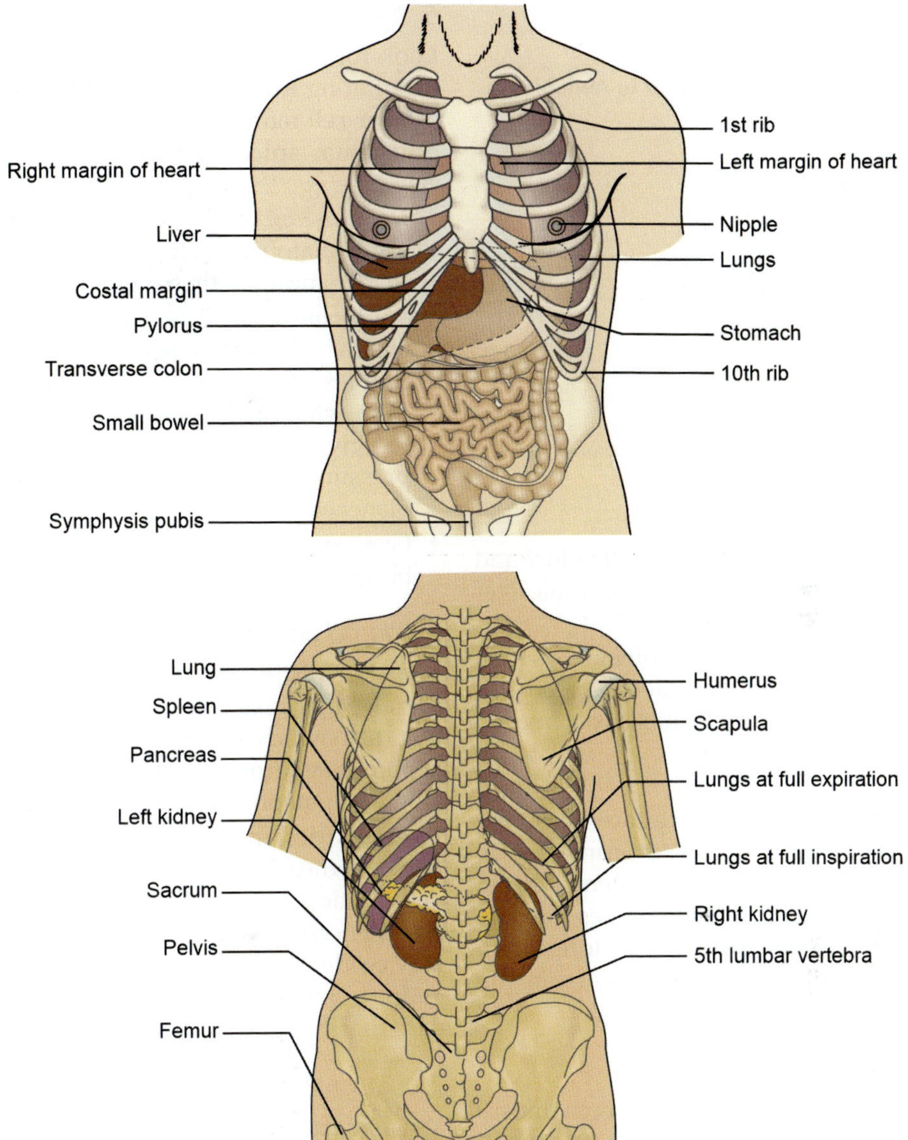

Fig. 10.2: Relationship of the various abdominal organs and the areas they occupy in the abdomen.

- Tachycardia is present in children with fever, appendicitis, perforation; or those with fluid overload (acute glomerulonephritis or acute renal failure).
- Bradycardia may be present in children with jaundice.

3. Blood Pressure

Record the blood pressure, and compare it with the normal for the child's age and sex. Hypertension may suggest renal involvement, the most common being acute glomerulonephritis or acute renal failure. On the other hand, children with intestinal perforation and peritonitis may be in shock and hypotensive.

B. General Examination

Before starting the systemic examination, perform a careful and thorough general examination. A good general examination will give you a rough idea about the patient's problem, and prove to be groundwork before you start the actual abdominal examination. Emphasize on the points listed in **Key Box 8**.

Key Box 8

General Examination Relevant to Abdomen

1. Jaundice
2. Pallor
3. Cutaneous bleeds
4. Lymphadenopathy
5. Signs of liver cell failure
6. Edema and dehydration
7. Jugular venous pressure
8. Clubbing
9. Bony tenderness
10. Nutritional status

1. Jaundice

It is an important sign of liver cell failure and present both in acute hepatitis or chronic liver disease.

10 Unconjugated hyperbilirubinemia as seen in cases of hemolysis is not deep. Absence of jaundice does rule out hepatic involvement.

2. Pallor

It is a significant finding in children suffering from chronic renal or liver disease, malabsorption syndromes, or hemolytic anemia. It can also be a significant and sometimes the only finding in children with worm infestation or in case of occult blood loss from the gastrointestinal tract.

3. Cutaneous Bleeds

Look for petechiae, purpura, or ecchymosis. Hepatosplenomegaly associated with cutaneous bleed may be suggestive of infection (typhoid, bacterial endocarditis, malaria, infectious mononucleosis, etc.), liver disease (chronic hepatitis) or malignancy (leukemia, lymphoma).

4. Lymphadenopathy

Generalized lymphadenopathy suggests disseminated tuberculosis, leukemia, or lymphoma. Abdominal or mesenteric lymph nodes are not usually palpable, and are detected only on an ultrasound examination. Inguinal lymph nodes are very commonly enlarged as they drain the perineum and the perianal area which are often infected in children.

5. Signs of Liver Cell Failure

Look for these signs in children suspected of suffering from chronic liver disease. Signs of liver cell failure include jaundice, palmar erythema, spider angioma, and parotid swelling.

- ***Palmar erythema:*** The palms are warm, erythematous, or bright red; especially on thenar and hypothenar eminences.
- ***Spider angioma:*** It is seen in the drainage area of superior vena cava, i.e. above the nipples. It consists of a central arteriole from which numerous capillaries radiate out giving an appearance of a spider. On pressing at the center, the whole lesion blanches.
- Gynecomastia and testicular atrophy may be seen in adolescent boys.

6. Edema and Dehydration

Look for pitting pedal edema **(Fig. 10.3)**, facial puffiness, or generalized edema **(Fig. 10.4)** which may be evident in patients of nephrotic syndrome, acute renal failure, acute glomerulo- nephritis, or chronic liver disease.

Assess for signs of dehydration in any child with diarrhea. It is also important to look for dehydration in patients suspected of having prerenal cause of acute renal failure. A child may get dehydrated due to inadequate intake or due to vomiting alone even if not associated with diarrhea.

7. Jugular Venous Pressure (JVP)

You may find the JVP to be raised in patients of acute glomerulonephritis, acute renal failure, or congestive cardiac failure.

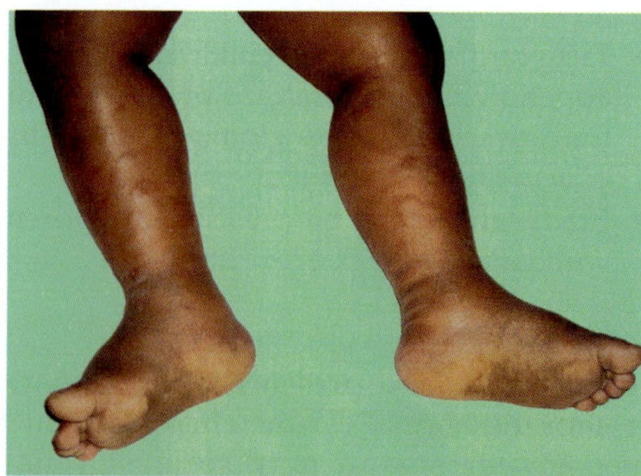

Fig. 10.3: Pedal edema in a child with nephrotic syndrome.

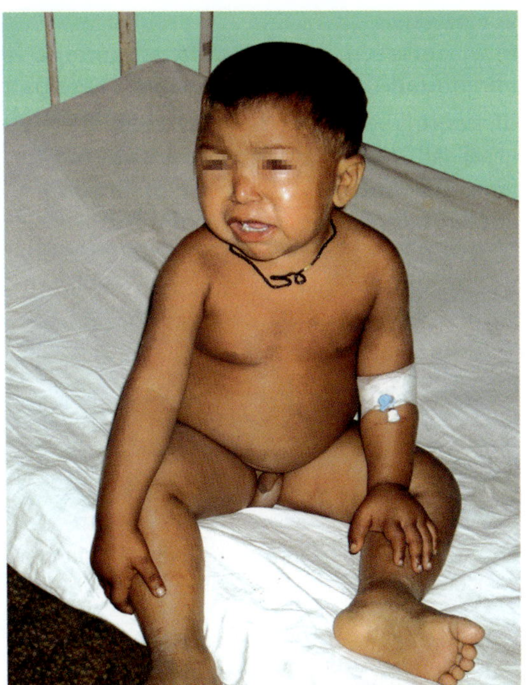

Fig. 10.4: A child with anasarca.

8. Clubbing

It is the bulbous enlargement of soft parts of the terminal phalanges. It is an important clinical sign in some abdominal conditions, like ulcerative colitis, Crohn disease, and primary biliary cirrhosis.

9. Bony Tenderness

Press over the midpoint of the sternum to elicit bony tenderness. This is the hallmark of malignant infiltration of the marrow—as seen in leukemia or lymphoma.

10. Nutritional Status

Assessment of the nutritional status is very important in any pediatric case. Perform a thorough anthropometric examination as described earlier. Look for various signs of malnutrition and multivitamin deficiency. The disease the child is suffering from may be a reason or a consequence of malnutrition. A chronic problem, like tuberculosis, renal or liver disorder, malabsorption syndrome, or chronic diarrhea, will lead to malnutrition. Malnutrition itself can lead to problems, like tuberculosis, diarrhea, or hypokalemia leading to abdominal signs and symptoms.

11. Eyes

Eyes should be examined for cataract, Kayser-Fleischer ring (best visible under a slit-lamp), chorioretinitis, and signs of vitamin A deficiency.

12. Oral Cavity

Oral cavity should be examined for angular cheilosis, stomatitis, loss of papillae (signs of vitamin B deficiency). Presence of oral candidiasis beyond neonatal period may be suggestive of an immunodeficiency states. Cleft palate is often missed unless specifically looked for. It can explain nasal regurgitation of feeds, difficulty in accepting feeds, and failure to thrive with no other attributable cause. Gingival hypertrophy may be seen in children with acute myeloid leukemia or on phenytoin therapy.

10.5 EXAMINATION OF THE ABDOMEN

A. Inspection (Key Box 9)

Where to examine?

Examine young children (<2 yr) in the mother's lap (Fig. 10.5) as the child may be too apprehensive to lie down on the examination couch. A very young infant till the age of 6–7 months may not show any anxiety as she has not developed stranger anxiety. If baby is crying or irritable, she can be put to the mother's breast to pacify her so that the abdominal muscles are relaxed.

A toddler is also afraid of lying down on the couch. Examining a resisting and constantly crying child is fruitless as most of the findings will be missed. Talk politely to the child

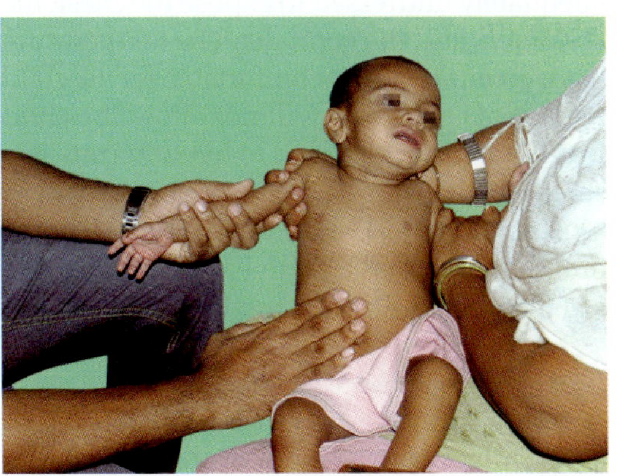

Fig. 10.5: Examining an infant in the mother's lap.

Key Box 9

Inspection of the Abdomen

1. Shape of the abdomen
2. Abdominal movements
3. Umbilicus: Position and shape
4. Skin scars or incision
5. Superficial dilated veins
6. Visible peristalsis
7. Visible pulsations
8. Groins and scrotum

explaining what you are about to do and that it will not be a painful experience. It is always better to make the mother or the attendant stand near the child to get full cooperation from the child. The child can be engaged with a toy or an attractive object and while the child plays with the toy you can examine the abdomen.

An older child or an adolescent will be more receptive, but still may be afraid. You can talk to the child throughout the examination to divert attention so that abdominal muscles are relaxed and your job becomes easier.

Position

The child should ideally be lying supine on a firm couch with the arms by the side and the lower limbs should be flexed at the hip joint to relax abdominal muscles. A toddler can also be examined in a standing position (Fig. 10.6).

Pre-requisites

You should stand on the right side of the patient. The room should be properly illuminated and warm. The child should be adequately undressed to expose the chest, the abdomen, and the genitalia. The temperature of the room should be comfortable for the child because a cold room will not allow the child to relax and can also lead to hypothermia in a small infant. Your hands should be warm as touching the child with cold hands will make him/her tighten the abdominal muscles.

Finally, stand-by the child and observe.

Points to Remember

1. In some very irritable and overanxious children, it may be impossible to pacify the child, and it may be wise to wait for the child to fall asleep to thoroughly examine the abdomen for finer details or confirm a doubtful finding.
2. While exposing the abdomen and genitalia of children, you should be careful about their privacy, a male examiner when examining a female child should have another female attendant or nurse in the room.

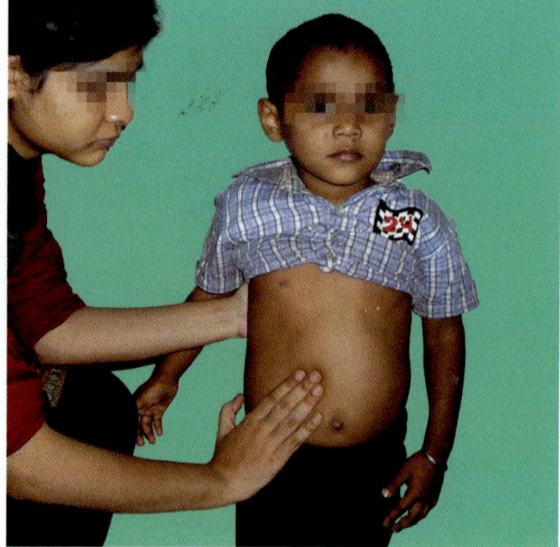

Fig. 10.6: Examination of a toddler in standing position.

1. Shape

Look for fullness, obvious visible swelling, distention, or a scaphoid abdomen. It is normally slightly full without any localized distention. Symmetry of the abdomen should be assessed while you are standing at the foot end with your eyes at the level of abdomen of the child.

- ***Fullness*** may be due to fat, fluid, flatus, or feces. The abdomen of an infant appears full or distended immediately after a feed. The abdomen of a toddler normally looks protuberant. The abdomen looks protuberant in hypotonia as seen in protein energy malnutrition and rickets. Fullness can also be due to an organomegaly, intestinal obstruction (Fig. 10.7), or presence of fluid (ascites) (Fig. 10.8). The lower abdomen appears full and distended in children on long-term steroids because of redistribution of fat (e.g. nephrotic syndrome). Distension is central in small bowel obstruction; and peripheral in large bowel obstruction.

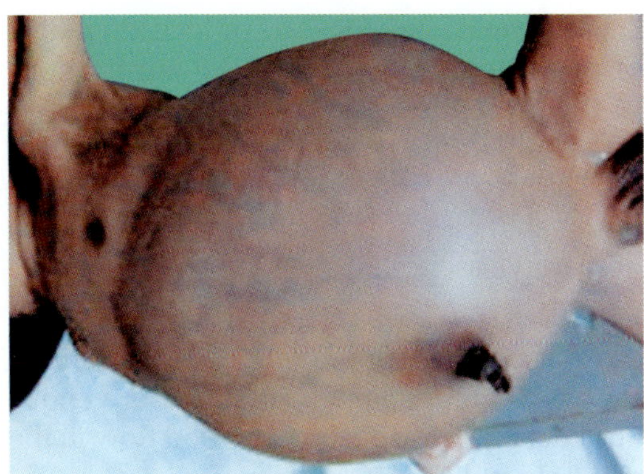

Fig. 10.7: Abdominal distention secondary to lower intestinal obstruction.

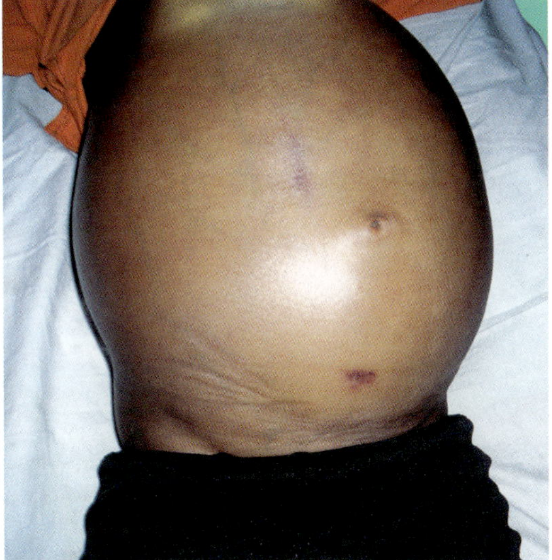

Fig. 10.8: Abdominal distention due to ascites.

- ***Localized distention:*** It may be seen in: (i) small bowel obstruction; (ii) organomegaly; or (iii) abnormal lump. A full bladder appears as a globular suprapubic lump which disappears when the child passes urine. A lump is seen transiently after feeds in congenital pyloric stenosis in the epigastrium just right to the midline.
- ***Scaphoid abdomen*** is seen in an extremely malnourished child or in a newborn with intrauterine growth retardation, congenital diaphragmatic hernia, or duodenal atresia.

2. Abdominal movements: These should be observed with each breath. Normally, there is gentle rise of the abdomen with each inspiration. In diaphragmatic paralysis, the rise may be seen with each expiration rather than inspiration. Sluggish or no respiratory movements of the abdominal wall indicates peritoneal irritation as seen in diffuse peritonitis.

3. Umbilicus: Umbilicus is normally placed at the midpoint of the line joining the tip of xiphoid and symphysis pubis. It is retracted and inverted.

- ***Umbilicus appears everted*** (Fig. 10.9) in the presence of gross distention of the abdomen—like ascites or visceromegaly.
- The umbilicus may become ***transverse*** due to gross abdominal distension which is also known as the smiling umbilicus (Fig. 10.10).
- ***Umbilical hernia*** is a very common finding in children less than 2 years which becomes ballooned when the child cries (Fig. 10.11). The umbilical hernia may also be pathological (Fig. 10.12).
- In young infants, look for signs of inflammation around the umbilicus, i.e. redness or

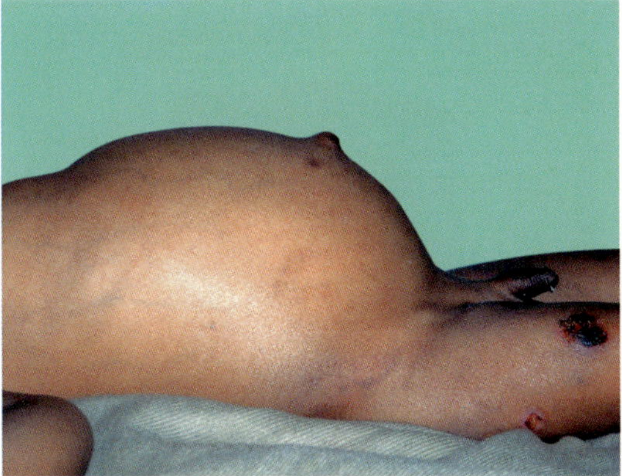

Fig. 10.9: Everted umbilicus because of ascites.

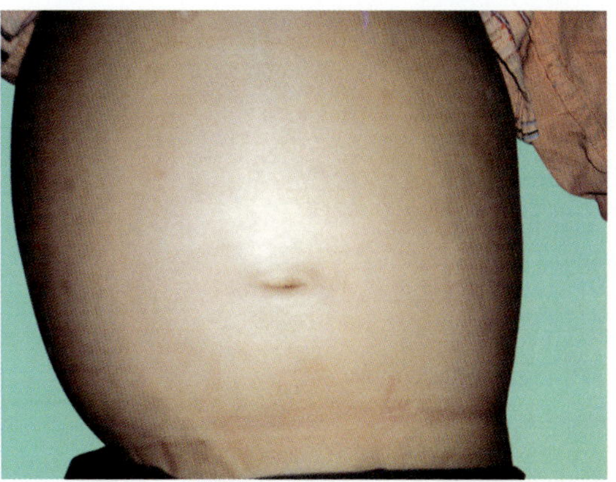

Fig. 10.10: A smiling umbilicus and impression of tight clothes indicating abdominal wall edema.

pus discharge to rule out umbilical sepsis (Fig. 10.13).

- A bright red nodular mass may be seen in the umbilicus with serosanguineous discharge in some infants due to the presence of *umbilical granuloma* (Fig. 10.14).

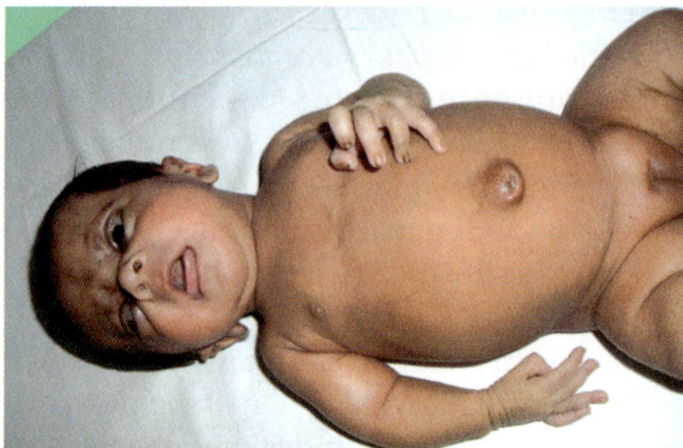

Fig. 10.11: An infant with physiological umbilical hernia.

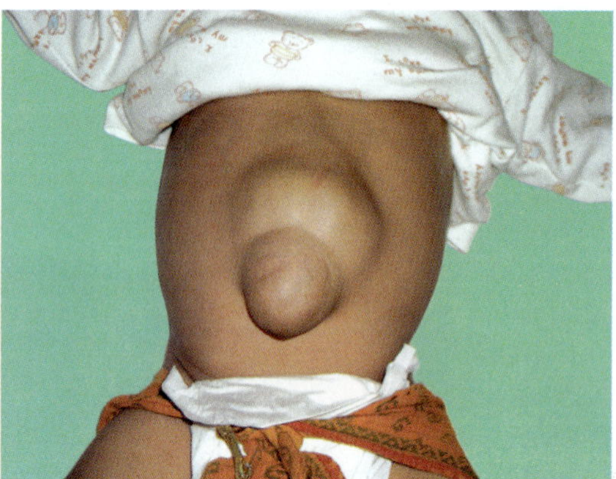

Fig. 10.12 An infant with pathological umbilical hernia.

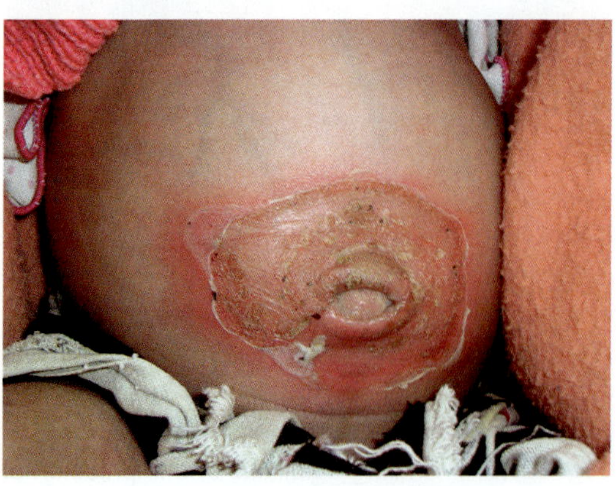

Fig. 10.13: Umbilical sepsis

4. Skin scars: Look for scars or incision marks of prior surgery that may have implications in the presenting illness. Skin may be tense and shiny in the presence of gross ascites or distention (Fig. 10.15). There can be ulceration in the skin because of stretching in presence of massive ascites.

5. Superficial veins: Small superficial veins are normally visible over the abdomen. If the veins are distended, it suggests venous obstruction. The direction of blood flow in the veins should be checked:

- Empty the vein of blood by placing two fingers side by side over the vein.
- Move one finger away while keeping the other fixed (also known as milking).
- Now, release the finger one by one to see the direction through which the blood fills the vein (Fig. 10.16).
- Direction of flow of blood is below upwards in inferior vena cava obstruction.

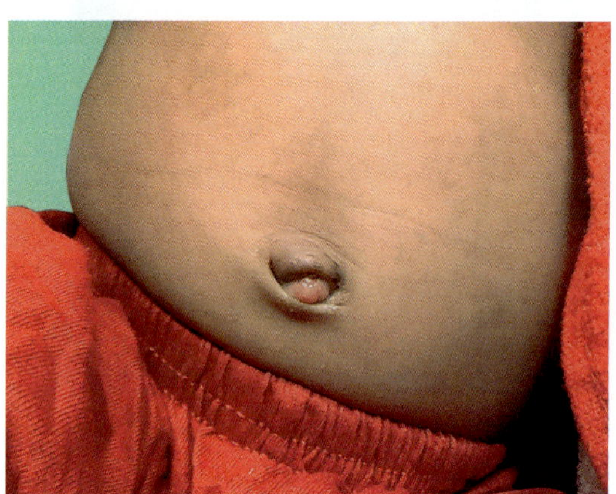

Fig. 10.14: Umbilical granuloma

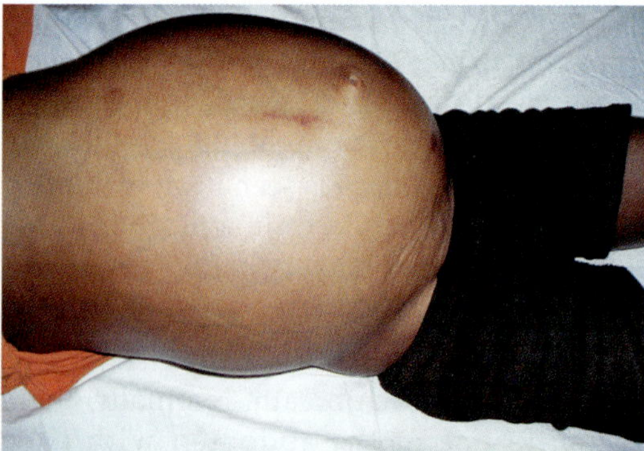

Fig. 10.15: Tense and shiny skin with visible dilated veins in a child with gross ascites.

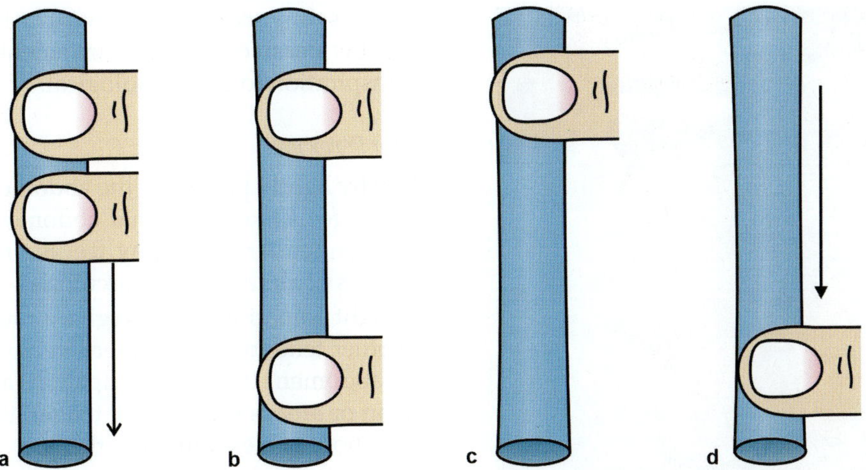

Fig. 10.16: Method of detecting the direction of blood flow: (a, b) Empty the vein of blood then (c) lift the lower finger but vein remains empty due to the venous valve which prevents retrograde flow then (d) the upper finger is lifted and the vein fills in the direction of flow.

- In superior vena cava obstruction, the veins fill from *above downwards*.
- In portal hypertension, the veins form a cluster around the umbilicus (caput medusa) and the direction of blood flow in the veins is *away from the umbilicus*.

6. Visible peristalsis: Look for movement of the intestine, visible on the abdominal wall. The usual direction of intestinal peristalsis is from left to right. Visible peristalsis is characteristic of obstruction in the large bowel or distal part of the small bowel.

7. Pulsations: These may be seen in the epigastrium in right ventricular hypertrophy. Also look for pulsations over the liver.

8. Groin and scrotum: The groin area and scrotum in boys must be examined for any swelling which may be a hernia. A hernia is an abnormal protrusion of an organ or tissue through a defect in the surrounding walls. In abdominal hernia, there is protrusion of the gut, mostly the intestines, through the defect. Depending on the site of defect, hernia is classified as inguinal **(Fig. 10.17)**, lumbar **(Fig. 10.18)**, umbilical, epigastric, femoral, or incisional.

The inguinal and femoral hernia are most common, they are seen in the groin region. Inguinal hernia is mostly seen in boys, while femoral hernia is more common in girls. There may be symptoms of pain and dragging sensation in the region, or the parents may just complain of a lump in the groin. Many times, it may be a chance finding during an abdominal examination.

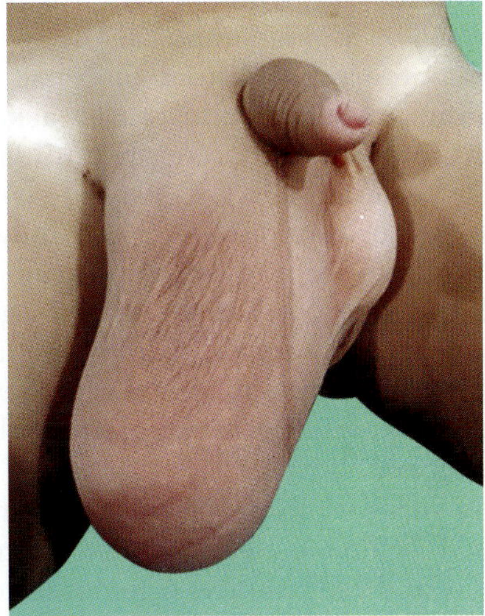

Fig. 10.17: Inguinal hernia presenting as scrotal swelling

An inguinal hernia is seen above and medial to the pubic tubercle and the femoral hernia is seen below and lateral to the pubic tubercle. A hernia may also present as a surgical emergency in which case the hernia may be tender, there may be associated nausea and vomiting. This can be because of an obstructed (the contents of the hernia cannot be reduced back into the abdominal cavity) or strangulated hernia (gangrene of the gut due to compromised blood supply).

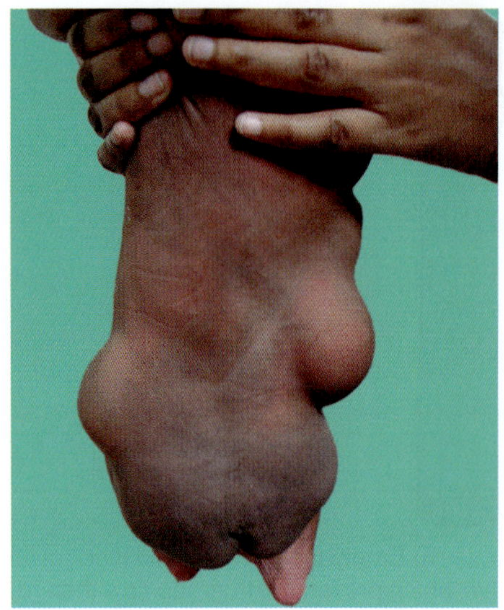

Fig. 10.18: Lumbar hernia

Confirmation of hernia: A hernia is mostly confirmed by a cough impulse. The swelling becomes more prominent or tense with coughing. An older child can be asked to cough, to observe the cough impulse. In younger children and infants, the swelling becomes more prominent when they cry, as it increases the abdominal pressure. It is usually possible to reduce the hernia by gently pushing the contents with the examining finger back into the abdominal cavity except when the hernia is obstructed or strangulated, as mentioned above.

Any mass or lump seen or felt in the inguinal region must be examined for cough impulse and reducibility. A femoral hernia may not show a cough impulse and it may not be possible to reduce it completely. If a hernia is suspected, detailed evaluation should be done by a surgeon.

Differential diagnosis: Inguinal hernia needs to be differentiated from lipoma, hydrocele, varicocele, inguinal lymphadenitis, epididymitis, and ectopic testis.

B. Palpation

- Ask the child to lie supine with the hip joints flexed and arms by the side.
- Ask the child to relax, if he is old enough to understand.
- Position your forearm horizontally along the abdomen and place the fingers flat on the abdominal wall.
- Press inwards during expiration and allow passive outward movement during inspiration to be physiological.

Light Palpation

Start by lightly palpating the abdomen to see how it feels like. A normal abdomen is soft and non-tender. A doughy feel is present in patients of abdominal tuberculosis.

Light palpation will also give a rough idea whether tenderness is present in any part of the abdomen. If, during palpation, a certain organ or area is found to be tender, then that area should be examined in the last.

Rigidity and guarding will be felt in children with peritonitis or perforation, this is due to the irritation of the parietal peritoneum. It is a part of the protective mechanism to prevent the spread of infection.

A ***tense abdomen*** is present in huge distention due to gas or fluid.

Rebound tenderness is a sign of peritonitis; due to presence of an inflamed organ underneath the peritoneum. The hand is pressed down gradually on the abdomen. The hand is now withdrawn suddenly and completely. The patient immediately winces in pain. This is due to the inflamed parietal peritoneum springing back along with the abdominal muscles.

Deep Palpation

In a obese child, palpate by dipping the hands deep into the abdomen. If the child is not relaxed or is crying, the abdomen will be rigid and tense.

1. Liver

There are two ways of palpating the liver:

a. Place the right hand over the right iliac fossa such that your fingers are parallel to the ribs, then ask the patient to take deep breaths (Fig. 10.19). Wait for the liver edge to come and strike the lateral border of the index finger with inspiration. The fingers should be placed gently over the abdomen and not dug deep which (Fig. 10.20) may lead to missing a soft liver or a small liver.
b. Another method of palpation is by keeping your hand parallel to the lateral rectus muscle (Fig. 10.21) so that the tips of the fingers are pointing towards the ribs. At the

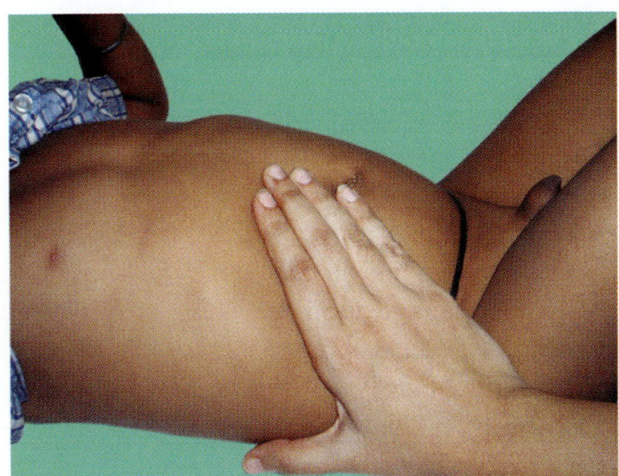

Fig. 10.19: Correct method of palpating the liver by keeping the fingers parallel to the subcostal margin.

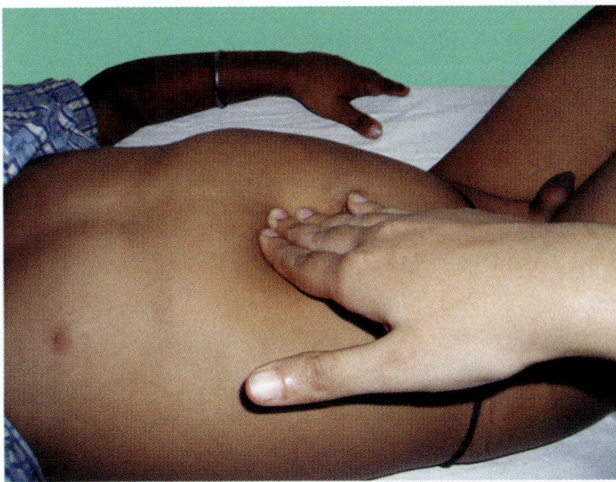

Fig. 10.20: Wrong method of palpating the liver by digging the fingers into the abdomen.

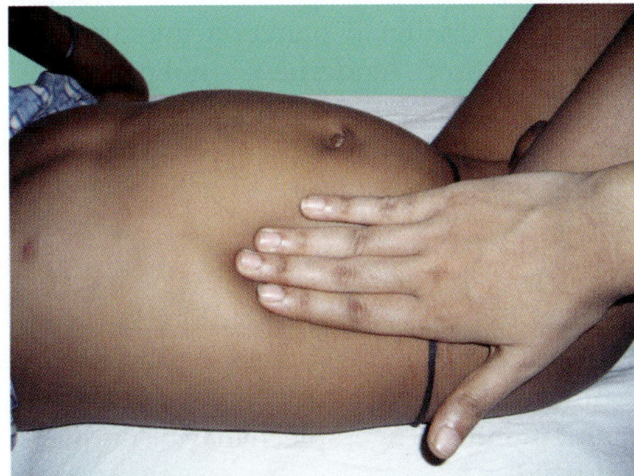

Fig. 10.21: Alternative method of palpating the liver by keeping the fingers perpendicular to the subcostal margin.

height of each inspiration, press the fingers firmly inwards and upwards to feel, for the liver edge. If the edge is not felt keep moving up towards the subcostal margin till the liver edge is palpable.

Right lobe: The *right lobe of liver* is palpable in the right hypochondrium or lumbar region depending upon the extent of enlargement.

Left lobe: The *left lobe of liver* is palpable in the epigastrium, and it must be looked for as it indicates a chronic hepatomegaly. You should start palpating the liver from the right iliac fossa and move upwards otherwise you may miss massive hepatomegaly extending up to the right iliac fossa.

You will feel the liver moving with respiration. The dictum is that "do not go for the liver; let the liver come to you". Liver is normally just palpable below the costal margin. Once the margins are palpated, look for the points listed in **Key Box 10**. A normal liver is soft, smooth, has rounded margins, and is non-tender. The presence and extent of hepatomegaly can also be confirmed by percussion.

Liver size: The liver is usually described in centimeters palpable below the right costal margin in the mid-clavicular line **(Fig. 10.22)**.

Key Box 10

Characteristics of Liver

1. Size
2. Surface
3. Consistency
4. Margins
5. Tenderness

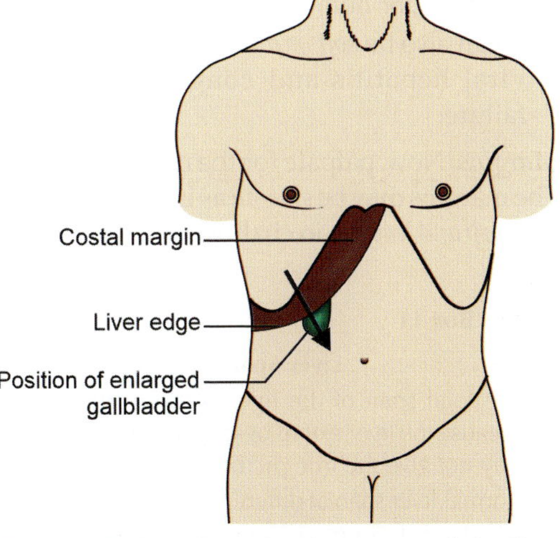

Fig. 10.22: Direction of enlargement of the liver and its relation to the subcostal margin.

Liver span is the distance measured between the upper and lower borders of the liver. The lower border of the liver is determined by palpation as described above. The upper border lies in the thorax and can be defined by percussion, which will be discussed in the next section on percussion.

The liver span varies according to the age of the child **(Key Box 11)**, therefore, a comment on the presence of hepatomegaly should be made only after comparing it with the normal for age. In children with pneumothorax, emphysema, or respiratory distress; the liver is pushed down by the diaphragm and will be palpable below the costal margin; giving a false impression of hepatomegaly. However, the total liver span is normal.

In another situation, liver may be palpable below costal margin, but when the total span is measured, it is reduced suggesting cirrhosis. In all these situations, you will miss the actual diagnosis, if you only examine the liver below the costal margins.

Common causes of hepatomegaly in children are listed in **Table 10.5**.

Surface: Feel for the surface of the liver. This is done by gently rolling the fingers over the surface of liver. The surface may be nodular in cirrhosis and malignancy; or smooth as in other causes of hepatomegaly.

Consistency: Feel for the consistency of liver.

- It is as hard as a bone in hepatic malignancy.
- It may be firm as the tip of nose in chronic conditions, like obstructive jaundice, cirrhosis, or hemolytic anemia.
- It can also be *soft as an ear cartilage* in acute viral hepatitis and congestive cardiac failure.

Margins: Now, palpate for the margins of liver. The margins may be *smooth* as in a normal liver or *sharp and leafy* as in cirrhosis or malignancy.

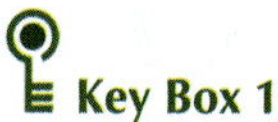

Key Box 11

Liver Span

1. The total span of the liver is more important because the liver extent below the costal margin may not give the true picture.
2. Normal liver span at different ages is as follows: Infants: 5–6.5 cm; 1–5 years: 6–7 cm; 5–10 years: 7–9 cm; and 10–15 years: 8–10 cm.

Table 10.5: Common causes of hepatomegaly

Infants

- Intrauterine infections, like TORCH group of infections
- Septicemia
- Neonatal hepatitis
- Extrahepatic biliary obstruction
- Glycogen storage disorder
- Galactosemia
- Alpha-1-antitrypsin deficiency
- Congestive cardiac failure

Older children

- *Fatty liver*—as in malnutrition
- *Hepatic abscess:* Bacterial or amebic
- *Lipid storage disorders:* Gaucher, Niemann-Pick disease
- Glycogen storage disorders
- Hepatitis (acute or chronic)
- Tuberculosis
- *Malignancies:* Leukemia, lymphoma, neuroblastoma, and hepatoblastoma
- *Metabolic diseases:* Alpha-1-antitrypsin deficiency, cystic fibrosis, Wilson disease
- Congestive cardiac failure, constrictive pericarditis, cardiac tamponade
- Hemolytic anemia
- Veno-occlusive disease, Budd-Chiari malformation
- Extrahepatic obstruction

Tenderness: While palpating the liver, note whether the child winces or not. Do not ask the child whether it pains on touching the liver. Sometimes tenderness is not present on light palpation, but may become evident on deep palpation. A liver of acute viral hepatitis, congestive cardiac failure, and liver abscess is tender.

2. *Spleen:* An enlarged spleen is palpable in the left hypochondrium. Unlike the liver, spleen is not palpable unless it is more than 2 times enlarged. But in young infants less than 3 months of age, spleen may be normally palpable.

- Start feeling for the spleen from the right iliac fossa otherwise you may miss a massive spleen.
- Keep the right hand over the abdomen with fingers pointing towards the left subcostal margin and press the fingers a little into the abdomen with each breath **(Fig. 10.23)**.

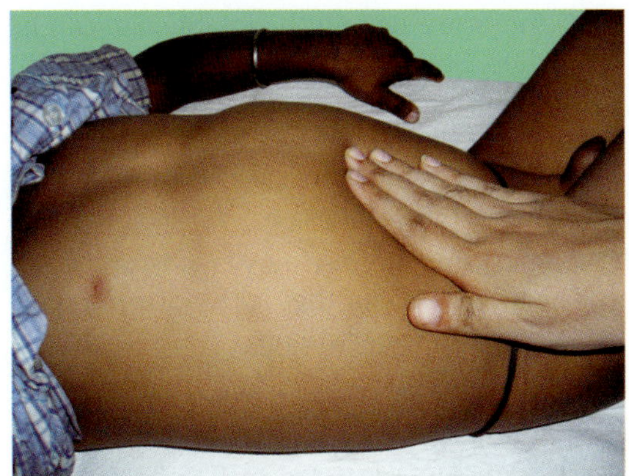

Fig. 10.23: Palpation of spleen.

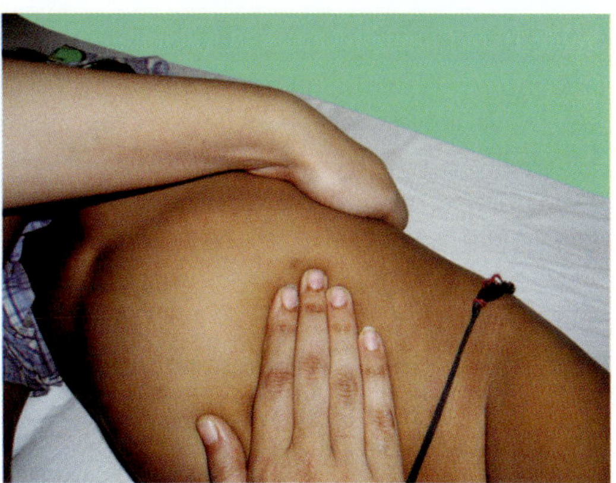

Fig. 10.24: Palpation of spleen in right lateral position.

- You can keep the palm of the left hand over the tenth, eleventh, and the twelfth ribs posterolaterally to support them from below.
- Try and feel for the splenic tip as it comes and strikes your fingers with the peak of inspiration.
- If not palpable, move your hands towards the left hypochondrium through the umbilicus till the tips of the fingers reach the left subcostal margin.
- If the spleen is not palpable, try and feel for it a little more medially along the left subcostal margin.
- The direction of splenic enlargement is downwards and towards the right iliac fossa.
- To palpate a *just palpable spleen*, turn the patient towards the right (in right lateral position). Support the left lower ribcage by your left hand and dip the right hand under the subcostal margin; the splenic tip may slip over the fingertips (Fig. 10.24).
- The patient should be inhaling deeply to facilitate the palpation of spleen.
- It will not be possible to insert the fingers between the spleen and the subcostal margin, and it will move with respiration.
- After the spleen has been identified—note its size, splenic notch, consistency, and tenderness.

Spleen size: The size of the spleen is measured from the left subcostal margin in the mid-clavicular line to the tip along the direction of enlargement. The usual direction of enlargement is towards the right iliac fossa. The size is described in cm below the left costal margin, towards right iliac fossa.

- The spleen is said to be *mildly enlarged*, if only the tip is palpable or it is palpable just 1–2 cm below the costal margin.
- It is *moderately enlarged*, if it is palpable 3–7 cm below the costal margin.
- There is *massive enlargement*, if it is palpable more than 7 cm below the costal margin or crosses the umbilicus (Fig. 10.25).

Consistency: Gently feel for the consistency of the spleen. It may be soft as in enteric fever, or firm as in hemolytic anemia. A moderate to severely enlarged spleen is usually firm.

Splenic notch: A notch is felt as an indentation on the lower medial border of spleen. It is easy to feel the notch in a firm and a moderately or massively enlarged spleen. It helps us to confirm that the lump we are palpating is an enlarged spleen.

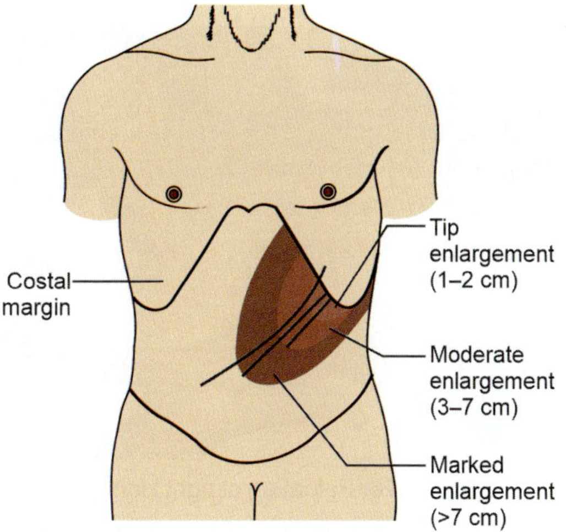

Fig. 10.25: Direction of enlargement of spleen.

Table 10.6: Common causes of splenomegaly
Infectious: Typhoid, malaria, endocarditis, septicemia, abscess, toxoplasma, cytomegalovirus, kala azar
Hematologic: Hemolytic anemias, leukemia, lymphoma, hemangioma
Infilterative: Lipid storage disorders (Niemann-Pick and Gaucher)
Congestive: Cirrhosis, portal hypertension, congestive cardiac failure
Miscellaneous: SLE

Common causes of splenomegaly in children are listed in **Table 10.6**.

*3. **Right kidney:*** Kidneys are palpated bimanually.

- To palpate the right kidney, keep the right hand over the right lumbar region and the left hand behind the right loin at the renal angle **(Fig. 10.26)**.
- Renal angle The renal angle is formed in the back by the lower border of the twelfth rib and outer border of erector spinae muscle.
- Press the right hand deep into the abdomen to push the kidney posteriorly during expiration when the abdominal muscles are relaxed.
- The left hand is used to push the kidney anteriorly.
- Try to feel for the lower pole of kidney as the child takes deep breaths.
- The kidney is felt as a smooth rounded swelling.
- Kidneys are usually ballotable, i.e. can be pushed between the two hands. To elicit ballotability, push the kidney down with the right hand, and feel by your left hand kept in the loin when it strikes the posterior surface of the abdomen.
- A renal lump will also move with respiration. The lower pole of the right kidney may be palpable in thin patients.

*4. **Left kidney:*** Palpate the left kidney in a similar way by keeping the right hand in the left lumbar region and the left hand posteriorly in the left loin **(Fig. 10.27)**. You can stand either on the right or the left side of the patient.

Renal lump: The kidneys are not as readily palpable as liver or spleen as the kidneys are placed deeper into the abdomen. Therefore, it may be difficult to appreciate a renal lump by an inexperienced examiner. A renal lump may also be difficult to appreciate, if the liver or spleen is also simultaneously enlarged and is extending up to the lumbar region. A renal lump also needs to be differentiated from an enlarged spleen **(Key Box 12)**.

A renal lump is palpable in following situations: Wilms tumor, perinephric abscess, hydronephrosis, renal cysts, congenital anomalies, and ectopic kidney.

Renal tenderness: To elicit renal tenderness, press your thumb at the renal angle with the patient sitting and bending forwards so that the back is outstretched.

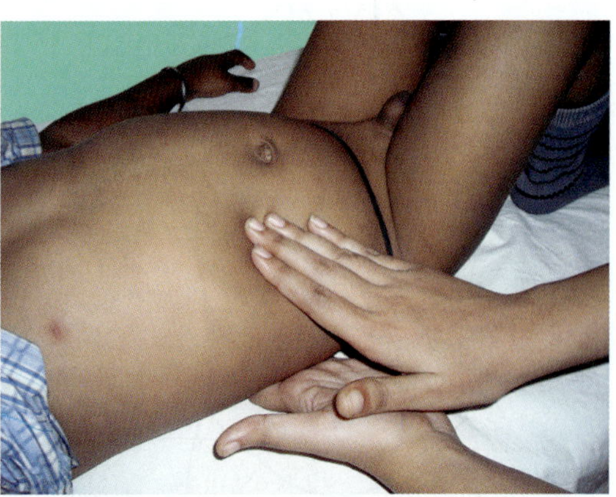

Fig. 10.26: Palpation of right kidney.

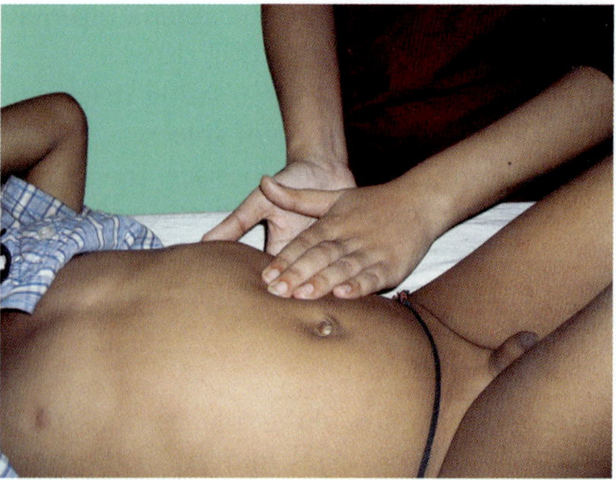

Fig. 10.27: Palpation of left kidney.

Key Box 12

Differentiating between the Renal Lump and Spleen

1. A spleen is not bimanually palpable.
2. The upper border of spleen cannot be reached, i.e. you will not be able to insinuate your fingers between the spleen and the left subcostal margin, whereas the upper border can be felt in a renal lump.
3. The direction of enlargement of spleen is towards the right iliac fossa.
4. A massive spleen can cross the midline, but a renal lump will not cross the umbilicus.
5. A splenic notch, if felt, will confirm the presence of a spleen.

Key Box 13

Description of an Abdominal Lump

1. *Site:* Which regions are being occupied by the lump?
2. *Origin:* Intra-abdominal or parietal
3. *Size:* Both in vertical and horizontal planes
4. *Shape:* Round, elongated, or irregular
5. *Margins:* Feel if the margins are well or ill-defined
6. *Surface:* Smooth or nodular
7. *Consistency:* Cystic, firm, or hard
8. *Mobility:* Moving with respiration or otherwise
9. *Ballotability*
10. *Signs of inflammation:* Whether present

5. Urinary bladder: It is not normally palpable. It may be felt as a smooth oval lump in the suprapubic region when it is full. A bladder lump may be palpable in patients with bladder neck obstruction, e.g. posterior urethral valve, bladder diverticula, urethral strictures, meatal stenosis, phimosis, or patients with voiding dysfunction. The upper border may reach the umbilicus. The lump will disappear when the patient passes urine and evacuates the bladder. But in patients of bladder neck obstruction, the bladder after micturition may still have residual urine and may still be palpable.

6. Fecoliths: Fecoliths, which are hard dried stool retained in the rectum, may be palpable in a constipated patient in the left iliac fossa as firm to hard lumps. They are usually multiple, and can be indented by pressing a finger into them.

7. Abdominal lump: Whenever a swelling or a mass is palpable in the abdomen, make sure that it is not a liver, spleen, kidney, or a bladder lump. If not, then try to find out the following details that may help you to decide on the origin and nature of the lump. Describe the lump in terms of characters outlined in **Key Box 13**.

Site and origin: See whether the lump is *intra-abdominal* or *parietal*.

Ask the child to lift his shoulders off the couch while you are pressing firmly against the forehead. You can also ask him to raise both the extended legs from the couch **(Fig. 10.28)**. If the swelling becomes less obvious due to the tautness of the abdominal muscles or disappears, then it is an intra-abdominal swelling. But, if it remains the same, then it is a parietal swelling.

Also note the region of the abdomen that the swelling is occupying. This will give you some idea about the organ of origin. Swelling over a hernial site may not necessarily be a hernia.

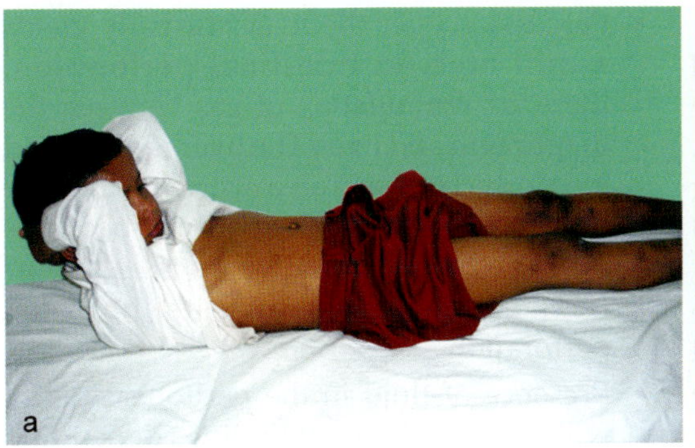

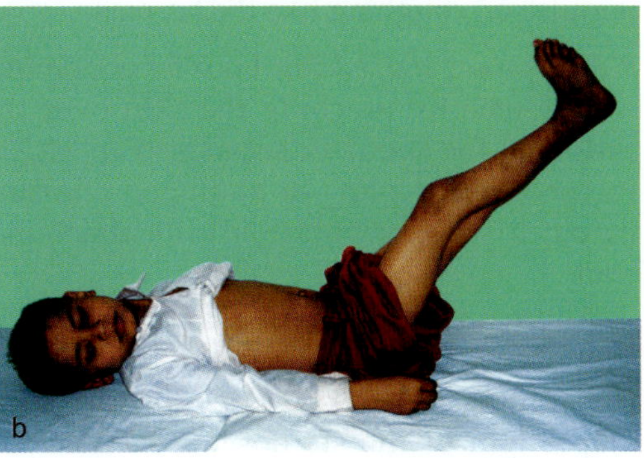

Fig. 10.28: (a) Patient lifting his shoulders off the couch; (b) straight leg raising test.

Size: Note the size of the swelling by measuring it in the two dimensions perpendicular to each other. Describe the size of the swelling in cm.

Shape: Note the shape of the swelling, whether it is round, elongated, or irregular.

Margins: Feel if the margins are well-defined or ill-defined.

Surface: Gently feel over the surface of the swelling and see if the surface is smooth or nodular.

Consistency: A hard swelling is suggestive of neoplasm. A firm swelling can be a benign tumor. The swelling may be cystic in nature.

Mobility

- If the swelling is moving with respiration, it could be arising from liver, spleen, kidneys, or stomach. But, they do not freely move with palpation.
- A swelling, such as a mesenteric cyst, may not move with respiration at all, but may move freely by palpation.
- A swelling which is firmly adherent to the surrounding structures, and is not mobile at all may either be a retroperitoneal mass, an advanced malignancy, or secondary to chronic inflammation.

Ballotability: A renal lump is ballotable. Method of eliciting ballotability has already been described.

Signs of inflammation: Note any signs of inflammation like redness, induration, and raised temperature which will suggest an inflammatory swelling. A strangulated hernia will present as an inflammatory inguinal swelling with severe pain abdomen.

Impulse on coughing: Swellings in continuity with the abdominal cavity will give rise to impulse on coughing like the hernias.

8. Abdominal wall edema: Look for abdominal wall edema by pinching the skin over the abdomen for about 10 seconds **(Fig. 10.29)**. Presence of indenting or pitting on releasing the pinch is suggestive of fluid in the abdominal wall.

Alternatively, press the diaphragm of the stethoscope against the lateral abdominal wall; pitting can be seen along the rim of the diaphragm of the stethoscope, when you release the pressure.

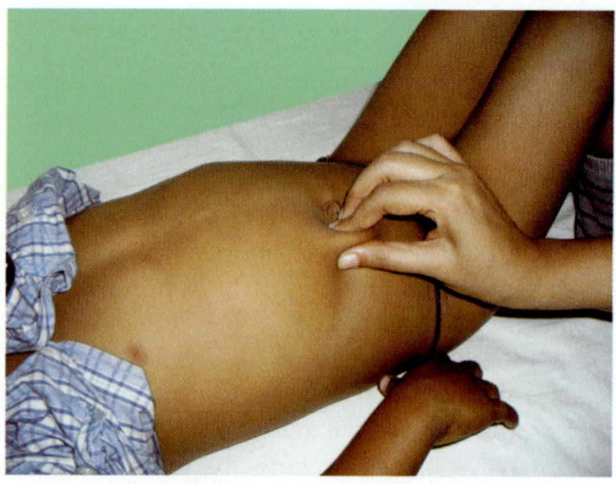

Fig. 10.29: Demonstration of abdominal wall edema.

Abdominal wall edema is a part of generalized anasarca (e.g. in nephrotic syndrome). It is also evident when you remove a tight cloth around the waist like a pant, etc. which leaves indentation on the abdominal wall (*see* **Fig. 10.10**).

Abdominal circumference: It is measured with a measuring tape at the level of the umbilicus. Monitoring of abdominal girth is important to assess the progression or reduction in abdominal distention due to any cause.

C. Percussion

Percussion of the abdomen is done with the child in the supine position and the lower limbs flexed at the hip joints. It not only confirms some of our findings of palpation, but also tells us more:

- *Gaseous distension:* Percussion over the abdomen helps to differentiate whether the abdominal distention is due to gas or fluid. In presence of gas in the abdomen, the overlying percussion note will be resonant or tympanic.
- Percussion over the liver normally yields a dull note. In intestinal perforation, there is accumulation of gas between the diaphragm and liver. The liver is displaced inferiorly. The usual area overlying the liver (which should have been dull) becomes resonant. This is known as *masking of liver dullness* and suggests intestinal perforation.
- Presence of fluid in the peritoneal cavity will result in different findings depending upon the amount of fluid present.

1. *Puddle sign:* If the fluid in the peritoneal cavity is minimal, it can be detected only by making patient prone so that he bears weight on his knees and hands. The abdomen is off the couch. When the patient assumes this posture, the fluid gravitates down around the center and percussion over the umbilicus will give a dull note **(Fig. 10.30)**.

2. *Shifting dullness:* If the amount of peritoneal fluid is moderate, it results in shifting of dullness to the dependent area.

- Ask the child to lie supine. Expose the abdomen, and stand on the right side of the child.
- Keep the pleximeter finger perpendicular to the midline at a point between the xiphisternum and umbilicus. Percuss here; this should normally elicit a resonant note.
- From this point, percuss downwards towards the umbilicus up to suprapubic region. The note should remain resonant. A dullness may indicate an underlying full urinary bladder. Ask the child to void so that the bladder becomes empty and does not interfere with the examination.
- After ensuring that the percussion note at the umbilicus is resonant, keep the pleximeter finger at the umbilicus in the midline.
- Start percussing from the umbilicus and go laterally towards the right or the left flank.
- If the note remains resonant throughout up to the flanks, this indicates absence of significant fluid in the peritoneal cavity.
- A dull note in the dependent flanks suggests presence of fluid because of gravitation.

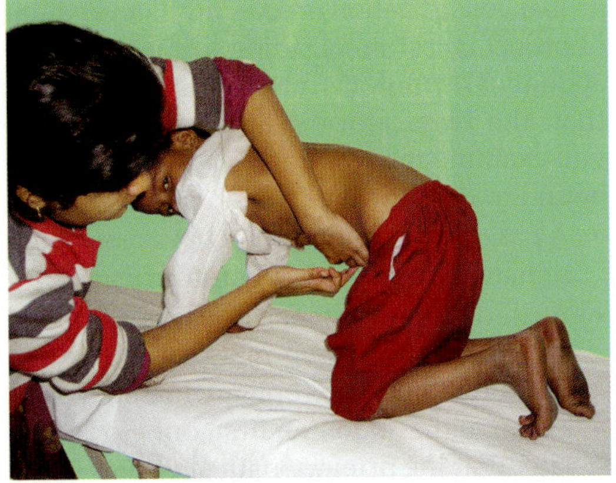

Fig. 10.30: Puddle sign.

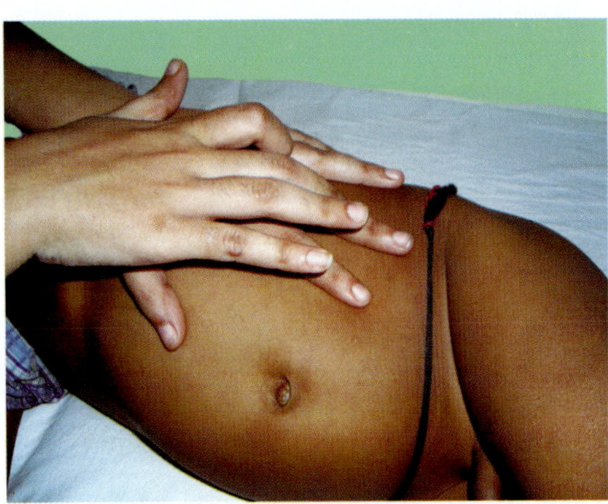

Fig. 10.31: Demonstration of shifting dullness.

- If the flanks are dull, turn the patient to the opposite side **(Fig. 10.31)** without displacing your pleximeter finger. In this position, the umbilicus becomes dependent and the flank is now on top. Wait for some time to let the fluid shift to the umbilicus and the other flank because of gravity. Percuss again over the same area. A resonant note now confirms that the fluid has shifted to the dependent area.
- The dullness also shifts to the umbilicus and the flank becomes resonant.
- The shifting can be confirmed by making the patient supine again, the dullness will shift back to the flanks and the umbilicus will become resonant.
- Avoid testing for shifting on the side that is already occupied by enlarged viscera.

3. *Fluid thrill:* If the amount of fluid in the peritoneal cavity becomes massive, it is not possible for it to shift with gravity, therefore, shifting dullness cannot be elicited. In such a patient, the whole abdomen will be dull.

To demonstrate fluid thrill, ask an assistant or a nurse to keep her hand longitudinally in the midline such that the ulnar border of her hand touches the abdomen, and press it firmly. Keep your left hand over the right flank and with the right hand give a flick over the left flank **(Fig. 10.32)**. You will feel a thrill that gets transmitted through the fluid under the left hand.

4. *Hepatosplenomegaly:* Percussion can also be used to demarcate the liver and spleen or confirm their presence.

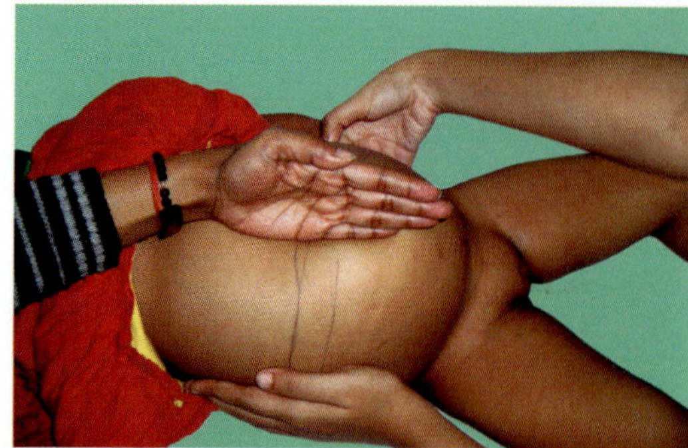

Fig. 10.32: Demonstration of fluid thrill.

Liver: You will be able to define the upper border of liver only by percussion as it lies in the thoracic cavity. Start percussing the right intercostal spaces from above downwards. The intercostal spaces will be resonant till the upper border of liver is reached, when the note will become dull. The upper border of liver usually lies in the 4th intercostal space. Note the space in which the dullness begins. Continue the percussion down the subcostal region keeping your fingers parallel to the ribs. The note will remain dull till the lower margin of liver is reached, and turning resonant beyond it. Distance between the upper and the lower border of the liver will give you the actual span of liver.

If the liver is pushed down as in case of emphysema or pneumothorax, the dullness will be present in a space lower than the fourth space. Liver dullness will be masked, i.e. the area over liver will remain resonant, if there is free gas in the peritoneal cavity subsequent to intestinal perforation.

Spleen: Area over spleen will also elicit a dull note on percussion. A normal spleen will result in dullness in the 9th, 10th and the 11th left intercostal spaces laterally. But, in case of an enlarged spleen, the dullness will be present all over the splenic surface below the costal margin.

D. Auscultation

- Auscultation over the abdomen is done to hear the *bowel sounds*. They are exaggerated in intestinal obstruction. The abdomen will be silent in patients of ileus or peritonitis.
- A *renal bruit* should be heard for, in children in whom you suspect renal artery stenosis like hypertension or arteritits. Press the bell of stethoscope deep into abdomen over both the lumbar regions, and try to hear for a bruit.
- A *venous hum* may be audible over liver or spleen in case of vascular tumors.

E. Genitalia

After a complete examination of the abdomen, genitalia must be examined. Look for hernial sites, undescended or retractile testis, ambiguous genitalia, testicular swelling, and inflammation.

The urethral opening (normally located at the tip of the penis) should be examined for stenosis, hypospadias, epispadias, chordee (shaft of penis is curved), phimosis, and penile length. Phimosis is inability to retract the prepuce and may be physiological till 18–24 months of age. If the urethra opens on the dorsal surface of the penis, this is called epispadias and if it opens on the ventral surface, it is known as hypospadias. Hypospadias may be associated with a chordee.

10.6 RELEVANT SYSTEMIC EXAMINATION

After you have done the abdominal examina-tion, take care to examine chest and cardiovascular system in detail. These may be concurrently involved by the same pathology or sometimes the main pathology involves some other system primarily, involving the abdomen secondarily.

Respiratory System

A patient presenting with abdominal pain may not have any abdominal pathology at all, but a lobar consolidation or an acute exacerbation of bronchial asthma leading to the pain. The abdominal symptoms may be more prominent than the respiratory symptoms, so unless you examine the respiratory system; you are bound to miss the diagnosis.

- A patient with ascites may have associated unilateral or bilateral pleural effusion.
- A child with tachypnea or dyspnea due to any reason can have marked abdominal distention due to aerophagy forcing you to examine the abdomen first, only to realize later that the primary pathology lies in the lungs.

- A liver palpable more than normal below the left costal margin giving a false impression of hepatomegaly may actually be normal when you measure the total liver span.
- A pneumothorax or hyperinflation of the right lung may push down the liver.
- In a child with disseminated tuberculosis, predominant symptoms may be those due to abdominal involvement, but when you examine the respiratory system you may find crepts or bronchial breathing or any other finding suggesting a pulmonary involvement as well.

Cardiovascular System

A child with ascites as a part of hypoalbuminemia or polyserositis can have pericardial effusion giving rise to a pericardial rub and other relevant findings.

A child with congestive cardiac failure will have hepatomegaly although acute failure will give rise to predominant respiratory symptoms. The hepatomegaly is tender. A patient with chronic congestive cardiac failure (chronic mitral regurgitation or cardiomyopathy) may sometimes present with firm non-tender hepatomegaly as a predominant sign.

Radiographs

Figures 10.33 to 10.36 depict some important radiographs characteristic of duodenal atresia (*double bubble appearance*), jejunal atresia (*triple bubble appearance*), intestinal obstruction (*multiple air fluid levels*), and pneumoperitoneum (*gas under the diaphragm*), respectively.

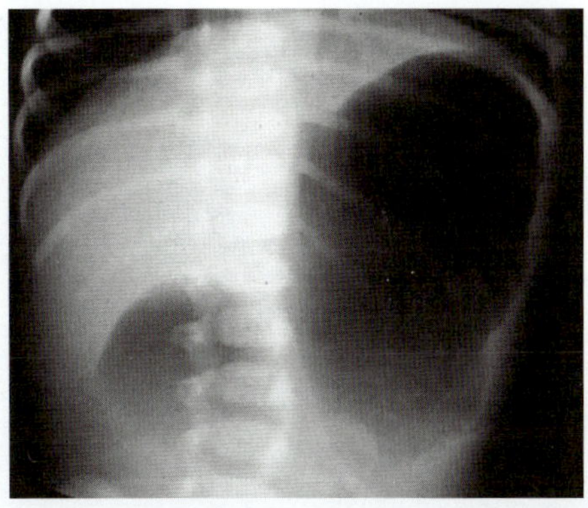

Fig. 10.33: Duodenal atresia. Note the typical double bubble appearance.

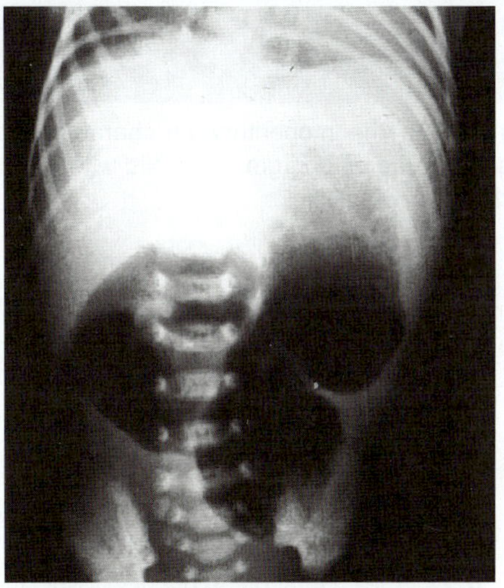

Fig. 10.34: Jejunal atresia. Note the typical triple bubble appearance.

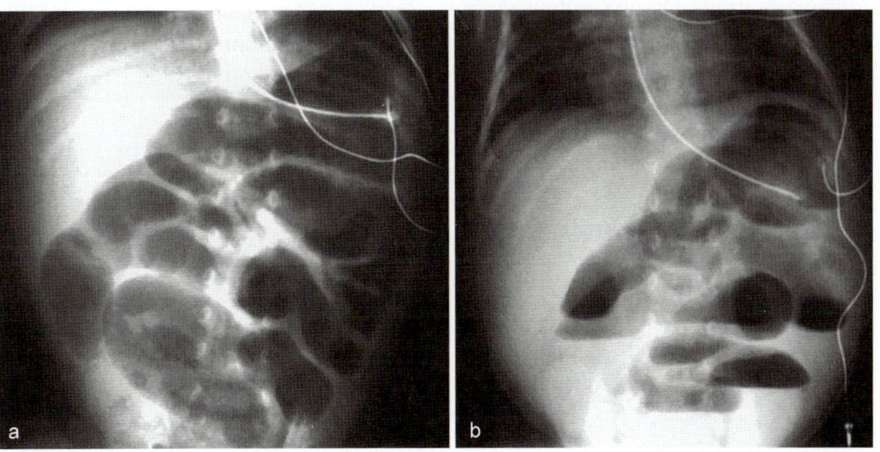

Fig. 10.35: Intestinal obstruction: (a) Supine film showing septate gaseous distension; (b) erect showing multiple air fluid levels.

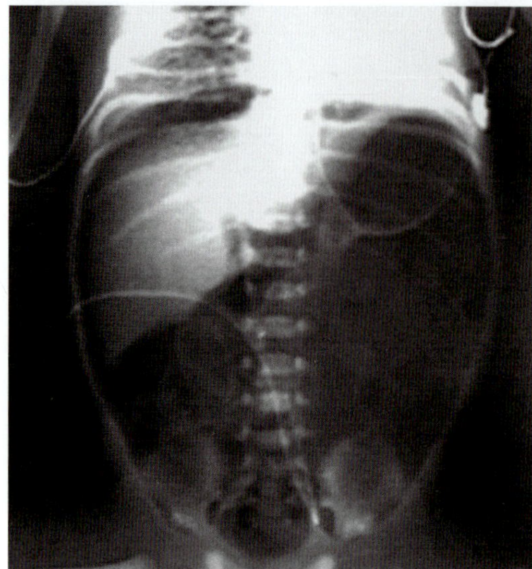

Fig. 10.36: Pneumoperitoneum characterized by gas under the diaphragm, in a child with intestinal perforation. Erect film.

Model checklist for abdominal examination

A. History

1. *Pain abdomen:* Site, radiation, timing, intensity, character
2. *Vomiting:* Bilious or not, timing, color, projectile or not
3. *Constipation:* Duration, associated with bleeding or not
4. *Diarrhea:* Duration, frequency, association with blood or mucous, urine output
5. Jaundice
6. Abdominal distention
7. *Bleeding from any site:* Hematuria, bleeding per rectum, hematemesis, melena
8. *Urinary complaints:* Dysuria, output, color
9. Alteration in appetite
10. *Scrotal swelling:* Painful or painless

B. Examination

1. Inspection
   - i. Shape
   - ii. Abdominal movements
   - iii. Umbilicus
   - iv. Skin scars
   - v. Superficial veins
   - vi. Visible peristalsis
   - vii. Pulsations
   - viii. Genitalia
2. Palpation
   - i. Light palpation
   - ii. *Liver:* Right/left lobe: Size, surface, consistency, margins, tenderness, pulsations
   - iii. *Spleen:* Size, consistency, notch
   - iv. Right kidney
   - v. Left kidney
   - vi. Urinary bladder
   - vii. Fecoliths
   - viii. *Any other lump:* Site and origin, size, shape, margins, surface, consistency, mobility, ballotability, signs of inflammation, impulse on coughing
   - ix. Abdominal wall edema
   - x. Abdominal circumference
3. Percussion
   - i. *Free fluid:* Puddle sign, shifting dullness, fluid thrill
   - ii. *Liver:* Upper border, total span
   - iii. Spleen
4. Auscultation
   - i. Bowel sounds
   - ii. Renal bruit
   - iii. Venous hum
5. Genitalia
   - i. Hernial sites
   - ii. Ambiguity
   - iii. Scrotum
   - iv. Urethral opening

Chapter 11

Examination of the Nervous System

❍ Suvasini Sharma ❍ Naveen Sankhyan ❍ Jaya Shankar Kaushik ❍ Piyush Gupta

Structure

11.1 AIM AND SCHEME OF NEUROLOGICAL EXAMINATION

The neurological examination is an intimidating task for many medical students and postgraduate residents. This belief stems from the fact that they find it hard to remember the relevant neuroanatomy or to do the examination systematically or to correctly interpret what they have found. Additionally, this examination seems exceptionally difficult in infants and young children. Conventional neurological examination **(Table 11.1)** is often applicable to older children (>5 years). In younger children, play techniques and observation are essential for monitoring intellectual and motor functioning. Hence, among toddlers, it is functional assessment rather than individual assessment of each function.

Table 11.1: Scheme of neurological examination
1. **Mental status** (appearance, behavior, communication, delusion/hallucination and emotions) and higher mental function (consciousness, orientation, memory, attention span, spatial perception, insight, abstract thinking, fund of information, calculation, released reflexes)
2. **Cranial nerve examination** (I–XII)
3. **Motor system examination** (gait/posture, bulk, tone, muscle power, deep tendon reflexes, superficial reflexes, abnormal movement)
4. **Sensory system examination** (lateral spinothalamic tract (pain/temperature), posterior spinothalamic tract (fine touch, vibration, joint position), cortical sensation (two-point discrimination, tactile localization)
5. **Cerebellar system examination**
6. **Meningeal signs** (neck rigidity, Kernig sign, Brudzinski sign)
7. **Skull and spine examination** (Macewen sign, transillumination)

11.2 COMMON SYMPTOMS RELATED TO CENTRAL NERVOUS SYSTEM

Common symptoms related to central and peripheral nervous system include headache, vomiting, altered sensorium, hemiparesis, flaccid paralysis, seizures, etc.

1. Headache

Headache is one of the most frequent presenting complaints among children. It is one of the symptoms where diagnosis lies in history. Examination and investigations have limited role in evaluating a child with headache. Headache often results from stretching or dilatation of pain sensitive intracranial blood vessels that are supplied by three divisions of trigeminal nerves. Hence, the pain is referred to eye, forehead, and temple. Other pain sensitive structures that may cause headache include extracranial blood vessels, pain from inflamed periosteum, and muscles attached to skull.

Common Causes

Common causes of headache in children include migraine, tension headache, headache secondary to analgesic abuse, meningitis, intracranial space occupying lesion (ICSOL), secondary to systemic illness.

- Recent onset severe headache associated with multiple episodes of projectile vomiting is ominous considering the possibility of ICSOL.
- Dull aching, mild headache through the entire day is more likely to be *tension headache.*
- Headache which is often severe in intensity where child prefers to sleep in a quiet and dark room and returns to normal activity once headache subsides is more likely to be *migraine.*
- Points in history that can help in characterizing the type of headache are listed in **Key Box 1**.

Key Box 1

History-taking for Headache: The 10 Points

1. Nature of headache (*dull aching, severe throbbing*)
2. Location of headache (*forehead, around eyes, occipital, diffuse*)
3. Duration of headache (*approximate*)
4. Frequency of headache (*daily, weekly, monthly*)
5. Severity of headache (*mild, moderate, severe*)
6. Activities during headache (*whether he/she continues with his/her routine activities or prefers to sleep*)
7. Any associated nausea, vomiting (*projectile*)
8. Any associated *photophobia* (irritation towards bright lights/prefers dark room during the headache) or *phonophobia* (prefers silence and gets irritated when someone makes noise during his/her headache)
9. Need for medications and any response to them
10. Does the headache require school absenteeism

2. Seizure

Paroxysmal clinical event (motor, sensory, autonomic) that results from abnormal electric discharge from the brain is a seizure. As a first step, it is imperative to delineate whether the paroxysmal event was an epileptic seizure or not. If it was true seizure, characterize the type of seizure by describing its semiology. Then final step is to ascertain whether there were any provoking factors like fever, head trauma, previous CNS infection or tumor, hypoglycemia, electrolyte imbalance (hyponatremia, hypernatremia, hypocalcemia), or history of toxic or drug ingestion.

Provoked Seizure

Seizure episodes could be provoked by prolonged fasting (hypoglycemic seizure) or following a diarrheal illness (dyselectrolytemia). Episodes provoked by fever could be either due to febrile seizures or CNS infection (meningitis). **Key Box 2** highlights the points in history that would help analyze the type of seizure and possible etiology for the seizure.

- Presence of fever (temperature >38°C), generalized seizures, seizure duration of less than 15 minutes, with no postictal loss of consciousness, in a child between 6 months and 5 years age is more likely to be *simple febrile seizures.*
- Children with history of fever, seizure, and encephalopathy are likely to have *meningoencephalitis.*

Unprovoked Seizure

History of developmental delay, perinatal asphyxia or other perinatal or postnatal injury, and a positive family history of epilepsy or febrile convulsion are more likely to be associated with an unprovoked epileptic seizure.

Key Box 2

History-taking for a Child with Seizure

1. Age at onset and presentation (neonate, infancy, childhood)
2. Provocation factors (head trauma, fever, preceding diarrheal illness)
3. Frequency of seizure (Is it first episode?)
4. Preceding events (awake, sleep, playing, exercise, following cry)
5. Presence of aura (somatosensory, auditory, visual, abdominal) (child >5 years)
6. Ictal manifestations (motor, sensory, autonomic, cognitive, behavioral)
7. Postictal period (postictal dizziness, loss of consciousness, immediate return to normal)
8. Does the semiology suggest a non-epileptic event rather than epileptic seizure
9. History of perinatal insult (birth asphyxia, neonatal seizures, neonatal meningitis, intracranial bleed)
10. Presence of developmental delay prior to onset of seizures
11. Non-attainment of milestones or regression of attained milestones with onset of seizure
12. Family history of epilepsy and febrile convulsions

Examination must focus on presence of neurocutaneous markers like café au lait macules (Fig. 11.1), ash leaf macules/shagreen patch (Fig. 11.2), port wine stain (Fig. 11.3), whorled hypopigmented lesions (Fig. 11.4) or hypopigmented scanty curly hair (Fig. 11.5). Also, look for injury marks on forehead or other body parts that may indicate falls due to myoclonic jerks or tonic jerks.

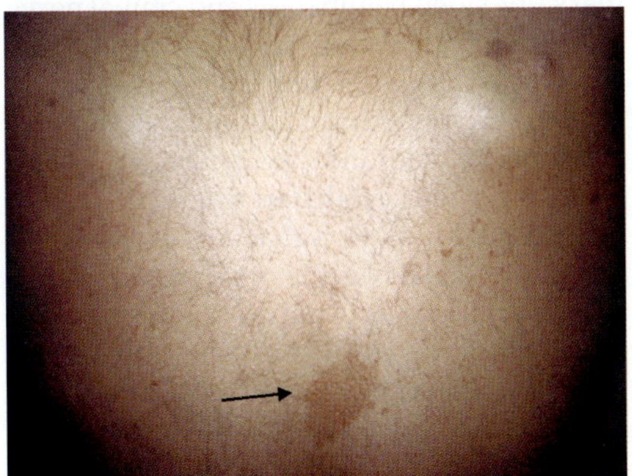

Fig. 11.1: Café au lait macule in a child with neurofibromatosis.

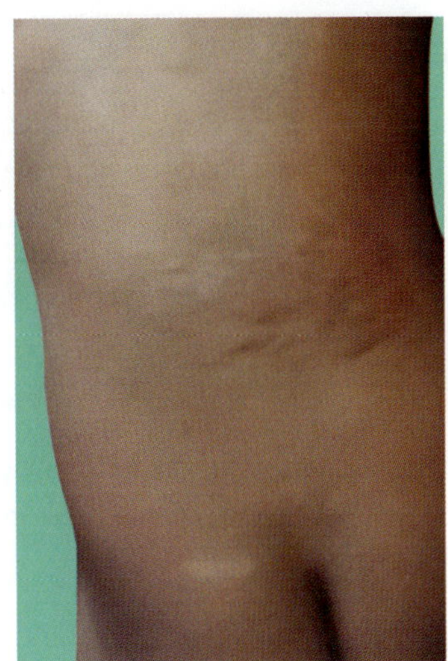

Fig. 11.2: Shagreen patch and ash leaf macule in a child with tuberous sclerosis.

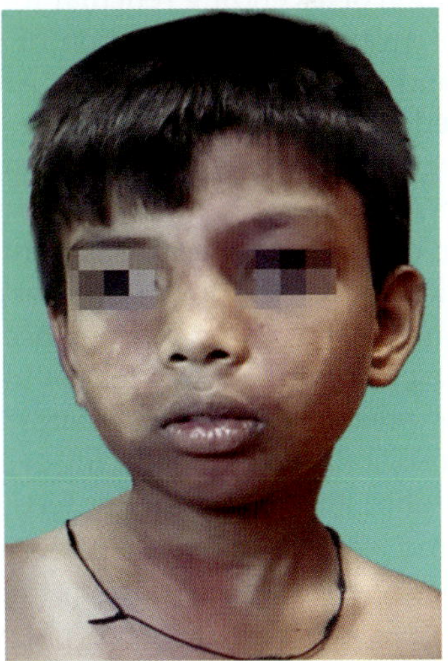

Fig. 11.3 Port wine stain in a child with Sturge-Weber syndrome.

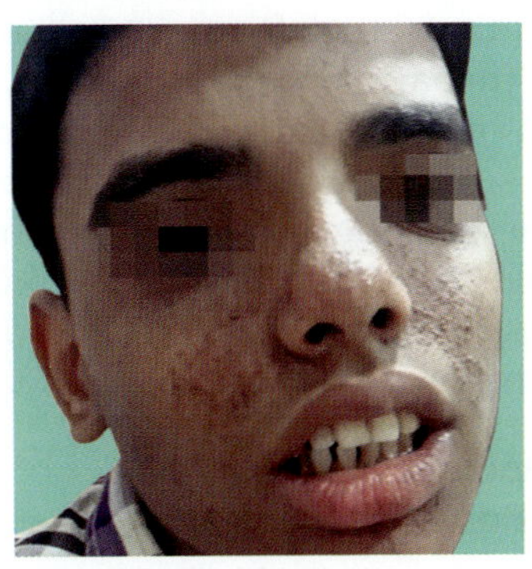

Fig. 11.4: Adenoma sebaceum in a child with tuberous sclerosis.

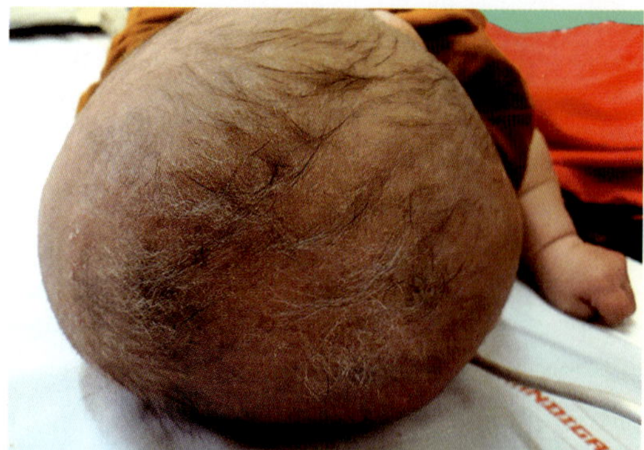

Fig. 11.5: Sparse, hypopigmented hair in a child with Menkes disease.

3. Altered Consciousness

Alteration in the level of consciousness (sensorium) is described as impairment in arousal and awareness. Arousal or wakefulness is a function of ascending reticular formation, whereas awareness is a function of cerebral cortex and subcortical structures. Arousal is described in terms of whether the sleep–wake cycle is preserved or not. Absence of sleep–wake cycle indicates "coma". Awareness in older children is expressed as interest in surroundings; recognition of his/her parents, indicating for bowel or bladder needs, and indicating for hunger. Awareness in infants can be expressed in terms of interest in their toys, consolability of child, placing eye contact with parents, and indicating for feed.

Altered sensorium may be associated with focal neurological deficits including hemiparesis or cranial nerve palsy. They may also be associated with features of raised intracranial pressure like headache or vomiting **(Key Box 3)**. Apart from a thorough systemic examination, general examination must focus on presence of icterus (hepatic encephalopathy), pallor (cerebral malaria, intracranial bleed), rash (measles, meningococcemia, rickettsial), petechiae (meningococcemia), cyanosis and clubbing (underlying cyanotic congenital heart disease), scalp hematoma (head injury) and dysmorphism (syndromic baby).

4. Hemiparesis: Weakness of One-Half of the Body

Weakness of one-half of body (upper limb and lower limb) is called **hemiparesis**, *whereas complete inability to move one half of the body is called* **hemiplegia**. This may or may not be associated with history suggestive of cranial nerve palsy **(Key Box 4)**.

By convention, neurological site of localization in hemiplegia or hemiparesis is central nervous system anywhere along the corticospinal tract (cortex, subcortical structure, brainstem). It is essential to know that same sided hemiparesis and cranial nerve palsy point to cortical or subcortical lesion. In contrast, crossed hemiplegia (weakness on one side of body and cranial nerve palsy on opposite side) indicate brainstem lesion. It is important to differentiate the onset of weakness (acute, subacute, or chronic). Common causes of acute onset of hemiplegia would include arterial or venous stroke secondary to prothrombotic condition, infection, congenital heart disease, intracranial bleed, Moya-Moya disease or focal cerebral arteriopathy.

A typical case of hemiparesis with approach to diagnosis is described in detail in Chapter 17.

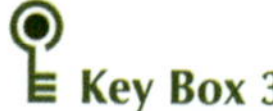

Key Box 3

History-taking in a Child with Altered Sensorium

1. Impairment of arousal and awareness
2. *History of cranial nerve palsy:* Malalignment of eyes, jerky movement of eyes *(3/4/6CN)*, visual fixation and following *(2nd CN)*, deviation of angle of mouth with drooling of saliva with preserved ability to close eyes *(7th CN)*, nasal regurgitation of feeds, alteration in speech or difficulty in deglutition *(9th–10th CN)*
3. *History of raised intracranial pressure:* Headache *(older children)*, repeated head banging or irritability *(younger child)*, projectile vomiting *(brain abscess, tumor, meningoencephalitis)*
4. *Etiological history:*
   a. History of head trauma *(subdural hematoma)*
   b. History of fever *(meningoencephalitis)*
   c. Bleeding from any site *(intracranial bleed)*
   d. History of diarrhea *(enteroviral encephalitis, cerebral venous sinus thrombosis, dyselectrolytemia)*
   e. History of yellowish discoloration of eyes and urine *(hepatic encephalopathy)*
   f. History of prior infection or vaccination *(acute disseminated encephalomyelitis)*
   g. History of seizures

Key Box 4

Key points in taking History for a Child with Acute Hemiparesis

1. **Description of weakness**
   - *Proximal upper limb:* Ability to lift arm to pick up an object in shelf, ability to comb hair, ability to remove shirt by self
   - *Distal upper limb:* Ability to hold pen/any other object, clumsiness in holding objects, ability to button/unbutton shirt, ability to break *chapatti*
   - *Proximal lower limb:* Inability to climb up/downstairs, ability to get up from the floor
   - *Distal lower limb:* Clumsiness while walking, repeated fall with twisting of ankles, slipping of *chappals*
2. **History of cranial nerve palsy:** Malalignment of eyes, jerky movement of eyes (3/4/6 CN), visual fixation and following (2 CN), deviation of angle of mouth with drooling of saliva with preserved ability to close eyes (7th CN), nasal regurgitation of feeds, alteration in speech or difficulty in deglutition (9th–10th CN)
3. **History of raised intracranial pressure:** Headache (older children), repeated head banging or irritability (*younger child*), projectile vomiting
4. **History pertaining to etiology of hemiparesis** Trauma to neck/head (*post-traumatic vascular insult*)
   - History of bluish discoloration of body (*cyanotic congenital heart disease*)
   - History of fast breathing, swelling in feet, palpitation (*acyanotic congenital heart disease*)
   - History of bleeding from any site (*intracranial bleed*)
   - History of preceding focal seizure (*Todd's palsy*)
   - History of associated headache (*hemiplegic migraine*)

5. Paraparesis: Weakness of Both Lower Limbs

Weakness of both lower limbs with sparing of upper limbs is called paraplegia. This may result from (a) spinal cord pathology; (b) anterior horn cell involvement; or (c) peripheral nerve involvement. It can be upper motor neuron type (spinal cord) or lower motor neuron type (peripheral nerve).

- Presence of distal weakness, atrophy, areflexia, or hyporeflexia and sensory loss points to *nerve pathology*.
- Presence of sensory level, hypertonia, hyperreflexia, bladder involvement, extensor plantar response points to *spinal cord pathology*.
- *Parasagittal region involvement in brain* as in cases with bilateral anterior cerebral artery stroke can also rarely result in weakness of bilateral lower limbs.

Common causes of acute onset paraplegia include Guillain-Barré syndrome, transverse myelitis, traumatic neuropathy, spinal cord concussion, epidural abscess, or spinal cord malignancy.

Evaluation of Paraplegia

Look for spinal tenderness. Many chronic paraparesis often have associated scoliosis, dimple or tuft of hair over skin of back, and foot deformities like pes cavus. Common presenting complaints include clumsiness in gait, refusal to stand or walk, refusal to bear weight on his/her legs, loss of bladder and bowel control. Uncommon presentation also includes random shock like jerk involving limbs (upper and lower) called spinal myoclonus **(Key Box 5)**.

Congenital malformation like atlantoaxial dislocation, Chiari malformation, meningomyelocele, familial spastic paraplegia, metabolic disorders like adrenoleukodystrophy can present with long-standing paraparesis.

6. Quadriparesis: Weakness of All the Four Limbs

Weakness of all four limbs is called quadriparesis. When weakness of arms exceeds legs in all four limbs involvement, it is termed double hemiplegia. Most common cause of spastic quadriparesis is secondary to perinatal asphyxia (cystic encephalomalacia) and neonatal intracranial bleed. Acute onset of flaccid quadriparesis is often secondary to cervical spinal trauma, Guillain-Barré syndrome, acute transverse myelitis, or traumatic neuritis. Scheme of history taking is similar to that described for paraplegia. Progression of weakness is most important parameter to be described in the history of presenting illness. **Figure 11.6** shows a diagrammatic representation of the onset and progression of weakness in a child with quadriplegia. The figure depicts that weakness

Key Box 5

Key Points in Taking History in a Child with Paraplegia

1. **Extent of weakness:** *Proximal lower limb:* Inability to climb up/downstairs, ability to get up from the floor
   Distal lower limb: Clumsiness while walking, repeated fall with twisting of ankles, slipping of *chappals*
2. **Onset of weakness:** Acute onset, subacute onset, chronic/slowly progressive weakness
3. **Progression:** Weakness improving with time (resolving), weakness slowly progressive or weakness has been static since its onset
4. **Involvement of sensory system:** Presence of paraesthesia or loss of sensation below one vertebral level with or without pain girdle sensation along a vertebral spinal level points to spinal cord pathology
5. **Involvement of bladder:** Presence of symptoms of small capacity hyperactive bladder (*urgency and frequency*), or severe hyperactive bladder (*urge incontinence*) points to UMN type of bladder involvement as seen in spinal cord disease. Presence of bladder retention points to spinal shock
6. **History of raised intracranial tension:** Loss of consciousness, seizures, headache, multiple episodes of projectile vomiting (central nervous system involvement as in case of bilateral anterior cerebral artery involvement)
7. **Pointers to etiology:** History of injection (*traumatic neuritis*), trauma to spine (*traumatic concussion injury or vertebral fracture*), history of preceding fever (*Guillain-Barré syndrome*), history of associated fever (*transverse myelitis*), presence of radicular pain (*compressive myelopathy*), and pain in muscles and fever (*viral myositis*)

started on day 4 of illness, reached its nadir on day 6. The weakness remained static till day 10 followed by gradual recovery.

7. Ataxia: Inability to Walk Properly or Wobbly Gait

Ataxia usually refers to disturbance in fine control of posture and movement or inability to perform smooth, coordinated and voluntary movement. Inability to walk properly can result from variety of neurological conditions including ataxia (cerebellar ataxia, sensory ataxia or vestibular ataxia), myoclonus (jerk followed by loss of stance), or neuromuscular weakness (Guillain-Barré syndrome or Miller Fisher syndrome).

Common causes of acute ataxia include drug-induced, post-infectious acute cerebellar ataxia, trauma, acute labrynthitis, and benign paroxysmal vertigo. Chronic ataxia usually has a genetic basis and includes both progressive causes (ataxia telangiectasia, Friedreich ataxia, abetalipoproteinemia) and static causes (congenital Dandy-Walker malformation). **Key Box 6** summarizes the key points for eliciting history in a child with ataxia.

Examination should focus on presence of ocular telangiectasia **(Fig. 11.7)**, ichthyoses (Refsum disease), angiokeratoma (Fabry disease) **(Fig. 11.8)**, pellagra-like rash (Hartnup disease), abnormal fat distribution (congenital disorders of glycosylation), short stature (Kearns-Sayre syndrome), cataract (cerebrotendinous xanthomatosis) and retinitis pigmentosa (abetalipoproteinemia).

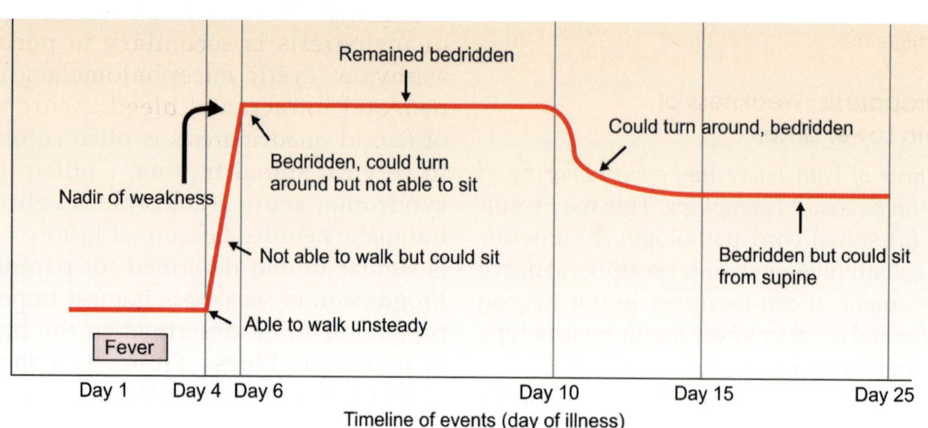

Fig. 11.6: Timeline of events for a child who presented with acute onset of flaccid quadriparesis.

Key Box 6

Key History Points in a Child with Ataxia

1. **Description of unsteady gait:** Unsteadiness or swaying while standing (stance), or on attempt to walk, distance to which he/she is able to walk with or without assistance
2. **Determining the type of ataxia:**
   a. Swaying while standing, inability to walk unassisted, overshooting of objects while trying to hold them, tremulous movement of hands while trying to reach for the object (*cerebellar ataxia*)
   b. Stability of stance and gait but starts swaying when he closes his eyes (*sensory ataxia*)
   c. Worsening of unsteadiness with sudden change of posture like sitting from supine position (*vestibular ataxia*)
   d. Sudden shock like jerky movement preceding loss of stance (*myoclonic seizures that result in falls, and in children with subacute sclerosing panencephalitis*)
   e. Buckling of knees while walking (quadriceps weakness), twisting of ankles with child taking high steps while walking with feet thumping on the floor with repeated slippage of chappals (*distal weakness of foot muscles as in hereditary motor sensory neuropathy*)
3. **Age at onset:** Infancy (metabolic causes like mitochondrial), childhood (ataxia telangiectasia), adolescent (spinocerebellar ataxia)
4. **Cognition:** Development of cognitive decline with onset of ataxia often points to progressive neurodegenerative disease
5. **Etiological history for acute ataxia**
   a. History suggestive of ipsilateral cranial nerve involvement, contralateral weakness with headache and altered sensorium suggests intracranial space occupying lesion of cerebellum (brain tumor)
   b. History of drug intake (anticonvulsants, antihistaminic)
   c. History of head trauma (traumatic causes)
   d. History of sport injury/injury to neck (vertebrobasilar injury)
   e. Presence of severe throbbing headache associated with abrupt and transient loss of consciousness, visual loss, vertigo, tinnitus (basilar migraine)
   f. Family history of migraine (basilar migraine)
   g. History of preceding viral infection suggests post-infective/immune causes
6. **Etiological history for chronic ataxia:** Recurrent sinopulmonary infections (*ataxia telangiectasia*), dry skin patches (*Refsum disease*), hearing loss (*Kearns-Sayre syndrome*), vision difficulties (*abetalipoproteinemia*), recurrent diarrheal illness (*abetalipoproteinemia*), difficulty in following objects with eyes (*ataxia with oculomotor apraxia*)

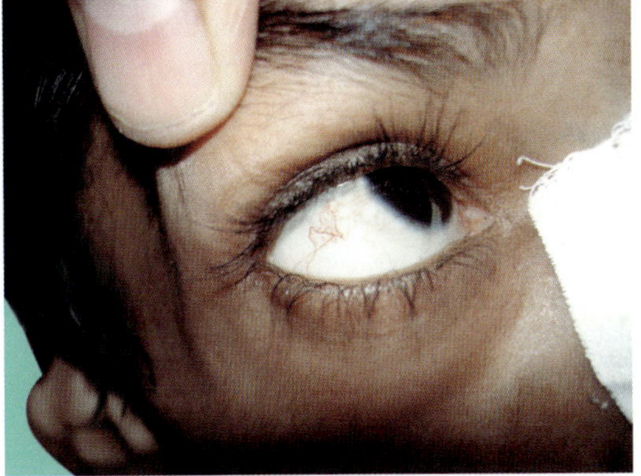

Fig. 11.7: Conjunctival telangiectasia in a child with ataxia telangiectasia.

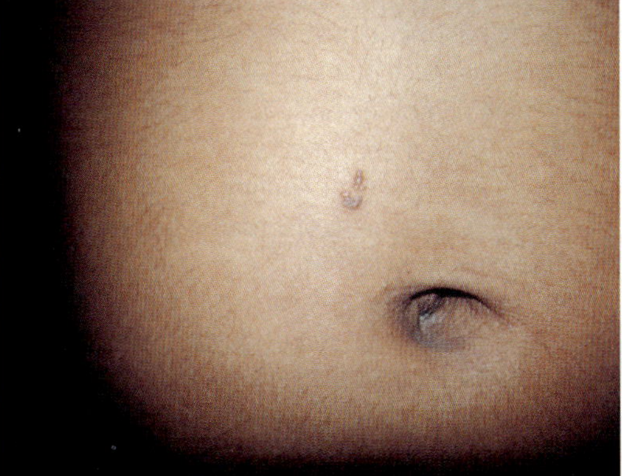

Fig. 11.8: Angiokeratoma in child with Fabry disease.

8. Abnormal Body Movements

Smooth coordination of movement requires normal muscle power along with normal inputs from eyes, cerebellum, posterior column, and vestibular system. Movement disorders are characterized by abnormal involuntary movement or impaired performance of voluntary movement, not resulting from neuromuscular weakness or abnormality of tone. Detailed description of movement as described by parents often needs to be supplemented with video recording of the event to precisely understand the nature of movement and characterize it accordingly.

Movement disorders can be broadly categorized into *hyperkinetic* and *hypokinetic* disorders.

- *Hyperkinetic movement disorders* include chorea, athetosis, ballismus, myoclonus, dystonia, tremors, tics, and stereotypies.
- *Hypokinetic movement disorders* include paucity of movement with fixed facial expressions (parkinsonian features).

Key Box 7 summarizes the clues in history that may help characterize the type of movement disorder.

9. Neuromuscular Weakness

Presenting complaints of neuromuscular weakness will depend on the extent of involvement **(Table 11.2)**. Clinical signs that may help in arriving at a diagnosis in children presenting with neuromuscular weakness are described in **Table 11.3**.

10. Difficulty in Vision

Vision loss is often one of the common presenting complaints in children. **Key Box 8** summarizes points that need to be elicited among children presenting with visual loss. Causes of visual loss and detailed history and examination of eyes are discussed in Chapter 12.

11.3 KEY CONCEPTS IN ANATOMY AND PHYSIOLOGY

A. Neuroaxis

The term "Localization" in neurology refers to site of lesion in the neuroaxis that could probably explain the symptoms and clinical signs of the child. Nervous system can be divided into central nervous system and peripheral nervous system. Neuroaxis refers to structures including cerebral cortex, subcortical brain structure, brainstem, cerebellum, spinal cord, nerve root, peripheral nerve, neuromuscular junction, and muscle **(Fig. 11.9)**.

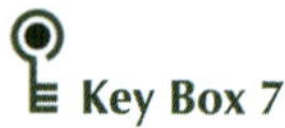

Key Box 7

Clues in History for Diagnosis of Movement Disorder

1. Is the pattern of movements normal (developmental movement disorder) or abnormal for age?
2. Are there excessive movements (hyperkinetic) or is there a paucity of movement (hypokinetic)?
3. Which part of the body is involved (mouth, face, head, neck, upper limb, lower limb)?
4. Is the movement paroxysmal (sudden onset for brief period which may recur), continual (repeated again and again), or continuous (without stop)?
5. Has the movement disorder changed over time (started with one movement and evolved to other movement types)?
6. Is the movement present over the rest/specific action/specific posture?
7. Do environmental stimuli or emotional stress modulate (increase or decrease) the movement disorder?
8. Does the movement abate with sleep?
9. Is the child aware of movement?
10. Can the movements be suppressed voluntarily?
11. Is the abnormal movement preceded by a premonitory sensation or urge?
12. Are there findings on the examination suggestive of focal neurologic deficit or systemic disease?
13. Is the child development normal for age?
14. Is there a family history of similar movement disorder?

Table 11.2: Diagnosing the site of neuromuscular weakness from presenting complaints	
Site of weakness	**Presenting complaints**
Hip girdle	Difficulty in getting up from floor, difficulty in raising from low chair, difficulty in climbing up and downstairs, alteration in gait (waddling gait)
Distal foot muscle	Slippage of sandals, repeated falls with twisting of ankles, wasting of foot muscles (stork leg-like appearance), walking with foot raising high and then slapping on the floor with a thump (high steppage gait)
Shoulder girdle	Difficulty in raising arms above the shoulder to lift object lying in the shelf, difficulty in combing the hair, difficulty in changing clothes independently
Distal hand muscles	Change in handwriting, clumsiness while holding the objects, difficulty in opening the key, difficulty in holding heavy objects
Trunk muscles	Difficulty in getting up from lying down position, turning around in the bed
Neck flexor/extensor	Difficulty in lifting head from the bed
Bulbar muscles	Difficulty in deglutition, nasal regurgitation of feeds and fluids, alteration in voice or hoarseness of voice
Extraocular muscles	Misalignment of eyes, diplopia (double vision), difficulty in following fast moving objects

Table 11.3: Clinical signs in children presenting with neuromuscular weakness	
Clinical sign	**Clinical significance**
Hepatomegaly	Acid maltase deficiency (Pompe disease)
Cataract	Myotonic dystrophy
Heliotrope rash, Gottron papule	Dermatomyositis
Optic atrophy	Mitochondrial myopathy
Early elbow contractures	Emery-Dreifuss muscular dystrophy
Intellectual disability	Duchenne muscular dystrophy

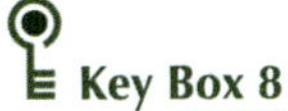

Key Box 8

Description of Vision Loss

1. *Onset and progression of vision loss:* Sudden onset and non-progressive (vascular or traumatic etiology), insidious onset and progressive (optic neuritis).
2. *Description of vision loss:* Difficulty in reading letters written in blackboard, reading cricket scores in television, blurring or distortion of words.
3. *Associated complaints:* Double vision (ophthalmoplegia), redness of eyes or eye discharge (conjunctivitis), haloes around bright light (glaucoma), headache (refractory error), floating spots (retinal detachment), pain in moving eyes (optic neuritis), not able to judge the periphery and bumps into objects (visual field defects).

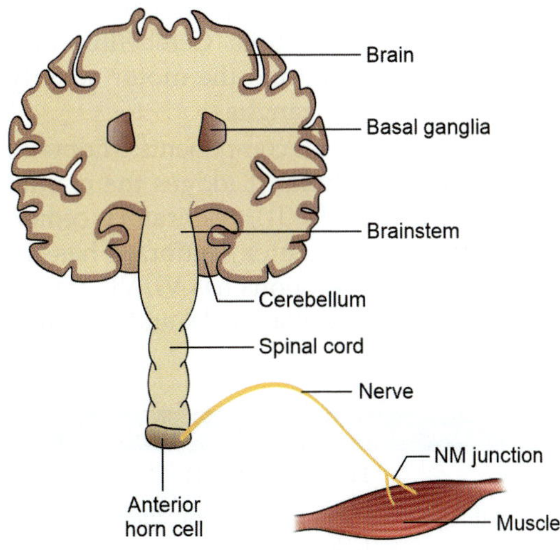

Fig. 11.9: The neurological axis.

- Cerebral cortex consists of four lobes—frontal lobe, temporal lobe, parietal lobe and occipital lobe. Precentral gyrus lodges motor cortex and postcentral gyrus lodges

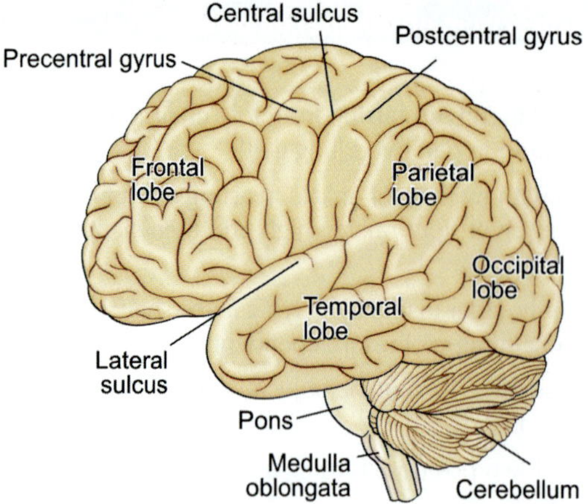

Fig. 11.10: Lobes of cerebrum with precentral gyrus lodging motor cortex and postcentral gyrus lodging the sensory cortex.

sensory cortex (Fig. 11.10). Function of each lobe is summarized in **Table 11.4**. Major functions of cerebral cortex include motor, sensory, speech and consciousness. There are two hemispheres: Right and left which are connected by corpus callosum. Right hemisphere controls left half of body and left hemisphere controls the right half of body.

- Subcortical structures refer to basal ganglia, internal capsule, and thalamus. Basal ganglia control the fine adjustments of movement, thalamus acts as a sensory relay station, and internal capsule transmits the motor and sensory signals from cortex to brainstem structures. Cerebellum also functions to fine tune the motor activity along with basal ganglia.
- Brainstem has three components: Midbrain, pons, and medulla. It lodges the cranial nerve nucleus (I–XII), respiratory center, and vasomotor center. Midbrain has III, IV cranial nerves, pons has VI, VII cranial nerves, and medulla has IX and X cranial nerves.

B. Motor System

Motor activity is governed by pyramidal system and extrapyramidal system.

1. Corticospinal Tract

The corticospinal tract mediates the voluntary skilled motor activity. The fibers of the corticospinal pathway arise mainly from the primary motor cortex, lateral premotor cortex, and the supplementary motor cortex (Fig. 11.11).

These fibers descend through the corona radiata, the posterior limb of the internal capsule, and the ventral portion of the midbrain and pons down to the ventral portion of the medulla, where they form two large pyramids. When they reach the caudal portion of the medulla, approximately 90% of fibers of each pyramid cross over to descend

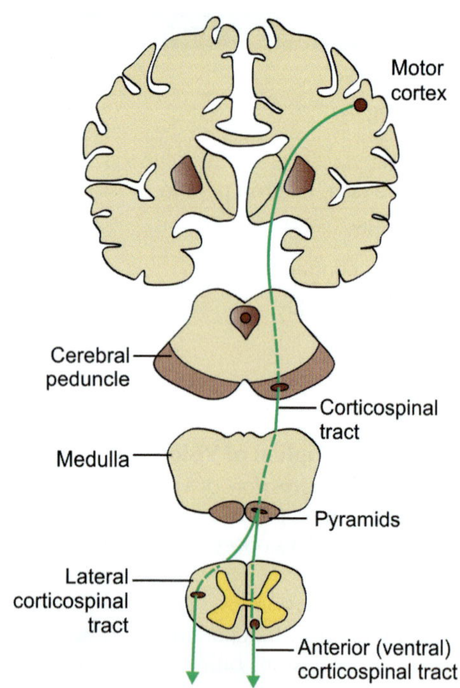

Fig. 11.11: The corticospinal tract.

Table 11.4: Major functions of each lobe of cerebral cortex

Lobe	Function (major)
Frontal lobe	Executive function, judgment, thinking, planning, problem solving, emotions, personality, behavior, voluntary motor functions (motor cortex), language production (Broca area)
Parietal lobe	Sensory input processing, sensory discrimination, calculation
Occipital lobe	Visual reception and interpretation
Temporal lobe	Auditory reception, smelling, memory retrieval, language comprehension (Wernicke area)

as the lateral corticospinal tract the lateral funiculus of the spinal cord. This is known as the pyramidal decussation. The other 10% of the fibers that do not decussate descend in the ipsilateral ventral funiculus as the anterior (ventral) corticospinal tract.

2. Extrapyramidal System

Extrapyramidal system consists of corticobulbar tract (controls the cranial nerve nucleus), reticulospinal tract (supplies trunk and proximal limb muscles), rubrospinal tract (stimulates the flexors of upper limb), vestibulospinal tract (position the head and neck in response to body tilting), tectospinal tract (control head, neck and eye movement), and olivospinal tract (facilitate muscle tone).

3. Corticobulbar Tract

Corticobulbar tracts control the cranial nerve nucleus. These tracts project bilaterally except for 7th cranial nerve (lower face) and 12th cranial nerve. Hence, in lesions of right- sided corticobulbar tract, we observe left-sided facial palsy (lower face involved but since forehead is supplied bilaterally, it remains spared) and deviation of tongue to left side. Face deviates to opposite side and tongue deviates to same side of palsy. Other cranial nerves are spared in unilateral corticobulbar lesion as they have bilateral innervations.

Pseudobulbar palsy results from upper motor neuron lesion to corticobulbar pathway in pyramidal tract. It is called "pseudo" because clinically child will have cranial nerve palsy (cranial nerve nuclei are located in brainstem or bulbus) but the lesion is not in brainstem but in the corticobulbar fibers.

4. Applied Anatomy of Motor System

Spasticity: *Lesions of pyramidal system result in spasticity.* Spasticity is a velocity-dependent hypertonia, i.e. when the speed of passive resistance increases, more resistance is felt. When passive movement is made across spastic limb, an initial catch followed by sudden release is felt. Spasticity generally involves flexors and pronator muscle group of upper limb and extensor of hip, knee, and ankle.

Rigidity: In contrast, *lesions of extrapyramidal tract result in rigidity.* Rigidity involves both agonist and antagonist; and both flexor and extensor muscles. This resistance is encountered from the start to end and it will not vary with speed of movement. This is known as typical *lead pipe rigidity.* The term *cogwheel rigidity* refers to tremors superimposed on *lead pipe* rigidity. This often involves neck muscles, trunk muscles, and proximal limb muscles.

Normal motor function involves integrated muscle activity that is modulated by the activity of the cerebral cortex, basal ganglia, cerebellum, and spinal cord. Motor system dysfunction leads to weakness or paralysis, or to ataxia or abnormal movements. Two basic patterns of weakness must be recognized: The upper and lower motor neuron type of weakness.

A. Upper motor neuron weakness: Upper motor neuron (UMN) lesions are characterized by spasticity, exaggerated deep tendon reflexes, and extensor plantar response. Spasticity may not be present in certain UMN lesions in the acute phase (e.g. spinal shock phase in spinal cord injuries and acute transverse myelitis).

This pattern of weakness results from disorders that affect the upper motor neurons (pyramidal cells in the motor area which give rise to the corticospinal tract) or their axons in the cerebral cortex, subcortical white matter, internal capsule, brainstem, or spinal cord. UMN lesions produce weakness through decreased activation of the lower motor neurons.

Distal muscle groups are affected more severely than proximal ones, and axial movements are spared unless the lesion is severe and bilateral.

B. Lower motor neuron weakness: Lower motor neuron lesions are generally associated with significant weakness, hypotonia, depressed reflexes, and flexor plantar responses. This pattern results from disorders of cell bodies of lower motor neurons in the brainstem motor nuclei and the anterior horn of the spinal cord, or from dysfunction of peripheral nerves, neuromuscular junction, or muscle **(Table 11.5)**.

- *Anterior horn cell involvement* (e.g. spinal muscular atrophy) is associated with wasting, fasciculation, and hyporeflexia.

Table 11.5: Clinical features depending on the site of lesion in lower motor neuron lesions

Site of lesion	Anterior horn cell	Nerve	Neuromuscular junction	Muscle
Bulk	Atrophy	Atrophy	Preserved	Atrophy only in late stages
Weakness	Generalized	Distal	Facial and extra-ocular muscle	Proximal
Deep tendon reflexes	Absent	Decreased or absent	Normal	Normal or decreased
Fasciculations	Present	Absent	Absent	Absent
Sensory system	Spared	May be affected	Spared	Spared
Fluctuations in weakness and diurnal variation	Absent	Absent	Present	Absent

- *Peripheral nerve involvement* (e.g. hereditary sensory and motor neuropathies) is associated with predominant distal weakness, distal wasting, hyporeflexia and sensory involvement.
- *Neuromuscular junction involvement* (e.g. myasthenia gravis) is associated with fatigable and fluctuating weakness. Facial and extraocular group of muscles are often affected in disorders of neuromuscular junction as in myasthenia gravis.
- *Muscle disease* (e.g. muscular dystrophies) is associated with proximal weakness and normal to decreased deep tendon reflexes. Atrophy of muscles in myopathy often occurs in late stages. Selective atrophy of one group of muscle with selective hypertrophy of other group of muscles strongly suggests a possibility of muscular dystrophy.

Key differences between upper and lower motor neurons are outlined in **Table 11.6**.

C. Basal Ganglia

Basal ganglia include the corpus striatum, the substantia nigra (pars compacta and a pars reticularis), and the subthalamic nucleus of Luys **(Fig. 11.12)**. The corpus striatum comprises the putamen, caudate nucleus, and the globus pallidus. The basal ganglia play a major role in the control of posture and movement.

Table 11.6: Key differences between upper motor and lower motor neuron lesions

Features	Upper motor neuron	Lower motor neuron
Site of lesion	Between cerebral cortex and motor neuron	Between spinal motor neuron and muscle
Weakness	Antigravity muscles: Flexors of upper limb and extensors of lower limb	Both flexors and extensors
Voluntary activity and reflex activity	Voluntary motor activity is lost but reflex activity is preserved	Both voluntary and reflex motor activities are lost
Tone	Spasticity	Hypotonia
Deep tendon reflex	Brisk	Diminished or absent
Plantar response	Extensor	Flexor or mute
Superficial reflex	Absent	May be normal
Muscle atrophy	Absent	May be present (neuropathy)
Fasciculations of muscle	Absent	May be present (anterior horn cell involvement)

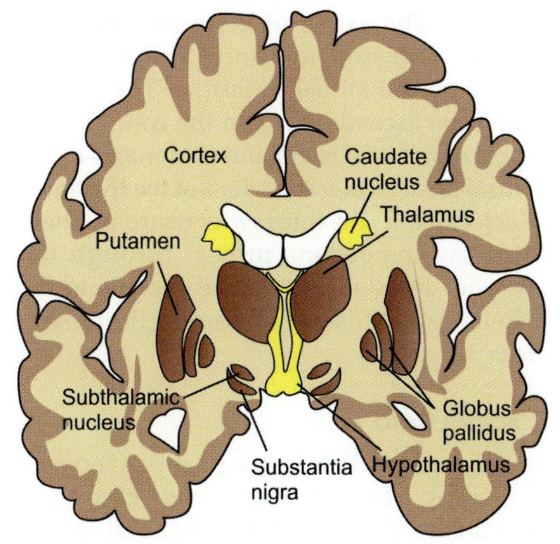

Fig. 11.12: Structure of basal ganglia.

The basal ganglia are involved in the planning and programming of initiation, sequencing, and modulation of movement, or more broadly, in the processes by which an abstract thought is converted into voluntary action. They discharge via the thalamus to areas related to the motor cortex, and the corticospinal pathways provide the final common pathway to the motor neurons. The basal ganglia are also involved in automatic stereotyped postural and reflex motor activity, such as swinging of arms while walking.

D. Sensory System

Sensory system relays sensations from periphery to the spinal cord and then up the thalamus and then to sensory cortex. There are two major sensory tracts: (a) Lateral spinothalamic tract that carries pain and temperature; and (b) posterior column that carries vibration and proprioception.

The Lateral Spinothalamic Tract (Fig. 11.13)

The lateral spinothalamic tract mediates pain and temperature sensation. The receptors for these sensations are free nerve endings. The lateral

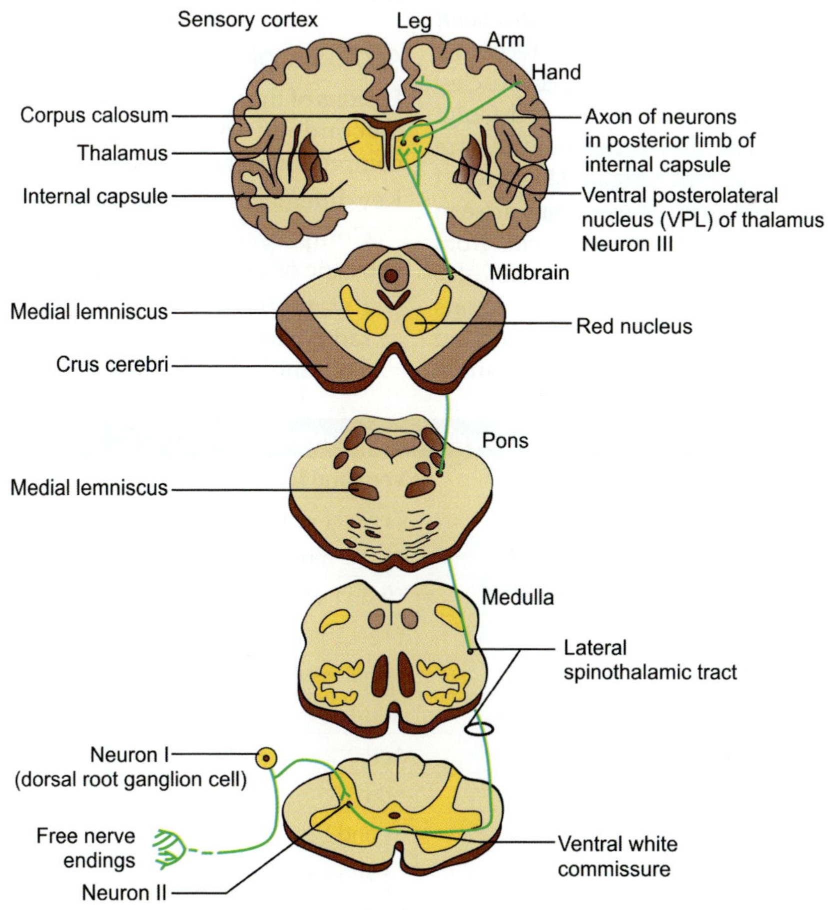

Fig. 11.13: Lateral spinothalamic tract.

spinothalamic tract receives input from the fast and slow conducting pain fibers. The efferent from these pain fibers reach the dorsal root ganglia. The dorsal root ganglia contain the first order neurons of the lateral spinothalamic tract. They project axons to the second order neurons within the dorsal horn of the spinal cord. The axons of these second order neurons decussate in the ventral white commisure and ascend in the contralateral lateral funiculus. These axons terminate in the ventral posterosuperior nucleus of the thalamus, which contains the third order neurons. These third order neurons project through the posterior limb of the internal capsule to the primary somatosensory cortex (Brodmann areas 3, 1 and 2).

The Dorsal Column-medial Lemniscus Pathway

The fibers of this tract carry information concerning discriminative senses which include joint position sense, vibration sense, weight perception, discriminative touch, pressure touch, two-point discrimination, and stereognosis. The receptors include Pacini and Meissner tactile corpuscles, joint receptors, muscle spindles and Golgi tendon organs. The first order neurons are located in the dorsal root ganglia. They project axons to the spinal cord. These axons arise in the spinal cord as the *fasciculus gracilis* from the lower extremities and *fasciculus cuneatus* from the upper extremities. These axons terminate in the second order neurons located in the gracile and cuneate nuclei of the caudal medulla. The axons of these second order neurons decussate and form a fiber bundle known as the *medial lemniscus*. The medial lemniscus ascends through the contralateral aspect of the brainstem and terminates in the ventral posterolateral nucleus of the thalamus which contains the third order neurons. These third order neurons project through the posterior limb of the internal capsule to the primary somatosensory cortex (Brodmann areas 3, 1 and 2).

E. Spinal Cord

Spinal cord has 31 spinal segments: 8 cervical, 12 thoracic, 5 lumbar, 5 sacral and 1 coccygeal. Spinal cord ends at L2–L3 level. **Table 11.7** highlights the corresponding vertebral and spinal cord levels. Hence if there is a lesion at T10 spinal cord level, clinically, it will correspond to T7–T8 vertebral level. Similarly, if there is compression at T8 level, we add 3, hence this compression will affect T11 spinal cord level.

Applied Anatomy

Lesions of the spinal cord may be compressive (secondary to tumor, trauma) or non-compressive (transverse myelitis, etc.).

Key differences are summarized in **Table 11.8**.

Compression of spinal cord could be extrinsic or intrinsic.

- *Extrinsic compression* will result in radicular pain (entrapment of nerve roots), asymmetric weakness (only one side of

Table 11.7: Level of spinal cord and their corresponding vertebral level

Spinal cord level	Vertebral level
Cervical spinal cord	Cervical vertebra
Thoracic spinal cord	T1–T8 vertebrae
Lumbar spinal cord	T9–T11 vertebrae
Sacral spinal cord	T12–L2 vertebrae
Vertebral level	**Spinal cord level**
Cervical vertebra	Add 1
Thoracic vertebrae 1–6	Add 2
Thoracic vertebrae 7–9	Add 3
Thoracic vertebra 10th	L1 and L2
Thoracic vertebra 11th	L3 and L4
Thoracic vertebra 12th	L5 and sacral segments

Table 11.8: Key differences between compressive and non-compressive myelopathy

Features	Compressive	Non-compressive
Bony deformity	May be present	Absent
Bony tenderness	Present	Absent
Girdle-like sensation	Present	Absent
Zone of hyperesthesia	Present	Absent
Root pain	Present	Absent
Onset	Gradual	May be acute
Symmetry	Asymmetrical	Symmetrical

spinal cord is compressed), ipsilateral hemiplegia (involvement of ipsilateral corticospinal tract), and ipsilateral loss of joint position and vibration (posterior spinothalamic tract ascends ipsilaterally and cross at medullary level).

- *Intrinsic cord lesion* will result in dissociative pain loss, anterior horn cell involvement and bladder involvement, considering the proximity of these tracts near the central canal of spinal cord.

Key differences between extramedullary and intramedullary lesions are given in **Table 11.9**.

Representation of cervical fibers is medial and sacral fibers are lateral in lateral spinothalamic tract. Hence, extrinsic compressive myelopathy will affect sacral sensory fibers before affecting cervical fibers. Reverse is true in dorsal column sensation with cervical being lateral and sacral being medial.

F. Blood Supply of the Brain

The brain is supplied by branches of the internal carotid and vertebral arteries. The internal carotid artery arises from the common carotid artery. The common carotid artery arises from aortic arch on the left side and from brachiocephalic trunk on the right side. Each internal carotid artery gives off 2 major branches: The anterior cerebral artery and the middle cerebral artery.

The two vertebral arteries arise from subclavian arteries and join to form the basilar artery. The two vertebral arteries ascend on the anterolateral aspect of medulla. At the lower border of the pons, they unite to form basilar artery. The basilar artery lies in the midline, ventral to the pons. The basilar artery begins at or slightly below the pontomedullary junction and stretches the length of the pons, tapering to its termination at the pons-midbrain junction where it bifurcates into its two terminal branches, the right and left posterior cerebral arteries.

The carotid and vertebral artery systems join at the base of the brain to form the circle of Willis **(Fig. 11.14)**.

1. The Anterior Cerebral Artery (ACA)

The ACA supplies the medial surface of the hemisphere from the frontal pole to the parieto-occipital sulcus **(Fig. 11.15)**. Here, the ACA supplies the paracentral lobule, which

Table 11.9: Key differences between extramedullary and intramedullary lesion

Extramedullary lesion	Intramedullary lesion
Root pains present (intradural)	Painless or burning pain
Vertebral body tenderness (extradural)	Absent
Motor involvement asymmetrical and early	Late and symmetrical motor weakness
Late sensory loss	Dissociative sensory loss
Bladder involvement late	Early bladder involvement
Sacrum involved	Sacral sparing is classical
No trophic changes	Trophic changes are common

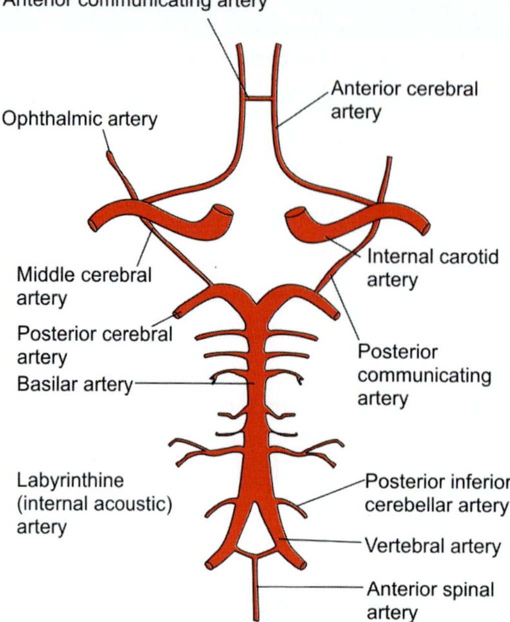

Fig. 11.14: Circle of Willis which consists of anterior circulation (anterior communicating artery, anterior cerebral artery) and posterior circulation (posterior communicating artery, posterior cerebral artery).

contains the leg-foot area of the motor-sensory cortices. The anterior communicating artery connects the two anterior cerebral arteries. The medial striate arteries are the penetrating branches of the ACA, which supply the anterior portion of the putamen and caudate nucleus and the anteroinferior portion of the internal capsule.

2. The Middle Cerebral Artery (MCA)

The middle cerebral artery (MCA), the largest branch of the ICA, arises below the medial part of the anterior perforated substance. It supplies most of the lateral surface of the cerebral hemisphere and the deep structures of the frontal and parietal lobes. Important areas in this region include: the Broca and Wernicke speech areas, the face and arm areas of the motor and sensory cortices, and the frontal eye field.

3. Posterior Cerebral Artery

The PCA are the terminal branches of the basilar artery, and supply the occipital lobes and the inferomedial portions of the temporal lobes. It also provides the major blood supply to the midbrain and supplies the thalamus, medial and lateral geniculate bodies.

Tables 11.10 and 11.11 outline the key differences in clinical features of anterior and posterior circulation strokes depending on the areas supplied by respective arteries.

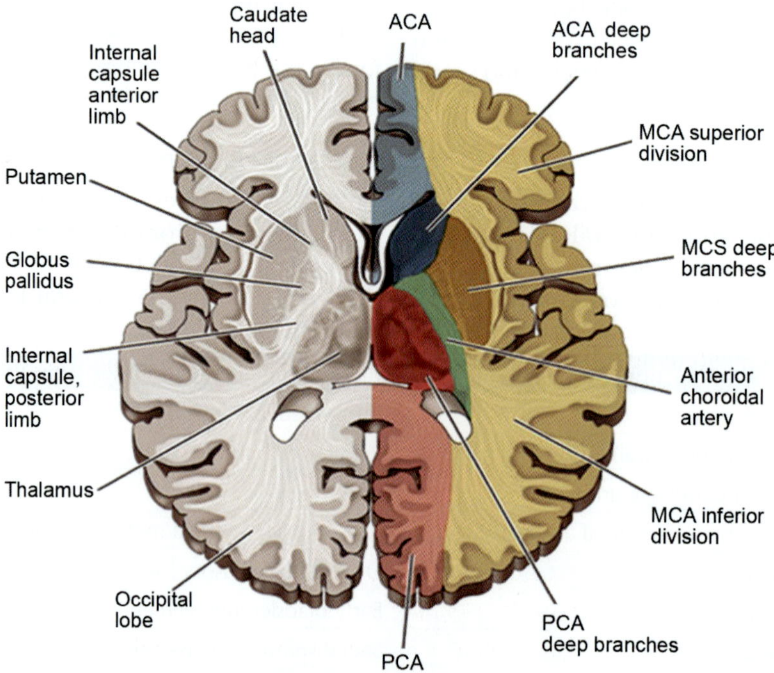

Fig. 11.15: Areas of brain supplied by anterior and posterior circulation arteries.

Table 11.10: Differences in clinical features of anterior circulation and posterior circulation stroke	
Anterior circulation stroke	**Posterior circulation stroke**
Weakness of contralateral side of face and limbs (contralateral hemiparesis and facial palsy)	Ataxia (loss of balance), vertigo more common than weakness and sensory loss
Sensory loss on contralateral side of arms/legs (hemianesthesia)	Sensory loss may occur
Language difficulty (aphasia)	Dysarthria (9th/10th cranial nerve involvement)
Visual disturbances (field defects and gaze palsy)	Visual disturbances (occipital lobe involvement resulting in cortical blindness)

Table 11.11: Clinical features of cerebral artery involvement	
Cerebral artery	**Clinical signs**
Anterior cerebral artery	Contralateral leg weakness, sensory loss
Middle cerebral artery	Contralateral face, arm, leg with or without visual field and gaze palsy • Right: Left hemineglect, apathy, spatial disorientation • Left: Aphasia frontal expressive
Posterior cerebral artery	Visual field loss with macular sparing, alexia without agraphia (right+CC)

11.4 EXAMINATION IN NEUROLOGICAL DISORDERS

A. Vital Signs

1. Temperature

Presence of fever points to an infective etiology like meningitis, encephalitis, brain abscess. Hypothermia is significant among neonates and children with protein energy malnutrition. Among children with altered sensorium, it is better to avoid temperature recording in oral mucosa for the fear of aspiration.

2. Heart Rate

Presence of tachycardia along with fever often indicates infective etiology. However, presence of tachycardia in absence of fever should alert the physician to look for early signs of septic shock (meningococcemia). Bradycardia in neurological child could point to sign of raised intracranial pressure especially when associated with hypertension and altered breathing pattern.

3. Respiratory Rate

Among patients with neurological disorders, presence of tachypnea with respiratory distress could point towards underlying bronchopneumonia. However, if a child presents with tachypnea without respiratory distress, one should always think of acidotic breathing pattern as in diabetic ketoacidosis. **Table 11.12** summarizes the abnormal patterns of respiration in neurological disorders. The odor of breath is also important in a comatose child.

Table 11.12: Abnormal respiratory patterns in CNS dysfunction		
Type of respiration	**Description**	**Site of lesion**
Cheyne-Stokes respiration	Periods of hyperventilation followed by apnea followed by hyperventilation	Bilateral hemispheric or diencephalic lesion
Central neurogenic hyperventilation	Continuous, rapid and deep breathing	Injury to midbrain tegmentum
Apneustic breathing	Prolonged inspiratory phase with shortened expiratory phase	Mid and caudal portion of pons
Cluster breathing	Long inspiration followed by pause	Lower pontine or high medulla
Ataxic breathing	Jerky breathing pattern	Medullary lesion

4. Blood Pressure

Hypotension with tachycardia is marker of septic shock (e.g. meningococcemia). Hypertension could be primary reason for encephalopathy (hypertensive encephalopathy and posterior reversible encephalopathy syndrome) or could be secondary to raised intracranial pressure.

B. General Physical Examination

In addition to routine head to toe general physical examination (as detailed in Chapter 6), a few important clinical signs that may point to underlying diagnosis must be looked **(Table 11.13)**. Presence of neurocutaneous markers could indicate neurocutaneous syndromes **(Table 11.14)**. One should always comment on presence or absence of BCG scar. Look for evidence of bed sores, contractures, poor hygiene, extravasation in cannula site, evidence of thrombophlebitis.

- Look on the back for a nevus, a dimple, or a lipoma.
- Coarse facies are seen in mucopolysaccharidosis, GM1 gangliosidosis, and mucolipidosis.
- Angiokeratomas are skin lesions seen in Fabry disease **(*see* Fig. 11.8)**.
- Hair abnormalities must also be looked for. In Menkes disease, the hair is sparse, hypopigmented, and kinky **(*see* Fig. 11.5)**.
- Eye examination must be done to look for cataract (galactosemia), Kayser-Fleischer rings (Wilson disease), and telangiectasia (ataxia telangiectasia) **(*see* Fig. 11.7)**. Icterus may point to underlying chronic liver disease, Wilson disease, tyrosinemia, and Niemann-Pick disease type I.

C. Relevant Physical Examination

Specifically look for consciousness, behavior, gait, posture, obvious abnormal movements, asymmetry of face or limbs, contractures, and callosities.

- Persistent fisting of hands after 3 months of age is suggestive of hypertonia or cortical spinal tract dysfunction.
- Presence of abnormal involuntary movements other than seizures—like chorea, athetosis, ballismus, nystagmus, or tremor—may suggest an injury to the basal ganglia/cerebellum. These will be discussed in detail in a later section.
- Marked hip abduction when lying supine is indicative of axial hypotonia.

A child with peripheral neuropathy must be examined for pallor (anemia), knuckle

Table 11.13: Clinical signs on general physical examination and neurological correlate

Physical sign	Neurological illness
Pallor	Intracranial bleed, cerebral malaria
Icterus	Hepatic encephalopathy, leptospirosis, complicated malaria
Rash	Meningococcemia, measles, rickettsia
Petechiae	Dengue, viral hemorrhagic fever
Head and scalp hematoma	Head trauma

Table 11.14: Neurocutaneous stigmata to look for in the CNS examination

Skin lesions	Neurocutaneous syndrome
Ash leaf macule, shagreen patch, subungal fibroma and adenoma sebaceum	Tuberous sclerosis
Unilateral cutaneous hemangioma (port wine stain) in face and presence of glaucoma	Sturge-Weber syndrome
Raised verrucous skin lesions in ovoid or linear plaques	Epidermal nevus syndrome
Café au lait macules, neurofibromatosis	Neurofibromatosis
Evolution of erythematous skin lesions to crusted, pigmented then hypopigmented lesions	Incontinentia pigmenti
Multiple hairy pigmented nevi	Neurocutaneous melanosis

pigmentation (vitamin B12 deficiency), palpable thickened nerves (hereditary peripheral neuropathies), posture, hypo- and hyperpigmented patches on the skin, local examination of the spine (for scoliosis), and presence of pes cavus (Friedreich ataxia).

Examine the other systems to look for relevant associated findings. For example, look for a carotid bruit, atrial fibrillation, or signs of infective endocarditis in a child with stroke.

Organomegaly should be sought in suspected inborn errors of metabolism, or in the intrauterine infections.

D. Neurological Assessment

To examine the neurological system, equip yourself with some basic tools, shown in Fig. 11.16. Follow the scheme given in **Key Box 9** for examination of the nervous system.

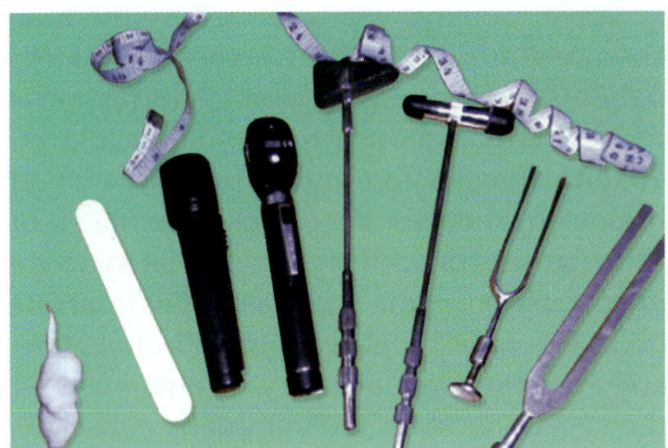

Fig. 11.16: Common tools for neurological examination.

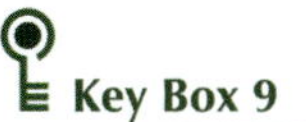

Key Box 9

Scheme of Neurological Examination

1. Higher mental functions (including consciousness)
2. Cranial nerves
3. Motor system examination:
   - Bulk of the muscles
   - Tone of muscles
   - Power of the muscles
   - Deep tendon and superficial reflexes
   - Gait, co-ordination
   - Abnormal movements
4. Sensory system examination
5. Cerebellar signs
6. Signs of meningeal irritation
7. Skull and spine

The neurological examination has to be tailored to child's condition, age, and setting (OPD/ward). It is neither *necessary* nor *possible* to do all aspects of neurological examination in all children. The traditional neurological examination can be done in older children and adolescents; however, the scheme and detail of examination needs to be modified for infants and young children.

11.5 CONSCIOUSNESS AND HIGHER MENTAL FUNCTION

Components of mental state examination and higher mental function (HMF) examination can be remembered easily by Mnemonic shown in Table 11.15. The mnemonic does not

Table 11.15: Checklist for higher mental function

Mental status	Higher mental function
Mnemonic: **ABCDE**	Mnemonic: **COMA-PIFAC**
Appearance	**C**onsciousness
Behavior	**O**rientation
Communication (speech and language)	**M**emory
Delusions and hallucinations	**A**ttention span
Emotion/mood	**P**erception
	Insight
	Fund of information
	Abstract thought
	Calculation
	Individual lobe functions
	Released reflex

provide the sequence for performing higher mental function examination, but will ensure that all components of higher mental functions are examined. Assessment of consciousness, orientation and attention will often determine the rest of the examination. *Hence, assessment of consciousness is the first step*. In a comatose child, HMF examination will be limited to assessment of consciousness; rest of it cannot be assessed. Similarly, in young infant, delirious child, uncooperative older child, HMF examination remains limited.

Assessment of HMF is particularly important for those presenting with unusual behavior, poor social judgment, poor attention and concentration, reading/writing/calculation difficulties, and memory difficulties.

I. Consciousness

Consciousness refers to the state of awareness of self and environment. Consciousness has two dimensions: Wakefulness and awareness.

- *Wakefulness* or arousal is mediated by the ascending reticular activating system, a network of diffuse neurons originating in the tegmentum of the pons and midbrain and projecting to diencephalic and cortical structures (medial hemispheric wall and basal forebrain).
- *Awareness* is dependent on the integrity of the cerebral cortex and its subcortical connections. **Figure 11.17** shows the various pathways responsible for consciousness in brain.

Impaired consciousness implies a significant impairment in the awareness of self and of the environment, with variable degrees of wakefulness. Evaluation of consciousness in infants and children must take into account the age and appropriate developmental level.

Descriptive terms such as *somnolence, stupor, obtundation*, and lethargy, used to denote different levels of consciousness, are best avoided; given the lack of uniformity in the way these states are defined in the literature.

It is best to describe all the components used in the assessment of consciousness, e.g. eye opening, motor and verbal responses, awareness of self and environment and presence of sleep–wake cycles. The chief characteristics of coma and other states of impaired consciousness are summarized in **Table 11.16**.

A. States of Consciousness

1. Coma: Coma is characterized by the total absence of arousal and of awareness. Comatose patients have no eye opening, no response to verbal command, no visual tracking, absent sleep–wake cycle but preserved brainstem reflexes. As opposed to states of transient unconsciousness such as syncope or concussion, coma must last for at least one hour. Coma is typically a transitional state, and evolves toward recovery of consciousness, the vegetative state, the minimally conscious state, or brain death. Coma is produced by conditions causing bilateral cerebral cortical

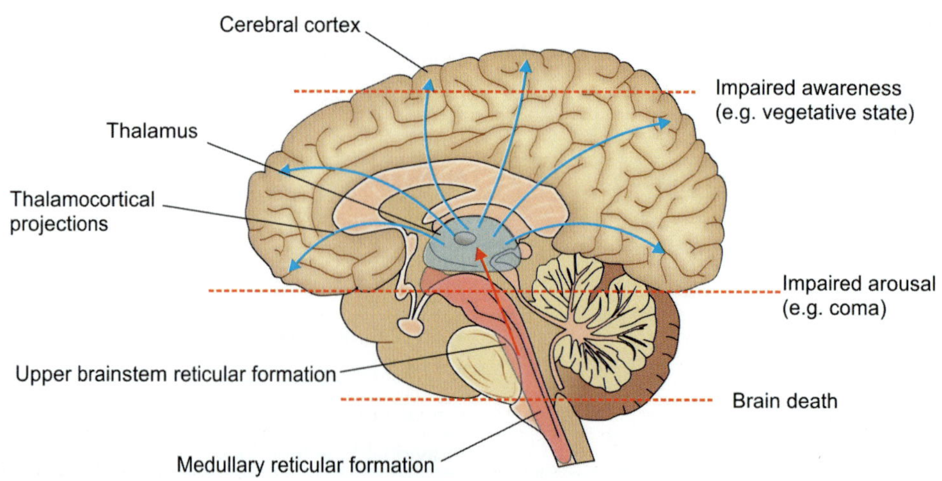

Fig. 11.17: Pathways for consciousness in brain.

Table 11.16: Disorders of consciousness

Condition	Awareness of self/ environment	Sleep–wake cycles	Brainstem function	Respiration
Coma	Absent	Absent	Variably preserved	Variably depressed
Brain death	Absent	Absent	Absent	Absent
Vegetative state	Absent	Preserved	Variably preserved	Normal
Minimally conscious state	Present (minimal but definite)	Preserved	Preserved	Normal
Locked-in state	Normal	Normal	Preserved	Normal to variably depressed
Akinetic mutism	Limited	Normal	Preserved	Normal to variably depressed

dysfunction, ascending reticular activating system dysfunction or both.

2. Vegetative state: This describes a condition of complete unawareness of the self and the environment characterized by no response to verbal command (may startle to loud sound), no visual fixation or following, no voluntary motor response. The sleep–wake cycle is preserved with patient showing intermittent eye opening. The vegetative state is deemed to be permanent—12 months after traumatic brain injury; and 3 months after non-traumatic injury.

3. Minimally conscious state: This is defined as a condition of severely altered consciousness in which the child demonstrates minimal but definite behavioural evidence of self- or environmental awareness. Children in this state are able to do any or all of the following:

- Follow simple commands
- Gesturally or verbally give yes/no responses (regardless of accuracy)
- Verbalize intelligibly
- Perform movements or affective behaviors in contingent relation to environmental stimuli (and not due to reflexive activity).

4. Locked-in syndrome: Refers to a condition in which the child retains consciousness and cognition but is unable to move or communicate, because of severe paralysis. The locked-in syndrome occurs due to bilateral ventral pontine lesion involving damage to the corticospinal, corticopontine, and corticobulbar tracts. The child has total paralysis below the level of the third nerve nuclei and only vertical eye movements are possible.

5. Akinetic mutism: This is a rare condition consisting of pathologically slowed or nearly absent bodily movement. Wakefulness and self-awareness are usually preserved in most patients, but the level of mental function is reduced. This condition results from bilateral frontal lobe lesions, diffuse cortical lesions or lesions, of the deep grey matter.

6. Delirium: It is an acute confusional state characterized by changes in the level of consciousness, impaired attention, disconnected thoughts, agitation and a fluctuating course. It may occur with toxic-metabolic encephalopathy, focal lesions, or seizures.

7. Brain death: Brain death is defined as the permanent absence of all brain functions including those of the brainstem. Brain-dead patients are irreversibly comatose and apneic with absent brainstem reflexes.

B. Level of Consciousness

The child should be inspected for spontaneous body position, motor activity, eye opening, or verbalization. The response to stimuli of graded intensity should then be observed, starting with verbal commands, progressing to tactile cues and finally to painful stimulus. Look for the presence of sleep–wake cycles. Look for evidence of interaction with environment such as following commands, appropriate smiling or crying, gestural responses, reaching for objects, fixation, and following.

Painful stimuli should be delivered without inducing tissue trauma and with regard to the possibility of conscious pain perception; preferable sites are the nail bed and the notch of the supraorbital nerve. Supraorbital pressure evokes a response even in children who may have lost afferent pain pathways as a result of peripheral neuropathy or spinal cord lesions. Asymmetrical withdrawal responses may indicate weakness of one side. Finally, the level of consciousness must be recorded in the form of an objective scale, such as the Glasgow Coma Scale (GCS) **(Table 11.17)**.

Glasgow coma scale (GCS): The GCS was initially devised for adults with traumatic brain injury, but it has been widely used in children in both traumatic and non-traumatic coma. GCS works well for children >5 years, but for children <5 years, modifications for verbal component are needed.

The verbal score of GCS also needs to be modified in intubated children, using grimace response. The minimum score of GCS is three and NOT zero. Maximum score is 15. It is pertinent to note that the best response score must be recorded. For example, eye opening to verbal command (E3) and then pain (E2) must be tested before labeling it as no eye opening (E1).

Four score: One of the other commonly used scales is FOUR (Full Outline UnResponsiveness) scores **(Fig. 11.18)**. There are four components to FOUR scores: Eye response, motor response, brainstem reflexes, and respiratory pattern. FOUR scores were introduced considering difficulties in scoring the verbal component of GCS among intubated children and non-representation of brainstem reflexes and breathing pattern in assessment of coma in GCS. FOUR scores are simple to administer and information derived from FOUR scores allows accurate assessment of children with altered sensorium.

II. Higher Mental Function

After determining that the child is conscious, the higher mental functions should be tested, preferably in the order given in **Key Box 10**. Remember that a detailed higher mental function testing is neither needed nor feasible in each and every child with a neurological problem. Higher mental function testing is a must in children who present with cognitive decline, stroke, language, and memory

Table 11.17: Glasgow Coma Scale with modification for children and intubated patients

Best eye response		
1. No eye opening		
2. Eye opening to pain		
3. Eye opening to verbal command		
4. Eyes open spontaneously		
Best verbal response		
Adult version (>5 y)	**Children's modification**	**Grimace response for preverbal or intubated patients**
1. No verbal response	No vocal response	No response to pain
2. Incomprehensible sounds	Occasionally whimpers and/or moans	Mild grimace to pain
3. Inappropriate words	Cries inappropriately	Vigorous grimace to pain
4. Confused	Less than usual ability and/or spontaneous irritable cry	Less than usual spontaneous ability or only response to touch stimuli
5. Oriented	Alert, babbles, coos, words or sentences to usual ability	Spontaneous normal facial/oromotor activity
Best motor response		
1. No motor response to pain		
2. Abnormal extension to pain		
3. Abnormal flexion to pain		
4. Withdrawal to painful stimuli		
5. Localizes to painful stimuli or withdraws to touch		
6. Obeys commands or performs normal spontaneous movements		

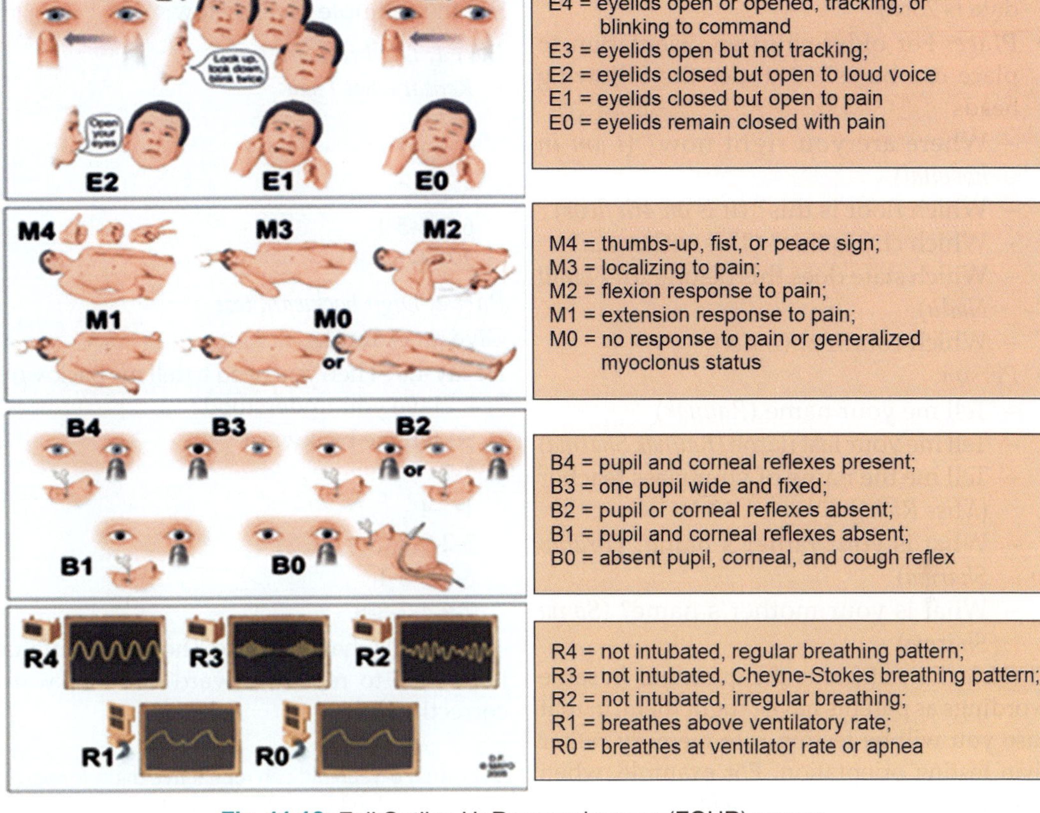

Fig. 11.18: Full Outline UnResponsiveness (FOUR) scores.

Key Box 10

Higher Mental Function—10 Components

1. Appearance and behavior
2. Delusion, hallucination and emotions
3. Orientation
4. Attention span
5. Speech and language
6. Memory
7. Higher cognitive functions
8. Spatial perception and construction
9. Lobe functions
10. Release reflexes

problems. If a child comes with only muscular weakness, and there is no cognitive decline or altered sensorium as per history, then a detailed higher mental function testing is not necessary.

1. Appearance and Behavior

Observe the child when you are taking the history from the parents. Look for personal cleanliness (hair, teeth, dress). Is the child interested in the surroundings? Look for his facial expressions. Does he make a good eye contact with his parents and with you? Did he cooperate with you during the examination? Is he hyperactive or aggressive during the examination? Does he appear anxious, lethargic, or indifferent?

2. Delusion, Hallucination, and Emotion

Look for evidence of delusion or hallucinations while talking to the child and parents. Note if there is any evidence of emotional outburst or emotional lability.

3. Orientation

Check the orientation of the child to time, place, and person. This should be appropriate to the developmental level of the child. Ask the child following questions for children >7 years:

- ***Time:*** What year? Season? Month? Day of week? Date? (*The year is 2024, season is* *winter, it is month of January, today is* Tuesday, date is 23rd)

- ***Place:*** For older children orientation to place can be asked under the following heads
  - Where are you right now? (*I am in hospital*)
  - Which floor is this? (*It is on 4th floor*)
  - Which city is this? (*This is Chennai*)
  - Which state does this belong to? (*Tamil Nadu*)
  - Which country? (*India*)
- ***Person:***
  - Tell me your name (*Raunak*)
  - Tell me your last name (*Raunak Sharma*)
  - Tell me the name of your class teacher (*Miss Richa*)
  - What is your father's name? (*Pratap Sharma*)
  - What is your mother's name? (*Sonia Sharma*)

(*Note:* Do not frame the questions in same wordings as parents have taught them, in that case you will be testing rote memory rather than testing orientation. For example, when you ask *"How is your dad addressed?"* child might not reply but he might answer the question *"What is your father's name"*).

In infants and younger children, also look for stranger anxiety/familiarity with parents.

4. Attention Span

Establish the child's ability to *sustain* attention before evaluating complex functions—such as memory, language, and abstract thinking. *Attention* is defined as the child's ability to attend to a specific stimulus without being distracted by extraneous internal or environmental stimuli. Attention is assessed using the "Digit repetition test".

Digit repetition test or digit span test: Tell the child "I am going to say some numbers. Listen carefully and repeat after me". Say the digits in a normal tone of voice at a rate of one digit per second. Take care not to group digits either in pairs (e.g. 1-3, 2-6) or in sequences such as telephone numbers (2-6-5-2, 3-1-6-7). Numbers should be presented randomly without natural sequences (e.g. not 2-4-6-8). Begin with a two-number sequence, and continue till the child fails to repeat all the numbers correctly. See the example given below:

Part 1: Digit forward test

Repeat what I say

3-7

1-7-4

5-2-9-7

6-3-8-5-1

2-9-4-7-3-8

Part 2: Digit backward test

Give an example:

If I say 4, 7: Then you need to tell me backward 7, 4. Have you understood?

So tell me backward

3-7

1-7-4

5-2-9-7

6-3-8-5-1

2-9-4-7-3-8

Note till what level (up to how many digits) is he able to repeat forward and backward correctly.

A normal 6-year-old can repeat five digits forward and 3 digits backward. A normal 10-year-old child can repeat 6 digits forward and 4 digits backward.

Other methods to test attention span among children >7 years are as follows:

1. Tell the months of year (Jan, Feb, March, April…)..Good…Now tell them backward (Dec, Nov, Oct, Sept…)
2. Start with 100, now subtract 7 (93),..now further subtract 7 (86)…now further subtract 7 (79)…..till 65 [*serial 7s*]

The basic anatomic structures that are responsible for maintaining an alert state are the brainstem reticular formation and the diffuse thalamic projection system. The mechanism of focused attention with screening out of extraneous distraction is by cortical and limbic influences.

5. Speech and Language

- *Language* is defined as use of conventional system of symbols (spoken word, sign language, written words, pictures) for communication. Components of language are enumerated in **Key Box 11**.

Key Box 11

Components of Language
- Comprehension
- Naming object
- Repetition
- Reading
- Writing
- Articulation
- Fluency

- *Speech* is defined as expressive production of sound that includes articulation, fluency, voice, and resonance quality. Assess the following components of speech: (a) articulation, (b) volume of speech; and (c) fluency. Identify the child's first/native language (mother tongue).

Cerebral dominance: If the child is over 4 years of age, establish whether he/she is right- or left-handed. Handedness is important to understand the cerebral dominance. Approximately, 90% of the population is right handed. Of this 90%, more than 99% are strongly left hemisphere-dominant for language. Because of this strong language dominance in right-handed individuals, left hemisphere lesions frequently cause aphasia. Amongst left-handed individuals, approximately 70% are left hemisphere dominant, 13% are right hemisphere dominant, and the remainder are mixed.

Language areas in brain: Sounds are recognized in the Wernicke's area in the superior temporal gyrus, which is then connected to a *concept area* where the meaning of the words is understood. The 'concept area' is connected to *Broca's area* in the inferior frontal gyrus,

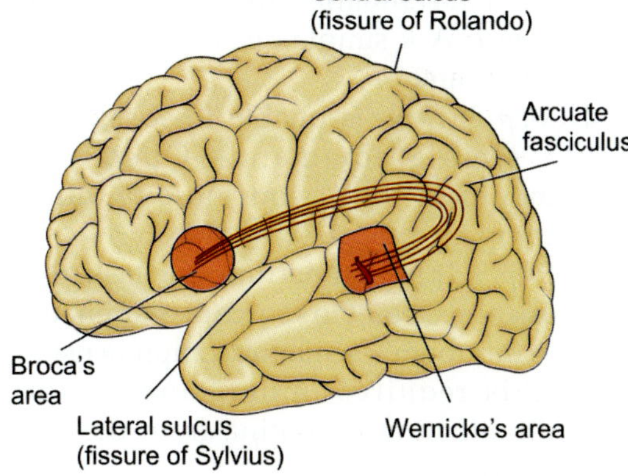

Fig. 11.19: Language areas in brain.

where speech output is generated **(Fig. 11.19)**. Wernicke's area is also connected directly to the Broca's area by the arcuate fasciculus.

A. Definitions

Aphasia: It implies the inability to understand or express words for the purpose of communication, even though the primary sensorimotor pathways to receive and express language and the mental status are relatively intact.

Dysarthria: It is defined as a defect of articulation or enunciation of speech.

Dysphonia: It refers to abnormality in volume of voice. This usually occurs due to local vocal cord pathology, e.g. laryngitis, abnormality of nerve supply via vagus, or occasionally a psychological disorder. As voice production occurs during expiration, disorders which cause respiratory muscle weakness, e.g. Guillain-Barré syndrome may also lead to reduced volume of voice.

B. Testing language functions (Table 11.18)

Language function is tested by the following steps.

Table 11.18: Language testing: What you find and what it means

Type of aphasia	Understanding	Fluency	Repetition	Naming
Global aphasia	–	–	–	–
Wernicke's aphasia	–	+	–	–
Broca's aphasia	+	–	–	–
Transcortical sensory	–	+	+	–
Transcortical motor	+	–	+	–
Conduction aphasia	+	+	–	–
Nominal aphasia	+	+	+	–

1. ***Assess understanding and comprehension***
   a. *Step 1:* Ask simple questions—What is your name?
   b. *Step 2:* If he is unable to speak, give a simple command—Open your mouth or touch your nose (auditory comprehension).
   c. *Step 3:* If he can perform the task, then ask him: "point to source of illumination in this room" (semantic comprehension) (this requires understanding that illumination is coming from the tube light).
2. ***Assess articulation:*** Look for articulation of words during spontaneous speech. Ask the child to repeat some difficult phrases, e.g. 'yellow lorry' and 'baby hippopotamus'. Listen carefully for (i) the rhythm of the speech, (ii) any slurred words, and (iii) which sounds cause the greatest difficulty. Sounds that are generated from lips (labials) are "pa", tip of tongue (linguals) "ta", throat (guttural) "kha". In children with dysarthria, there will be difficulty in articulation. You can ask the child to say: "pa pa pa pa pa" "ta ta ta ta" "kha kha kha kha". It is easy to remember patakha (crackers are called "पटाखा" in Hindi).
3. ***Assess fluency:*** Assess the spontaneous speech. Observe if the speech is fluent and the child is using the words correctly. Is the child using meaningless words (jargon)? Assess the word finding ability by asking the child to name all the animals he/she can think of in one minute.
4. ***Assess repetition:*** Ask the child to repeat a simple phrase. Sentences like "No ifs and buts" or in Hindi "*Billi doodh peeti hai*" can be used to test repetition.
5. ***Assess naming:*** Show some familiar objects (e.g. watch, pen, etc.) and ask the child to name the objects.
6. ***Assess reading:*** Write a line that says "touch your nose". Show this paper to the child and ask the child to perform the action written in the paper.
7. ***Assess writing:*** Ask the child to write his/her name, address, and school name on paper.

Interpretation of aphasia

Global aphasia: Lesion is in dominant hemisphere affecting both Wernicke's and Broca's area. This usually occurs with a *massive left middle cerebral artery infarction.*

Wernicke's aphasia: Poor comprehension, fluent but often meaningless speech (may contain neologisms and paraphasia), no repetition. *The lesion is in the Wernicke's area.*

Broca's aphasia: Preserved comprehension; nonfluent speech, no repetition; *lesion in Broca's area* (inferior frontal gyrus). This may be associated with hemiplegia.

Conductive aphasia: Loss of repetition with preserved comprehension and output. *Lesion is in arcuate fasciculus.*

Transcortical sensory aphasia: As in Wernicke's aphasia but with preserved repetition. *Lesion is in posterior parieto-occipital region.*

Transcortical motor aphasia: As in Broca's aphasia but with preserved repetition. *It is an incomplete lesion in Broca's area.*

Nominal aphasia: Inability to name objects. *Lesion is in the angular gyrus.*

Interpretation of dysarthria

Cerebellar dysarthria (scanning or staccato speech): The child speaks slowly or deliberately as if scanning a line of poetry. The speech sounds slurred as if drunk. Sometimes, each syllable is given equal emphasis, e.g. artillery pronounced as ar-til-ler-y.

Pseudobulbar or spastic dysarthria: This type of dysarthria is seen in children with upper motor neuron lesions, such as cerebral palsy. This occurs due to bilateral lesion in corticospinal fibers supplying muscles of face, larynx, tongue, and respiration. Individual syllables are slurred. The precision of consonant production is lost. The child is hardly able to open the mouth, and the speech sounds as if the child is trying to speak from the back of the mouth. Associated findings may include brisk jaw jerk, extensor plantar response, dysphagia, and drooling.

Extrapyramidal dysarthria: This kind of speech is characteristic of basal ganglia lesions such as Wilson disease and dyskinetic cerebral palsy. Dysarthria may be hypokinetic or hyperkinetic. In the *hypokinetic type*, the speech is monotonous, without rhythm and intonations. The sentences start and stop suddenly. In the hyperkinetic type, the speech is jerky, uncontrolled in loudness, harsh, and poorly coordinated with breathing. It is frequently associated with orofacial-lingual dyskinesias.

Bulbar dysarthria: This type of dysarthria occurs due to lower motor neuron lesions affecting speech musculature. Causes include bulbar palsy due to diphtheria, Guillain-Barré syndrome, and brainstem encephalitis. The speech appears nasal as with a bad cold. There may be associated nasal regurgitation of fluids, dysphagia to solids, and nasal twang of sound due to palatal air escape during phonation. The gag reflex is weak.

6. Memory Testing

Memory is a general term for a mental process that allows the individual to store information for later recall. Clinically, memory is subdivided into three types: Immediate, recent, and remote.

Immediate memory: It is used to recall a memory after an interval of a few seconds, e.g. the digit repetition test. Ask "Can you repeat what I said (immediate memory)".

Recent memory: It is the capacity to remember current day-to-day events, e.g. "what did you have for breakfast today?" Recent memory is the retrieval of material after interval of minutes, hours, or days.

Remote memory: This traditionally refers to the recall of facts or events that occurred months to years ago. Ask the following questions to test remote memory.

- What is your teacher's name?
- Which school do you study?
- What are your father's and mother's name?
- How many brothers and sisters you have? What are their names?

7. Higher Cognitive Function (Intelligence)

A. Calculation: The calculation ability needs to be checked according to the age and level of schooling of the child. Start first with simple additions. Then move on to subtraction, multiplication and division.

You may consider asking, if i give you two pencils and she gives you four, how many will you have? Now, if i take 3 from you, how much you are left with?

Do not ask questions like 2 + 2, 4 + 4, as they are often answered by rote memory.

The nodal point for calculation is in the left angular gyrus.

B. Abstract thinking: Ask the child to explain well-known proverbs. Ask the child to explain the difference between pair of objects, e.g. a skirt and a pair of trousers. An older child (>7 years of age) may be asked the similarity between a tree and a cat (both are living things). One can test the analogy by asking "leg is to table, so .... is to car". Fill in the blank.

8. Spatial Perception and Constructional Ability

This tests parietal and occipital lobe function. Ask the child to draw a clock face and to fill in the numbers **(Fig. 11.20)**. Ask him then to draw the hands on at a given time. Ask the child to copy a five-pointed star **(Fig. 11.21)**.

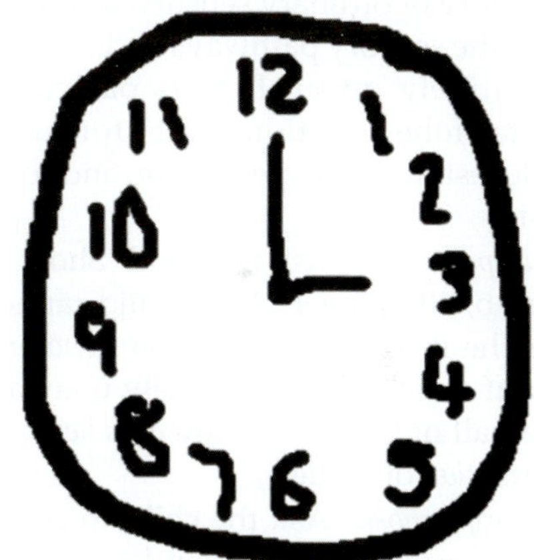

Fig. 11.20: Ask child to draw clock, write the number and then ask him to make 3'o clock position.

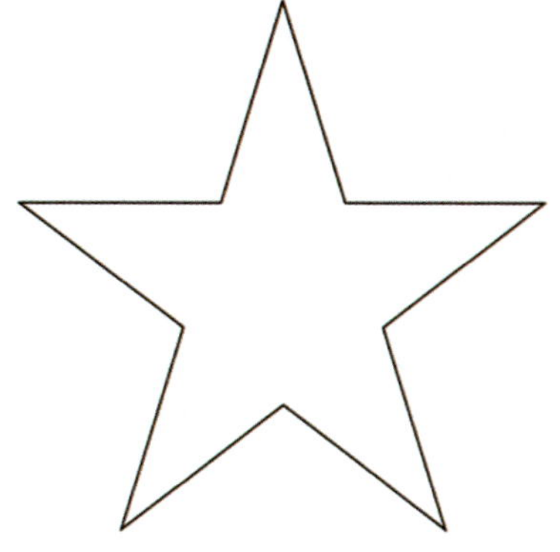

Fig. 11.21: Ask the child to copy this five- pointed star.

A. Apraxia: Apraxia is the inability to accomplish previously learned and performed complex motor actions even though motor system, sensory system, understanding, and co-ordination are relatively intact. Apraxia occurs whenever there is parietal lobe dysfunction. Ask the child 'show how you will comb your hair/wear your shoes/drink a cup of tea' Ideational apraxia. If difficulty, give appropriate object or demonstrate.

B. Right and left orientation (parietal lobe function): Right-left orientation occurs by 4 years of age. Ask the child to do the following to test it:

1. Show your left hand?
2. Touch your left ear with your right hand?
3. Show my right hand?
4. Touch my left hand with your right hand?

C. Agnosia: Agnosia is the inability to understand the meaning or symbolic significance of ordinary sensory stimuli even though the sensory pathways and sensorium are relatively intact. It tests parietal and occipital lobe function. Tests for agnosia include tests for body perception and sensory agnosia.

1. *Body perception:* Ask the child 'Show your thumb, little finger'. If the child cannot do this, he is said to have *finger agnosia*. See also if the child is completely unaware of one-half of the body, known as *hemispatial inattention* or neglect.
2. *Sensory agnosia:* Ask the child to close his eyes. Place an object, e.g. coin, key in his hand and ask him what it is. Inability to recognize the object is known as astereognosis. With the eyes of the child closed, write a number or letter on hand of the child and ask to identify. Inability to perform this task is known as agraphaesthesia.

Lesions of either parietal lobe may cause contralateral loss of astereognosis and other discriminative modalities, but hemispatial inattention is more common with right parietal lobe lesions. Finger agnosia and right-left disorientation are more common with left posterior perisylvian lesions.

D. Frontal lobe functions: Assess these functions by asking the following (for children more than 7 years)

1. How did you come to this place (I took bus and then a auto-rickshaw).
2. Why have you come to this place (insight) (I am sick so papa brought me here!).
3. Judgment (what will you do if you see a house on fire?).
4. Fist edge palm test (keep your hand on the table, make a fist, now make a edge and now make palm on the surface of table... now do this fast) **(Fig. 11.22)**.

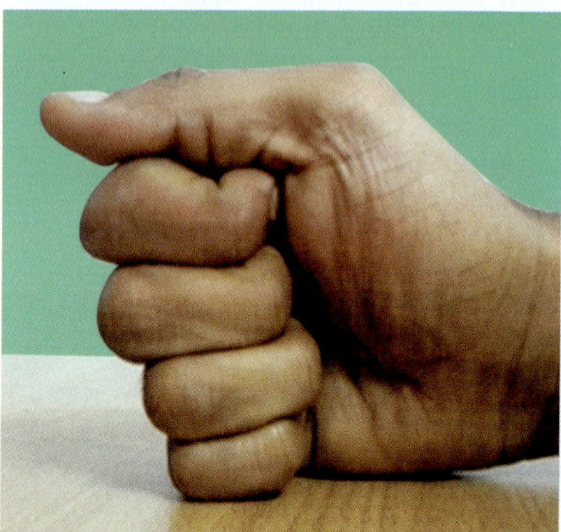

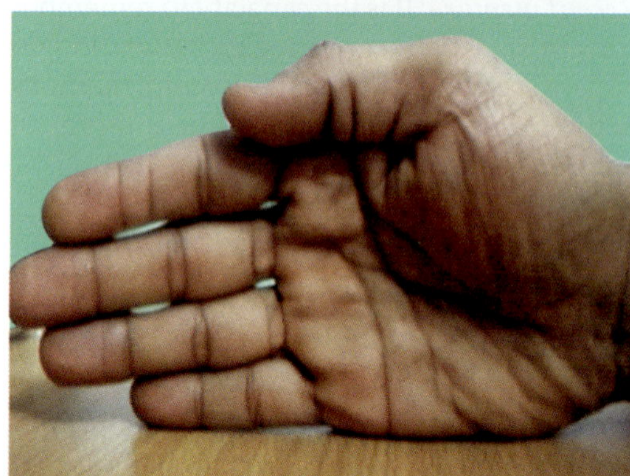

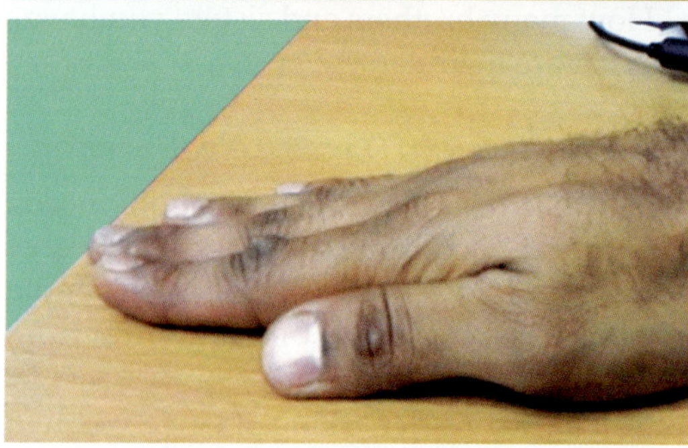

Fig. 11.22: Demonstrate to child the sequence of fist, edge and palm and ask him to do this sequence of fist-edge-palm as fast as possible.

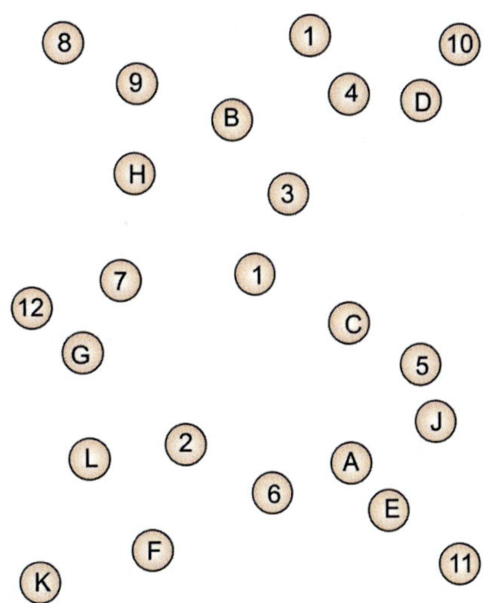

Fig. 11.23: Ask the child to complete trail of numbers starting from 1.

PURPLE YELLOW RED
BLACK RED GREEN
RED YELLOW ORANGE
BLUE PURPLE BLACK
RED GREEN ORANGE

Fig. 11.24: Ask the child to name the color and NOT to read out the letter.

5. Trail making test (ask the child make a trail of numbers) **(Fig. 11.23)**.
6. Stroop test (to identify the color of word and NOT to read the letter **(Fig. 11.24)** (it assesses disinhibition which is frontal lobe function).

10. Release Reflexes

These are also known as "frontal release signs." Frontal release signs are responses that get inhibited as the infant cortex matures and the myelination proceeds. Cortical/ subcortical damage particularly frontal lobe damage releases these signs and hence the name. These are seen with frontal lobe disease. These must be tested for children with suspected neurodegenerative disorders.

a. *Grasp reflex:* Stroke the palm on radial aspect preferably between palm and forefinger and a palmar grasp is elicited.
b. *Palmomental reflex:* On scratching the thenar eminence with a key/pin, there is brief contraction of the mentalis muscle causing puckering of the chin.
c. *Glabellar tap:* A series of sharp finger taps to the glabella normally elicits 2–3 blinks before it gets inhibited. A positive test is when a blink follows each stimulus as there is no habituation.
d. *Snout reflex:* A gentle pressure on the child's lips causes reflex puckering of orbicularis oris. It is caused by impairment of the corticobulbar projection.
e. *Suck reflex:* Stimulation of the perioral region is followed by sucking movements of the lips, tongue, and jaw.

11.6 CRANIAL NERVE EXAMINATION

The cranial nerve examination is an excellent tool to localize a brainstem lesion. There are 12 cranial nerves and they can be categorized as sensory, motor, or mixed nerves. Overall, sensory nerve nuclei tend to be located in the lateral brainstem, while motor nuclei tend to be located medially. All cranial nerves except 1st and 2nd, originate in the brainstem **(Key Box 12)**.

A. Olfactory Nerve

Anatomy

The olfactory epithelium consisting of bipolar sensory cells (basal cells) is located in the superior part of nasal septum, nasal attic and superior part of lateral wall of nasal cavity. The central processes of these cells

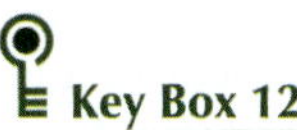

Key Box 12

Cranial Nerves

1. Olfactory: Sensory nerve
2. Optic: Sensory nerve
3. Oculomotor: Motor nerve
4. Trochlear: Motor nerve
5. Trigeminal: Mixed nerve
6. Abducens: Motor nerve
7. Facial: Mixed nerve
8. Vestibulocochlear: Sensory nerve
9. Glossopharyngeal: Mixed nerve
10. Vagus: Mixed nerve
11. Accessory: Motor nerve
12. Hypoglossal: Motor nerve

are the olfactory nerves (around 20 on each side) which penetrate the cribriform plate of ethmoid to synapse in the olfactory bulb. The cells of olfactory bulb course posteriorly as medial and lateral olfactory striae. Median olfactory striae connects to the olfactory tract of opposite side, while the lateral striae terminate in the primary olfactory cortex in temporal lobe.

Function

Olfactory nerve is a sensory nerve whose only function is perception (olfactory pathway) and identification (olfactory cortex) of smell. Olfaction is functional even during prenatal life. At birth, newborns have highly efficient olfactory abilities, allowing them to discriminate the odor of their mother's skin or milk from those of other mothers and to modify their feeding behavior according to the milk flavor. The human neonatal olfaction probably plays a role both in mother–child bonding and in newborn feeding behavior. Healthy infants and toddlers (3 months to 3 years) have good olfaction abilities. Objectively, olfactory discrimination is testable from the age of 5 years onwards.

Disorders

Impairment of olfactory nerve is rare in childhood. *Anosmia* refers to loss of sense of smell; *Hyposmia/hyperosmia*—decreased/increased ability to smell; and Parosmia—distorted sense of smell.

Common causes of anosmia include upper respiratory tract infection (including COVID-19), nasal trauma, nasal and sinus disease, and idiopathic. Anosmia of neurological origin include meningioma of sphenoidal ridge/olfactory groove and frontal lobe gliomas.

Clinical Examination

- Ensure that nasal passages are patent. Ask the child to close one nostril and blow air through the other one; feel the air by keeping your finger in front of child's open nostril. This can also be checked to ask the child to breathe out through alternative nares on a glass slide, and looking for misting.
- Use non-irritating substances (coffee powder, toothpaste, soap, chocolate, etc.) for testing smell. Use substances that the child is likely to be familiar with. Irritants will stimulate trigeminal nerve endings rather than olfactory nerve.
- The test substances are kept in small plastic/glass bottles.
- Examine each nostril separately.
- With child's eyes closed and one nostril occluded, bring the test substance near the open nostril; first ask if the child can perceive any smell; if yes, then ask what is this smell.
- Repeat the same procedure for opposite nostril.
- Perception of smell indicates intact olfactory pathway. Correct identification of smell indicates intact cortical center for smell.

Testable age for olfaction: Olfaction identification and discrimination can be reliably tested in children from 5 years onwards using standard tools. But, in younger children behavioral responses can be used to test for the intactness of olfactory sensation although olfactory differentiation may not be possible.

B. Optic Nerve: 2nd Cranial Nerve

The two main functions of optic nerve are (a) vision; and (b) afferent for pupilloconstriction.

Anatomy

The optic nerve consists of fibers derived from the ganglionic cells of the retina. Optic nerves from both eyes join to form optic chiasma in middle cranial fossa. At optic chiasma, fibers from nasal side cross over to temporal side and vice versa to form optic tract. Each optic tract passes backward and outward from the optic chiasma to reach lateral geniculate body. Fibers from lateral geniculate body carry visual information through optic radiations (upper and lower) to reach visual cortex. Some of the fibers in the optic tract end in the pretectal nucleus (for pupillary reflexes) and superior colliculus (for extraocular movements).

Examination

Testing of optic nerve involves five components listed in **Key Box 13**.

1. Visual acuity: It is the ability of eye to resolve details. At birth—20/2000, 2 months of age—20/200, one year—20/60, four years—20/40;

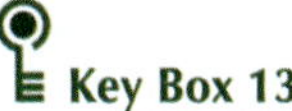
Key Box 13

Testing of Optic Nerve

1. Visual acuity
2. Color vision
3. Field of vision
4. Pupillary reactions
5. Fundus

it reaches adult range by 5 years. Test charts include Snellen chart for distant vision and near card (Rosenbaum pocket vision screener held at 14 inches) for near vision (*see* Chapter 11 for details on vision testing).

- If the child cannot read, ask the child to count fingers kept at 1 meter.
- If the child is unable to do finger counting, ask him to show the direction of bright light shown from different directions (*projection of rays*).
- If the child still cannot see, shine bright light just in front of the eyes, and ask if he can see something (*perception of light*).
- In newborns and infants, behavioral responses to light, faces of parents or brightly colored toys can be observed: Blinking, turning eyes and/or head towards light or becoming calm suddenly, fixation on an object. The *menace response* is a useful test in young children. Bring your hand from the side in front of the child's eye. The child should blink to avoid the 'menacing stimulus', if he has vision.
- Infant with poor vision will fail to fix and follow the light. They often develop nystagmus (wandering eyes) by 2 months of age. These infants might also have associated rhythmic head movement and disturbed circadian rhythm resulting in disturbed sleep–wake cycle.
- Blindness without a primary eye disease is termed *amaurosis*, whereas impaired vision due to any organic cause like cataract, strabismus, or anisometropia is termed *amblyopia*.

2. Color vision: This is tested using Ishihara color vision charts (*see* Chapter 12 for details). Color testing should be performed in children with acute or chronic vision loss, and suspected color blindness. Children with optic nerve injury (e.g. optic neuritis) will have decreased color vision.

3. Fields of vision: The visual pathways are organized in such a way that different patterns of visual field abnormality result from lesions at different sites **(Fig. 11.25)**. The visual fields are divided vertically through the point of fixation into the temporal and nasal fields. Something on your right as you look ahead is the temporal field of your right eye and the nasal field of your left eye. The visual fields are described from the child's point of view.

- Field defects are said to be *homonymous* if the same part of the field is affected in eyes, e.g. a right homonymous hemianopia means there is a field defect in the temporal field of the right eye and nasal field of the left eye. Whereas a bitemporal hemianopia would be a *heteronymous* field defect.
- Homonymous field defects are called *congruous*, if the field defects in both eyes match exactly or *incongruous* if the field defects do not match exactly.

Localize the lesion according to the field defect **(Table 11.19)**. Visual fields are clinically tested by the confrontation test.

Confrontation test

- Sit in front of the child (confront) at a distance of about 50 cm with your eyes at the same level as the child's eyes **(Fig. 11.26)**.

Table 11.19: Localization of field defects

Type of field defect	Localization
Mono-ocular	Lesion anterior to optic chiasma
Bitemporal	Lesion at the optic chiasma
Homonymous field defect	Lesion behind the optic chiasma
Incongruous homonymous	Lesion in optic tract
Congruous homonymous	Lesion behind lateral geniculate bodies

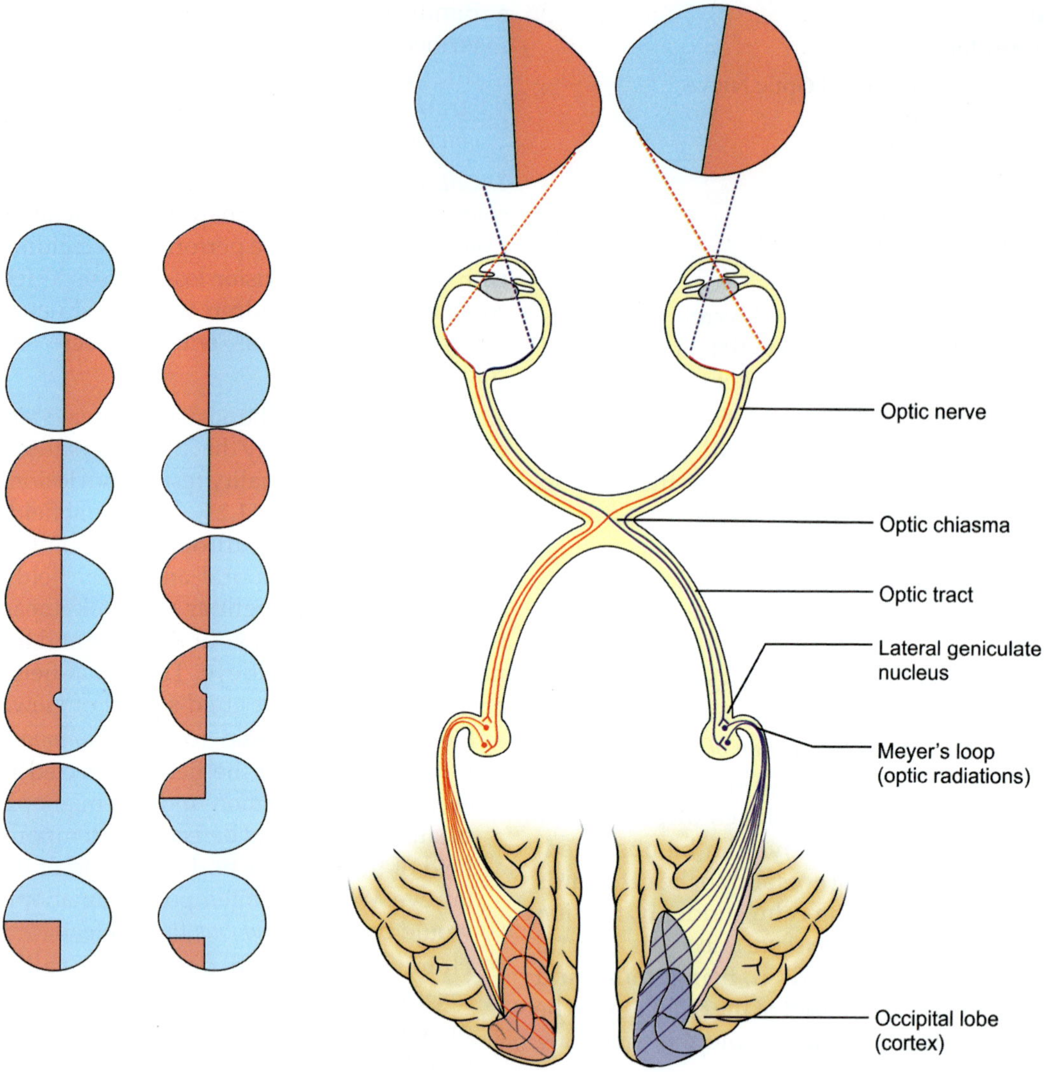

Optic nerve

Optic chiasma

Optic tract

Lateral geniculate nucleus

Meyer's loop (optic radiations)

Occipital lobe (cortex)

Fig. 11.25: Visual pathway and visual field defects.

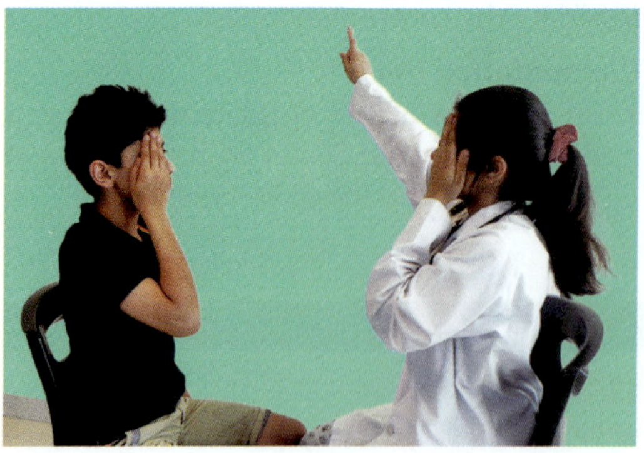

Fig. 11.26: Confrontation test.

- Instructions to the child:
  - Look directly into my eye; don't look away; don't look at my nose
  - I want to check how far you can see; say "yes" (or raise your hand) as soon as you see my finger
- For testing the child's left eye, occlude his right eye and occlude your left eye.
- Hold up your finger outside your own visual field in the middle of one quadrant; wiggle your finger and move slowly towards the central field; ask the child to raise his hand or say "yes" when he first sees your wiggling finger; match your field with the child's field of vision; A red pin/white pin of 10 mm can also be used instead of finger
- Test the field in all four quadrants and both eyes separately

Testing visual fields in infants: In infants and young children, a rough assessment of the fields can be performed by bringing a bright colorful object into the various quadrants of the child's visual field, and observing whether the child looks and follows the object.

A two persons examination technique is also described for testing visual field in infants. Infant is held in parents lap and first examiner sits in front of the child and engages him with toys. The second examiner comes from behind the child and introduces toy in field of vision. We look for saccades in infant's eyes.

4. Pupillary light reflex: Evaluation of the pupillary light reflex is one of the most important aspect of the neurological examination. This is critical in children with coma, head injury, stroke, and brain tumor. You must know the pathway of this reflex very well.

The normal pupil constricts promptly in response to light. Pupillary constriction also occurs as a part of the accommodation reflex (also called the near response), along with medial convergence and change in the curvature of the lens (rounding up of the lens for efficient near vision).

Anatomy: The pupillary light reaction is mediated by the macula, optic nerve, chiasm, and optic tract (Fig. 11.27). Before reaching the lateral geniculate body, pupil afferents leave the optic tract to synapse in the pretectum. In addition to the decussation of bilateral nasal fibers, extensive crossing occurs through the posterior commissure with pupillary afferents synapsing both ipsilaterally and contralaterally. This is the mechanism for the direct and consensual light reflex. Fibers project from the pretectum to the Edinger-Westphal nucleus (which is a part of the oculomotor nuclear complex in the midbrain).

Parasympathetic pupillary efferents from the Edinger-Westphal nucleus enter the third nerve and enter the orbit. These fibers travel to the ciliary ganglion, then through the short ciliary nerves to the sphincter papillae muscle.

Cortical visual impairment is one of the common causes of blindness in neurological children like hypoxic–ischemic encephalopathy or neonatal hypoglycemia. Absence of visual regard with poor fixation

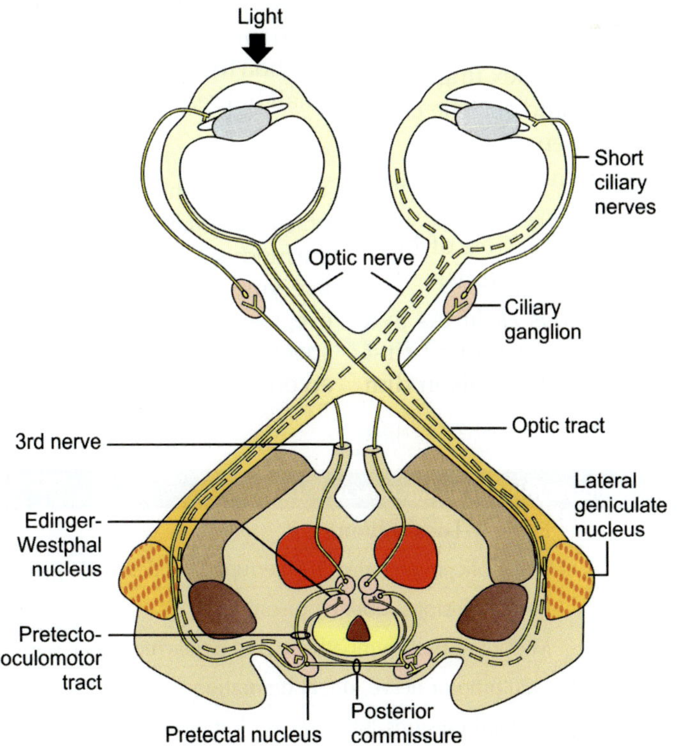

Fig. 11.27: Pathway of the pupillary reflex.

but normal pupillary response (as pupillary reflex pathway skips occipital cortex) points to cortical blindness especially when there is radiological and clinical correlation of neonatal insult.

Testing pupillary reactions in a conscious child

- Ask the child to look at a distant object
- Check pupils—size, shape, and symmetry between the two sides. The ambient light in the room should be a little dim, to observe the pupils in their resting state.
- Beam a bright light into the eye from side; observe whether both pupils constrict briskly and equally.
- *Direct light reflex:* There is constriction of pupil in the eye stimulated by light.
- *Indirect/consensual reflex:* There is constriction of pupil in the opposite eye.
- *Swinging flash light test:* Swing light alternately from one eye to the other eye for 3–5 seconds. If there is optic nerve pathology on one side, the pupil will dilate when the light shifts from normal to affected eye (Marcus Gunn pupil/afferent pupillary defect). This test is useful, only if there is unilateral pathology.
- Accommodation reaction
  - Ask the child to look at a distant object.
  - Suddenly bring your index finger or a pen in front of eyes and ask the child to fixate on finger/pen.
  - Observe the movement of eyeballs and pupils.
  - *Normal response:* Adduction of both eyes and constriction of pupils.

Testing pupils in unconscious child: As in a conscious child, pupils are examined first by observing the size of both pupils in dim light and then by assessing reactivity to a bright light shined in each eye. Topical administration of mydriatics must be avoided, but if done, should be documented in the case records to avoid confusion in interpretation. Pupillary size, shape, symmetry and response to light provide valuable clues to brainstem and third nerve dysfunction. The pupillary light reflex is very resistant to metabolic dysfunction. Abnormalities especially when unilateral, indicate structural lesions of the midbrain or oculomotor nerve.

Asymmetric pupils are caused either by disruption of the oculomotor nerve (cranial nerve III) or impairment of sympathetic fibers (Horner syndrome). *Unilateral pupillary dilatation in the comatose child should be considered as evidence of oculomotor nerve compression from ipsilateral uncal herniation, unless proved otherwise.*

Drugs and toxins which may rarely cause unreactive pupils include barbiturates, succinylcholine, lidocaine, phenothiazines, and aminoglycoside antibiotics. Hypothermia and acute anoxia may also cause unreactive pupils, which, if persistent, carry a poor prognosis. Hypothalamic damage causes unilateral papillary constriction and a Horner syndrome. Midbrain lesions cause mid-position fixed pupils and pontine lesions cause small but reactive pupils **(Table 11.20)**.

5. Fundus examination (also see Chapter 12)

You should have an ophthalmoscope and practice regularly to get confidence in examining the fundus. For the child's right eye, you should use your right eye, and for the child's left eye, use your left eye **(Fig. 11.28)**. If you wear spectacles, adjust the ophthalmoscope lens according to your refractory error.

Table 11.20: Pupillary abnormalities in an unconscious patient

Pupil appearance	Etiology/Localization
Small, reactive	Metabolic, hypothalamic (interruption of descending sympathetic pathway)
Pinpoint, reactive	Pontine lesions, opiate poisoning
Mid-position, fixed	Midbrain (both sympathetic and parasympathetic paralysis)
Ipsilateral pupil dilated, fixed	Oculomotor nerve, uncal herniation
Bilateral dilated, fixed	Midbrain lesions, bilateral oculomotor nerve paralysis, severe hypoxic–ischemic encephalopathy

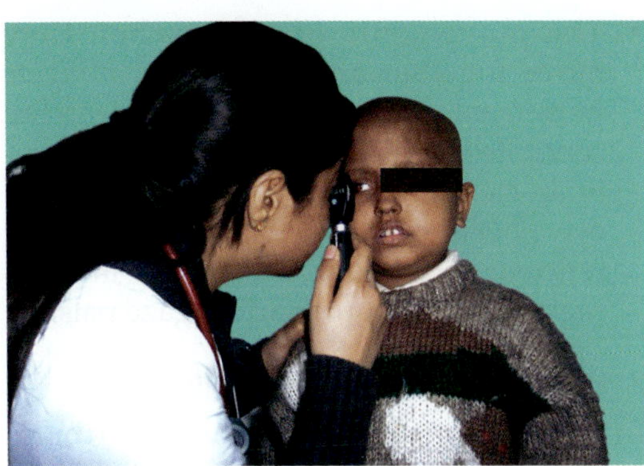

Fig. 11.28: Fundus examination.

- Ask the child to fixate on a fixed point far away.
- Bring the ophthalmoscope from a far distance, and look for the red reflex.
- *Look for the retinal vessels:* Arteries are bright and thin with central silver line, veins are dull looking, thicker and pulsate; severe attenuation/narrowing of vessels is an early sign of retinitis pigmentosa **(Fig. 11.29)**.
- Locate a vessel and follow it till the optic disc.
- *Optic disc:* Note color (yellow/light pink/red/chalky white), disc margins (well defined or blurred), and optic cup. Loss of venous pulsations, disc hyperemia, blurred disc margins, and disc hemorrhages are serial signs of papilledema.
- Nasal margin of optic disc is slightly blurred in some normal individuals also.
- *Look at the macula:* This is a little yellow area in the darker peripheral retina, and is located 2 disc diameters temporal to the disc. Look for a *cherry red spot*.
- Look at rest of the retina. Look for hemorrhages/exudates/bony spicules/granulomas.

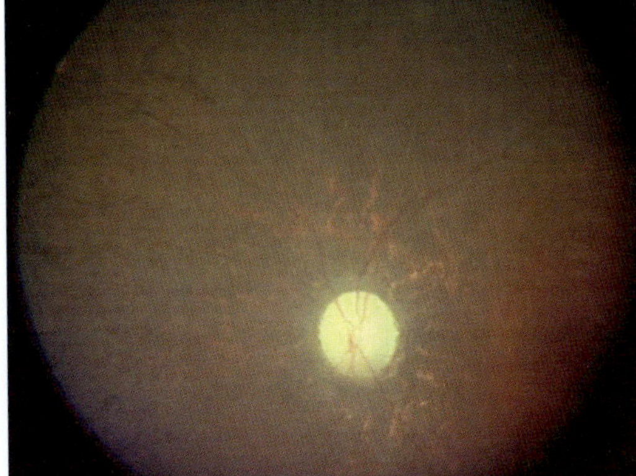

Fig. 11.29: Retinitis pigmentosa. Note the pale disc, peripheral pigment deposition, and attenuated retinal vessels.

Papilledema: Papilledema means a blurred or elevated optic nerve head or disc **(Fig. 11.30)**. Most often, papilledema results from transmission of increased intracranial pressure into the eye via the subarachnoid space, which extends out along the optic nerve. The retinal veins converge on the optic papilla to form the ophthalmic vein, which enters the retinal end of the optic nerve. If the pressure around the vein increases, it collapses, obstructing the retinal veins. The retinal veins distend and leak fluid into the nerve fibers on the optic papilla and into the surrounding retina. Severity of papilledema is staged as in **Key Box 14**. The veins may rupture, causing visible hemorrhages on or around the papilla.

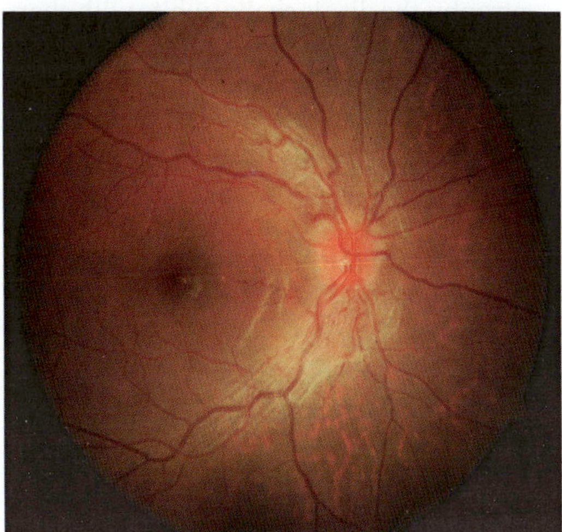

Fig. 11.30: Papilledema.

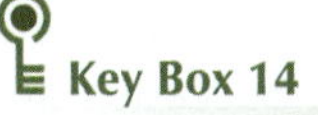

Key Box 14

Staging of Papilledema

Stage 1: Engorged veins and loss of venous pulsations

Stage 2: Nasal blurring, the physiological cup obliterates

Stage 3: Swollen optic cup, temporal blurring

Stage 4: Linear peripapillary hemorrhages, vessels disappear into the disc, retinal exudates

Papilledema needs to be differentiated from papillitis which is unilateral, degree of cup swelling is less, veins are not engorged, humping of veins is only slight, disc area not greatly enlarged and clinically vision is often affected (in contrast to papilledema where vision is not affected until late stage). It is important to know that when only optic nerve head is elevated without any surrounding edema, one should also think of pseudopapilledema. This can be correlated clinically when the child does not have any clinical or radiological evidence of raised intracranial pressure.

Optic atrophy: In optic atrophy, the disc is paler than normal and more sharply demarcated from the surrounding retina. The physiological cup may be abnormally prominent. Loss of myelinated axons and their surrounding capillaries with replacement by gliotic scar produce the lack of color. Optic atrophy may be primary or secondary.

- *Primary optic atrophy* results from lesions of the optic nerve or retina. In primary optic atrophy, the disc is chalky white with sharp margins.
- *Secondary optic atrophy* results due to long-standing papilledema or papillitis. In secondary optic atrophy, the disc is gray with shaggy margins.

C. Oculomotor (3rd), Trochlear (4th) and Abducens (6th) Nerves

The 3rd, 4th, and 6th cranial nerves control the movements of upper eyelid, eyeball, and pupils. They help in finding, fixating, focusing, and following a visual target. These three nerves are tested together.

1. Eye Movements

Eye movements can be divided into various types.

- *Saccades* are rapid eye movements from one point of fixation to another. Saccades are mediated by the frontal lobe.
- *Pursuit* eye movements are slow eye movements that are used to maintain fixation on a moving target. They are mediated by parieto-occipital temporal lobe.
- *Vestibulo-ocular* eye movements are eye movements that compensate for movement of the head to maintain fixation.
- The movements of eyes, when they move together are known as *conjugate* movements. The conjugate movements are controlled by centers in the frontal lobe and brain-stem (pons and midbrain). Vertical eye movements are mediated by midbrain reticular formation. Any lesions in these regions lead to supranuclear gaze palsies.

2. Physiology of Eye Movements

In the brainstem, inputs from the frontal and occipital lobes and the cerebellum and vestibular nuclei are integrated so that both the eyes move together. These are mediated by the center for the lateral gaze in the pons and the medial longitudinal fasciculus which connects the nuclei of 3rd, 4th, and 6th cranial nerves. Different pathways mediate conjugate vertical and horizontal eye movements.

Horizontal eye movements: The pathway for voluntary conjugate horizontal eye movements begins in the frontal lobe cortex (posterior inferior part) and runs to the pontine tegmentum. This cortical pathway terminates in the opposite paramedian pontine reticular formation (PPRF). The medial longitudinal fasciculus connects the PPRF to the 3rd, and 6th nerve nuclei. This pathway mediates lateral gaze to the opposite side. Therefore, the right frontal lobe center will mediate the lateral gaze to the left and vice versa (Fig. 11.31).

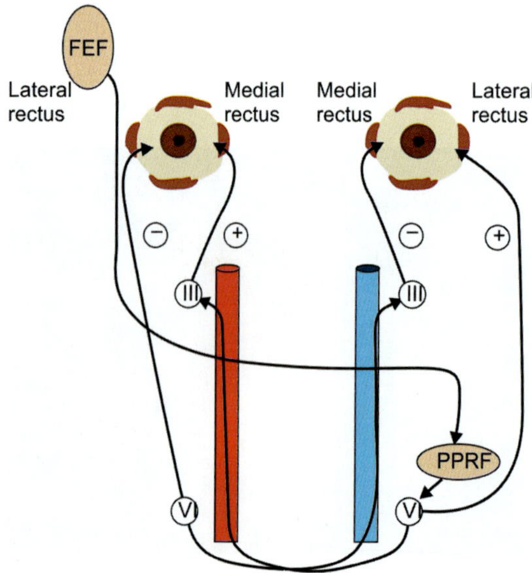

Fig. 11.31: Supranuclear control of horizontal eye movement.

- ***Supranuclear vs. infranuclear gaze palsy:*** Inability to move eyes in one direction of the gaze is called gaze palsy. For example, inability to move the eyes to left side but able to move the eyes to right side is left-sided gaze palsy. As we learnt that gaze centers have supranuclear control, they can also result from lesion at the level of brainstem as in PPRF/MLF (*nuclear gaze palsy*). Clinically, the two can be differentiated from each other by testing for other brainstem reflexes (e.g. corneal reflex, pupil reaction). If brainstem reflexes are intact, then gaze palsy is supranuclear and if absent, it indicates nuclear or infranuclear lesion.
- ***Direction of gaze:*** Interruption of the cortical efferent pathway for horizontal gaze above the decussation results in eye deviation as the same side as the lesion, because the opposite pathways are intact. For example, a destructive frontal lobe lesion on the left side affecting the gaze center will result in eye deviation towards the left. In contrast, an irritative left-sided frontal lesion will result in tonic deviation of eyes to right side. Hence destructive lesion = same side and irritative cortical lesion = opposite side. It is easy to remember "we tend to look away from irritative people and we look towards people who got destroyed". However, a pontine lesion on the left side will lead to gaze deviation towards the right.
- ***Other lesions:*** Interruption of the medial longitudinal fasciculus leads to internuclear ophthalmoplegia. In this condition, during horizontal gaze, the child cannot adduct the eye ipsilateral to the lesion, and develops nystagmus of the contralateral abducting eye. Interruption of both medial longitudinal fasciculus and PPRF on one side leads to gaze palsy on that side and loss of adduction of ipsilateral eye to opposite side. Hence the only movement possible is abduction to opposite side, or in other words, rest of 1½ movements are not possible (one and half syndrome). Other eye movements including vertical gaze and pupillary responses remain normal.

Vertical eye movements: Pathways for vertical eye movements arise diffusely from parieto-temporal and occipital cortices and project to the midbrain. The pathway for upward eye movements runs dorsal to the pathway for downward movements.

3. Extraocular Muscles

All the extraocular muscles are supplied by 3rd nerve except lateral rectus (which is supplied by the sixth nerve) and superior oblique (which is supplied by the 4th nerve). All muscles have their origin at annulus of Zinn at the apex of orbit except inferior oblique which originates from inferomedial rim of the bony orbit **(Fig. 11.32)**.

- The 3rd cranial nerve emerges between the cerebral peduncles of the midbrain.
- The 4th cranial nerve courses posteriorly and decussates a short distance from its

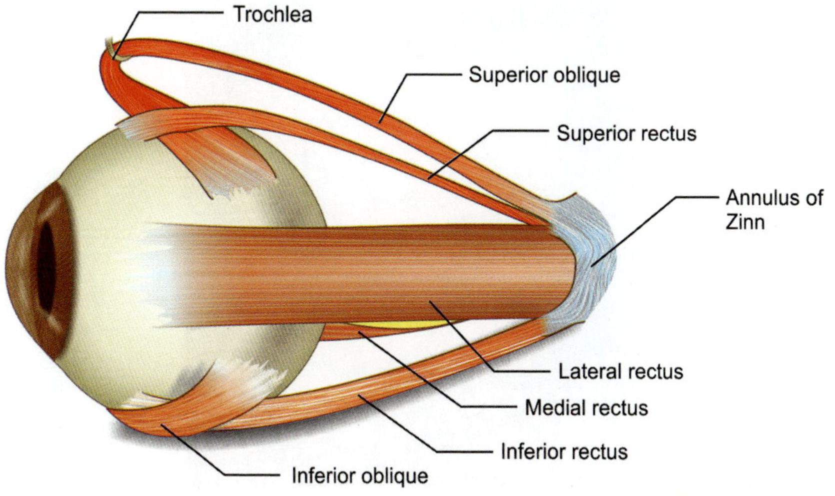

Fig. 11.32: Muscles of the eyeball.

origin before emerging from the dorsal surface of the brainstem, just caudal to the inferior colliculi. It, therefore, innervates the contralateral superior oblique muscle.

- The 6th cranial nerve arises at the level of the lower pons. It has a very long intracranial course, and may get affected by any lesion causing raised intracranial pressure. Therefore, a 6th nerve palsy is frequently a false localizing sign in children with raised intracranial pressure.

4. Principle of Testing

Actions of extraocular muscles are summarized in **Table 11.21**. The medial and lateral recti have only the primary actions of adduction and abduction, respectively. However, the other muscles (superior and inferior recti, and superior and inferior obliques) have multiple actions, because of their oblique attachments on the eyeball, and consequent direction of pull **(Figs 11.33 and 11.34)**. For example, the superior rectus elevates (primary action) and adducts (secondary action). Hence to test the pure elevation action of the superior rectus, you should first ask the child to abduct his eye (so that the secondary adduction action is counteracted) and then elevate. In the abducted position, superior and inferior recti act as pure elevators and depressors, respectively. Similarly, in the adducted eye, the superior and inferior obliques act as pure depressors and elevators, respectively.

5. Examination of Eye Movements

- ***Eyeball position:*** See if there is any enophthalmos or exophthalmos.

Table 11.21: Actions of extraocular muscles

Muscle	Primary action	Secondary action	Tertiary action
Medial rectus	Adduction	—	—
Lateral rectus	Abduction	—	—
Superior rectus	Elevation	Adduction	Intorsion
Inferior rectus	Depression	Adduction	Extorsion
Superior oblique	Depression	Abduction	Intorsion
Inferior oblique	Elevation	Abduction	Extorsion
Levator palpebrae superioris	Elevation of eyelid		

*Remember the mnemonics SIn and RAd (Superiors are Intortors, and Recti are Adductors)

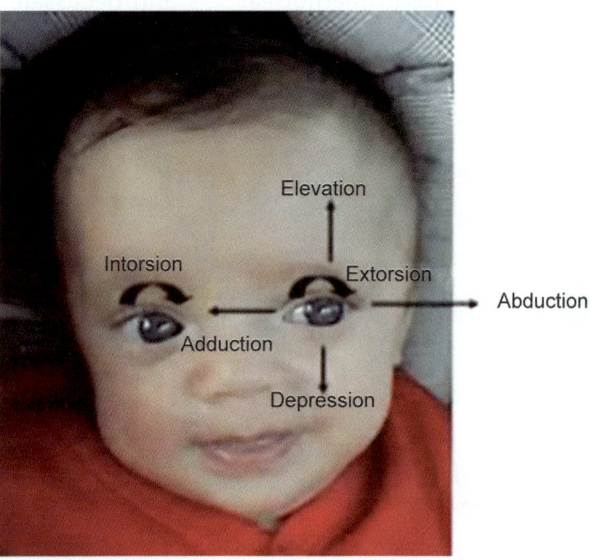

Fig. 11.33: Eye movement terminology.

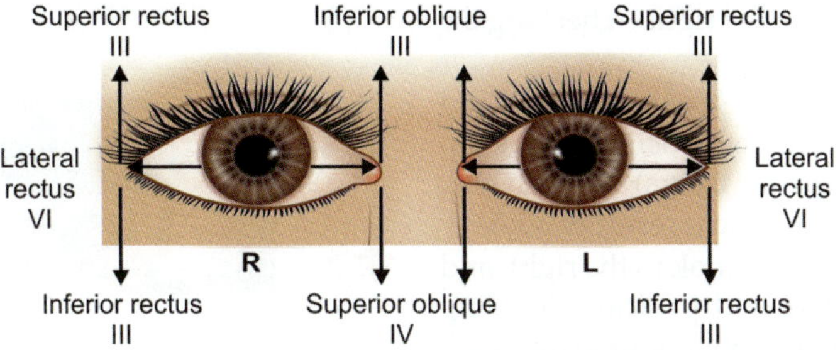

Fig. 11.34: Actions of extraocular muscles.

- ***For ptosis:*** Compare the distance between lid margin and corneal light reflection (margin-reflex distance). This is decreased in ptosis with drooping of eye lid **(Fig. 11.35)**. Most common cause of unilateral complete ptosis is 3rd CN palsy. Unilateral partial ptosis is seen in Horner syndrome. Bilateral mild ptosis is often seen in myasthenia gravis, or ocular myopathy.
- ***Ocular alignment***
  - ***Hirschberg test* (Fig. 11.36):** This is a test for manifest squint. Beam a torch light into the eyes and observe the position of corneal light reflection. The reflection is normally at the center of cornea; in case of ocular misalignment (as in squint), the position changes (shift to nasal, temporal, upwards or downwards). Manifest squint can be esotropia (eye is adducted at neutral position) or exotropia (eye is abducted at neutral position) **(Fig. 11.37)**.
  - ***Cover test:*** This is a test for latent squint, where the squint is not evident on neutral gaze. Ask the child to look with both eyes at your right eye. Cover his left eye. Then uncover his left eye rapidly and cover the right eye. Look to see if the left eye has to correct to look back at your eye. Repeat covering the left eye and watching the right eye. If one eye has to correct as it is uncovered, this indicates that the child has a latent squint. *See* Chapter 12 for pictorial depiction.
- ***Testing the extraocular muscles* (Fig. 11.37):**
  - Test one eye at a time.
  - Fix the position of head; ask the child not to move the head when moving the eyes.
  - Testing the left eye:
    - Ask the child to look to the left—checking lateral rectus, and then ask

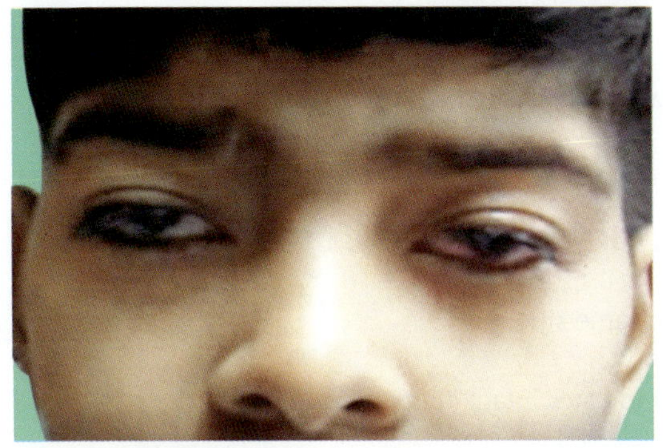

Fig. 11.35: Bilateral ptosis in a child with myasthenia gravis.

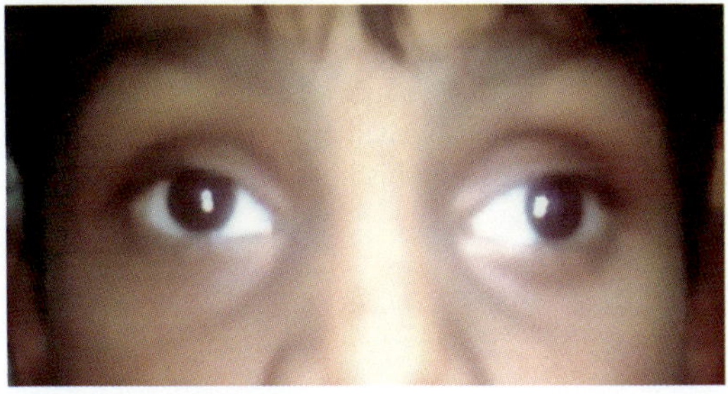

Fig. 11.36: Hirschberg test.

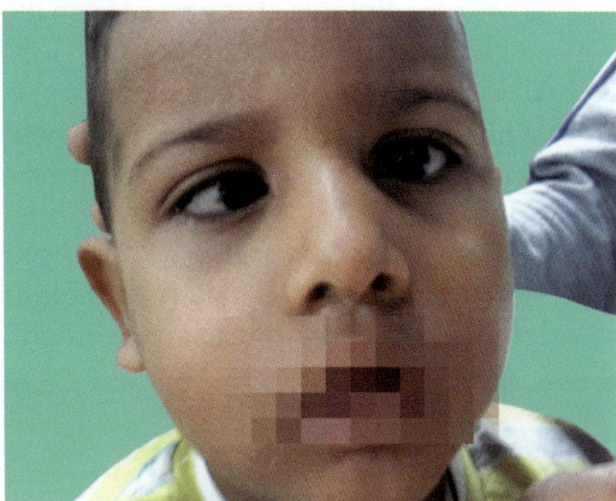

Fig. 11.37: Manifest squint in a child.

him to look to the right—checking the medial rectus.

- Then ask him to look to the left, and in that abducted position, look up (testing superior rectus) and then look down (testing the inferior rectus).
- Then ask him to look to the right, and in that adducted position, look up (testing inferior oblique) and then look down (testing the superior oblique).
- Ask for diplopia at any point from the child ("do you see two fingers?").
- Repeat the procedure in the right eye.

– While testing for extraocular movement of each eye examiner's fingers forms a English letter "H" (Fig. 11.38).

– If there is 6th CN palsy on the right side: When child is asked to look at left, there is conjugate eye movement; when child is asked to look at right, there is lack of abduction of right eye but normal adduction of left eye suggestive of right 6th cranial nerve palsy (Fig. 11.39).

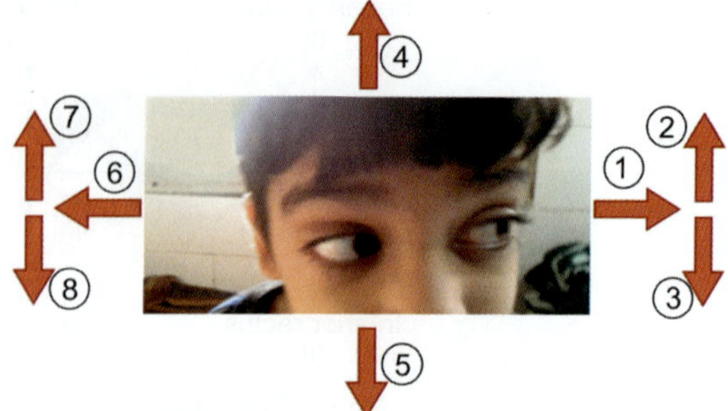

Fig. 11.38: Testing extraocular movement.

Key Box 15 summarizes the features suggestive of 3rd and 4th cranial nerve palsy also.

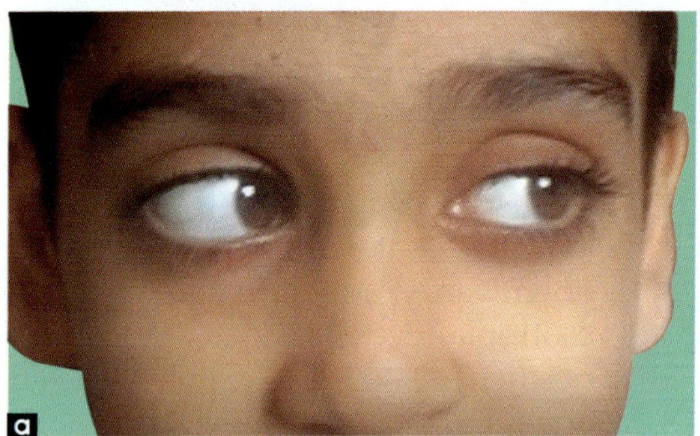

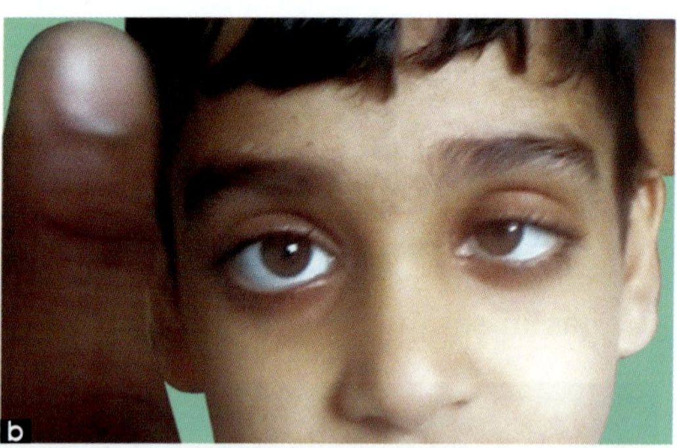

Fig. 11.39: Right sixth cranial nerve palsy evident when child is asked to look at left (a) and right (b).

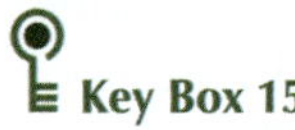

Key Box 15

Features of 3rd, 4th, 6th Nerve Palsy

A. 3rd Nerve Palsy

- Ptosis (Margin-reflex distance decreased) on the same side
- Eyeball—down (SO) and out (LR)
- Intorsion of the globe in attempted downgaze (indicates intact 4th nerve)
- Mydriasis (affected pupil is dilated)
- Pupils can be reactive to light (pupil sparing 3rd CN palsy) or not reactive to light (as seen in posterior communicating artery (PCOM) aneurysm as it compresses the 3rd CN at its exit)

B. 4th Nerve Palsy

- Superior oblique paralyzed (depress, intorts, abducts), SO is strongest depressor in adducted position. Hence, if there is right 4th CN palsy, on looking at right side, both eyes move conjugate but when asked to look at left, left eye will move but right eye which adducting eye will move up as depression at adducted position is lost. Hence to compensate, this patient will tilt his head to right side.
- Very subtle diplopia when walking downstairs or reading book

C. 6th Nerve Palsy (Fig. 11.38)

- Inability to abduct the eye to the side of lesion
- Paralytic squint worse in the direction of action
- Esotropia in primary position

- ***Testing oculomotor apraxia:*** Ask the child not to move his head or you may ask the parents to hold the head. Stand in front of the child and keeps both your hands wide apart and flicker the fingers. Instructs the child to look immediately at the side of flickering of fingers. Change the side of flickering finger rapidly. Look for saccadic movement of eyes trying to catch flickering finger from right side to left side and back.

Lack of saccadic pursuit movements is called oculomotor apraxia. The child, instead of moving the eyes to fix on rapidly changing direction, will move the head to follow that object **(Fig. 11.40)**.

- Look for evidence of nystagmus.
- Look for direction of nystagmus, do they increase or decrease with any direction of gaze (gaze-evoked nystagmus), does the child achieve any head tilt to achieve a null point in which nystagmus is least.

Congenital nystagmus is usually horizontal, never gaze evoked, they achieve a null point by turning/tilting their head, decreases with convergence. In contrast, in acquired lesions like cerebellar/brainstem, nystagmus are gaze evoked nystagmus.

Ophthalmoplegia: Paralysis of muscles of eye.

- ***External ophthalmoplegia:*** Paralysis of extraocular muscles with resultant restricted eye movements. Child will move the entire head to follow the fingers instead of eyes alone while testing for extraocular muscle movement.
- ***Internal ophthalmoplegia:*** Paralysis of muscles responsible for pupillary reactions.

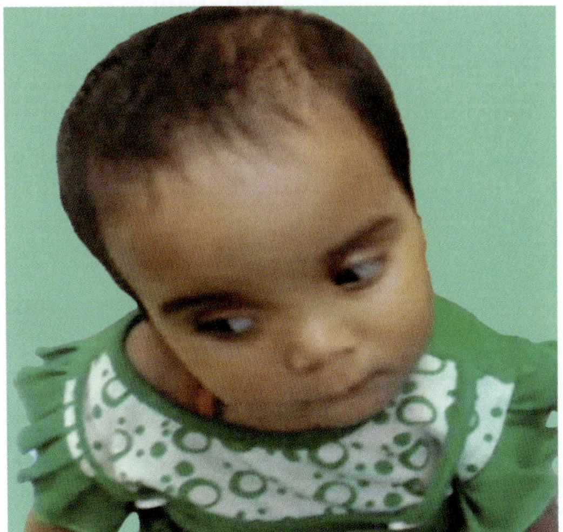

Fig. 11.40: Oculomotor apraxia where the child tilts the head and follows the object by moving her head instead of moving her eyes.

Examination of Eye Movements in Unconscious Children

- Conjugate lateral deviation of the eyes is a sign either of an ipsilateral hemisphere lesion, a contralateral hemisphere seizure focus, or damage involving the contralateral pontine horizontal gaze center (parapontine reticular formation).
- Lateral gaze palsy may signal central herniation with compression of bilateral sixth nerves.
- Tonic upward gaze has been associated with bilateral hemispheric damage.
- Ocular bobbing, a rapid downward jerk followed by a slow return to midposition, is indicative of pontine lesions.
- Rapid intermittent horizontal eye movements suggest seizure activity.

Doll's Eye Movements

The oculocephalic or doll's eye maneuver **(Fig. 11.41)** is performed by moving the head side-to-side or vertically, and should only be performed when it is certain that there is no cervical spine injury. A positive response in a

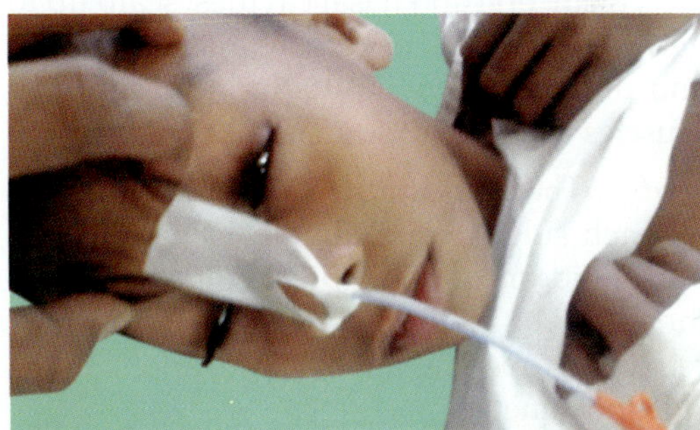

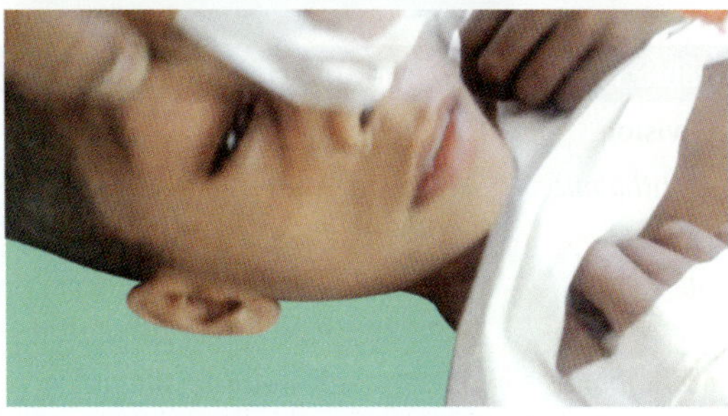

Fig. 11.41: Oculocephalic maneuver in an unconscious child.

comatose child consists of conjugate deviation of the eyes in the direction opposite head movement. Absent response may be seen in structural brainstem abnormalities, where it may be asymmetric, and in metabolic-toxic encephalopathies, where it is almost always symmetrical.

D. Trigeminal Nerve

This is the largest of the cranial nerves. It has both motor and sensory components.

Anatomy

There are one motor nucleus and three sensory (chief sensory nucleus, mesencephalic nucleus, and nucleus of descending tract) nuclei.

- The motor and chief sensory (touch and pressure) nuclei are located in mid-pons.
- Mesencephalic nucleus is located in the mid- brain. Mesencephalic root receives proprioceptive inputs from masticatory muscles.
- The spinal tract and nucleus (pain and temperature) extend from pons down to upper cervical cord.

Functions

Sensory: The three divisions of the fifth cranial nerve (ophthalmic, maxillary, and mandibular) arise from Gasserian ganglion and innervate face, teeth, oral and nasal cavities, scalp up to vertex, intracranial dura, cerebral vasculature and proprioceptive inputs from masticatory muscles **(Table 11.22, Fig. 11.42)**.

Motor: There are four masticatory muscles on each side: Temporalis, masseter, medial pterygoid and lateral pterygoid. Chewing movements include: Jaw protrusion and retraction, opening and closure, and side-to-side movement.

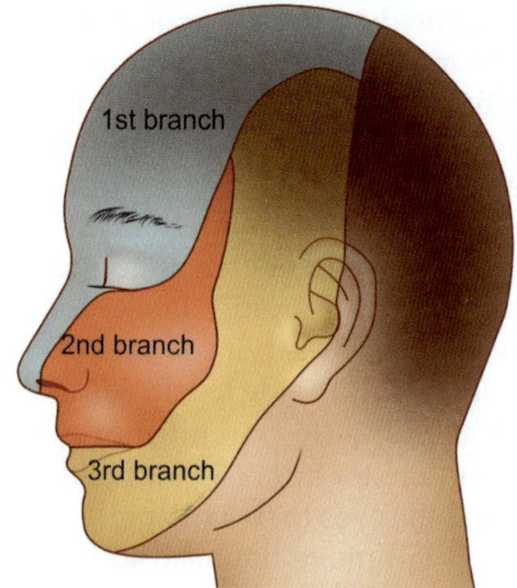

Fig. 11.42: Divisions of the trigeminal nerve with their areas of cutaneous innervations.

- **T**emporalis: **R**etracts the jaw; all others protrude
- Lateral pterygoids: **O**pen the jaw; all others close
- Medial and lateral pterygoids of one side "**push**" the jaw to opposite side

Therefore, in trigeminal nerve palsy, there will be jaw deviation towards the affected side.

These actions can be remembered by a mnemonic "**Push..TR..OLey**".

Examination

- ***Look:*** Look for hollow temple, flattened cheek, deviation of jaw and dangling jaw. Bilateral 5th CN lesion as seen in bilateral supranuclear lesion will result in dangling jaw.
- ***Feel:*** Keep the fingers across the anterior border of masseter and ask the child to clench teeth and feel the bulk of masseter.
- ***Do:*** Ask the child to perform these maneuvers to test the masticatory muscles:

Table 11.22: Divisions of the trigeminal nerve with their cutaneous innervations

Division	Cutaneous innervations
Ophthalmic	Bridge and side of nose, upper eyelid, cornea, forehead, scalp up to vertex, eyeball, lacrimal gland, nasal septum, lateral wall of nasal cavity, ethmoid sinus
Maxillary	Cheek, lateral forehead, side of nose, upper lip, upper teeth and gums, palate, nasopharynx, meninges of anterior and middle cranial fossa
Mandibular	Inner cheek, temple, lateral scalp, external auditory meatus, tympanic membrane, temporomandibular joint, mandible except angle, lower teeth and gums, anterior 2/3rd of tongue, lower lip, chin, meninges of anterior and middle cranial fossa

i. Open and close jaw (with and without resistance)
ii. Protrude and retract the jaw (with and without resistance)
iii. Move the jaw from side to side against resistance

If there is right 5th CN palsy, jaw will deviate to right side on spontaneous jaw opening and he cannot move the jaw to left side on command. While looking for jaw deviation, look at incisors rather than looking at lips to judge presence or absence of deviation.

Sensations

- With a wisp of cotton, test the touch sensation in all three divisions of trigeminal nerve on both the sides (Fig. 11.43).
- Remember the question to child is NOT Do you feel the cotton sensation? It should be does it feel the same on both sides?
- Cold and hot water (30°C and 44°C, respectively) are used to test temperature.
- Pain is tested using a pin. This can be omitted in children, if the temperature sensation is normal, because both these sensations are carried in the spinal tract of the trigeminal nerve.

Jaw Jerk

Tapping the chin with the jaw muscles relaxed stimulates proprioceptive afferents that terminate in the mesencephalic nucleus of the midbrain, which sends collaterals to the motor nucleus of the fifth nerve and causes the masseters to contract.

Ask the child to open his mouth a little. Place your finger on the child's chin. Strike your finger with a reflex hammer. Normally, there is no appreciable movement. Jaw jerk is exaggerated when there is clearly visible movement of jaw (closure), indicating an upper motor neuron lesion of the 5th cranial nerve as in pseudobulbar palsy.

Corneal Reflex

Be very careful of asepsis when you perform this test. The eyes should be open. Touch the limbus of the cornea with a strand of cotton from side and below (Fig. 11.44). Do NOT go near the center. Normally, blink response is observed on both ipsilateral and contralateral side.

This test must first be explained to the child, otherwise he will undoubtedly flinch if some object is brought near his eye (menace response). Also remember that it must be the cornea, and not the lids, lashes or conjunctiva that should be touched!

Observe the reflex blink of both eyes. Corneal reflex is absent in 5th nerve lesion (afferent) affecting ophthalmic division; and in lower motor neuron type of 5th nerve paralysis (efferent) as the orbicularis oculi muscle is paralyzed.

- *If there is a 5th cranial nerve lesion*, there will be no response from either lid when the abnormal side is stimulated, and a normal response from both lids when the normal side is stimulated.
- *In 7th cranial nerve lesions*, there will be no response from the side of the facial paralysis

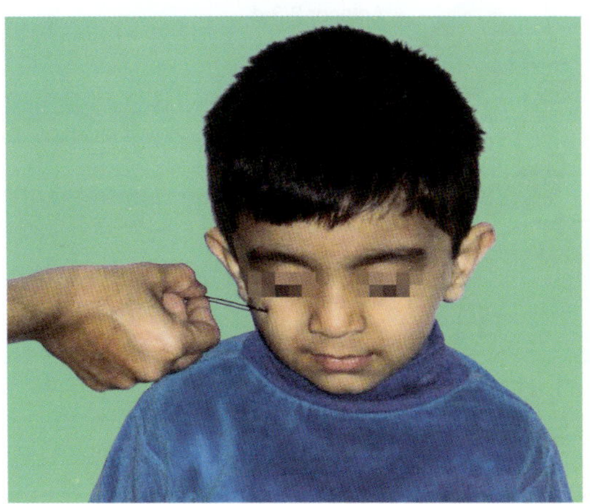

Fig. 11.43: Testing sensations of face.

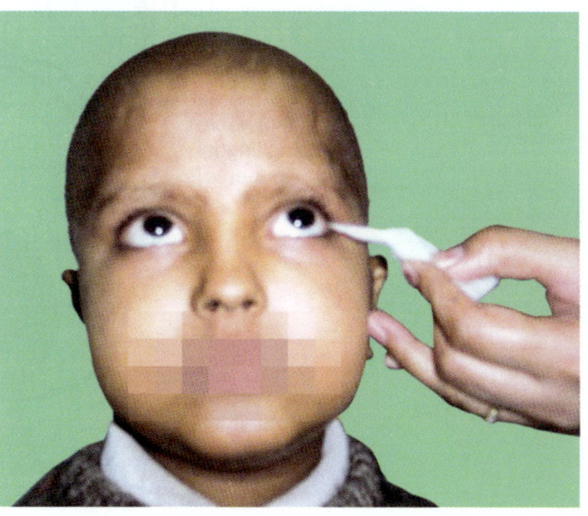

Fig. 11.44: Testing corneal reflex.

no matter which side is stimulated, but if the 5th nerve is intact, there will be a blink on the normal side even when the abnormal side is stimulated.

E. Facial Nerve

1. Anatomy

The seventh nerve is mainly a motor nerve, supplying all the muscles concerned with facial expression on one side.

- ***Taste sensation anterior 2/3rd of tongue:*** The sensory component is small; it conveys taste sensation from the anterior two-thirds of the tongue through the chorda tympani, which conveys taste sensation via the facial nerve to the nucleus of the tractus solitarius.
- ***Secretomotor fibers:*** These fibers innervate the lacrimal gland through the greater superficial petrosal nerve and the sublingual and submaxillary glands through the chorda tympani.
- ***Motor supply to facial muscles:*** The motor nucleus of the seventh nerve lies ventral and lateral to the abducens nucleus in the pons. Facial nerve emerges and enters the internal auditory meatus with the acoustic nerve and then bends sharply forward and downward around the anterior boundary of the vestibule of the inner ear. At this angle (*genu*) lies the sensory ganglion (named *geniculate* because of its proximity to the genu). The nerve continues in its own bony channel, the facial canal, within which, just distal to the geniculate ganglion, it provides a branch to the pterygopalatine ganglion, i.e. the greater superficial petrosal nerve; somewhat more distally, it gives off a small branch to the stapedius muscle (nerve to stapedius) and is joined by the chorda tympani. It makes its exit from the skull at the stylomastoid foramen and then passes through the parotid gland and subdivides into 5 branches that supply the facial muscles, the stylomastoid muscle, the platysma, and the posterior belly of the digastric muscle (Fig. 11.45).

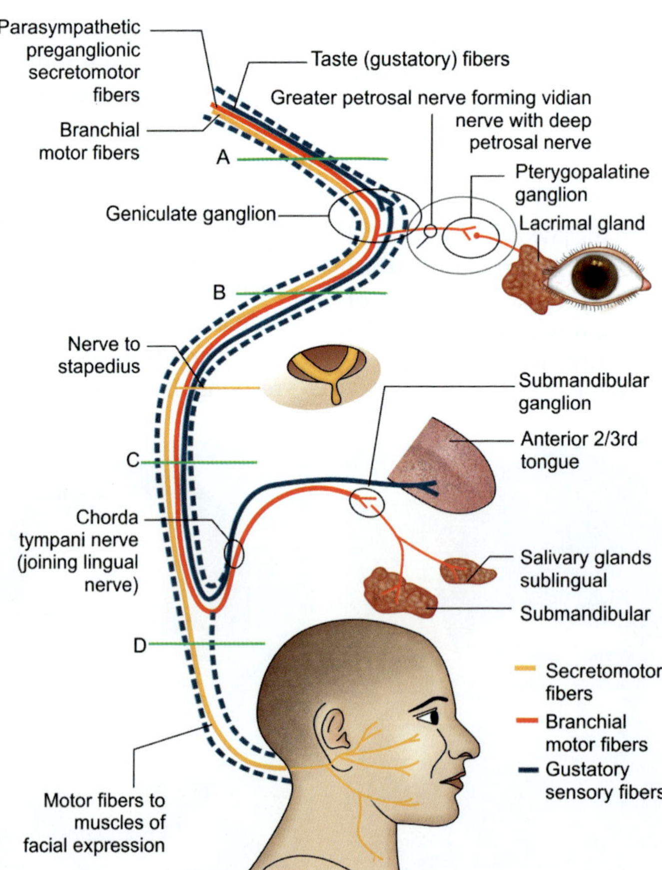

Fig. 11.45 Branches of facial nerve.

2. Functions and Lesion of the Facial Nerve

The functions of facial nerve are summarized in **Key Box 16**. A complete interruption of the facial nerve at the stylomastoid foramen paralyzes all muscles of facial expression **[Fig. 11.45(D)]**. The corner of the mouth droops, the creases and skin folds are effaced, the forehead is unfurrowed, the palpebral fissure is widened, and the eyelids will not close **(Fig. 11.46)**. Upon attempted closure of the lids, both eyes roll upward (Bell phenomenon), but the one on the paralyzed side remains visible because of lack of eyelid closure. The lower lid sags also, and the punctum falls away from the conjunctiva, permitting tears to spill over the cheek. Food collects between the teeth and cheek, and saliva may dribble from the corner of the mouth. The child complains of heaviness or numbness and sometimes an aching pain in the face, but sensory loss can usually not be demonstrated. Taste, however, is intact because the lesion is beyond the site where the chorda tympani has separated from the main trunk of the facial nerve.

If the lesion is in the facial canal above the junction with the chorda tympani but below the geniculate ganglion, all the preceding symptoms are present but in addition, taste is lost over the anterior two-thirds of the tongue on the same side **[Fig. 11.45(C)]**. The nerve to the stapedius muscle is also usually involved with a lesion at this site and there is hyperaccusis (painful sensitivity to loud sounds) **[Fig. 11.45(B)]**. If the geniculate ganglion or the motor root proximal to it is damaged, lacrimation and salivation may be reduced **[Fig. 11.45(A)]**. Lesions at this point may also affect the adjacent eighth nerve, causing deafness, tinnitus, or dizziness.

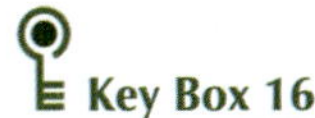

Key Box 16

Functions of Facial Nerve

1. Motor to all the muscles of facial expression and facial movements
2. Taste from the anterior 2/3rd of the tongue
3. Secretory fibers to the lacrimal and salivary glands

3. Motor Examination of the Facial Nerve

Inspection

- Examine the facial symmetry at rest and during spontaneous movements (e.g. talking, smiling, crying).
- Look at the folds in the forehead, eyelid position, width of palpebral fissure.
- Depth and symmetry of nasolabial folds.
- Look and notice the angle of the mouth.

Maneuvers: Ask the child to do the following **(Fig. 11.46)**:

- ***Shut the eyes tightly:*** Assess the strength of orbicularis oculi on the two sides. Normally it would be difficult to force open the eyes. Also look for Bell's phenomenon! (It's a normal phenomenon when one closes his eyes; it becomes visible due to inability to close the eyes).
- 'Blow out' the cheeks; whistle.
- Show the teeth; pout the lips. Look for any asymmetry.
- Retract the chin (to make platysma prominent).

Interpretation

- ***Unilateral lesions***
  - *Lower motor neuron lesions:* These are seen in Bell's palsy, pontine/cerebellopontine angle tumors;

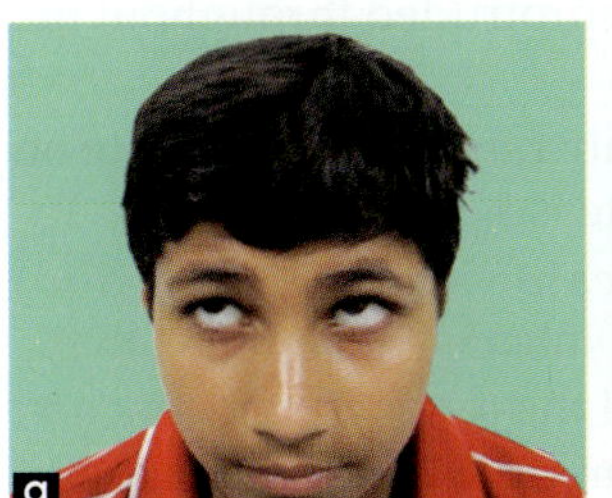

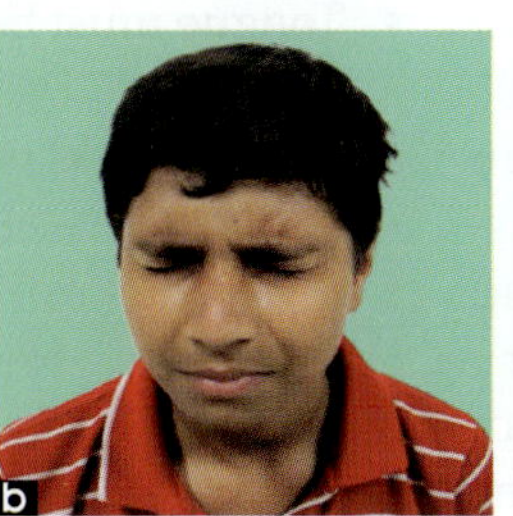

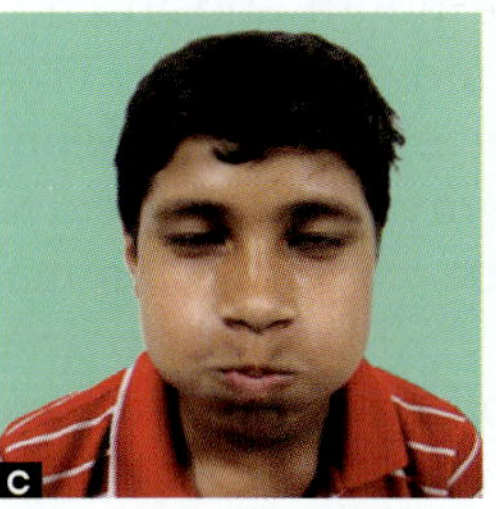

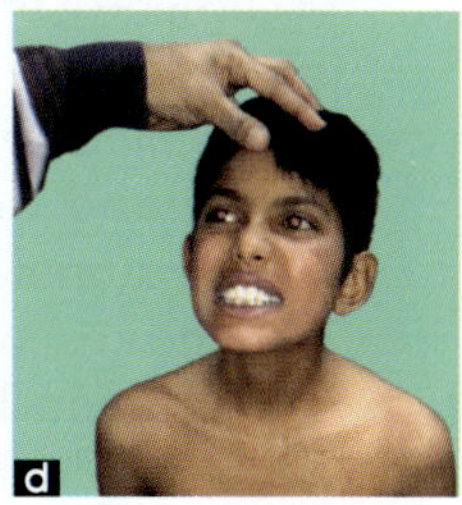

Fig. 11.46: Testing facial nerve motor function: a. Wrinkling the forehead, b. Close eyes, c. Holding air in the mouth, d. Looking for symmetry of nasolabial folds on both sides and lack of deviation of angle to mouth to either side suggestive of normal facial nerve.

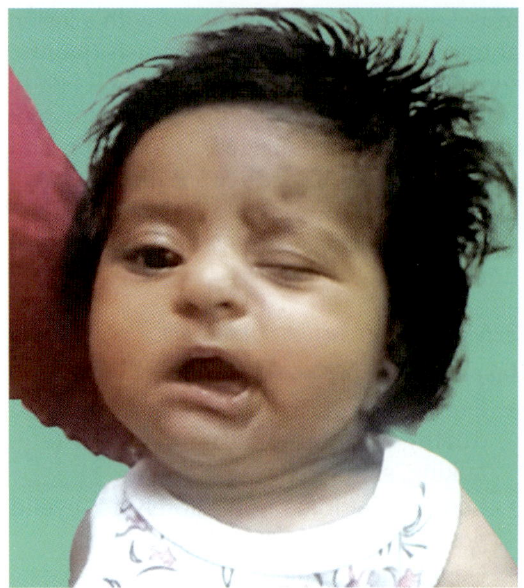

Fig. 11.47: Lower motor neuron type of facial palsy.

infections/tumors/trauma of the middle ear, and parotid tumors. Unilateral LMN lesions of the facial nerve are characterized by complete lack of ipsilateral facial movements. Eye closure is impaired, ipsilateral palpebral fissure is widened, ipsilateral nasolabial fold gets obliterated and the angle of the mouth deviates towards the opposite unaffected side as child tries to smile (Fig. 11.47).
  - *Upper motor neuron lesion (stroke):* Only the lower half of the face is affected and that too on the opposite side.
- ***Bilateral lesions (facial symmetry may be maintained)***
  - *Lower motor neuron lesion:* Seen in myopathies, myasthenia gravis, and Guillain-Barré syndrome. There is flattening of all normal folds, sagging of corners of the mouth, and absence of any voluntary movement (Fig. 11.48).
  - *Upper motor neuron lesions:* Seen in stroke and demyelinating lesions. Mouth cannot be moved on command but moves well during ordinary conversation, blinking is less affected. There can be fixed facial expressions among children with extrapyramidal involvement as in dyskinetic cerebral palsy (Fig. 11.49).

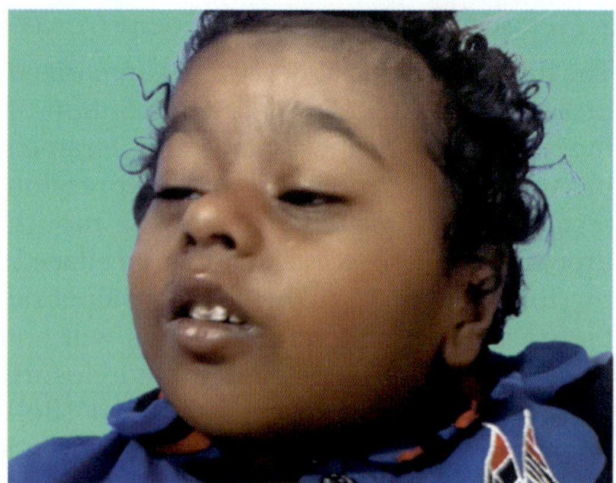

Fig. 11.48: Myopathic facies with bilateral ptosis in a child with congenital myasthenia.

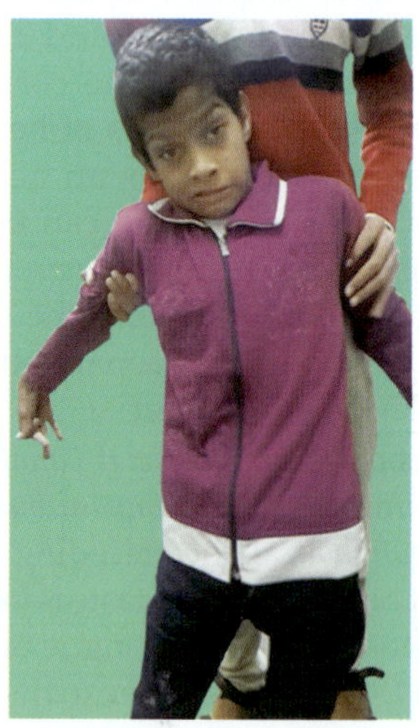

Fig. 11.49: Fixed facial expressions with oromandibular and generalized dystonia in a child with dyskinetic cerebral palsy secondary to kernicterus sequelae.

4. Sensory Component Examination

Taste from anterior 2/3rd of the tongue:

- *4 primary tastes are tested:* Bitter, sour, sweet, and salt.
- Tongue must be protruded throughout the testing.
- Child should only raise his hand/write on paper when taste is perceived.
- A damp applicator stick (e.g. earbud) coated with test substance is applied to the dorsal surface of the tongue at the junction of anterior and middle 2/3rd of tongue.
- Taste should be tested bilaterally.
- Mouth must be rinsed between the tests.
- Bitter should be tested in the end!

Interpretation
- Most children identify the taste in <10 seconds.
- If the child with LMN facial palsy has loss of taste, then the lesion is proximal to the origin of chorda tympani. A lesion at/distal to stylomastoid foramen does not affect taste.

F. Vestibulocochlear Nerve (8th Cranial Nerve)

The vestibulocochlear nerve has two components, the vestibular and cochlear, blended into a single trunk. The cochlear portion subserves hearing; the vestibular nerve subserves equilibrium, coordination, and orientation in space. The two components originate in separate peripheral receptors and have distinct central connections. Although they are united along their course through the skull, they differ so much both in their anatomical connections and their function, that they are considered separately.

I. The Cochlear Nerve

Anatomy: The cochlea contains the receptor (the organ of Corti) and the spiral ganglion, from which the cochlear nerve originates. The spiral ganglion contains the primary neurons for hearing. The cochlear and vestibular divisions of the 8th nerve run through the internal auditory canal, accompanied by the facial nerve. The 7th and 8th cranial nerves attach to the brainstem at the pontomedullary sulcus. The cochlear nerve fibers bifurcate to synapse in both dorsal and ventral cochlear nuclei. Fibers from dorsal cochlear nuclei and some fibers from ventral nucleus (intermediate acoustic stria) cross to the opposite side and join the contralateral lateral leminiscus. Fibers from the ventral nucleus (ventral acoustic stria) synapse in the superior olivary nucleus and then ascend as lateral leminiscus. Some fibers also synapse in the contralateral superior olivary complex. Fibers from the lateral leminiscus ascend to the medial geniculate body through the inferior colliculus. From the medial geniculate body, fibers pass through the posterior limb of internal capsule, through auditory radiations, and terminate in the cortex in the superior surface of the temporal lobe.

In ascending through the brainstem, as explained above, the auditory pathway disperses about equally ipsilaterally and bilaterally. Therefore if a child has a profound unilateral hearing loss, the lesion will most likely affect the auditory nerve, and not the auditory pathway or the auditory cortex.

Examination
- Ask the child if he has any problems in hearing. Young children with hearing problems present with speech delay.
- Perform otoscopy to ensure that the external auditory canals are open and the tympanic membrane is normal.
- *Free field test* (for screening purposes):
  - Examiner stands to the side of the ear to be tested.
  - Non-test ear is masked using tragal pressure.
  - Test the hearing for the following:
    - ❑ Whispered voice at 6 cm (15 dB)
    - ❑ Whispered voice at 15 cm (35 dB)
    - ❑ Conventional voice at 60 cm (50 dB)
    - ❑ Conventional voice at 15 cm (55–60 dB)
  - You can use a watch or crumpling of paper for screening.
  - Compare in both ears

Tuning fork tests: A 512 Hz tuning fork is used. Basically in these tests, air conduction (AC) and bone conduction (BC) are assessed.

1. *Rinne test* (Fig. 11.50)

First keep the vibrating tuning fork on the mastoid process (bone conduction) and ask the child to inform you when he stops hearing the sound. Then move it besides the ear (air conduction), and ask him if he can still hear it. It should still be audible.
- Normally, air conduction is better than bone conduction—*Rinne positive.*
- In conductive hearing loss, bone conduction is better than air conduction—*Rinne negative.*
- In sensorineural hearing loss, both air conduction and bone conduction are impaired while retaining their normal relationship of air conduction better than bone conduction—*Rinne positive.*

2. *Weber test* (Fig. 11.51)

The vibrating tuning fork is placed in the midline (vertex, nasal bridge, forehead, or

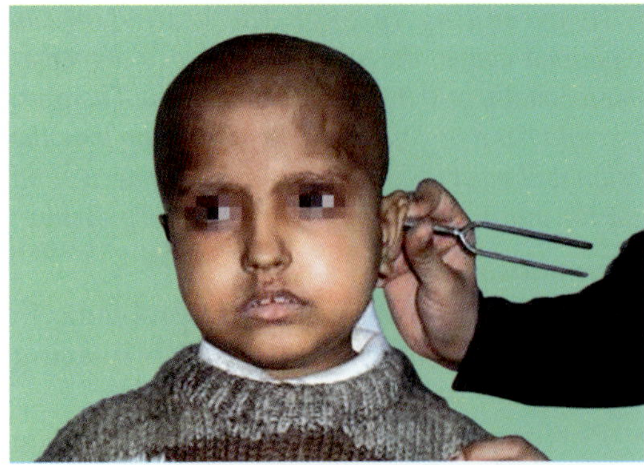

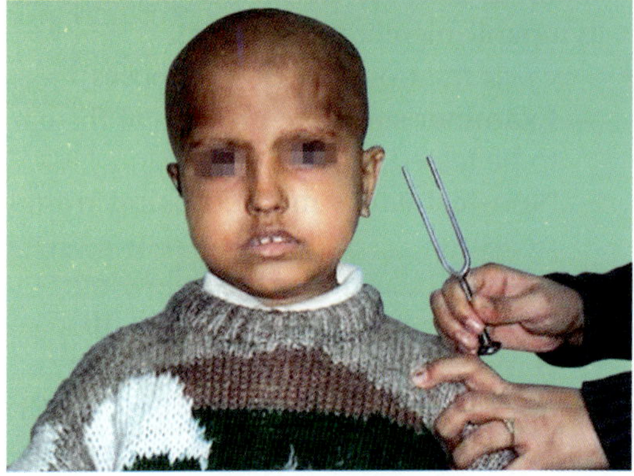

Fig. 11.50: Rinne test.

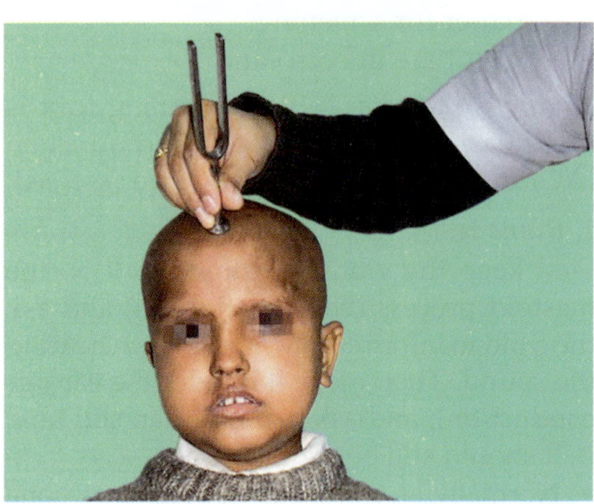

Fig. 11.51: Weber test.

maxilla) and child is asked 'In which ear is the fork better heard?'

- Normally the sound is equally heard in both the ears.
- In conducting hearing loss, sound is better heard in the involved ear. *Lateralized to the worse ear.*
- In sensorineural hearing loss, sound is heard best in the normal ear. *Lateralized to the normal side.*

3. Absolute bone conduction

Tuning fork is placed over the mastoid process of the child (after occlusion of external auditory canal). When the child is unable to hear the sound anymore, the fork is transferred to the mastoid process of the examiner (after occlusion of EAC).

- Normally, the examiner must not be able to hear the fork.
- In sensorineural hearing loss, examiner will be able to hear the sound. It is assumed that examiner's hearing is normal.

II. The Vestibular Nerve

Anatomy: The vestibule of the labyrinth connects with 5 structures that are involved in vestibular function: Utricle, saccule and the three semicircular canals. Each of these components lie in membranous labyrinth, is bathed in endolymph, and contains sensory neuroepithelium.

The central processes of the vestibular ganglion cells form the vestibular nerve. It joins the cochlear nerve and passes through the internal auditory canal, crosses cerebellopontine angle and enters the brainstem. The vestibular nuclei make connections with four primary areas: Cerebellum, spinal cord, oculomotor system and cortex.

Function

- Utricle and saccule (static labyrinth) detect gravitational effects and linear acceleration.
- Semicircular canals (dynamic labyrinth) detect the angular acceleration or rotation.

This information is relayed to cerebellum, cortex, spinal cord and oculomotor system and helps in maintaining balance and posture of the body.

Examination: Vestibular functions are not routinely tested. Indications include symptoms like dizziness, vertigo, tinnitus; and assessment of brainstem function in critically ill children.

Vestibulo-ocular reflexes

1. Oculocephalic test
    - Used for evaluation of comatose children.
    - Turning the head in one direction causes the eye to turn in the opposite direction.
    - This response indicates that brainstem is intact (pathways connecting the

vestibular nuclei to the extraocular nuclei are functioning).

2. Caloric test
   - Frequently used in comatose children to assess the brainstem integrity.
   - Instillation of cold water in one ear canal causes tonic deviation of eyes towards the side of irrigation in a comatose child with intact brainstem function.
   - Nystagmus is seen only when the cortex is functioning normally.
   - In an awake child, instillation of cold water (30°C) causes nystagmus with fast component away from the irrigated side.
   - Warm water (44°C) has the opposite effect. However, it is the slow component that is often appreciated clinically.

Remember the mnemonic 'COWS' for direction of fast component—Cold Opposite Warm Same.

Caloric Abnormalities

If there is no response, or a decreased response, to both warm and cold water on one side, this is termed *canal paresis*. It is caused by lesions of one labyrinth (Meniere disease), or vestibular nerve (e.g. acoustic nerve tumor), or lesions of the vestibular nuclei.

If the response is always reduced for irrigations producing nystagmus in the same direction (e.g. cold water in the right ear and warm water in the left), this is known as *directional preponderance*. This is a sign of imbalance between the two sides of the vestibular system, normally held in a state of equilibrium. This balance can be disturbed by lesions of the peripheral or central vestibular apparatus or of the cerebellum and corticofugal fibers deep in the temporal lobe.

G. The Glossopharyngeal (9th) and Vagus (10th) Nerves

Anatomy

The glossopharyngeal or the 9th cranial nerve arises from medulla as 3–6 rootlets which unite to form a single nerve, which leaves the skull through the jugular foramen. Subsequently, it enters the carotid sheath and reaches the lateral pharyngeal wall. It divides into its terminal branches under the hyoglossus muscle. Most of the pharyngeal muscles are supplied by both the 9th and the 10th cranial nerves except stylopharyngeus which is supplied by the 9th cranial nerve alone.

The vagus or the 10th cranial nerve also arises as a series of rootlets just below those of the glossopharyngeal nerve. It leaves the skull through jugular foramen, descends the neck in the carotid sheath and finally enters the thorax.

Functions

- To carry common sensations from the pharynx, tonsils, soft palate and posterior one-third of the tongue.
- To carry sense of taste from posterior one-third of the tongue (almost purely by the 9th cranial nerve).
- To give motor supply to the palatal and pharyngeal muscles.
- To give motor supply to the vocal cords (purely by the 10th cranial nerve).

Examination

The glossopharyngeal nerve is difficult to examine in isolation as most of its functions are shared by other nerves. It is not possible to isolate the motor functions from those of the vagus. Bedside testing of taste on the posterior third of the tongue is seldom attempted. So examination of both the nerves is done together.

- Note the pitch and quality of the child's voice.
- Note any nasal twang.
- Ask and observe for any difficulty in swallowing the saliva, and coughing.
- Observe and ask for nasal regurgitation of fluids (Fig. 11.52).
- Ask the child to open his mouth wide. Visualize the oropharynx.
- Ask the child to say 'Ah'
- Note the movements of palate, uvula and pharynx.

Interpretation

- High-pitched hoarse voice may indicate vocal cord palsy.
- Nasal tone, that increases if the head is bent forwards, signifies palatal paralysis.
- If the child chokes on his saliva, there may be both palatal and pharyngeal weakness.

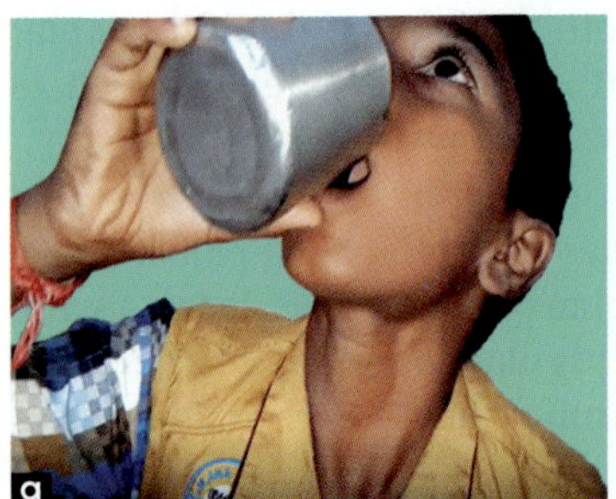

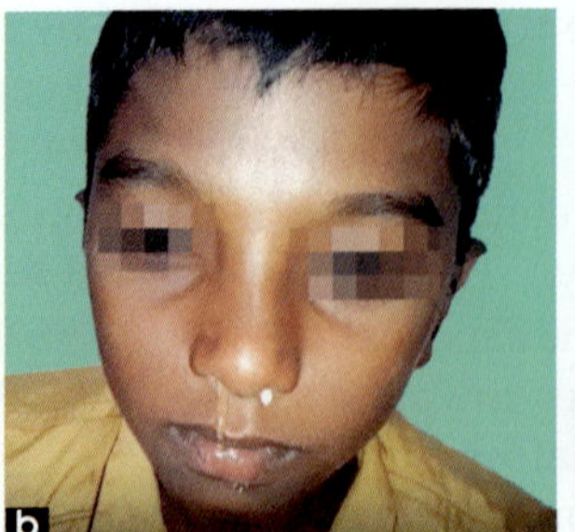

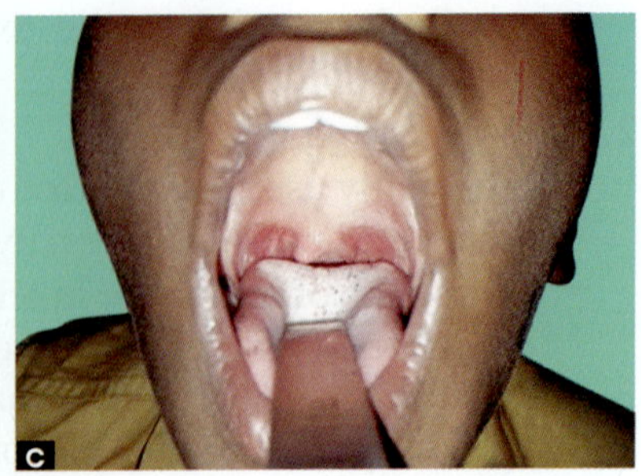

Fig. 11.52: (a, b) Nasal regurgitation of water in a child with 9/10th CN palsy. (c) Deviation of uvula to right side on phonation, suggestive of right-sided 9th/10th CN palsy.

- Flattening of the palatal arch (at rest) may be seen on the affected side in case of unilateral weakness.
- Normally, on phonation, palate moves symmetrically upwards and backwards, uvula remains in the midline and both sides of the pharynx contract symmetrically. Note any asymmetry.
  - *With unilateral lesion*, on phonation, medial raphe and uvula deviates towards the normal side; pharyngeal muscles also appear to move towards the normal side.
  - *Bilateral lesions:* No movement of palate and pharynx but may not droop on both sides owing to intact 5th cranial nerve.

Gag Reflex

This test is uncomfortable and should be done at the end of examination. In infants and young children, a feed can be observed. If the child appears to be swallowing well without any choking or drooling, testing for the gag reflex can be omitted.

The afferent limb of the reflex is mediated by 9th cranial nerve and the efferent limb through both 9th and 10th cranial nerves. The reflex center is in the medulla. Gag reflex has three motor components: Elevation of the soft palate, closure of the glottis, and constriction of the pharynx. Reflex is elicited by touching the lateral oropharynx in the region of anterior faucial pillar (*pharyngeal reflex*), one side of soft palate or uvula (*palatal reflex*), base of the tongue, or posterior pharyngeal wall. Observe all the three components; look for any asymmetry.

The gag reflex is a protective reflex. It is designed to prevent noxious substances or foreign objects from going beyond the oral cavity.

Interpretation

- Unilateral absence of the gag reflex may be due to loss of sensation, or motor power, or both. If due to loss of sensation alone, stimulation of the normal side will produce a normal symmetric reflex. This would be because of a lower motor neuron type of isolated 9th nerve palsy, which is extremely rare. It is important to remember that corticobulbar fibers to 9th cranial nerve has bilateral innervations, hence unilateral cortical lesion rarely produces clinical weakness.
- If the defect is due to combined motor and sensory paralysis, stimulation of the normal side will cause the palate to be pulled towards that side. This is a much more common scenario than the one mentioned above. This indicates a combined lesion of the 9th and 10th nerves.
- Hyperactive gag reflex may be seen in pseudobulbar palsy in children with cerebral palsy. This often results in retching and vomiting.

H. The Spinal Accessory Nerve

Anatomy

This is a purely motor nerve, of spinal rather than cranial origin. Its fibers arise from the anterior horn cells of the upper four or five cervical segments and enter the skull through the foramen magnum. Intracranially, the accessory nerve travels for a short distance with the part of the tenth nerve that is

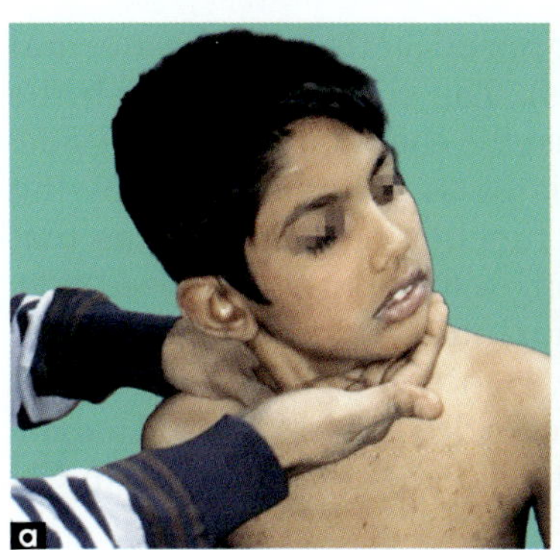
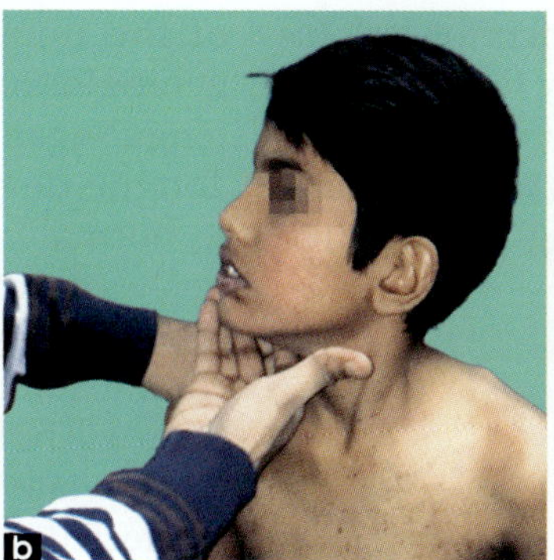
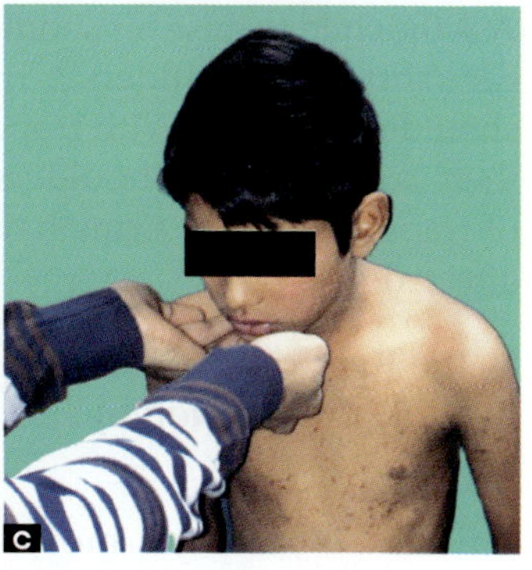

Fig. 11.53: Testing sternocleidomastoid (a) right (b) left and (c) both sides simultaneously.

derived from the caudal-most cells of the nucleus ambiguus. The two roots together leave the skull through the jugular foramen. The vagal fibers then rejoin the main trunk of the vagus. The motor fibers derived from the upper cervical segments of the spinal cord form an "external ramus" and innervate the ipsilateral sternocleidomastoid and trapezius muscles.

Functions

To supply motor power to sternocleidomastoid and trapezius.

Sternocleidomastoid: When one sternocleidomastoid muscle contracts, the occiput is pulled to the ipsilateral shoulder and face turns in the opposite direction and upward. Both sternocleidomastoid acting together flex the neck and bring the head forward and downward. With the head fixed, they help in elevation of thorax in forced inspiration.

Trapezius: When one muscle contracts (with shoulder fixed), head is drawn to that side. When both muscles contract, head is drawn backward and face is deviated upward. When head is fixed, trapezius elevates, retracts and rotates the scapula and assists in abduction of arm above horizontal.

Both sternocleidomastoid (SCM) and trapezius have bilateral supranuclear innervations. However, input to SCM motor neuron pool is predominantly unilateral, whereas that for trazepius is predominantly contralateral. Hence right cerebral hemispheric lesion will affect right SCM, hence will turn the head to left-side, not to right-side (SCM turns head to opposite side).

Examination

***Sternocleidomastoid* (Fig. 11.53):** Place one hand against right-side of child's face and ask him to turn his head against it. Observe for the prominence of left sternocleidomastoid muscle. Repeat this in opposite direction and compare the two sides for bulk and strength. Rest a hand on child's forehead and ask him to bend his head forwards. Observe for the prominence of both the sternocleidomastoid muscles.

In unilateral sternocleidomastoid weakness, the child will fail to turn the head against resistance to the opposite side. Unilateral paresis causes a little change in the resting position of the head. When you flex the head against resistance, head deviates to paralyzed side. In bilateral weakness, child may not be able to lift his head off the couch.

***Trapezius* (Fig. 11.54):** Observe the contour of trapezii and position of scapula from behind.

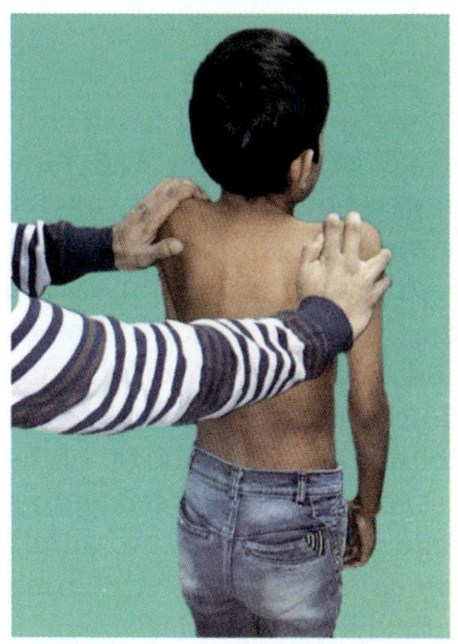

Fig. 11.54: Testing trapezius by asking patient to shrug his shoulders against resistance.

Ask the child to raise his shoulders towards his ear ('shrug his shoulders'). Try to depress the shoulders forcibly. With trapezius weakness, there is drooping of shoulders with flattening of trapezius ridge. Arms hang lower on the affected side.

I. The Hypoglossal Nerve (12th Cranial Nerve)

Anatomy

This is also a pure motor nerve, which supplies the musculature of the tongue. The nerve innervates (a) the genioglossus muscle, which acts to protrude the tongue; (b) the styloglossus, which retracts and elevates its root; and (c) the hypoglossus, which causes the upper surface to become convex.

Complete interruption of the nerve results in paralysis of one side of the tongue. The tongue curves slightly to the healthy side as it lies in the mouth, but on protrusion it deviates to the affected side, owing to the unopposed contraction of the healthy genioglossus muscle. By pushing against the tongue in the cheek, one can judge the degree of weakness. The tongue also cannot be moved with natural facility, causing difficulty with handling food in the mouth. The denervated side becomes wrinkled and atrophied, and fasciculation and fibrillations can be seen.

Functions

- To control all the movements of the tongue.
- To aid in certain movements of hyoid bone and larynx during and after deglutition.

Examination

Ask the child to open his mouth and observe the surface, size, shape and position of the tongue. Look for any fasciculation. Fasciculations are common in anterior horn cell disease such as spinal muscular atrophy.

- Ask the child to protrude the tongue, move it in and out, from side to side and upward and downward.
- Ask the child to press the tip of the tongue against each cheek as the examiner tries to dislodge it with finger pressure. Normal tongue cannot be moved. Compare the strength on the two sides.

In unilateral weakness, tongue deviates towards the weak side on protrusion (because of the unopposed action of the normal genioglossus). The child cannot push the tongue against the cheek on the normal side. Tongue deviates to paralyzed side owing to normally functioning genioglossus that pushes the tongue to opposite paralyzed side. Moreover, supranuclear control of 12th CN is contralateral. Hence in right cortical lesion, there will be left-sided hemiparesis and tongue will deviate to left-side as left-sided 12th CN is affected.

11.7 MOTOR SYSTEM

Key Box 17 summarizes the components of motor examination.

A. Muscle Bulk

Observe the bulk of the muscles. Look for any atrophy or hypertrophy. Look for any asymmetries. Observe general muscular development of individual muscles and muscle groups; compare symmetric parts on two sides. Note any flattening, hollowing, bulging. Specifically look for shoulder, pelvic girdle, thenar and hypothenar eminences (Fig. 11.55). There can be an overall reduction in the muscle bulk in systemic illness including malnutrition.

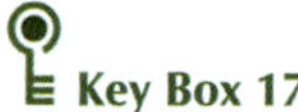

Key Box 17

Components of Motor System Examination

1. Muscle bulk
2. Tone of the muscle
3. Power (strength) of the muscle
4. Deep tendon reflexes
5. Superficial reflexes
6. Gait
7. Abnormal movements

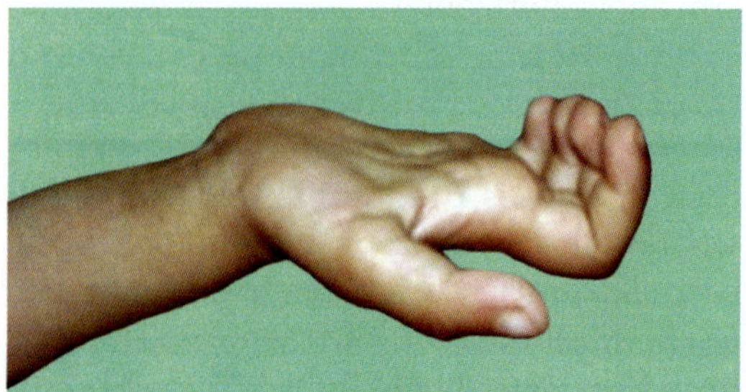

Fig. 11.55: Atrophy of intrinsic hand muscles.

Look for asymmetry on both sides. If asymmetry is present, measure the muscle bulk on both sides and compare. For measurement, use fixed points or bony landmarks (e.g. medial malleolus, olecranon, etc.) with identical parts in similar position on two sides.

If hypertrophy or atrophy is present, note its distribution. The distribution of the muscle hypertrophy can give important clues to the underlying etiology. For example, in Duchenne muscular dystrophy (DMD), there is prominent hypertrophy of the calf muscles (Fig. 11.56). Calf enlargement is also seen in Pompe disease and spinal muscular atrophy type III. Also there is hypertrophy of the posterior fibers of the deltoid and the infraspinatus leading to the "valley sign" (Fig. 11.57). In DMD, apart from calf muscles, there is selective hypertrophy of tibialis anterior, deltoid, infraspinatus, and brachioradialis muscles. In neuropathies, there is early atrophy of the extensor digitorum brevis muscle (Fig. 11.58).

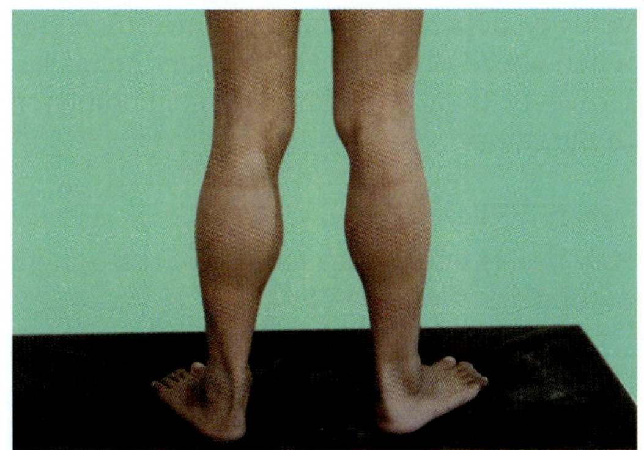

Fig. 11.56: Pseudohypertrophy in child with Duchenne muscular dystrophy.

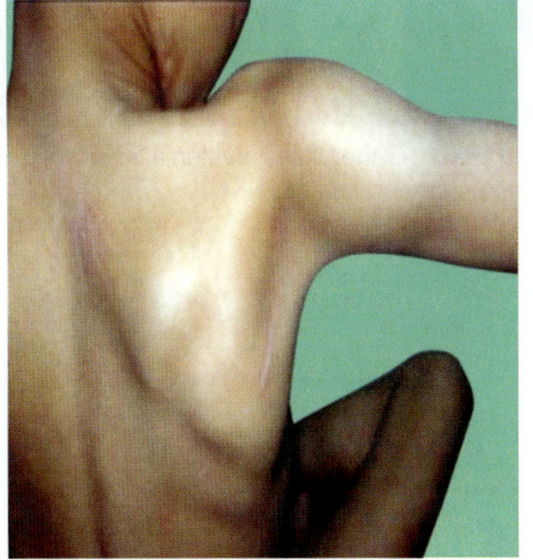

Fig. 11.57: Valley sign in child with Duchenne muscular dystrophy.

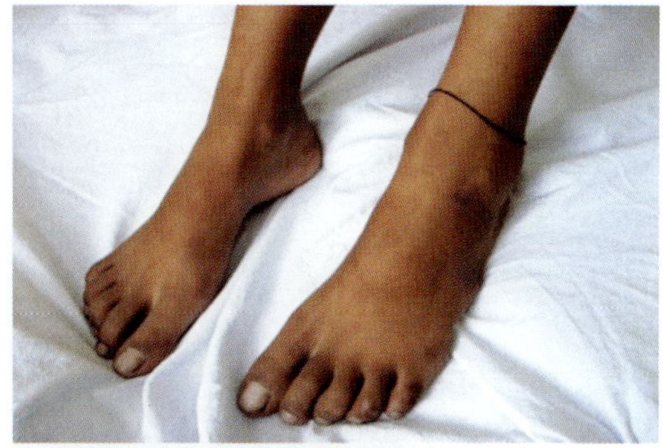

Fig. 11.58: Atrophy of extensor digitorum brevis (EDB) in peripheral neuropathy.

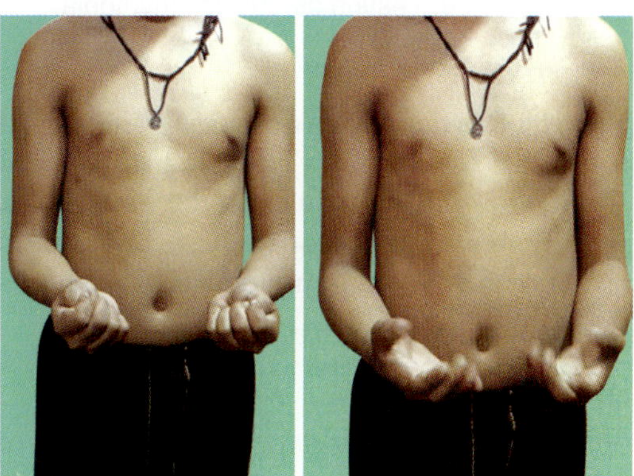

Fig. 11.59: Testing grip myotonia.

Although not a part of bulk assessment, among clinically suspected neuromuscular disorder one should look for evidence of myotonia: *Grip myotonia and percussion myotonia.* Ask the child to make a tight fist and release it suddenly: Inability to open it suddenly is evidence of grip myotonia (Fig. 11.59). Percussing thenar muscles using knee hammer to elicit presence of sustained muscle contraction is percussion myotonia (Fig. 11.60). Myotonia can be elicited in myotonia congenita and mothers of children with congenital myotonic dystrophy.

B. Muscle Tone

Tone is defined as resistance to passive stretching. It excludes resistance as a result of joint, ligament, or bone problems. The muscle may have a normal tone, hypotonia, or hypertonia.

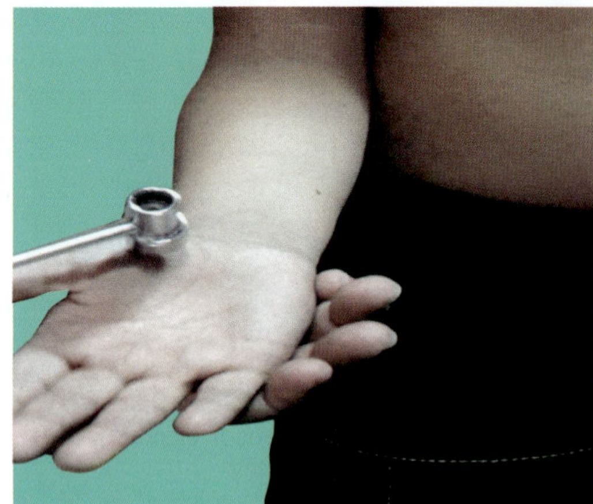

Fig. 11.60: Testing percussion myotonia.

Abnormalities of Tone

Hypertonia is defined as abnormally increased resistance to externally imposed movement about a joint. It may be caused by spasticity, rigidity, or a combination of these. Dystonia is an abnormal twisting movement of the limbs that mimics hypertonia.

Spasticity

Spasticity is a velocity-dependent resistance of a muscle to stretch. In spasticity, if the passive movement is made slowly, there may be a little resistance. If, however, the movement is made quickly, there may be an initial increased resistance followed by a 'catch'. This is also known as clasp-knife spasticity because of the feeding of suddenly giving way after an initial resistance.

Spasticity can vary depending on a child's state of alertness, activity, or posture. Spasticity can be increased by anxiety, emotional state, pain, surface contact, or other non-noxious sensory input. *Spasticity is caused by lesions in the corticospinal pathways (the pyramidal system).*

Rigidity

Rigidity is a diffuse increase in resistance to passive stretching that occurs primarily with lesions that involve the basal ganglia (the extrapyramidal system). The increased tone affects both agonist and antagonist muscles and is equally present throughout the range of motion at a given joint. The increased tone is constant from beginning to the end of the movement and does not vary with the speed of the movement. It has been classically described as *cog-wheel* (stepwise) or *lead-pipe* (uniform) resistance to passive movement.

Dystonia

Dystonia is the term used to describe spontaneous, involuntary, sustained muscle contractions that force the affected part of the body into abnormal twisted movements or postures, sometimes with co-contraction of agonists and antagonists **(Fig. 11.61)**. Dystonia occurs because of disturbance in the extrapyramidal system. *It is essential to realize that dystonia is a movement disorder and NOT an abnormality of tone.*

Paratonia

Inability to relax during a passive movement is called paratonia. It is more common in adults with dementia. Paratonia is often misinterpreted as spasticity as both are velocity dependent; the resistance increases when speed of passive movement increases. However, there is no clasp knife phenomenon in paratonia.

Assessment of Tone

Key Box 18 enlists the methods of assessment of tone.

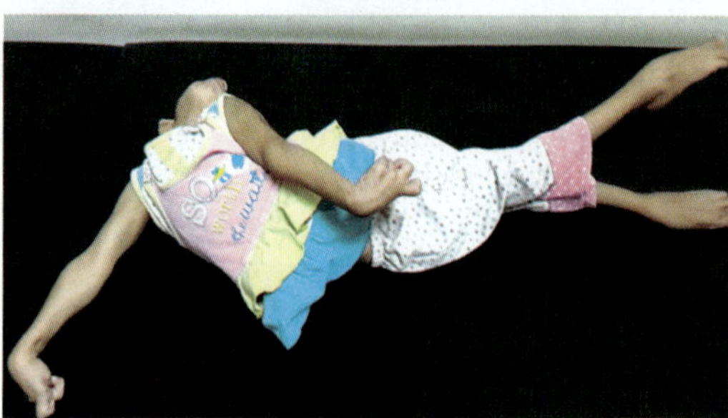

Fig. 11.61: Generalized dystonia in a child with dystonic cerebral palsy.

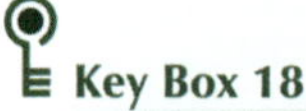

Key Box 18

Methods of Tone Assessment

1. *Inspection:* Observe the posture
2. *Palpation:* Feel the muscles
3. Movement at joint: Assess the resistance to passive stretching
4. Assess the flappability
5. Range of movements

1. ***Posture:*** Observe the spontaneous posture of the child when lying down in bed. A floppy hypotonic baby will lie in a frog-like position (abduction at hip and flexion at knee). A hypertonic child may have extended lower limbs and scissoring of the legs.
2. ***Feel the muscles:*** Normal muscles feel firm. Hypotonic muscles feel flabby and soft. Hypertonic muscles feel stiff.
3. ***Resistance to passive stretching:*** Move the limbs passively at each joint to assess the resistance to passive stretching. Examine this in all four limbs. This maneuver tests the resting tone and must always be examined in quiet environment with minimal sensory stimulations. One must look for asymmetries. If the tone appears increased, see if this increase is there throughout the range of motion, or there is an initial catch, and later give-way. If the tone is increased throughout the range, it is rigidity. If there is an initial catch, and then the tone reduces, it is spasticity. In spasticity, you will also find that the tone varies with the speed of stretching (velocity dependent). This means that tone will appear to be reduced when you test with low speed and increase (you feel the catch followed by release) when you test it in a fast speed. Hence, tone must be always assessed in slow speed to detect rigidity and in fast speed to detect spasticity.
   In infants also look for the truncal tone. Young infants with evolving cerebral palsy may have axial hypertonia with limb hypotonia and *vice versa*.
4. ***Flappability:*** Shake the limb to and fro and observe the movement at the distal joint. For example, shake the forearm, and observe the movement at the wrist. If there is hypotonia, the movement at the wrist (i.e. flappability) will be increased. If there is hypertonia, the movement at the wrist will be decreased. In ambulatory children, arm swing while walking can give a clue. Stiff arms that do not swing while child is walking are an indicator of hypertonia. Increased arm swing is an indicator of hypotonic limb.

Tone Assessment in Infants

Apart from the methods mentioned above, in infants, the range of motion can be quantified using angles as described by the Amiel-Tison method. Also, some maneuvers are useful in demonstrating the hypotonia in floppy infants.

Angles: The angles are evaluated by visual assessment. There are some prerequisites. The infant should be calm and not crying. Note the angle, and compare with the age norms **(Table 11.23)**. Do not use forcible strength to stretch as much as possible. You should stop when the child starts crying. The head should be in the midline, otherwise you will find asymmetries. Angles are an indicator of range of motion (ROM) used in assessment of passive tone. Lesser the angle, lesser is the ROM and hence an indicator of hypertonia (increased passive tone).

1. ***Adductor angle*** **(Fig. 11.62)**: Place a finger on femoral diaphysis and abduct both the lower limbs as far as possible.
2. ***Popliteal angle*** **(Fig. 11.63)**: Flex both the thighs by the side of the abdomen and extend both the knees simultaneously. The popliteal angle, which is formed by the calf and thigh, is estimated in both legs simultaneously. Compare the angles on both sides. Significant asymmetry is indicated by a difference of 10–20° between both the sides.

Table 11.23: Normal ranges of angles in infancy (Amiel-Tison)

	0–3 months	4–6 months	7–9 months	10–12 months
Adductor angle	40°–80°	70°–110°	100°–140°	140°–170°
Popliteal angle	80°–100°	90°–120°	110°–160°	150°–170°
Dorsiflexion angle	60°–70°	60°–70°	60°–70°	60°–70°
Scarf sign	Does not reach midline	Reaches midline	Crosses midline	Reaches opposite shoulder

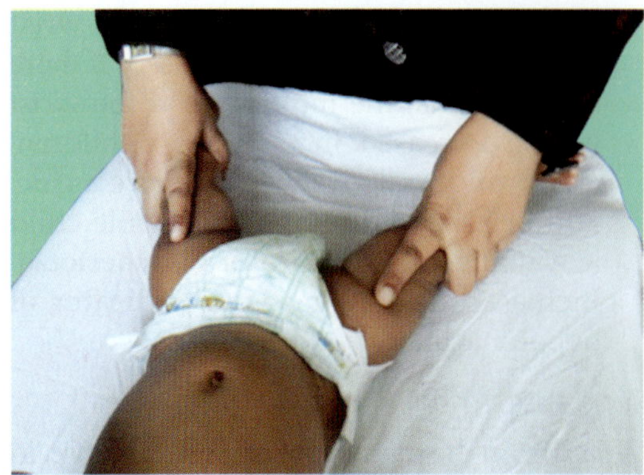

Fig. 11.62: Assessing the adductor angle.

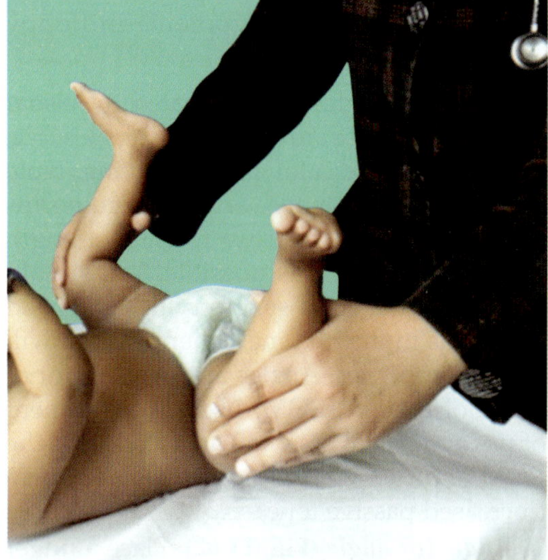

Fig. 11.63: Assessing the popliteal angle.

3. ***Dorsiflexion angle of the foot*** (Fig. 11.64): Hold the infant's leg straight and flex the foot towards the leg. The dorsiflexion angle is formed between the dorsum of the foot and the anterior aspect of the leg. This is a two-phase maneuver: First, a slow moderate pressure is applied to measure smallest dorsiflexion angle (slow angle). Then, sudden quick flexion is performed and the angle is measured (rapid angle). Normally, both angles are equal. A difference between the rapid and slow angles of >10 degrees indicates an abnormally exaggerated stretch reflex.

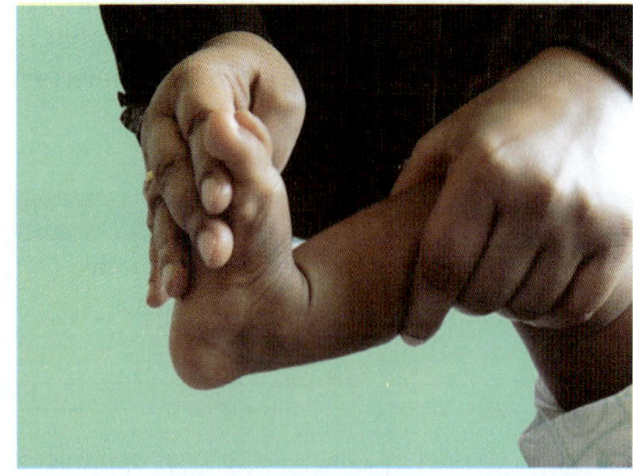

Fig. 11.64: Assessing the dorsiflexor angle.

4. ***Scarf sign:*** Hold the infant in semi-reclining position. Pull the infants arm as far as possible across the chest towards opposite shoulder. Note whether elbow does not reach midline, or crosses midline or it reaches the opposite shoulder.

Maneuvers for Assessment of Active Tone

- *Pull to sit:* Grasp with thumb and pull to sitting position. There will be complete head lag (Fig. 11.65).
- *Vertical and ventral suspension:* The hypotonic infant will slip through on vertical suspension. A floppy child will hang like a rag doll on ventral suspension (Fig. 11.66). However, a hypertonic infant will exhibit scissoring on vertical suspension (Fig. 11.67).

C. Testing for Muscle Power

Principles of Muscle Testing

- ***Positioning:*** The child should be seated comfortably on firm surface and appropriately undressed to allow visualization of the

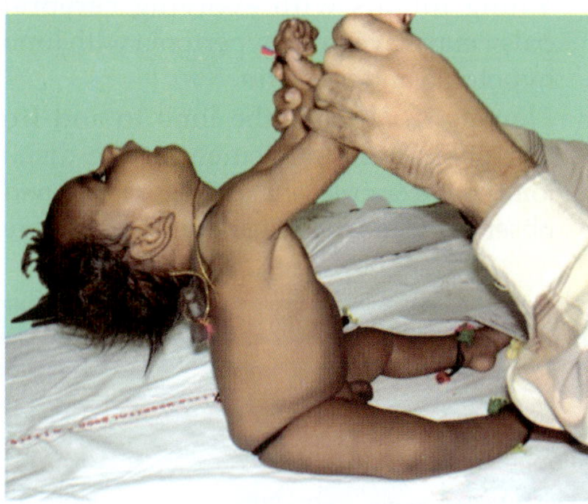

Fig. 11.65: Complete head lag in a floppy infant evident on "pull-to-sit" maneuver. Also, note position of the lower limbs.

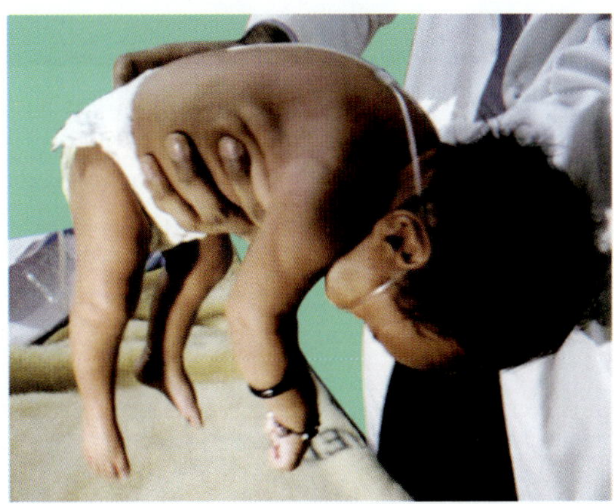

Fig. 11.66: Rag doll appearance on ventral suspension of a child with spinal muscular atrophy.

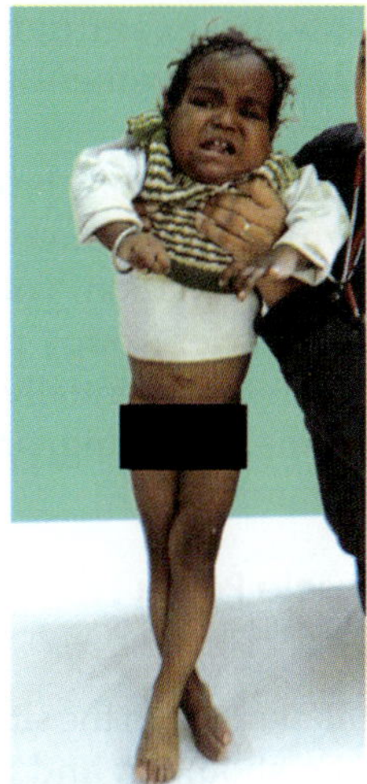

Fig. 11.67: Scissoring of the lower limbs in a hypertonic infant on vertical suspension.

muscle. In bedridden children, power grades can be approximated.

- *Assess range of motion:* Ask the child to move the body part actively. Note the quality of the movement. Is there any bradykinesia, ataxia, or tremor? If the range of motion is restricted, see if there is pain, joint swelling or adhesions, or contractures.
- *Fixation:* To test distal muscle, the proximal limb should be stabilized.
- *Grading:* The most frequently used is Medical Research Council (MRC) scale **(Table 11.24)**. This is based on gravity resistance techniques.
- Many clinicians have subdivided the power between 3 and 5 by using "+" to indicate a little more than that grade and "–" to indicate little less than that grade. So, this makes this 5-point grading into 9-point grades. Hence, 3+ will indicate he can easily perform that movement against gravity and 3– will indicate that he is able to do it against gravity with a lot of difficulty. Hence, this introduces lot of subjectivity within the assessment of muscle strength beyond a power of 2/5.

Table 11.24: Muscle power grading

Grade	Definition
5	Normal strength
4	Muscle holds the joint against a combination of gravity and resistance
3	Muscle cannot sustain the joint against resistance, but moves the joint fully against gravity
2	Muscle moves the joint when gravity is eliminated
1	A flicker of movement is seen or felt in the muscle
0	No movement

- Do not test the child's power against your power. You should apply resistance which is appropriate to the child's age. Normal children of various age groups have a wide variation in their power, therefore, you should practice with a lot of normal children to get a feel of the normal power for that particular age group.
- To get the child's best effort, make it a game for the child. Challenge the child as in a game "I'm trying to see who is stronger—you or me! Don't let me win". Encourage the child's efforts with praise.
- Power is tested in various muscle groups (e.g. shoulder abductors, hip flexors, etc.); and not joints. So, you should not say "the power in the hip joint is 3/5". Rather, you must mention that power is 3/5 in the hip flexion. We know that muscles that cause hip flexion are iliacus and psoas major. Hence, it is a group of muscle that is tested rather than power of individual muscles. Although, you can test individual muscle strength as well but it is very time consuming and often difficult in children.
- You should first test the power in any muscle group against gravity. If the child

Table 11.25: Position for testing various muscle groups

Sitting position	Supine	Side lying	Prone
1. Shoulder abductors	1. Neck flexors	1. Hip abductors	1. Neck extensors
2. Elbow flexors	2. Abdominals	2. Hip adductors	2. Shoulder extensors
3. Elbow extensors	3. Shoulder flexors		3. Hip extensors
4. Wrist dorsiflexors			4. Knee flexors
5. Wrist extensors			
6. Hip flexors	**Standing**		
7. Knee extensors	1. Ankle plantar flexors		
8. Ankle dorsiflexors			
9. Finger flexors			
10. Intrinsic muscles of hands			

is able to perform this movement, then apply resistance in the same position (against gravity) and check if the child is able to perform the movement. If the child is not able to perform the movement, then eliminate gravity and see if the child is able to perform the movement. Elimination of gravity is essential to receive a grade of 2/5 or less. For example, hip abductors are traditionally tested in side lying position. With gravity eliminated, the same would be tested in supine position.

- While examining for ability to move against resistance, avoid applying resistance at the start of the movement. The child might just refuse to move further, thus falsely underscoring the muscle power. It is always good to apply resistance at a position where the muscle will be strongest.
- Test the various muscle groups in various positions (sitting, supine, etc.) so that movements against gravity can be tested. For example, if the hip joint is to be tested, you should test the hip flexors in the sitting or supine position, hip extensors in the prone position, and hip abductors and adductors in the side-lying position. It is essential to test full range of motion and against gravity (3/5) before applying resistance. The resistance needs to be applied against movement. There are two ways in which resistance can be applied. Resistance can be applied at the end of the movement and child maintains that end-movement position and the examiner tries to break it (breaking the resistance). In another way, examiner resists the performance of movement (fighting the resistance).
- In order that the child may be comfortable, and not be made to change position for every joint's examination, you should test the various muscle groups position wise **(Table 11.25)**. Test sequentially in the sitting position, supine, side lying, prone position and finally standing.

Testing for Muscle Power

Sitting Position

1. ***Shoulder abductors:*** In the sitting position, stabilize the shoulder, and ask the child to lift the arm. Apply resistance in the downward direction and ask the child to resist that movement of yours **(Fig. 11.68)**.

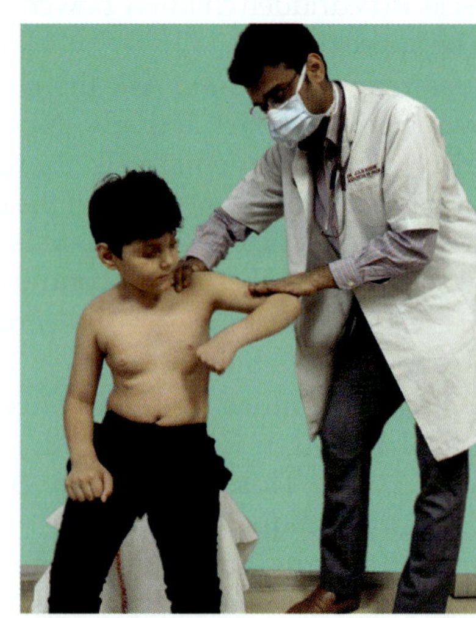

Fig. 11.68: Testing shoulder abduction.

You can tell the child "I am going to push it down; you hold it and don't let me do that".

2. ***Shoulder adductors:*** They can be tested simultaneously on both the sides by asking child to abduct both the arms and flex the elbow. Ask the child to apply pressure downward.
3. ***Elbow flexors* (Fig. 11.69)*:*** In the sitting position with the arm adducted, stabilize the elbow by holding it against the child's body. Then ask the child to flex the elbow and instruct him that "I will try to pull it, don't let me do that". Hence, you are trying to extend the elbow and child is resisting that movement.
4. ***Elbow extensors* (Fig. 11.70)*:*** Ask the child to flex the elbow and hold the arm perpendicular to trunk as shown in Fig. 11.70. Then ask him to extend the elbow and you apply pressure resisting that extension. By this position, child will be extending the elbow against gravity and against resistance.
5. ***Wrist flexors:*** Keep the forearm in the supinated position and ask the child to flex the wrist. Apply resistance in the downward direction.
6. ***Wrist extensors* (Fig. 11.71):** Keep the forearm in the pronated position and ask the child to extend the wrist. Apply resistance in the downward direction and tell him to resist that movement.

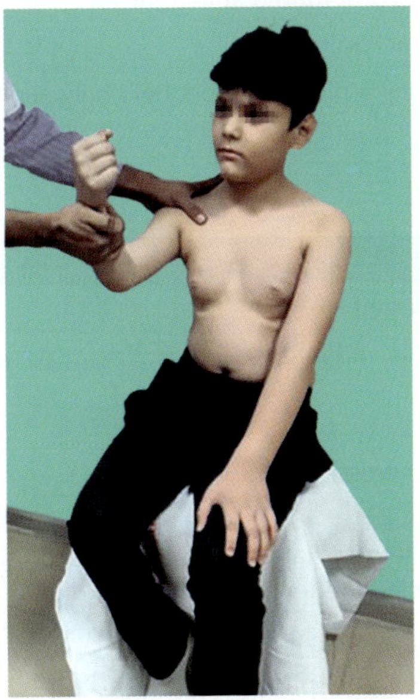

Fig.11.69: Testing elbow flexor.

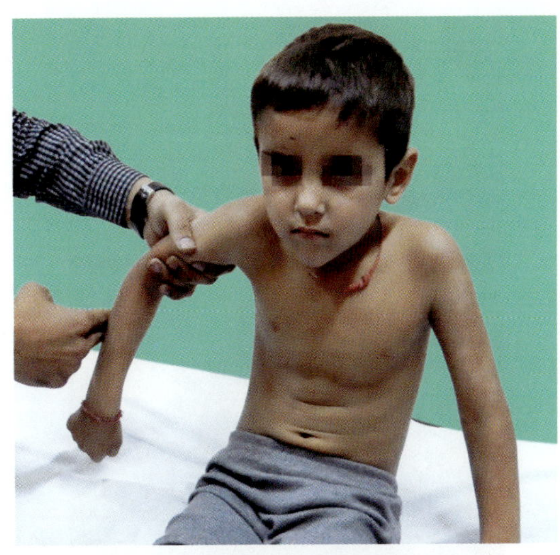

Fig. 11.70: Testing elbow extensor.

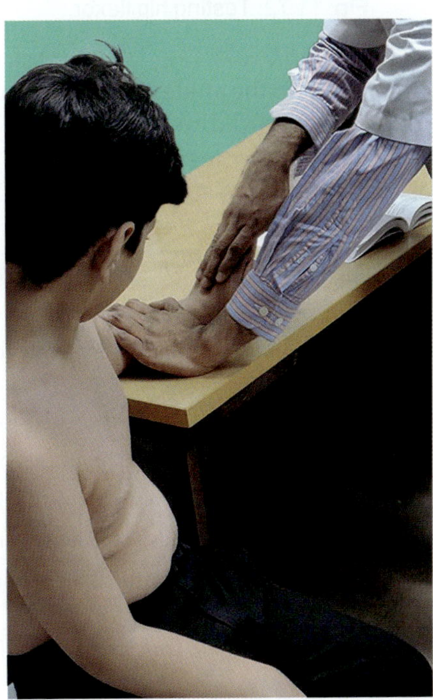

Fig. 11.71: Testing wrist extensor.

7. ***Hip flexors* (Fig. 11.72):** Stabilize the hip joint and then ask the child to lift up the thigh. Apply resistance in the downward direction and tell him "don't let me push it down".
8. ***Knee extensors* (Fig. 11.73):** Ask the child to extend the knee. Apply resistance in the downward direction. "Keep it straight, don't let me bend your knee".

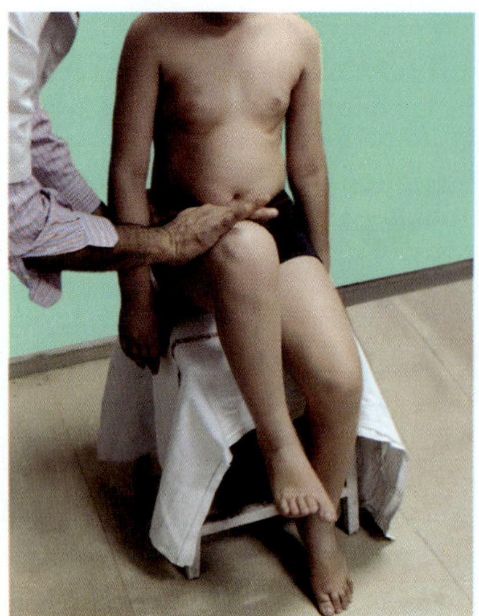

Fig. 11.72: Testing hip flexor.

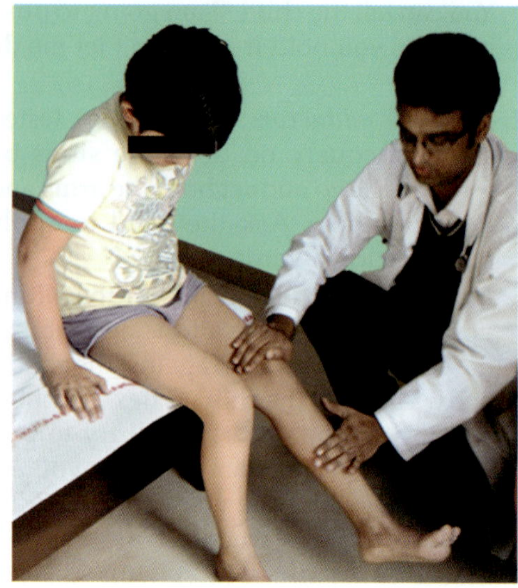

Fig. 11.73: Testing knee extensor.

9. *Ankle dorsiflexors* (Fig. 11.74): Ask the child to lift up the ankle. Apply resistance in the downward direction.
   Another way to test dorsiflexor is by asking the child to stand on the heel.

10. *Hand muscles:* Small muscles of hand including the movement of thumb needs to be tested separately, as shown in **Tables 11.26 and 11.27**. A detailed pictorial description for testing of the muscles of

Table 11.26: Testing small muscles of thumb

Muscle	How to test?
Abductor pollicis brevis	Keep the thumb abducted, examiner tries to force the thumb down towards the palm
Flexor pollicis longus	Resist the extension of distal phalanx of thumb at IP joint
Flexor pollicis brevis	Resist the extension of thumb at MP joint
Extensor pollicis longus	Resist passive flexion of distal phalnx of thumb at IP joint
Extensor pollicis brevis	Resist passive flexion of thumb at MP joint
Adductor pollicis	Ask the patient to resist withdrawing a piece of paper held between thumb and index finger
Opponens pollicis	Touch tip of little finger to thumb

Table 11.27: Testing small muscles of hand

Movement	Muscle tested
Flexion at MCP and extension at interphalangeal joint by asking patient to maintain this position against resistance	Lumbricals and interossei
Adduction of fingers tested by ability to retain the piece of paper held between the two fingers	Palmar interossei
Resist fanning of fingers	Dorsal interossei (at index finger: First dorsal interossei and little finger: Abductor digiti minimi)
Flexion of four fingers at PIP joint	Flexor digitorum sublimus
Flexion of four fingers at DIP joint	Flexor digitorum profundus

PIP: Proximal interphalangeal; DIP: Distal interphalangeal; MCP: Metacarpophalangeal joint.

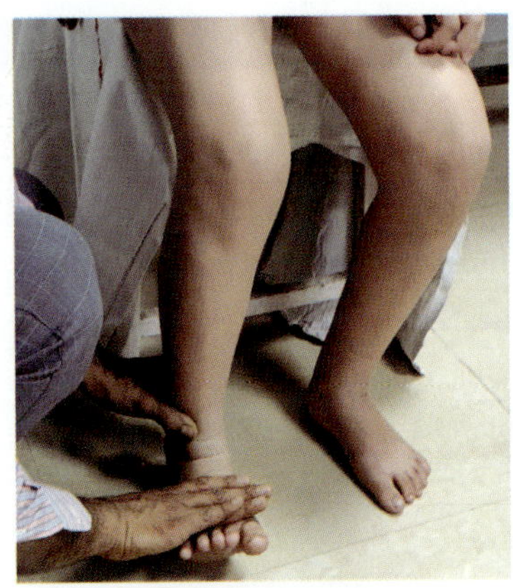

Fig. 11.74: Testing ankle dorsiflexor in sitting position.

thumb and hand is provided in **Fig. 11.75**. Shoulder girdle muscle assessment is summarized in **Table 11.28** and **Fig. 11.76**.

Supine Position

1. ***Neck flexors* (Fig. 11.77)**: Make the child lie supine with head supported on the table and ask him to keep the head raised. Ask the child to raise head off the table. Apply resistance in downward direction and instruct him not to let me do that.

   Remember: Neck flexors are the earliest muscle group to be affected in children with Duchenne muscular dystrophy. So, if

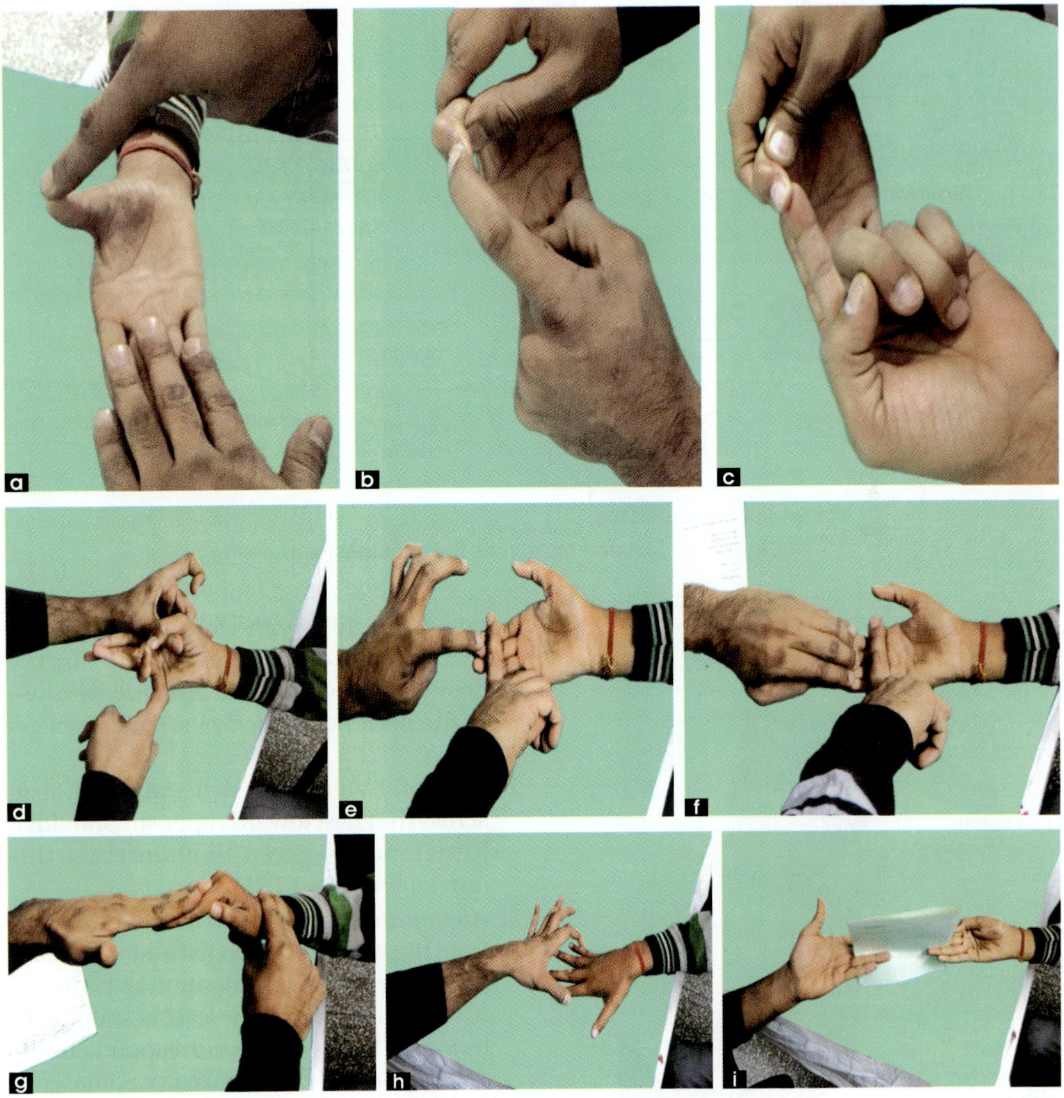

Fig. 11.75: Testing hand muscles: Abductor pollicis brevis (a), extensor pollicis longus (b), flexor pollicis longus (c), opponens pollicis (d), flexor digitorum profundus (e), flexor digitorum sublimus (f), lumbricals (g), finger abductors (h), and finger adductors (i).

Table 11.28: Testing muscles of shoulder girdle

Movement at shoulder	Muscles
Abduction of arm	Supraspinatus (first 15°), deltoid (up to 90°)
Adduction of arm	Pectoralis major, teres major
Flexion of arm	Anterior fibres of deltoid, pectoralis major
Extension of arm	Triceps, posterior fibres of deltoid
Rotate outward (external rotation)	Infraspinatus, teres minor
Rotate inward (internal rotation)	Subscapularis, teres major

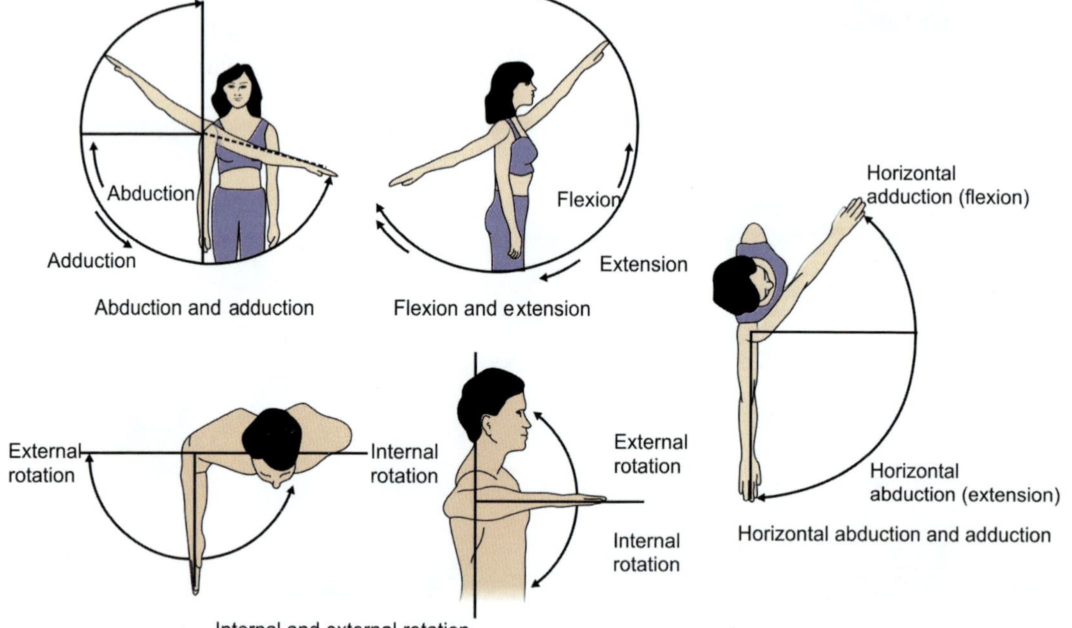

Fig. 11.76: Movements across the shoulder joint.

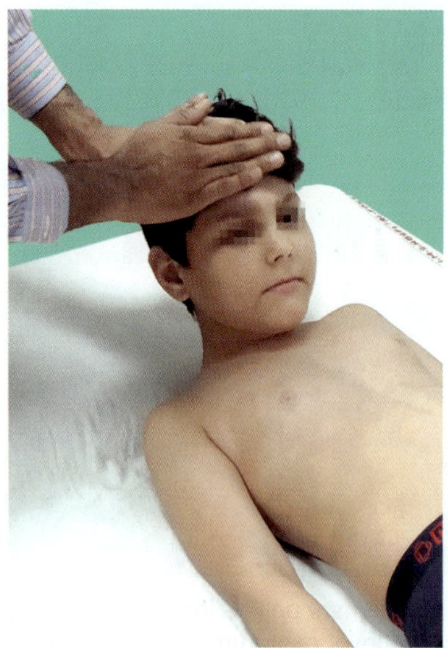

Fig. 11.77: Testing neck flexor muscles.

you ask a child with Duchenne muscular dystrophy to sit up from the supine position, he will turn to one side (because of the neck flexor weakness) and then get up.

2. ***Shoulder flexors:*** Ask to pull the arm across the chest towards opposite shoulder. Resistance is given to counteract this movement **(Fig. 11.78)**.
3. ***Abdominal muscles:*** Ask the child to sit up from the supine position with hands behind head. The umbilical migration test is a very useful test to localize the level of spinal cord lesions. The umbilicus corresponds to the T10 segment of the spinal cord. Spinal cord transaction at the T10 level paralyzes all the muscles below that level. We usually do not grade strength of abdominal muscles.

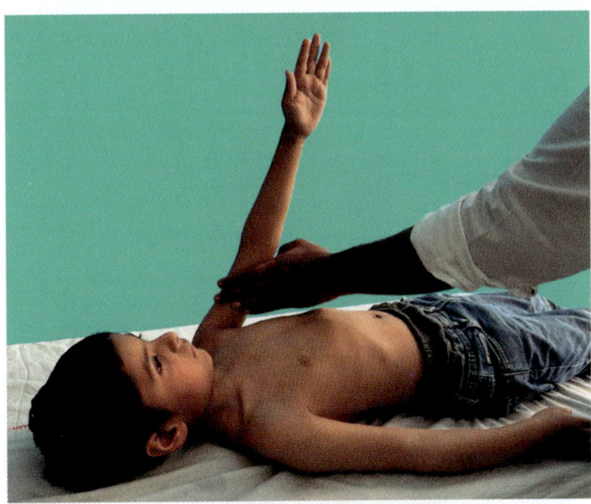

Fig. 11.78: Testing shoulder flexors.

- ***Paralysis of the lower abdominal muscles*** when a child with a T10 level cord lesion contracts the abdominal muscles, the umbilicus moves upward.
- ***Weakness of the upper abdominal muscles:*** The umbilicus will move downwards when the child attempts to rise up. This is called Beevor sign. The Beevor sign is also present in facioscapulohumeral muscular dystrophy.

Side-lying Position

1. ***Hip abductors*** **(Fig. 11.79)**: Ask the child to lie on the side opposite the side you want to test. Knee and hip should be in extension. Stabilize the pelvis. Ask the child to abduct the hip and ask him to maintain that position and you apply resistance downwards.
2. ***Hip adductors*** **(Fig. 11.80)**: Ask the child to lie on the side you want to test. Fully support the upper leg. Ask the child to raise the lower leg (which you want to test) and apply resistance to lower leg.

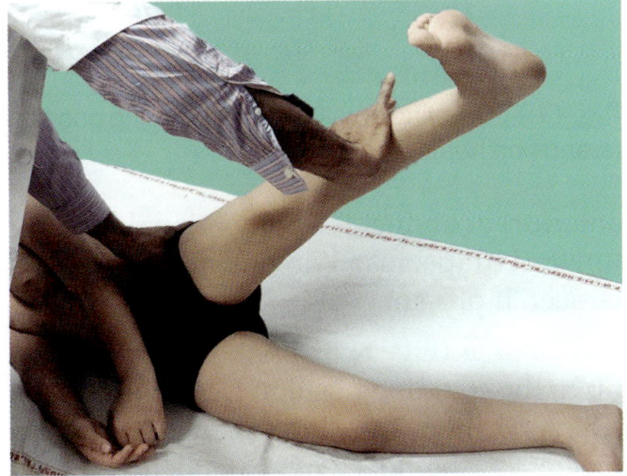

Fig. 11.79: Testing hip abductor of left side.

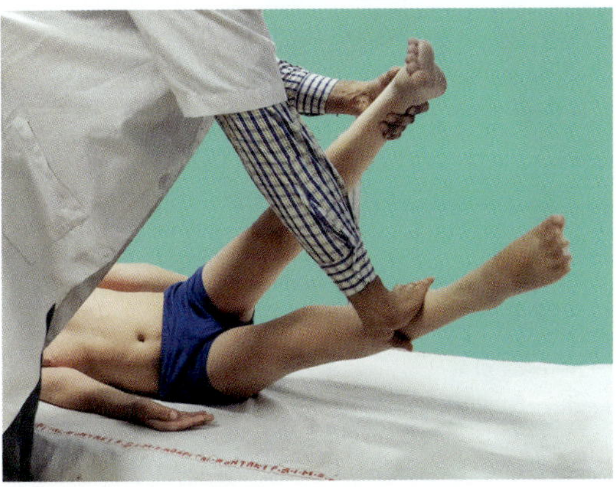

Fig. 11.80: Testing hip adductor of right side.

Prone Position

Ask the child to lie prone.

1. ***Neck extensors*** **(Fig. 11.81)**: Ask the child to lift up the head and hold it up there. Apply resistance in downward direction.
2. ***Hip extensors*** **(Fig. 11.82)**: Stabilize the hip. Ask the child to extend (will test gluteus maximus and hamstrings) or flex (will test gluteus maximus alone) the thigh. Ask him

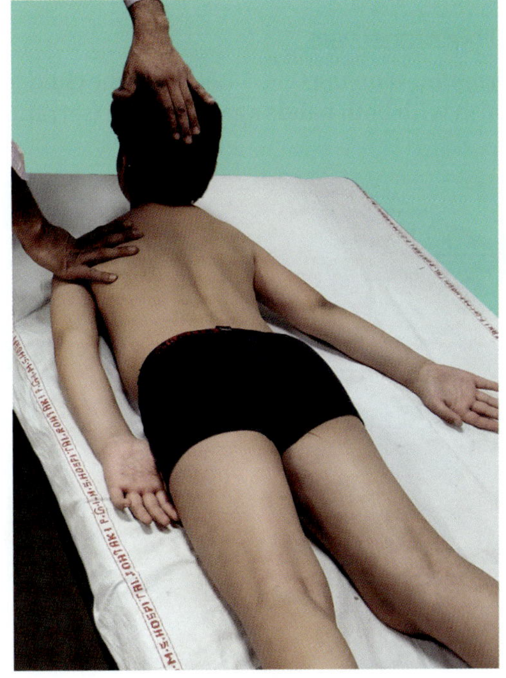

Fig. 11.81: Testing neck extensor.

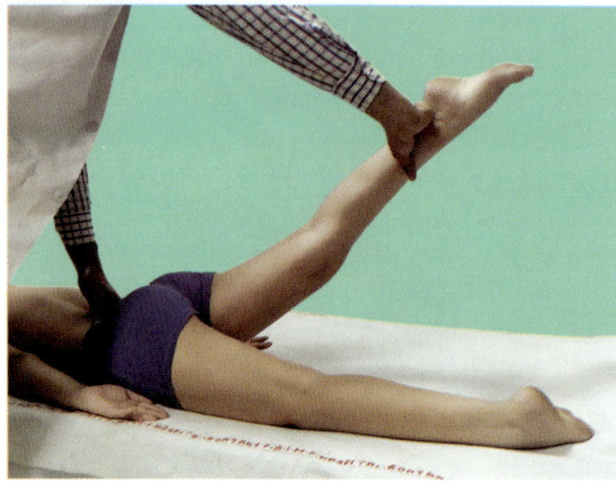

Fig. 11.82: Testing hip extensor.

to hold it in the air. Apply resistance at the thigh in downward direction.

3. *Knee flexors* (Fig. 11.83): Stabilize the hip. Ask the child to flex the knee to 45° and maintain that position while you are applying resistance to extend.

Standing Position

Plantar flexors (gastrocnemius, soleus): Ask the child to stand on his toes. The plantar flexors are tested well by this maneuver (Fig. 11.84). Dorsiflexors of foot can be tested by asking child to stand on heels (Fig. 11.85).

Key Box 19 describes the various patterns of muscle weakness.

Other Maneuvers

Scapular winging (Fig. 11.86)*:* Ask the child to push with both hands against a wall (serratus

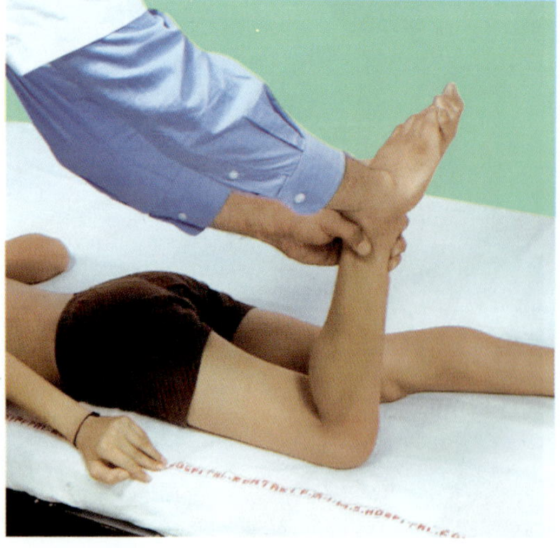

Fig. 11.83: Testing knee flexor.

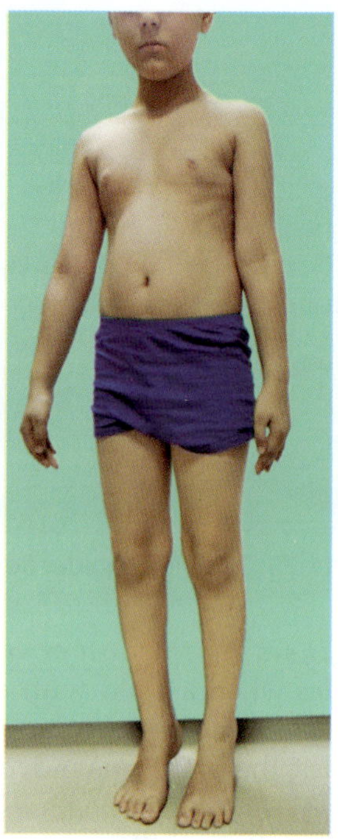

Fig. 11.84: Testing for plantar flexion by asking the child to stand on toes.

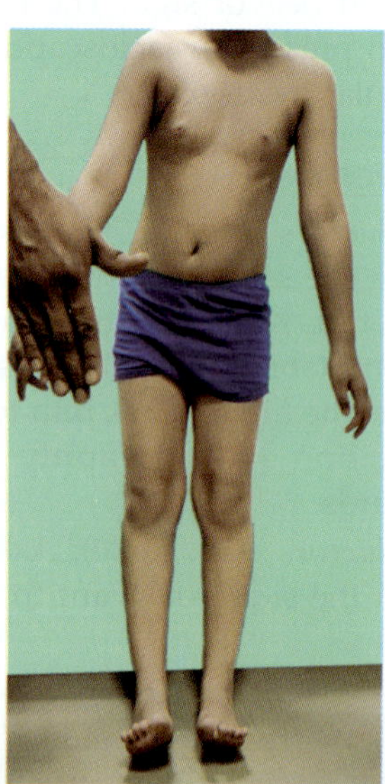

Fig. 11.85: Testing dorsiflexors in standing position (stands on heels).

anterior) or abduct the arm with palm facing upward (trapezius). Winging of scapulae can be seen if present.

Gower sign (Fig. 11.87)*:* Ask the child to get up to the standing position from the supine/ sitting position. The child will first turn prone, pushes on the floor with extended elbow to raise the hips and extends his knees, thus

Key Box 19

Patterns of Muscle Weakness in Various Lesions

1. *Upper motor neuron type:* Weaker extensors than flexors, with increased tone.
2. *Lower motor neuron:* Global weakness with flaccidity and wasting.
3. *Peripheral neuropathy:* Usually distal wasting and weakness.
4. *Mononeuropathy:* Local muscle wasting or weakness.

forming a triangle (apex is hip, two bases are hands and feet). Then the child will 'climb on himself', i.e. get up with the support of his hands on his legs. The Gower sign indicates proximal hip girdle muscle weakness.

Power Testing in Upper Motor Neuron Lesions

The detailed testing mentioned above can be done only in older co-operative children. It needs to be done in children with neuromuscular disorders such as muscular dystrophies, spinal muscular atrophy, congenital myopathies, etc. In upper motor neuron lesions such as stroke and cerebral palsy, gross power assessments need to be done. The emphasis is on comparing the power in the upper limbs versus lower limbs, proximal versus distal joints and to look for any asymmetries.

Power Testing in Infants and Young Children

- Detailed power testing is not possible in infants and young children.
- Watch for spontaneous limb movements.
- Watch if infant has anti-gravity movements.
- Tickle, or give mildly painful stimulus like a pinch, and watch for the limb movements and power.
- Toddlers can be asked to do play items like jump, hop.

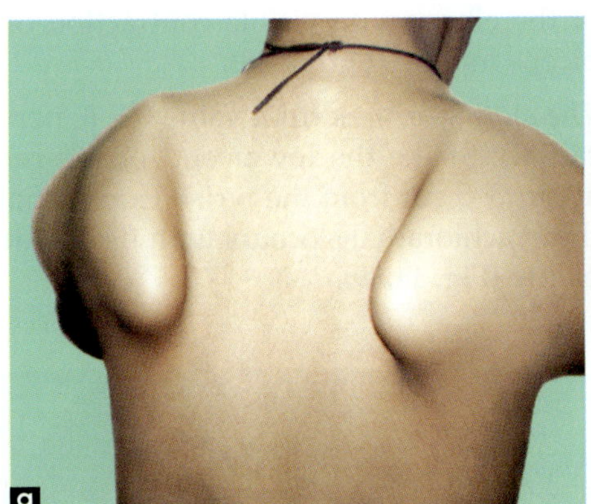

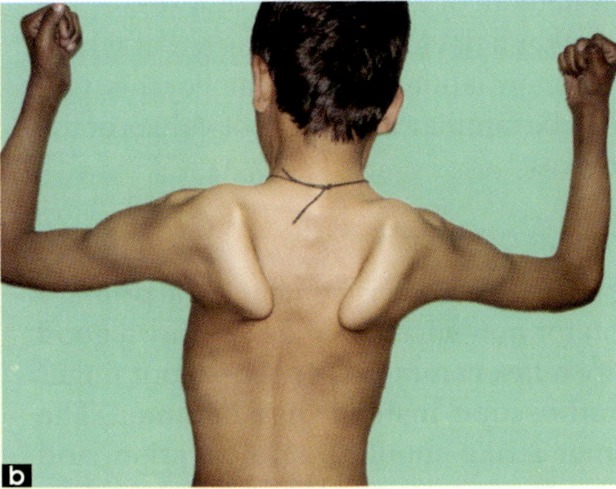

Fig. 11.86: (a) Note the scapular winging exaggerated by asking the child to push against the wall (serratus anterior). (b) The other method is by asking the child to abduct arms (trapezius).

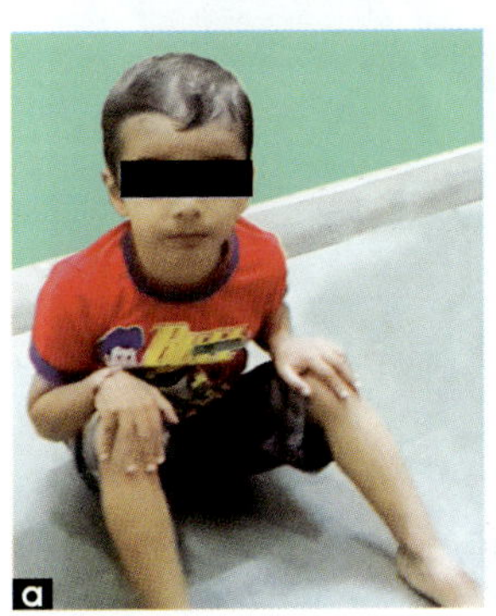

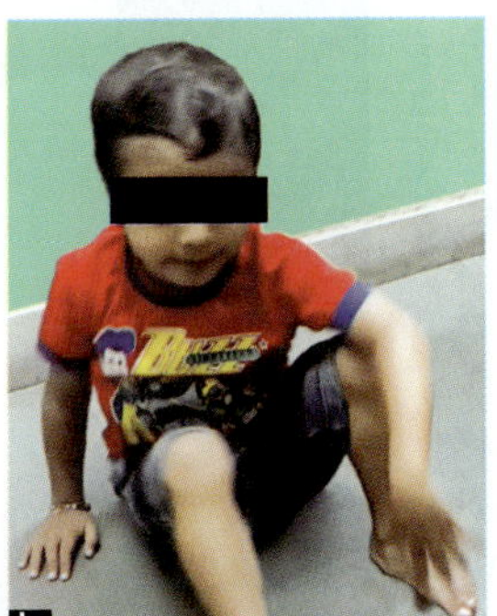

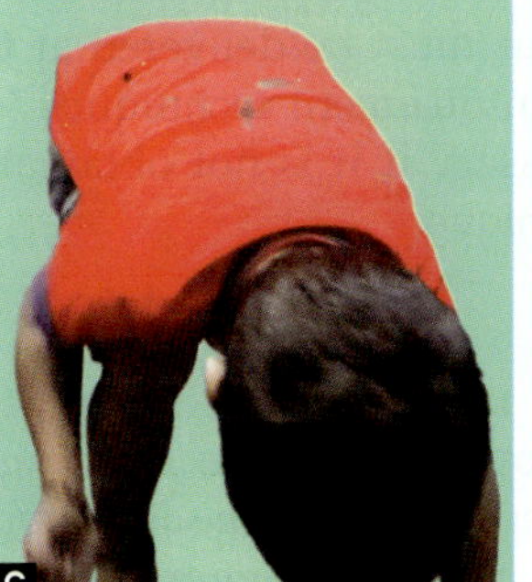

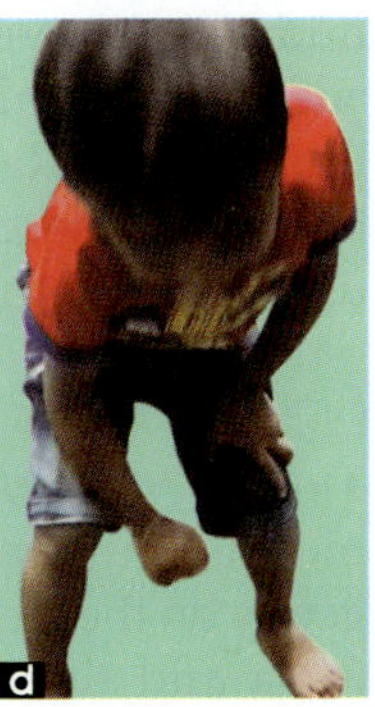

Fig. 11.87: Gower sign.

Physiology of Deep Tendon Reflexes

The purpose of striking the tendon is to stretch the muscle. When a normal muscle is passively stretched, its fibers resist the stretch by contracting. In the monosynaptic stretch reflex, sudden lengthening stretches the muscle spindles, which send impulses via the primary spindle afferents into the spinal cord. The spindle afferents synapse directly on the alpha motor neurons, innervating the muscle, causing a reflex contraction of the muscle.

Purpose of Examining Deep Tendon Reflexes

1. Determine whether the reflex is present or absent.
2. If present, whether it is normal, or abnormal (abnormal supraspinal control).
3. If absent, whether the arc is breached on the motor or sensory side.
4. DTRs are useful for localization of lesion. Whether the abnormalities are unilateral, or bilateral, or affect all the reflexes.
5. Whether a 'level' can be detected at which the abnormalities first appear. For this, you must be familiar with the root values of the reflexes.

Technique of Examination

Poor technique and instrument is the primary reason for non-elicitable reflexes. Buy a good quality reflex hammer. Do not use your finger or stethoscope instead of a hammer. The hammer strike should be quick, crisp, and forceful (as necessary). The child should be comfortable, relaxed, and properly positioned. The muscle should be exposed. Look for the muscle contraction, not just the movement at the joint. The optimal position is usually midway between range of motion. The adequate stimulus must be delivered at the proper spot. Reinforcement techniques (*see* below) are necessary if it is not obtainable using usual technique.

Eliciting the DTRs

The biceps jerk (root value: C5; nerve—musculocutaneous): Press the forefinger gently on the biceps tendon in the antecubital fossa and then strike the finger with the hammer. A normal reflex consists of flexion of the elbow with visible contraction of the biceps muscle (Fig. 11.88).

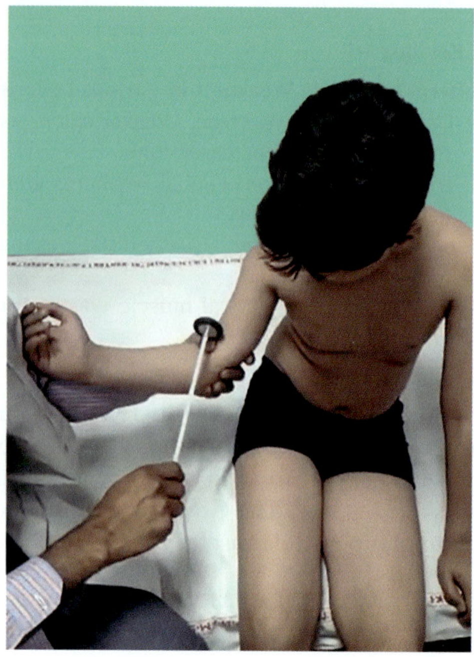

Fig. 11.88: Biceps jerk.

The supinator jerk (root value C5, 6; nerve—radial): Strike the lower end of the radius about 3–5 cm from the wrist. Contraction of the brachioradialis occurs with flexion at the elbow (Fig. 11.89).

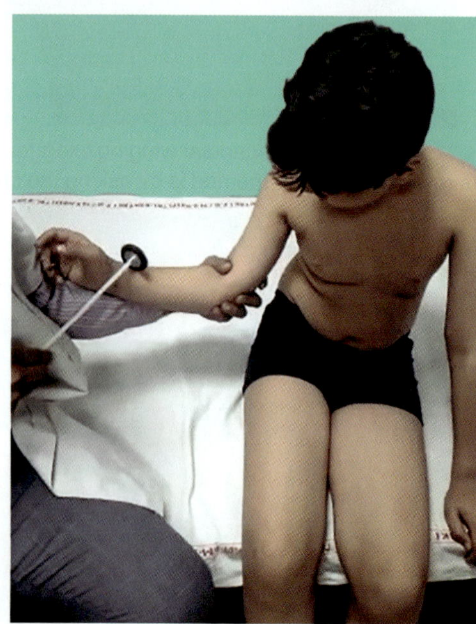

Fig. 11.89: Supinator jerk.

The triceps jerk (C 6, 7; nerve—radial): Keep the forearm semiflexed across the child's abdomen. Strike the triceps tendon above the elbow. There will be extension of the elbow and visible contraction of the triceps **(Fig. 11.90)**.

The knee jerk (root value L3, 4; nerve—femoral): Examine with the child lying supine **(Fig. 11.91)**. Keep the knee partially flexed.

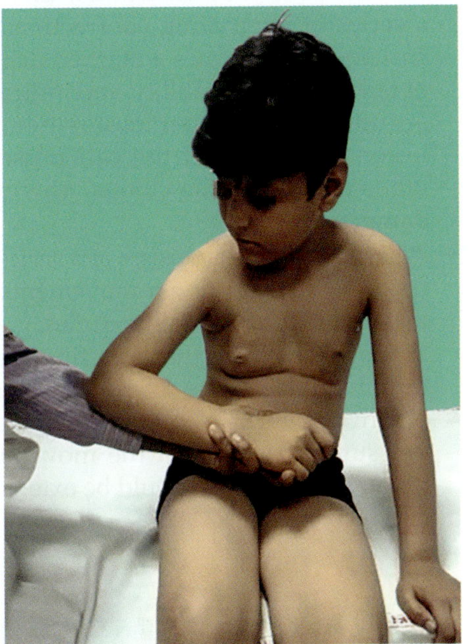

Fig. 11.90: Triceps jerk.

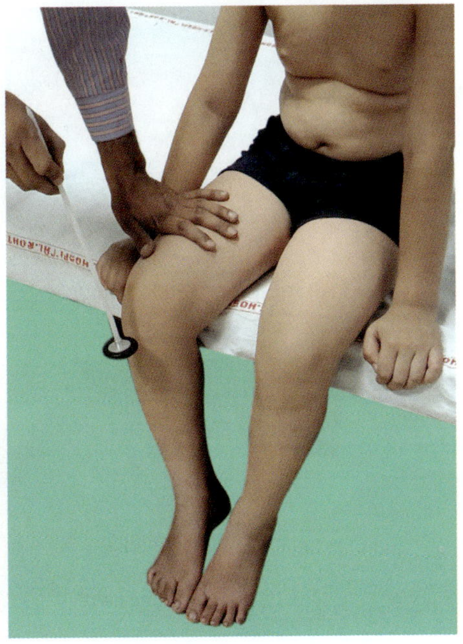

Fig. 11.91: Knee jerk.

Strike the patellar tendon lightly. There is extension of the knee and visible contraction of the quadriceps.

The ankle jerk (root value S1; nerve—medial popliteal): The child's leg should be externally rotated and slightly flexed **(Fig. 11.92)**. Slightly dorsiflex the foot, and strike the tendoachilles. There will be contraction of the foot and contraction of the gastrocnemius.

An alternative method is to make the child kneel on a chair with his back to the examiner **(Fig. 11.93)**. The tendoachilles can then be struck from above, and it is also easy to compare the responses on both sides.

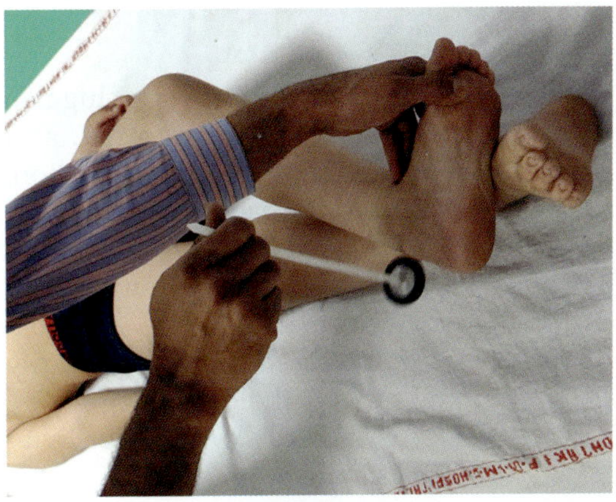

Fig. 11.92: Ankle jerk.

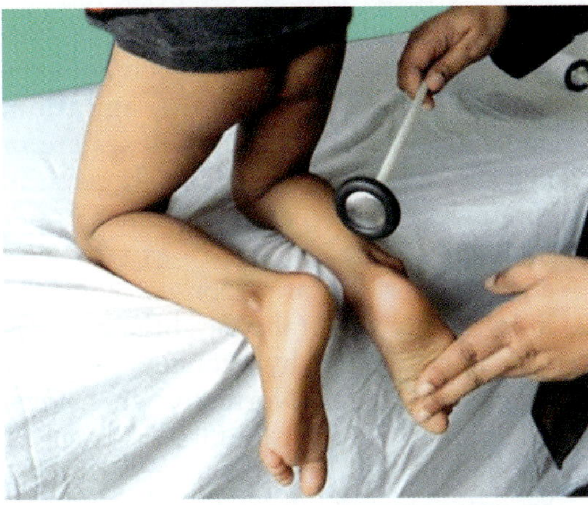

Fig. 11.93: Alternative method of ankle jerk.

Reinforcement Techniques

If a tendon reflex appears absent or reduced, this need not necessarily be pathological. This situation is often found in tense children, and those who are very relaxed. If other muscles

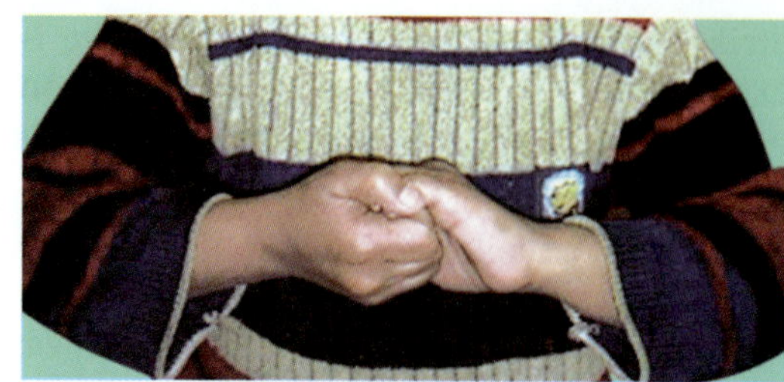

Fig. 11.94: Jendrassik maneuver.

are placed under strain, the reflex may then be elicitable. The child may be asked to clench his teeth. The *Jendrassik maneuver* may be tried. In this, the child interlocks the flexed fingers of his two hands and pulls one against the other at the moment the reflex is elicited (Fig. 11.94).

Grading of Reflexes

Reflexes may be graded as absent, sluggish or diminished, normal, exaggerated, and markedly hyperactive. For documentation, the following numerical grading may be used:

0	Absent
1+ (or +)	Present but diminished
2+ (or ++)	Normal
3+ (or +++)	Increased but not necessarily to a pathological degree
4+ (or ++++)	Markedly hyperactive, with clonus

Abnormalities

1. ***Brisk reflexes:*** Excessively brisk reflexes occur with upper motor neuron lesions. Remember however that such reflexes may also occur with fright, agitation, and anxiety. Hence, brisk reflexes are of pathological significance only if taken in conjunction with features of other upper motor neuron disease such as spasticity and extensor plantar responses. However, in hypotonic cerebral palsy, brisk reflexes are associated with hypotonia.
2. ***Pendular reflexes:*** Normally when knee DTR is elicited, after the first response of knee extension, further response is halted by antagonist, i.e. hamstring muscle. In cerebellar lesion, this antagonist fails to dampen the response. This makes the kene swing to and fro like a pendulum. These occur in cerebellar disease.
3. ***Hung-up reflexes:*** This is the term used when the relaxation phase is prolonged. Such reflexes occur in acquired hypothyroidism.
4. ***Clonus:*** The muscle that has been stretched goes into clonic contractions until the stretch is relieved. This is most commonly seen with knee and ankle jerks.
   - ***Ankle clonus:*** The child should be relaxed with hips flexed, with knee and ankle in moderate flexion (Fig. 11.95). Support the child's leg with one hand under the knee, grasp the foot from below, quickly dorsiflex the foot. In clonus, there is a series of alternating contractions. If sustained, it indicates a marked degree of reflex hyperexcitability, and indicates an underlying upper motor neuron lesion. Do not hold the calf muscles while eliciting ankle clonus. This will dampen the response.
   - ***Patellar clonus:*** It consists of a series of rhythmic up and down movements of the patella. To elicit patellar clonus, grasp the patella between the index finger and thumb, and execute a sudden, sharp, downward thrust, holding downward pressure at the end of the movement (Fig. 11.96). The leg should be extended and relaxed.

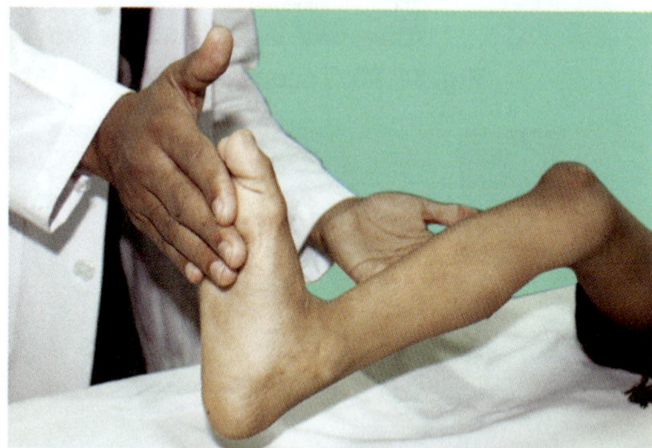

Fig. 11.95: Eliciting ankle clonus.

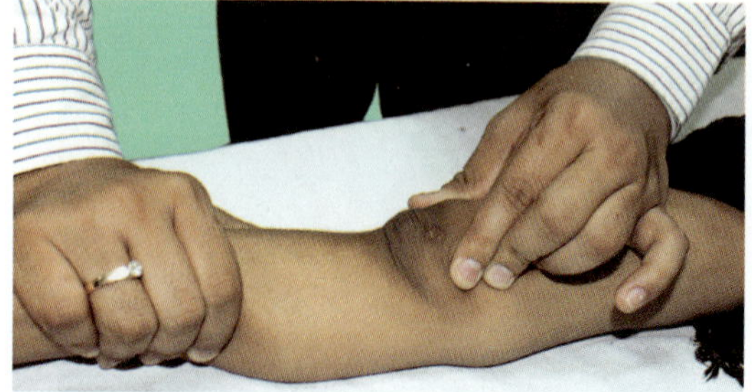

Fig. 11.96 Eliciting patellar clonus.

5. ***Pathological spread of reflexes:*** Ideally only the muscle that is stretched or group of muscle that performs the same action must contract while eliciting DTR. However, if other muscles also contract, then it is a sign of reflex hyperactivity. For example, one eliciting knee DTR if the hip adductors also contract, then it is pathological spread.
6. ***Absent or reduced reflexes:*** Reflexes may be absent or reduced in lower motor neuron lesions, and peripheral neuropathy. Reflexes may also be absent in the 'spinal shock' phase after spinal injury or acute transverse myelitis. An extensor plantar response often appears long before the reflexes return, in spinal shock.

Caveats with Deep Tendon Reflex Examination in Children

To classify the reflexes as normal, exaggerated, or depressed, you must be familiar with the standard of normal for the various reflexes, some of which are naturally more brisk compared to the others. You must also be familiar with reflexes in various age groups in normal children, so that you can identify which are pathological. For this you must practice on a large number of normal children in various age groups. In young infants, the predominant flexor tone of early infancy almost invariably suppresses the triceps jerk entirely, and the ankle jerk may be difficult to elicit. Young children are often relatively hypotonic and their reflexes may be depressed by adult standards.

E. Superficial Reflexes

Corneal reflex: This reflex is dependent on the 5th and 7th cranial nerves. It has been already discussed in the section on cranial nerves.

Abdominal reflexes (segmental innervations—epigastric T7–9, upper abdominals T9–11, lower abdominals T11–12): The child should lie supine. Explain that something is about to be drawn across the abdomen. Lightly stroke the abdomen with a pencil or key (Fig. 11.97). Do not use a sharp object such as a pin and do not leave scratch marks on the child's abdomen. Stroke from without inwards, towards the umbilicus. Stimulate each of the four quadrants of the abdomen. The muscles in the quadrant stimulated contract and the umbilicus moves in that direction.

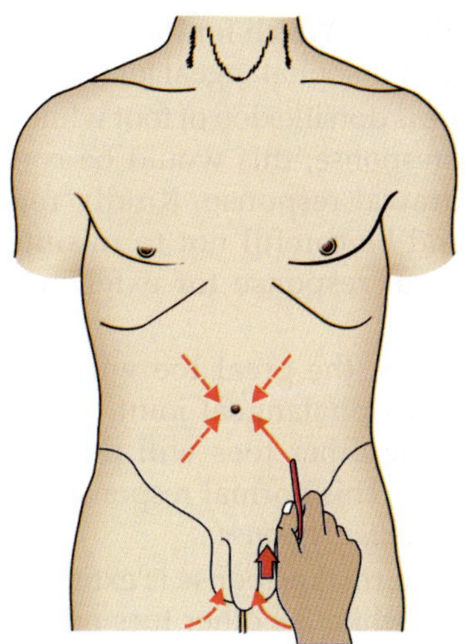

Fig. 11.97: Method of elicitation of abdominal and cremastric reflexes.

Absent abdominal reflexes may be due to upper motor neuron lesion above the upper level of the segmental innervations. They may also be absent in the hemiplegic side in children with acute stroke.

Cremastric reflex (segmental innervations L1–L2): Stroke on medial-aspect of thigh (Fig. 11.97). There is contraction of cremastric muscle with elevation of ipsilateral testicle. Innervation is ilioinguinal and genitofemoral nerves. Absence indicates upper motor neuron disease.

Anal reflex (segmental innervations S4–5): Lightly scratch the perianal skin. There should be contraction of the external anal sphincter.

Plantar reflex (segmental innervations L4–S2): The lower limb should be extended at the hip and knee (i.e. with the child fully supine). The stimulus should be firm and noxious. Stroke the sole of the foot with the blunt handle of the reflex hammer, or with a key. In infants and young children, use your finger. Start at the heel on the lateral aspect and move the stimulus toward the toes. Stop the stimulus when a response is obtained. The big toe may move after the stimulus has moved 3 cm or less. The total movement of the stimulus can be up the lateral edge of the foot to the little toe and then across the sole to the head of the metatarsal of the big toe. The *response* has usually appeared before the stimulus has moved this far. Watch for the first movement of the metatarsophalangeal joint.

If there is dorsiflexion of foot while eliciting plantar response, this would be considered a withdrawal response. Kindly repeat the reflex and be careful not to misinterpret a withdrawal response for extensor plantar response.

- Normally, the great toe will flex at the metatarsophalangeal joint. At the same time, the other toes will flex and close together. This normal response is called a *flexor plantar response*.
- The abnormal response is extension of the big toe while the other toes open out in a fan-wise manner and are dorsiflexed. This is the *extensor plantar response* **(Fig. 11.98)**.
- This is also called the Babinski response. Remember that the Babinski response means an extensor plantar response. Do not use wrong terms such as a positive or negative Babinski response, or a Babinski flexor response.

The Babinski response indicates disturbance in the upper motor neuron system. Remember however, that the plantar response may be normally extensor in infants under 1 year of age.

Other methods of eliciting an extensor plantar response are described below (these methods will not elicit any response if plantar reflex is flexor).

- ***Chaddock sign:*** Apply the stimulus along the lateral aspect of the foot, below the external malleolus. Results in extension of toes.

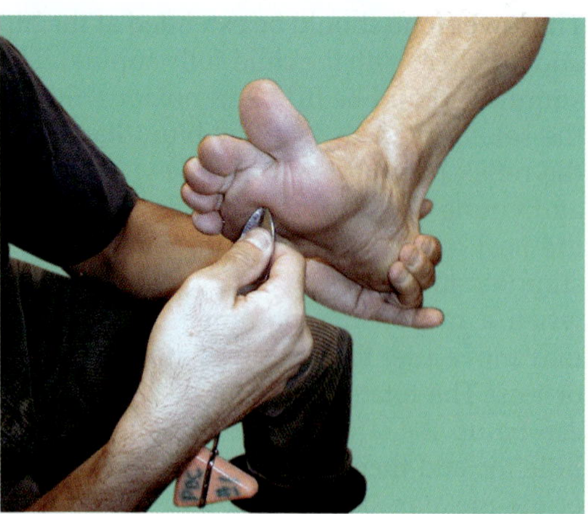

Fig. 11.98 The extensor plantar response.

- ***Oppenheim reflex:*** Apply firm pressure along the shin of the tibia from below the knee up to the ankle with knuckles of your index and middle finger. There is extension of toes.
- ***Gordon reflex:*** Squeeze the calf muscle and look for extension of great toe.
- ***Schaefer sign:*** Squeeze the achilles tendon and observe for extension of toes.

F. Gait (Key Box 20)

Ask the child to get out of the chair, walk away from you (9–10 m or so), turn quickly to his/her left, and without a pause walk back towards you. When the child reaches you, have him turn quickly to his right and repeat the process. Ensure that the child's arms and legs are adequately exposed.

- Assess with shoes on (to hear the gait) and bare feet to assess components.
- Ask the child to walk on tiptoes forward across the examining room.
- Ask the child to walk on his heels backward across the examining room.
- Ask the child to hop across the room on one foot and then the other.
- Test Tandem walking **(Fig. 11.99)**.

1. Hemiparetic Gait

This gait is seen in children with hemiparesis.

Upper limb: The affected upper limb is relatively immobile and has a reduced swing, is held close to body. The upper limb is held adducted and internally rotated at shoulder, flexed at elbow and wrist, and pronated.

Lower limb: The lower limb is relatively stiff and extended, at knee joint with plantar flexion (foot drop). Hence, the foot is dragged, and circumducted. There is scrapping of toes

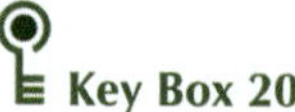

Gait: What to Observe and Describe

1. Stance/posture
2. Distance between feet
3. Ankle/knee/hip position
4. Pelvis
5. Shoulder and arms
6. Look at the whole movement
7. Look for any asymmetries

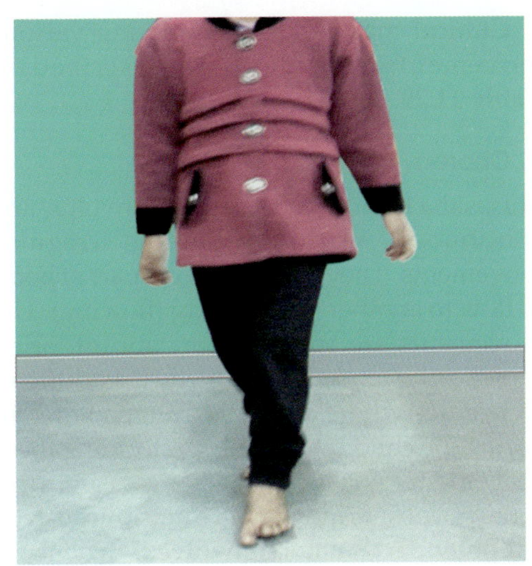
Fig. 11.99: Tandem walking.

as the limb moves in a semicircle outward and forward. In mild hemiparesis, these abnormalities may be as subtle as just reduced arm swing.

2. Spastic Diplegic Gait

In bilateral upper motor neuron disease the legs are stiff and the steps are small with the knees adducted and a tendency to walk on toes, irrespective of which foot is holding the weight or is coming forward. There is *scissoring* of the legs (crossing over one another). Walking requires a lot of effort, and the toes are often dragged on the floor. There is often a compensating movement of the trunk or upper limbs with each labored movement of the lower limbs. When the child walks, there is partial flexion at the hips and knees with weight bearing on the toes. Walking is slow and difficult with dragging of foot with short steps and narrow base.

Remember: Appears as if the child is trying to walk in water (hip deep).

3. Myopathic Gait

This gait is also known as the waddling gait. Hip girdle muscles keep the pelvis at level. When there is weakness on one side, that side of pelvis tilts upward causing the patient to lurch to opposite side while walking (Trendelenburg gait). So, when there is weakness of both sides, the child will waddle on both the sides. It commonly results from bilateral hip girdle weakness (remember that it is not specific for Duchenne muscular dystrophy) but can also occur in other causes of hip girdle weakness or disease of the hip joints.

The characteristics of this gait are: (a) Stance with exaggerated lordosis and protruded abdomen, (b) side to side rotation of the hips and shoulder, and (c) a broad base. In those with advanced muscular dystrophy, there may be additional toe walking due to contractures.

Remember: Appears "Like a Duck"

4. Extrapyramidal Gait

These gaits can be either hypokinetic gait or hyperkinetic.

The hypokinetic gait is typically seen in parkinsonism. The walking is slower than normal, cautious, and contained. The steps get smaller and the child will eventually shuffle. In more advanced disease, there is flexion at the knees and hips and the child walks on her toes while sliding the feet forward. The arms are adducted and flexed at the elbow, with hands held in front of thighs or abdomen.

The hyperkinetic gait is seen in children with chorea/choreoathetosis with or without associated dystonia. It is characterized by jerky dance like movements, the movements are irregular, non-directional, and lack any pattern. Involuntary movements may be visible. The gait is best be described as bizarre or very clumsy.

5. Ataxic Gait

This gait most commonly results from cerebellar disease or rarely from sensory neuropathies or posterior column disease. It is characterized by wide based stance and walk, staggering, unsteadiness, lurching from side to side, difficulty turning. Their gait is irregular in that there will be a short step followed by a long step, a lurch to the right, a long step, a short step, and so on. They often are helped by holding onto another person or a piece of furniture.

Remember: Appears as if the child is trying to walk in a moving train.

Additionally in those with sensory ataxia, the child watches the ground to guide steps and the gait and stance worsens with the eye closed.

The heel-to-toe or tandem walking maneuvers, and standing on one leg may bring out mild dysfunction.

6. Steppage or Neuropathic Gait

A child with neuropathic gait who has foot drop will raise the foot high to overcome dragging of the foot on the floor; the toe hits the ground first. There is no ataxia. He has to flex the limb as a whole at hip and knee so that the foot will clear the ground. This type of gait occurs in peripheral neuropathies causing foot drop (e.g. traumatic neuritis, hereditary sensory motor neuropathy).

Remember: It appears as if the child is "walking upstairs".

11.8 INVOLUNTARY MOVEMENTS

Watch the child at rest as well as when he is doing some activities, e.g. holding objects, writing, etc. to see whether if he has any abnormal movements **(Key Box 21)**. Dystonia has been described earlier. Other important abnormal movements are described below.

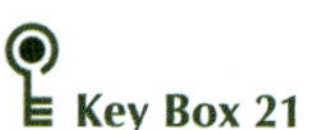

Key Box 21

Abnormal Movements

1. Dystonia
2. Chorea
3. Ballism
4. Athetosis
5. Tremors
6. Tics
7. Myoclonus
8. Stereotypies

Clinical markers for identifying various movements disorders are described in **Table 11.29**.

1. Chorea

This is the term used to describe involuntary, continuous, writhing, flowing, irregular movements. They start from one part of body to flow to another part of body (flowing). The movements are spontaneous, abrupt, brief, rapid, jerky, and unsustained. It is difficult to predict where the next movement will occur. The child often while performing these movements enacts as if trying to perform some purposive movement (quasipurposive). All body parts may be involved. Sydenham chorea as seen in rheumatic fever is a classic example.

2. Ballism

This is defined as involuntary high-amplitude, flinging movements typically generated proximally. Ballismus is often considered high amplitude chorea. If only one side of the body is involved, this is called hemiballism.

3. Athetosis

This is defined as slow, writhing, or continuous, involuntary movement. These most often affect the distal joints. They often occur in association with chorea, hence the term choreoathetosis.

4. Tremor

Tremor is defined as oscillating, rhythmic movements about a fixed point, axis or plane that occur when antagonist muscles contract alternately. Tremors can be elicited by asking

Table 11.29: Clinical markers for identification of movement disorder

Characteristics	Movement disorder
1. Movement that is evident at rest	Chorea, athetosis, myoclonus
2. Movement that is more evident with action (semipurposive)	Dystonia (abnormal twisting posture), chorea
3. Movement that is evident with certain posture (like outstretched hands)	Tremors
4. Movement that subsides with sleep	Most of movement disorders subside with sleep
5. Presence of premonitory urge, voluntarily suppressible for brief period, exacerbation with emotional stress	Tics

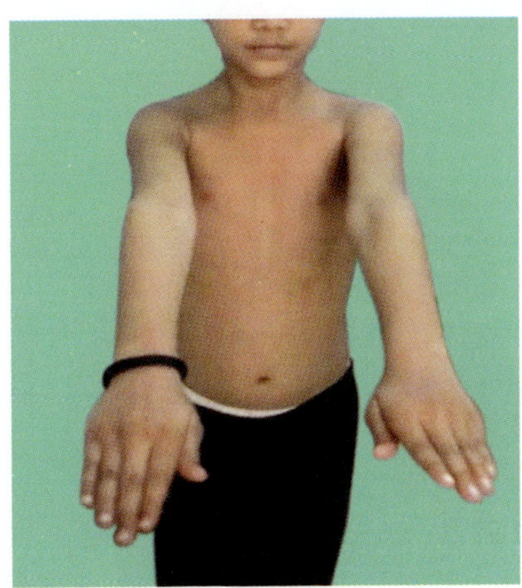

Fig. 11.100: Tremors on outstretched hand (action tremors).

child to outstretch the hand (*action tremor*) (Fig. 11.100). Action tremors can be postural-elicited when maintaining certain posture like *wing beating tremors* of Wilson disease.

5. Tics

Tics are defined as involuntary, rapid, abrupt, repetitive, nonrhythmic, simple or complex movements or vocalizations.

6. Myoclonus

Rapid, very brief, electric shock-like contraction of muscle would be considered myoclonus. It can involve any part of the body. Myoclonus in the body may result in loss of stance (astatic component) and is often difficult to predict. Action mycoclonus can be provoked or elicited.

11.9 THE SENSORY SYSTEM

Sensory system examination requires cooperation from the child. There is a lot of subjectivity in this testing. Remember that detailed sensory testing is not needed in each and every child. You will definitely need this while searching for a level of lesion in a child with suspected spinal cord disease, child with suspected syringomyelia, or in delineating a peripheral nerve or plexus lesion. However, it will not be of much use in a child with hemiplegia or neurodegenerative disorder.

Explain to the child about the procedure. Demonstrate the test with eyes open. Then the child should be requested to close his/her eyes during the actual testing.

There are three steps in examination of sensory system:

1. Determine, if the child can perceive the sensory modality.
2. Determine, whether the child perceives the sensory modality similarly on both sides.
3. Determine, if the child can interpret the sensation.

Two ascending tracts are important components of sensory system. These are:

- ***Spinothalamic tract:*** Pain, light touch, and temperature.
- ***Dorsal column:*** Vibratory sensation, joint position sense and discriminative sensation (must have intact dorsal column plus intact contralateral parietal cortex).

Distribution of Sensory Deficit

Sensory deficit from a spinal nerve lesion is distributed in a dermatome pattern. Sensory deficit from a peripheral nerve lesion is in the distribution of that peripheral nerve. Sensory deficit from a polyneuropathy will have a *stocking* and *glove* distribution because the longest axons are the most affected.

Sensory Dermatomes

You must have a clear picture in your mind of the sensory dermatomes; the spinal segmental supply to each area under stimulation, the shape and the extent of the dermatome in which it lies, and which peripheral nerves supply it (Fig. 11.101). Avoid testing at the fringes (edges) of the dermatomes because sometimes overlaps occur.

Remember these important landmarks for dermatomes:

- C1 gives no supply to the skin.
- The occiput is supplied by C2.
- C7 supplies the middle finger.
- T3 dermatome lies in the axilla.
- T10 supplies the umbilicus.
- L3 dermatome supplies the knee.
- L5 runs diagonally from the outer aspect of the tibia to the inner aspect of the foot.
- S1 supplies the little toe.
- S3, 4, 5 are in concentric rings around the anus.

Sensory level: A sensory level is valuable in determining at which level spinal cord lesion

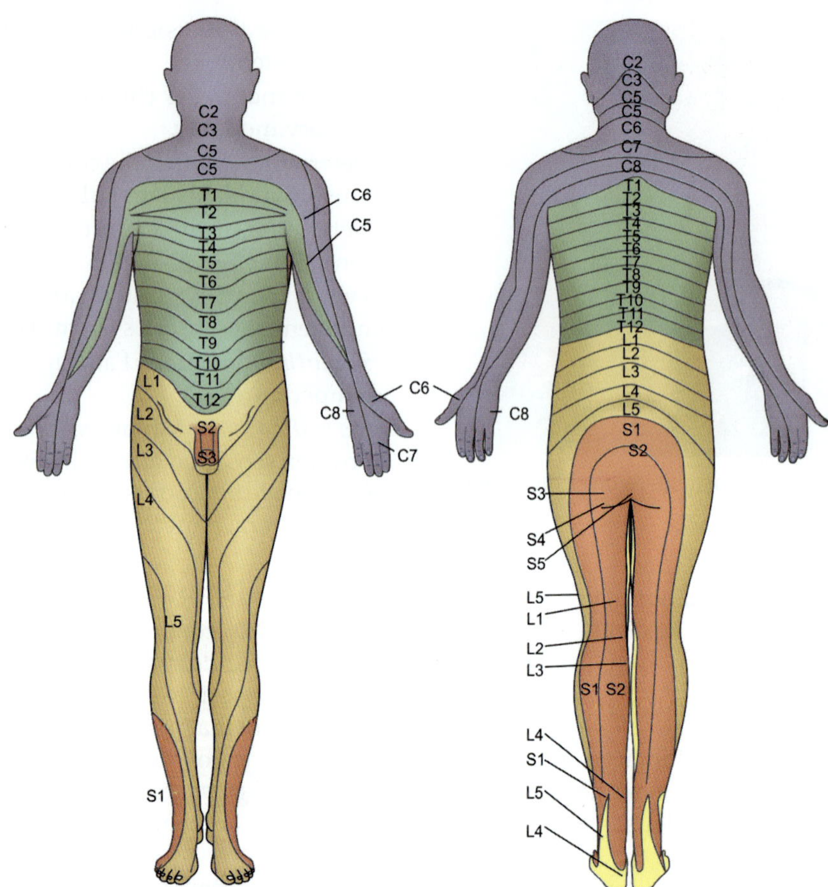

Fig. 11.101: The sensory dermatomes.

is present. The sensory level on examination is usually 1–2 spinal cord segments below the actual spinal cord lesion.

A. Examination of Major Sensations

Test first, and then compare distal and proximal sites on the extremities; and then the right side with the left.

1. Light Touch Sensation

For screening purposes, test only the dorsum of the hands and feet, in addition to the face using wisp of cotton or a tissue paper or a soft brush. The history determines how far to extend the sensory examination. Move the touch stimulus up and down the trunk to discover a dermatomal loss or spinal cord sensory level.

2. Pain Sensation

- Show the child a straight pin with its sharp and dull ends. Ask the child to respond (*sharp* or *dull*) when you apply the pin. Then have the child shut the eyes to prevent visual cues.
- ***Use of the pin:*** Touch the child with the two ends of the pin randomly to monitor the child's attentiveness and reliability. Hold the shaft of the pin lightly between the thumb and the index finger, as if to allow it to slip a little, thus applying the stimulus with the same pressure. Start with a normal area to establish communication, so that the child knows what to expect.

3. Temperature Discrimination

This need not be tested routinely, as the same pathways which carry pain sensation (lateral spinothalamic tract) carry the temperature sensation as well.

- ***Warm and cold tube test:*** Fill one tube with warm water (44°C) and one with cold water (30°C). Avoid extremes of temperature.

- *Instruction to the child:* "I want to see how well you can differentiate warm from cool. Please close your eyes, and I will place something on your cheek. Tell me whether it is warm or cool."

4. Joint Position Sense

With one hand, support the child's hand or foot and ask the child to remain completely relaxed. With the other hand, grasp the digit by its side and wiggle it up and down, stopping randomly in one direction or the other. Separate the digit being tested so that you do not touch other digits. Ideally all the digits should be tested but testing 4th digit is most useful as 1st, 2nd and 5th digits have largest cortical representation and only large lesions will have impairment.

- While the child watches, stop the digit at one position or the other and instruct him to report whether the finger is up or down. This step communicates what you expect of the child.
- Then, for the actual testing, ask the child to close his eyes. Test this 3–5 times. Do not routinely alternate 'up' and 'down' else the child may get the answers right by guesswork. Test the digits of all four extremities.

5. Romberg Test

Ask the child to stand with the feet together. Note whether the child sways. Then ask the child to close the eyes, and note whether the swaying increases. Reassure the child that you will catch him and not let him fall. Stand behind the child with arms held up ready to catch him/her, but do not touch the child **(Fig. 11.102)**.

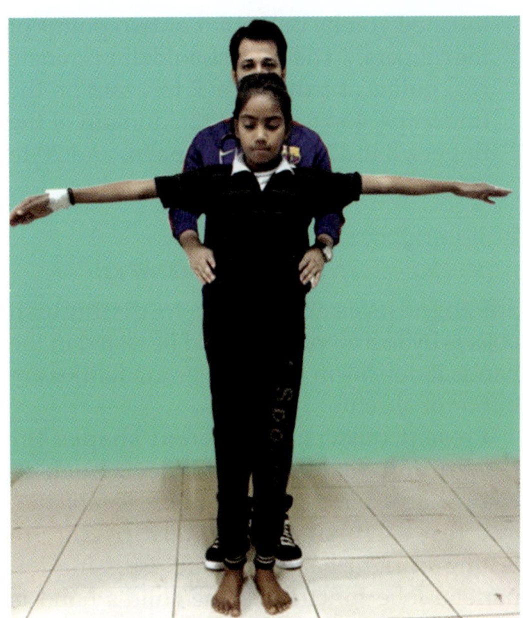

Fig. 11.102: Testing for Romberg sign. Ensure that examiner stands at the back so that child does not fall once she closes her eyes.

Interpretation: Children with dorsal column lesions, such as tabes dorsalis, sway much more with eyes closed and may fall unless supported. Children with severe sensory polyneuropathies also sway more with eyes closed.

Remember that the Romberg sign is a test for posterior column sensation, and not a cerebellar sign!

6. Vibration Sense

Start with the child's eyes open. Show the child what you will do, but do the test with the child's eyes closed. This should be tested over the small joints of the fingers and toes. If impaired, move proximally up to the level of normal perception.

- *Test procedure:* Hold a tuning fork (128 cps) by the round shaft and strike the tines a crisp blow against the ulnar side of your palm to set the fork vibrating. Apply the free end of the shaft to the child's distal interphalangeal joint of finger or toe just proximal to the nail bed.
- Inquire, "Do you feel the buzz?" If the child fails to feel vibration at the nails for as long as you can, apply the fork to proximal bony prominences: Ulnar styloid process or distal radius and internal malleolus or shin.

Tests for Dorsal Column and Intact Parietal Lobe (Cortical Association Area)

1. Two-point Discrimination

- *Test items:* Use a calipers or a device called a Discriminator. This test is applicable only for children >7 years age.
- *Technique:* Start with the device wider than the expected distance to establish communication and gain the child's cooperation. Randomly alternate touching one or two points of the calipers. Ask him "close your eyes, now tell me have i

touched you by one point or two points of the calipers?" The child should discriminate two points at a distance: 2 to 4 mm on the fingertips, 4 to 6 mm on the dorsum of the fingers, 8 to 12 mm on the palm, and 20 to 30 mm on the dorsum of the hand.

2. Stereognosis (stereo = form, gnosis = knowing)

Stereognosis is the ability to distinguish objects by feel alone. It should be tested in the hands if deficits in the simpler modalities are minor or absent.

Present objects of different shapes for recognition. Use familiar objects such as coin, sharpener, pencil, buttons, safety pin, etc. Test each hand separately. If you are testing in right hand, you are assessing left parietal lobe function. If the child's hand is paralyzed, examiner may move the fingers of child's hand. Absence of stereognosis is called *astereognosis* which is observed in parietal lobe lesion.

3. Graphasthesia

It is the ability to recognize numbers or letters traced out on the palm with eyes closed. By 8 years, a child can identify all the numbers.

- Ask the child to close the eyes.
- Trace a number over his/her palm.
- Ask the child to identify the number.

Significant defects in graphasthesia and stereognosis occur with contralateral hemispheric disease, particularly in the parietal lobe (since this is the somatosensory association area that interprets sensation). It is difficult or impossible to test cortical sensory function when there are deficits of the primary sensory functions.

4. Tactile Localization

Ability to localize the area touched with eyes closed on face, arm, hand, leg and foot. The child is asked to point to area being touched or tell the area verbally. This is parietal lobe function.

11.10 CEREBELLAR SIGNS

A. Anatomy and Physiology of the Cerebellum

The cerebellum is divided into three main subdivisions.

- The *flocculonodular lobe,* located inferiorly, controls vestibular functions and regulates the vestibulo-ocular reflex.
- The *anterior lobe,* or *paleocerebellum,* is the portion of the corpus cerebelli rostral to the primary fissure. In lower animals, the anterior lobe constitutes most of the cerebellum, but in humans it is relatively small, consisting of the anterosuperior vermis and the contiguous paravermian cortex. Vermis controls axial functions, the voice and eye movements.
- The *posterior lobe,* or *neocerebellum,* consisting of the middle divisions of the vermis and their large lateral extensions. The major portions of the human cerebellar hemispheres fall into this, the largest, subdivision. The cerebellar hemispheres control distal limb movement of the ipsilateral limbs.

B. Clinical Manifestations of Cerebellar Dysfunction

Children with cerebellar dysfunction suffer from various combinations of tremor, incoordination, difficulty walking, dysarthria, and nystagmus, depending on the parts of the cerebellum involved **(Key Box 22)**. Cerebellar disease may also cause hypotonia and slowness of movement. Cerebellar hemispheric lesions result in limb ataxia ipsilateral to the side of lesion.

1. Dysarthria

Dysarthria in children with cerebellar disease consists of slowness, slurring of words, and scanning speech. In scanning speech, the child's voice varies from a low volume to a high volume as if scanning from peak to peak. Cerebellar disease produces a spluttering staccato speech. For example, the word "artillery" will be spoken as "ar-til-lery".

Key Box 22

Clinical Manifestations of Cerebellar Disease

Part of cerebellum involved	Clinical manifestation
Flocculonodular lobe	Nystagmus
Vermis	Gait ataxia
Cerebellar hemisphere	Limb ataxia and incoordination

11

2. Eye Signs

Cerebellar lesions result in nystagmus, dysmetria of saccades, jerky pursuit eye movements. Cerebellar nystagmus occurs predominantly during volitional use of the eyes and thus is gaze evoked. Smoothness of eye movements (both saccades and pursuit) is affected in cerebellar lesions. Hemispheric lesions will result in gaze provoke nystagmus on involved side.

3. Gait Ataxia

Cerebellar lesions impair the gait and stance (the standing posture). To compensate for unsteadiness of stance and gait, the child assumes a broad-based stance and a broad-based gait. There will be tendency to fall forward or backward in vermis lesion and ipsilateral to side of cerebellar hemispheric lesion. Subtle abnormalities may be better picked by asking child to do tandem walking.

4. Dysmetria (Past Pointing)

The child, in seeking a specific end point, such as the nose on the finger-to-nose test, frequently undershoots or overshoots the target because of failure to control, or meter, the muscular contractions that set the distance.

5. Intention Tremor

The tremor is of a particular type, consisting of rhythmic, variably 3–8 Hz oscillations that occur predominantly on voluntary activity and the tremor reaches its peak of oscillation toward the end of the movement in an attempt to reach for the object. It disappears at rest (Fig. 11.103).

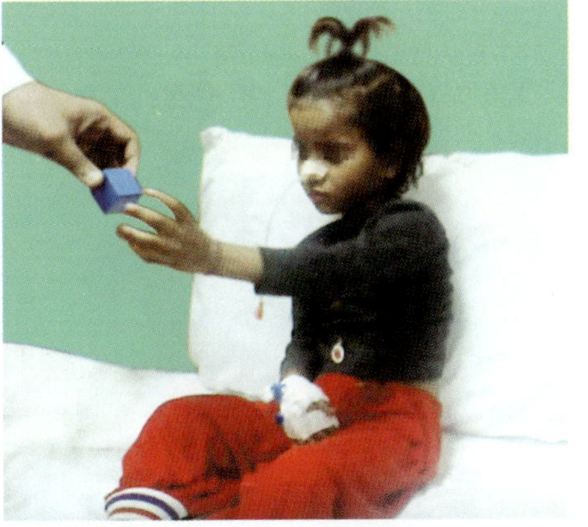

Fig. 11.103: Testing for intentional tremor.

6. Dysdiadochokinesia

This is a technical term for difficulty in performing of rapid alternating movements. It means only incoordination of muscular contractions during rapid alternating movements. Cerebellar lesions produce inaccuracies in rapidly repeated movements.

7. Overshooting

The child has difficulty in maintaining a posture or position against a sudden, unexpected displacement. Cerebellar children lack the normal rebound response.

8. Incoordination of Limbs

This is tested by the finger nose test for the upper limb and heel-shin test for the lower limbs. The heel-to-shin test for incoordination supplements gait testing in bedridden children.

9. Hypotonia

Children with cerebellar disease are often hypotonic. Hypotonia is much more apparent with acute than with chronic lesions.

10. Pendular Reflexes

These result because of the presence of cerebellar hypotonia. In a normal child, the leg normally stops swinging after one or two excursions during the knee jerk. In a child with cerebellar disease, the leg swings to and fro several times, like a pendulum, without the normal checking of the excursions by muscle tone.

Presence of cerebellar signs should be cautiously interpreted in presence of weakness, spasticity, rigidity, or sensory loss.

C. Examination for Cerebellar Signs

1. Speech

Listen for disordered speech rhythm, scanning character, and slurring.

2. Eye Signs

Look at the eyes for nystagmus. Test for smoothness of saccadic and pursuit eye movements.

3. Stance and Gait

Inspect the child for swaying when standing, which involves volitional posture, and for

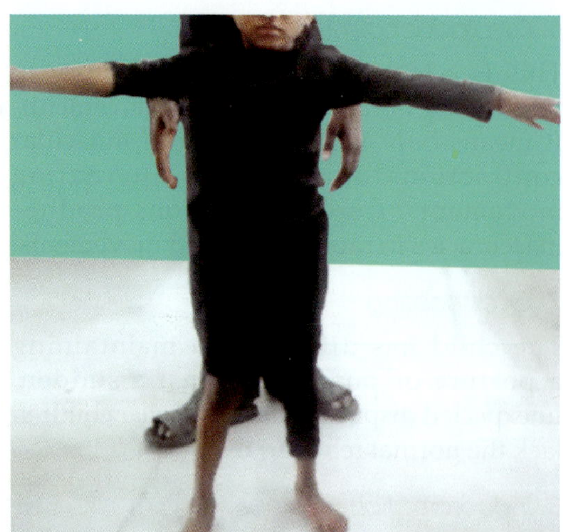

Fig. 11.104: Wide based stance in a child with acute cerebellar ataxia.

gait ataxia. Ask the child to walk up and down looking for inability to succeed with heel-toe walking and broad-based, ataxic gait (Fig. 11.104).

Tandem walking: To expose gait incoordination, ask the child to step along a straight line, placing the heel of one foot directly in front of the toe of the other, the so-called tandem walking.

4. Finger-Finger-Nose Test

Ask the child to alternately touch (with his index finger) his nose, your finger, and his nose (finger-finger-nose test) several times. Ask the child to extend the arms straight out in front. Instruct him to touch your finger tip placed in front of him and then to place his index finger over the tip of his nose (Fig. 11.105). Start slowly, then ask the child to do fast. Once he is able to perform the task smoothly and accurately, keep moving the target on the horizontal axis to look for presence of dysmetria. Observe for following:

a. ***Ataxia*** of the finger movement in progress
b. ***Intention tremor:*** Frank tremor that increases as the finger approaches the nose.
c. ***Dysmetria*** (past pointing): The child fails to precisely place the tip of the finger to the tip of the nose (overshoots or undershoots the target). He might overshoot the target or pause for a little while before slowly reaching the target.

5. Dysdiadochokinesia (for children >7 years)

Ask the child to hold out his hands and pronate and supinate them as rapidly as possible (Fig. 11.106). Test the two hands separately and together. Ask the child to touch alternately dorsum and palm of one hand on the other hand. Next, ask to touch all the fingers one by one to thumb.

6. Overshooting and Rebound Phenomenon

This is tested by the wrist tapping test. Have the child hold the arms extended out front. Grasp the wrists and ask the child to try to hold them in place as you pull down on them. Suddenly release your grip. The normal arm will fly upward a small distance, check and rebound, and quickly resume the resting position. A child with cerebellar involvement specifically overshoots by flying upward a greater distance and then overshoots up and down position several times.

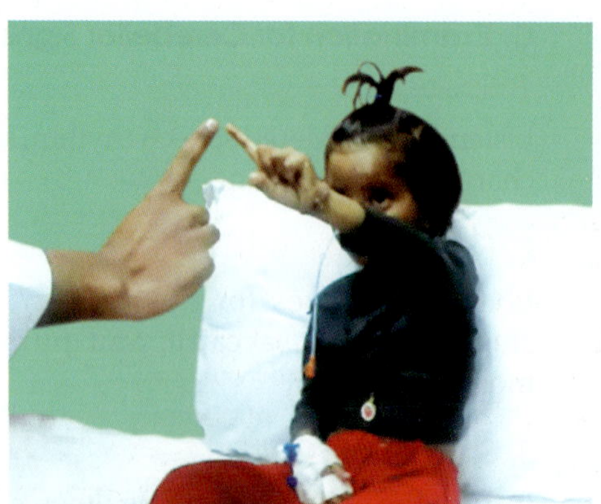

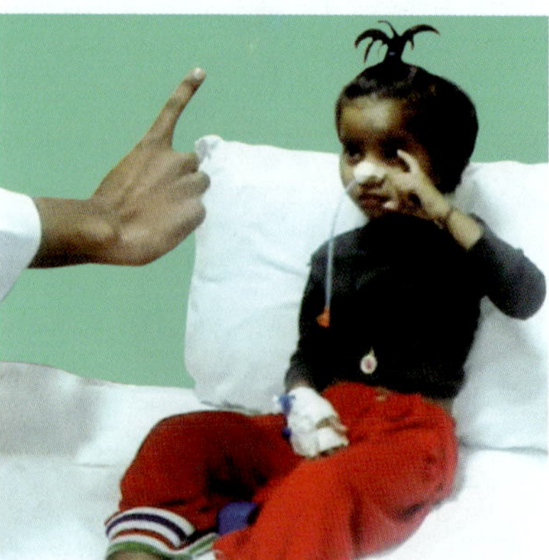

Fig. 11.105: Finger–nose test.

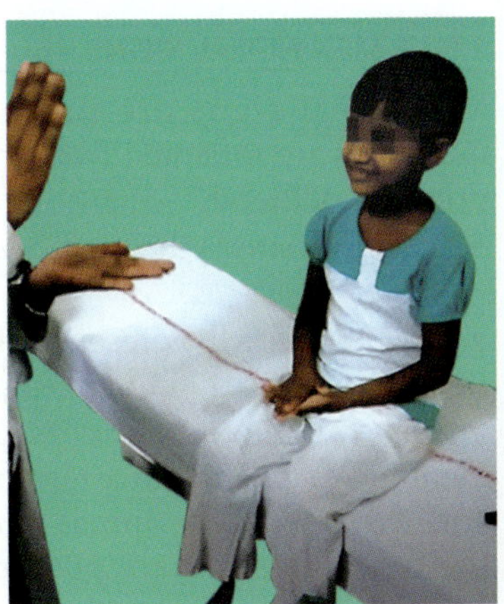
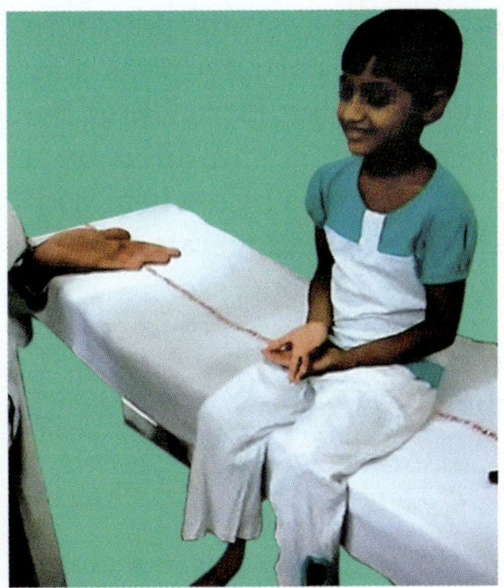

Fig. 11.106: Rapid alternating movement.

7. Heel-to-shin Test

Have the child supine or sitting. Instruct him to place one heel precisely on the opposite knee, and ask to run the heel in a straight line precisely down the shin. Cerebellar lesions result in dyssynergia and child is not able to perform this test.

8. Hypotonia

Test muscle tone in the usual way as described for motor examination.

9. Pendular Knee Jerk

The child is asked to sit with his legs swinging freely over a table edge. After the knee jerk is elicited, the leg normally stops swinging after one or two excursions. In a child with cerebellar involvement, leg swings to and from several times, like a pendulum.

11.11 AUTONOMIC NERVOUS SYSTEM

The autonomic nervous system controls non-striated muscles and glands. It has three divisions—sympathetic (dorsolumbar), parasympathetic (craniosacral), and enteric. The first two divisions consist of a preganglionic neuron in the central nervous system (amygdala, hypothalamus, basal forebrain, ventral striatum, brainstem and spinal cord) which terminates in a ganglion outside CNS and a postganglionic neuron which terminates in the concerned viscera. The enteric division is present in the gastrointestinal tract walls. In addition, there are dorsal root ganglia which convey afferent visceral impulses. The autonomic functions are beyond voluntary control and most part beneath consciousness.

A. Symptoms of Autonomic Dysfunction

Children with autonomic insufficiency may complain of symptoms related to (a) orthostatic hypotension; (b) abnormalities of sweating; or (c) dysfunction of the gastrointestinal or genitourinary tracts.

- The *symptoms of orthostasis* include lightheadedness, syncope, and palpitations, which become worse with standing.
- *Sweating abnormalities* produce dry areas with excessive sweating in the uninvolved regions.
- *Other symptoms* include constipation, early satiety, anorexia, diarrhea, urinary retention, urinary urgency, recurrent urinary tract infections, and urinary/fecal incontinence.

Some of the common disorders with autonomic insufficiency that we encounter in pediatric age group are Guillain-Barré syndrome, acute transverse myelitis, hereditary sensory autonomic neuropathies, chronic renal failure, chronic liver disease, and those induced by cancer chemotherapy.

B. General Examination

Note the color of the skin, especially extremities. Look for local or general flushing or cyanosis, and feel the temperature of the skin in different parts of the body. Acute sympathetic lesions produce warmth and redness in the affected areas. Note whether sweating is normal, increased, or decreased.

Complete sympathetic lesions result in absence of sweating, but partial lesions may produce excessive sweating. Scratching the skin will produce a line surrounded by a spreading flare and followed by a wheal with central pallor. This is often exaggerated below the level of a transverse cord lesion.

C. Examination of the Cardiovascular Reflexes

1. Postural Hypotension (Sympathetic Function)

The child is made to lie quietly on a couch for 15 minutes with sphygmomanometer and cardiac rate meter/lead 1 of ECG attached. Then he is asked to stand/elevate the head by 60 degrees in children with neurological deficits and measure the BP at 1 and 3 minutes. In normal subjects, the systolic BP should not decrease by >10 mmHg. In children with autonomic dysfunction it falls by >30 mmHg. The pulse rate is noted from 15th and 30th beat after standing, the 30th/15th ratio is normally >1.03 but in children with autonomic dysfunction it is 1.0.

2. BP Response to Pressor Stimuli (Sympathetic Function)

The child is subjected to mental arithmetic, sustained handgrip, or exposure to cold. Commonly we measure maximal handgrip, using sphygmomanometer. Measure the rise in diastolic BP after 30% sustained handgrip for 5 minutes. Normally it rises >16 mmHg but in autonomic dysfunction it rises <10 mmHg.

3. Deep Breathing Test (Parasympathetic Function)

The child is asked to lie supine and relax. When the pulse has steadied, record pulse rate during 6 maximal deep breathes. Normally pulse falls by >15/min., with autonomic dysfunction it slows <10 per min.

4. Valsalva Test (Both Sympathetic and Parasympathetic Functions)

The child is made to blow into a sphygmomanometer maintaining a pressure of 40 mmHg for 15 seconds. The ratio of highest pulse rate during rest to the lowest pulse rate during test is normally >1.5 but in autonomic dysfunction it is <1.1.

11.12 MENINGEAL SIGNS

Meningeal signs are present when the meninges are inflamed from infection or the presence of blood.

- *Meningismus* is the presence of meningeal signs.
- *Meningism* is the presence of neck stiffness in the absence of meningeal inflammation.

The various maneuvers used to elicit meningeal signs produce tension on inflamed and hypersensitive spinal nerve roots and the resulting signs are postures, protective muscle contractions or other movements that minimize the stretch and distortion of the meninges and roots.

1. Nuchal Rigidity (Neck Stiffness)

It is characterized by stiffness and spasm of neck muscles resulting in pain on attempted voluntary movement as well as resistance to passive movement. Resistance to passive neck flexion is an early finding. Extreme rigidity causes retraction of the neck into opisthotonus position. Meningeal irritation may also cause resistance to movements of legs and back with the child lying with legs drawn up and resists passive extension.

During the range of movement from neck extension to neck flexion, the cord and nerve roots change from a relaxed state to a stretched state. When there is meningeal inflammation, this stretching puts tension on the inflamed structures. This initiates a protective muscle spasm to inhibit the painful movement.

How to Elicit Neck Rigidity

Older children can be asked to touch their chin on the sternum to look for evidence of neck stiffness (Fig. 11.107). Many young children voluntarily resist their neck being passively flexed.

A good way to look for neck stiffness is to see if the child moves or bends his neck spontaneously when you are talking to the mother. Draw the child's attention to his toes. For example, you can shine a torch on the toes or tickle the toes to encourage the child to look down. Look to see if the child can bend his or her neck when looking down at his or her umbilicus or toes.

If you still have not seen the child bend

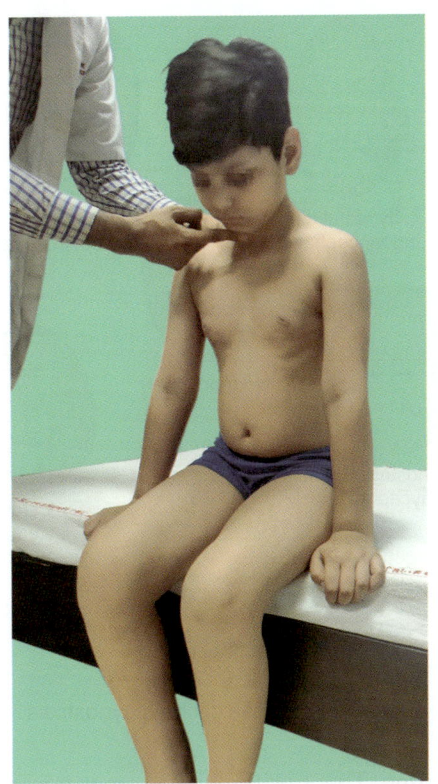

Fig. 11.107: Testing neck rigidity in older child.

his or her neck himself, make the child lie supine. Gently support the child's back and shoulders with one hand. With the other hand, hold the child's head. Then carefully bend the head forward towards the child's chest (Fig. 11.108). If the neck bends easily, the child does not have neck stiffness. If the neck feels stiff and there is resistance to bending, the child has neck stiffness. This maneuver is useful in uncooperative young children who tend to extend their neck resisting our attempt to flex the neck. When you bring the child to the edge of the couch, the child would want to flex his neck so that he does not fall. This will ensure that voluntary resistance is abolished by this method.

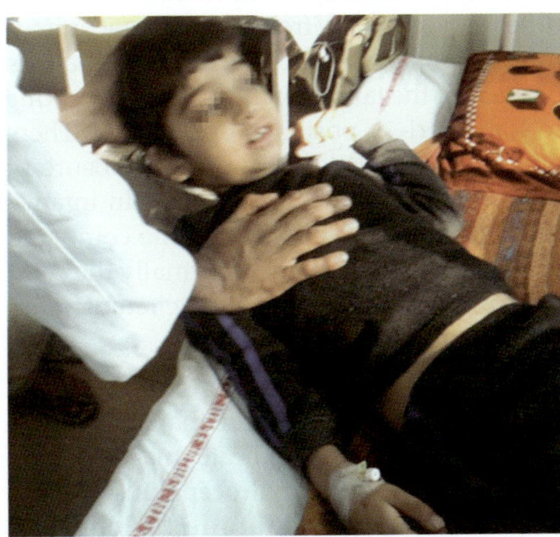

Fig. 11.108: Eliciting neck stiffness by bringing head to the edge of bed.

2. Kernig Sign

Flex the child's hip and knee to 90°, and attempt to extend the knee (Fig. 11.109). In children with meningeal irritation, on attempted passive extension of knee, there is pain, resistance, and inability to fully extend the knee. Usually there is inability to extend the knee beyond 135° while the hip is flexed.

Brudzinski Sign

When one hand is placed under child's head and the neck is flexed while holding down the chest with the other hand, there is flexion of the hips and knees bilaterally. This sign can be observed when looking for neck rigidity (Brudzinski neck sign) (Fig. 11.110).

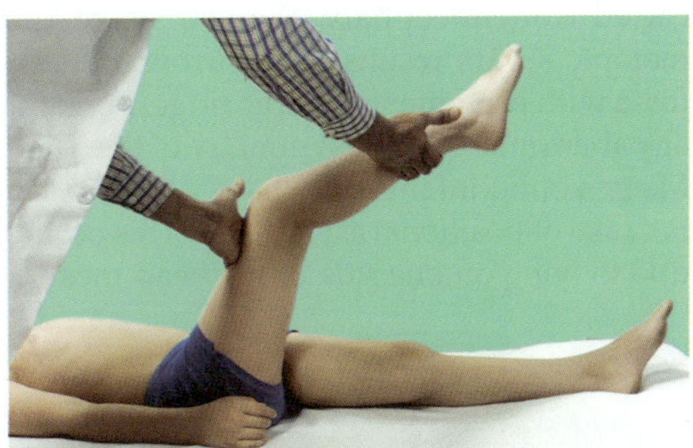

Fig. 11.109: The Kernig sign.

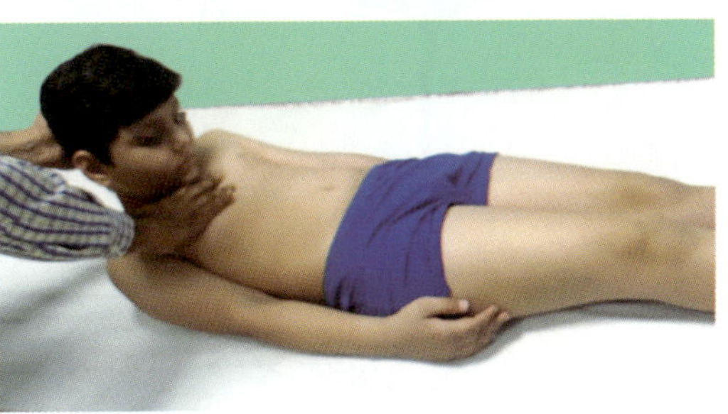

Fig. 11.110: The Brudzinski neck sign.

A. Examination of Head

1. Head Shape

- Look for presence of encephalocele (occipital or frontal).
- Feel for any bony depressions. These may indicate old depressed fractures or congenital anomalies such as biparietal foramina.
- Look for prominent and distended scalp veins.
- Feel for anterior and posterior fontanel. Presence of tense bulging fontanel with absence of normal pulsations is an indicator of raised intracranial pressure. Examine the fontanel in a calm baby in erect posture.
- Feel the sutures—metopic, sagittal, coronal, and lambdoid **(Fig. 11.111)**.

Craniosynostosis occurs because of premature closure of the sutures and results in abnormally shaped head **(Fig. 11.112)**. Premature closure of the coronal suture prevents growth of the skull in the anteroposterior direction, and leads to a flattened appearing head called brachycephaly. Closure of the sagittal suture prevents growth in the lateral direction, resulting in a long narrow skull, called dolichocephaly. Synostosis of the metopic suture results in a narrow anterior fossa with prominent metopic ridge. Look for any abnormal shape or symmetry of the head. Many young infants may have *plagiocephaly* because of positional asymmetry. This occurs due to lying on one side of the head most of the time. This positional asymmetry is often exaggerated in hypotonic babies and in those with motor developmental delay.

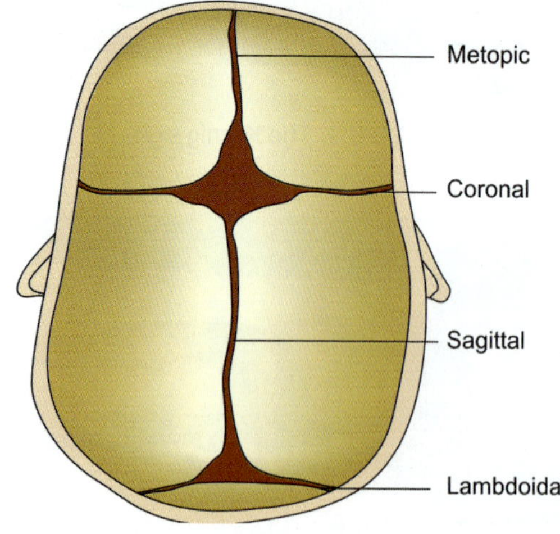

Fig. 11.111: Sutures of skull.

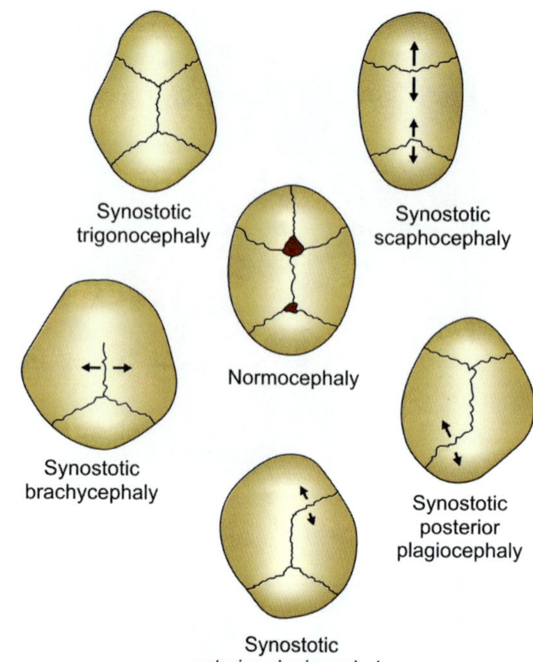

Fig. 11.112: Types of craniosynostosis.

2. Head Size

Measure the head circumference (*see* Chapter 5).

Microcephaly: It is defined as head circumference more than –3SD below the median for the child's age and gender. See also the shape of the head. Is it uniformly small? Careful examination of the head may help to differentiate *primary* from *secondary* (acquired) microcephaly. Secondary microcephaly is because of the failure of the brain to grow due to some peri- or postnatal brain insult. There will be sutural ridging and early closure of the anterior fontanel in this case. In infants, the head circumference should be compared to the chest circumference; normally the chest circumference exceeds the head circumference by 12 months of age.

Macrocephaly: Head circumference which exceeds the median by more than 2SD for the child's age and gender indicates macrocephaly. It may occur due to hydrocephalus, rickets, megalencephaly, subdural effusions, and intracranial tumors. Megalencephaly occurs in storage disorder. Look for sutural diastasis.

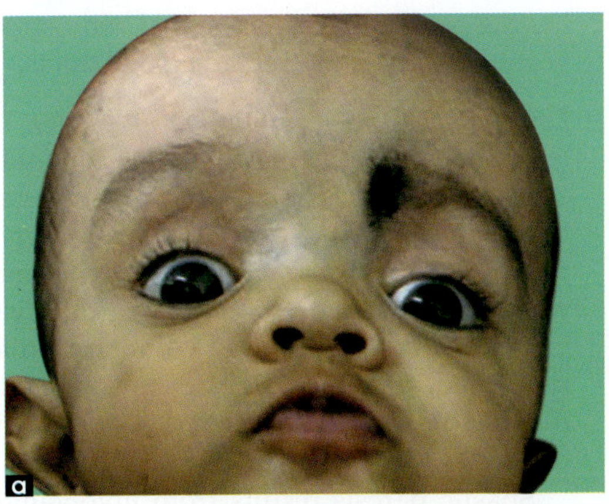
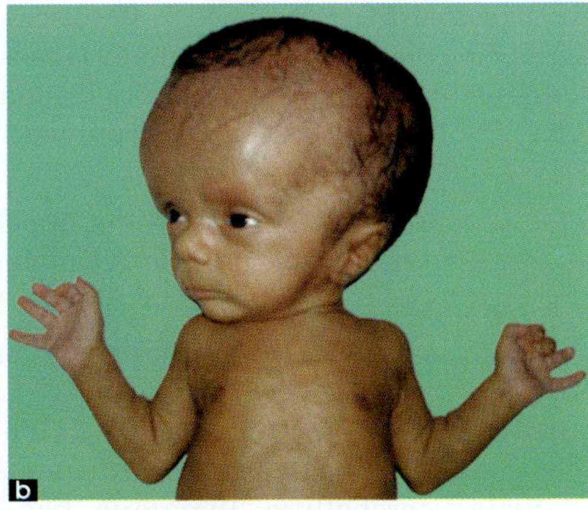

Fig. 11.113: Hydrocephalus with (a) sun setting sign and (b) large head.

Children with hydrocephalus often have sun setting sign in their eyes and distended scalp veins **(Fig. 11.113)**.

3. Transillumination Sign

Place a beam of bright torch light on the skull in a darkened room to look for halo around the light. In a normal infant skull, small rim of bright light is seen around the beam. However, if there is hydrocephalus, there will be generalized transillumination in entire skull. Transillumination may also be positive in subdural effusion.

4. Macewen Sign or Crackpot Sign

Details of this clinical sign are described in Chapter 6 (General physical examination). Percussion of normal skull will not elicit resonant note (since the pot is not broken). However, in children with raised intracranial pressure (where the pot will start getting cracked from within), percussion of skull will elicit a resonant note. Be careful not to hold the head, while eliciting crackpot sign (obviously you cannot hold the pot to see and hear if it is cracked, you need to hold it by its neck).

B. Examination of the Spine (Also See Chapter 16)

The spine must be examined in all children with neurological illness, but this is especially important in children with paraplegia.

- Look for any meningocele or meningomyelocele.
- A tuft of hair or dimple may indicate an underlying neural tune defect.
- Look for any localized vertebral tenderness.
- Look for any kyphosis, lordosis, or scoliosis.
  - Kyphosis is the term used for excessive backward convexity of the spine.
  - Lordosis is the excessive concavity which most commonly occurs in the lumbar region that results from proximal hip girdle weakness. Lumbar lordosis is common in neuromuscular disorders such as Duchenne muscular dystrophy. Scoliosis is the sideways curvature of the spine. This may be congenital or acquired. Scoliosis may be seen in non-ambulatory children with Duchenne muscular dystrophy and children with Friedrich ataxia and cerebral palsy.
- Feel the spinous processes by standing behind the child and asking him to stand and then bend forward to touch his extended hands to feet. The spinous processes are used for localizing the level of the vertebral segment. Remember some important landmarks which help to localize the vertebral level. The most prominent spinous process at the base of the neck corresponds to the C7 vertebra. D7 is at the level of the lower angle of the scapula. L4 is at the level of the iliac crest. You must also be aware of the spinal segments which correspond to the vertebral levels.

11.14 LOCALIZATION OF NEUROLOGICAL LESION

Localization is the process of determining, from the clinical evaluation, the area in the nervous system that is involved by the disease process. Knowledge of neuroanatomy is basic to formulating any hypothesis of localization. We suggest the following stepwise approach for localization of motor weakness:

Step 1: Whether the lesion is in the upper motor neuron (UMN) or in the lower motor neuron (LMN)?

Step 2: If the lesion is in the upper motor neuron, is it in the brain or spinal cord?

- ***Step 2a:*** If the lesion is in the brain, is it in the cerebral cortex, the subcortex (corona radiata), cerebellum, thalamus, basal ganglia, internal capsule, mid-brain, pons, or medulla?
- ***Step 2b:*** If the lesion is in the spinal cord, find out the spinal level at which this lesion is occurring. Next, translate the spinal level to a vertebral level.

Step 3: If the lesion is in the lower motor neuron, where is it exactly located—starting from the anterior horn cell to the nerve, neuromuscular junction, or muscle?

Let us discuss these steps one by one.

Step 1: Upper *vs* Lower Motor Neuron

The first question to address is whether it is upper motor neuron (UMN) or a lower motor neuron (LMN) involvement. UMN involvement is characterized by spasticity, brisk reflexes, extensor plantar, preserved bulk, and a UMN pattern of weakness. Weakness secondary to LMN is characterized by reduced tone, hyporeflexia, atrophy, and fasciculation.

A common expression of UMN involvement is *hemiparesis* (weakness of one-half of the body), which results from lesions in the motor tract. There are four major sites causing hemiparesis: Cortex, corona radiata, internal capsule, and brainstem. Paraparesis (weakness of both lower limbs), on the other hand, can be both due to UMN or LMN lesions.

1. Upper Motor Neuron (UMN)

An upper motor neuron consists of the neural pathways: (i) Above the motor nuclei of the cranial nerves; and (ii) above the anterior horn cell in the spinal cord. Upper motor neurons travel mainly in the corticospinal tract; besides corticobulbar, tectospinal, rubrospinal, vestibulospinal, and reticulospinal tracts.

Lesion of the upper motor neuron (UMN): The lesion may be a pure pyramidal lesion (of the corticospinal tract) or may involve damage to tracts other than the corticospinal tract. A *pure pyramidal lesion* is characterized by hypertonia, weakness that is predominant in the distal muscles and compromised voluntary skilled movement, Babinski sign (extensor plantar response), and absence of the superficial reflexes.

Spastic paresis results from involvement of corticospinal tract, reticulospinal and vestibulospinal tract. It results in clasp knife spastic paralysis, hyperreflexia, preserved muscle bulk and Babinski sign. Atrophy, if present, will be late and mild. The power in the limb will be usually at least grade 3 unless the lesion is acute and severe in which case, the patient will be in state of neuronal shock. During this phase, there is reduced tone of the affected limb. The spasticity and flexor spasms of the UMN syndrome are due to hyperactive spinal reflexes owing to loss of supraspinal inhibitory control. This reflex hyperexcitability develops over a variable period of time following the primary lesion in brain or spinal cord.

Distribution of muscle weakness: In an upper motor neuron lesion, there is a particular pattern of muscle weakness.

- *In the upper extremity,* the shoulder abductors, the external rotators and the extensors of the elbow, and the wrist are primarily affected with weakness. In contrast, antagonist muscles will develop spasticity. Hence hemiplegic patient will have shoulder adducted and internal rotated with elbow and wrist being flexed and pronated. However, when the weakness is minimal, UMN signs in upper limb can be elicited when both the upper limb is held out in front of the body. Classically one observes a pronator drift with the affected limb going into pronation due to the relative supinator weakness and that limb drifts down.
- *In the lower extremity,* the flexors, the internal rotators, and the dorsiflexors are primarily affected. Usually, the muscle paralysis is unilateral, the opposite side being

affected if the lesion is above the pyramidal decussation, and ipsilateral if the lesion is below the pyramidal decussation. Hence in hemiplegia, lower limb is extended at hip and knee with plantar flexion of foot and while walking these children will have circumduction gait. However, in a spinal cord lesion the deficits may be bilateral.

2. Lower Motor Neuron (LMN)

The lower motor neuron constitutes the nervous system at and beyond the anterior horn cell. A motor unit consists of the anterior horn cell, the spinal roots, the peripheral nerve, the neuromuscular junction and the muscle. LMN lesion thus affects nerve fibers traveling from the anterior horn of the spinal cord to the relevant muscle.

In an LMN disease, hypotonia is the rule, the muscle bulk may be decreased, and the deep tendon reflexes (DTR) are diminished. The distribution of weakness depends on the tissue affected and type of pathology. The limb that is affected offers a little or no resistance to passive movement; this is due to the loss of the stretch reflex.

Long-standing anterior horn cell pathology will result in areflexia, presence of fasciculations and severe muscle atrophy. In contrast, neuropathy has a distal weakness and atrophy with loss of DTRs. Myopathy will have proximal weakness with sluggish DTRs.

Salient differences between UMN and LMN lesions have been tabulated earlier in **Table 11.6**.

Step 2: Localizing an Upper Motor Neuron Lesion

In a child presenting with features of an UMN lesion (spasticity, hyperreflexia, positive Babinski sign), the next step is to decide whether the lesion is in the cord or above the spinal level.

A common expression of UMN involvement is hemiparesis. Associated features that can help to clinch an *upper motor neuron lesion above the spinal cord* are: Cranial nerve involvement (usually unilateral), higher mental function involvement (like mood changes, loss of memory, behavioral changes, speech involvement), seizures, ataxia, movement disorders or impaired consciousness. Further localization can be attempted based on the characteristics described below:

Step 2a

If the lesion is in the brain, is it in the cerebral cortex, the subcortex (corona radiata), cerebellum, thalamus, basal ganglia, internal capsule, mid-brain, pons or medulla?

1. Cortex: Cortical lesions cause contralateral hemiparesis with contralateral facial weakness. Both impaired consciousness and seizures are common. The weak limb is flaccid. Owing to larger representation of hand in the cortex, upper limb is more involved as compared to lower limb. There is a loss of cortical sensation (2-point discrimination, graphasthesia, and stereognosis). There can be aphasia (if dominant hemisphere is affected) and/or presence of a homonymous hemianopia.

When there are unusual, uncoordinated movements such as choreoathetosis (involuntary jerky movements), dystonia (abnormal twisting postures), and hemiballismus (violent flinging movement of one-half of the body considered high amplitude chorea) it may point to an associated basal ganglia lesion.

2. Corona radiata: In hemiparesis due to corona radiata involvement, the findings are same as cortical lesions except that seizures and impaired consciousness are less common. The visual radiations traverse the occipital lobe well beneath the cortex. Therefore, a visual field cut usually signifies a subcortical lesion.

3. Internal capsule: In hemiparesis due to internal capsule involvement there is contralateral hemiparesis with contralateral facial weakness. The hemiplegia is dense-arm and leg affected equally, often severely weak. There may be associated hemisensory deficit. Importantly, there is no aphasia and homonymous hemianopia is rare. Both impaired consciousness and seizures are uncommon.

4. Brainstem: Midbrain, pons and medulla.

Like the spinal cord, lesions of the brainstem cause lower motor neuron disturbance on the level where the lesion is and long tract signs below the lesion. There is contralateral hemiparesis along with ipsilateral cranial nerve involvement. The involvement of brainstem is characterized by crossed findings.

- There are LMN disturbances on the level of the lesion and UMN signs below the lesion.
- The cranial nerves will be affected on the same side (ipsilateral), while the extremity motor deficits are on the other (contralateral) side, because the motor tract decussates (cross) just above the spinal cord.
- Involvement of 3rd and 4th cranial nerves suggests mid-brain involvement, that of 6th and 7th cranial nerve suggests lesion in the pons; and involvement of 9th to 12th cranial nerves is characteristic of involvement of the medulla.

Step 2b

If the lesion is in the spinal cord, find out the spinal level at which this lesion is occurring. Next, translate the spinal level to a vertebral level.

Spinal cord lesion: The hallmark of spinal cord involvement is a 'level' on chest or abdomen, below which the patient has sensory, motor, or reflex abnormalities; and above which the sensory, motor, and reflex functions are normal.

Spinal shock: Acute paralysis as a result of spinal cord disease is accompanied by flaccidity and the loss of tendon and cutaneous reflexes, caused by the sudden withdrawal of activity descending to anterior horn cells from the cerebral cortex and the brain stem. This syndrome of areflexia and hypotonia is known as the spinal shock. Over several days to several weeks, muscle tone and reflexes return. Later muscles become hypertonic and tendon reflexes become hyperactive (spasticity).

In more slowly progressive weakness of spinal origin, there is no intervening stage of spinal shock. The child develops a gradually progressive spasticity without an intervening phase of hypotonia and hyporeflexia.

Muscle spasms are another phenomenon seen with spinal cord injury and result in sudden spontaneous contraction of synergistic muscles. The most common types of spasms are flexor, adductor, or extensor spasms in the legs of patients with paraplegia or quadriplegia. Spastic paralysis is usually associated with the presence of an extensor plantar response (Babinski sign) and loss of superficial reflexes.

Selected patterns in spinal cord lesion

Complete transection: It results in paralysis (LMN type at the level and UMN type below the lesion) and loss of all sensations below the level of lesion, along with loss of bladder and bowel control.

Hemicord lesion (Brown-Sequard syndrome): It results in ipsilateral motor weakness (LMN type at the level and UMN type below the lesion), and loss of vibration and joint position sense (posterior columns) below the level of the lesion. There is additionally contralateral loss of light touch, pin prick and temperature sense (spinothalamic tract).

Posterior column disease: Pathologic processes involving the dorsal columns cause gait ataxia, because of loss of proprioception. There is loss of position and vibration sense in the feet with preserved ankle jerk. Rhomberg sign can be elicited among patients with posterior column involvement. If the lesion affects the cervical cord, there is also upper extremity ataxia. Vision is able to compensate for loss of position sense to a great degree and thus minimize sensory ataxia. Dorsal column disease also causes paresthesias, which are described as tingling, numbness, crawling, or deadness, and which are felt mainly in the distal parts of the extremities.

A thoracic cord lesion results in bilateral loss of position and vibration sense in the feet with a definite level of pinprick loss on the abdomen or chest.

Anterior cord disease: This pattern of injury results most commonly from ischemia or infarction in the distribution of the anterior spinal artery, which supplies the anterior two-thirds of the spinal cord and medulla. Clinical features include a complete motor paralysis below the level of the lesion and loss of pain and temperature sensation at and below the level of the lesion. Proprioception and vibratory sensation is preserved, as it is in the dorsal side of the spinal cord. Areflexia, flaccid anal sphincter, and urinary retention may also be present in individuals with anterior cord syndrome.

Central cord syndrome: Such injury usually results due to traumatic injury to cord due to hyperextension of the cervical region of spine. At the level of injury there is bilateral LMN weakness and muscular atrophy. Below the level there is prominent spastic arm weakness out of proportion to leg weakness (cervical cord) with sacral sparing. Early and prominent bladder involvement is seen. Bilateral loss of pain, temperature, light touch and pressure sensations below the level of lesion with sacral sparing.

Intramedullary lesion: Loss of pinprick sensation over legs and trunk with normal perianal sensation. This is due to the lamination of the spinothalamic tracts with the sacral sensory fibers situated laterally.

Cauda equina lesion: Loss of pinprick sensation in the perianal area and in the upper part of both posterior thighs—saddle anesthesia.

Step 3: Localizing a Lesion in the Motor Unit

The signs and symptoms of lower motor neuron diseases vary depending upon the etiology, pathology and the part of the motor unit affected. Diminished deep tendon reflexes are a constant and characteristic feature of all peripheral neuropathies.

Muscle wasting is a characteristic feature of lower motor neuron disease except the pseudohypertrophy (seen in Ducchene muscular dystrophy) or hypertrophy seen in congenital myotonic dystrophy. Other features of LMN lesion include muscle weakness, loss of reflexes (however, may not be seen in myopathies), fasciculation, and sensory signs and symptoms due to neuropathy.

1. Anterior Horn Cells

A pure motor syndrome is the hallmark of anterior horn cell involvement. Fasciculation is the most characteristic finding in chronic disorders. There is no sensory loss. There is gross muscle wasting. Hereditary disorders (such as spinal muscular atrophy) are characterized by hypotonia, generalized weakness, fasciculation, areflexia, and muscle atrophy and no sensory loss or UMN signs. Acquired involvement is commonly due to viral infection, polio being the prototype. Such involvement results in a typical asymmetric, patchy flaccid weakness, muscle atrophy and areflexia. Anterior horn cell disorders typically produce significant muscle atrophy.

2. Root Disease (Radiculopathy)

Root pain is the clue, it occurs in the involved dermatome and may radiate to the limbs. The pain can be provoked by particular movements or positions (such as straight leg raise). There are associated sensory symptoms in the form of hyperesthesia, tingling, and numbness. Neurological findings are usually asymmetric and involve muscle atrophy, weakness, loss of deep tendon reflexes, and sensory loss only in the concerned dermatomes and myotomes. However, for acute polyradiculopathy, as seen in Gullain Barre Syndrome, the sensory manifestations are minimal and symmetric weakness is characteristic.

3. Peripheral Neuropathy

Peripheral neuropathy is characterized by sensory, motor or mixed deficits. It may be a mononeuropathy or a polyneuropathy.

- Sensory symptoms are usually the presenting symptoms of neuropathy and include positive (burning, pain, walking on cotton wool, band-like sensation on feet or trunk, stumbling, tingling, pins and needles) and negative symptoms (numbness, loss of sensation) in hands and feet (glove and stalking distribution). These manifestations are very rare in children.
- In case of a nerve root and peripheral nerve disease, with monoradiculopathies and mononeuropathies, the weakness is limited to the muscles which that nerve or nerve root innervates.
- In case of axonal polyneuropathy, the affection is bilateral, symmetrical, and distal.
- Motor symptoms include distal muscle weakness and child may complain of difficulty in turning keys in locks, unfasten button, and opening bottles and jars.
- Usually, the motor weakness in peripheral neuropathy is distal; however, early proximal weakness is a feature of demyelinating polyneuropathy.

4. Neuromuscular Junction

Neuromuscular junction disorders may result from drugs and toxins or from diseases such as myasthenia gravis. Neuromuscular junction disorders most commonly involve the ocular and pharyngeal involvement. The hallmark of the weakness is fluctuation and easy fatigability. The weakness improves after a period of rest. Deep tendon reflexes and muscle bulk are generally preserved despite the weakness.

5. Muscle Diseases

Muscle diseases most often produce a pattern of proximal and symmetrical weakness. Muscle disease may result from primary causes within the muscle or secondary to systemic diseases. Primary myopathies can be broadly categorized as muscle dystrophies, congenital myopathies, inflammatory myopathies, and metabolic myopathies. The dystrophies and metabolic myopathies tend to be slowly progressive. Importantly, muscular dystrophies usually present with a specific pattern of weakness and differential muscular atrophy and hypertrophy. Meaning, some muscles will atrophy and some will hypertrophy.

11.15 THE FINAL DIAGNOSIS

A few important questions that need to be answered after the clinical evaluation are:

- At what age did the problem start?
- Is the onset acute or insidious?
- Is the process static or recurrent or progressive?
- Is the process focal/multifocal/diffuse/neuronal group disorder?
- What parts of the neuraxis are involved?
- What is the likely pathophysiological process and etiology **(Table 11.30)**?

After you complete your history, try to write a summary of the important points in history. The summary should generally be maximum 4–5 lines long. The whole exercise of writing a summary enables you to focus on the salient features in the history and plan the examination in its perspective. This is the time when you should have a hypothesis going on the anatomical involvement, nature of pathophysiological process, and the possible etiology. Finally the management plan is prepared; remember that management would involve systematic investigations and treatment of primary illness and the co-morbidities.

Example: In a 3-year-old boy having tubercular meningitis, the summary of the history may be expressed as follows:

A 3-year-old, partially immunized boy, presented to us with fever for 1 month, vomiting for 15 days, 2 episodes of right focal motor seizures on day 20 and 25 of illness, and rapidly progressive altered sensorium for 2 days. There was a significant history of contact with an adult with pulmonary tuberculosis 6 months back.

Similarly, the examination should also end with a short summary of positive findings and important negative findings.

On examination, the child is wasted, stunted, and has moderate pallor. Neurological examination revealed a GCS of 10, bilateral papilledema, left 6th nerve palsy, right UMN facial nerve palsy, right hemiparesis, neck stiffness, and Kernig sign.

This step is followed by formulating a clinical synopsis derived from a combined summary of history and examination.

A 3-year-old boy presented with prolonged pyrexia, seizures, altered sensorium, features of raised intracranial pressure, left 6th nerve palsy, right UMN facial nerve palsy, right hemiparesis (upper limb predominant), and meningeal signs. The child was chronically malnourished and there was a positive history of tubercular contact.

Table 11.30: Etiological categories in neurological disorders

Infections	Trauma
• Perinatal brain insult • Neurodevelopmental disorders • Immune mediated • Vascular • Metabolic • Neurological complications of systemic diseases • Toxins	• Nutritional • Neurodegenerative disorders • Congenital anomalies • Genetic disorders • Psychiatric/psychogenic disorders

The next step is to attempt and localize the disease process on the neuraxis. Localization would first involve to ascertain if this is a focal, multifocal, or diffuse disease. Further, the areas involved need to be outlined. Look for features of involvement of spinal cord, brain stem, cranial nerve, cerebellum, basal ganglia, and cortical, or subcortical structures.

Summary outlined above suggests involvement of cerebral cortex (seizures, raised ICP, altered sensorium), and meninges (meningeal signs). The neurological deficit (right hemiparesis with upper limb predominant) suggests a disease of middle cerebral artery (most probably, infarction).

The next step is to formulate a pathophysiological hypothesis.

The prolonged pyrexia and meningeal signs suggests chronic meningitis process. Meningitis and hydrocephalus have resulted in raised ICP. The altered sensorium may have resulted from raised ICP and infarction of MCA. The left 6th nerve palsy may have resulted from raised ICP or entrapment of the nerve in the basal exudates. The right UMN facial nerve palsy and right hemiparesis (upper limb predominant) are likely secondary to arterial stroke due to entrapped vessels in basal exudates. Anemia, wasting and stunting—indicate nutritional deprivation with secondary worsening by recent infection.

The final component of the diagnostic process is the etiological possibilities.

In this case the likely etiology is infective (tubercular meningitis) with hydrocephalus and arterial stroke on a background of chronic malnutrition, incomplete immunization, and contact with TB patient. The other causes of chronic meningitis need exclusion in the appropriate clinical context.

Chapter

12

Examination of the Eye

○ Payal Gupta

Structure

12.1 AIM AND SCHEME OF EYE EXAMINATION

Examination of the eyes in infants and children is of critical importance since they most often do not report ocular complaints. They are brought to the ophthalmologist only if an alert parent notices something not quite right with the child's vision or eyes. Visual problems at this age, if ignored, might mean a lifetime of visual deprivation. Also, eye problems can sometimes be the sole presentation/manifestation of a systemic disease. For example, tuberculosis may present as a phlycten in the conjunctiva or cornea.

In this chapter, we will introduce you to common eye symptoms and signs that you can expect to encounter in a pediatric set-up **(Key Box 1)**. Further, we will familiarize you with important eye examination techniques; these can be challenging since you will be dealing with an uncooperative population.

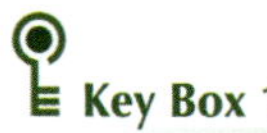

Key Box 1

Goals for Eye Examination in a Child

1. Assessment of the functional status of the eyes, particularly vision and binocularity
2. Assessment of ocular health, particularly in reference to the systemic condition
3. Counseling of caregivers and referring to an ophthalmologist where appropriate

12.2 COMMON SYMPTOMS RELATED TO THE EYE

A. Eye Discharge

Any discharge from the eyes of a child should be viewed with suspicion.

- In a newborn, it could indicate ophthalmia neonatorum, congenital glaucoma, or congenital dacryocystitis.
- In older children, it may be due to allergic or infective conjunctivitis, trauma, or chronic dacryocystitis.

You should be able to broadly ascribe an etiology based on the type of discharge **(Table 12.1)**.

B. Red Eye

Congestion in the eye is always pathological. The cause may be as trivial as rubbing due to itching, but may be a portent of visually threatening conditions. Redness may result from dilation of superficial (conjunctival) or deep (ciliary) vessels. The causes are tabulated in **Table 12.2**.

C. Itching

Itching is the hallmark of allergic conjunctivitis, but may be seen in blepharitis.

Table 12.1: Types and causes of eye discharge

Type of discharge	Possible etiology
Watery (Fig. 12.1)	Viral, chlamydial or allergic conjunctivitis, refractive errors
Mucoid	Allergic or chlamydial conjunctivitis, congenital or chronic dacryocystitis
Mucopurulent	Bacterial conjunctivitis, congenital or chronic dacryocystitis
Purulent	Ophthalmia neonatorum, bacterial conjunctivitis, acute dacryocystitis
Hemorrhagic	Membranous conjunctivitis, ocular trauma, bleeding disorder

Table 12.2: Types of congestion and clinical features of red eye

Type of congestion	Clinical features	Etiology
Conjunctival	Superficial, red, branching vessels, running from conjunctival fornices to the limbus	Conjunctivitis, conjunctival injury or foreign body
Ciliary	Deep, dull red flush surrounding the limbus	Keratitis, uveitis, glaucoma, ocular trauma, contact lens related

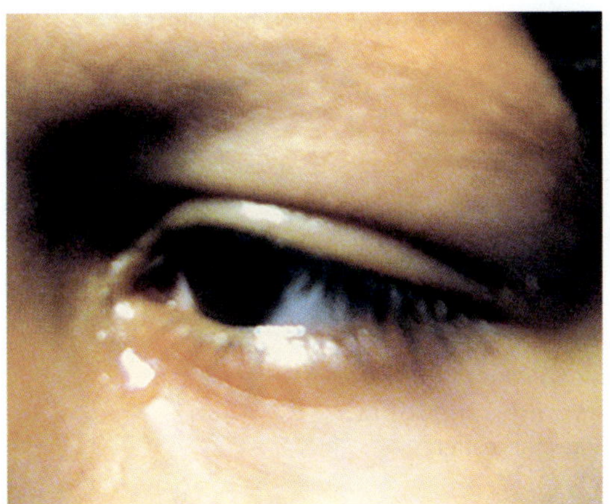

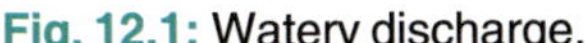

Fig. 12.1: Watery discharge.

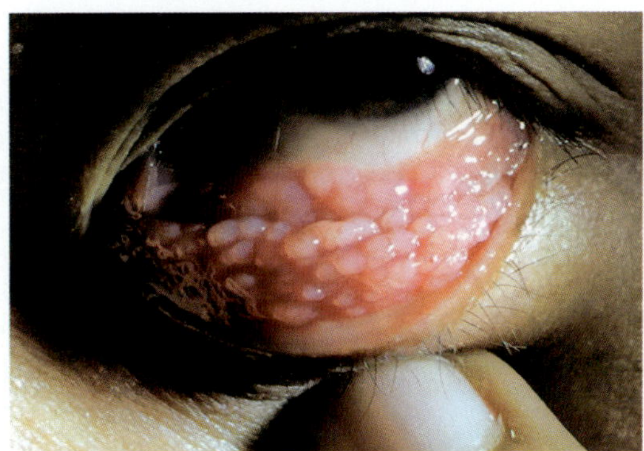

Fig. 12.2: Giant papillary conjunctivitis.

- Allergy may be seasonal due to pollens; it is usually difficult to pinpoint the allergen.
- Allergy may be related to animal hair, so that it appears on every exposure to the animal.
- It may be due to topical or systemic drugs, cosmetics, or contact lens solutions (Fig. 12.2).

A careful history should elicit the offending agent.

D. Mass Lesions in the Vicinity of the Eyelid

Table 12.3 shows the differentiating features of the more common mass lesions. Chalazion and stye usually occur in older children, while dermoid is congenital, and hemangioma presents within the first few months of birth.

E. Reduced Vision

1. Older Children

They may report difficulty in copying off the blackboard, reading bus numbers, viewing cricket scores on the television, etc. The child and the parents may not notice when only one eye has poor vision; the child, though monocular, manages tasks of daily living satisfactorily.

2. Preschool Children

You should suspect reduced vision in a preschooler when he tends to sit too close to the television, holds toys/books close to the eyes, or complains of eye ache. When only one eye has poor vision, it may pass unnoticed, since the child manages well using the other eye.

Table 12.3: Mass lesions around the eyelids

Mass lesions around the eyelids	Cause	Clinical features	Look for the following clues
Chalazion	Blockage of meibomian gland opening with a granulomatous reaction to the lipid content in the gland	Firm, painless, slow growing swelling in the tarsoconjunctiva, free from overlying skin	Bluish or yellowish discoloration on the conjunctival side of the lesion
Stye	Blockage of the duct of glands of Moll or Zeis with bacterial superinfection, usually staphylococcal	Acutely tender, inflamed swelling of one of the glands associated with eyelashes	A pus point at the root of the lash
Distension of the lacrimal sac	Incomplete canalization of the nasolacrimal duct	Soft swelling in the medial canthal region	Pressure over the swelling causes mucopus regurgitation into the conjunctival sac
Dermoid	• Congenital; arises from areas of ectoderm pinched off along bone suture lines; may be seen at the limbus **(Fig. 12.3)** • Dermoid is the commonest orbital mass in children	• Firm to soft cystic mass in relation to a bony suture, usually the fronto-zygomatic • May be connected to an orbital or intracranial dermoid (rare)	Subcutaneous, with normal overlying skin, fixed to periosteum
Hemangioma	Hamartomatous proliferation of vascular endothelial cells	Soft, red mass, presents within 6 months of birth, usually medial side of upper eyelid. Grows rapidly during infancy to produce ptosis and amblyopia. Involutes thereafter	Blanches with pressure

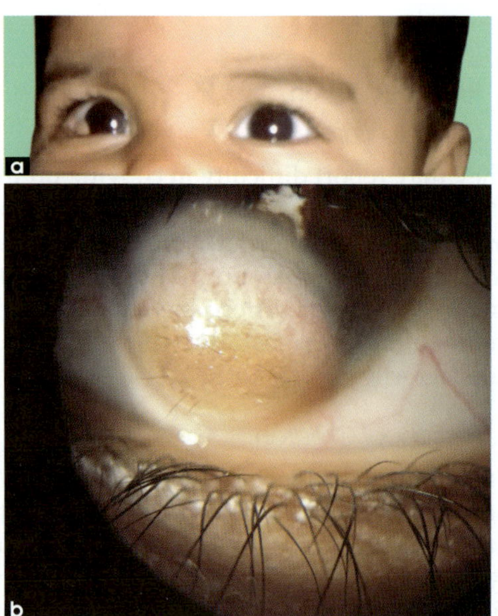

Fig. 12.3: (a) Limbal dermoid, right eye; (b) Slit lamp photo of a limbal dermoid with hair.

3. Infants

Parents may or may not notice the indirect clues to reduced vision like poor response to bright light, not reaching out to play with toys, not recognizing mother, deviation of the eye or abnormal eye movements. In the absence of gross eye abnormality, reduced vision is rarely noticed in infants.

In the section on ocular examination techniques, we have described signs that give a clue to subnormal vision in infants.

F. Pain in the Eye or Orbit

Uncorrected refractive errors in school going children may cause eyeache, especially on near work, and which tends to get worse as the day progresses. The eyeache is improved by resting the eyes or sleeping. Orbital pain is suggestive of ethmoidal or frontal

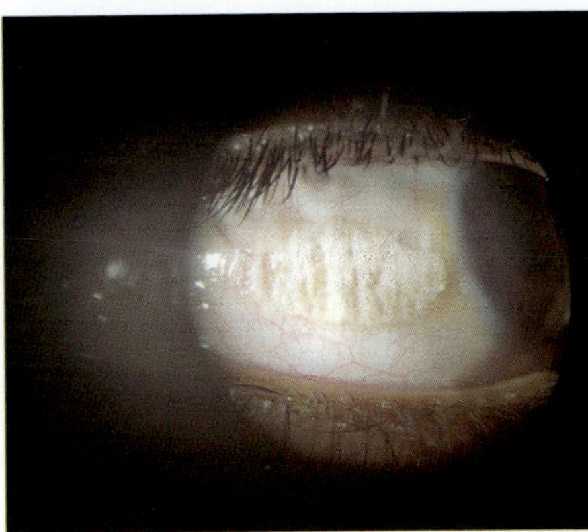

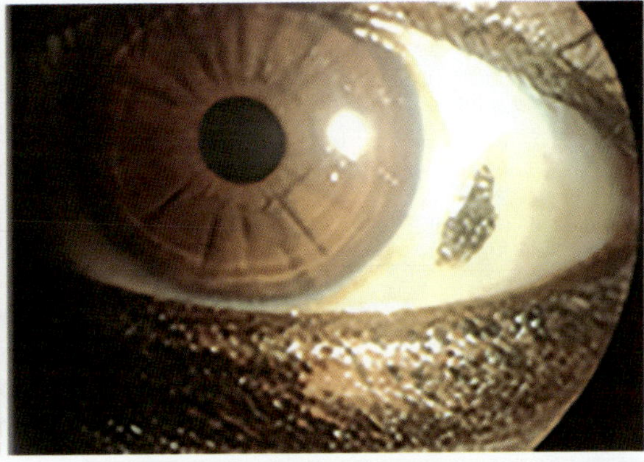

Fig. 12.4: Left: Bitot's spot with conjunctival xerosis; Right: Bitot's spot with *kajal* deposits on the surface

sinusitis and is associated with signs of upper respiratory infection.

G. Headache

Uncorrected refractive errors may infrequently cause headache. Headaches from refractive errors are differentiated from migraine and secondary headaches in that they are non-acute, and are related to prolonged reading or near work. Further, headaches due to refractive errors are not associated with features like aura (migraine), projectile vomiting (intracranial space occupying lesions), fever (sinusitis, meningitis), etc. Vision assessment and refraction testing will clinch the diagnosis of refractive error; spectacle use will relieve the symptoms. Although only a small proportion has refractive errors, you should advise ophthalmic assessment for children with headache. Papilledema, optic atrophy, or oculomotor disorders may be detected, suggesting secondary (central nervous system) causes for the headache. Early detection and intervention may save vision and life.

H. Abnormalities in Color or Shape of Eyeball

1. Discoloration of Conjunctiva

In older children, some degree of pigmentation around the limbus and in the exposed bulbar conjunctiva (between upper and lower lids) is normal and it corelates with the degree of pigmentation of the skin. Nevi are not unusual; they may appear soon after birth, in the first year, and may grow as the eyeball grows. They are asymptomatic, flat, avascular, and localized. Bitot's spots due to vitamin A deficiency are triangular keratinized areas with deposits of epithelium and sebaceous secretion on the surface; they lie on one or both sides of the cornea in the inter-palpebral fissure (Fig. 12.4). The surface deposits (cellular, oily, or cosmetics) can usually be swept off, but recur.

2. White Cornea

A white cornea is indicative of corneal edema/ opacity (Fig. 12.5).

- In infants, you should suspect congenital glaucoma, particularly if the eyeball is enlarged. It may also be due to corneal infections or inflammation (keratitis), keratomalacia (in top-fed infants), and birth or other trauma.
- In older children, you should rule out keratomalacia (especially if bilateral), keratitis, and trauma.

3. White Reflex in Pupil

This is also known as amaurotic cat's eye reflex or leucocoria, and has ominous implications (Fig. 12.6). Causes are listed in **Table 12.4**

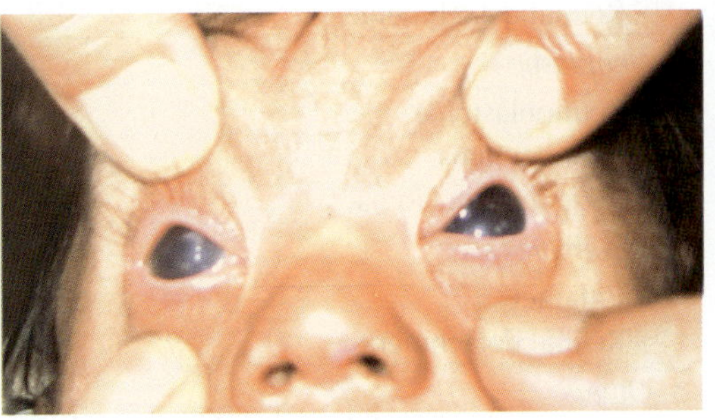

Fig. 12.5: White cornea in keratomalacia.

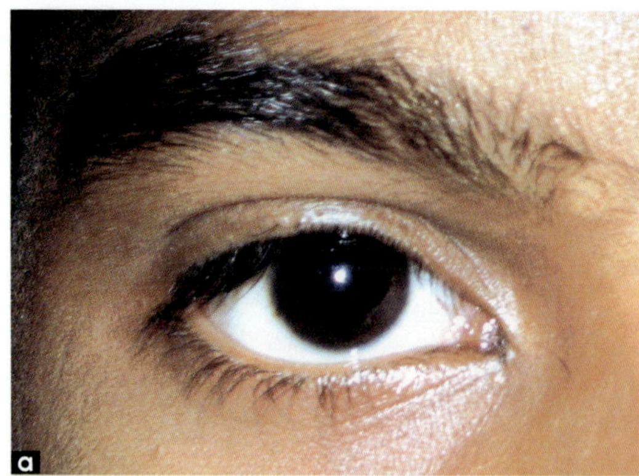

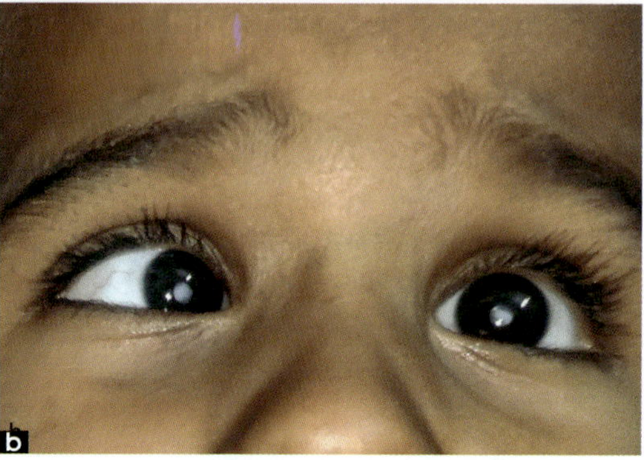

Fig. 12.6: (a) Normal color of the pupil; (b) White reflex in the pupil due to bilateral cataract.

Table 12.4: Causes of white reflex
1. *Congenital* • Cataract • Persistent hyperplastic primary vitreous • Coats' disease • Choroidal coloboma • Retinal detachment • Vitreoretinal dysplasias: Norrie disease, incontinentia pigmenti, Walker-Warburg syndrome
2. *Inflammatory* • Cyclitic membrane • Endophthalmitis • Toxocariasis • Retinal detachment
3. *Neoplastic* • Retinoblastoma • Retinocytoma • Retinal astrocytoma
4. *Traumatic* • Cataract • Retinal detachment
5. *Others* • Retinopathy of prematurity (ROP)

- In neonates, it could indicate congenital cataract, congenital abnormalities of retina, choroid or vitreous, retinoblastoma, or endophthalmitis. Retinoblastoma is rare after the age of 7 years.
- In older children, white reflex may be due to congenital or traumatic cataract, retinal detachment, or endophthalmitis.

White reflex in pupil is indicative of a serious vision threatening condition, and you should immediately refer the child to an ophthalmologist.

4. Large Eyeball

A large eyeball is seen in congenital glaucoma. The sclera of children under the age of 3 years is susceptible to stretching in response to raised intraocular pressure. You should look for the hallmark symptoms of watering, photophobia, and blepharospasm (Fig. 12.7).

5. Small Eyeball

A small eyeball could be due to congenital microphthalmos or phthisis bulbi.

- *Microphthalmos* is congenital, and depending on severity, variable eyeball details are visible; some vision may be present.
- *Microphthalmos* may be unilateral or bilateral, and may be associated with other ocular (coloboma of iris) (Fig. 12.8) or systemic (rubella embryopathy) abnormalities.
- Phthisis bulbi is acquired because of severe infection/trauma. The eyeball is completely disorganized and blind. A careful history of mode of onset should elucidate the cause.

6. Absent Eyeball (Anophthalmos)

This may be congenital or acquired. Primary congenital anophthalmos is rare; it is more

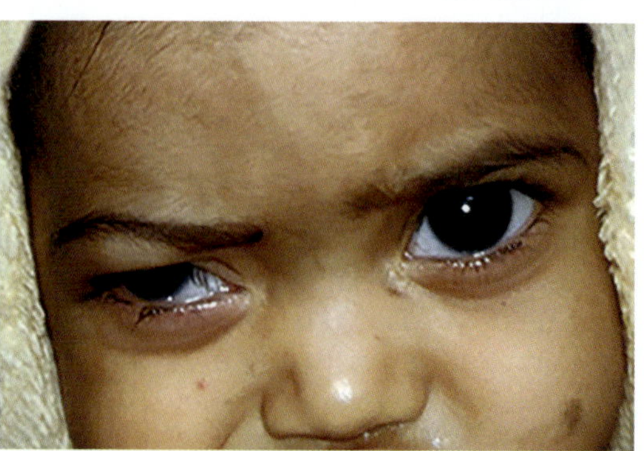

Fig. 12.7: Buphthalmos.

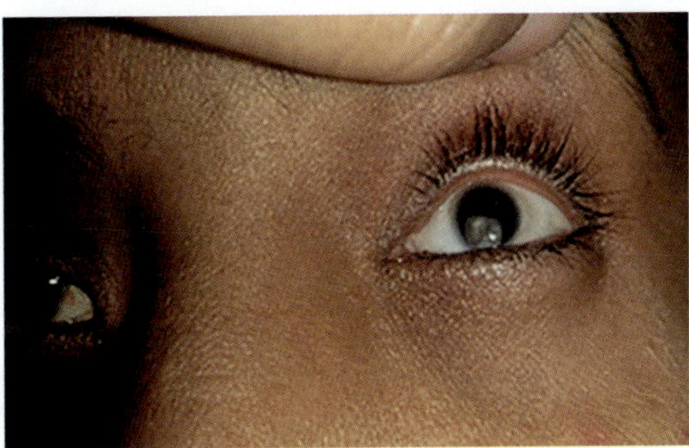

Fig. 12.8: Microphthalmos with coloboma of iris with cataract.

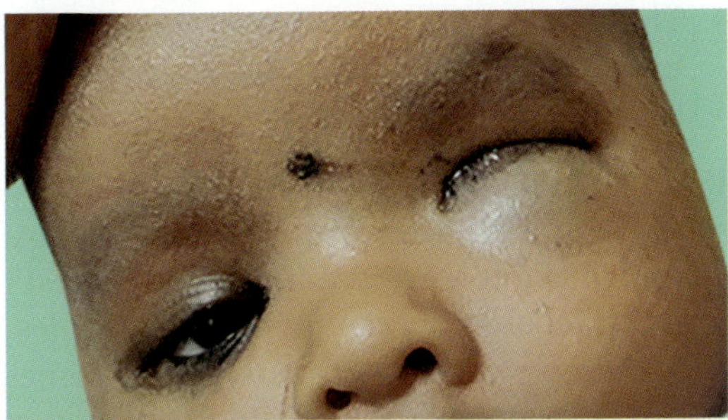

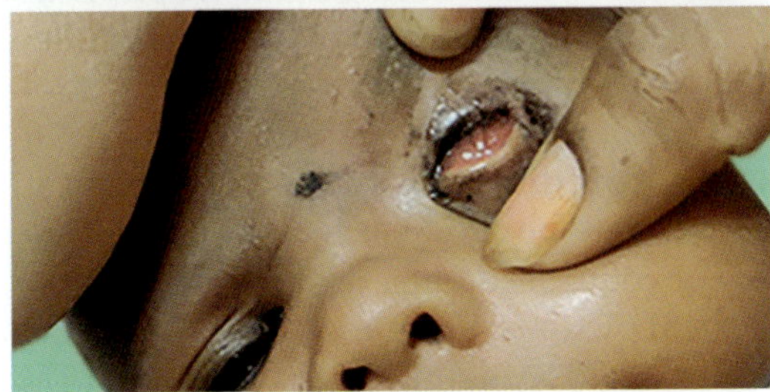

Fig. 12.9: Absent left eyeball (congenital anophthalmos).

usually extreme microphthalmos. Acquired cases are due to removal of eyeball for intraocular tumor, blind painful eye, or severe destructive eyeball trauma (Fig. 12.9).

12.3 EXAMINATION OF THE EYE

A sequential examination will ensure that you do not miss important findings. We recommend the scheme of examination highlighted in **Key Box 2**.

The first three components must be assessed during your first contact with every child even when no ocular complaints are reported. Remember, you may be the first to pick up a potentially sight-threatening condition in an infant or child.

- Screening of babies' eyes at birth by the pediatrician is important, and should be reinforced with examination by an ophthalmologist at 6 months, 2 years, and 4 years of age.
- The visual system at this time is highly susceptible to both insult and therapeutic intervention; this protocol will enhance prevention, early detection and treatment of visual and non-visual ocular problems in children.
- Opt for objective assessment methods for infants and preverbal children.
- Examine them after a nap or while feeding, when they are likely to be cooperative and alert.
- Perform all tests considerably more rapidly than you would in older children, since they are easily distracted and will stop co-operating.

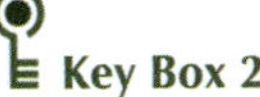

Key Box 2

Scheme of Examination

1. Assess for obvious abnormality of eye or asymmetry
2. Evaluate the visual acuity of each eye separately
3. Assess the visual axes and ocular movements
4. Examine the eyelids and lacrimal sac
5. Examine the conjunctivae and sclera
6. Examine the cornea
7. Examine pupils, lens and fundus oculi
8. Finally, measure the intraocular pressure and assess color vision, if required

Prerequisites for Vision Testing

- Vision testing should comprise the first step of ocular examination, prior to torch light being shone in the eye and inducing glare.
- Both eyes are to be examined separately.
- Make sure the other eye is covered without undue pressure (to avoid transient corneal edema which can result in underestimation of visual acuity). You may use the child's or the parent's palm as cover, if a plastic occluder is not available.
- You should ask the child to stand 6 meters from the vision chart (Fig. 12.10), or 3 meters from a mirror in which the chart is reflected.
- The minimal illumination of the chart should be 480 lux. This can be easily achieved by directing a spotlight at the

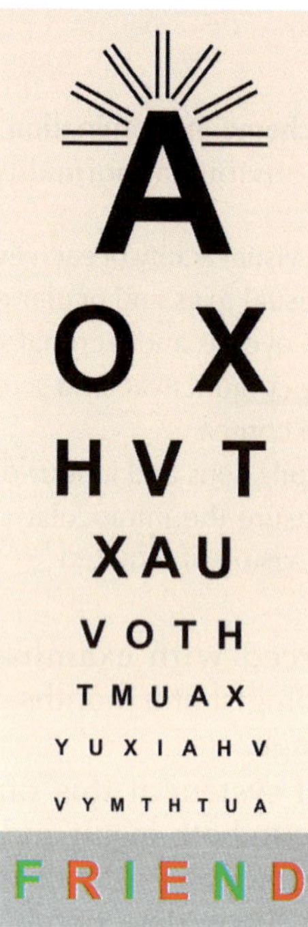

Fig. 12.10: Self-illuminated Snellen chart.

chart or using a self-illuminating one (a well-lit room generally provides more than 480 lux of illumination).

A. Visual Acuity Assessment

1. Snellen Chart (Fig. 12.10)

You will have seen the chart sometime during your ophthalmology posting.

- It comprises a series of letters arranged in rows of varying sizes in descending order. The letters are constructed keeping in mind that the minimal visual angle at which a normal person can resolve objects is 1 minute.
- Thus, the components making up each letter subtend an angle of 1 minute at the retina, the whole letter subtending an angle of 5 minutes, when seen from the reference distance.
- Conventionally, letters in the top row subtend that angle when viewed from a distance of 60 meters, while letters in subsequent rows make the same angle at distances of 36, 24, 18, 12, 9 and 6 meters, respectively. Some charts have a line beneath the 6 meters line which makes a 5-minute angle at the retina when viewed from 5 meters.
- Thus, a child with normal vision should be able to read the last line from a distance of 6 meters.

How to Use?

- Ask the child to start reading from the topmost letter down to the smallest that he can read clearly.
- Visual acuity is notated as a fraction with the numerator indicating the distance between the child and the chart, and the denominator indicating the smallest line that the child could read clearly.
- Thus, normal vision is 6/6. If only the topmost letter is clear, vision is designated as 6/60.

What should you do if the child cannot read?

- Preverbal children can be examined by forced-choice preferential-looking tests using Teller acuity charts and Leah paddles.
- Children who do not know the alphabet can be examined using Landolt open rings (Fig. 12.11) which are based on Snellen optotypes.
- The rings have open ends pointing in different directions (up, down, right and left) that the child has to indicate.
- For younger children, letters can be replaced with pictures of common objects that they are asked to identify or match (Fig. 12.12).

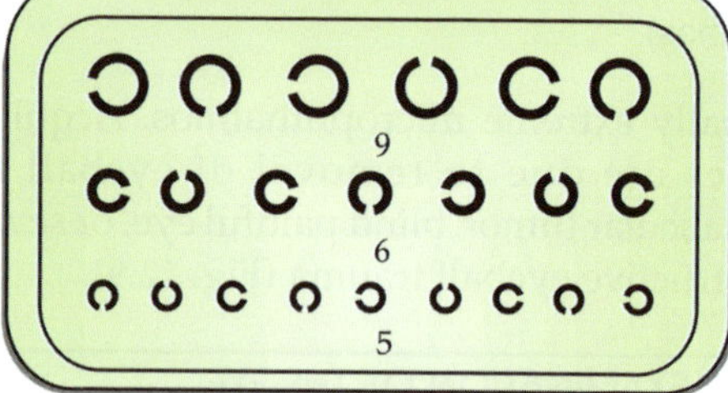

Fig. 12.11: Landolt open rings chart.

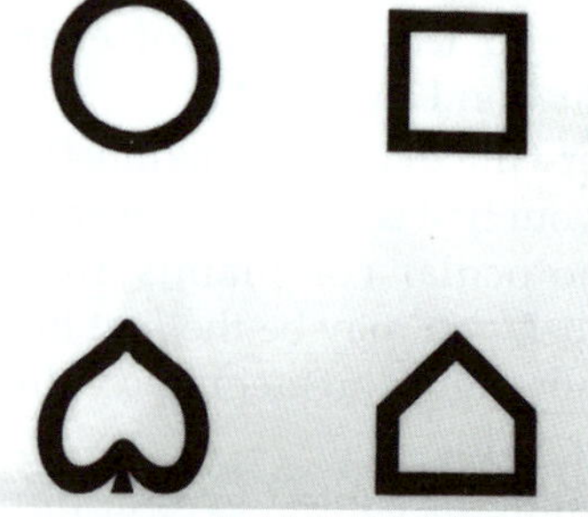

Fig. 12.12: Picture chart.

What should you do if the child cannot identify the topmost letter on the chart?

- Bring the child closer to the chart until he can read the topmost letter. The visual acuity will then be designated as $x/60$, where x is the distance (in meters) between the child and the chart.
- Visual acuity of less than 1/60 can be recorded as *'counting fingers'* (CF) if the child is able to count them from a meter or so.
- If he cannot, you should check if he can perceive waving movements of your hand–*'hand movements'* (HM).
- When hand movements are also not perceived, you should check for *'perception of light'* (PL) by throwing a bright light on the child's eye and asking whether he can perceive it. Do not forget to cover the other eye properly, preferably with your own palm, to prevent stray light stimulating the retina of the other eye.
- Thereafter, you should check the functional integrity of different quadrants of the retina by projecting light from the superior, inferior, temporal, and nasal fields with the child staring straight ahead. The child should be able to accurately indicate the position of the torch ('Projection of rays'; PR). It is represented with a cross dividing the visual field into four quadrants. A plus sign in a quadrant indicates normal projection in that quadrant; a minus sign indicates absent projection in that quadrant (Fig. 12.13).
- The other eye is to be examined similarly. If the child is wearing spectacles, check his aided visual acuity also.

How can you tell if a child's glasses are hypermetropic or myopic?

Look at a distant object through the lens. If it magnifies the object and it moves opposite to the movement of lens, the child is wearing convex lenses and is hypermetropic. If objects appeared minified on looking through the glasses and move in the same direction, the child is using concave lenses and is myopic.

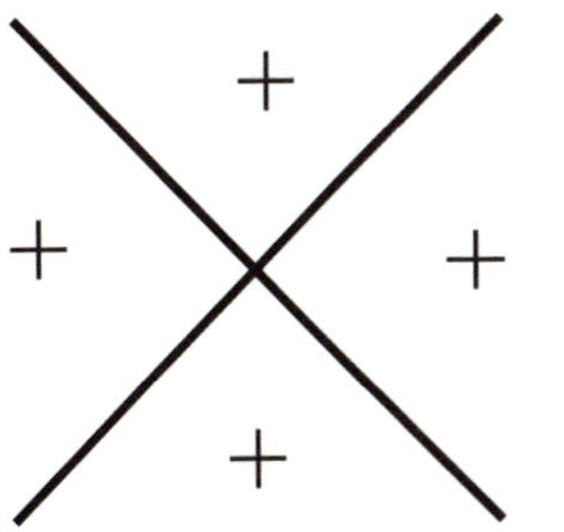

Fig. 12.13: Representation of projection of rays.

How will you check the visual status of infants and uncooperative preschoolers?

You cannot use Snellen's chart but must rely on indirect clues and objective methods to determine if vision is subnormal or not. Assessment of visually evoked response and optokinetic nystagmus can reliably predict visual acuity. However, they are complicated and may not be available in your set-up.

Clinical clues to determine subnormal vision in an infant **(Key Box 3)**

- Presence of squint or nystagmus should immediately alert you to the possibility of reduced vision in this age group. Nystagmus may have an ocular origin, when the child cannot fixate light because of media opacity (cataract) or macular disease (toxoplasmosis, ROP, retinoblastoma); when it is of central origin, the rapid eye movements do not allow the macula to fix long enough to allow good vision.
- Another useful sign is the resistance shown to occlusion of one eye. While you may occlude the eye with reduced vision without incident, the child will protest when you attempt to occlude the eye with normal vision.
- Most children above the age of 3 months (about the time when the fixation reflex develops) will move the eyes to fixate a torchlight shone at them; disinclination to do so is indicative of poor vision.
- A sluggish or absent pupillary reaction to direct light is indicative of serious

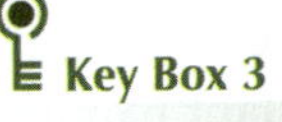

Clinical Clues to Determine Subnormal Vision in an Infant

1. Presence of squint or nystagmus
2. Resistance shown to occlusion of one eye
3. Inability to follow a moving light source
4. Sluggish or absent pupillary reaction to direct light
5. Absent red reflex in the pupil

pathology and mandates immediate referral to an ophthalmologist.

View the infant's pupil through a direct ophthalmoscope held about 25 cm away. The light is reflected back from the vascular choroid into your eye and you see a red reflex in the pupil. Absence or obscuration of the red reflex is indicative of media opacity (cataract, ROP, retinoblastoma, etc.).

2. Pinhole Examination

- Children with subnormal visual acuity can be asked to read the Snellen's test types through a pinhole of diameter 0.75–1 mm.
- Improvement of vision using the pinhole indicates uncorrected refractive error. If vision does not improve, or worsens, it is probably an organic abnormality.
- If a preformed pinhole is not available, you can make it by piercing a dark-colored cardboard with the tip of a standard ballpoint pen.

Principle of the pinhole: Peripheral rays are cut off by the pinhole allowing only a narrow pencil of rays to enter the eye. As it enters along the principal axis, it undergoes minimal refraction. In addition, the pinhole also cuts off spherical aberrations induced by peripheral cornea and lens. Thus, regardless of type of refractive error, vision improves.

B. Assessment of Visual Axis

The visual axes of the two eyes should be parallel to each other in all gazes except in convergence and divergence.

You can examine the relative direction of both visual axes by the **Hirschberg test**.

- Make the child sit straight keeping the head straight.
- Throw torchlight at his glabella from arm's length distance (approximately 25–33 cm).
- Ask the child to look at a distant fixation target and examine the corneal reflections of the torchlight on the two corneas.
- If the reflection is central in one eye and eccentric in the other, the child has manifest squint. If the eccentric reflection is nasal to the center, the child has divergent squint (Fig. 12.14); and if it is temporal, the child has convergent squint.

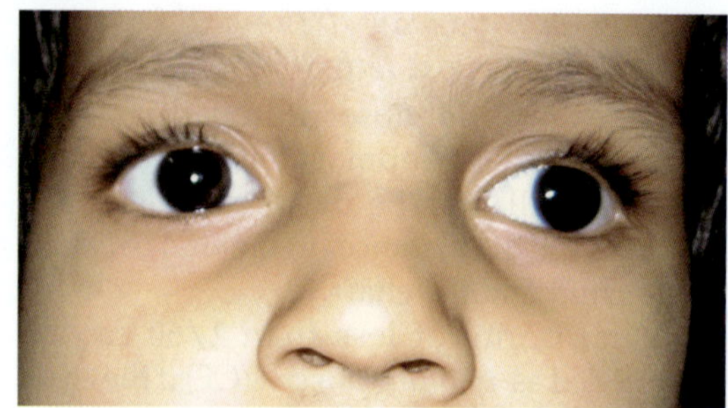

Fig. 12.14: Divergent squint left eye, 30°.

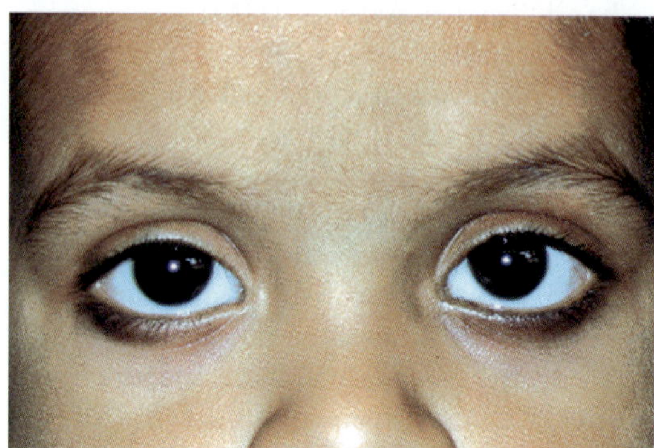

Fig. 12.15: Corneal reflections in the center of both pupils: no squint.

- If the reflections are exactly in the center of both pupils (Fig. 12.15), then the child either has no squint, or has a latent squint.

Latent Squint

Sometimes children can keep their eyes aligned by excessive use of accommodation or of their binocular reflexes. Thus, squint is not obvious on the Hirschberg test; however, when the child is tired, daydreaming, or ill, the eyes tend to dissociate from each other, and latent squint becomes manifest. Thus, if you find that the corneal reflections are exactly in the center of both pupils on Hirschberg test, simply cover one eye (the **cover test:** it breaks the binocular association between the two eyes). If the child has a latent squint, the eye behind cover will deviate; when you remove the cover (the cover-uncover test), that eye makes a movement to re-fixate since the two eyes are associated again. This recovery movement confirms the presence of latent squint. If there is no movement of the eye behind cover, there is no squint.

How will you determine the degree of squint?

A 1 mm deviation of corneal reflection is equal to 7° of squint. Thus, you can roughly assess the amount of squint from the position of the corneal reflection. If the eccentric reflection is at the pupillary margin, the amount of squint is approximately 15°. If it lies at the corneal limbus, the amount of squint is approximately 45°.

How will you determine if squint is paralytic or non-paralytic?

The symptom of diplopia is usually indicative of paralytic squint; however, young children often suppress the image from the squinting eye, so that diplopia disappears.

The child may adopt a head posture in the direction of the paralyzed muscle to overcome the diplopia.

The alternate cover test: The cover is moved from one eye to the other alternately, thus forcing first one eye and then the other to fixate. In this way, you can measure the deviation (of left eye) when the right eye fixates, and of the right eye, when the left eye fixates. In non-paralytic squint, the deviation is the same regardless of which eye is fixing; however, if a muscle is paralyzed, the deviation demonstrated when the eye with the paralyzed muscle fixates (secondary deviation) is greater than when the other eye fixates (primary deviation). The reason for this is that greater innervation is sent to the paralyzed muscle in an attempt to move the eye to enable it to fixate; simultaneously, the yoke muscle in the other eye also receives enhanced innervation, resulting in increased deviation **(Hering's law of equal innervation of yoke muscles)**.

You should test ocular movements as described below; these will be defective in a particular direction in case of paralytic squint.

C. Examination of Ocular Movements

It is important to assess ocular movements both uniocularly and binocularly.

- Uniocular assessment alone will fail to give you an idea of the binocular interactions between the two eyes.
- Binocular assessment alone may mislead you into thinking that movements in a particular direction are paralyzed.

Let us illustrate this with an example: In a child with a large non-paralytic divergent squint **(Fig. 12.16a)**, the divergence between the two visual axes will be maintained in all directions of gaze. When you ask the child to fix a target to the left you will notice that while the left eye looks at the target, the right eye is relatively divergent, so that it appears that there is a paralysis of medial movement in that eye **(Fig. 12.16b)**. However, if you now cover the left eye, the child moves the right eye medially in order to fixate the object **(Fig. 12.16c)**. Thus, uniocular testing rules out a paralysis of medial movement.

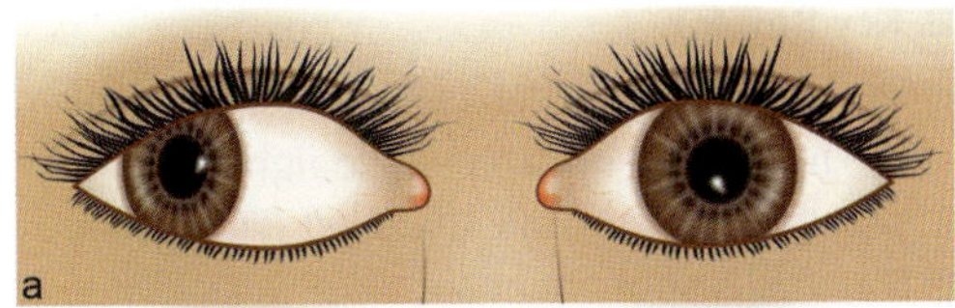

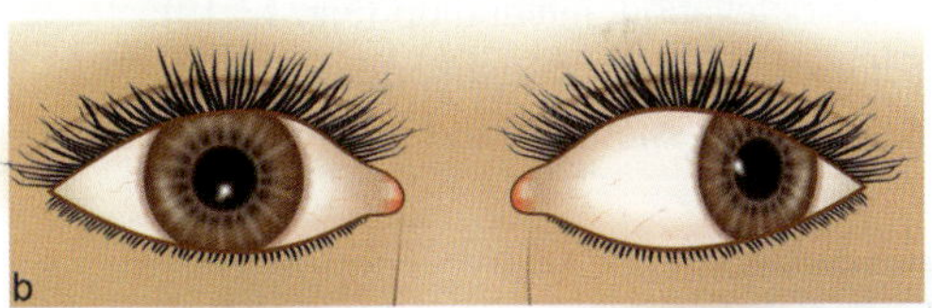

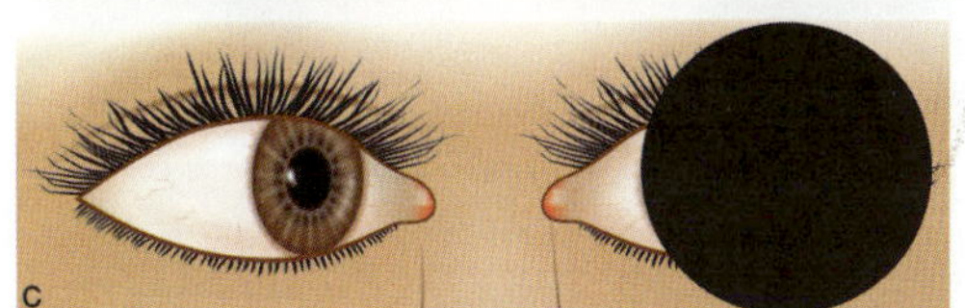

Fig. 12.16: (a) Right divergent squint, looking straight; (b) Right divergent squint, looking left; (c) Right divergent squint, looking left, left eye covered.

Method of Assessment

Binocular movements are called versions. To check them, ask the child to keep both eyes open and look towards a fixation target, without moving the head. The fixation target is moved in six cardinal gazes, usually starting with the horizontal **(Fig. 12.17)**. Six cardinal gaze positions are listed in **Key Box 4**. The range of movement is assessed by comparing the relative position of both corneas in different directions of gaze.

What is the Importance of Testing in the Six Cardinal Directions of Gaze?

- There are six extraocular muscles in each eye (medial rectus, lateral rectus, superior rectus, inferior rectus, and superior and inferior oblique muscles).

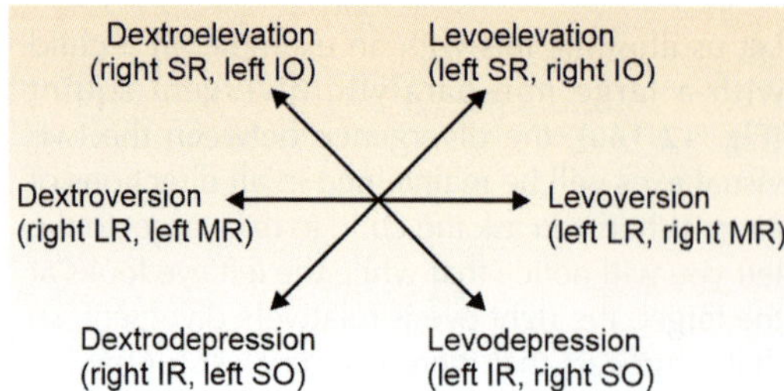

Fig. 12.17: Six cardinal directions of gaze for assessing binocular ocular movements and the muscles responsible for these movements.

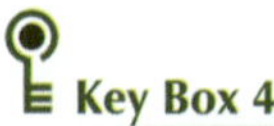

Key Box 4

Six Cardinal Positions for Assessing Gaze

1. Dextroversion, horizontally to right
2. Levoversion, horizontally to left (Fig. 12.18)
3. Dextroelevation, right and up
4. Levoelevation, left and up (Fig. 12.19)
5. Dextrodepression, right and down
6. Levodepression, left and down (Fig. 12.20)

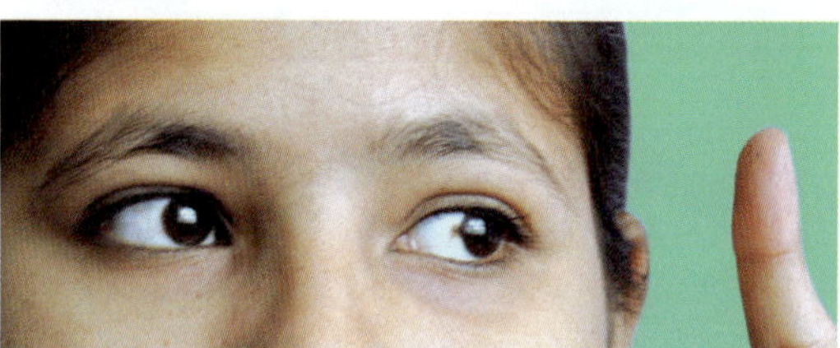

Fig. 12.18: Checking horizontal movements.

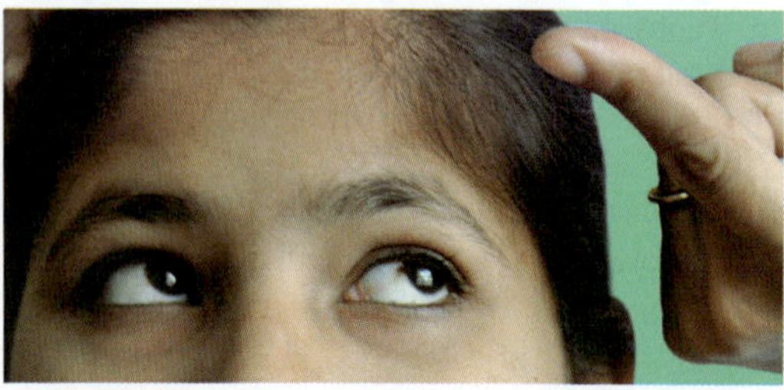

Fig. 12.19: Checking levoelevation.

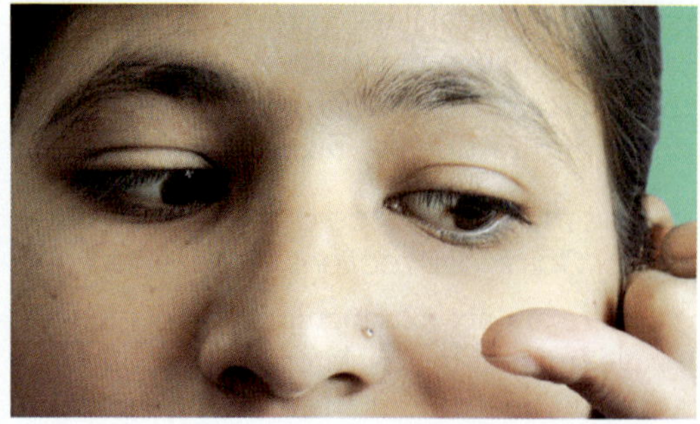

Fig. 12.20: Checking levodepression.

- Owing to their peculiar origins and insertions, each is primarily responsible for movement in only one of the six cardinal positions of gaze.
- Thus, depending on the direction of movement restriction, it becomes easy to identify the involved muscles in a child with paralytic squint.
- You may find it easy to remember the nerve supply of the extraocular muscles with this mnemonic LR_6 SO_4REST_3. Here, LR = lateral rectus, SO= superior oblique, and REST are the other four muscles.
- Uniocular movements (*ductions*) are checked by covering one eye and asking the child to follow the target in four diagnostic positions (laterally, medially, up, and down).

How can You Tell if Ocular Movements are Normal?

- In the full range of adduction (medial movement), the nasal one-third of the cornea should lie medial to an imaginary vertical line through the lower lacrimal punctum.
- In the full range of abduction (lateral movement), the temporal limbus just touches the lateral canthus.
- For elevation and depression, the excursions of the two corneas are compared relative to each other. Normally, the eyeball should move comfortably to the extremes of gaze. You might need to lift the upper eyelid to view vertical movements in their entirety.

When Should You Look for Ocular Movements?

- At your first interaction with a child, especially in a well baby clinic; early identification of squint and early treatment will prevent amblyopia. Amblyopia results when there is inadequate foveal stimulation early in life (due to uncorrected refractive error, cataract, ptosis, etc.), or from abnormal binocular interactions (as in squint). If intervention is delayed, the fovea and the corresponding occipital cortex fail to develop to their full visual potential. Thus, vision remains poor even after the original cause has been successfully treated. If you suspect that the child squints, you should counsel the parents to visit an ophthalmologist for evaluation.

- Squinting is not uncommon up to the age of 3 months (before fixation and binocular reflexes develop). However, squint may be the result of a serious ocular disorder—like retinoblastoma or congenital cataract. Early ophthalmic intervention may be life saving in the former and will prevent amblyopia in the latter.
- When you suspect neurological illness like meningitis, where 6th nerve palsy is not unusual.
- In children with head injury, multiple cranial nerve injuries may coexist.

How will You Assess Ocular Movements in a Child who is too Young to Cooperate?

Use an interesting object, preferably one that makes a noise, to engage the child. While the parent holds the head gently to prevent head movement, move the object into the six cardinal directions of gaze.

How will You Assess Ocular Movements of a Child in Coma?

Use Doll's head maneuver

- Use both hands to open the eyelids so that you can see the corneas. Now rapidly but gently turn the head from side-to-side, watching the eyes.
- When the head is turned to one side, both eyes should move to the opposite side due to the oculocephalic reflex.
- If the eyes remain fixed in mid-position, Doll's eye movements are said to be absent. It indicates a lesion in the mid-brain or pons with involvement of the third and sixth cranial nerves.
- When the Doll's head maneuver reveals gaze deviation to one side, but not to the other, it indicates a unilateral brainstem lesion on the side opposite to the direction of gaze.

> Never attempt the Doll's head maneuver in a child with trauma unless cervical spine injury has been ruled out.

D. Examination of the Ocular Adnexa

The ocular adnexa include the eyelids and related structures.

1. Position of the Eyelid

Drooping (ptosis): Ptosis can be identified by a narrow aperture between the upper and lower lids (palpebral aperture). If *unilateral*, it can be easily detected by comparison with the other side (Fig. 12.21). When *bilateral*, the degree of ptosis is determined by comparison with a normogram. Normal vertical height of the palpebral aperture is 10 mm.

Ptosis may be congenital, or acquired as a part of third cranial nerve palsy. Causes are listed in **Table 12.5**.

Amblyopia may result if ptosis is severe and the lid covers the pupillary area. This is particularly true for children below 5 years of age. Early diagnosis and treatment of ptosis is the key to prevent amblyopia.

Lid retraction: Lid retraction from lagophthalmos can cause exposure of the cornea with subsequent drying and ulceration (exposure keratopathy). In children with seventh cranial nerve palsy, you must check for *Bell's phenomenon* (when you try to open forcefully closed eyelids, the corneas should roll up). A good Bell's phenomenon is protective against exposure keratopathy. You should advise frequent lubrication with antibiotic and artificial tear formulations during the day, and antibiotic eye ointment and eye padding at night. Ask the careproviders to ensure that the eyelids are closed before applying the pad, as the pad itself can abrade the cornea.

In addition, at every follow-up of such patients, you should check the eye for conjunctival redness, corneal dryness, and frank ulceration. If such signs appear in spite of medication, a tarsorrhaphy will be required. Tarsorrhaphy is usually not advised in the

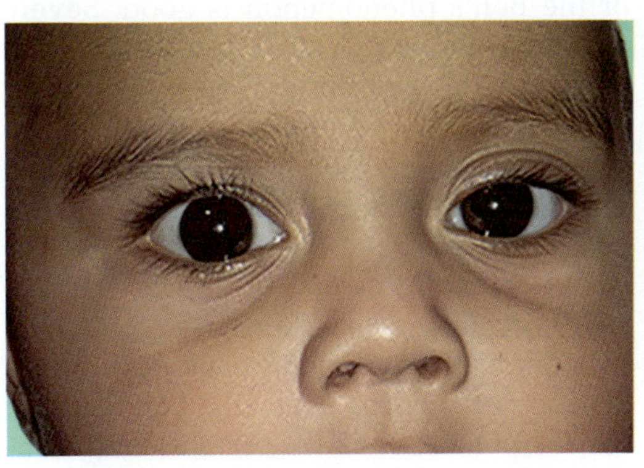

Fig. 12.21: Ptosis of the left upper lid.

Table 12.5: Causes of ptosis

	Unilateral	Bilateral
Congenital	• Congenital ptosis • Marcus Gunn ptosis	Blepharophimosis syndrome (Fig. 12.22)
Acquired	• Edema (stye, trauma) • Tumor (Fig. 12.23) • 3rd cranial nerve palsy • Horner syndrome • Trauma to levator palpebrae superioris • Postoperative: After extraocular surgery	• Horner syndrome • Myotonic dystrophy

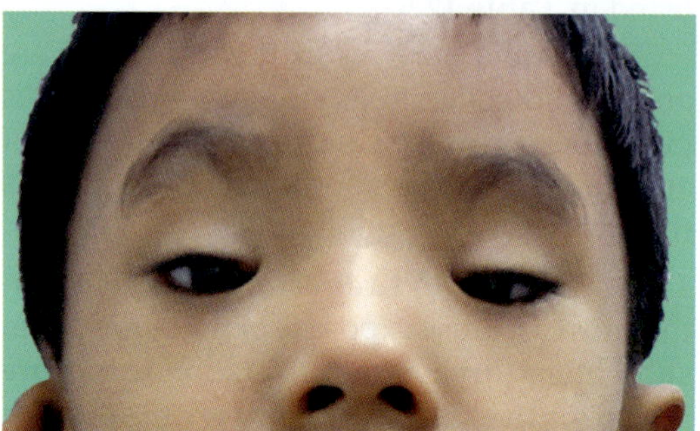

Fig. 12.22: Blepharophimosissyndrome with bilateral ptosis.

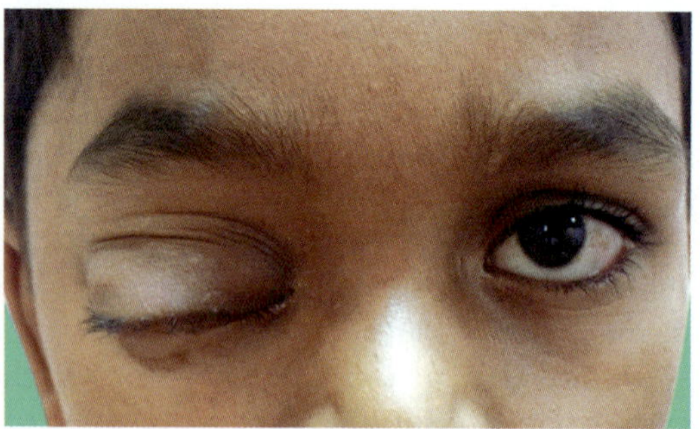

Fig. 12.23: Plexiform neurofibromatosis, right side, with unilateral severe ptosis.

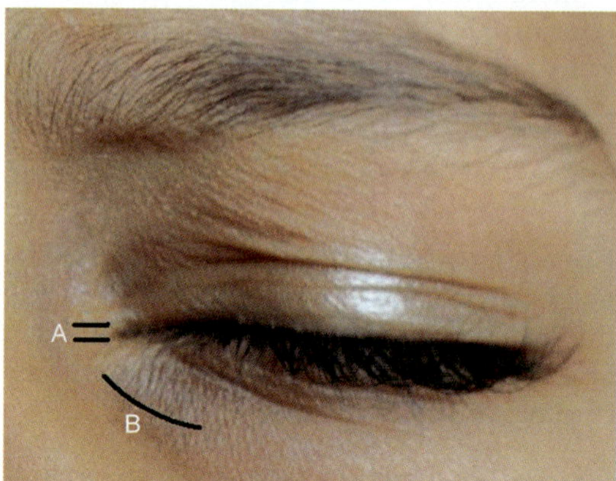

Fig. 12.24: Surface landmarks to correctly locate the lacrimal fossa; (A) Medial canthal ligament; (B) anterior lacrimal crest.

first instance when the palsy is expected to be temporary, the lagophthalmos is not severe, or the Bell's phenomenon is good. Severe scarring of the eyelid skin (trauma, burns) can also cause lid retraction.

2. Examination of Lacrimal Sac

You need to examine the lacrimal sac in neonates who have watering from one or both eyes. While watering may be due to sight-threatening conditions, like congenital glaucoma or ophthalmia neonatorum, the absence of corneal haze and conjunctival redness point towards *congenital dacryocystitis*. In the latter condition, epithelial debris or membranous valves block the nasolacrimal duct, resulting in stasis of tears. The lacrimal sac distends with mucopus. Two important landmarks (Fig. 12.24) will help you to identify if a swelling in the medial canthal region is due to dacryocystitis.

a. ***Medial canthal ligament:*** This is palpable as a thin band running from the medial angle to the side of the nose; the fundus of the sac lies just behind and partly above the medial canthal ligament.
b. ***Anterior lacrimal crest:*** It is the edge of the inferomedial orbital rim. The anterior lacrimal crest is the anterior boundary of the fossa which houses the lacrimal sac.

These landmarks are of particular importance in the diagnosis and management of congenital dacryocystitis.

Congenital dacryocystitis: *For diagnosis,* press the area just below the medial canthal ligament. Regurgitation of fluid or mucus into the conjunctival sac indicates presence of congenital dacryocystitis.

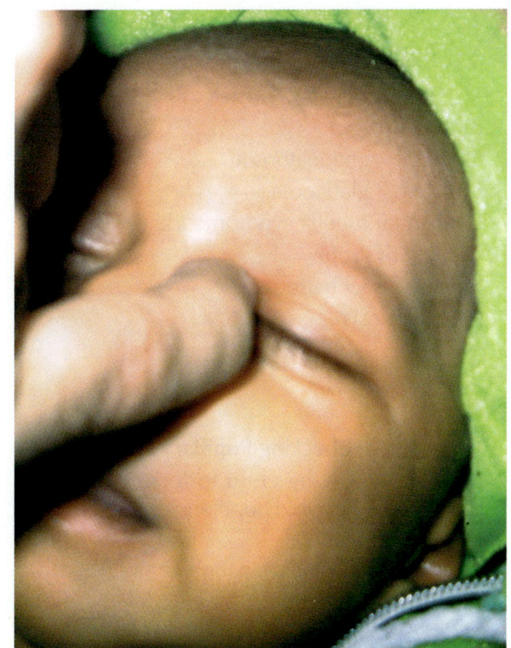

Fig. 12.25: Correct area for applying pressure for hydrostatic lacrimal sac massage.

For management, advise the mother to perform hydrostatic massage over the sac. Sustained pressure should be applied just below the ligament and just behind the crest (Fig. 12.25). This maneuver closes the common canaliculus and increases the hydrostatic pressure in the sac (which is already distended with accumulated mucopus due to the obstruction in the nasolacrimal duct). Note that the aim of the massage is not to express the contents of the sac into the conjunctival sac, but to push them down the nasolacrimal sac, thus forcing the obstructing debris into the nose.

E. Examination of the Conjunctiva

Your most frequent reason for examination of the conjunctiva in a child will be to rule out anemia or jaundice.

- Look for anemia in the pink and vascular inferior palpebral conjunctiva.
- Look for jaundice in the superior bulbar conjunctiva; it is covered by the upper lid and thus, less susceptible to color changes induced by environmental factors.

How will You Examine?

- ***To examine the lower palpebral conjunctiva and fornix:*** Ask the child to look up, while

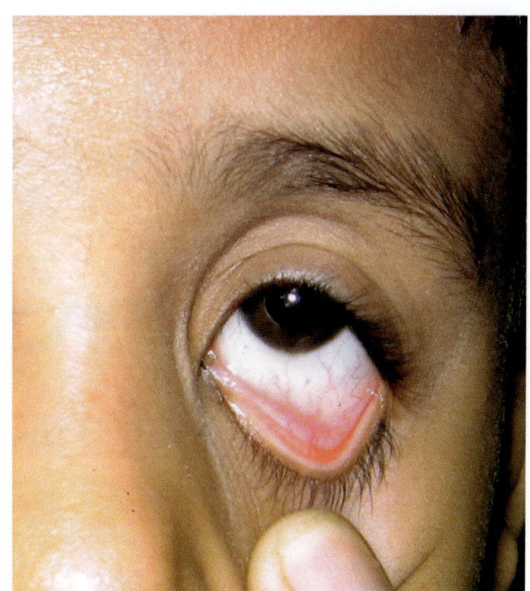

Fig. 12.26: Examining the lower palpebral conjunctiva. Ask the child to look up and pull the lower eyelid downward with your finger.

you pull the lower eyelid downwards **(Fig. 12.26)**.
- ***To examine the upper palpebral conjunctiva:*** You will have to evert the upper eyelid. This is a bit tricky and takes a few attempts to master.
    - i. Ask the child to look down and grasp the eyelashes and lid margin of the upper lid between your thumb and forefinger **(Fig. 12.27a)**.
    - ii. Place the cotton tip of a swab stick over the eyelid skin approximately at the level of lid crease, and evert the lid over the swab stick **(Fig. 12.27b)**.
- ***To examine the upper fornix:*** This is a critically important step when you want to look for, and remove particles of lime. You will have to double evert the upper eyelid. To do this, first evert as we have demonstrated, then apply a Desmarre's lid retractor from the skin side, and evert again.

F. Examination of the Cornea

1. Corneal Size

The horizontal diameter should be approximately 10 mm at birth, and between 11 and 12 mm by 3 years of age. A larger than normal cornea may be seen in congenital glaucoma (buphthalmos) or megalocornea. The cornea is

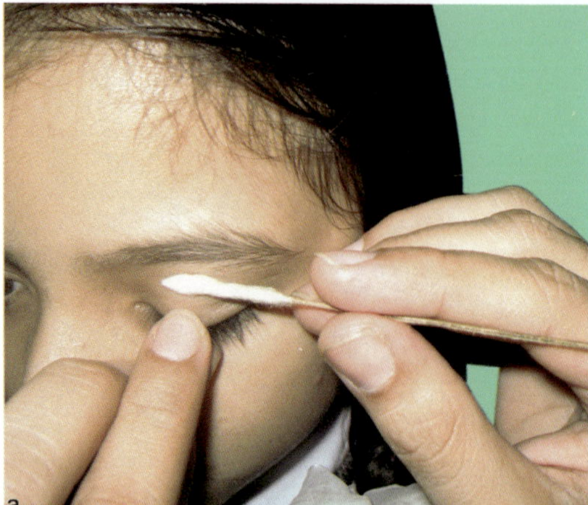

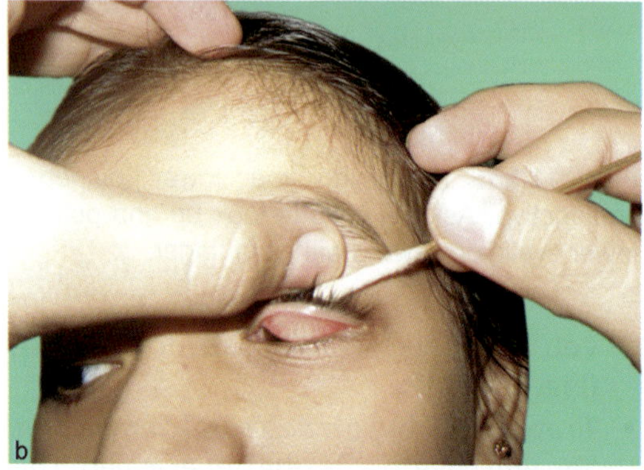

Fig. 12.27: Everting the upper eyelid; (a) Grasping the eyelid margin with forefinger and thumb; (b) Everting the lid over the swab stick.

hazy in the former and transparent in the latter condition. A smaller than normal cornea is seen in microcornea or microphthalmos, both usually not commensurate with normal vision.

2. Corneal Transparency

Loss of corneal transparency will manifest as a gray-white cornea, through which the details of iris and pupil may be difficult to view. It is a serious condition, and may result from infective or non-infective causes. You should consider ophthalmia neonatorum, congenital glaucoma, or birth trauma in infants **(Key Box 5)**. Corneal haze in older children may result from injury, vitamin A deficiency, or infective keratitis.

G. Examination of the Pupil

Use a bright torchlight in a dimly illuminated room, and look for pupil size, shape, and reaction to light **(Key Box 6)**.

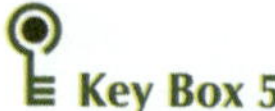

Key Box 5

Causes of Hazy Cornea in Neonates

1. Birth trauma
2. Ophthalmia neonatorum
3. Congenital glaucoma
4. Congenital rubella syndrome (due to keratitis)
5. Corneal dystrophy
6. Mucopolysaccharidosis
7. Mucolipidosis

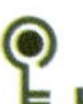

Key Box 6

Tips While Checking Pupillary Reactions

1. If possible, ask the child to look at a distant target. This will avoid pupillary constriction due to accommodation.
2. Keep the ambient illumination dimmed to avoid pupillary constriction from light falling on the other eye. However, there should be sufficient light to permit evaluation in the eye that is **not** being stimulated with light (consensual response).
3. For checking the direct response, ensure that the other eye is completely occluded so no stray light enters it. You should securely occlude the eye with your own palm, as the child may inadvertently peek.
4. For the consensual response, the flashlight should fall on the other eye only, while you look for a reaction in the eye under investigation. To avoid stray light stimulating the direct reflex, keep your palm or a small dark cardboard in between both eyes.
5. You must remember to assess pupillary reaction to light **before** dilating the pupils for fundus examination. In comatose or uncooperative children, pupillary reaction is the only clue that helps in differentiating disk edema due to raised intracranial pressure (papilledema) from that due to optic neuritis. The direct reaction will be sluggish or absent in the latter.

1. Pupil Size

The normal pupil is about 3 mm in diameter. Compare the pupils of the two eyes. They should be equal in size. A larger pupil may result from bilateral optic atrophy or third nerve palsy. You may recall that pupillary fibers from one eye connect to the Edinger-Westphal nucleus of ***both*** sides. Thus, unilateral optic atrophy will not change the size of the pupil on that side since it can constrict due to ambient light falling in the other eye.

Ask the patient to fix a distant target so that accommodation does not cause miosis, thus misleading you into imagining a smaller than normal pupil.

2. Pupil Shape

The pupils should be round and regular. Misshapen pupils (dyscoria) may signify uveitis or traumatic sphincter tears.

3. Pupillary Reaction to Light

The pupil being examined should constrict to light being shone directly into that eye (*direct light* or *direct response*) as well as to light being shone into the other eye (*consensual light* or *consensual response*). This is due to the fact that stimulation of the afferent (optic nerve) in one eye will trigger the efferent (oculomotor nerve) on both sides resulting in constriction of both pupils.

Swinging flashlight test: It is a useful test to elicit pupillary reaction to light. The torchlight is rapidly alternated between the two eyes.

1. Normally, on swinging the torchlight from one to the other, both pupils will remain constricted, regardless of which eye is stimulated with light.
2. On swinging the torchlight to the affected eye, pupil of that eye will dilate (due to absent direct reflex, and an intact consensual reflex from the other eye).
3. On swinging back the torchlight to normal eye, the pupil of that eye will constrict (due to intact direct reflex pathway but an absent consensual reflex from the affected eye).

Diseases affecting the afferent limb of the reflex (optic atrophy, optic neuritis, retinal detachment, glaucoma, retinoblastoma) will result in an absent response to direct light, but a normal response to consensual light. The other pupil, on the other hand, will react normally to direct light, but not to consensual light.

In diseases that affect the efferent limb of the reflex (meningitis, encephalitis, brain tumors, head or orbital trauma), the pupil will respond neither to direct nor to consensual light. Thus, the pupil will be dilated and fixed. The other pupil will respond normally to both direct and consensual lights.

12.4 EXAMINATION OF THE FUNDUS OCULI

Retina is the only structure in the body where you can directly visualize blood vessels and part of a cranial nerve (optic nerve). Examination of the retina can detect several systemic disorders affecting the CNS, hematological, and cardiovascular systems. The etiology could be infective, vascular, nutritional, or metabolic. Fundus findings will give you an idea of what is occurring elsewhere in the body.

A. Direct Ophthalmoscopy

You can view the central part of the retina, up to the retinal equator using direct ophthalmoscopy through a dilated pupil. The optic disk, major retinal blood vessels, posterior retina, and macula lutea can be visualized by this method. You require an ophthalmoscope to see the fundus (Fig. 12.28). However, to examine the retinal periphery, particularly in cases of retinopathy of prematurity and degenerative myopia, indirect ophthalmoscopy is required. The instrumentation and technique for indirect ophthalmoscopy is sophisticated, and these children should be referred to an ophthalmologist.

Method of Direct Ophthalmoscopy (Key Box 7)

- You should use your right eye to examine the child's right eye, holding

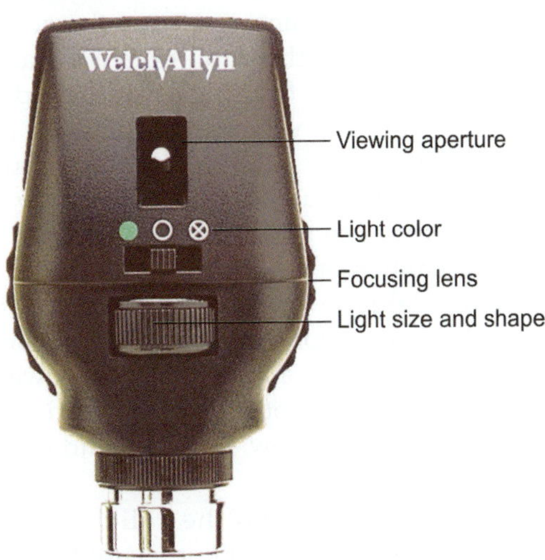

Fig. 12.28: Direct ophthalmoscope from patient's side.

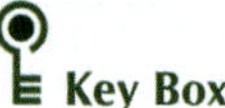

Key Box 7

Prerequisites for Direct Ophthalmoscopy

1. Dilate pupils with a short-acting mydriatic, like tropicamide 1% eyedrops, after evaluating pupillary reaction to light.
2. The room lights should be dimmed.
3. Ensure that both you and the child are comfortable.
4. You should always wear a mask.
5. Remove the child's spectacles, if any. However, you may or may not remove your own spectacles.
6. Make sure that infant is not hungry. Hold the infant's head between your knees, while the parent holds the supine body in his/her lap, holding the arms against the body.
7. Older children can be made to lie down supine, or if cooperative may agree to an examination sitting on the parent's lap or on a stool.

the ophthalmoscope in your right hand. Likewise, use left eye and left hand for the child's left eye. This will prevent obstruction by the child's nose, as you must move very close to examine the fundus in greater detail.

- Look through the viewing aperture and center the ophthalmoscope light on the eye to be examined. You will find this easier to perform if you keep both eyes open. With experience, you will be able to center the light with the other eye closed.
- The first step is to perform a *distant direct ophthalmoscopy* (DDO) which will give you an idea of the transparency of the ocular media. Look at the pupil from a distance of 25–33 cm. The focusing lenses should be rotated first one way then the other till the pupil is in focus. At this point, you should be able to see a reddish-orange glow in the pupil. The glow is a reflection of the ophthalmoscope light from the vascular choroidal layer of the eye. It is absent or dull in conditions like cataract, vitreous hemorrhage, and endophthalmitis. Always compare with the other eye when in doubt. An absent red glow should mandate an ophthalmic referral.
- Next, go as close to the child's eye as possible, keeping the light focused on the pupil. Eventually, the middle finger of the hand holding the ophthalmoscope will be close to or resting on the child's cheek. The fingers of your other hand should rest on the child's forehead, and the thumb used to gently pull up the upper eyelid. You should be angled slightly temporal of center while the child looks straight ahead. In this way, you can avoid throwing light on the macula and dazzling the child. Rotate the focusing lenses with your index finger, clockwise, and then counter-clockwise, till you see some retinal structure. The appropriate lens is usually found by trial and error and will vary from patient to patient. It depends on the refractive error of the examiner's and patient's eyes, and on the accommodation being exerted by both.
- The retina has a refractile, orange-red appearance, varying a bit with the skin color and age of the patient. You will only see a small segment of the retina at any one time. Usually, you will see retinal vessels; trace them till you come to the optic disk.
- To view different areas, you will have to keep changing the angle of view by small degrees at a time, in a systematic manner, i.e. up, down, left, and right. It is a good idea to give the child a break now and then, since it is hard for him to keep looking in one direction while a bright light is being shone in the eye. Keep reminding the child to look straight ahead, otherwise it will be impossible for you to focus on anything long enough to make a judgment.
- A general scheme should be followed for examination of retina **(Key Box 8)**.

1. Optic nerve head: It should be examined for size, shape, color, and margins. It is a vertically oval to round disk, pink in color with a pale center (optic cup) from which emerge the central retinal artery and vein. It has distinct margins **(Fig. 12.29)**.

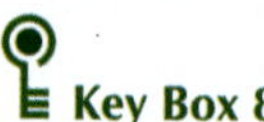

Key Box 8

Normal Scheme for Retinal Examination

1. The optic nerve head is examined first. It has no rods and cones, so is insensitive to light; the child is not likely to be uncomfortable
2. The major retinal vessels
3. The general retina
4. The macula lutea (most sensitive to light, so should be examined last)

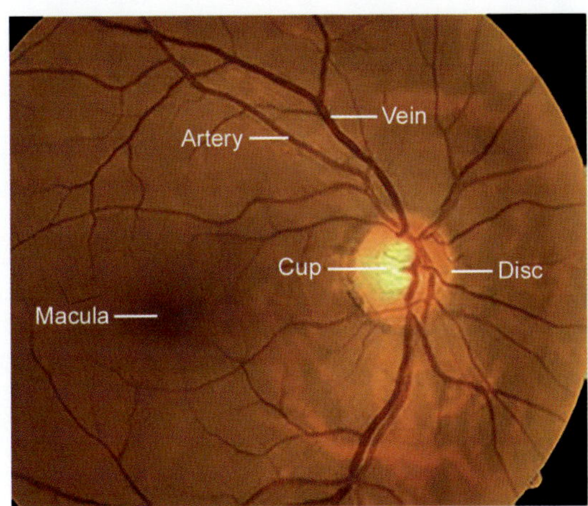

Fig. 12.29: Normal fundus.

In papilledema, the optic nerve head is hyperemic, the cup is full, the margins blurred with peripapillary retinal edema, and hemorrhages, the retinal veins at the disk are tortuous and dilated (Fig. 12.30).

2. *Retinal vessels:* The retinal vessels should be examined next for their caliber, tortuosity, and any changes at the sites where arterioles and venules cross each other. Arterioles are bright, pinkish-red, with a shiny reflex running down their center. They are thinner, being approximately two-thirds of the thickness of venules. The latter are dark red vessels.

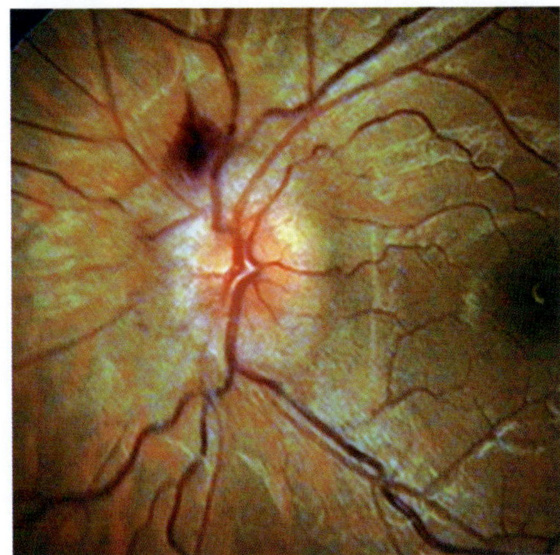

Fig. 12.30: Papilledema, with superficial retinal hemorrhages.

In children with hypertension and diabetes, the caliber of the vessels may change, there may be hemorrhages and exudation from leaky vessels; in malignant hypertension, there may be disk edema. Disk edema is also seen in optic neuritis when the involvement is mainly of the optic nerve head (papillitis). In retrobulbar neuritis, on the other hand, the disk will not be edematous, but may show pallor on the temporal side in later stages.

3. *Background of the retina:* It should be orange-reddish in color, the color depending on the degree of pigmentation in the choroid and retina. It is pale in anemic patients and when there is retinal edema. You may also find superficial retinal hemorrhages and Roth's spots in patients with severe anemia.

- Superficial hemorrhages are flame-shaped as they lie in the superficial nerve fiber layer.
- Roth's spots, also seen in leukemia and subacute bacterial endocarditis, are small superficial hemorrhages with pale centers.

4. *Macula lutea:* Lastly, ask the patient to look directly into the light of ophthalmoscope and you will see the macula lutea, the central retina, which is darker in color due to luteal pigment. In its center, there is a small depression called the foveola. The light reflects off the walls of the foveola to produce a bright light reflex that helps in identifying this area.

In children who cannot cooperate, the macula is located by moving temporal to the disk by approximately two disk diameters (3 mm). Absence of the foveolar reflex should suggest a macular lesion. Subhyaloid hemorrhage is a characteristic boat-shaped hemorrhage in the macular area. It is seen in severe anemia due to any cause. The hemorrhage breaks into the space between the macula and the vitreous. Since the posterior vitreous is attached to the retina around the macula, the hemorrhage tends to remain confined to a circular area; the red blood cells settle due to gravity so that a horizontal level is achieved, giving the hemorrhage its boat shape. These hemorrhages immediately reduce visual acuity and take a longer time to resolve since the macula is relatively avascular.

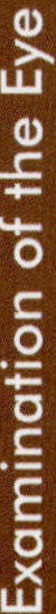

B. Screening a Neonate for ROP (Retinopathy of Prematurity)

Target Group

As per the National Neonatology Foundation's Evidence Based Clinical Practice Guidelines 2010: Preterm neonates born at <34 weeks of gestation and/or weighing less than 1750 grams at birth; also in older (34–36 weeks gestational age) or larger (1750–2000 grams birth weight) babies who have risk factors for ROP.

Recent ROP Operational guidelines suggest that all babies less than 34 weeks and/or less than 2 kg or babies with risk factors, irrespective of age or birth weight should be screened at discharge from NICU or within 30 days of life, whichever is earlier.

Risk factors include sepsis, respiratory distress syndrome, blood transfusions, exchange transfusions, intraventricular hemorrhage, apnea and need for cardio-respiratory support.

Age at First Examination

The NNF recommendation for first screening is within 4 weeks of birth in infants born at ≥28 weeks of gestational age and a little sooner (within 2–3 weeks of age) in infants born at <28 weeks or weighing <1200 grams at birth.

Preparation for Indirect Ophthalmoscopy

- Dilate the pupils with tropicamide 0.5% eyedrops (instill twice at an interval of 15 minutes) and phenylephrine 2.5% eyedrops (one instillation only).
- Darken the room or provide a screen around the baby to reduce light.
- The baby's head should be stabilized with one hand and her hands and body with the other. A pediatric wire speculum is used to keep the eyelids apart; a scleral indenter helps in rotating the eyeball and in indenting sclera to bring peripheral retina into view.
- Look first at the posterior pole to identify any plus disease or straightening of the vascular arcades.
- Then, rotate the eye so that peripheral quadrants of the retina can be examined one by one, right up to the periphery.

Complications

- Eye manipulations in very premature and low birth weight infants can produce respiratory and cardiac problems, so both functions should be monitored during the examination.
- Hypothermia should be prevented by keeping the baby wrapped up.
- The eyedrops used for dilating the pupil (parasympatholytic and sympathomimetic drugs) are absorbed into the systemic circulation and can cause cardiac and gastrointestinal complications. Therefore, infants should never be overdosed.

Definitions

Plus disease indicates evidence of vascular activity, an ominous sign. It includes one or more of the following signs: Arteriolar tortuosity and venous dilatation at the posterior pole, iris vascular engorgement, pupillary rigidity, and vitreous haze.

Aggressive posterior ROP (AP-ROP; previously called Rush disease) is a very rapidly progressive ROP; chances of AP-ROP are higher when retinal vascularization ends in zone I or very early in zone II, and there is plus disease.

Threshold disease is the stage at which treatment is invariably recommended since delaying treatment has serious blinding potential. Threshold disease is defined, by the Cryo-therapy for Retinopathy of Prematurity Cooperative Group (CRYO-ROP), as five contiguous or eight non-contiguous clock hours of retina showing stage 3 ROP, with plus disease, in zone I or II.

High-risk prethreshold ROP type-1 also requires treatment. It is defined by the Early Treatment for Retinopathy of Prematurity (ETROP) Group as any stage of ROP in zone I with plus disease; or stage 3 ROP in zone I without plus disease; or stage 2 to 3 ROP in zone II with plus disease (Fig. 12.31).

In prethreshold ROP, type 2 (stage 1 or 2 ROP in zone I without plus disease; or stage 3 ROP in zone II without plus disease), babies are followed up and treated only if progression occurs.

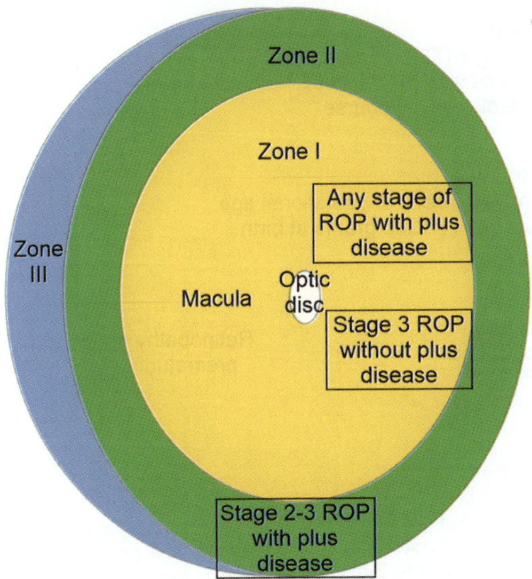

Fig. 12.31: Indications according to zone and stage of ROP for starting treatment [Early Treatment for Retinopathy of Prematurity (ETROP) Group Guidelines].

How will You Interpret the Zones of ROP Involvement?

Zone I extends in a circle, the center of which is the optic nerve, and the diameter of which is twice the distance from the optic nerve to the macula. If the optic disk and signs of ROP are present in the same view on ophthalmoscopy with a 28-dioptre lens, it is taken to be zone I disease. Zone I disease is extremely labile and changes occur within days. Any stage (even stage 0) in zone one requires treatment, so these babies should be seen as soon as possible by an ophthalmologist.

Zone II is a circle surrounding zone I with the nasal ora serrata as its nasal limit. If you notice that nasal vessels have not yet reached the nasal ora serrata, this is taken to be zone II. The disease may progress over 1–2 weeks, so screening is done every 15 days; however, if plus disease appears, or a thickened red three-dimensional ridge of tissue (hot dog) forms in the involved area, you should follow-up every week or sooner.

Zone III is the crescent, temporally, that zone II leaves out. If you find that the nasal vessels have reached the nasal ora serrata, but not the temporal, then it is zone III. Aggressive disease is rarely seen in this zone; two or three weekly evaluations are adequate, unless there are signs of plus disease.

How will You Recognize the Stages of ROP?

Stage 0: The mildest form of ROP, with immature retinal vasculature, but you will not see any clear demarcation between vascularized and non-vascularized parts of the retina.

Stage 1: A fine, thin demarcation line will be seen between the vascular and avascular parts of the retina. The line has no height or thickness.

Stage 2: The demarcation line transforms into a broad, thick ridge separating the vascular and avascular parts of the retina.

Stage 3: Neovascularization appears, giving the ridge a velvety appearance and ragged borders.

Stage 4: The fibrovascular ridge contracts, pulling the retina towards the vitreous; you will find a subtotal retinal detachment beginning at the ridge. Stage 4A does not include the fovea; in stage 4B, the fovea is also detached.

Stage 5: The entire retina is completely detached, resembling a funnel; the funnel may be open (stage 5A) or closed (stage 5B).

Follow-up

- It depends on the presence, extent and severity of ROP and is detailed in Fig. 12.32.
- You should remember that any stage of ROP in zone I requires more frequent follow- up than usual, at weekly or shorter intervals. The appearance of plus disease, or of neovascularization, in zone I mandates treatment within 72 hours.
- Any premature infant should continue to be monitored until active disease has subsided.
- Even without intervention, premature babies may develop squint or refractive errors, or rarely glaucoma; thus, you should refer to an ophthalmologist for screening every 6 months, until age 3 years, and annually thereafter.
- Even with aggressive treatment, babies with ROP may become blind due to retinal detachment and glaucoma; they should be referred to blindness rehabilitation services early enough to benefit fully.

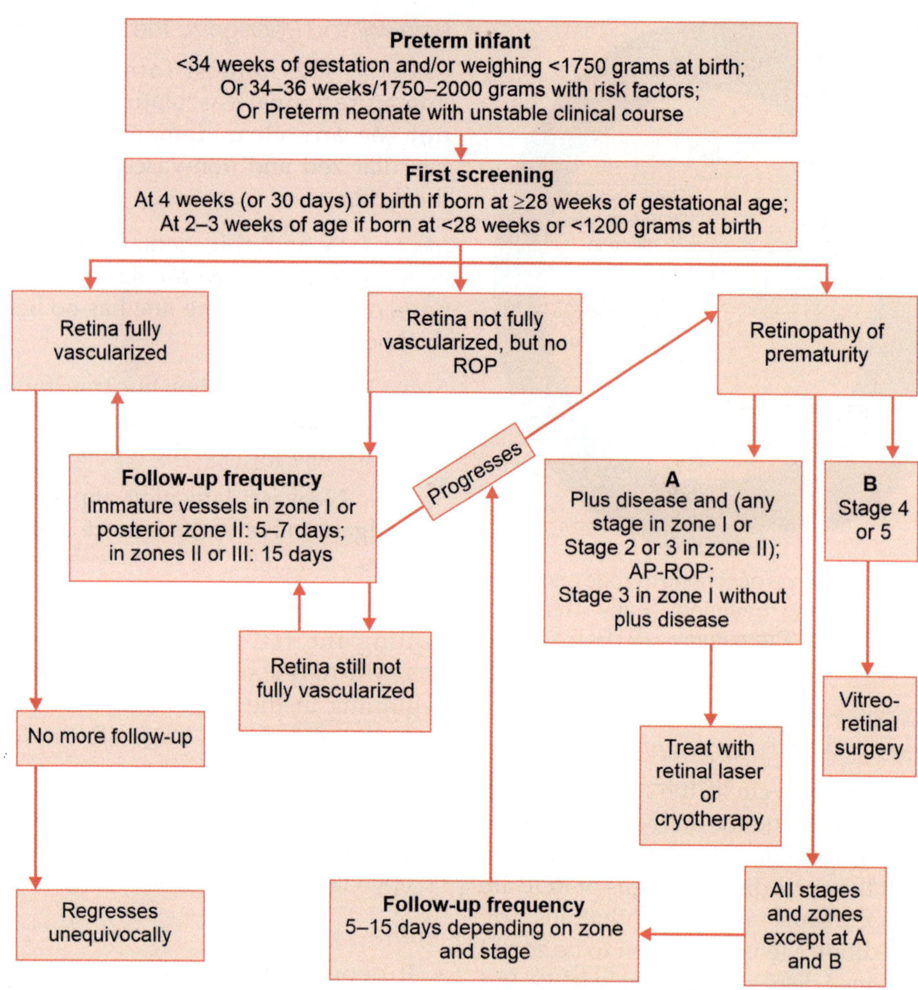

Fig. 12.32: Protocol for screening of retinopathy of prematurity (ROP).

12.5 ASSESSMENT OF INTRAOCULAR PRESSURE

You can get an approximate idea of the intraocular pressure by digital palpation. Ask the child to look downwards, without closing the eyelids. Ballot the eyeball with the index fingers of both hands while resting the other fingers on the child's forehead. Compare with the other eye. *The more ballotable the eye, the lower the pressure.*

You should assess intraocular pressure in babies with enlarged eyeball and/or corneal haze, where you suspect congenital glaucoma. The method described here is subjective; objective methods using tonometers should be preferred.

Never attempt to measure intraocular pressure if you suspect a ruptured globe.

12.6 ASSESSMENT OF COLOR VISION

Color vision defects are not uncommon, affecting 4–10% of males and 0.4% of females. They are most commonly congenital, inherited as X-linked defects. The commonest defect results in the child confusing reds and greens. Problems with colors in the blue-yellow range are less common.

Color vision defects do not usually result in visual problems. The child learns to use hue and texture to differentiate between objects of the confusing colors. However, diagnosed early, the affected children can make sensible career choices. Persons with color vision deficiency in India cannot join the armed or police force, drive public transport, or take up mining engineering.

Diagnosis

The standard method for diagnosing color vision defects is using Ishihara's pseudoisochromatic plates. These plates are composed of numbers or a winding path made up of colored dots that vary in hue and brightness from dots in the background (Fig. 12.33). The colors of the dots in the number and the background are chosen such that they are confusing to persons with deficiency of color vision. Thus, they either cannot decipher any number, or see an entirely different number from that seen by a person who is not color blind.

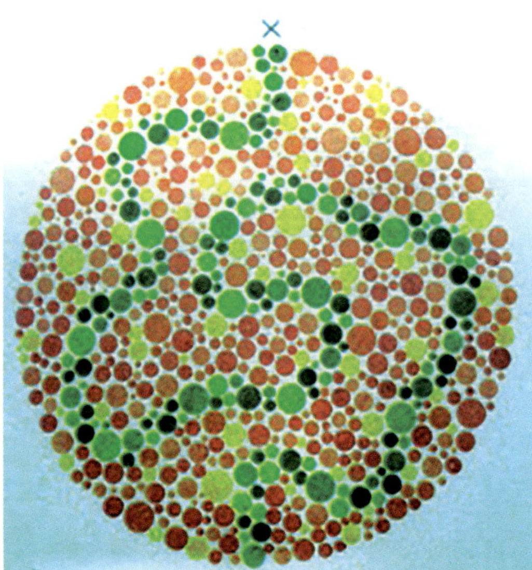

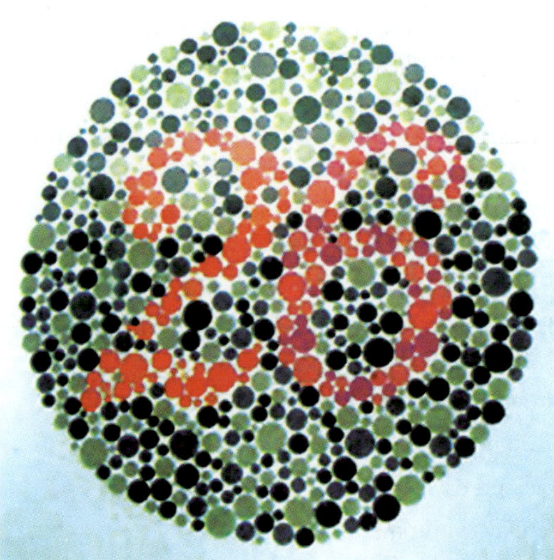

Fig. 12.33: Ishihara chart for testing color vision.

12.7 ASSESSMENT OF VISUAL FIELDS

The normal visual field extends outwards in all directions in each eye. Field defects refer to specific regions in the field where the child cannot see. This signifies that the visual impulse is interrupted in its path from the retina to the visual cortex.

The ideal method to assess visual fields is by automated perimeter. However, the confrontation method is a good technique for identifying neurological defects.

Method of Examination

- In a well-lit room, both examiner and child should sit comfortably facing each other about 1 m apart, with eyes at the same level.
- For testing the right eye, close the left eye of the child with an eye pad. Since you are the reference point, you should close your right eye, asking the child to stare continuously into your left eye. This method ensures that you monitor the child's cooperation.
- Explain to the child that he is to indicate to you as soon as he sees your index finger anywhere in the visual field.
- Take your hand to one side where it is just visible to you, making sure it is about equidistant from you and the child. Then bring it in slowly towards your nose till the child says that he can see it. Repeat this in the horizontal, vertical, and oblique meridians. If the child's field compares well with yours, it should be considered normal. If not, make a note of the areas that are not visualized.
- The other eye is tested similarly.
- In children who can count fingers, you may hold out variable number of fingers in different areas of the visual field and ask the child to count. This must be done quickly to prevent the child from sneaking a look at the fingers before replying.
- For very young children and infants, keep their focus on your face by talking to them, and flash a toy or brightly colored object in the peripheral field. If the peripheral field is normal, the child will change focus to look at the object of interest.

Remember that there is a physiologic blind spot in each eye. It is an area in the temporal visual field which marks the position of the optic disk where there are no photoreceptors.

Field Defects

Various types of field defects that may be uncovered by the confrontation method include the following. Note that the confrontation test is crude and is likely to miss small visual field defects.

Hemianopia

One-half of the vertical visual field (nasal or temporal) is defective. It signifies visual pathway defect that is at or distal to the optic chiasma.

- A lesion ***at the chiasma*** may result in a bitemporal (temporal half of field in both eyes) or binasal (nasal half of field in both eyes) visual field defect.
- A lesion ***distal to the chiasma*** will cause a homonymous (the same side in both eyes, i.e. both left half or both right half of fields) hemianopia.

Congruous Defect

The defect is symmetrical in the two eyes. The more congruous a field defect, the closer the lesion is to the occipital cortex.

Altitudinal Defect

One-half of the horizontal visual field (top or bottom) is defective. This usually results from vascular lesions at the optic nerve head. It is rare.

12.8 OCULAR MANIFESTATIONS OF SYSTEMIC DISORDERS

Eye examination can provide vital information regarding the underlying systemic disorder. **Table 12.6** summarizes the common childhood illnesses that can be suspected from an ocular manifestation.

Table 12.6: Ocular manifestations of systemic disorders of childhood

Eye finding	Suspected disorder
Proptosis (Fig. 12.34)	Hyperthyroidism, cranial dysostosis, capillary hemangioma, metastatic neuroblastoma, neurofibromatosis, hydatid cyst, lymphocytic leukemia, cavernous sinus thrombosis **Fig. 12.34:** Proptosis.
Enophthalmos	Horner syndrome
Microphthalmos	Congenital CMV, rubella, or toxoplasmosis
Hypertelorism	Down syndrome
Ptosis	Myasthenia gravis, muscular dystrophy, neurofibromatosis, Horner syndrome, Sturge-Weber syndrome
Dacryoadenitis	*Acute:* Influenza, mumps, infectious mononucleosis *Chronic:* Syphilis, tuberculosis, sarcoidosis
Dry eyes	Stevens-Johnson syndrome, dehydration, Riley-Day syndrome, ectodermal dysplasia, muscular dystrophy, rheumatoid arthritis, Sjögren syndrome
Conjunctivitis	Tuberculosis (phlyctenular), allergic eosinophilia, Reiter disease, Stevens-Johnson syndrome, viral illness, infectious mononucleosis
Episcleritis/scleritis	Rheumatoid arthritis, SLE
Corneal opacification/ pigment	Mucopolysaccharidosis, glycogen storage disease, lipidosis, cystinosis, Fanconi syndrome, Wilson disease, ariboflavinosis, vitamin A deficiency
Keratoconus	Down syndrome, Marfan syndrome, osteogenesis imperfecta
Megalocornea	Marfan syndrome, osteogenesis imperfecta
Interstitial keratitis	Congenital syphilis, tuberculosis, leprosy
Dendritic ulcers of cornea	Herpes simplex infection, Riley-Day syndrome

(Contd...)

Table 12.6: Ocular manifestations of systemic disorders of childhood (*Contd...*)	
Eye finding	**Suspected disorder**
Discoloration of sclera	Jaundice, Marfan syndrome, osteogenesis imperfecta, cutis hyperelastica, alcaptonuria (black)
Uveitis	Connective tissue disorders, brucellosis, viral infection (mumps, infectious mononucleosis), sarcoidosis
Chorioretinitis	Congenital cytomegalovirus, toxoplasmosis, or rubella infection; tuberculosis
Dilated non-reactive pupil	Atropine poisoning, transtentorial herniations due to subdural hematoma or raised intracranial tension, tonic pupil of Riley-Day syndrome
Small pupil	Pontine hemorrhage, opium poisoning, barbiturate poisoning, Horner syndrome
Cataract	• *Congenital:* Syphilis, toxoplasmosis, rubella • *Metabolic:* Galactosemia, diabetes mellitus, Wilson disease, hypocalcemia, cretinism, phenylketonuria, homocystinuria • *Chromosomal disease:* Down syndrome, trisomy 18, Turner syndrome • *Trauma/irradiation/drugs:* Corticosteroid, chlorpromazine, tetracycline • *Others:* Lowe syndrome, Marfan syndrome, Alport syndrome, myotonic dystrophy, Kartagener syndrome
Ectopia lentis	Homocystinuria, Marfan syndrome, Weill-Marchesani syndrome
Nystagmus	Albinism, internal ear lesions, posterior fossa tumors, vestibular disorders
Extraocular muscle palsies	Diabetes mellitus, myasthenia gravis, polioencephalitis, cavernous sinus thrombosis, lead toxicity, botulism, thiamine deficiency, fracture of base of skull
Buphthalmos	Congenital rubella, trisomy 18, trisomy 21, Marfan syndrome, homocystinuria, mucopolysaccharidosis, neurocutaneous syndromes, prolonged steroid therapy
Papilledema	Intracranial tumors, brain abscess, meningitis/encephalitis, intracranial hemorrhage, hydrocephalus, pseudotumor cerebri (benign intracranial hypertension), craniostenosis, hypertensions, anemia/polycythemia/leukemia
Optic atrophy	Microcephaly, hydrocephalus, pituitary tumors, osteoporosis, homocystinuria

Chapter 13

Evaluation of the Ear, Nose, and Throat

○ Neelima Gupta ○ Richa Saha

Structure

13.1 AIM AND SCHEME OF EAR, NOSE, THROAT EXAMINATION

Diseases of the ear, nose, and throat are fairly common in the pediatric age group. Often, these disorders are associated with systemic manifestations. Usually, children with a problem of ear, nose, or throat are first brought to a general practitioner or a pediatrician before being taken to an ENT specialist. It is, therefore, important that you are aware of the common signs and symptoms of diseases of ear, nose, and throat; and their methods of examination.

13.2 COMMON SYMPTOMS RELATED TO THE EAR

The common presenting symptoms of ear diseases in children are listed in **Key Box 1**.

Key Box 1

Common Symptoms of Ear Disease

1. Pain in the ear
2. Itching in the ear
3. Discharge from the ear
4. Hearing loss
5. Swelling in/around ear
6. Others—ringing sensation in the ear, giddiness, nausea, and vomiting

1. Pain in the Ear

Common causes of ear pain are listed in the **Key Box 2**. Pain in the ear can also be due to referred pain from larynx, pharynx, teeth, or the temporomandibular joint. Common causes of referred pain include acute tonsillitis, peritonsillar abscess, and dental caries.

Key Box 2

Common Causes of Pain in the Ear

1. Impacted wax in the external auditory canal
2. Foreign body in the ear
3. Acute suppurative otitis media (ASOM)
4. Acute otitis externa/furuncle in the canal
5. Acute mastoiditis
6. Viral myringitis
7. Chronic suppurative otitis media (CSOM) associated with otitis externa

The pain is usually inside the ear and is continuous and severe. Young children may present with excessive crying or history of tugging at the ear. Infants may present with history of diarrhea, refusal to take feeds, and vomiting. You should ask for associated complaints of running nose, fever, and sore throat. History of pain in any tooth, specially molars and premolars, should be elicited to rule out referred otalgia. In children less than three years of age, acute otitis media is a common cause of earache, while impacted wax is found to be more common in older children. Pain in the ear associated with complaint of impaired hearing may be seen in cases with impacted wax. Children with otitis externa may also have associated swelling of the ear canal.

2. Itching in the Ear

Itching in the ear may or may not be associated with pain and/or discharge from the ear. Common causes of itching in the ear are wax, fungal infection, otitis externa, and CSOM. Pain with itching in the ear may be seen in children with wax and otitis externa. There is associated ear discharge in children with CSOM.

Continuous scratching because of itching may cause excoriations over the pinna or in the external auditory canal. This may also lead to superimposed infection and swelling around the ear.

3. Discharge from the Ear

A discharging ear is also a common presenting symptom in children. Children with poor nutritional status, poor hygiene, and those from a low socioeconomic background have a higher incidence of CSOM. Incorrect feeding practices and low level of awareness in parents also contribute to the high incidence of CSOM in our population. So, make it a point to elicit appropriate nutritional, socioeconomic, personal, and family history.

The parents may give a history of acute upper respiratory tract infection preceding onset of ear discharge. There may be a history of earache preceding the discharge from the ear. This is the stage of acute otitis media when the pain is relieved after the tympanic membrane ruptures and the pus is released.

You should ask for the characteristics of the discharge, i.e. the (i) consistency; (ii) color; (iii) smell; (iv) amount; and (v) associated features such as blood staining and remission on treatment. Also ask for associated history of pain in the ear and decreased hearing.

- Mucoid or mucopurulent, non-foul smelling and profuse discharge indicates *tubotympanic* type of CSOM or *mucosal* CSOM with a central perforation in the tympanic membrane.
- Purulent, foul smelling, occasionally blood-stained and scanty discharge indicates *atticoantral* type of CSOM or *squamosal* CSOM. This is associated with findings of cholesteatoma, granulations, or polyps and requires an early surgical management.

> Ask for associated symptoms of fever, headache, nausea, vomiting, giddiness, or convulsions. Any complaint of inability to close the eye and deviation of angle of mouth, or swelling behind the ear or in the neck should also be asked for. Any of these symptoms, if present along with ear discharge, would indicate a complication of CSOM and requires an urgent referral to ENT specialist.

4. Hearing Loss

Hearing loss in infants and children presenting as an isolated symptom requires a detailed evaluation. Profound hearing loss or decreased hearing in infants leads to a defective speech development. Often the parents are unable to identify the problem till the age of 12 months or even later. It is important to recognize these infants early, for a timely intervention. See section on newborn hearing screening.

It is important to be aware of the non-hereditary causes of hearing loss, such as; (a) rubella and other maternal infections in the antenatal period; (b) premature birth, low birth weight, hyperbilirubinemia, neonatal ICU stay and (c) meningitis, measles, mumps and (d) trauma. All infants with any of the above high-risk factors or any child presenting with decreased hearing causing parental concern should be referred for specialist consultation.

Hearing impairment is associated with discharge from the ear in children with CSOM. Other associated symptoms may be fullness or heaviness in the ear in children with serous otitis media, impacted wax, or otomycosis.

5. Giddiness

Symptoms like giddiness are rare in children, unless it is associated with a complication of CSOM. Children are unable to explain what

Key Box 3

Causes of Giddiness

1. Conditions with hearing loss—CSOM, otitis media with effusion
2. Migraine
3. Epilepsy
4. Post-traumatic vertigo
5. Benign paroxysmal vertigo
6. Meniere disease
7. Central causes

they are experiencing and may present with symptoms, such as history of falls or vomiting. After the age of five years, a child may be able to complain of episodes of dizziness. The main differentials to be considered in children with giddiness are listed in **Key Box 3**.

While taking the history it will be important to establish the true nature of symptoms, duration of episode, associated symptoms, such as headache and vomiting, preceding illness or trauma, drug history, and detailed neurological and developmental history. Examination will include otoscopy, nystagmus assessment, and standard balance assesssment such as the gait test, Romberg test; cerebellar function tests, etc.

Tinnitus

Some children may occasionally report abnormal sounds in the ear. This may be due to wax, conductive hearing loss due to any pathology in middle ear, or following head trauma. Further examination and investigations can elucidate the cause. However, tinnitus as an isolated symptom is rare in children.

13.3 EXAMINATION OF THE EAR

A. Method of Examination

Position

Proper positioning and stabilizing the child is of utmost importance for examination of ear, nose, and throat.

- *Infants* are better examined in a lying down position with the parent or a nurse steadying the head and holding the legs of the baby.
- *Toddlers* can be examined while sitting in the parent's lap. The legs of the child are held between the parent's legs; one hand of the parent steadies the head while the other hand grasps the arms of the child, as shown in Fig. 13.1.

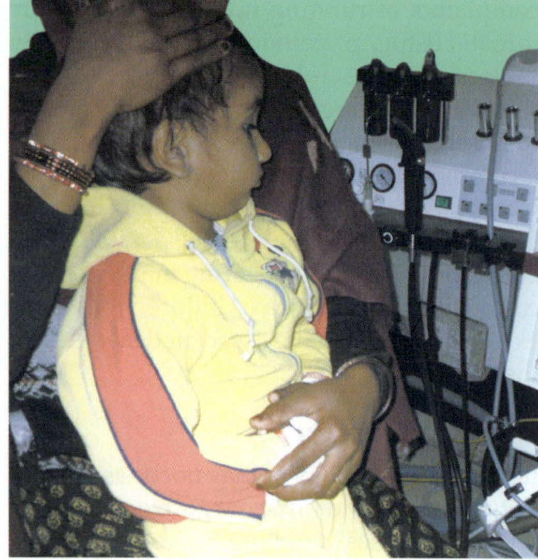

Fig. 13.1: Patient position of a toddler for ear examination.

- *Older children* can be seated comfortably opposite the examiner. The height of the seat can be adjusted, and the child can be examined after explaining the procedure.

Process of Ear Examination

For examination of the ear, you need a torch or a headlight and an otoscope. An ear speculum can be used while examining with the headlight as shown in Fig. 13.2.

- Hold the otoscope in your one hand (Fig. 13.3) and pull the pinna backwards

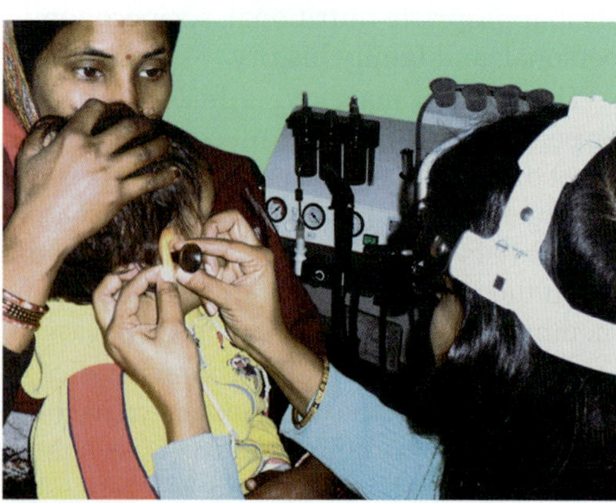

Fig. 13.2: Examination of ear using speculum and headlight.

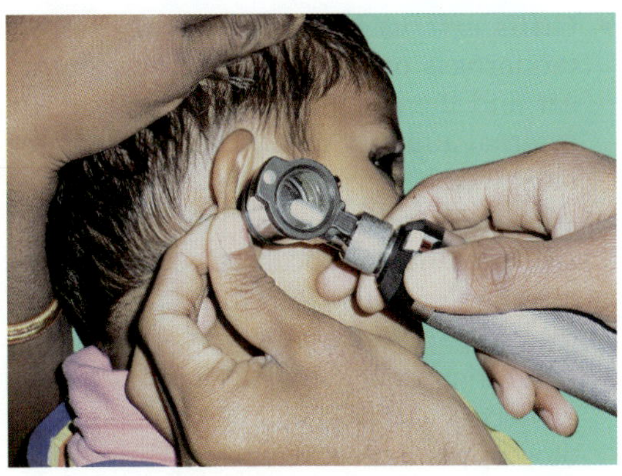

Fig. 13.3: Examination of ear using the otoscope.

and upwards with the other hand, so as to straighten the external auditory canal.

- Hold the otoscope in the right hand while examining the right ear and in the left hand while examining the left ear.
- Ensure that the head of the child is kept stable, and you are introducing the correct size speculum in a gentle and controlled manner.
- The speculum is inserted into the external auditory canal, and the canal and tympanic membrane are examined.

B. Examination of Specific Parts

1. External Ear

- Examine the external ear for any congenital anomaly in terms of shape and size.
- Look for the presence of accessory auricles, pre-auricular skin tags (Fig. 13.4) and pre-auricular sinus (a small opening at the root of helix).

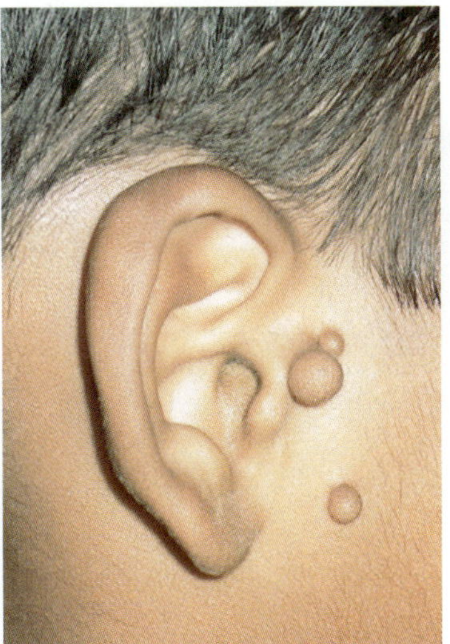

Fig. 13.4: Pre-auricular skin tag.

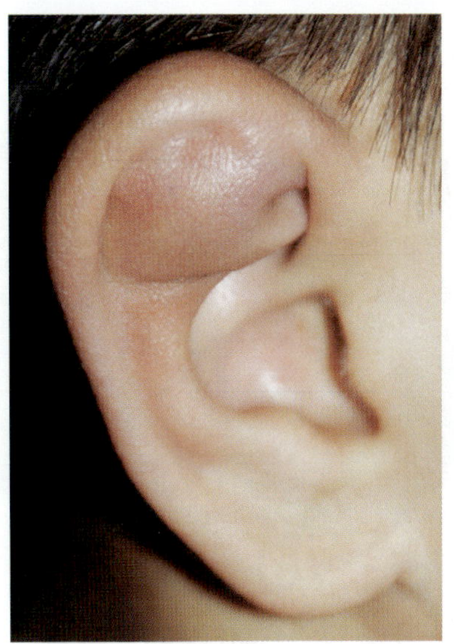

Fig. 13.5: Hematoma on auricle.

- Palpate the ear for any tenderness, which may be present in otitis externa. Any swelling over the auricle may be due to collection of blood after trauma (Fig. 13.5).
- Palpate the mastoid process for any fullness or tenderness. Tenderness over the mastoid is seen in mastoiditis. A fistula may be present over the mastoid in CSOM (Fig. 13.6).

2. External Auditory Canal

The external auditory canal is narrow and more tortuous in children. The bony part

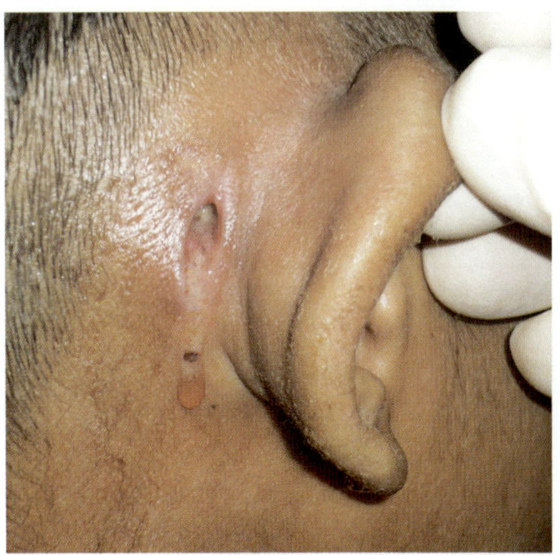

Fig. 13.6: Post-auricular fistula.

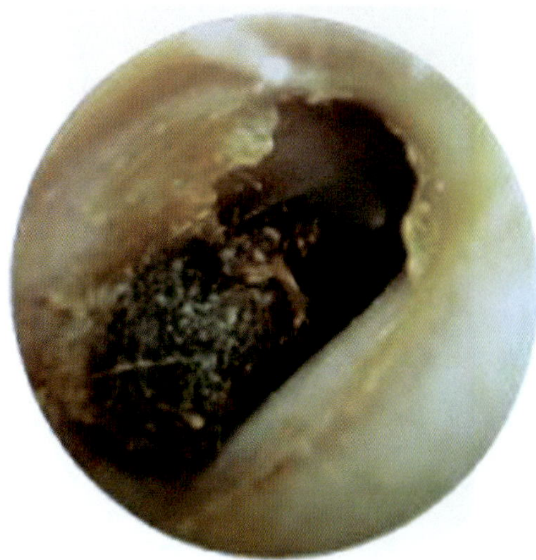

Fig. 13.7: Wax in the ear canal.

of canal is not fully developed, so it is a collapsed structure. The meatus may be stenosed or canal may be atretic in children with congenital anomaly of the ear.

- Examine the external auditory canal for wax which appears as brown or black debris **(Fig. 13.7)**. If wax is hard and impacted it will be almost completely occupying the canal, obscuring the view of the tympanic membrane. This is a frequent cause of decreased hearing and earache.
- Toddlers can put small objects, like beads, eraser pieces, pieces of paper, seeds, pulses, small stones, etc. into the canal **(Fig. 13.8)**. If a *foreign body* or impacted wax is seen on examination, the child needs referral to a specialist.

Fig. 13.8: Foreign body in the canal.

- *Otitis externa* is suspected, if there is tenderness on palpation of the external ear and there is a diffuse swelling of the external auditory canal. The canal may be narrowed because of the swelling.
- A *furuncle* in the external auditory canal will present as a localized swelling. The infection may also lead to enlargement of the pre-parotid lymph nodes.
- A whitish debris like a wet newspaper or debris with visible blackish spores on otoscopy is indicative of *otomycosis*.
- Often the canal is full of discharge, due to *chronic suppurative otitis media*. You should examine the discharge for its color, quantity, consistency, and odor. If it is a foul smelling discharge or if it is blood-tinged, then you should think in terms of atticoantral type of CSOM.

3. Tympanic Membrane

It is difficult to examine the tympanic membrane in small children because the child keeps on shaking the head and the canal is narrow and collapsed. Normal tympanic membrane is a pearly gray translucent structure **(Fig. 13.9)**.

- Look for congestion of the membrane or bulging of the membrane; indicative of acute otitis media **(Fig. 13.10)**.
- A retracted tympanic membrane or a dull membrane with fluid bubbles behind it is indicative of serous otitis media **(Fig. 13.11)**.

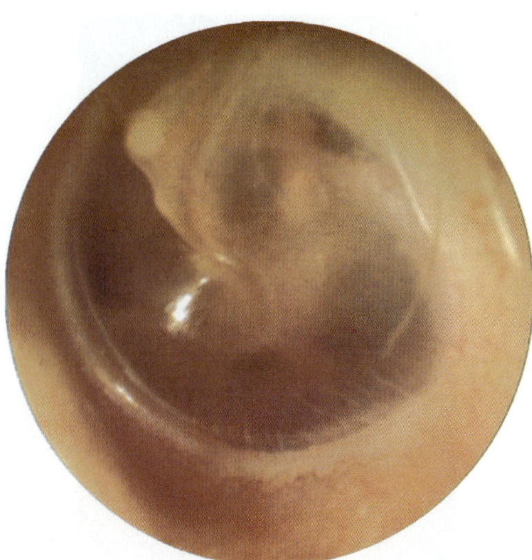

Fig. 13.9: Normal tympanic membrane.

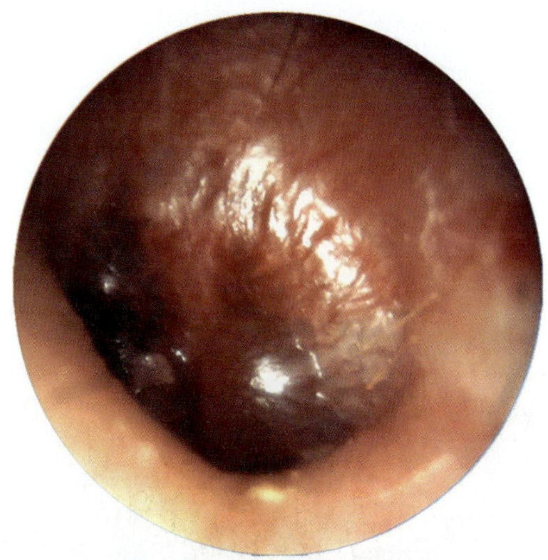

Fig. 13.10: Acute otitis media showing a bulging tympanic membrane.

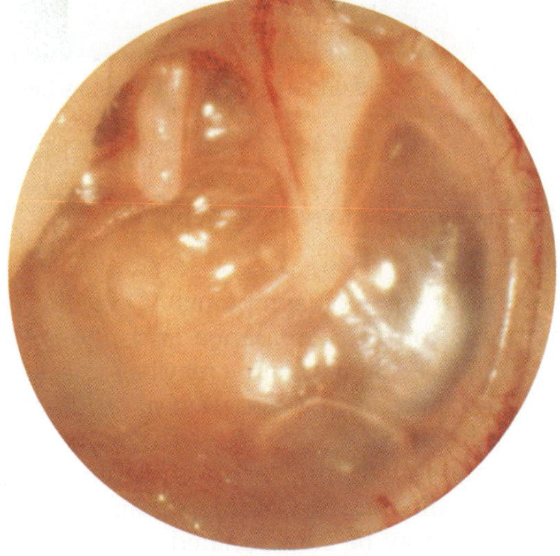

Fig. 13.11: Serous otitis media.

- A perforation in the membrane will be visible as a defect in the membrane with smooth edges (Fig. 13.12).
- Look for granulations, polyp, and whitish flakes along with a foul smelling discharge. If present, you must be alerted to the possibility of unsafe CSOM. This may need surgical management. So patient should be referred to a specialist.

C. Assessment of Hearing

Early detection of hearing loss is important to avoid delay in speech development of the child because these initial years of life are crucial for development of speech.

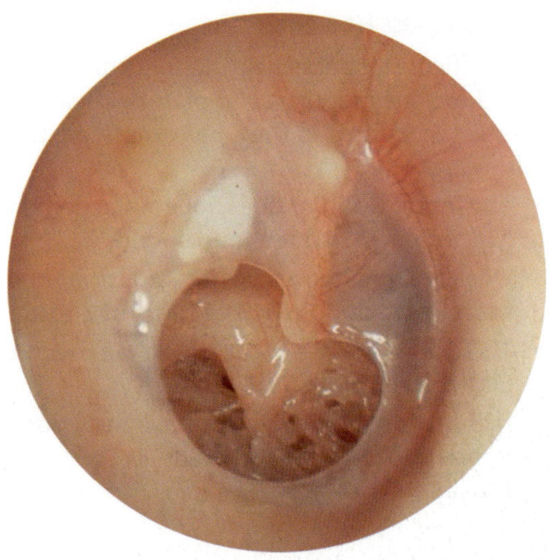

Fig. 13.12: Chronic suppurative otitis media showing a central perforation.

Hearing loss can be congenital or acquired. It can be either:

i. *Conductive*—due to defect in the sound conduction pathway; or
ii. *Sensorineural*—due to a defect in the perception mechanism of the sound. Common causes are enumerated in **Key Box 4**.

Key Box 4

Common Causes of Hearing Loss

1. Conductive
   a. *Congenital:* Meatal atresia, fixation of ossicles, congenital cholesteatoma.
   b. *Acquired:* Obstruction in the external auditory canal (due to wax, foreign body, acute inflammatory swelling or stenosis of the canal), tympanic membrane perforation, acute otitis media, serous otitis media (glue ear), ossicular discontinuity (due to trauma, CSOM, cholesteatoma).
2. Sensorineural
   a. *Congenital:* Genetic anomalies of the inner ear, prenatal or perinatal factors contributing to damage to hearing apparatus.
   b. *Acquired:* Delayed onset genetic syndromes, infections of the inner ear, traumatic injury to inner ear due to temporal bone fractures, noise-induced hearing loss, ototoxic drugs.

How to Assess Hearing?

It is difficult to assess hearing in a child. The guardians may report a complaint of hearing loss in an infant, if they have noticed the following:

- The infant/toddler does not get startled on exposure to a sudden loud sound;
- Does not look around to try and locate the source of sound, such as a rattle or a toy;
- Toddlers may be reported as being inattentive; and
- Inability to understand simple instructions unless spoken in a loud voice.
- Delayed speech development

Newborn

Presence or absence of hearing can be checked using otoacoustic emission (OAE) testing and brainstem evoked response audiometry (BERA). Behavioral observation audiometry can be done in a child between 0 and 6 months.

Infant

Assess the hearing status by presenting a loud sound to the infant, such as a loud clap and see if the child blinks his eyes (auropalpebral reflex). Alternatively, sound a bell or crumple a paper at around half a meter from child's ears and see whether the infant turns her head to locate the source of sound.

Toddler

A toddler's hearing can be assessed by giving him easy to understand instructions in a normal conversational voice and observing his reaction. Tuning fork tests can be done in a child who can follow instructions. For quantitative estimation, tests such as play audiometry may be used according to the age of the child.

Older Children

They can be assessed using the standard pure tone audiometry, because they can understand the instructions (Fig. 13.13). Methods of hearing testing used in children 1–5 years of age include behavioral response audiometry, play audiometry, and free field audiometry; where estimation of hearing thresholds can be done.

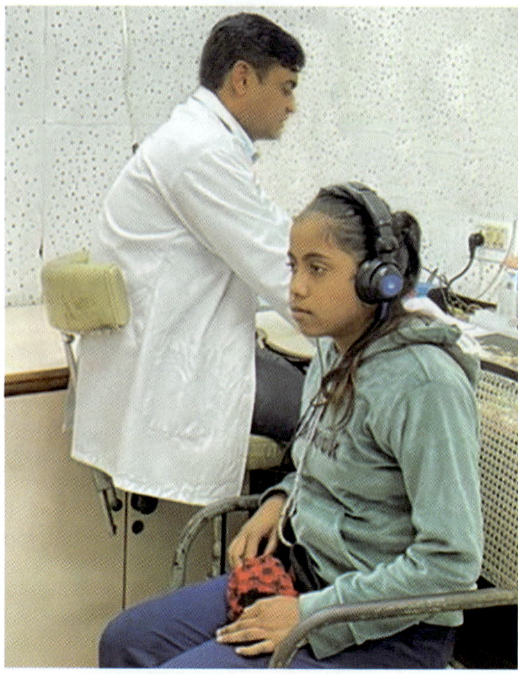

Fig. 13.13: A child undergoing standard pure tone audiometry.

D. Assessment of Vestibular Function

Indication

Two most common symptoms of vestibular dysfunction are imbalance and nausea/vomiting. Vestibular testing may be indicated in children reporting sensation of giddiness or imbalance, children with recurrent unexplained falling, or in children with learning difficulties. Giddiness, nausea, and vomiting may be an associated symptom in children suffering from atticoantral CSOM, if they develop a complication of labyrinthitis.

How to Assess?

The vestibular function can be assessed as per tests outlined in **Key Box 5**.

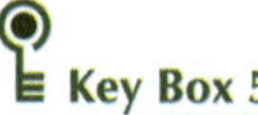

Key Box 5

Tests to Assess Vestibular Function

1. Spontaneous nystagmus
2. Gaze-evoked nystagmus
3. Tandem heel-toe gait test
4. Romberg test, Untenberger stepping test
5. Caloric testing
6. Electronystagmography

Spontaneous and Gaze-evoked Nystagmus

First ask the child to look straight, and observe for any nystagmus. Then, ask the child to follow your finger placed approximately 30 cm in front of the face. Move your finger on either side, and ask the child to follow it, without moving the head. Look for any sudden jerky movements of the eyes (nystagmus), specially in horizontal axis.

Gait Test

Ask the child to walk along a straight line (with heel following the toe) to a fixed point, first with eyes open and then closed. Note any swaying to either side.

Others

Caloric testing, electronystagmography, and rotational chair testing are the other tests which can be performed after taking the child in confidence to elicit cooperation. These tests require interpretation by a specialist.

13.4 COMMON SYMPTOMS RELATED TO THE NOSE

Key Box 6 summarizes the common symptoms related to nose in children.

A. Nasal Obstruction and Discharge

Nasal obstruction may be unilateral, bilateral, or periodically alternating. Infants and children may present with complaints of mouth breathing, feeding problems, sleep disturbance, and in severe cases with failure to thrive. Ask for any associated symptoms such as recurrent nasal discharge, snoring, sneezing, and headache. History of birth trauma, pain in the ear, and recurrent chest infection should be elicited. Family history of atopy and history of asthma are important while evaluating a child with nasal symptoms.

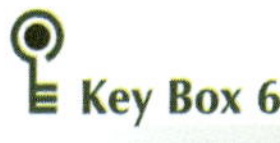

Key Box 6

Symptoms of Nasal Disease in Children

1. Nasal obstruction or nasal stuffiness
2. Discharge from the nose
3. Itching in the nose
4. Sneezing
5. Bleeding from the nose (epistaxis)

A watery discharge suggests allergic rhinitis; mucoid or mucopurulent discharge is characteristic of acute rhinitis or rhinosinusitis. A child presenting with a prolonged history of nasal obstruction, recurrent nasal discharge, and headache should be evaluated for chronic rhinosinusitis.

Causes

The common causes of nasal obstruction in children are listed in **Key Box 7**.

Choanal Atresia

An infant with bilateral complete atresia will have extreme difficulty in breathing because infants are obligate nose breathers and will require immediate measures to maintain breathing. Neonate may present with cyclical cyanosis (cyanotic spells relieved by crying). Unilateral choanal atresia may present with unilateral persistent nasal discharge without any history of foreign body insertion. Association with CHARGE (**C**oloboma, **H**eart defect, Choanal **A**tresia, Growth **R**etardation, **G**enital abnormalities, **E**ar abnormalities) must be evaluated in all cases of choanal atresia.

Deviated Nasal Septum

Child with a deviated nasal septum may have a history of trauma at birth or thereafter. Septal deviation may or may not be associated with an external nasal deformity. There may be a history of bleeding from the nose due to crusting on the deviated part of the nasal septum.

Adenoidal Hypertrophy

- Children with adenoidal hypertrophy may have an associated history of recurrent rhinitis, recurrent sore throat, and/or recurrent attacks of acute otitis media.

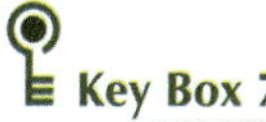

Key Box 7

Common Causes of Nasal Obstruction

1. Congenital, such as choanal atresia, or nasal masses
2. Deviated nasal septum
3. Foreign body in the nasal cavity
4. Inflammatory causes—allergy, infection
5. Nasal polyp
6. Hypertrophied adenoids

- The parents may give a specific history of mouth breathing, snoring while sleeping, and in severe cases history suggestive of short apneic attacks in sleep (*obstructive sleep apnea*).
- In older children, the facial features get modified to give the characteristic *adenoid* facies; consisting of open mouth, pinched up nose due to poorly developed alae nasi, high arched palate with crowding of teeth, and protruded upper jaw.
- Child may have an associated complaint of decreased hearing due to otitis media with effusion arising due to persistent Eustachian tube blockage because of enlarged adenoids.

Foreign Body

A child 3–5 years of age may present with unilateral nasal obstruction and unilateral mucopurulent discharge. This is most commonly due to a neglected foreign body in the nasal cavity.

Allergic Rhinitis

These children present with recurrent sneezing, watering from eyes, watery nasal discharge, itching in the nose, and associated nasal obstruction. There may be a history of co-existing atopic dermatitis and/or asthma.

Nasal Infections

Children are prone to attacks of viral cold, being exposed to viruses in the daycare and school environment. Viral rhinitis may be associated with malaise and fever. The color, consistency, and amount of the nasal secretions will guide you to the possible etiology.

Children with allergic rhinitis, immune defects, or gastroesophageal reflux disorder are predisposed to development of rhinosinusitis. A purulent or mucopurulent nasal discharge, facial pain, loss of sense of smell along with nasal congestion is usually indicative of rhinosinusitis. Ask for associated symptoms of fever, headache, post-nasal drip, and pain in the throat.

Nasal Mass

Children may present with nasal obstruction due to nasal polyp formation. This is commonly an antrochoanal polyp arising from the maxillary sinus, which is unilateral and may block the posterior choanae as well. Mass in the nasal cavity, or an infected nasal polyp, may present with blood-stained nasal discharge along with nasal obstruction.

B. Epistaxis

Bleeding from the nose is rare in children less than two years of age. It is more common in the age group of 3–8 years. It is found to be a more common complaint during the winter season due to increased frequency of upper respiratory tract infections.

Causes

The common causes of bleeding from the nose are listed in **Key Box 8**. The most common cause is frequent nose picking. Children may cause fingernail trauma to the anteroinferior part of the nasal septum which is the area of vascular anastomosis.

You must consider nasopharyngeal angiofibroma as a strong possibility, if the patient is an adolescent male with history of nasal obstruction and spontaneous bleeding from the nose.

Epistaxis may be the first presenting feature of a bleeding or coagulation disorder. Always look and ask for other features of hematological involvement, and a family history of similar episodes.

C. Other Symptoms

Other symptoms of nasal disease are headache, postnasal drip, and atypical facial pain. In the absence of any systemic cause of headache, the child will need detailed evaluation of nose and paranasal sinuses. Itching in the nose and frequent sneezing is indicative of allergic rhinitis.

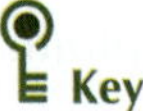

Key Box 8

Common Causes of Nasal Bleed

1. Digital trauma (fingernail trauma)
2. Deviated nasal septum
3. Infections
4. Allergic rhinitis
5. Foreign body
6. Nasopharyngeal angiofibroma
7. Trauma to the face and nose
8. Idiopathic

13.5 EXAMINATION OF THE NOSE

A. How to Examine

1. Position

- You will need a torch/headlight or an otoscope light. For detailed evaluation of the nasal cavities, a pediatric size nasal speculum will be valuable.
- Examine the nose with the child in sitting position. A small child needs to be sitting in the caregiver's lap with him/her holding the arms and steadying the head of the child.

2. Inspect and Palpate the External Nose

The external nose is inspected for the presence of any swelling, scar, or sinus. There may be a sinus opening in the midline of the dorsum of the nose which is commonly a dermoid sinus. This will need surgical excision, if there is discharge and recurrent infection.

Next, palpate the nasal framework: Both bony and cartilaginous, for any tenderness or swelling.

3. Examination of the Internal Nose

The nasal vestibule and the interior of the nose in children can be examined by gently pushing up the tip of the nose using a finger or thumb (**Fig. 13.14**). Alternatively, an appropriate size nasal speculum can be used, if the child is co-operative (**Fig. 13.15**). The otoscope can also be used to examine the anterior nasal cavity.

4. Examine the Nasal Cavity

The nasal cavity needs to be examined for the abnormalities listed in **Key Box 9**.

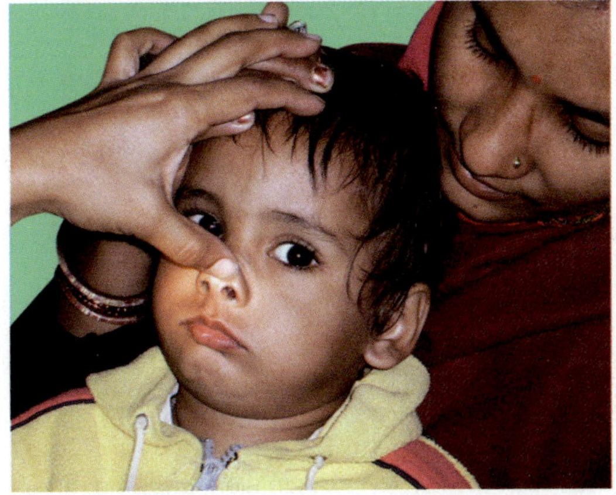

Fig. 13.14: Examination of the nose.

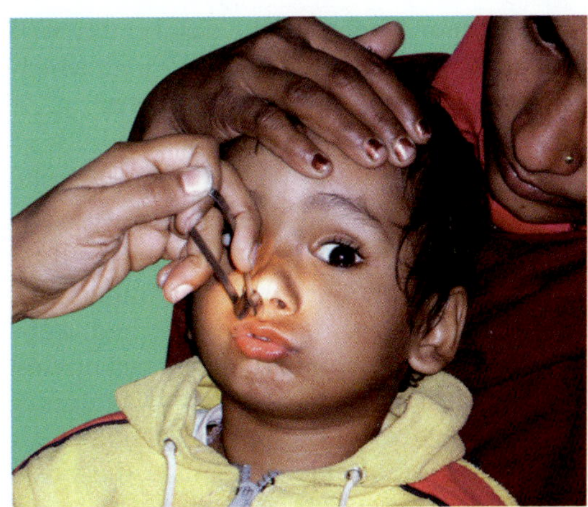

Fig. 13.15: Examination of the nose using nasal speculum.

Key Box 9

Examine the Nasal Cavity for Following

1. Type of nasal discharge: Watery, mucoid, or purulent
2. Condition of the nasal mucosa
3. Swelling of the inferior turbinates
4. Deviation of the nasal septum
5. Any mass in the nasal cavity

Nasal discharge: A little amount of thin, whitish nasal secretions are normal. If the discharge is thick and excessive, it is indicative of some pathology. A purulent discharge is indicative of infection in the nose and/or sinuses.

Nasal mucosa: The nasal mucosa is normally slightly pinkish. It is congested and the color changes to dark pink or red in acute rhinitis or rhinosinusitis. It may be pale in allergic rhinitis.

Turbinates: The turbinates are pinkish projections from the lateral nasal wall and are sensitive to touch.

Nasal septum: Normal septum is a midline structure. Slight deviations do not cause symptoms and can be ignored. A septal deviation may be visible as a sharp angulation of the midline nasal septum or as a smooth deviation towards the lateral nasal wall. If the deviation is significant and is causing symptoms, then you need to refer the child to ENT specialist for consultation.

Nasal polyp: A polyp in the nasal cavity will be a pale, smooth structure (Fig. 13.16) which can be confused with nasal secretions.

5. Adenoids

A child with adenoidal hypertrophy will have typical facial features. The face will be elongated, mouth open, with a vacant look on the face. The palate may be high arched, teeth crowded, and the nose may be pinched up due to disuse atrophy of the muscles. Diagnosis is assisted by X-ray of the nasopharynx, which shows adenoidal enlargement in the post-nasal space (Fig. 13.17).

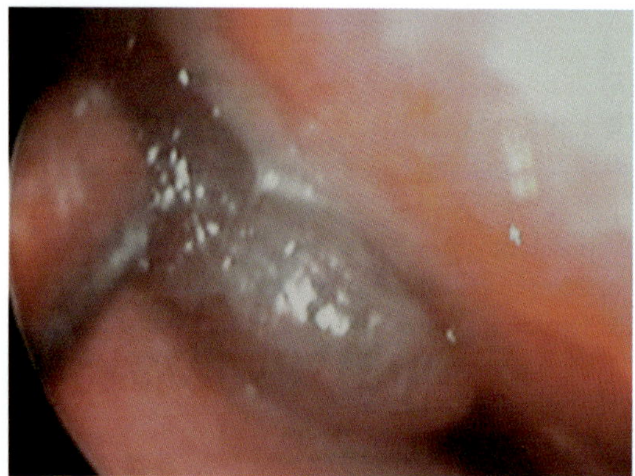

Fig. 13.16: Nasal polyp.

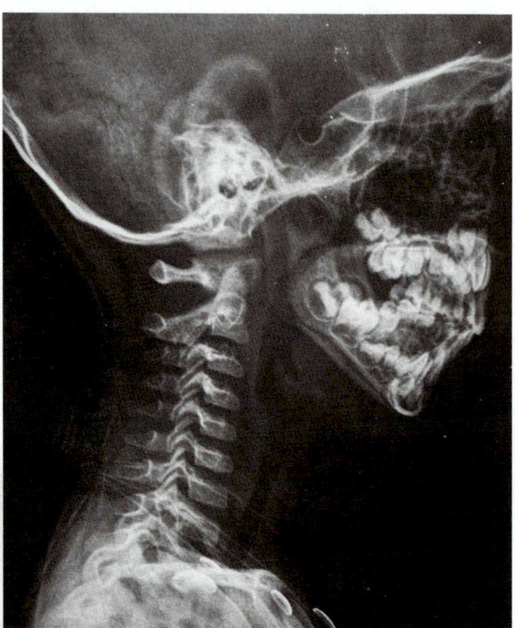

Fig. 13.17: X-ray of adenoids.

13.6 SYMPTOMS RELATED TO THE ORAL CAVITY AND OROPHARYNX

Symptoms related to oral cavity are listed in **Key Box 10**.

1. Throat Pain

The pain in throat is usually dull, continuous, and is aggravated during swallowing leading to refusal of feeds and excessive crying in toddlers. The pain may radiate towards the ears. Pain may be associated with fever and swelling in the neck.

Causes

Common causes of pain in the throat include tonsillitis (Fig. 13.18), peritonsillar abscess, dental caries, acute pharyngitis, retropharyngeal abscess, and acute epiglottitis.

If the child presents with history of frequent episodes of pain in the throat, ask for the frequency and severity of episodes, school

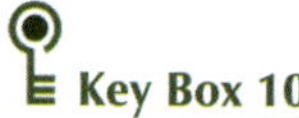

Key Box 10

Symptoms of Disorders of the Oral Cavity and Oropharynx

1. Pain in the throat
2. Difficulty in swallowing
3. Pain and swelling in the neck
4. Change in voice
5. Difficulty in breathing

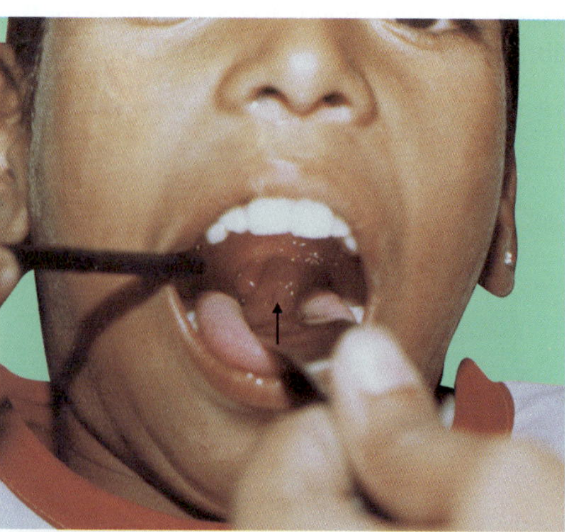

Fig. 13.18: Throat examination showing gross enlargement of tonsils.

absenteeism, difficulty in swallowing, and difficulty in breathing associated with fever. The commonest cause is tonsillar infection and this detail will help in deciding whether the child should be referred for surgical management.

Pain in the throat and difficulty in swallowing may also be due to a peritonsillar abscess, where the voice of the child also changes accompanied with fever and malaise.

Acute epiglottitis will also present with pain in the throat, severe dysphagia, drooling of saliva, and difficulty in breathing which increases on lying down. There may be associated stridor.

2. Neck Swelling

The child may present with complaint of swelling in the neck.

Lymph Nodes

- Recurrent attacks of tonsillitis are usually associated with enlarged jugulodigastric lymph nodes.
- Inflammatory conditions in the oral cavity and oropharynx, dental caries, etc. will lead to enlargement of submandibular lymph nodes.
- Small, single lymph nodes which are rubbery in consistency, non-tender, and have persisted for a long duration without increase in size, may be due to some infection in the past. These can be followed up without any active management.

Dysphagia with Neck Swelling

The differential diagnosis in these cases can be Ludwig angina, deep neck space infection, cervical lymphadenitis, and diphtheritic infection in the throat.

Diphtheria

In diphtheria, there may be bilateral swelling in the neck, grayish white dirty slough like membrane covering the tonsils and surrounding area, with the symptoms often rapidly progressing to difficulty in breathing and severe stridor. Such a child needs urgent confirmation of the diagnosis and specific management.

Abscess

A child with parapharyngeal/retropharyngeal abscess may also present with swelling in the neck; this will be associated with fever, dysphagia, and difficulty in breathing.

13.7 EXAMINATION OF THE ORAL CAVITY AND OROPHARYNX

You need a torch or headlight to examine the oral cavity and oropharynx. Child is best examined in a sitting position in the caregiver's lap.

Neck

Inspect the neck for any gross swellings, sinus openings, and use of accessory muscles of respiration. Palpate the neck gently with warm hands for enlarged lymph nodes, swellings, and any tenderness.

Mouth

Inspect the child's lips, teeth if present, buccal mucosa, tongue, and floor of mouth. Then, examine the hard palate and the soft palate. This examination is assisted by the use of a wooden tongue depressor or a metallic appropriate size spatula (Fig. 13.19). Care must be taken to be gentle and not to insert the spatula too inside so as to touch the uvula or the posterior pharyngeal wall because that will cause the child to gag, and then refusal to cooperate. Look for cleft lip and cleft palate, tongue swellings, retention cysts, dental caries, and swelling of the hard or the soft palate.

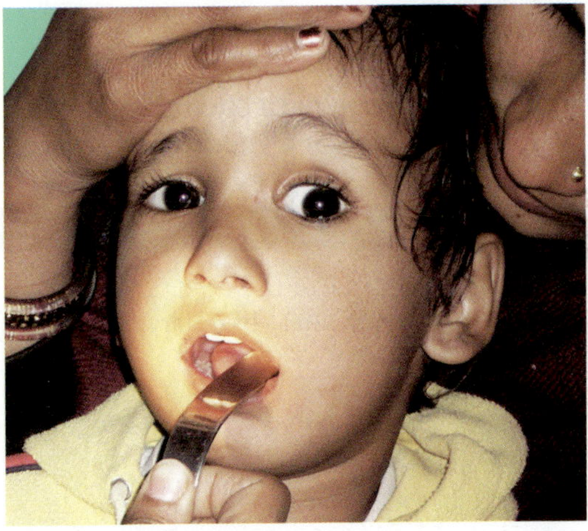

Fig. 13.19: Examination of the oral cavity using metallic tongue depressor.

Examination is then directed to the tonsillar pillars, tonsils, and posterior pharyngeal wall.

- Note any congestion of the tonsillar pillars; and congestion, inflammatory granular swellings or mucoid/mucopurulent discharge on the posterior pharyngeal wall.
- Also examine the posterior pharyngeal wall for any bulge or fullness which indicates retropharyngeal abscess.
- Examine the tonsils for enlargement, congestion, pus follicles, or any membrane formation on the surface.
- Also look for associated enlarged tender lymph nodes or pooling of saliva.

A child with chronic tonsillitis may have hypertrophied tonsils with no follicles/ membrane or congestion. A child with acute tonsillitis, however, will have angry looking enlarged tonsils, with or without pus follicles or a characteristic membrane.

13.8 SYMPTOMS OF LARYNGEAL INVOLVEMENT

Symptoms of laryngeal involvement are listed in **Key Box 11**.

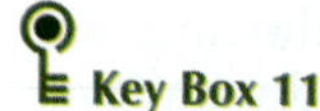

Key Box 11

Symptoms of Laryngeal Involvement

1. Change in voice (hoarseness)
2. Pain in the throat
3. *Stridor:* Noisy breathing
4. Choking or coughing while eating
5. Difficulty in swallowing

1. Hoarseness

A child may present with change in voice (hoarseness). This may or may not be associated with other symptoms, like dysphagia, fever, or neck swelling. The causes can be laryngotracheobronchitis, laryngitis, or even vocal nodules in children with a history of chronic voice abuse.

2. Stridor

Stridor (noisy breathing) is often a troublesome symptom in infants and children. It is caused by turbulent airflow due to partial obstruction of the airway. Causes of stridor are listed in **Table 13.1**. A detailed history regarding the onset, progression, duration, history of trauma, and aggravating and relieving factors of stridor is essential to point towards the site, cause, and severity of airway compromise.

- Stridor present at birth signifies a congenital narrowing of airway.
- Conditions, such as laryngomalacia, manifest in the first few weeks after birth. In this condition, typically, the stridor is worse when the child is taking feeds or is crying.
- Laryngeal obstruction produces an inspiratory stridor, while tracheal obstruction more often causes a biphasic stridor.
- Hoarseness along with stridor indicates a vocal cord palsy or recurrent respiratory papillomatosis.
- Cough with stridor is generally due to a tracheoesophageal fistula or tracheomalacia.
- Laryngotracheobronchitis is another common condition in children, which manifests with hoarseness, stridor and cough.

3. Foreign Body

A history of foreign body inhalation should alert you to the possibility of a foreign body lodged in the airway. A foreign body may get

Table 13.1: Causes of stridor

Infants	Older children
• Congenital anomalies like laryngeal web, laryngeal cysts, etc. • Congenital tumors • Laryngomalacia • Subglottic stenosis • Subglottic hemangioma • Any lesion causing intrinsic or extrinsic narrowing of the small airway	• Acute epiglottitis • Laryngotracheobronchitis • Foreign body aspiration • Laryngeal diphtheria • Vocal cord paralysis • Retropharyngeal abscess; intubation trauma • Injury to the larynx • Swellings in the neck, e.g. cystic hygroma

lodged in the nasopharynx (although rare), oropharynx, supraglottis, glottis, subglottis, or into the tracheobronchial tree. Symptoms are variable depending on the shape, size, and nature (organic/inorganic) of the foreign body.

The characteristic history of a foreign body aspiration is sudden episode of choking, followed by cough, difficulty in breathing, and sometimes a change in voice. The child is usually playing while eating or laughing while eating and suddenly aspirates food material or any other toy part, etc.

A large foreign body gets lodged in the supraglottis, and may precipitate severe laryngospasm and severe difficulty in breathing. If a foreign body gets stuck in the glottic region, it can cause a change in voice and stridor.

You must also think of a neglected long-standing foreign body, if a child presents with chronic history of cough, persistent mild difficulty in breathing, and recurrent pneumonia.

13.9 EXAMINATION OF THE LARYNX

Examination of the larynx is usually performed by otorhinolaryngologists. However, children with laryngeal involvement in various conditions may present to the pediatricians. In cases with noisy and labored breathing, the child or infant must be observed for use of accessory muscles, intercostal/suprasternal retraction, and the phase of respiration when stridor is maximum. Additional signs, such as wheeze, cough, change in voice or cry, and air entry in both the lungs must be evaluated.

1. External Examination of Larynx

Look for any swelling, displacement of the midline laryngeal structures, and any changes in overlying skin. Palpate the hyoid bone, thyroid cartilage, and the cricoid cartilage for any tenderness or change in contour.

2. Laryngoscopy

To examine the base of tongue, vallecula, epiglottis, and endolarynx; special procedures, like indirect laryngoscopy, fiberoptic laryngoscopy, or direct laryngoscopy are required.

Indirect Laryngoscopy

Older children may cooperate for indirect laryngoscopy which is done in the outpatient department with the child sitting in the examination chair and does not require any anesthesia.

Fiberoptic Laryngoscopy

In toddlers and in younger children, flexible fiberoptic nasopharyngoscopy and laryngoscopy is a useful, painless procedure and can be attempted after anesthetizing the nose of the child and explaining him the procedure. This can be done to rule out nasopharyngeal pathologies, like adenoid enlargement, laryngeal pathologies, and vocal cord lesions, etc.

Direct Laryngoscopy

If a child is uncooperative or the lesion requires a detailed evaluation, then you have to resort to direct laryngoscopy. This can be done in OPD for conditions, like suspected laryngomalacia in infants but mostly requires general anesthesia for detailed evaluation.

13.10 NEWBORN HEARING SCREENING

WHO estimates that 70% of hearing loss is preventable in developing countries. Neonatal hearing screening aims to offer hearing assessment tests to all the newborns regardless of presence or absence of any risk indicator or any ear symptoms, thus identifying newborns with hearing impairment. An early detection of hearing loss can lead to an early and timely intervention which helps in normal speech and language development, social and emotional growth, and cognitive development of the child.

Tests for Newborn Hearing Screening

Skilled observation of the child's response to speech and non-speech stimuli is referred to as behavioral hearing assessment. The two objective tests commonly used for neonatal hearing screening are:

1. Otoacoustic emission (OAE)
2. Brainstem evoked response audiometry (BERA)

Otoacoustic emission: OAE are forms of energy, measured as sound, generated by the healthy outer hair cells (OHCs) of cochlea, in response to received auditory input. A sound stimulus is sent via an ear probe placed in the external meatus. The probe simultaneously records signals returning from OHCs of the cochlea. It is an easy test and can be done bedside.

BERA: This is an electrophysiologic method which measures the neural activity of the brainstem in response to sounds presented to the child via earphones. Three electrodes are taped to the head to record the signals from the brainstem thus enabling us to diagnose auditory neuropathy. There is production of waves from the inner ear till the central auditory pathway. Both the instruments employ automated detection algorithms for the determination of presence or absence of any response, thus making it easier for the screening staff to record the response.

Universal Neonatal Hearing Screening (UNHS)

Identification of all newborns with hearing loss before 6 months of age has now become an attainable and realistic goal.

A two-step screening procedure has been implemented in most of the UNHS programs as a cost effective and accurate approach. In newborns with no risk factors, OAE is performed first, followed by BERA (if required) if the neonate does not pass the OAE. Newborns with risk factors (particularly with newborns requiring neonatal intensive unit care) are tested using BERA, as this population is at increased risk of auditory neuropathy. Risk factors for hearing loss are listed in **Key Box 12**.

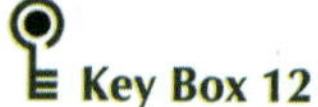

Key Box 12

Risk Factors for Hearing Loss

- Family history of permanent hearing loss
- Intrauterine infection (TORCH infections)
- Craniofacial anomalies including those involving the external ear
- Low birth weight babies less than 1500 g
- Apgar score less than 7 at 5 minutes
- Neonatal intensive care unit stay >2 days OR with any of the following regardless of duration of stay:
  - Hyperbilirubinemia at a serum level requiring exchange transfusion
  - Ototoxic drug use by mother during pregnancy
  - Assisted ventilation
  - Extracorporeal membrane oxygenation

This two-step screening has been found to be highly effective in identifying infants with hearing loss at the earliest thus leading to timely intervention. Neonates with high risk indicators should be followed up even after passing the screening to pick up progressive or late onset hearing loss.

- Any baby missing screening before hospital discharge is called for OAE test at the earliest or on the first immunization visit.
- All babies with abnormal BERA are recommended to undergo detailed ENT evaluation and auditory rehabilitation as early as possible. Systemic evaluation should be done to categorize hearing loss into syndromic or non-syndromic hearing loss.

Chapter

14

Examination of the Skin

Deepika Pandhi

Structure

14.1 AIM, IMPORTANCE, AND SCHEME OF SKIN EXAMINATION

In this chapter, we introduce you to the systematic process of examination of the cutaneous lesions. The skin is the most accessible and easily examined organ of the body. The recognition of morphologic patterns can help in diagnosis of common skin lesions, and provide clues to underlying systemic diseases. A pediatrician needs to be familiar with common dermatologic nomenclature, variation in disease presentation, and evolution of lesions in the course of the disease.

Follow the steps given in **Key Box 1** for assessment of cutaneous lesion.

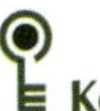

Key Box 1

Approach to Diagnosis of a Skin Lesion

1. **History**: Obtain brief history pertaining to onset, duration, symptoms, and relevant personal and family history.
2. **Primary lesion:** Identify the primary lesion and determine the secondary change, if any.
3. **Distribution:** Determine extent of lesional involvement by a complete and thorough muco-cutaneous evaluation.
4. Carry out relevant **systemic examination.**
5. Formulate **differential diagnoses.**
6. Perform relevant **laboratory investigations.**

14.2 HISTORY AND EXAMINATION OF CUTANEOUS LESIONS

It is more rewarding to obtain a preliminary history, examine the child, and subsequently ask leading questions as indicated by the physical findings. This is known as the 'sandwich format' for history-taking.

Preliminary History

Ask specifically for onset and evolution of the lesion and associated symptoms (itch, pain, burning sensation, paresthesias, etc.) and the treatment history including use of cosmetics. Pointed questions may now be asked depending on differential diagnoses considered including aggravating factors, e.g. flare up on photo-exposure. In a child with generalized maculopapular rash, ask for prior drug intake or systemic symptoms like fever, malaise, and upper respiratory tract infection to rule out viral etiology.

Past History

Ask for previous occurrence of similar illness, medications, allergies, and chronic illness including tuberculosis.

Family History

In an infant, the importance of prenatal and natal history is obvious. In addition, history of inherited disorders may be available (for example, in cases of tuberous sclerosis, neurofibromatosis, xeroderma pigmentosa). Family history may also be helpful in making a diagnosis of atopic dermatitis (family members may have atopic diathesis) or scabies.

Personal and Social History

This should include history of sexual behavior (in an adolescent), intravenous drug abuse, exposure to blood products, travel, and residence. History of clustering of cases in school or in playmates may point to an infectious etiology.

Cutaneous Examination

- You should conduct the examination under adequate illumination. While natural daylight is ideal, it may be substituted with fluorescent overhead lighting of adequate intensity and supplemented by a movable light source.
- You should examine the entire skin surface including hair, nails, palms, soles, and mucosae (including oral and anogenital) at the initial visit.
- Avoid separating an infant or toddler from parents and whenever possible examine the child in the lap or at least in close proximity with the caregiver. Sequential examination of body parts should be done in infants to prevent cooling.
- While eliciting history remain seated, maintain eye contact, and avoid sudden movements, which will alarm infants and younger children.
- To avoid embarrassment to adolescents, it is prudent to gain the trust of the patient by initial history-taking before proceeding to examination. Caution should be taken to cover the genitalia while the cutaneous examination is conducted.
- You will be able to pick up subtle elevation by tangential viewing of the lesion.
- After a careful inspection, palpate the lesion to evaluate consistency, depth, and tenderness.
- A hand-held magnifying lens (convex lens with 5 testing or 10 magnification) is useful in assessment of small lesions or to pick subtle surface alterations.
- We recommend that gloves should not be used initially while approaching the patient as that is likely to alarm a younger child. Palpation by bare hands also reassures patients and parents that the skin disease is not contagious. Gloves are recommended mostly for wet, oozing lesions, examination of orogenital mucosae, or for examination of the neonate in the nursery.

14.3 MORPHOLOGY OF SKIN LESIONS

This section will familiarize you with basic knowledge of terminology used to describe skin lesions. First differentiate whether this is a *primary* or *secondary* lesion.

- ***Primary lesion:*** A lesion that develops *de novo* and is characteristic of the disease is the primary lesion.
- ***Secondary lesion:*** These lesions develop during evolution of disease. They may sometimes be the only type of lesions present at the time of examination.

Then, note the points given in **Key Box 2**, in that order.

A. Primary Lesions

1. Macule

Macule is a flat, circumscribed area of altered skin color, with no change in skin consistency. The color may help in establishing differential diagnoses.

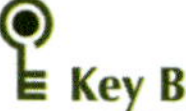

Key Box 2

Points to be Noted for Skin Lesion(s)

1. Identify whether primary or secondary
2. Characterize the morphology
3. Single or multiple
4. Note the color of the lesion
5. Note the edges: Sharpness of lesion—well-defined or ill-defined
6. Assessment of the shape of lesion/s, patterns, and distribution
7. Presence of specific signs (e.g. Koebner phenomenon, Nikolsky sign)

Hyperpigmented macules: Examples include café au lait macule, junctional nevi, ephelides (freckle), lentigo, melasma, and erythrasma.

i. ***Café au lait macules*** (Fig. 14.1) These are round or oval, uniformly light brown, pigmented lesions, which are found in up to 30% normal children. They do not regress with age. *Presence of 6 or more macules larger than 1.5 cm is pathognomonic of neurofibromatosis.* They can also be found in McCune-Albright syndrome (larger and darker macules), multiple lentigines syndrome, Fanconi anemia, and Gaucher disease.

ii. ***Lentigines:*** These are common, 1–10 mm, oval or circular, uniformly dark brown pigmented, sharply circumscribed macules. They may present at birth or during early childhood, and increase in adult life. They may be part of multiorgan syndromes, like Peutz-Jeghers syndrome, Leopard syndrome, and multiple lentigines syndrome.

iii. ***Ephelides*** (Freckles, Fig. 14.2): These are small, light brown, well-circumscribed macules that appear in light-skinned children in sun-exposed skin and tend to fade during winters. They may show variegated pigmentation. Freckles may be observed in neurofibromatosis or xeroderma pigmentosum.

iv. ***Melasma:*** It occurs primarily in pubertal girls and women but occasionally in adolescent boys. It presents as symmetric, patchy, facial hyperpigmented macules. It is often associated with intake of drugs like oral contraceptives and phenytoin.

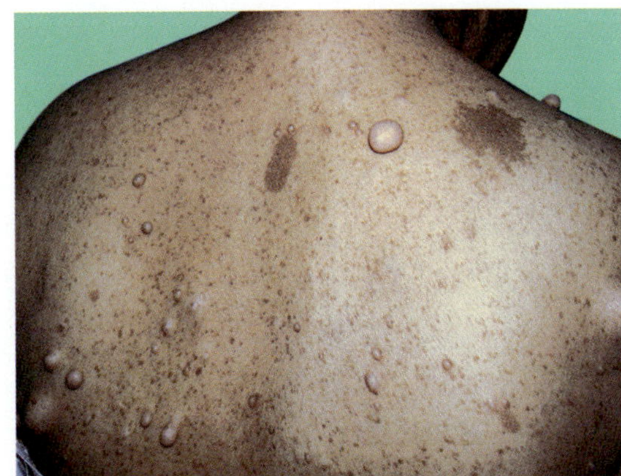

Fig. 14.1: Multiple, hyperpigmented macules over trunk. The larger macules range from 3 to 4.5 cm (café au lait macules), smaller are pinpoint to 0.5 cm (freckles). Skin-colored tumors are neurofibromas.

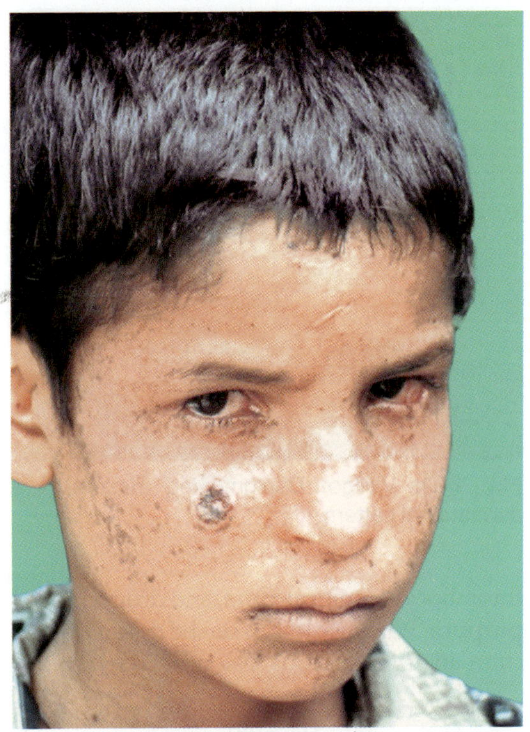

Fig. 14.2: Xeroderma pigmentosum with noduloulcerative basal cell carcinoma. Note the rolled out margins of the ulcer, facial scarring, ectropion and freckles (ephelides).

v. ***Nevi:*** Acquired nevi develop in early childhood as pigmented macules (1–2 mm). They enlarge to papules and darken during puberty.

Hypopigmented macules: Hypopigmented macules can be the primary lesions in leprosy, malnutrition, and tuberous sclerosis (ash leaf macule). Ash leaf macules are hypopigmented, lance ovate-shaped lesions, classically present on trunk at birth. They may appear in early childhood, be round or confetti-like in shape.

Depigmented macules: These are seen in vitiligo (Fig. 14.3) and piebaldism.

Erythematous macules: Reddish macules are seen in drug rash, rheumatic fever, viral exanthem, and juvenile rheumatoid arthritis. They usually result because of vascular dilatation.

Purpuric macules: Small red-colored spots (due to extravasation of red blood cells) are typically seen in viral exanthems, idiopathic

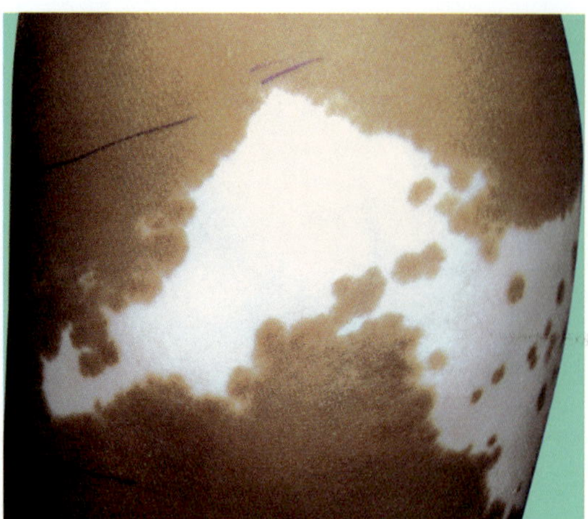

Fig. 14.3: Vitiligo: Depigmented macule in a dermatomal pattern.

thrombocytopenic purpura, and drug-induced purpura. Purpuric lesion can be differentiated from an erythematous lesion by diascopy.

Diascopy

Press the lesion with a glass slide. If redness disappears, it is due to vascular dilatation. If redness persists, it is due to extravasation of red blood cells.

Bluish or gray macules: Mongolian spots (Fig. 14.4) are a typical example. These are poorly circumscribed, slate-gray, congenital macules, ranging from 1 to 20 cm in size, over the trunk (lumbosacral predominantly) and proximal extremities. They fade by 5 years of age. Nevus of Ota (melanosis in trigeminal nerve distribution), and minocycline-induced rash also present as bluish or gray macules.

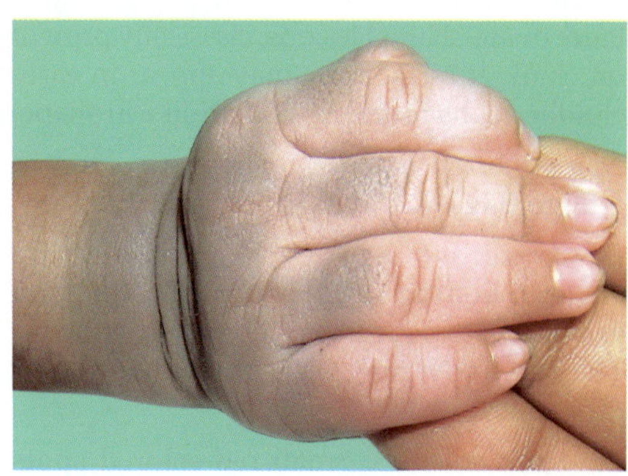

Fig. 14.4: Slate-gray macule (Mongolian spot) over the wrist, dorsum of hand, and digits.

2. Papule

Papule is a circumscribed elevation of skin less than 0.5 cm in diameter.

Look for the shape

- *Dome-shaped:* Trichoepithelioma.
- *Umblicated:* Molluscum contagiosum (Fig. 14.5), cryptococcosis.
- Verrucous Verruca vulgaris (Fig. 14.6); and mostly plaques in tuberculosis verrucosa cutis or hypertrophic lupus vulgaris (Fig. 14.7).
- *Pedunculated:* Skin tag.
- *Flat-topped:* Lichen planus (Fig. 14.8), verruca plana.

Look at the color of the papules

- *Red papules:* Acne, folliculitis, leukocytoclastic vasculitis (Fig. 14.9), milaria, scabies, psoriasis, insect bite.

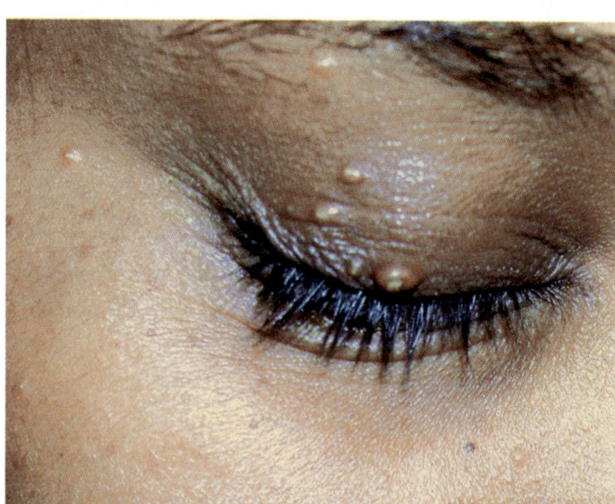

Fig. 14.5: Multiple, umbilicated papules of molluscum contagiosum over upper eyelids.

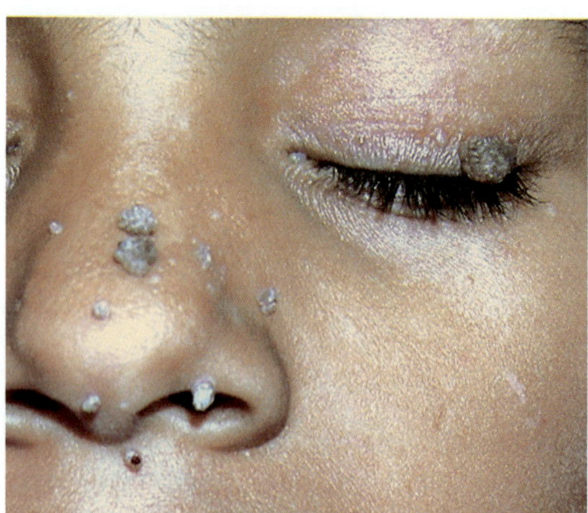

Fig. 14.6: Filiform warts (verrucous surface) on eyelids and nose.

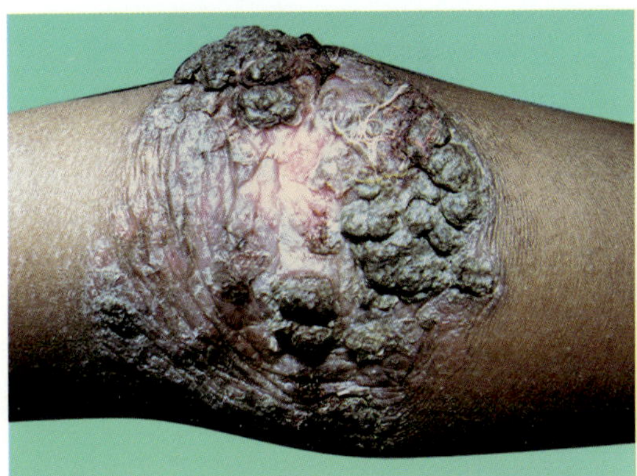

Fig. 14.7: Hypertrophic lupus vulgaris over the knee. Note the verrucous surface of the plaque.

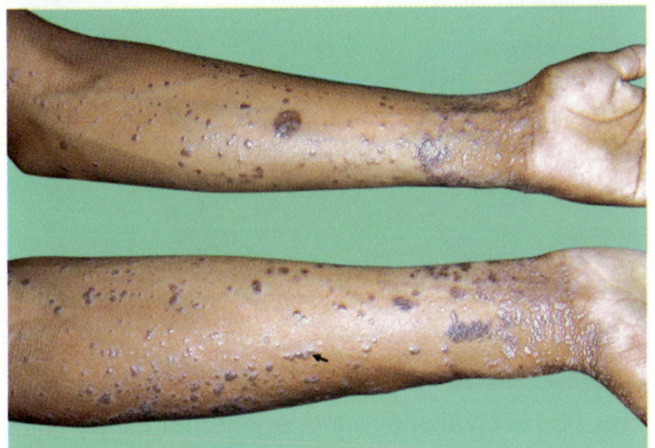

Fig. 14.8: Violaceous, shiny, flat-topped papules of lichen planus over flexor surface of forearms, arrow highlights Koebner's phenomenon (appearance of new lesions in linear fashion at the site of trauma scratch).

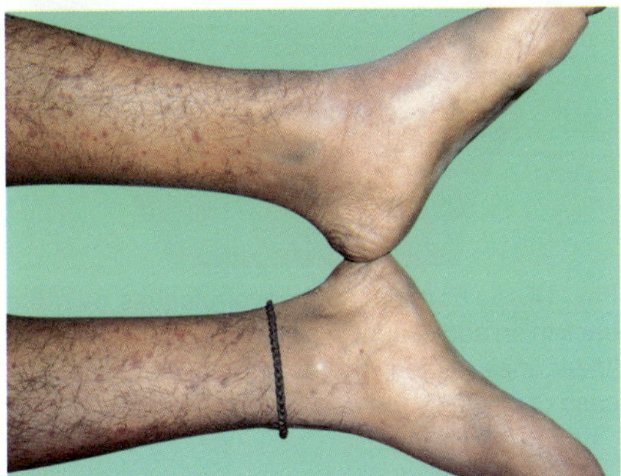

Fig. 14.9: Palpable purpura over the legs. Note pedal edema and left articular swelling. The lesions did not blanch on diascopy.

- *Brown or flesh-colored papules:* Skin tag, adenoma sebaceum (Fig. 14.10), verruca plana, dermal nevi.

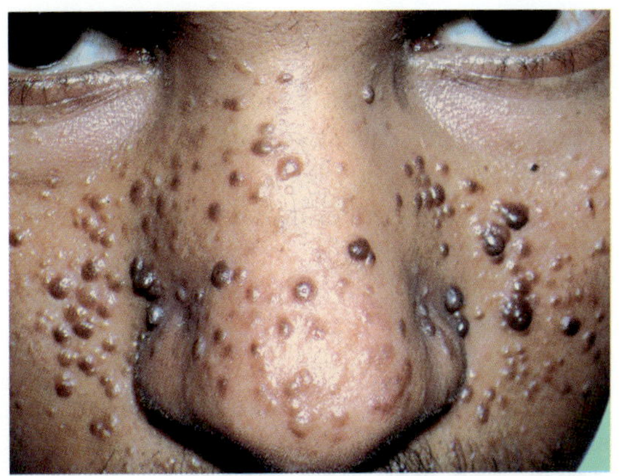

Fig. 14.10: Skin-colored to brown-red papules over central face in a case of tuberous sclerosis (adenoma sebaceum).

- *White or yellow papules:* Closed comedones, lichen nitidus, milia, molluscum contagiosum, sebaceous hyperplasia, xanthelasma palpebrum (Fig. 14.11).

Pearly penile papules (Fig. 14.12) are asymptomatic 1–3 mm, white, uniform

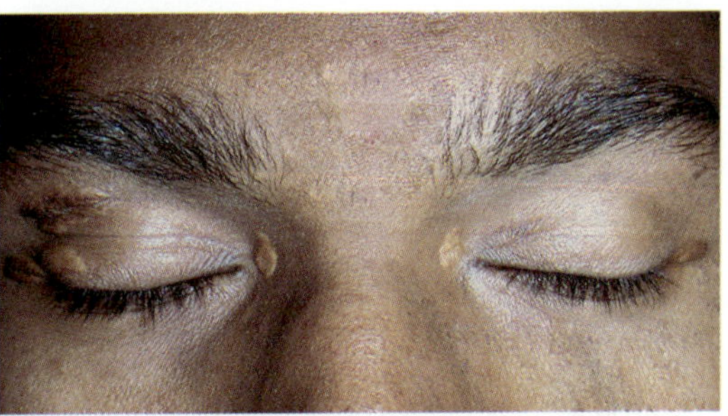

Fig. 14.11: Discrete and coalescent yellow papules of xanthelasma palpebrarum overlying bilateral eyelids. A biochemical and systemic examination for signs of hyperlipidemia should be carried out in such a patient.

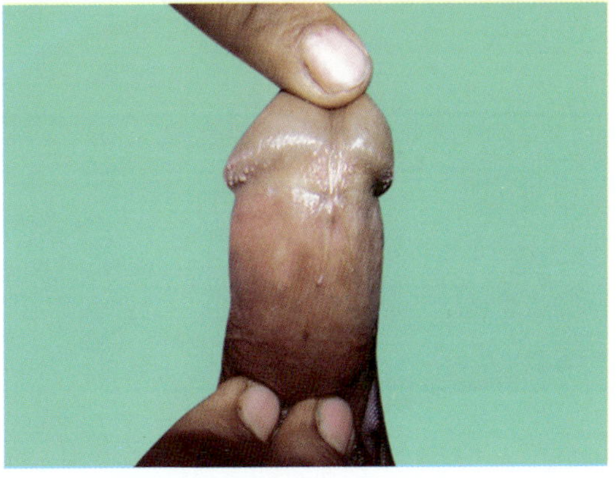

Fig. 14.12: White papules around corona of penis (pearly penile papules).

papules, forming a ring around corona of penis in adolescents. You must differentiate these normal variants from genital warts, which may indicate sexual activity.

- *Blue or violaceous papules:* Lichen planus (Fig. 14.8), angiokeratoma (Fig. 14.13), blue nevi, melanoma.

3. Plaque

Plaque is an elevated, flat, or depressed circumscribed area of change in consistency of skin greater than 0.5 cm. It is without substantial depth, and may form by enlargement or confluence of papules.

Plaques are seen in psoriasis vulgaris (Fig. 14.14), pityriasis rosea (Fig. 14.15), seborrheic dermatitis, secondary syphilis, discoid lupus erythematosus, nummular eczema, tinea corporis, tinea versicolor, lupus vulgaris, granuloma annulare, cutaneous sarcoidosis, cutaneous mastocytosis (Fig. 14.16), or congenital melanocytic nevi (Fig. 14.17).

You can demonstrate soft apple jelly nodules at the margins of the plaque in lupus vulgaris (cutaneous tuberculosis) by diascopy. Sarcoidal plaques have a sand grain-like consistency on diascopy.

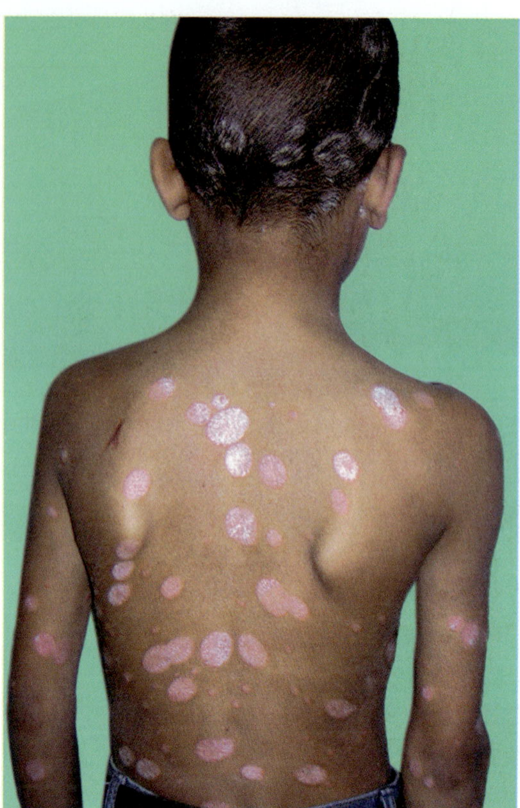

Fig. 14.14: Oval and round, erythematous plaques in psoriasis vulgaris.

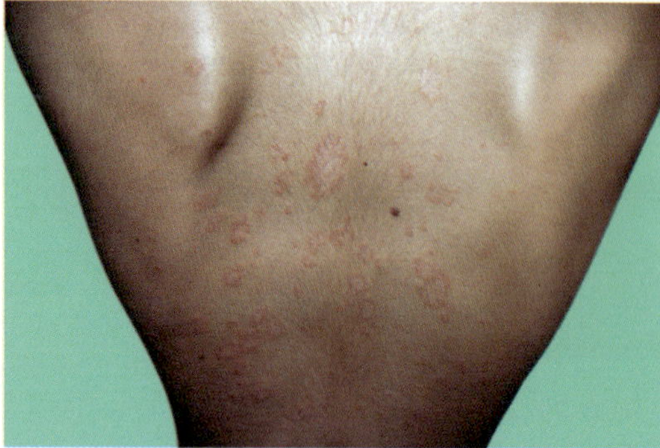

Fig. 14.15: Erythematous, oval plaques over the back in an adolescent in a fir tree pattern (following linear lines of cleavage) with collarette scaling. A case of pityriasis rosea.

Probable causes of lesions based on color

- *Red lesions:* Inflammatory or vascular.
- *Purple and blue lesions:* Vascular, tattoos, drug reactions like fixed drug reaction (Fig. 14.18) or deep dermal pigment.
- *Brown lesions:* Epidermal or superficial dermal pigment.

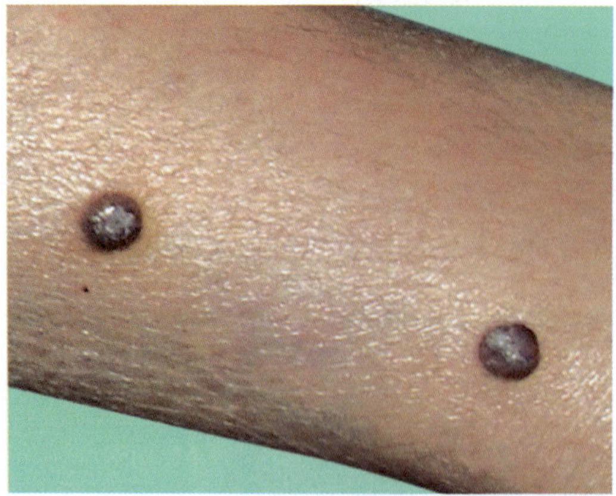

Fig. 14.13: Blue papules on the forearm (angiokeratoma).

- *Yellow lesions:* Lipid laden cells (of xanthelasma palpebrarum and xathomas, Fig. 14.11).
- *White lesions:* Loss of normal pigment.
- *Miscellaneous:* Tattoos, heavy metals, drugs, infectious agents (e.g. green due to *Pseudomonas aeruginosa*).

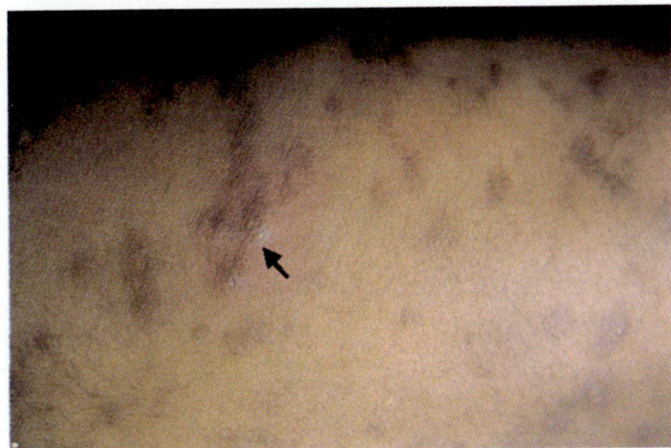

Fig. 14.16: Hyperpigmented minimally raised plaques (tangential viewing and palpation revealed they were minimally raised) of urticaria pigmentosa (cutaneous mastocytosis). Linear stroking of the lesion led to wheal and flare formation (Darier's sign, arrow).

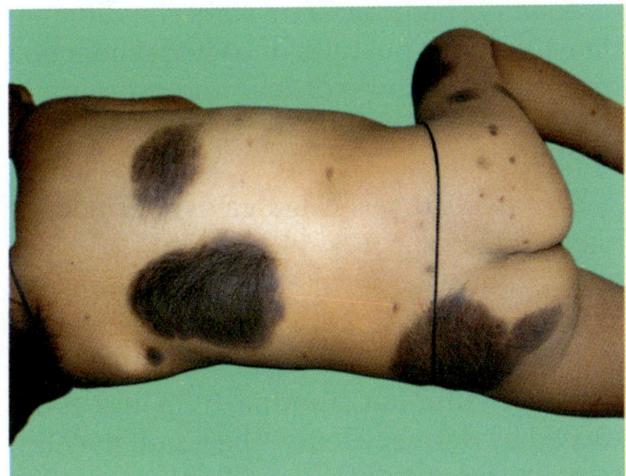

Fig. 14.17: Multiple plaques of variegated brown color with localized hypertrichosis in congenital melanocytic nevus.

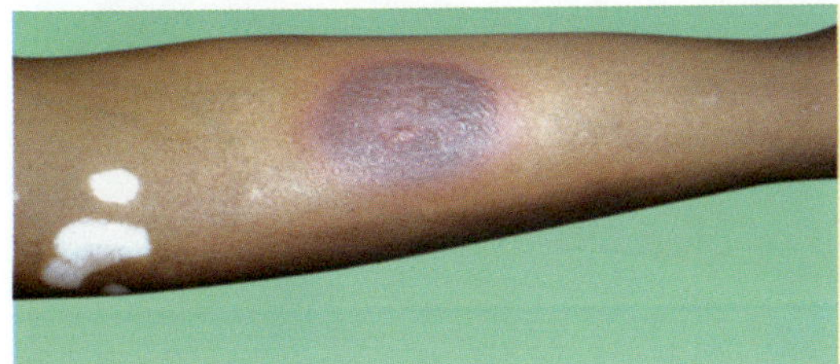

Fig. 14.18: Violaceous plaque (note minimal elevation) with erythematous halo (in a child with fixed drug eruption to sulfonamides).

4. Nodule

Nodule is an elevated skin lesion more than 0.5 cm. The depth of a nodule is even more than the surface elevation. Nodules are often more easily appreciated by palpation. Examples include erythema nodosum

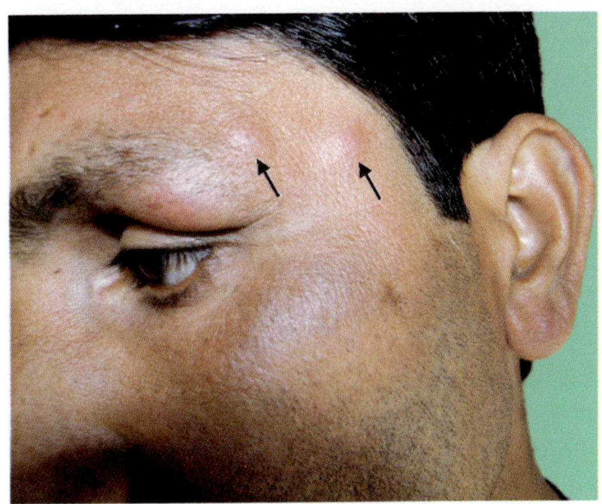

Fig. 14.19: Nodules of erythema nodosum.

(Fig. 14.19), cutaneous polyarteritis nodosa, xanthoma, lymphoma, and sporotrichosis.

5. Tumors

Tumor is the enlargement of tissues by normal or pathologic cells or material to form a mass: neurofibroma (Fig. 14.1), hemangioma, basal cell carcinoma (Fig. 14.2), and squamous cell carcinoma.

6. Vesicle and Bulla

Vesicle: Vesicle is a circumscribed collection of fluid less than 0.5 cm in diameter. Vesicles are characteristically seen in herpes simplex, herpes zoster (Fig. 14.20), chickenpox (Fig. 14.21), pemphigus, and acute eczema.

Bulla: Bulla is fluid-filled lesion greater than 0.5 cm. Lesions with subepidermal cleavage present as tense bullae. Common bullous lesions include staphylococcal skin-scalded syndrome, pemphigus vulgaris (Fig. 14.22),

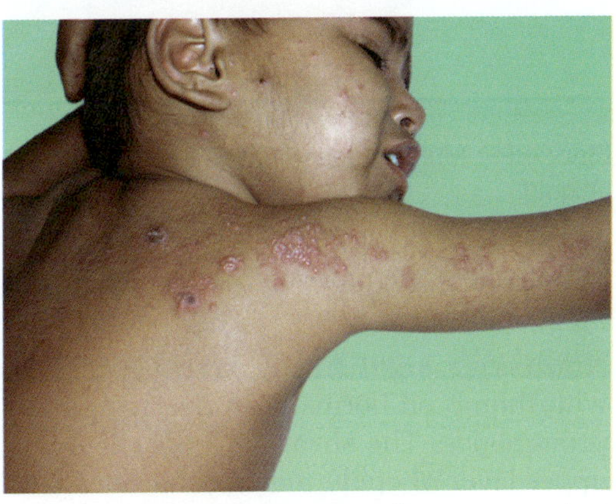

Fig. 14.20: Grouped vesicles (herpes zoster).

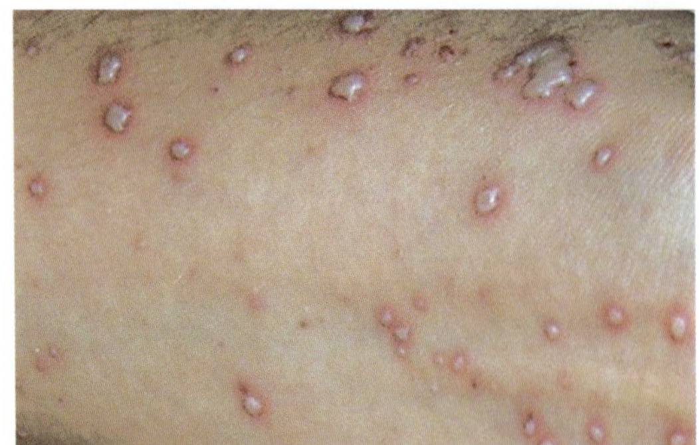

Fig. 14.21: Vesicles over hemorrhagic base (dew drops on rose petals sign in chickenpox).

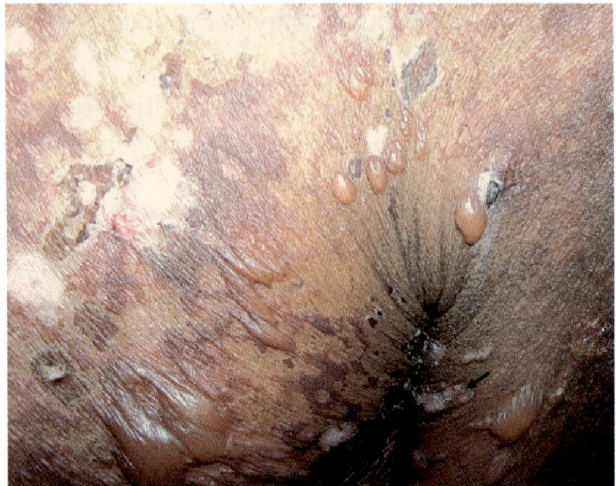

Fig. 14.22: Flaccid bullae in pemphigus vulgaris.

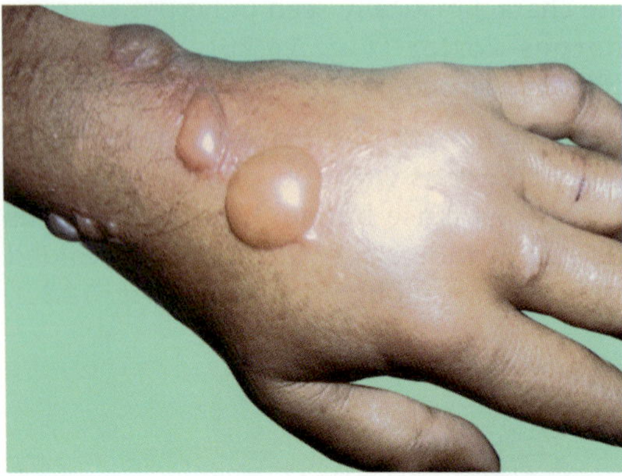

Fig. 14.23: Multiple, tense bullae in bullous pemphigoid.

bullous pemphigoid (Fig. 14.23), and linear IgA disease.

Nikolsky's sign: Apply lateral pressure with thumb on normal skin overlying bony prominence. The shearing force dislodges upper layer of epidermis in conditions with intra-epidermal cleavage (staphylococcal skin-scalded syndrome, pemphigus vulgaris). A positive result in normal looking skin close to the blister or at a distant site indicates disease activity.

Bulla spread sign: Mark the bulla with pen at margins. Apply slow careful, unidirectional pressure to the bulla causing extension beyond marked margins, again indicating intra-epidermal cleavage.

7. Pustule

Pustule is a circumscribed collection of leukocytes and free fluid. It can be seen in children with acne, chickenpox, superficial folliculitis, herpes simplex, herpes zoster, impetigo contagiosa, candidiasis, scabies, and pustular psoriasis (Fig. 14.24).

A simple bedside Gram stain can differentiate infectious pustules of bacterial infection from sterile pustules of acne and psoriasis.

8. Abscess

A thick-walled pus-filled cavity formed by necrosis of tissue (Fig. 14.25).

9. Wheal

Wheal is an evanescent, firm, elevated lesion, usually white surrounded by a red flare, caused by dermal edema. The lesion may last from few hours to 72 hours. Wheals presenting in a linear fashion (Fig. 14.26) is known as dermographism. Wheals are characteristic of urticaria.

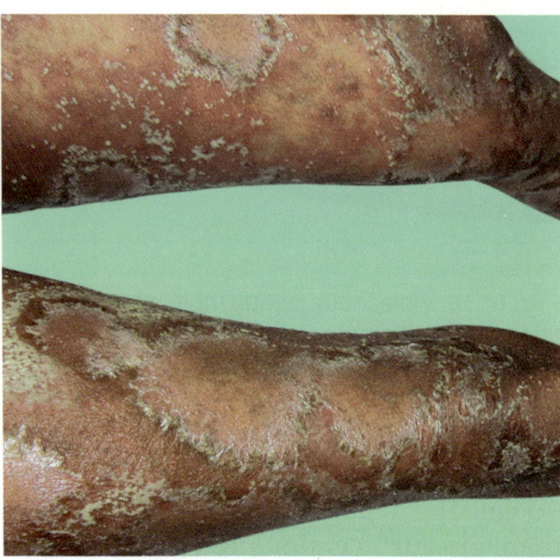

Fig. 14.24: Sterile pustules in annular fashion on the legs (pustular psoriasis).

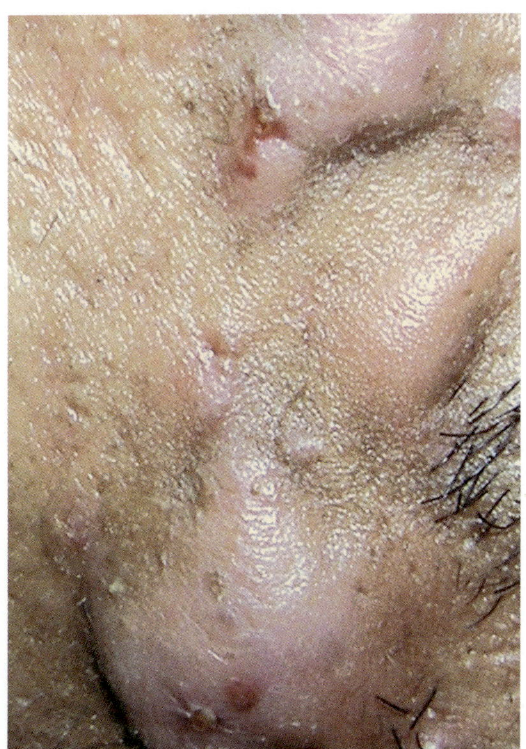

Fig. 14.25: Abscess over face. Note yellow crust.

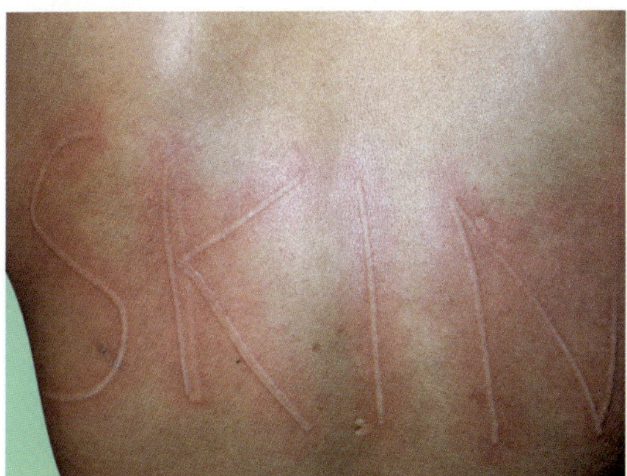

Fig. 14.26: Linear wheals (dermographism) over the trunk.

10. Petechiae and Purpura

These are maculopapular lesions formed due to extravasation of blood. The lesions do not blanch on diascopy.

- *Petechiae:* A circumscribed deposit of blood less than 0.5 cm in diameter.
- *Purpura:* A circumscribed deposit of blood greater than 0.5 cm (Fig. 14.9).

11. Telangiectasia

This is a visible dilatation of superficial blood vessels (Fig. 14.27). Cutaneous telangiectasia can be seen in lupus erythematosus, dermatomyositis, or systemic sclerosis.

12. Poikiloderma

It refers to a triad of atrophy of skin, reticulate pigmentation, and telangiectasias (Fig. 14.28); may be present in dermatomyositis, and cutaneous T cell lymphoma.

13. Cyst

Cyst is a circumscribed lesion with a wall and a lumen containing fluid or solid matter. Sebaceous cyst containing sebum is the most common example (Fig. 14.29). Dermoid cyst is another example.

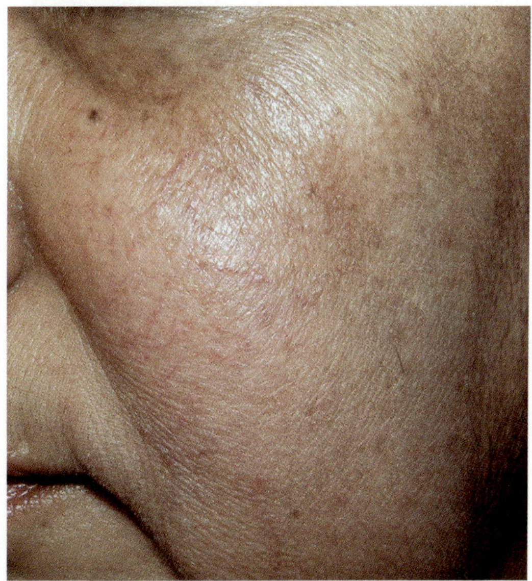

Fig. 14.27: Cutaneous telangiectasias.

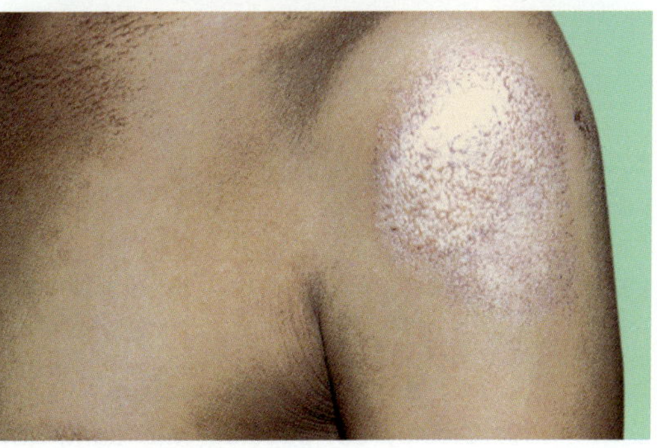

Fig. 14.28: Poikiloderma: Circumscribed, oval area of atrophy of skin with reticulate pigmentation and telangiectasias over upper arm.

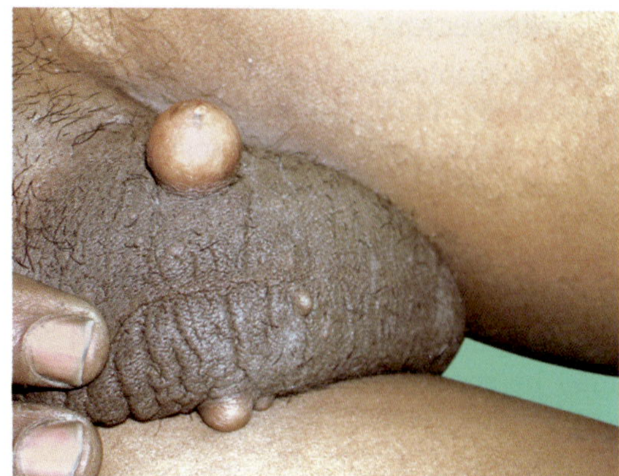

Fig. 14.29: Sebaceous cysts on scrotum.

14. Comedone

Comedone is the typical lesion found in acne vulgaris in adolescents. It is characterized by an inspissated plug of sebaceous and keratinous material lodged in a dilated pilosebaceous orifice. These may be open (black) or closed (white) (Fig. 14.30).

15. Milia

Milia is a small superficial, subepidermal keratin cyst. It is a normal finding in newborn infants or can be idiopathic (Fig. 14.31), or following deep inflammation in older children. Milia may also be seen in scars resulting from lesions crossing the dermoepidermal junction (Fig. 14.32).

16. Burrow

Burrow is a thread-like elevated, tortuous channel in the skin produced by a parasite. The open end usually has a papule. It is pathognomonic of scabies (Fig. 14.33).

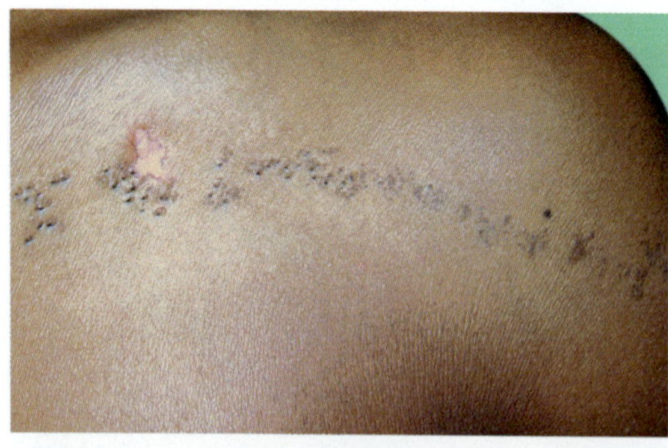

Fig. 14.30: Closely set papules with dark, firm hyperkeratotic plugs in center (comedone-like) in a case of linear nevus comedonicus. Note hypertrophic scar at biopsy site.

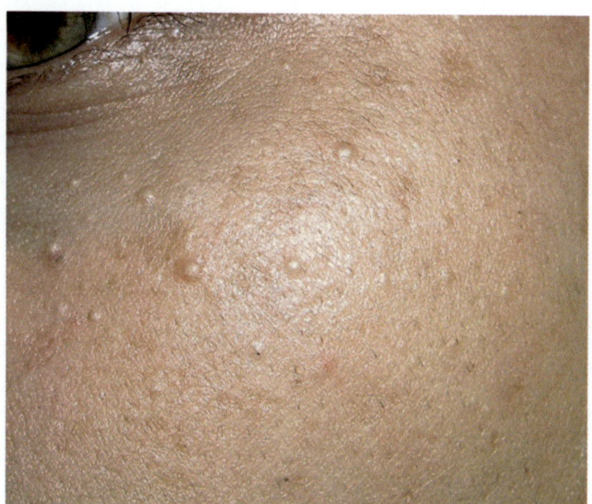

Fig. 14.31: Milia: White, globoid, firm, papules on face.

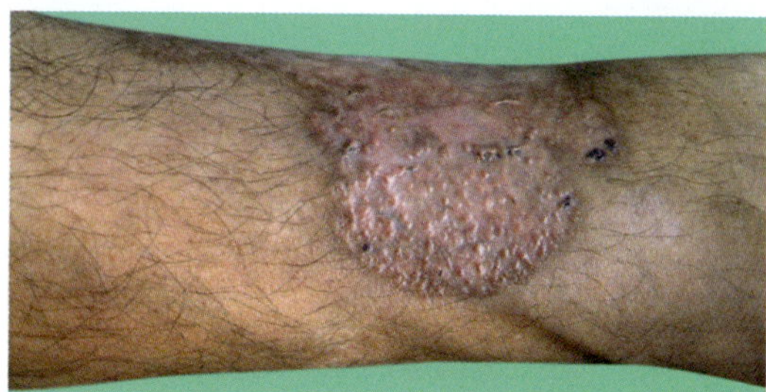

Fig. 14.32: Multiple milia in a scar following healing of pyoderma gangrenosum ulcer.

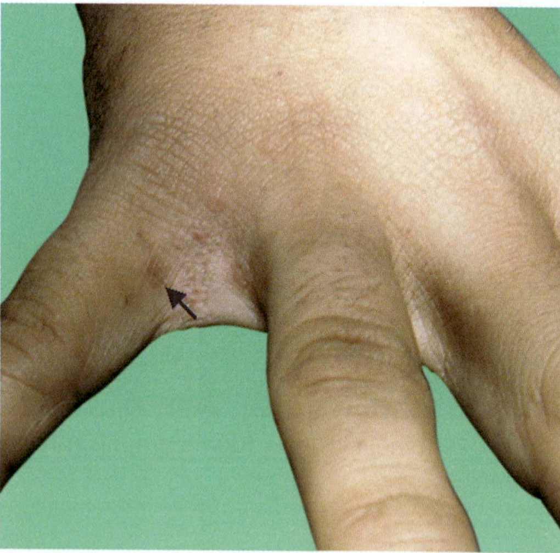

Fig. 14.33: Tortuous, irregular, burrow (arrow) in finger web with vesicle and erythematous papule in scabies.

B. Secondary Lesions

These lesions develop during evolution of disease. They may sometimes be the only type of lesions present at the time of examination.

1. Scale

A scale is a visible flake caused by shedding of the horny layer (stratum corneum) of the skin. Type of scale can often give a clue to the diagnosis:

- *Fine:* Tinea versicolor, xerosis.
- *Silvery:* Psoriasis vulgaris (Fig. 14.34).
- *Collarette:* Pityriasis rosea (Fig. 14.15).
- *Fish-like:* Ichthyosis (Fig. 14.35).
- *In sheets (desquamation):* Staphylococcal skin-scalded syndrome (Fig. 14.36), Kawasaki disease.

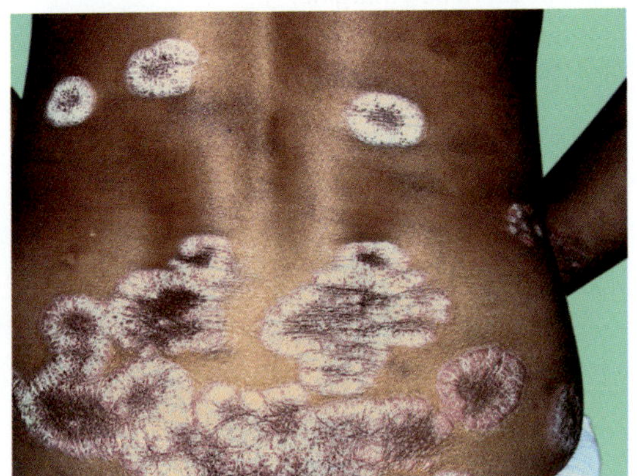

Fig. 14.34: Silvery scales: Annular lesions of psoriasis vulgaris over back

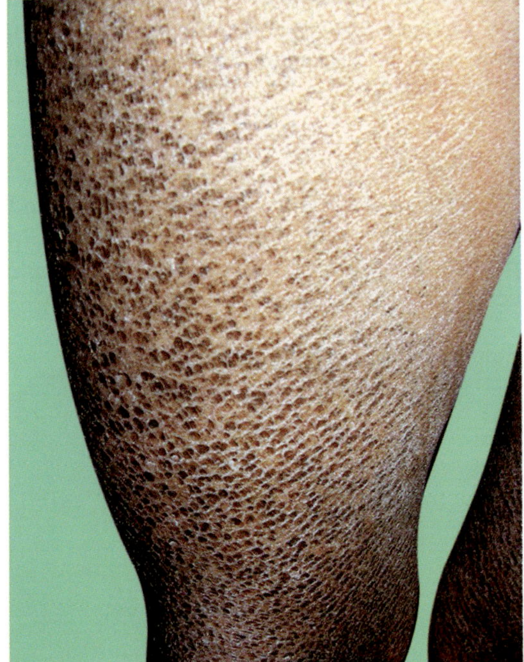

Fig. 14.35: Adherent, hyperpigmented, fish-like scaling over legs in X-linked ichthyosis.

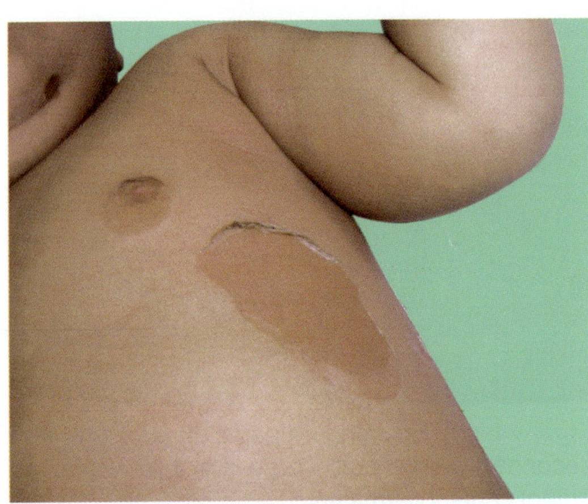

Fig. 14.36: Sheet-like desquamation in staphylococcal-scalded skin syndrome. Note diffuse erythema over upper chest and medial arm.

- *Carpet tack* (with an underlying plug) Discoid lupus erythematosus.
- *Greasy:* Seborrheic dermatitis.
- *Mica-like* Pityriasis lichenoides chronica.

2. Crust

Crust is a collection of dried serum and cellular debris. It may be yellow or brown due to the presence of dried blood. Conditions characterized by presence of crusts include acute eczema and tinea capitis. Honey-colored crusts are typical of impetigo contagiosa (Fig. 14.37).

3. Erosion

There is a focal loss of epidermis with no loss of dermis. There is no residual scarring upon healing. Erosive lesions are present in herpes

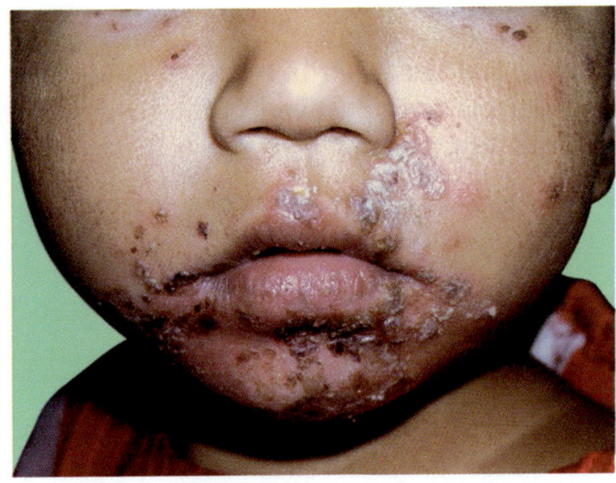

Fig. 14.37: Honey-colored and hemorrhagic crusts in impetigo contagiosa.

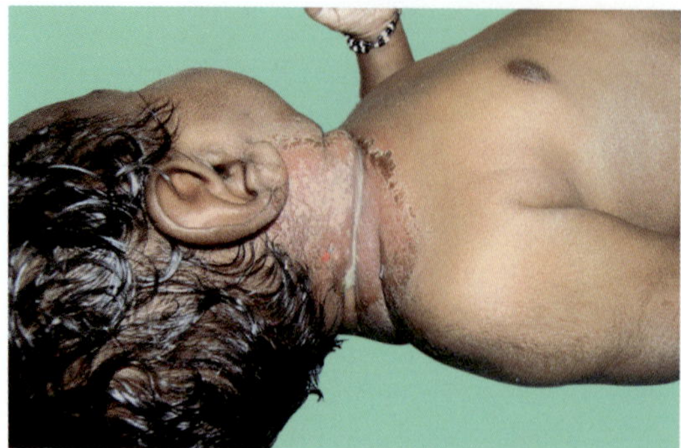

Fig. 14.38: Erosion: Superficial erosion with secondary purulent discharge in a child with acute irritant contact dermatitis.

simplex, candidiasis, tinea pedis, acute eczema (Fig. 14.38), and vesiculobullous disorders.

4. Ulcer

There is a focal loss of epidermis and also the upper dermis. *Inspect* the ulcer and describe the site, size, shape, floor, margin and the skin surrounding the ulcer. *Palpate* for presence of induration and attachment to underlying tissue.

- Undermined margin can be seen in tubercular ulcers (Fig. 14.39).
- Pyoderma gangrenosum (Fig. 14.40) is a chronic ulcer with hemorrhagic, purple, undermined or boggy border. Development of new lesions at site of trauma (*pathergy*) may be seen. You should carry out systemic evaluation for underlying diseases like inflammatory bowel disease, leukemia, rheumatoid arthritis, or cirrhosis.
- Rolled out margin is seen in basal cell carcinoma.

5. Fissures

Fissure is a linear slit-like loss of epidermis and dermis typically seen in intertrigo, and eczema (Fig. 14.41).

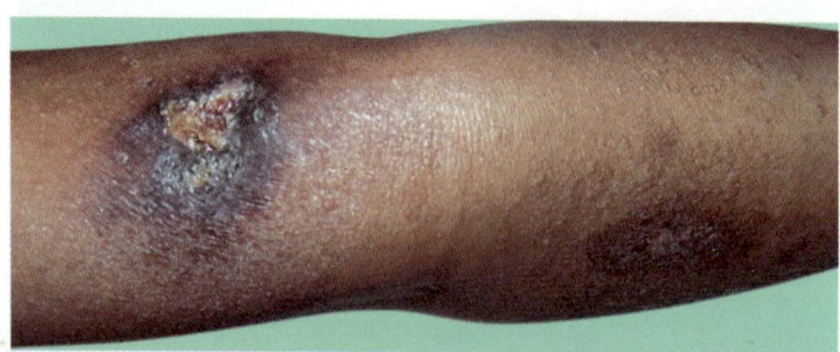

Fig. 14.39: Irregular, undermined margins in tubercular ulcer (scrofuloderma). The ulcer was attached to the underlying bone.

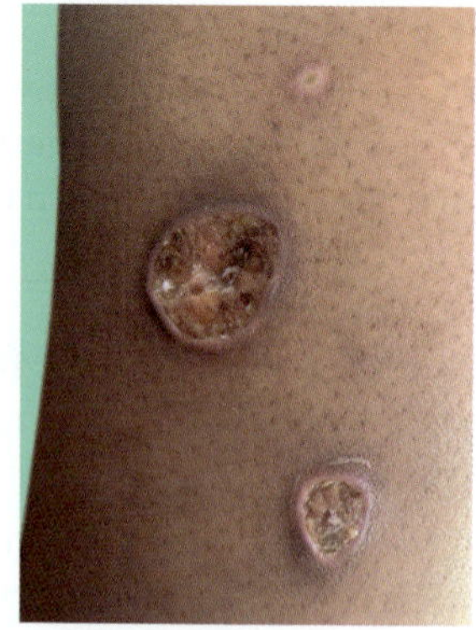

Fig. 14.40: Ulcers of pyoderma gangrenosum with violaceous, raised margins.

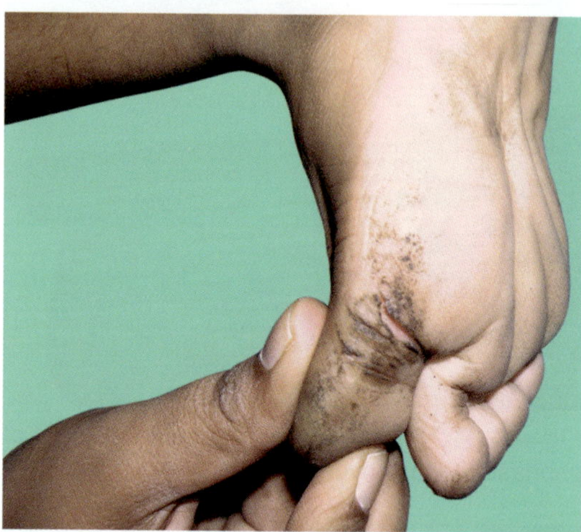

Fig. 14.41: Fissure in chronic eczema. The surrounding skin is thickened, hyperpigmented with lichenification.

6. Excoriation

Excoriation is a linear erosion or ulcer caused by scratching (Fig. 14.42). It is common in pruritic disorders including scabies and atopic eczema.

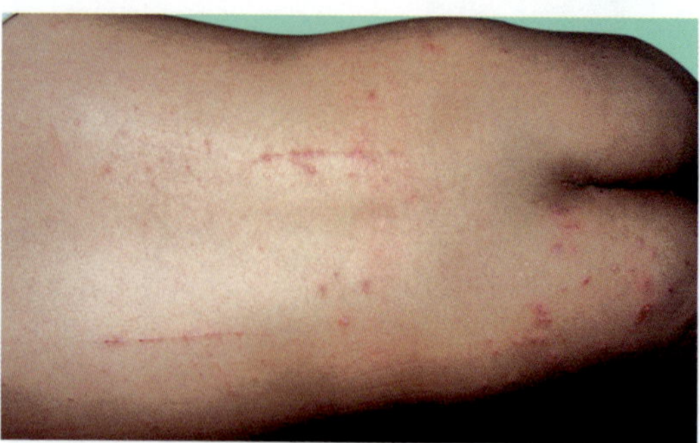

Fig. 14.42: Linear excoriations on trunk with multiple papules in a child with scabies.

7. Atrophy

There is thinning of epidermal, dermal or subcutaneous tissue (Fig. 14.43). *Epidermal atrophy* presents as shiny wrinkled skin and skin markings may be lost; for example, in leprosy. *Dermal atrophy* may present as depressed skin; as in morphea and discoid lupus erythematosus.

8. Scar

Scar is an abnormal formation of connective tissue, which replaces the normal structures in skin. The normal skin markings are lost. Scars can be *atrophic* (loss of tissue, example—acne, chickenpox) or *hypertrophic* (increased tissue—keloid, post-traumatic) (Fig. 14.44).

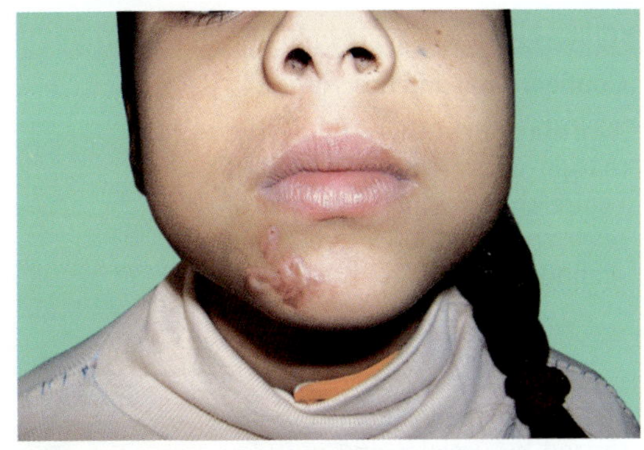

Fig. 14.44: Hypertrophic scar on chin due to self-application of caustic for verruca plana.

9. Sclerosis

Sclerosis is a circumscribed or diffuse area of induration and binding down of skin; typically seen in sclerosing disorders: for example—morphea (Fig. 14.45) and systemic sclerosis.

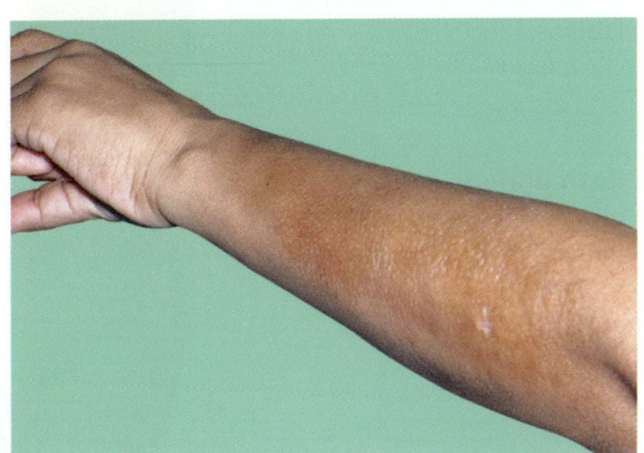

Fig. 14.45: Linear morphea showing induration and binding down of skin. Appendages are lost in lesional area.

10. Lichenification

This is an area of skin which is thickened due to repeated scratching. There is associated hyperpigmentation and increased skin markings (Fig. 14.46). It is seen in children with chronic eczema, atopic dermatitis, or as part of primary immunodeficiency syndromes, like hyper-IgE or Wiscott-Aldrich syndrome.

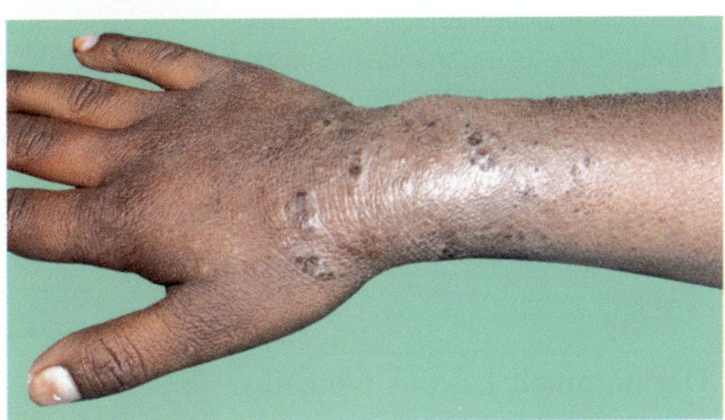

Fig. 14.46: Lichenification in atopic eczema.

C. Organization and Arrangement of Lesions

The shape and local relationship of the lesions to each other gives rise to a specific morphology. **Table 14.1** provides a detailed description of common configuration patterns in skin diseases.

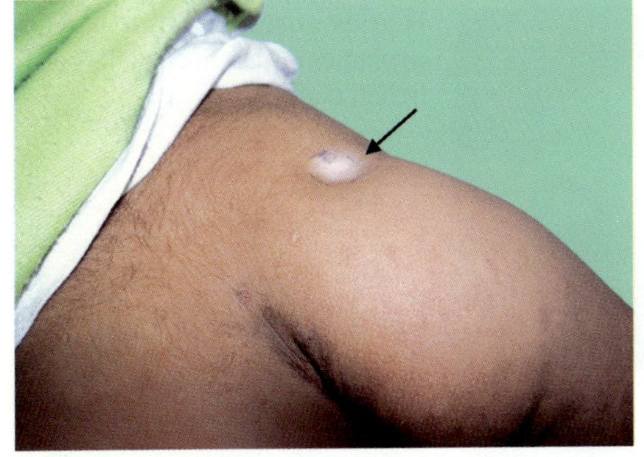

Fig. 14.43: Subcutaneous tissue atrophy secondary to corticosteroid injection.

You should also examine for the distribution and pattern of cutaneous involvement. The anatomic location or specific arrangement of skin lesions can often provide a clue to diagnosis. Some common patterns with examples of skin disease are given in **Table 14.2**.

Table 14.1: Shape and configuration pattern of skin lesions

Configuration and description		Examples
Annular: Lesion with active margin and clearing in center. Figure shows annular plaque of *tinea corporis* showing marginal scaling.	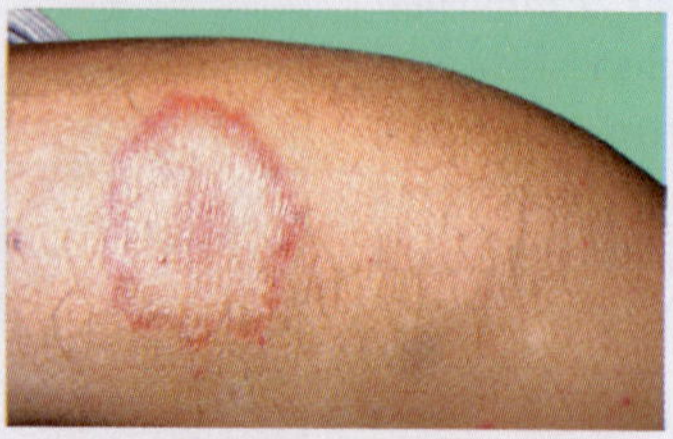	Tinea corporis, pityriasis rosea, seborrheic dermatitis, linear IgA disease of childhood, syphilis granuloma annulare, lichen planus, psoriasis, sarcoidosis, subacute lupus erythematosus
Herpetiform: Lesions characterized by vesicles and pustules in a grouped arrangement. Figure shows grouped pustules with honey-colored crusts in herpes labialis.	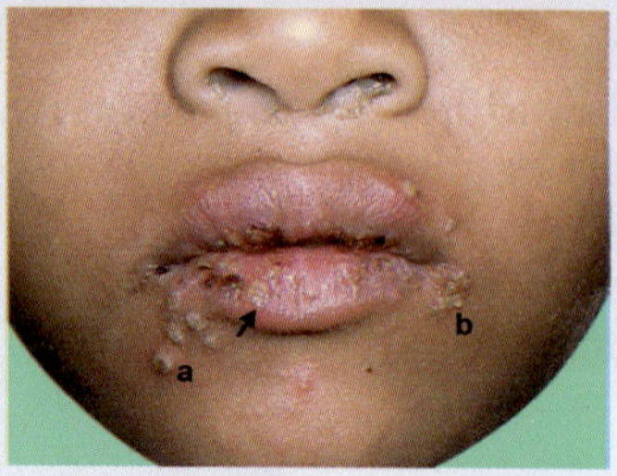	Herpes simplex, herpes zoster, dermatitis herpetiformis, lymphangioma circumscriptum
Reticulated: Net-like appearance. Figure shows reticulate pattern of cutis marmorata	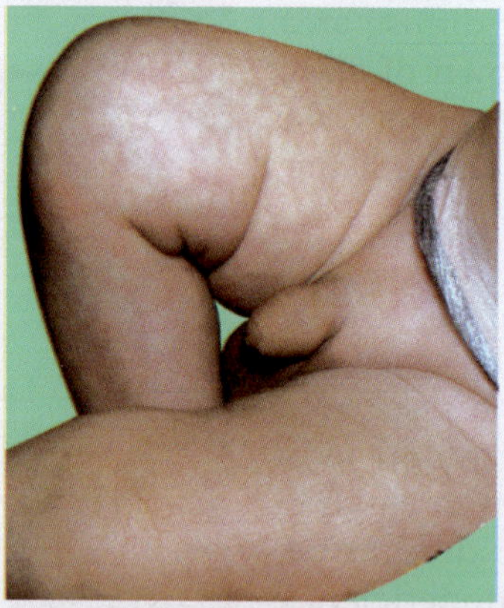	Cutis marmorata, livedo reticularis, erythema ab igne, reticulated and confluent papillomatosis, cutis marmorata telangiectatica congenita
Linear: Occurring in a line. Figure shows closely set papules in a line (linear nevus comedonicus).	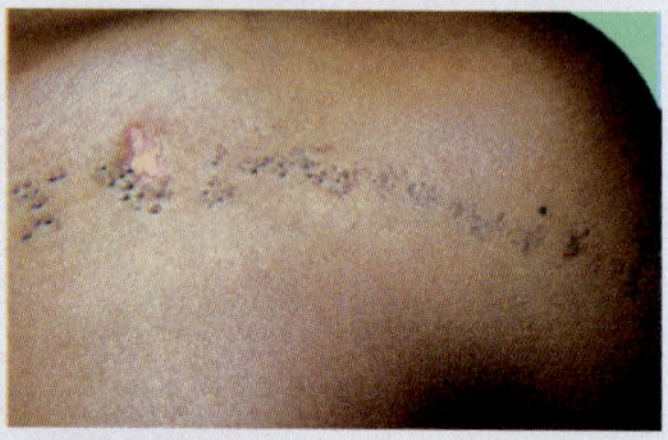	Lichen planus, lichen striatus, epidermal nevi, ichthyosis, warts, morphea, deep mycosis (sporotrichosis), contact dermatitis (plants), factitial
Dermatomal: Lesions typically follow a nerve or body segment. Figure shows depigmented macule of vitiligo in a dermatomal pattern	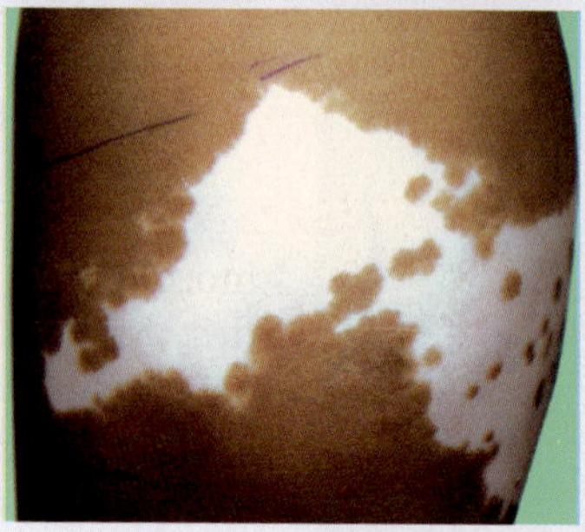	Herpes zoster, vitiligo, nevus depigmentosus, café au lait spots, lichen planus

(*Contd...*)

Configuration and description		Examples
Table 14.1: Shape and configuration pattern of skin lesions *(Contd...)*		
Guttate: Drop-like lesions. Figure shows erythematous papules and coalescent plaque with silvery scaling over extensors of forearms (guttate psoriasis) in a 7-year-old boy.	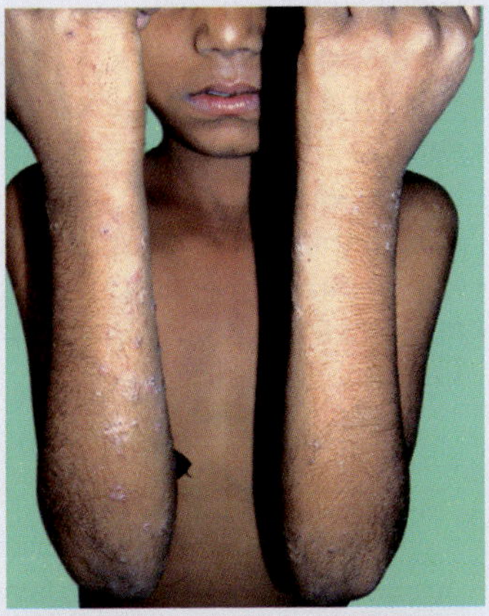	Psoriasis
Targetoid: Lesions with dark dusky center and erythematous halo. Figure shows targetoid lesions of erythema multiforme.	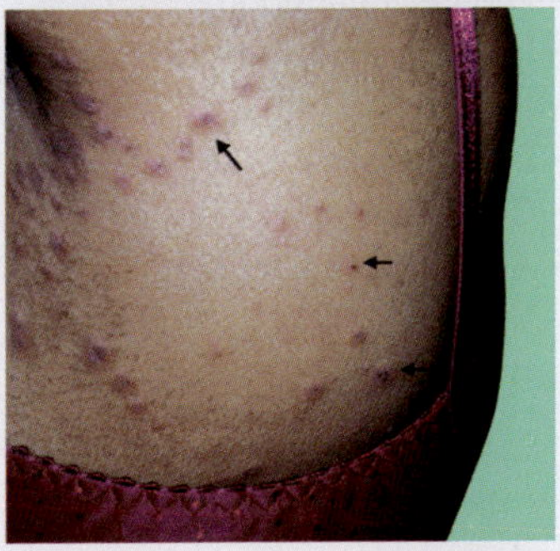	Erythema multiforme, Stevens-Johnson syndrome, lupus erythematosus, Rowell syndrome
Arciform: Semicircular lesions, arranged in an arc. Figure shows pityriasis rosea with semicircular margins of plaque.	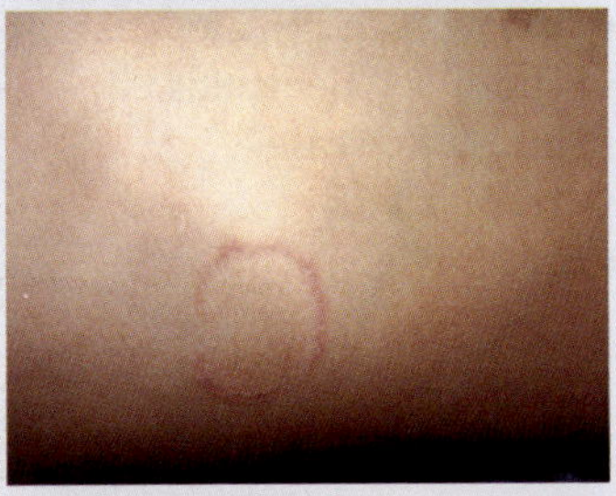	Urticaria, pityriasis rosea, erythema multiforme, granuloma annulare
Bizarre: Not following a pattern and conforming to possible articles of abuse. Lesions in the figure correspond to cigarette burns in a patient of child abuse.	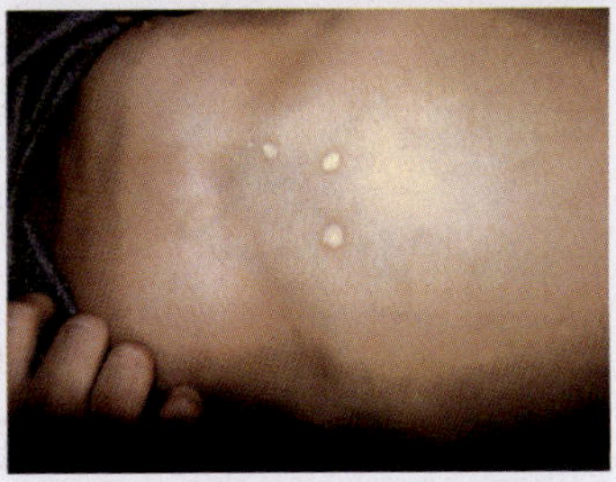	Factitial dermatoses, child abuse
Gyrate: Twisted, spiral lesion **Discoid:** Coin-shaped **Umbilicated**		Urticaria, erythema annulare centrifugum, erythema gyratum repens Nummular/discoid eczema Molluscum contagiosum

Table 14.2: Distribution and pattern of cutaneous involvement

Distribution	Disorders	Example
A. Photoexposed sites	• Lupus erythematosus • Dermatomyositis • Porphyria • Pellagra • Hydroa vacciniforme • Polymorphous light eruption • Xeroderma pigmentosa • Phototoxic reactions (drugs, sunburn, contact)	An adult case of pellagra with eczematous involvement of photo-exposed sites. Note involvement of neck in a V-shaped pattern.
B. Flexural rash	• Atopic dermatitis (adolescents and late childhood) • Infantile seborrheic dermatitis • Inverse psoriasis • Intertrigo • Candidiasis • Air-borne contact dermatitis	A case of flexural psoriasis. Scaling is usually absent and Auspitz sign may be negative.
C. Acrodermatitis (peripheral)	• Acrodermatitis enteropathica • Papular acrodermatitis • Kawasaki disease • Id reaction • Acral vitiligo	Chronic erythematous (eczematous) lesions over legs and anogenital areas in an infant with acrodermatitis enteropathica. The margins were irregular and necrotic.
D. Extensor rash 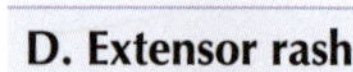 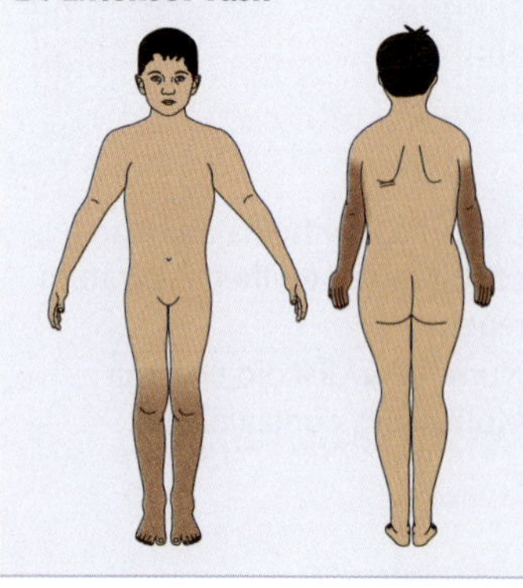	• Psoriasis • Atopic dermatitis (infantile and early childhood) • Dermatitis herpetiformis • Photo-aggravated skin diseases	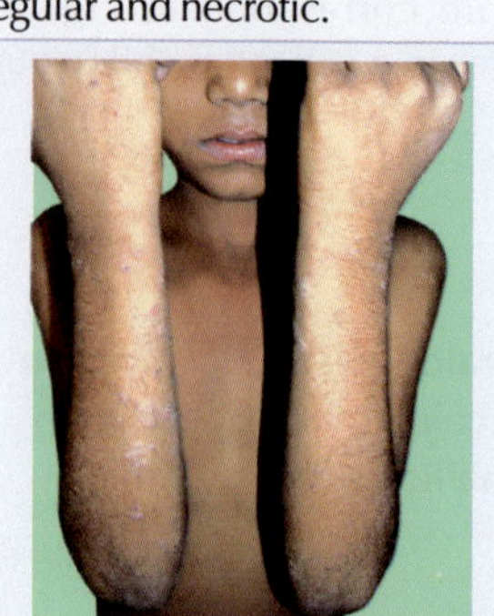 Involvement of extensors of arm in guttate psoriasis.

(Contd...)

Table 14.2: Distribution and pattern of cutaneous involvement (*Contd...*)

Distribution	Disorders	Example
E. Lines of Blaschko	• Verrucous epidermal nevus • Nevus sebaceous • Lichen striatus • Incontinentia pigmenti • Focal dermal hypoplasia • CHILD syndrome	Verrucous lesions following lines of Blaschko in verrucous epidermal nevus.
F. Acneiform rash	• Acne vulgaris • Cushing syndrome • Drug-induced acne (cortico-steroid, isoniazid) • Rosacea • Cosmetic acne • Chloracne • Pityrosporum folliculitis	Acneiform eruption over chest in an adolescent
G. Erythroderma 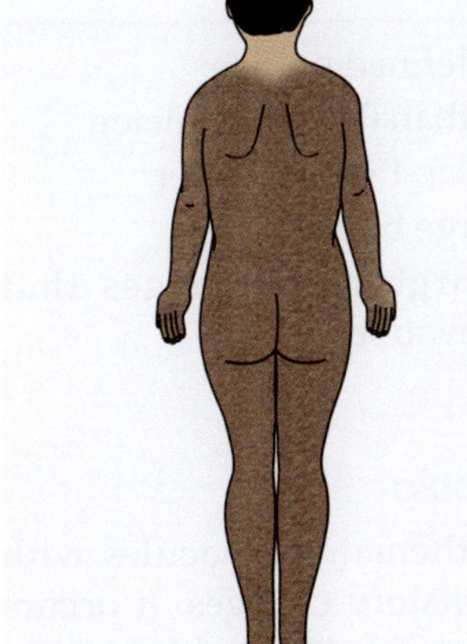	Ichthyosiform erythroderma • Atopic dermatitis • Infantile seborrheic dermatitis • Psoriasis • Drug Induced	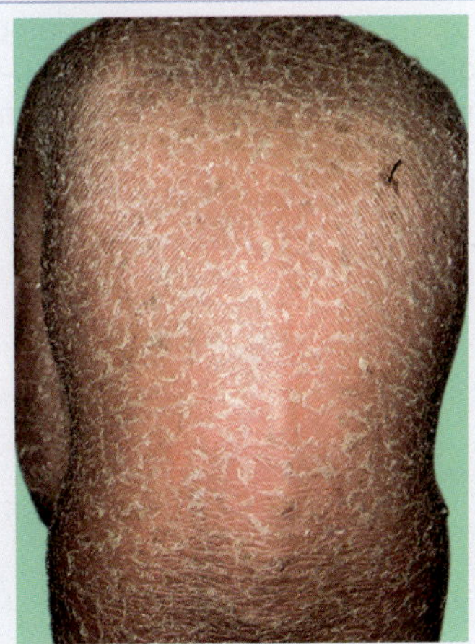 Psoriatic erythroderma in a 14 years old boy

The involvement of palms and soles may be the only cutaneous sign present as in inherited keratodermas (Fig. 14.47), psoriasis, or eczema (contact). Infections like warts; hand, foot and mouth disease (caused by coxsackievirus, Fig. 14.48), and herpetic whitlow may affect the palms and soles.

Lesions of palms and soles may help you in corroborating your diagnosis in certain systemic diseases including secondary syphilis (Fig. 14.49), pustular psoriasis, erythema multiforme, vasculitis, or liver diseases (presence of palmar erythema).

Desquamation of palms and soles is evident in Kawasaki disease and in post-streptococcal infection.

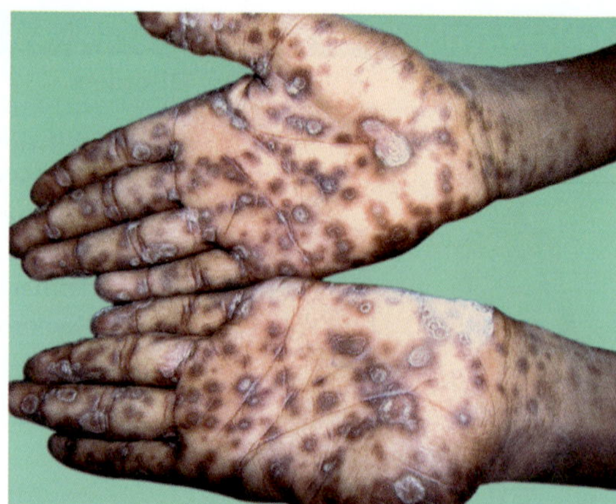

Fig. 14.49: Dusky, macular, scaly rash over palms in patient with secondary syphilis. Central pressure with a small blunt object will elicit tenderness (Buschke-Olendörf sign).

Mucous Membrane

Mucous membrane disorders may be categorized as having erosions and ulcerations as you will find in Behçet disease, herpes labialis, pemphigus, or immunodeficiency syn-dromes. White lesions can be seen in leukoplakia, oral candidiasis or lichen planus (Fig. 14.50; with violaceous papules and plaques).

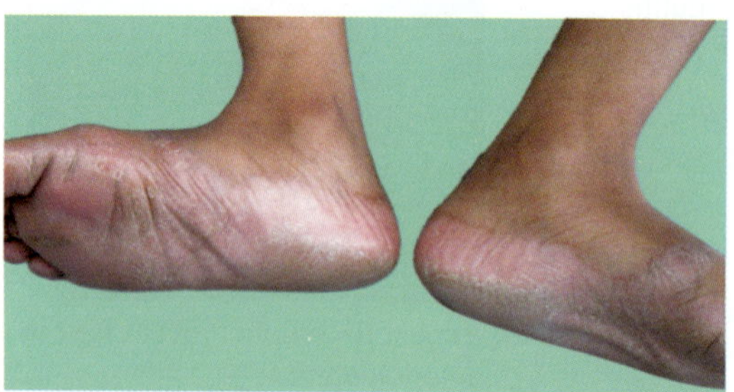

Fig. 14.47: Diffuse erythematous thickening of soles and dorsum of feet in a 10-year-old girl with inherited palmoplantar keratoderma.

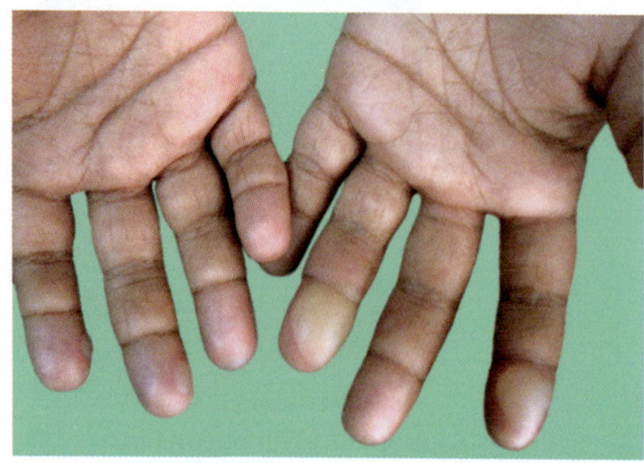

Fig. 14.48: Bullae of hand, foot and mouth disease in a 6-year-old boy.

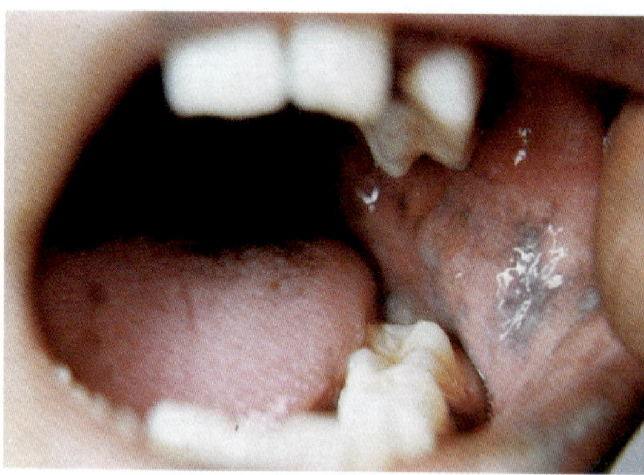

Fig. 14.50: Violaceous papules and plaque with white striae in oral lichen planus.

14.4 SKIN HEMORRHAGES AND VASCULAR LESIONS

Hemorrhages are defined by size:

- *Petechiae:* Less than 0.5 cm diameter.
- *Purpura:* From 0.5–1 cm diameter.
- *Ecchymoses:* Large bruises.
- *Hematoma:* Large hemorrhages that produce skin elevations.

1. Purpura

Non-palpable Purpura

It presents as erythematous macules with absence of inflammatory changes. It occurs due to (a) conditions associated with increase in capillary fragility, or (b) clotting defects.

Palpable Purpura

It is caused by disorders with inflammatory involvements of the vessels which may be immune mediated. Thus, these children will require relevant systemic examination. Important causes of both are listed in **Table 14.3**.

Henoch-Schönlein Purpura

It is the most common form of leukocytoclastic vasculitis in children with a peak incidence between 4 to 8 years of age. You will find lesions of palpable purpura **(Fig. 14.51)**, 5–10 mm in diameter; over the buttocks and extensors of arms and legs. It occurs in crops 2–4 weekly and lesions fade over 3–5 days. Less commonly you will find hemorrhagic bullae, ecchymoses, scalp edema, and periarticular edema. Look for systemic involvement in the form of abdominal colic with melena, or renal and central nervous system involvement.

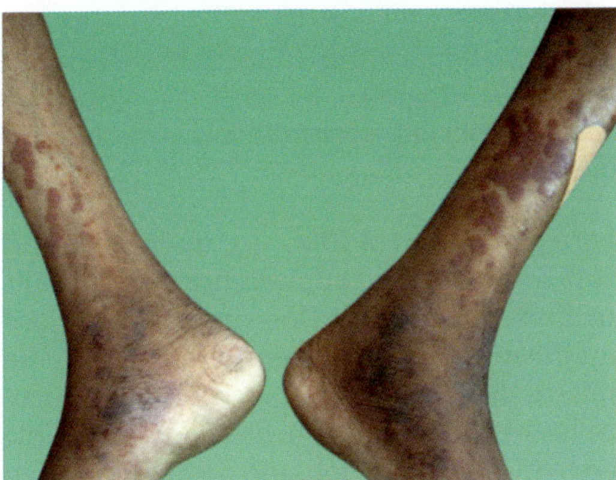

Fig. 14.51: Palpable purpura with necrotic lesions over lower legs in a boy with Henoch-Schönlein purpura who also had gastrointestinal bleed and proteinuria.

Table 14.3: Causes of purpura
Non-palpable purpura
• Measles, rubella, influenza, HIV infection
• Idiopathic thrombocytopenic purpura
• Acute leukemia
• Drugs—quinine, heparin, thiazides, NSAIDs
• Traumatic
• Endocarditis
Palpable purpura
• Meningococcemia
• Henoch-Schönlein purpura
• Lupus erythematosus
• Hepatitis B, and hepatitis C infection
• Leukocytoclastic vasculitis
• Endocarditis
• Drugs—quinine, antibiotics, phenytoin

2. Vascular Nevi

Vascular nevi can be categorized as (a) vascular malformations, and (b) hemangiomas. You must be able to distinguish between them as their treatment and prognosis is very different. Initially, examine whether the lesion is a macule which points to a vascular malformation.

Vascular Malformations

Salmon patch is commonly a pink macule present on the face, neck, and scalp in infants and it darkens during crying episodes. Systemic component is absent and regression occurs by 2 years of age.

Port-wine stain **(Fig. 14.52)** is congenital and presents as red macular (or plaque), non-blanchable lesion. In older children, nodulation and soft tissue hypertrophy may develop. Screening should be carried out for the many associated syndromes. Elicit history of seizures, hemiplegia, and measure intraocular tension, if there is involvement of first division of trigeminal nerve (Sturge-Weber syndrome). Limb hypertrophy with increased limb girth and length may be present in Klippel-Trenaunay-Weber syndrome.

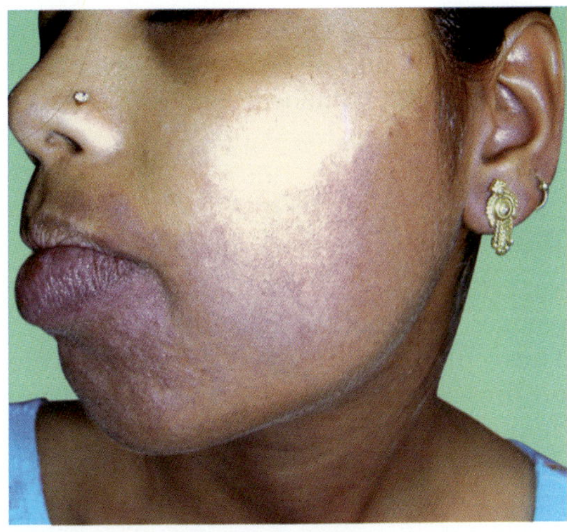

Fig. 14.52: Port-wine stain. Dusky, erythematous macule over face, involving left ear, lips and neck. The lesion was non-blanchable.

Key Box 3

How to Describe a Vascular Lesion

1. Macule/plaque/nodule
2. Overlying telangiectasias, varicosity, ecchymosis, purpura, ulceration, secondary infection
3. Blanchable on diascopy
4. Compressible
5. Temperature raised
6. Thrill, bruit
7. Limb length and girth
8. Systemic evaluation

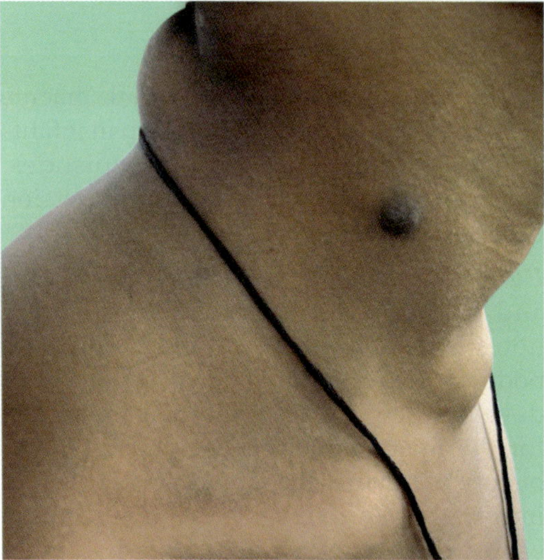

Fig. 14.53: An adolescent with bluish tumors and nodules of blue rubber bleb syndrome over neck. He also had gastrointestinal venous malformations.

In some patients, associated deep venous malformation may be present giving a bluish hue (Fig. 14.53). Prominent venous varicosities may be visible.

Infantile Hemangiomas

These may be superficial, deep or mixed.

Superficial hemangiomas are bright red plaques with lobulated surface (Fig. 14.54). These plaques are partially blanchable on diascopy but non-compressible. They demonstrate proliferation in infancy that distinguishes them from port-wine stain which proliferates in the older child.

Deep hemangiomas are nodular, partially compressible with increased local temperature, overlying telangiectasias, or venous varicosities. Involution occurs in 30% and 90% by 3 years and adolescence, respectively. In presence of high flow in arterial or AV malformations, local temperature may be raised, thrill may be palpated, and bruit may be heard on auscultation. Presence of multiple ecchymosis, induration, and deranged clotting profile may be seen in Kasabach-Merritt phenomenon. Hemangiomas occurring around eye may cause obstruction amblyopia in early infancy. Obstruction of urethral, anal opening, or airway should also be looked for and urgently treated.

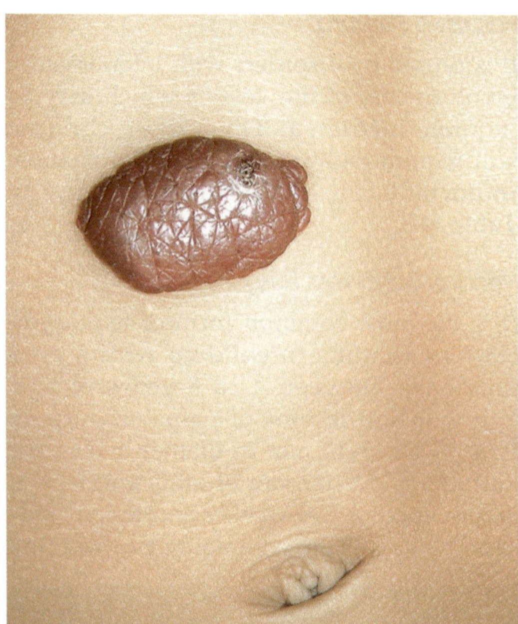

Fig. 14.54: Capillary hemangioma (strawberry nevus). Bright red, lobulated tumor is present over trunk.

14.5 HAIR AND NAILS

Hair and nails are of ectodermal origin and composed of keratin. Diseases of hair and nail may be associated with cutaneous and systemic disease. This emphasizes the importance of their thorough examination.

A. Hair

1. Amount of Hair

Hypertrichosis: Growth of excessive hair, at any site which is coarser and more profuse than normal for age, sex, or race of the individual, is designated as hypertrichosis. *Hirsutism* (Fig. 14.55) refers to growth of coarse

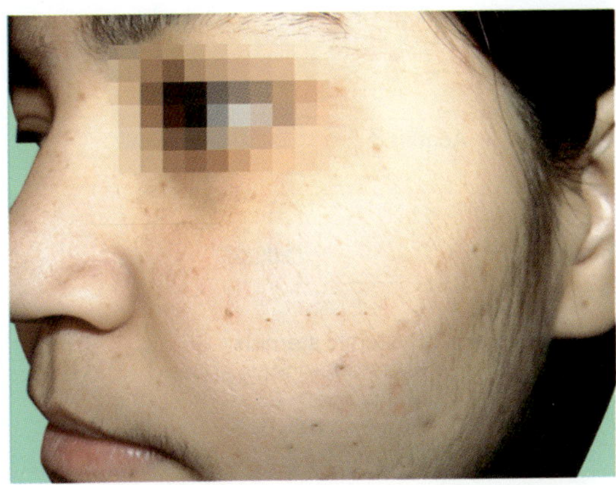

Fig. 14.55: Hirsutism over the face in a 15-year-old girl. Note black comedones, freckles over nose and post-inflammatory hyperpigmented macules on cheeks.

terminal hair in the adult male sexual pattern in females.

Alopecia: This refers to hair loss, which can be localized or diffuse. Alopecia areata is a common, autoimmune disorder, characterized by round or oval patches of circumscribed or diffuse hair loss **(Figs 14.56 and 14.57)**. It may be seen in infants and young children and generally occurs in 50% patients by 16 years of age. Association with other autoimmune disorders, especially thyroiditis, trisomy 21, and atopy is described.

Trichotillomania is usually seen in children above 5 years and most commonly involves the scalp and presents as a compulsive pulling

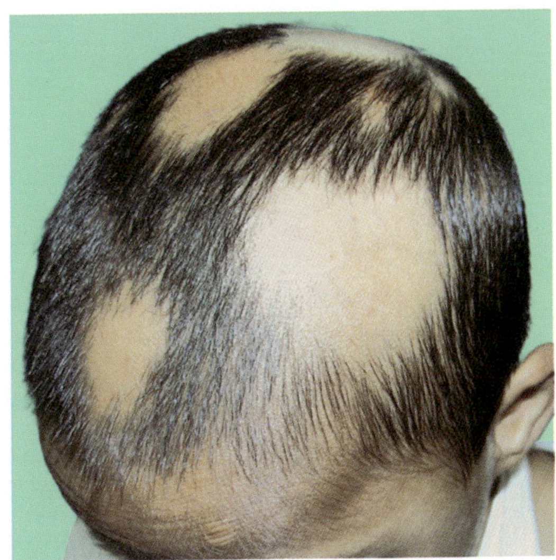

Fig. 14.56: Circumscribed areas of localized non-scarring alopecia (alopecia areata).

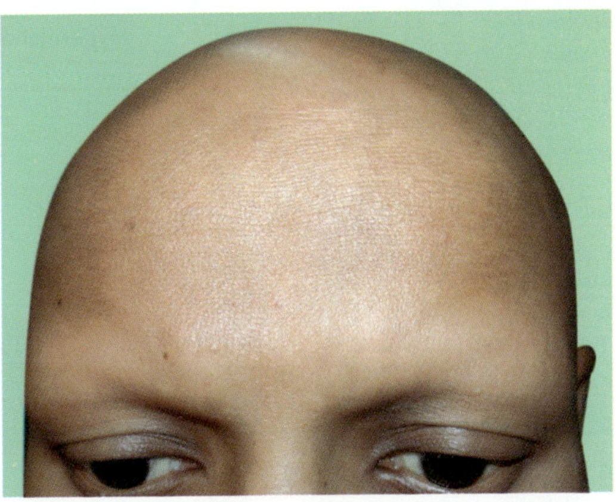

Fig. 14.57: Acquired, diffuse alopecia involving scalp, eyebrows in alopecia areata universalis. There was associated loss of body hair.

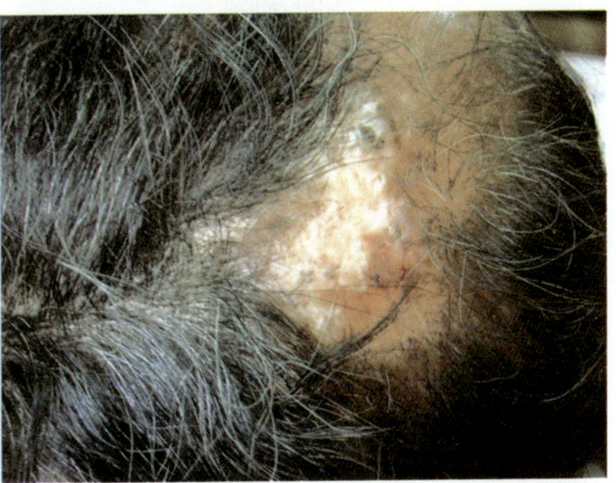

Fig. 14.58: Cicatricial alopecia. Note absence of follicular openings and crusting. Hair will not regrow in involved area.

of hair resulting in irregular areas of partial hair loss (mostly accessible sites). In scarring alopecia, the follicular openings are not visible **(Fig. 14.58)**.

Figure 14.59 provides you a brief scheme for diagnosis of hypertrichosis and alopecia.

2. Color of the Hair

Next evaluate the color of the hair. Premature graying of hair **(Fig. 14.60)**, especially of scalp hair, at an age earlier than physiologically accepted (20 years) can be seen in vitiligo and alopecia areata. It is also described in pernicious anemia, hyperthyroidism, ataxia telangiectasia, tuberous sclerosis, progeria, and with intake of a drug, like chloroquine. Differential diagnosis includes scalp involvement in vitiligo **(Fig. 14.61)**, and alopecia areata.

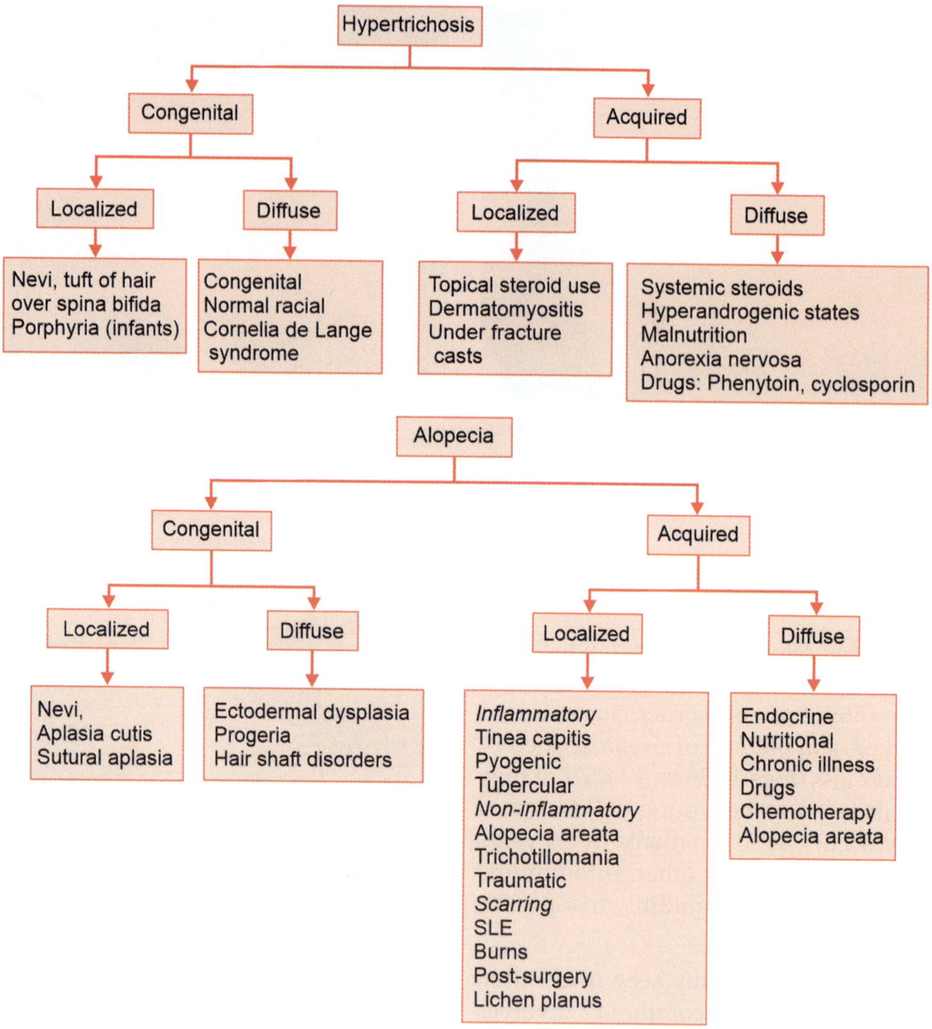

- Hypertrichosis
  - Congenital
    - Localized
      - Nevi, tuft of hair over spina bifida
      - Porphyria (infants)
    - Diffuse
      - Congenital
      - Normal racial
      - Cornelia de Lange syndrome
  - Acquired
    - Localized
      - Topical steroid use
      - Dermatomyositis
      - Under fracture casts
    - Diffuse
      - Systemic steroids
      - Hyperandrogenic states
      - Malnutrition
      - Anorexia nervosa
      - Drugs: Phenytoin, cyclosporin

- Alopecia
  - Congenital
    - Localized
      - Nevi,
      - Aplasia cutis
      - Sutural aplasia
    - Diffuse
      - Ectodermal dysplasia
      - Progeria
      - Hair shaft disorders
  - Acquired
    - Localized
      - *Inflammatory*
        - Tinea capitis
        - Pyogenic
        - Tubercular
      - *Non-inflammatory*
        - Alopecia areata
        - Trichotillomania
        - Traumatic
      - *Scarring*
        - SLE
        - Burns
        - Post-surgery
        - Lichen planus
    - Diffuse
      - Endocrine
      - Nutritional
      - Chronic illness
      - Drugs
      - Chemotherapy
      - Alopecia areata

Fig. 14.59: Causes of hypertrichosis and alopecia.

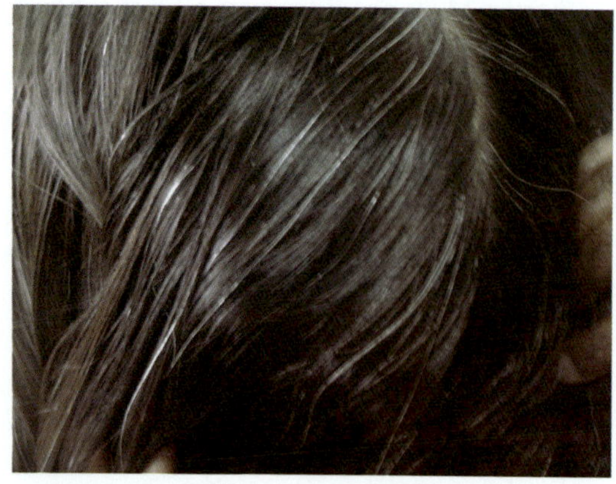

Fig. 14.60: Premature graying of hair in a 10-year-old girl.

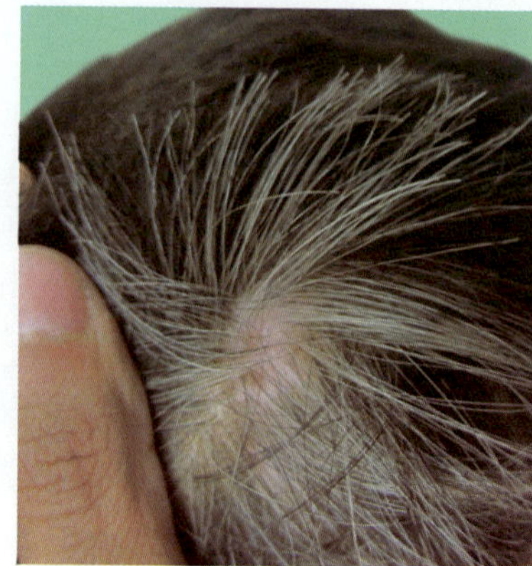

Fig. 14.61: Scalp vitiligo with associated graying of hair.

B. Nail

Examine the nail plate, nail folds and cuticle.

1. Nail Plate

- ***Nail pitting*** is a common problem and presents as small to large punctate depressions. Shallow, random, irregular, large pits are seen in psoriasis (Fig. 14.62) and atopic dermatitis. Regularly spaced, fine pits in rows are seen in alopecia areata.
- ***Beau's line*** is a transverse groove or furrow that develops as a reaction to stress that temporarily interrupts nail growth. They may occur due to trauma in infants (due to birth trauma) or due to chronic dermatoses in older children, acrodermatitis enteropathica and associated with periungual dermatitis (Fig. 14.63).
- ***Koilonychia*** is a thin, depressed, concave nail. It can be seen in infants (resolves with age), iron deficiency anemia, and lichen planus.

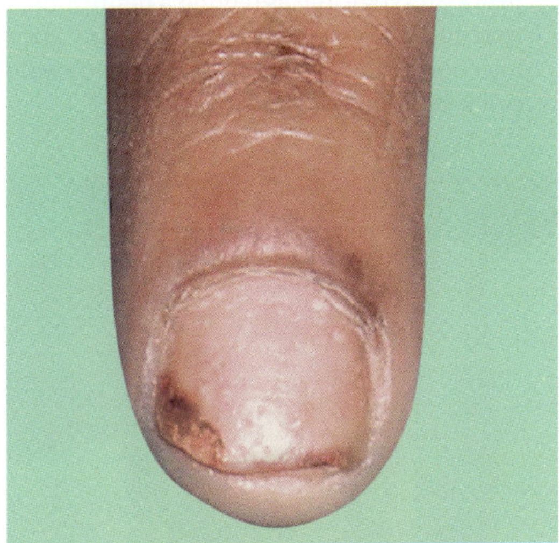

Fig. 14.62: Irregular, coarse pitting in nail psoriasis.

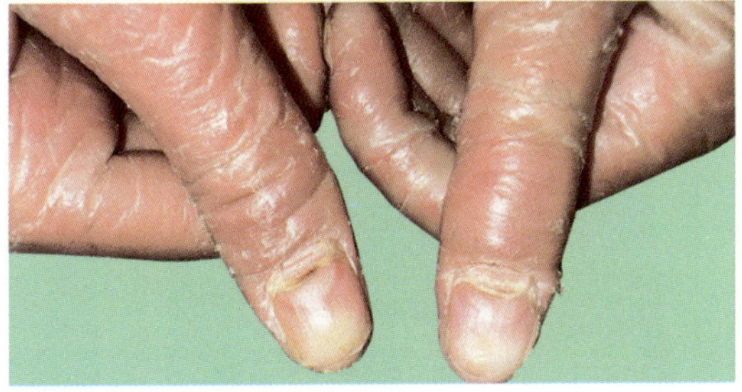

Fig. 14.63: Beau's line in a patient with psoriatic erythroderma

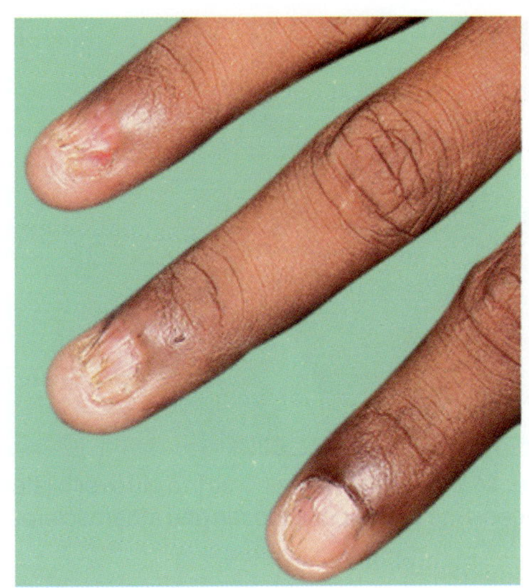

Fig. 14.64: Pterygium formation in lichen planus.

- ***Platyonychia*** or flattened nails are seen in cirrhosis.
- ***Clubbing*** of nails is seen in a variety of conditions: Pulmonary, cardiac, gastrointestinal, and others (familial, traumatic sarcoidosis, pachydermoperiostosis).
- ***Pterygium*** (Fig. 14.64) is an adhesion of the proximal nail fold to the proximal nail bed following inflammation that destroys the nail matrix. Scar formation occurs, leading to partial loss of the nail plate.

2. Nail Fold and Cuticle

Paronychia: It is the inflammation of the nail folds (skin surrounding nails) resulting from infection. The cuticle may be lost, and you may see nail dystrophy in chronic cases. The infection may be pyogenic (usually acute) or candidal. Ask parents for history of thumb or finger sucking by toddlers.

Cuticle is disrupted in children with lupus erythematosus and dermatomyositis (with nail bed hemorrhages), and those with history of chronic nail biting.

Nail color: The nail color can give you clues to underlying disease.

- *White nails* (leukonychia) may be punctate or present as white-paired bands in patients with cirrhosis, septicemia, renal failure, or hypoalbuminemia. In half and half nail, you will see that the proximal nail bed is white and distal is red or brown (seen in renal failure).

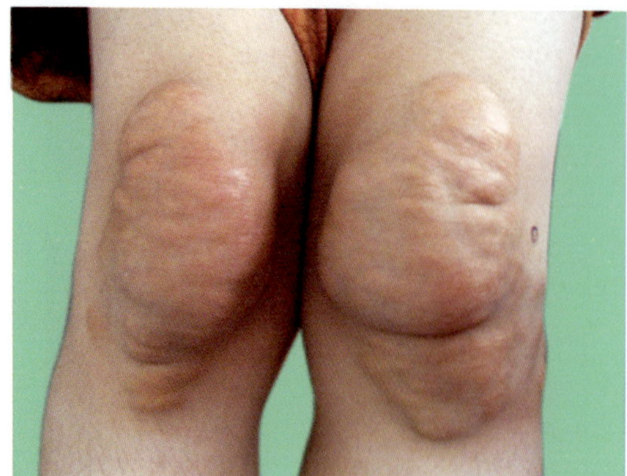

Fig. 14.65: Tuberous xanthoma in a girl over bilateral knees. She had hyperlipidemia and atherosclerosis.

- *Yellow nail* may be observed in hyperbilirubinemia, onychomycosis, chronic use of topical agents or drugs, like tetracyclines.
- *Brown or black pigment in the nail* can be seen in Addison disease, Peutz-Jeghers syndrome, and intake of antimalarials, lithium, or bleomycin.
- *Blue pigmented lunula* is visible in Wilson disease (hepatolenticular degeneration), argyria, and with intake of drugs, like phenothiazines.
- *Red lunula* can be appreciated in dermatomyositis, congestive heart failure, carbon monoxide poisoning, and bacterial endocarditis.

Therefore, as is evident, careful appreciation of the signs and symptoms of the diseases affecting skin will not only help in their correct diagnosis but also may help in diagnosis of underlying systemic disease (Fig. 14.65).

14.6 IMPORTANT CLINICAL SIGNS AND DIAGNOSTIC METHODS

Clinical Signs

1. ***Dermographism:*** The urticarial wheal response that appears after the skin is stroked (*see* Fig. 14.26). White dermatographism causes the development of a white line on stroking in patients of atopic dermatitis.
2. ***Koebner or isomorphic phenomenon:*** Characteristic lesions of the dermatoses appears at the site of trauma. It could be classified as true isomorphic phenomenon as is evident in inflammatory dermatoses like psoriasis and lichen planus (*see* Fig. 14.8) and pseudoisomorphic phenomenon is seen in infective conditions like warts or molluscum contagiosum and is due to trauma-induced autoinoculation.
3. ***Nikolsky sign:*** Gentle lateral pressure applied on the border of an intact blister results in the separation of the normal epidermis and extension of the blister. It is characteristically demonstrable in pemphigus vulgaris.
4. ***Bulla spread sign (Asboe Hansen sign):*** Vertical pressure on the roof of an intact bulla results in its enlargement and extension beyond the marked margin.
5. ***Darier sign:*** This is characterised by the appearance of an urticated wheal and flare reaction after rubbing a skin lesion that has mast cell activation, for example urticaria pigmentosa (*see* Fig. 14.16).
6. ***Pathergy:*** The appearance of a papule or a pustule (Fig 14.66), that is confirmed histopathologically as having a neutrophilic reaction or vasculitis, 24–48 hours after injection of saline on forearm or after needle prick or biopsy.

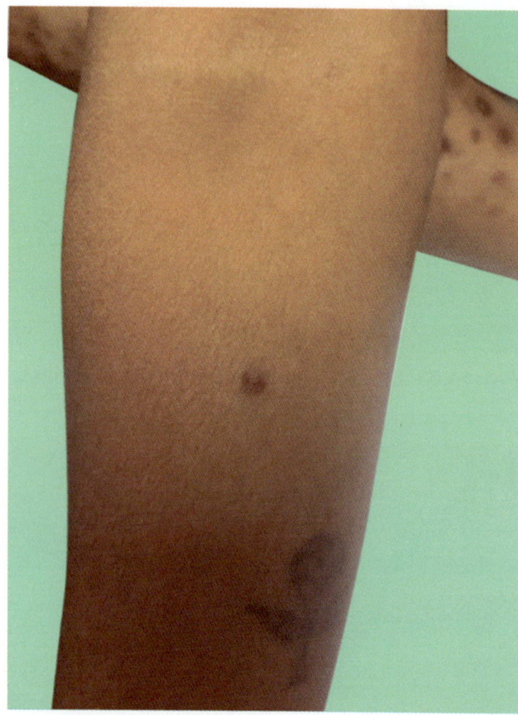

Fig. 14.66: Development of a papule (Pathergy) in a girl with Behcet's disease

Diagnostic Methods

1. *Magnifying lens* is the most important aid used for appreciating subtle changes of cutaneous lesions.
2. *Dermoscopy:* Dermatoscope, also known as epiluminescence microscope, is a device that enables 10x–200x magnification and has an in-built light source and crossed-polarizers. Dermoscopy allows for improved visualization of skin conditions and is a non-invasive, rapid diagnostic tool for dermatoses that obviates the need for a diagnostic skin biopsy. Therefore, including it in the examination of cutaneous, mucosal, hair and nail lesions is especially relevant in the pediatric age group. It is an important tool for the evaluation of melanocytic lesions, skin growths, infective conditions, vascular lesions and papulosquamous lesions in children.
3. *Diascopy:* It is used to differentiate the etiology of an erythematous lesion. A microscope slide is pressed against a lesion (diascopy) to see whether it blanches. Inflammatory, urticarial, or vascular lesions blanch, whereas petechiae or purpuras do not blanch. Diascopy can also help in evaluation of granulomatous conditions, for example in lupus vulgaris, apple jelly nodules become evident.
4. Smear examination can be performed to aid in the diagnosis. A potassium hydroxide smear could help in the diagnosis of dermatophytic or yeast infection. Other common stains include; Gram stain, Ziehl-Neelsen, and Tzanck staining.
5. Patch testing, histopathology, immunohistochemistry, and advanced molecular and imaging diagnostic methods are increasingly being employed for diagnosis of dermatological diseases.

Chapter 15

Examination of the Musculoskeletal System

❍ Anil Agarwal ❍ Prateek Rastogi

Structure

15.1 INTRODUCTION

The first step in the musculoskeletal examination of children is to develop a rapport with the child. Whether some playful activity or with the use of a toy, child should feel comfortable in the health care environment. Observing the child while playing or making him do some activity wilfully may be first steps of examination rather than following any rigid scheme of examination. For example, eliciting tenderness can be reserved for the last because if a child starts to cry due to pain, further examination becomes extremely difficult.

After undressing the child in a warm room, any birthmarks, abnormalities, swellings, deformities, abnormal or loss of movements should be observed. Head, neck, facial features should be examined for presence of any characteristic feature of skeletal dysplasia. Any abnormal posturing of back and positioning of limbs should be observed and active movements can be stimulated by gently stroking the limb. Examination of older children can be carried out similar to that of adults, still with the caution of not irritating the child making him uncooperative.

The age of the child is an important factor in the clinical examination and history. The chief complaints are different according to the age of the child. **Table 15.1** lists the common musculoskeletal disorders grouped according to child's age.

15.2 PEDIATRIC ASSESSMENT OF GAIT, ARMS, LEGS, AND SPINE (pGALS)—A SCREENING TOOL

pGALS is an excellent tool to detect musculoskeletal abnormalities by asking the child to do simple manoeuvres. The evaluation can be completed in 2 minutes.

- Three screening questions are asked, followed by assessment of gait, arms, legs, and spine as detailed in **Table 15.2**.
- Throughout pGALS, the sequence of 'look (inspection), feel (palpation), move (range of movements)' is followed.
- Verbal and non-verbal signs of discomfort (e.g. facial expression, withdrawal) are noted.
- Do the full screen as the extent of joint involvement may not be obvious from the history.
- Look for asymmetry (e.g. muscle bulk, joint swelling, range of joint movements).

Table 15.1: Age-wise distribution of common musculoskeletal problems in children

Newborn and infancy
• Developmental dysplasia of the hip (DDH) • Congenital talipes equinovarus (CTEV) • Arthrogryposis multiplex congenita (AMC) • Limb deficiencies and deformities (e.g. hemimelia) • Congenital syndromes • Cerebral palsy • Nutritional disorders (e.g. rickets) • Infections (e.g. septic arthritis, osteomyelitis)
Childhood (1–12 years)
• Juvenile idiopathic arthritis (JIA) • Nutritional disorders (e.g. rickets) • Infections (e.g. septic arthritis, osteomyelitis) • Osteochondroma, leukemia, Ewing sarcoma • Legg-Calve-Perthes disease • Varus/valgus deformities of elbow/ knee
Adolescence
• Slipped capital femoral epiphysis • Tumours (osteosarcoma and Ewing sarcoma) • Juvenile idiopathic arthritis • Idiopathic scoliosis • Osteochondromas
Any age
• Septic arthritis • Nutritional disorders (e.g. rickets) • Tuberculosis • Osteomyelitis • Trauma • Reactive arthritis

- Consider clinical patterns (e.g. non-benign hypermobility and Marfanoid habitus or skin elasticity) and association of leg length discrepancy and scoliosis.

Gait

The gait is assessed by asking the child to walk across in the room. Any limp, abnormal rhythm, difficulty in turning around is noted. Then the child is asked to walk on heels and then on tiptoes. Look for expression of pain and ask for discomfort.

Arms

For assessing arms (upper limbs), the upper limbs are scanned (look) for any skin problems or rashes such as psoriasis, nails, joint swelling, deformity and muscle bulk. Look for any atrophy. The child can be asked to do various manoeuvres (**Table 15.2**). It is often easier if the child is able to copy the examiner, hence the examiner can stand in front of the child and demonstrate the various manoeuvres. As the child copies these manoeuvres, the examiner asks for pain and looks for facial expression of discomfort. In a normal child, these manoeuvres are easy to perform. Clues to hypermobility with excessive range of motion can be picked up. Asymmetry/ reduction in range of movements may help localize a joint disease.

Legs

For assessment of legs (lower limbs), the lower limbs should be exposed appropriately (look). The muscle bulk and wasting are checked. Lower limb alignment and deformities like knock knee and bow legs are noted. Limb length discrepancy, if any, is noted. The feet, including soles should always be checked as they may be a cause of limp (e.g. sores, foreign body). The knees are checked for warmth and effusion (feel). Normally, a child of school age is able to raise the heel to their buttock (move).

Spine

For assessment of spine, look from the back for any scoliosis or cutaneous manifestations of spina bifida. Looking from the side will reveal the smooth curve of the spine or any kyphotic deformity. The movement of the spine can be checked by the simple manoeuvres outlined in **Table 15.2**.

15.3 PHYSIOLOGICAL PARAMETERS AND VARIATIONS IN CHILDREN

Knowledge of normal physiological parameters and variations in a child is of paramount importance.

- Some bowing of legs in a child till the age of 1–1.5 years of age **(Fig. 15.1)** and knock knees in 3–4 years age can be physiological and corrects gradually.
- Similarly, W-sitting **(Fig. 15.2)** in a child can be due to increased femoral anteversion and may correct on its own as the child grows.
- Mild degree of flat feet can be present in initial years of age and can resolve as the medial longitudinal arch develops.

Table 15.2: pGALS assessment

Screening questions • Do you have any pain or stiffness in your joints, muscles or your back? • Do you have any difficulty getting yourself dressed without any help? • Do you have any difficulty going upstairs and downstairs?	
Gait • Observe the child walking • "Walk on your tip-toes/walk on your heels"	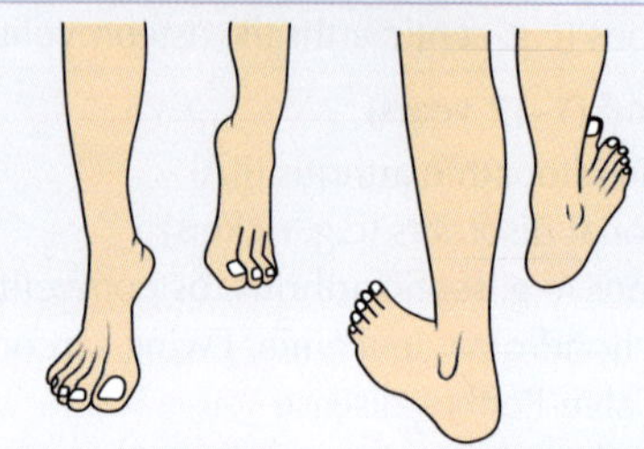
Arms • "Put your hands out in front of you" • "Turn your hands over and make a fist" • "Pinch your index finger and thumb together" • "Touch the tips of your fingers with your thumb" • "Squeeze the metacarpophalangeal joints of the examiner" • "Put your hands together/put your hands back-to-back" • "Reach up and touch the sky" • "Look at the ceiling" • "Put your hands behind your neck"	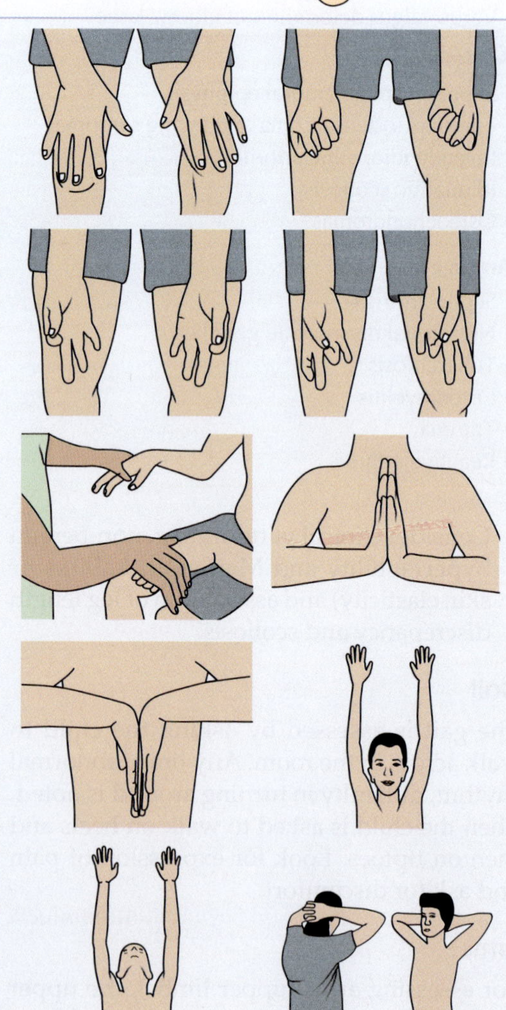

(Contd...)

Table 15.2: pGALS assessment (Contd...)

Legs • Feel for effusion at the knee • "Bend and then straighten your knee" (feel for crepitus during active movement of the knee) • Passive flexion (90 degrees) with internal rotation of hip	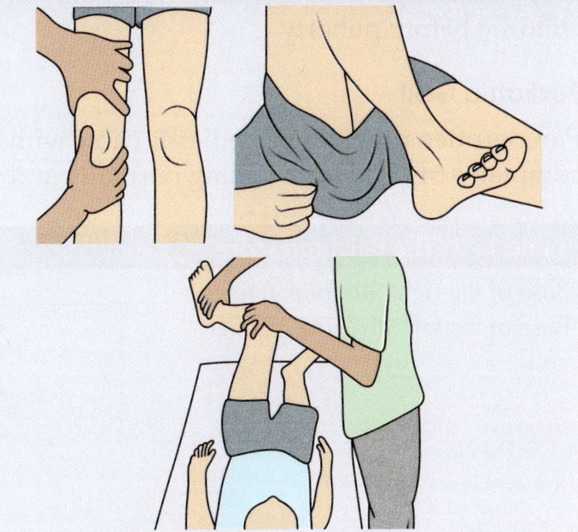 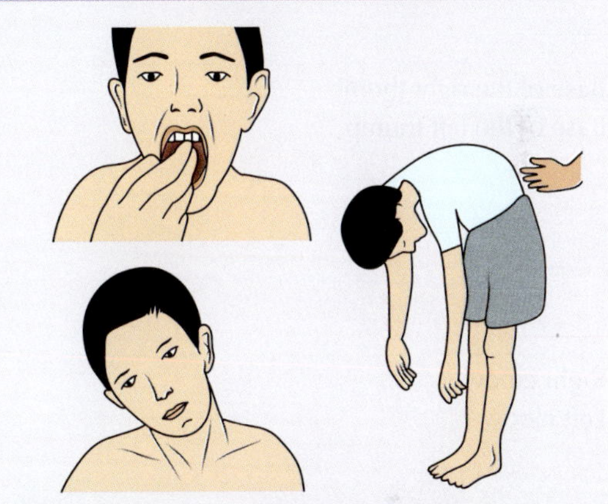
Spine • "Open your mouth and put 3 of your (child's own) fingers in your mouth" • Lateral flexion of cervical spine—"Try and touch your shoulder with your ear" • Observe the spine from behind • "Can you bend and touch your toes?" Observe curve of the spine from side and behind	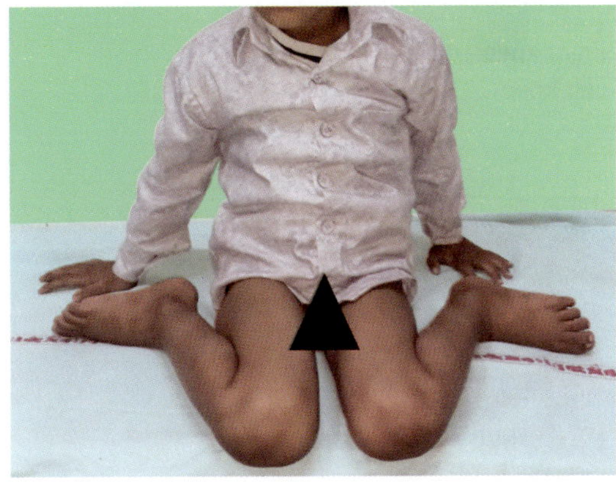

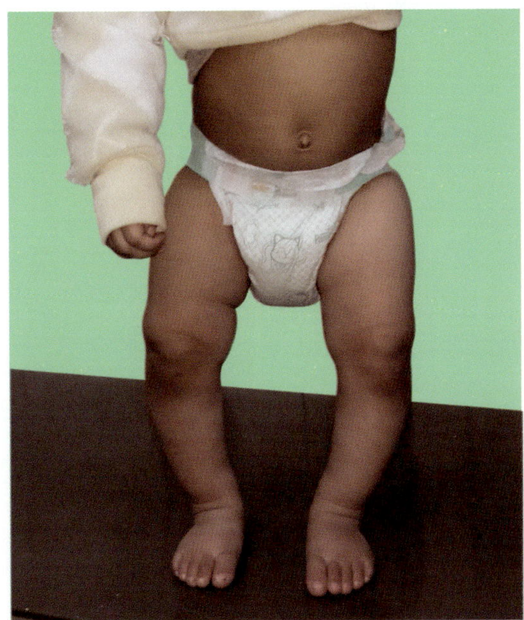

Fig. 15.1: Physiological bow legs: Bilateral, symmetrical, painless.

Fig. 15.2: 'W' sitting

Joint Laxity

Children's joints are more flexible as compared to adults but hyperlaxity should be evaluated and documented. The Beighton score assesses joint hypermobility on a 9-point scale. One point is given for each of the following joints* that show hypermobility on exam (Table 15.3). A

Beighton score greater than or equal to 6 points is evidence of generalized joint hyperlaxity in children before puberty.

Pediatric Gait

Parents often present in a pediatric clinic with complains of child not walking normally and most of the times they will point out some vague abnormity in the gait. A recent change in gait pattern noticed by a parent should be thoroughly evaluated. Child might not readily walk in the outpatient setup and thus a simple video made by parents outside the outpatient room may be of more use than trying to force

Table 15.3: The Beighton score

Base of the right 5th (pinky) finger Base of the left 5th (pinky) finger	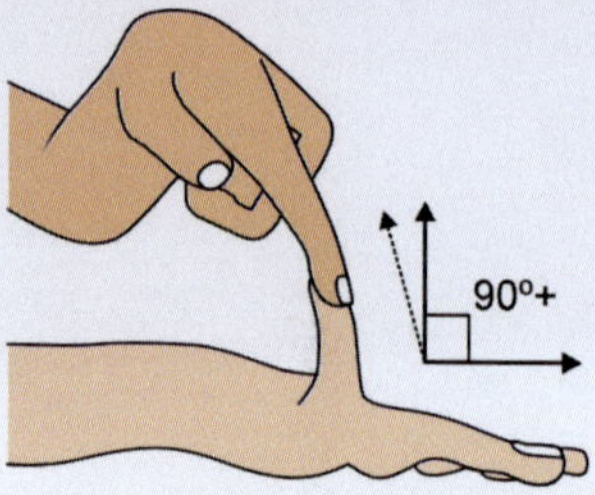 90°+
Base of the right thumb Base of the left thumb	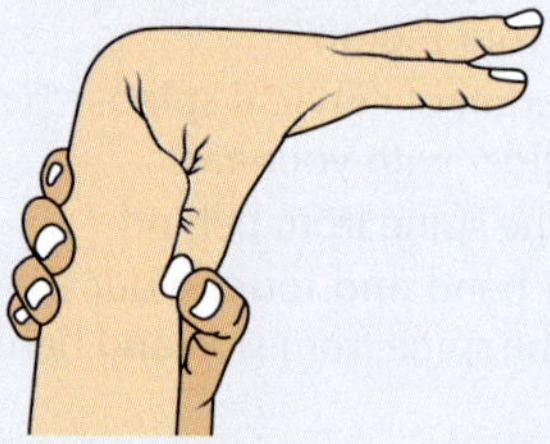
Right elbow Left elbow	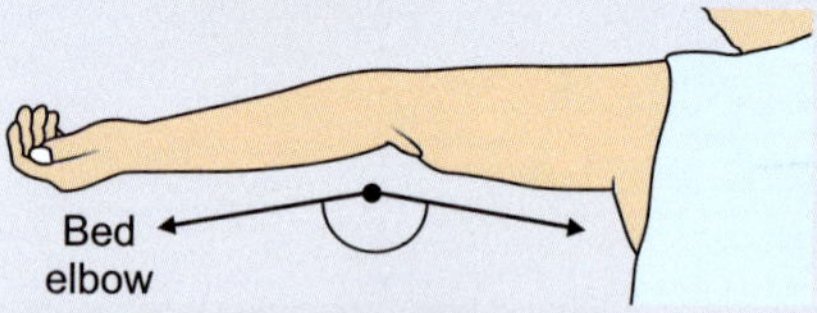 Bed elbow
Right knee Left knee	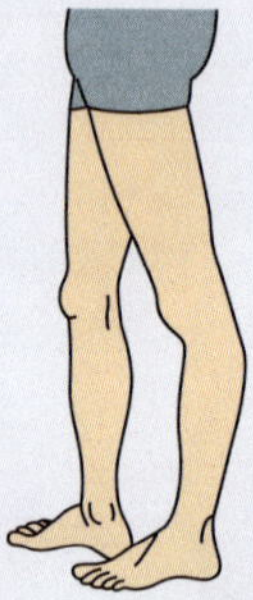
Lower spine	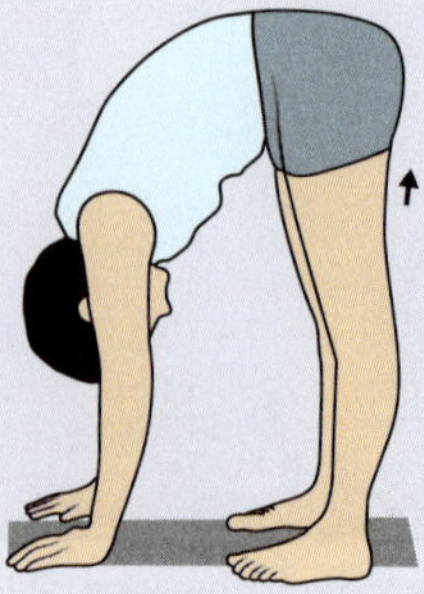

* Children may also have hypermobility in joints that are not measured by the Beighton score.

the child to walk. Comparison from a previous video, if available with the parents, helps in delineating any obvious change in the gait pattern.

Common gait patterns/problems noticed by parents are described below.

Toe Walking

When children start/learn to walk, many of them tend to walk on toes, i.e. with heels of the ground (Fig. 15.3). Bilateral and painless toe walking up to the age of 2 years can be considered normal and will eventually go as the child grows and his gait matures.

Unilateral toe walking could be due to a shorter lower limb as compared to other. Nevertheless, every child with a toe walking pattern should be clinically examined to rule out cerebral palsy with spastic diplegia, hereditary spastic paraplegia and Achilles contracture. Increased tone, exaggerated reflexes and positive Babinsky sign point towards an upper motor cause of spastic gastrocsoleus.

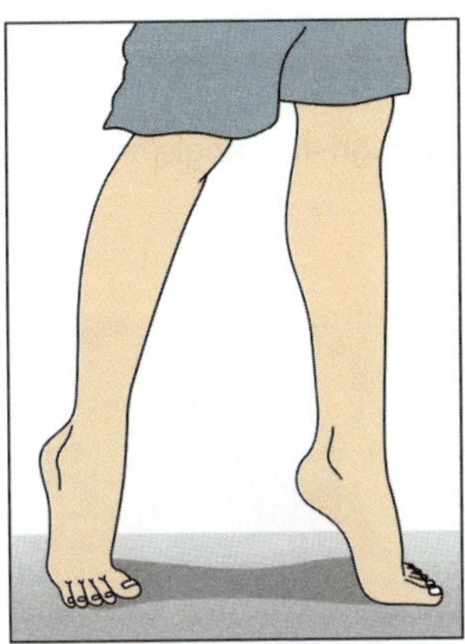

Fig. 15.3: Toe walking.

Intoeing Gait

Most common reason of painless, intoeing gait is increased femoral anteversion. The femur of the child is rotated inwards. For the same reason, the child sits in W-posture. This is benign and tends to correct as the child grows with age.

Examination of the hip movements palpating the trochanter provides idea about increased femoral anteversion (Fig. 15.4). Other causes can be increased tibial torsion (rotational abnormality of tibia) confirmed by checking the thigh–foot angle (Fig. 15.5), and metatarsus adductus (deformity of foot) confirmed by checking the heel–foot angle. In cases of unilateral intoeing, previous history of malunited fracture should be ruled out.

Out Toeing Gait

Out toeing up to 30 degrees (foot progression angle) can be considered normal and it may correct naturally. Persistence of out toeing warrants evaluation of rotational abnormalities of the tibia.

Specific Conditions

Cerebral Palsy

Cerebral palsy (CP) has been described as a group of disorders of the development of movement and posture that are attributed to nonprogressive disturbances that occurred in the developing fetal or infant brain. Although the presentations are varied, common contractures/deformities in spastic variety include adduction of lower limbs (sometimes severe enough to cause scissoring) (Fig. 15.6), flexion at hips and knees and ankle equinus.

With the patient in supine position, passive abduction of the hip is performed with the knee in extension and with the knee kept in 90° flexion (Phelp's Test). If abduction improves on knee flexion, the primary pathology lies in the medial hamstring muscles and gracilis (these are biarticular muscles and relaxed in knee flexion). If both the measurements are the same, the prime pathology is in the adductor muscles.

Thomas' hip flexion test: It is commonly used for measuring hip flexion contracture. The test is performed with the patient in supine position and the uninvolved limb is adequately flexed to eliminate exaggerated lumbar lordosis. The angle formed between the horizontal axis of the thigh and horizontal line parallel to the floor measures the hip flexion contracture.

Popliteal angle test: Knee flexion contracture is usually attributed to hamstring origin. The test used to test hamstring tightness is called popliteal angle test (Fig. 15.7). It is performed with the hip joint in 90° of flexion in supine position. The knee of the tested limb

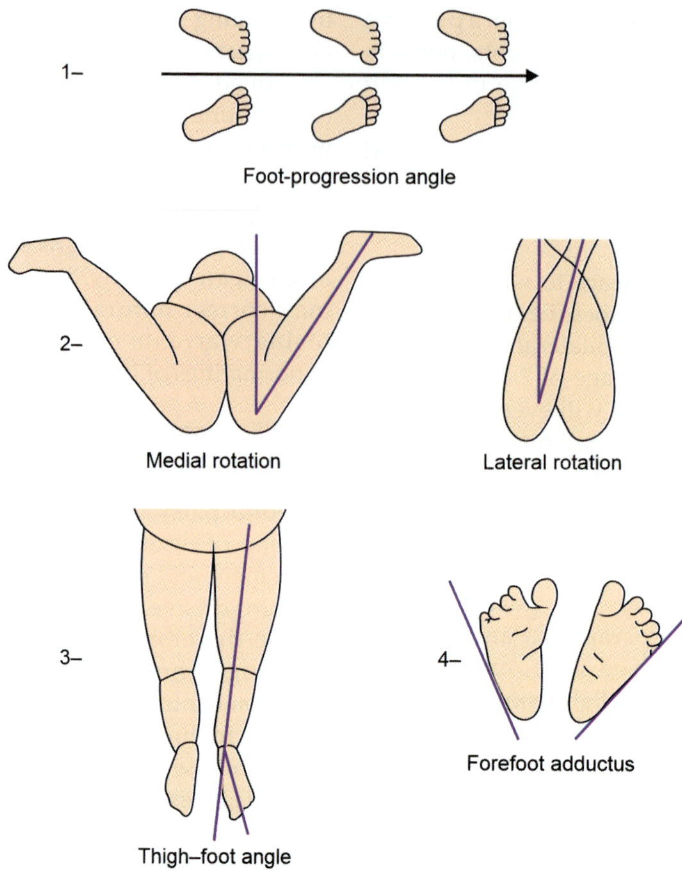

Fig. 15.4: In child with intoeing gait, examination of hip movements, thigh–foot angle and heel–foot angle are essential.

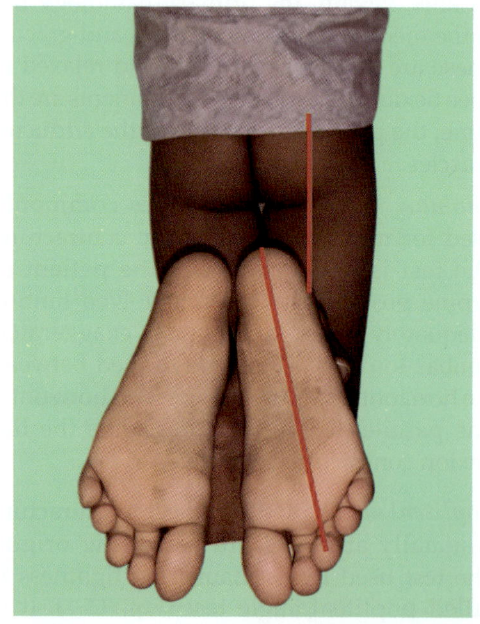

Fig. 15.5: Thigh–foot angle indicates the rotational abnormality of tibia.

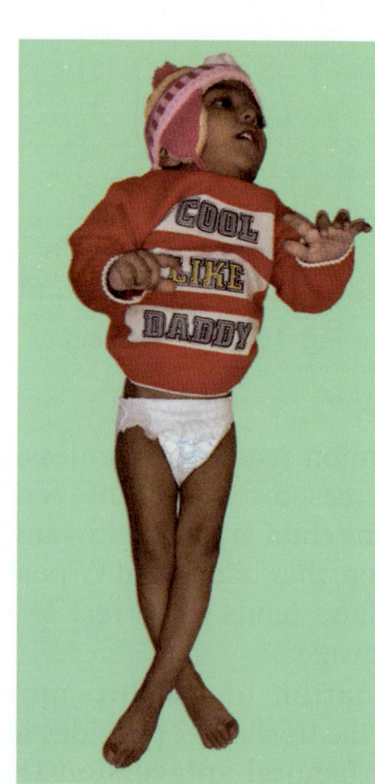

Fig. 15.6: Scissoring due to bilateral adductor contractures seen in cerebral palsy.

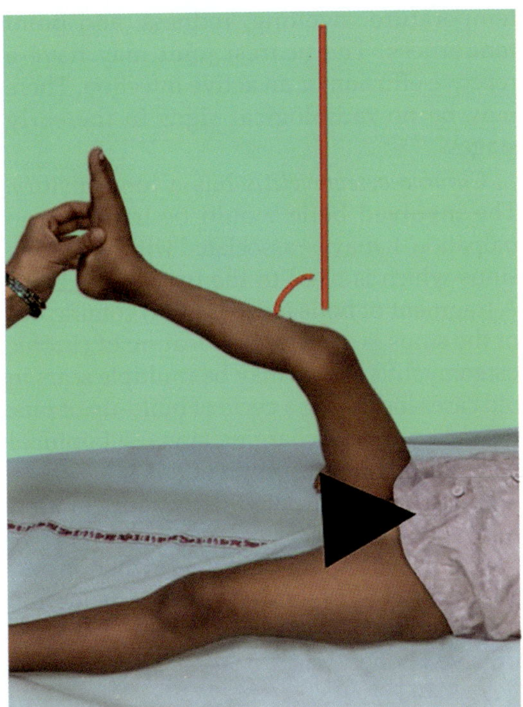

Fig. 15.7: Popliteal angle to assess hamstring tightness.

is extended until resistance and further loss of knee extension is measured and expressed as popliteal angle.

Silfverskiold test: Ankle equinus (gastrocsoleus spasticity/contracture) is assessed by passive dorsiflexion of ankle with knee in extension and then with the knee joint in 90° flexion (Silfverskiold test). Gastrocnemius being biarticular muscles partially relaxes with knee flexed position. Thus, differences in ankle dorsiflexion with knee flexed and extended indicates a gastrocnemius component (Fig. 15.8).

Musculoskeletal Infections

Septic Arthritis

Septic arthritis is an infection in the joint (synovial) fluid and joint tissues usually by a bacteria. The classical presentation of septic arthritis in children is a combination of a painful joint with limited range of movement, inability to bear weight on the involved limb and fever. If the joint is superficial, inflammation signs and joint tenderness can be appreciated. Fluid accumulates inside the affected joint and the same is most often held in a position that maximizes intracapsular volume. For example, the hip takes position of flexion, abduction, and externally rotation (Fig. 15.9).

During infancy, the clinical presentation differs from the older children. The younger child may present with irritability, failure to feed/suck or gain weight and reduced movement of the affected limb. Sometimes, the symptoms are as subtle as child crying on changing the diapers or decreased active movement of the joint (pseudoparalysis). Sometimes, the child presents when infection has been largely controlled but the joint suffered significant damage, e.g. septic sequelae hip. The findings can then be variable.

Osteomyelitis

Osteomyelitis is an infection in a bone again most commonly by bacteria. A child with an

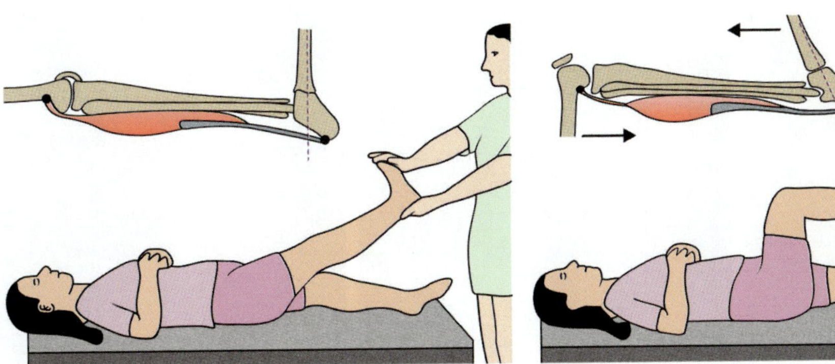

Fig. 15.8: Passive dorsiflexion of ankle with knee in extension and then with the knee joint in 90° flexion (Silfverskiold test).

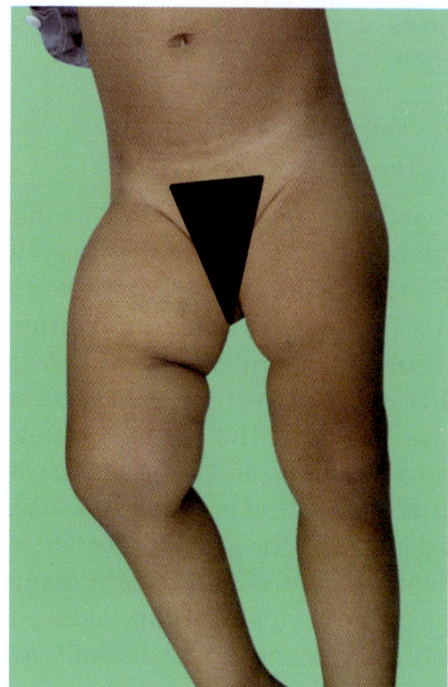

Fig. 15.9: Septic affection of the right hip. Note the flexion, abduction and external rotation attitude.

acute hematogenous osteomyelitis can present with a febrile episode, with the affected extremity kept in a state of pseudoparalysis due to the throbbing pain. Sometimes, septic arthritis and osteomyelitis coexist. The affected part would be inflamed with raised temperature, swelling, redness, and point tenderness. The nearest joint may have a reactive effusion or an active infection. There may be no radiological signs in the early stages.

Chronic osteomyelitis has a long history. The involved bone would be irregular on palpation. It may be associated with a draining sinus which is fixed to the underlying bone. A fragment of bone (sequestrum) coming out of the sinus is sometimes a feature of chronic osteomyelitis. There may be multiple scars in old cases indicating a cycle of build-up of pus, formation of a discharging sinus, suboptimal healing and build-up of pus again **(Fig. 15.10)**. There may be associated deformities around the adjoining joint or limb length discrepancy due to infective insult to the growing physis. Radiological signs consist of cloacae, sequestra, and involucra along with sclerosis of the involved bone.

Osteoarticular Tuberculosis

The symptoms will depend on the joint/bone involved and duration of symptoms. Spine is the commonest site. In children, hands, feet and elbows are other common sites. Symptoms can include back/joint/

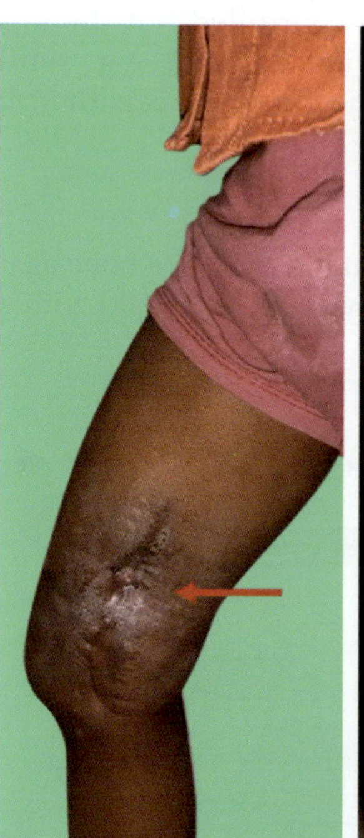

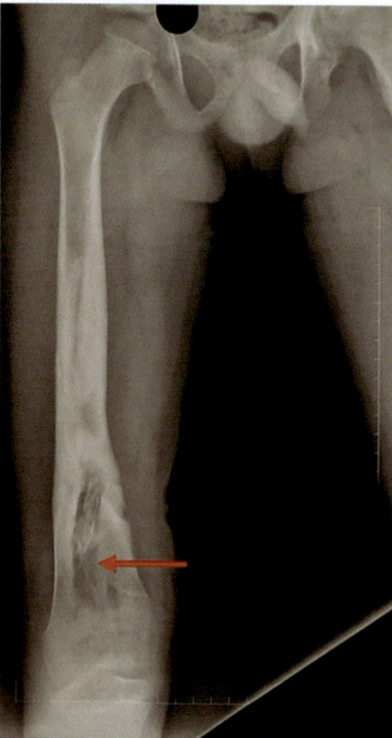

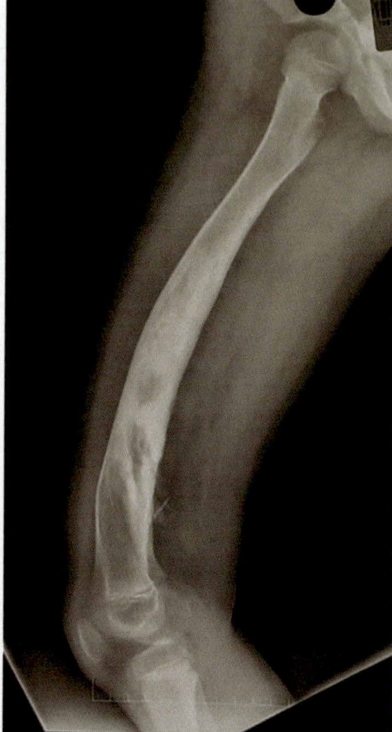

Fig. 15.10: Chronic osteomyelitis of right femur. The arrows indicate the discharging sinus and sequestrum in radiographs.

bone pain, spasms, muscle wasting, swellings, collections/abscess, discharging sinuses, stiffness/restriction of movements, weakness in upper and/or lower limbs, spinal or bone deformities, etc. Sometimes, the involvement is multifocal, i.e. more than one site is involved.

15.4 EXAMINATION OF THE SPINE

The common symptoms are pain, stiffness/ decreased range of movements, deformity or weakness in lower or upper limbs. Examination of both upper and lower limbs form part of spinal examination.

Inspection

Inspect the overlying skin for any scars from prior surgery or trauma, lipoma, or café au lait patches (neurofibromatosis). A tuft of hair (faun's beard), nevus, lipoma, sinus, or a dimple in the lumbar or cervical spine region may indicate a congenital structural abnormality, such as spina bifida occulta or diastematomyelia (Fig. 15.11).

With the child seated or standing, inspect the spine for posture, normal resting spinal curvatures, or any evidence of deformity.

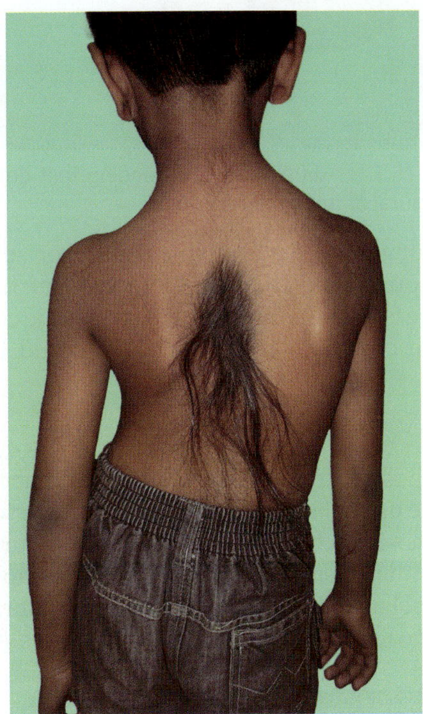

Fig. 15.11: A tuft of hair in the back generally indicates an underlying spinal deformity.

The normal dorsal spine is a smooth curve in the sagittal plane which is slightly convex posteriorly. This normal curvature of the thoracic spine is called kyphosis with a normal value of 20 to 40°. The standing posture and alignment are assessed for any asymmetry or deformity. Heel and toe walking are observed for any asymmetry or weakness.

Palpation

Run your hand over the spinous processes of the vertebral column. The normal vertebral column has 3 gentle curves—cervical lordosis, thoracic kyphosis, and lumbar lordosis. With the child sitting and the head supported, the external occipital protuberance is readily identified. The cervical spinous process below it is that of C2; the C1 spinous process is rudimentary or absent.

Each spinous process is palpated for tenderness, swelling, or deformity. The absence of a spinous process in the lower lumbar spine may indicate a spina bifida. Tenderness and paraspinal muscle spasm are best elicited by giving a rotatory strain to consecutive spinous processes in opposite directions.

Range of Movements

Flexion, extension, lateral flexion, and rotations are possible in the neck region. A proper assessment of spinal range of movements can only be made in school going children. Toddlers are less likely to be cooperative. Coin test is a simple test to check for spinal range of movements. Drop a coin or any other object on the floor and ask the child to bend down and pick it up.

Adam's Forward Bending Test

This is a reliable means of screening for scoliosis. View the patient from the back during the test. The child stands evenly on both legs with the knees straight, and then bends forward at the waist with the arms hanging free. The examiner evaluates the back for elevation of one hemithorax or flank relative to the other to determine the presence of a rotational deformity due to scoliosis. A detailed neurologic examination and palpation of pulses is mandatory in any disease involving the spine.

Sternomastoid Tumour and Torticollis

A neonate or young infant (usually at 2–4 weeks of life) presents as lump in the neck region located approximately over the sternomastoid muscle (Fig. 15.12) known as sternomastoid tumour. It is usually well defined and firm. The neck is neither twisted at this stage nor there is any restriction of movements. The benign lump has a tendency to disappear in few months' time. In some proportion of children, the neck gradually bends laterally resulting from fibrosis of sternomastoid muscle (torticollis or wry neck) (Fig 15.13). The sternomastoid tendon feels tight and cord-like, and the movements of the neck to opposite side (lateral bending and rotations) are restricted. Facial deformities often accompany long standing torticollis.

Scoliosis

A lateral curvature of the thoracic or lumbar spine is referred to as scoliosis. This is best observed from behind with the child standing. Scoliosis may be *nonstructural* (compensatory or postural) or *structural* (fixed).

Compensatory scoliosis results from limb length discrepancy or hip contractures. Typically, this type of scoliosis disappears when the patient sits.

Postural scoliosis is observed while standing. It typically disappears when the child bends forward.

Fixed or structural scoliosis may represent idiopathic adolescent scoliosis, or it may be secondary to neurologic disease (muscular dystrophy, neurofibromatosis, syringomyelia)

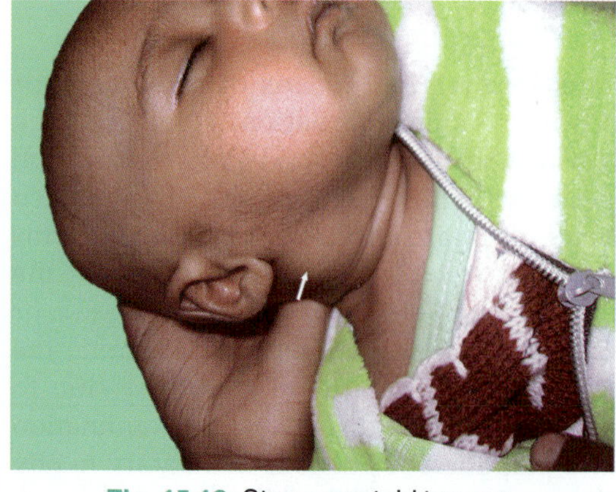

Fig. 15.12: Sternomastoid tumour.

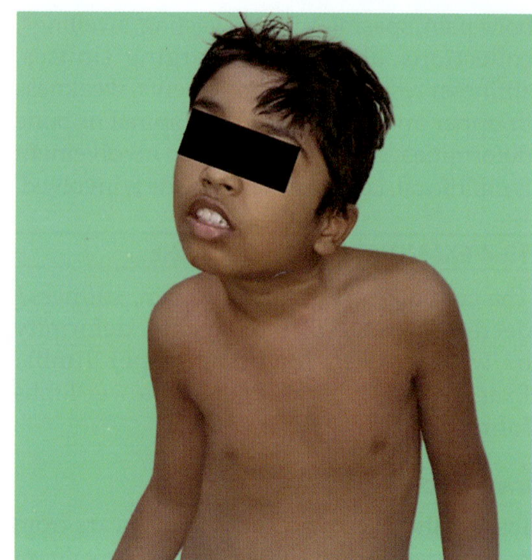

Fig. 15.13: Left-sided torticollis. Note the facial flattening on the affected side.

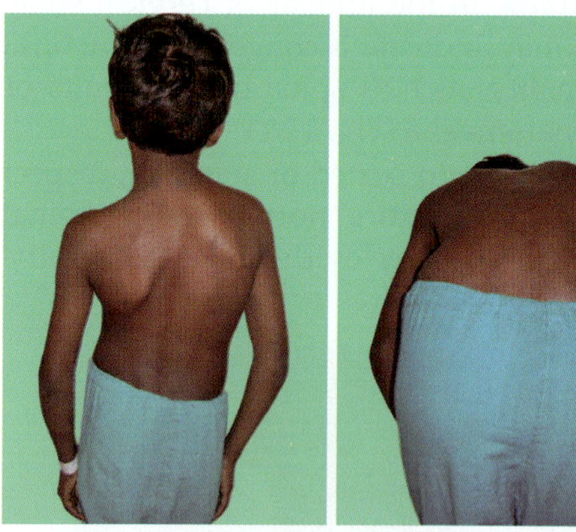

Fig. 15.14: Adam's forward bending test detects structural or functional scoliosis.

or congenital fused hemivertebra, or spinal tumours. The diagnostic feature of fixed curve is that forward bending makes the curve more obvious (Adam's forward bend test) (Fig. 15.14).

Kyphosis

Kyphosis is an exaggerated, forward rounding of the upper back. A unique form of adolescent kyphosis (Scheuermann's disease) occurs at around pubertal age. The child may complain of backache and fatigue. A smooth thoracic kyphosis extending multiple vertebrae is seen.

Pott's Spine

Pott's spine or tubercular spine is another common pathology. Although thoracic tuberculosis is commoner, involvement of lumbar or cervical vertebrae may occur as well. The history is generally insidious. Pain, muscle spasm, deformity **(Key Box 1)** are common presentations. Sometimes, abscess in the back or neurological deficits of lower limbs are the presenting symptoms. The back should be watched while the child attempts to bend forwards. The movements are typically restricted and the attempts results in pain and accompanying muscle spam.

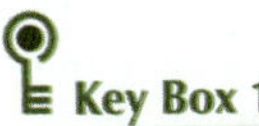

Key Box 1

Kyphotic deformities

- *Knuckle deformity* is a sharp kyphotic deformity of the spine usually involving 1–2 spinous processes (Fig. 15.15).
- *Angular kyphus* involves 2–4 spinous processes and is sharply angulated as compared to a knuckle.
- *Gibbus deformity* is a rounded kyphotic angulation of the spine, particularly the thoracic spine spanning more than 4–6 spinous processes. It may result from an infection, mostly, spinal tuberculosis; or less commonly from compression fractures.

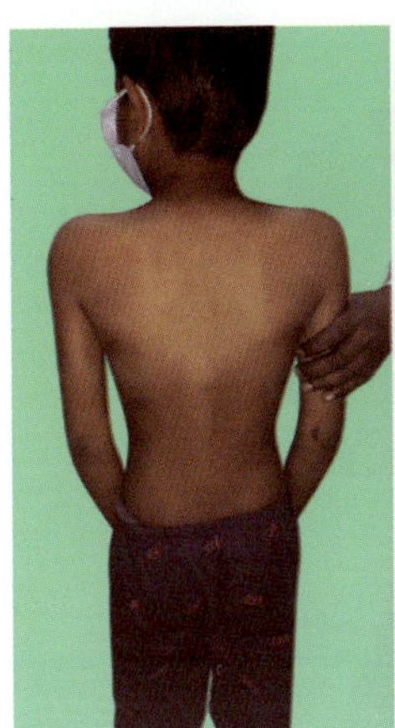

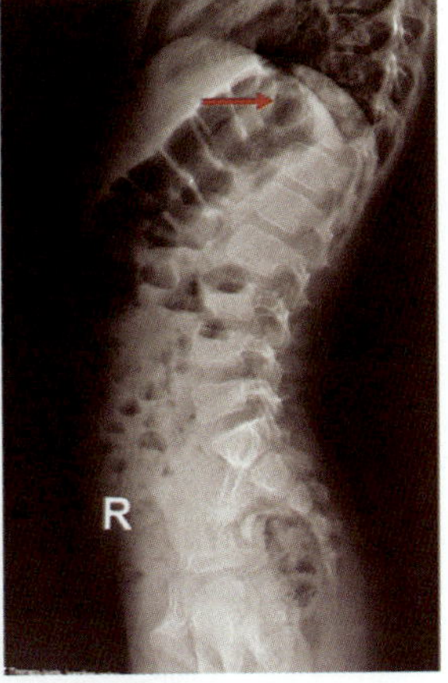

Fig. 15.15: Pott's spine with knuckle deformity.

15.5 EXAMINATION OF THE SHOULDER JOINT

The shoulder joint is relatively well covered with muscles. As such, obvious swellings are a less common presentation. The usual symptoms in the shoulder region can be pain, deformity or restriction of movements.

Inspection

The child is examined from the front and back exposing neck, chest and the entire upper limb. The axilla can also be inspected with the shoulder abducted. Asymmetry between the two shoulders and scapular pathologies can be appreciated better from back.

Palpation

The bony points palpable are almost whole of subcutaneous clavicle, acromion process and proximal humerus.

Range of Movements

The movements possible at the shoulder joint are abduction, adduction, flexion, extension, internal and external rotation.

- To test the abduction, the child's arm is raised by the side of the body until the finger tips point towards the ceiling.
- Adduction is the movement of the arm across the front of the body towards midline.
- Flexion is the arm movement in forward direction and vice versa for extension.
- *Rotations:* For testing rotations, the arm can be tucked by the side of trunk and elbow flexed 90 degrees. Another way to assess shoulder rotations is to abduct arm at right angles to the trunk and keep the elbow flexed 90 degrees (Fig. 15.16). In this position, the trunk does not interfere in the internal rotation component.
- For testing true glenohumeral movements, the scapula should be firmly stabilized at the acromion while the arm is abducted (Fig. 15.17).

Tests for Glenohumeral Instability

Laxity of the shoulder capsule and ligaments results in inferior subluxation of the humerus on downward traction of the arm, which produces a depression or hollow between the lateral edge of the acromion and the humeral head (positive sulcus sign) (Fig. 15.18). Sometimes, the condition is associated with generalized laxity of the other joints.

With the child supine, the shoulder is 90° abducted and 90° externally rotated; the examiner then applies forward pressure to the posterior aspect of the humeral head.

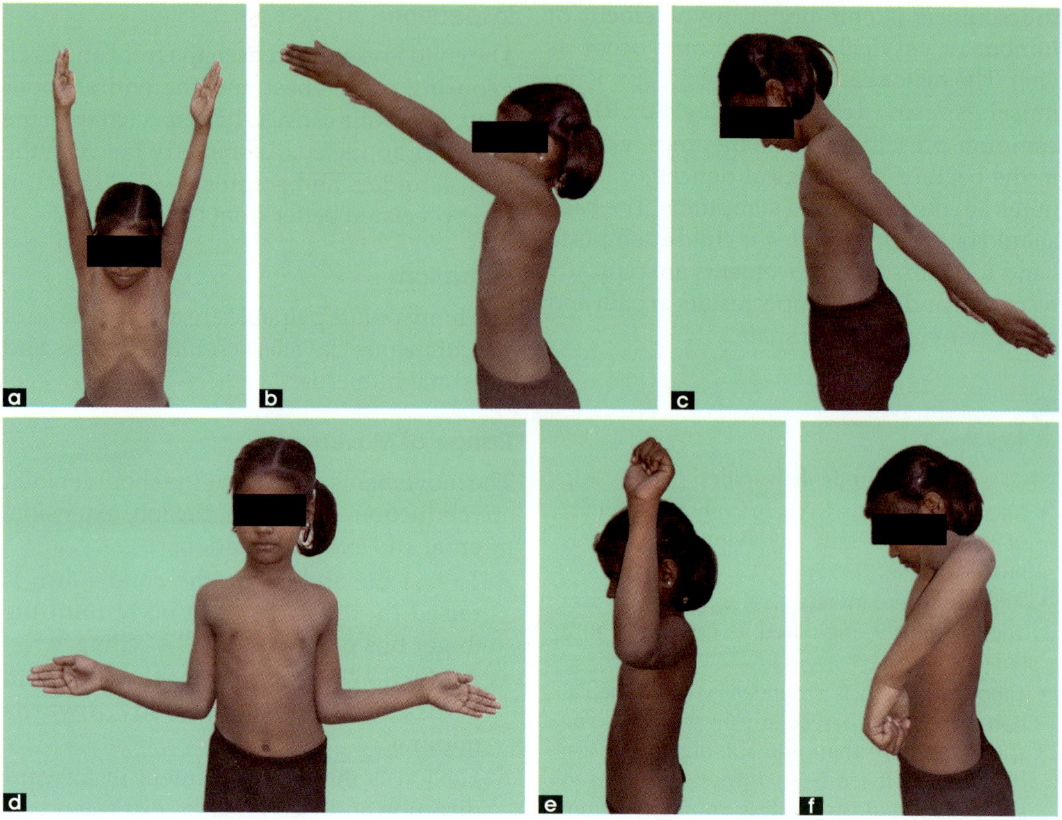

Fig. 15.16: Shoulder movements of abduction (a), flexion (b), extension (c). The external rotation can be checked either by arms tucked by side of trunk (d) or with the arms 90 degrees abducted and elbow 90 degrees flexed (e). Internal rotation (f).

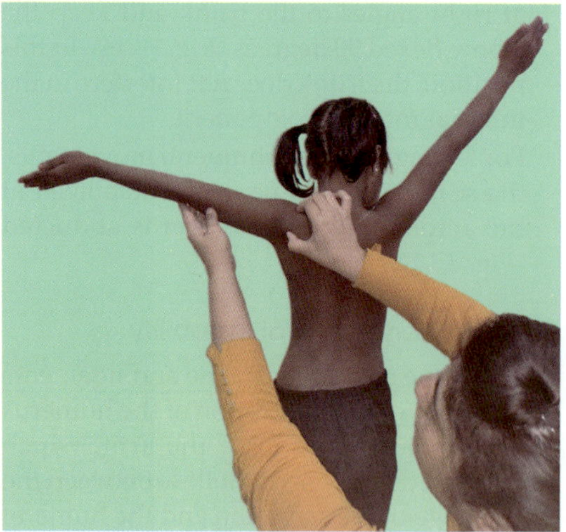

Fig. 15.17: For true glenohumeral movements, the scapula should be firmly stabilized at the acromion while the arm is abducted.

In the presence of glenohumeral instability and recurrent anterior subluxation, the child suddenly becomes apprehensive and

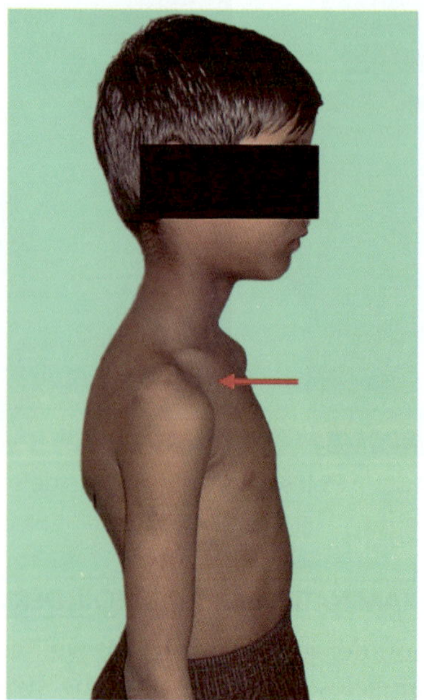

Fig. 15.18: Depression or hollow between the lateral edge of the acromion and the humeral head (positive sulcus sign).

complains of pain in the shoulder (positive anterior apprehension test or crank test).

Specific Conditions

Sprengel's Shoulder

Sprengel's shoulder (Fig. 15.19) is a congenital condition characterized by a small and undescended scapula. Clinically, the shoulder on the affected side is elevated to variable degrees. In severe varieties, the shoulder blades can be closer to the occipital region (near the neck). Although, the concerns are typically cosmetic, there may be restrictions of the affected shoulder abduction and flexion in some children.

The condition may be associated with anomalies of cervical or thoracic spine or opposite scapula. Occasionally, a bony or fibrous association may extend between the affected scapula and the cervical spine.

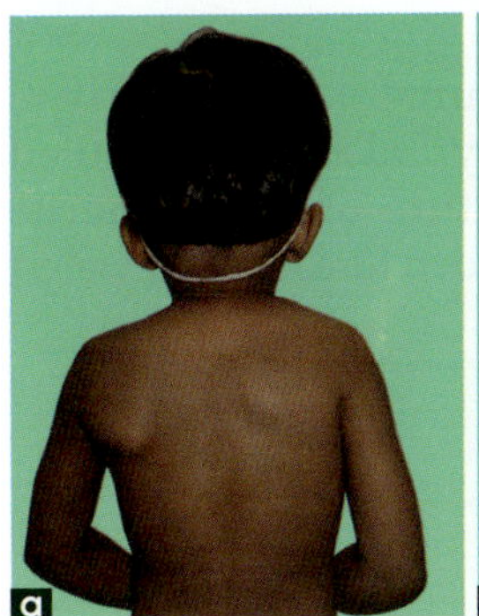

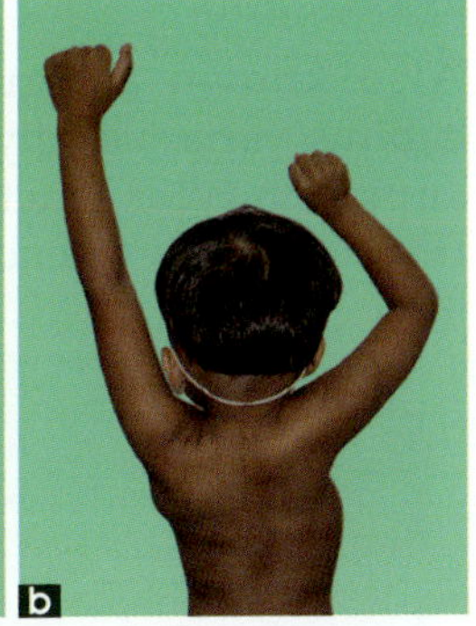

Fig. 15.19: Sprengel's shoulder on right side (a) was associated with restricted abduction of shoulder (b).

Klippel-Feil Syndrome

Klippel-Feil syndrome is a bone disorder characterized by abnormal fusion of 2 or more bones in the cervical spine. Bilateral failure of scapular descent is often associated. This creates a characteristic appearance of a short neck, low hairline, and gross restriction of neck movement (Fig. 15.20). Facial asymmetry and neck webbing is also seen. The fused vertebrae can limit the range of movement of the neck and back as well as lead to chronic headaches and muscle pain in the neck and back that range in severity.

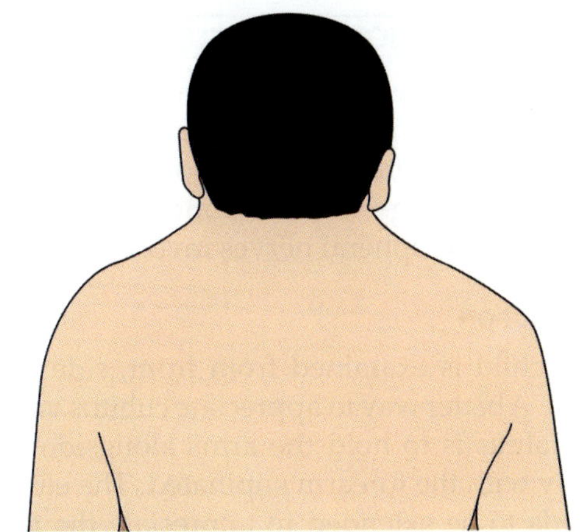

Fig. 15.20: Klippel-Feil syndrome. Observe the short neck and low hairline.

Osteochondroma of Proximal Humerus/Scapula

Osteochondromas are benign bone tumors that commonly affect the proximal humerus, but are rarely seen on flat bones like scapula. They are usually asymptomatic and present with cosmetic complaints. If the location is medial, neurovascular structures may be at risk of stretching. Scapular osteochondroma, if on undersurface, are sometimes cause of scapular malalignment and restricted abduction (Fig. 15.21). Osteochondroma follows course of bone growth until the closure of physis.

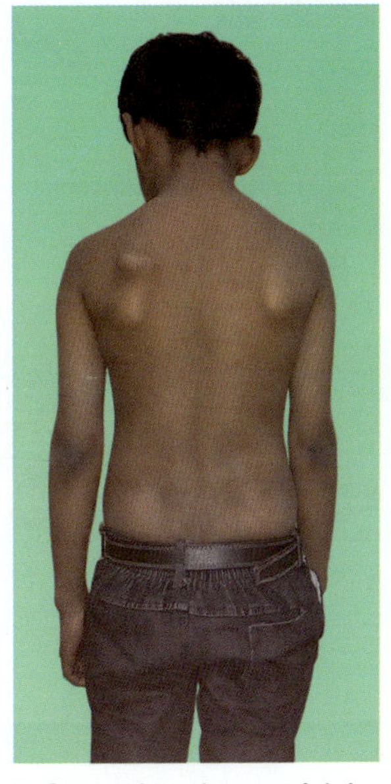

Fig. 15.21: Osteochondroma of right shoulder.

15.6 EXAMINATION OF THE ELBOW JOINT

The usual presenting symptoms in the elbow region can be pain, swelling, deformity or restriction of movements. Sometimes, the symptomatology manifests more distally in hand, e.g. peripheral nerves involvement.

Inspection

The child is examined from front, side and back. A better way to appreciate cubitus varus or valgus is to hold the arms alongside the body with the forearm supinated. The elbow needs to be extended to appreciate the true extent of deformity. A compliant child can be asked to hold the arms out sideways at right angle to the body keeping the elbows extended and forearm supinated. This will make any flexion deformity and hyperextension at elbows obvious. Comparison between two limbs and their range of movement is also easy in this position.

Palpation

The synovial thickening and effusion are best appreciated on the either side of olecranon. It is important to feel the supracondylar bony ridges for irregularities and compare the symmetry of bony points (the olecranon, the medial epicondyle, and the lateral epicondyle) between two elbows. Equally important is to establish the normal relationship between radial head and capitulum. The ulnar nerve passes just behind the medial epicondyle and should be palpated for any thickenings. The epitrochlear lymph nodes drain the forearm and hand. These are often inflamed in tuberculosis and other infective diseases. They are palpated along the medial supracondylar ridge of the humerus about 2 cm above the medial epicondyle.

Range of Movements

The movements possible at the elbow joint are flexion, extension, pronation and supination. Their passive and active ranges should be noted down.

Specific Conditions

Cubitus Varus

Also known as 'gunstock deformity', cubitus varus usually follows a malunited supracondylar fracture of the humerus (Fig. 15.22). The extended forearm is deviated

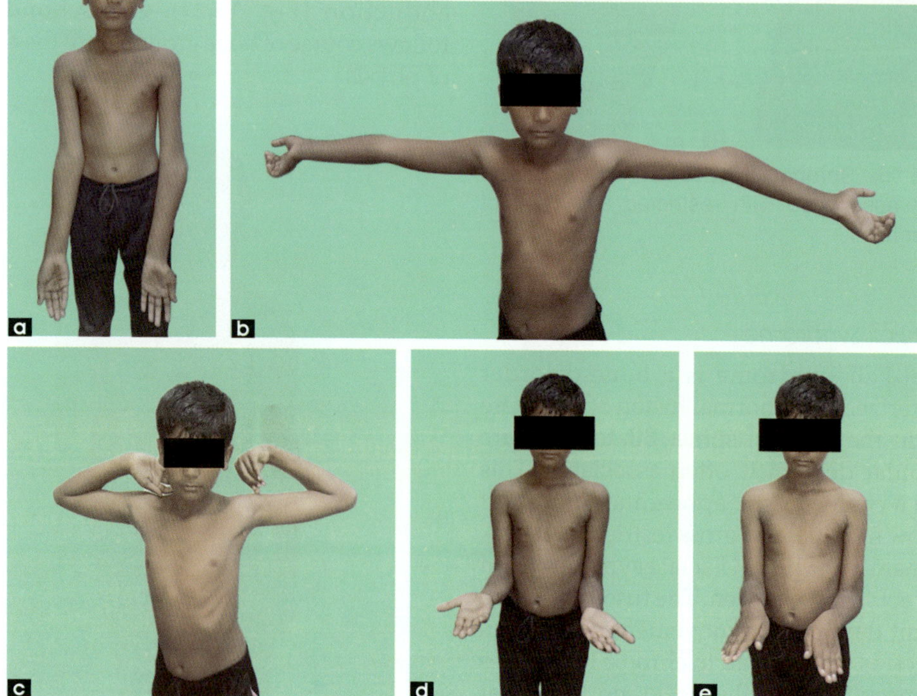

Fig. 15.22: Cubitus varus deformity left elbow (a). Note hyperextension of left elbow (b). Flexion (c), supination (d) and pronation (e). Note slight restriction of pronation on affected side.

towards midline of the body. The three-point bony relationship tested with elbow in 90° flexion usually remains unaltered in the pathology.

Cubitus Valgus

It is the moving of forearm away from midline of the body. The commonest cause is old fracture of lateral condyle humerus (Fig. 15.23). Unlike previous pathology, here the three-point bony relationship is not maintained because the pathology is intra-articular. There are chances of associated ulnar nerve palsy (tardy ulnar nerve palsy) in longstanding cases and hand examination therefore becomes important in these children.

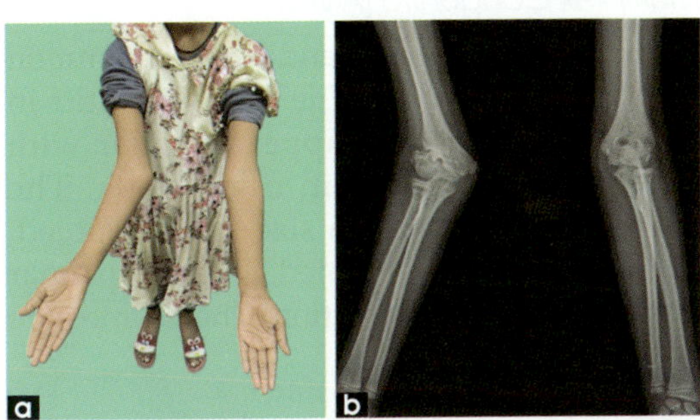

Fig. 15.23: Cubitus valgus deformity right elbow (a). The commonest cause is a non-united fracture lateral condyle of humerus (b).

Tuberculosis of the Elbow Joint

Elbow is a relatively superficial joint and therefore swelling and sinus formation is more obvious (Fig. 15.24). Marked wasting of arm and forearm muscles and restriction of joint movements are common. Often, there is an elbow effusion which can be appreciated as a fluctuant swelling or bulge in the lateral and medial paraolecranon grooves. Epitrochlear and axillary lymph nodes may be enlarged.

15.7 EXAMINATION OF THE WRIST JOINT

The usual symptomatology in the wrist region is pain, restriction of movements, swelling or deformity.

Inspection

While examining the wrist, exposure of elbow, forearm and hand is essential. Comparison of both wrists and forearms gives clue to deformity, swelling or restriction of movements.

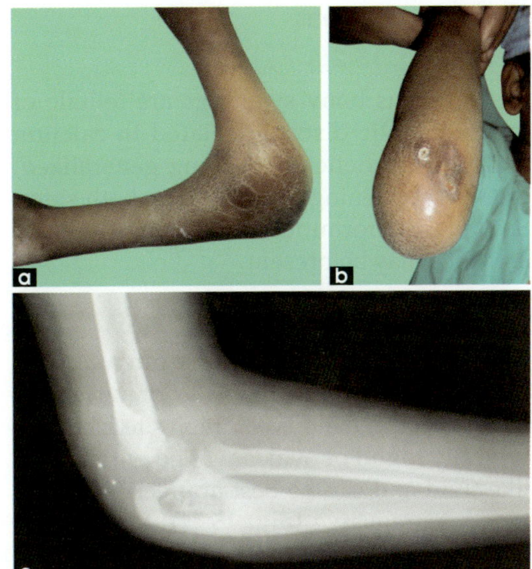

Fig. 15.24: Swelling and marked wasting associated with tuberculosis of the elbow joint (a). Being a superficial joint, sinus formation is common (b). Radiograph shows the coke sequestra (c).

Palpation

Points of tenderness should be localized. Characteristics of any swellings (e.g. ganglion) should be noted down. The bony landmarks palpable are the distal end of radius and ulna.

Range of Movements

The child can be asked to position the hands in form of 'Namaste' with elbows elevated to compare passive dorsiflexion at wrist. Reverse 'Namaste' with dorsum of hands touching each other is again a simple way to check and compare passive palmar flexion (Fig. 15.25). Other movements possible at wrist are radial and ulnar deviation.

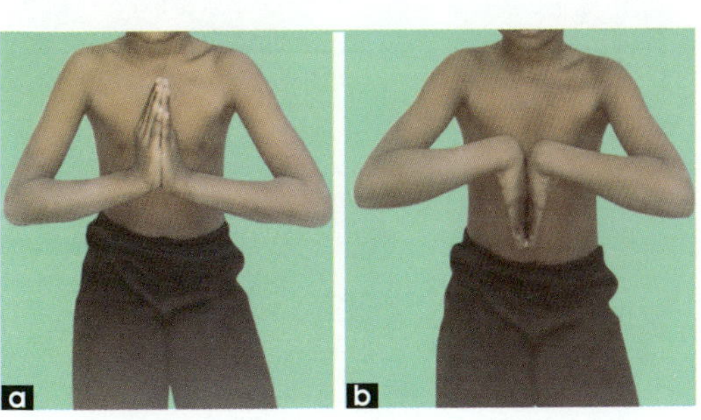

Fig. 15.25: 'Namaste' (a) and reverse 'Namaste' (b) is a quick way to check wrist dorsiflexion and palmar flexion.

Rickets (Fig. 15.26)

Distal radius bony swellings are telltale of this metabolic disorder related to calcium and vitamin deficiency. Being generalized, the wrist widening is obvious on both sides. Secondary deformities of other body regions, e.g. knee may be present.

Ganglion

Ganglia are lumps that most often appear along the tendons or joints of wrists or hands. Back of hand is common site. They are typically round or oval, are filled with a jelly-like fluid and can be best appreciated when tendons are active (Fig. 15.27). Most of the time they are painless and the main concern is cosmetic. At times, there can be dull ache in these cysts.

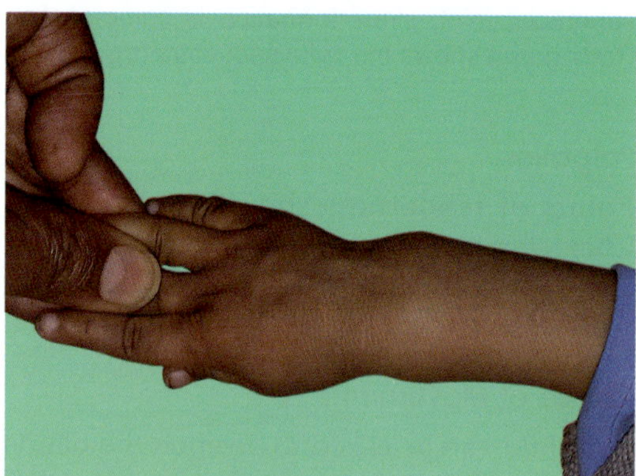

Fig. 15.26: Wrist widening resulting from changes in the distal end of radius are hallmark of metabolic disorder rickets. The disorder generally involves several joints and has bilateral presentation.

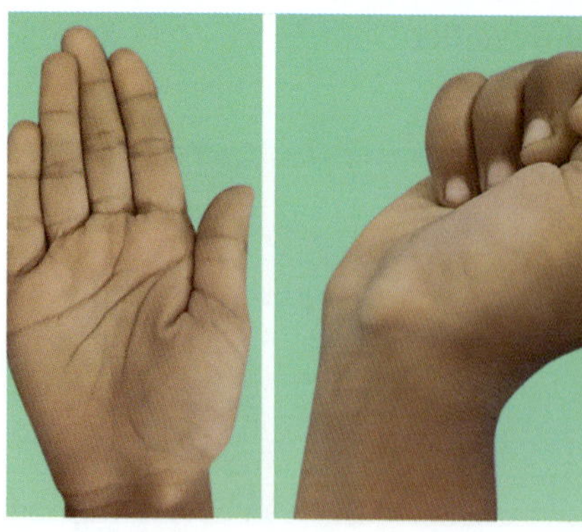

Fig. 15.27: Ganglion at volar aspect of wrist. The cyst becomes more prominent when tendons are contracted.

Radial Clubhand

The deformity is caused by deficiency of radius bone and underdevelopment of radial side of forearm and hand (Fig. 15.28). The severity may extend to complete absence of radius. Additionally, the thumb may be hypoplastic or absent. The wrist is palmar flexed and radially deviated, the forearm length is short and the elbow may be unstable. This condition is associated with various other anomalies, such as dextrocardia, VATER syndrome (affection of **v**ertebrae, **a**nus, **t**rachea, **e**sophagus, **r**enal), TAR (thrombocytopenia absent radius) syndrome, and Holt-Oram syndrome.

Arthrogryposis, also Called Arthrogryposis Multiplex Congenita (AMC)

Affection of upper limb and wrists is common in AMC (Fig. 15.29). The limbs are stiff in varying degrees and appear tubular with smooth creaseless skin over joints. The muscles are reduced in size and atrophied. Wrists are usually pronated, in severe palmar flexion and ulnar deviation. The thumbs are

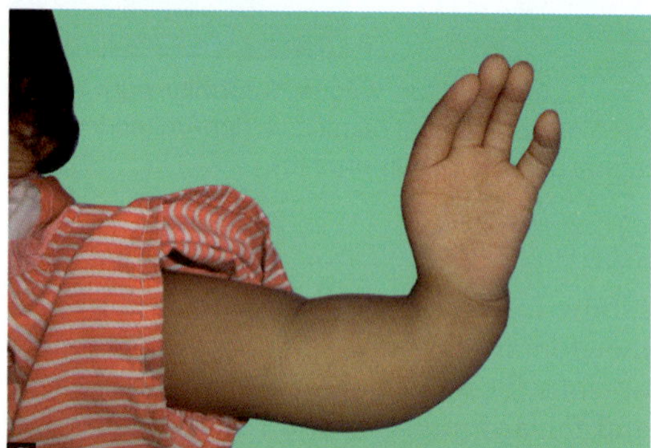

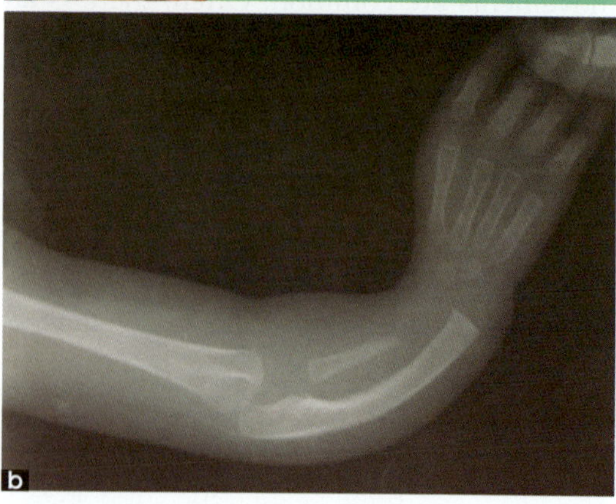

Fig. 15.28: Radial clubhand (a), radiograph showing hypoplastic radius, absent 1st ray and bowed ulna (b).

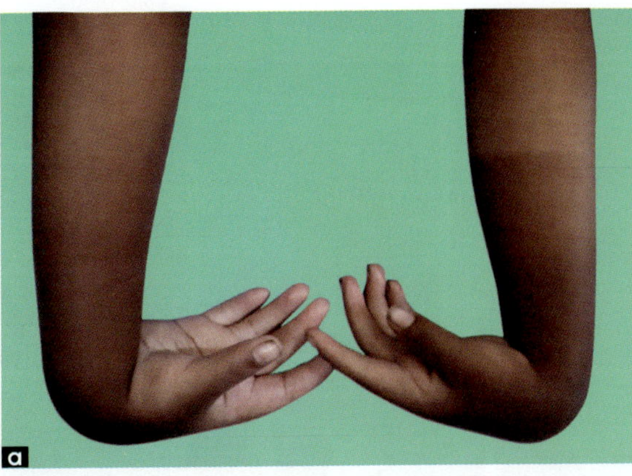

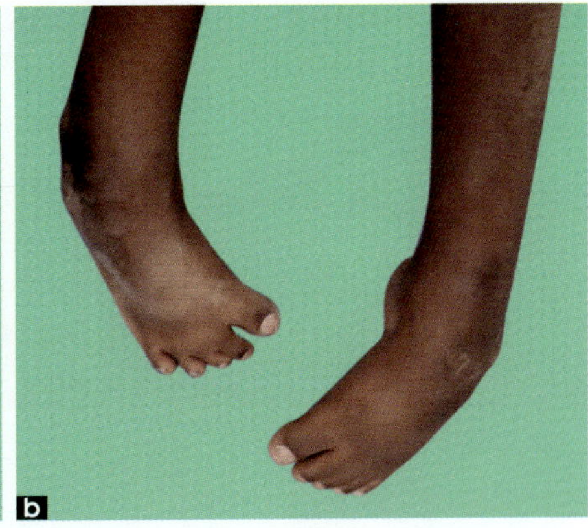

Fig. 15.29: AMC affection of both wrists (a), other joints are also involved (b). Note absence of elbow creases.

adducted across the palms (thumb-in-palm deformity) and the fingers are flexed and rigid.

15.8 EXAMINATION OF THE HIP JOINT

Typically, the common symptoms related to the hip joint are pain, decreased movements/ stiffness, and in a walking child, limp **(Key Box 2)**. Sometimes, the pain related to the hip joint is referred to the thigh region and knee. Warmth related to joint inflammation is seldom manifested externally, hip being a deep joint covered with muscles.

Inspection

Examination of the hip begins with watching the child walk. Hip should be examined in standing, sitting, and lying down positions from front, side and back.

- Observe the levels of shoulder and bony prominences like anterior superior iliac spine (ASIS), iliac crest and posterior superior iliac spine (PSIS, dimple of Venus) and compare with the normal side.
- Also observe spine for abnormal curvatures as in case of some spinal deformities, there can be compensatory pelvic abnormalities and vice-versa.
- Look for presence of any swelling or fullness in groin, thigh, or gluteal region.
- Observe for any quadriceps/gluteal wasting or asymmetry in the thigh/gluteal folds. Ask the child to sit cross-legged and squat to have idea about the functional status and gross range of movements.

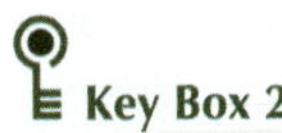

Key Box 2

The Irritable Hip

Irritable hip is non-specific term which indicates a variable combination of acute hip pain, joint stiffness, limp or non-weight bearing, indicative of an underlying disease. Septic arthritis, proximal femoral osteomyelitis, transient synovitis, tuberculosis, Perthes disease, SUFE are the common conditions leading to an irritable hip in a child. On examination, the hip is kept flexed, abducted and external rotated. Active and passive movements may be limited because of pain. Thorough general examination, relevant imaging and investigations help in arriving at the correct diagnosis.

Palpation

Tenderness over the joint line and bony prominences is elicited. Anterior hip joint line is palpated inferior and lateral to the mid inguinal point. Levels of greater trochanter and sacroiliac joints are compared on both sides. Also assess and compare the volume of femoral pulsations which may be weak or absent in case of posterior hip dislocation (*vascular sign of Narath*). A globular bony mass (femoral head) may be palpable in the gluteal region in these cases.

Range of Movements

First the child is asked to move the hip joint actively and then passive range of movements is elicited. To avoid pelvic movements while assessing hip movements, it is important to stabilize the pelvis with one hand by keeping thumb on ASIS and middle finger on PSIS. Normal range of movements of hip joint in all planes is described in the **Table 15.4 (Fig. 15.30)**.

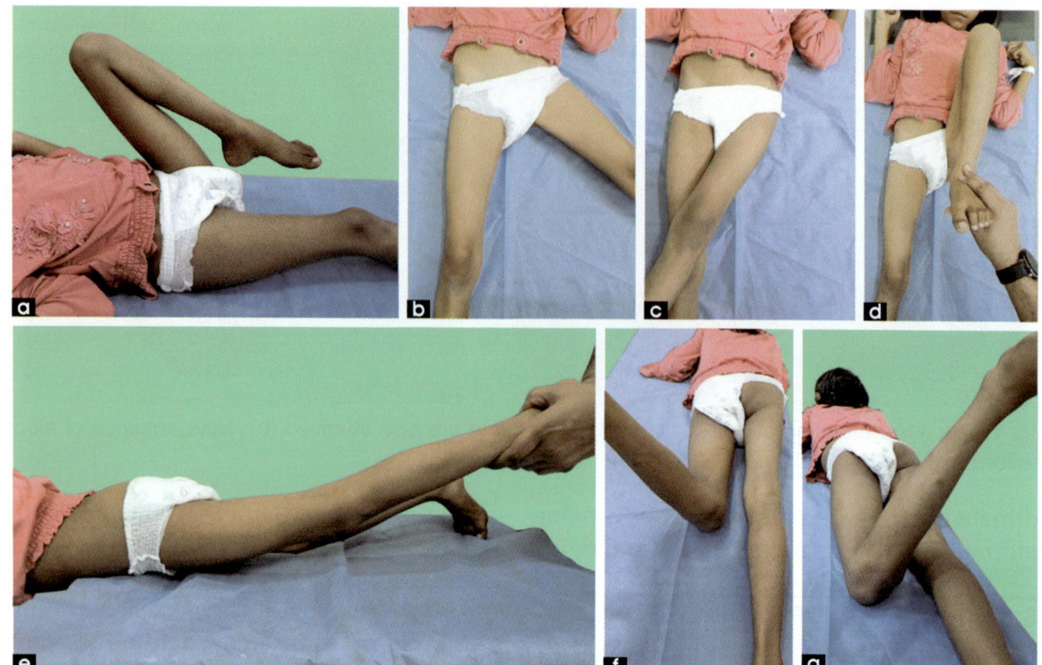

Fig. 15.30: While child is supine. Hip flexion (a), in normal children, it is possible to touch the front of thigh to abdomen; abduction (b), adduction (c), rotations with hip and knee in 90 degrees flexion. In prone position. Extension (e), another method of checking hip rotations, with hip neutral and knee flexed (f,g).

Table 15.4: Normal range of hip movements

Movements	Range in degrees
Flexion	0–130
Extension	0–20
Adduction	0–35 to 45
Abduction	0–45 to 55
Internal rotation	0–30 to 40
External rotation	0–40 to 50

- Rotational deformities are assessed by checking rotation arcs in both hip extension and 90° flexion. Range of movements are always compared with the normal side. Some pathologies have characteristic restriction of movements and should be kept in mind.
- Painless restriction of abduction is characteristic of developmental dysplasia of hip (DDH).
- Abduction and internal rotation are restricted in Perthes' disease.
- Abduction, internal rotation, and flexion can be decreased in slipped upper femoral epiphysis (SUFE).

Special Tests

Thomas Test

It is used to quantify the fixed flexion deformity. Patient lies supine on a hard surface. The unaffected hip is flexed till lumbar lordosis is obliterated. The flexion deformity at the hip is revealed as the diseased hip goes into flexion by itself (Fig. 15.31).

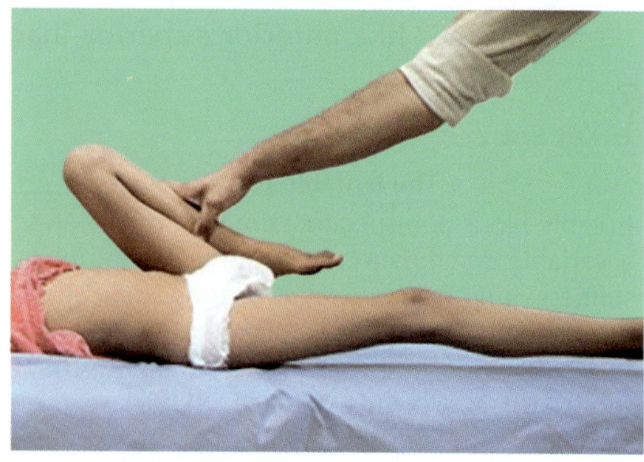

Fig. 15.31: Thomas test. The unaffected hip is flexed till low back and sacra are flat on the table. Avoid pulling unaffected hip into too much flexion, creating a posterior tilt of the pelvis which pulls the tested thigh off table. Flexion deformity, if present in the diseased hip, reveals itself.

Compensations

There are many compensations which body makes to bring both limbs parallel for standing/walking as well as lying down. In presence of shortening and deformity of one limb, these compensations can either accentuate or mask the true limb length discrepancy.

- *Apparent measurement* is done by placing both limbs parallel to each other and measuring the distance from a fixed midline bony prominence (xiphisternum) to tips of medial malleolus on both sides. To remove the effect of pelvic compensation one need to bring the level of both ASIS at the same level by abducting/adducting the limb.
- *True measurement* is now done by keeping the normal limb in identical mirror image position of the affected limb and measuring the distance between ASIS and medial malleolus on either side. While the child is standing, blocks can be added beneath the short foot till the pelvis is square. The total height of blocks gives the precise measurement of limb shortening (Fig. 15.32).

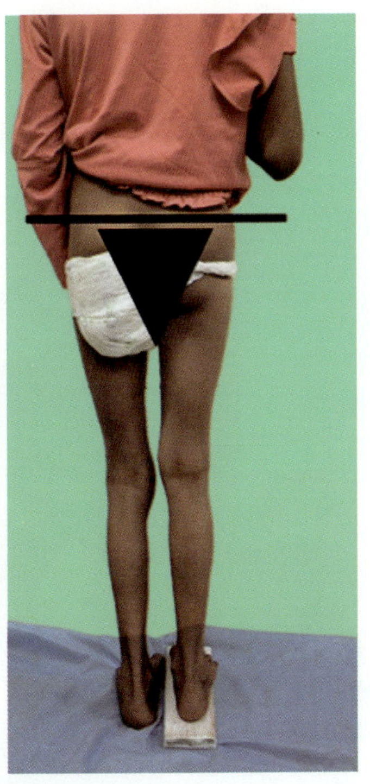

Fig. 15.32: Limb length discrepancy measurement using block method.

Allis Sign/Galeazzi Test (Fig. 15.33)

Further assessment includes, identifying whether the shortening is in the thigh section or leg. Allis sign/Galeazzi test is performed by flexing the hip and knee to rest both the feet together on the couch and checking the levels of knees. Modifications of the test can be used identify shortening in thigh/leg or both.

Trendelenburg Test

A pain-free hip with no adduction or abduction deformity is a prerequisite to perform this test. The examiner stands behind the child who is asked to stand on the affected side and lift the normal side above the ground for 30 seconds. Posterior superior iliac spines (PSIS) are observed.

- If the PSIS of opposite side (normal hip) remains at the same level or rather is slightly raised above the level as compared to the affected side, the test is said to be negative and abductor function on the affected side can be considered normal.
- But if abductor function is impaired or weakened, the child is not able to hold the pelvis for 30 seconds and there is drop in pelvis on the opposite (normal) side indicated by the lower level of PSIS. This is called positive Trendelenburg test (Fig. 15.34).

Telescopy Test

This test is done to evaluate the stability of hip. Child is placed supine with hip at 90° flexion and some adduction and held by one hand at knee/thigh. The other hand is placed with thenar eminence at ASIS and fingers palpating posteriorly. Gentle push/pull force is applied by first hand and excursion of greater trochanter is palpated and compared to other side. A greater excursion on the affected side indicates instability of hip (Fig. 15.35). This can also be positive in cases of sequelae of septic hip where head is partially or completely resorbed or in cases of non-united fracture of neck femur.

Ortolani and Barlow's Tests

These are described for DDH for children less than 3 months of age (Fig. 15.36).

Ortolani test: For a dislocated but reducible hip, Ortolani test is described. Both limbs

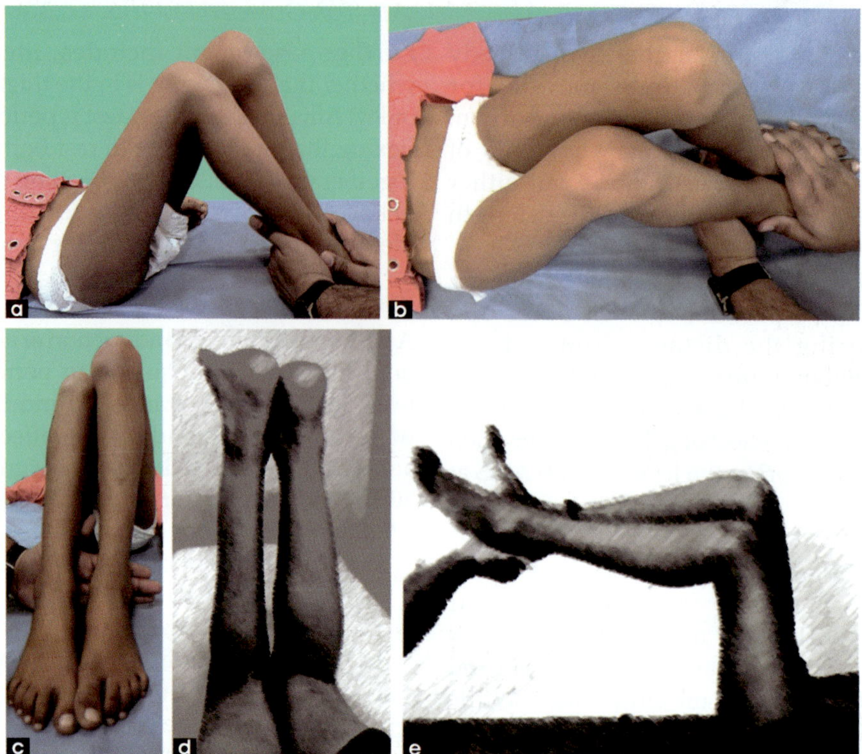

Fig. 15.33: Allis sign/Galeazzi test is performed by flexing the hip and knee to rest both the feet together on the couch and checking the levels of knees. The observations can be made from side (a), top (b) or from the side of feet (c). If tested in prone with thighs kept flat, differences in feet level indicated leg shortening (d). If the limbs are held with hip and knee flexed, thigh shortening can clearly be distinguished by comparing the knee levels.

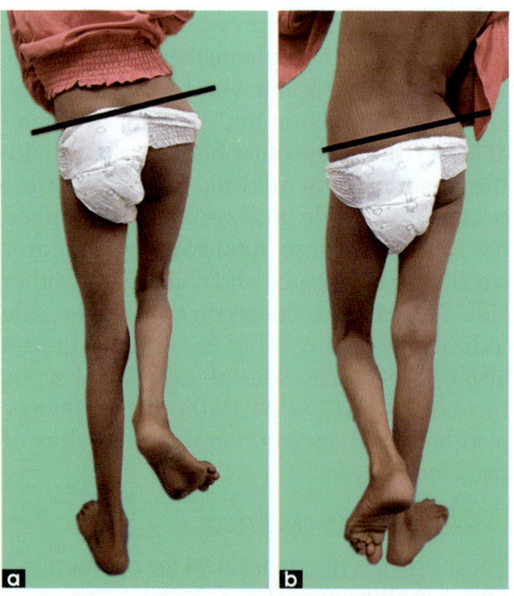

Fig. 15.34: Positive Trendelenburg test right side (a, b). Right hip is affected with impaired hip abduction mechanism.

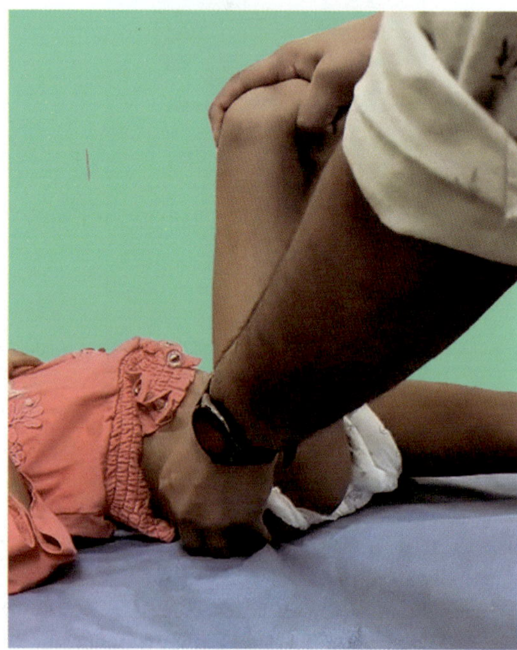

Fig. 15.35: Telescopy test.

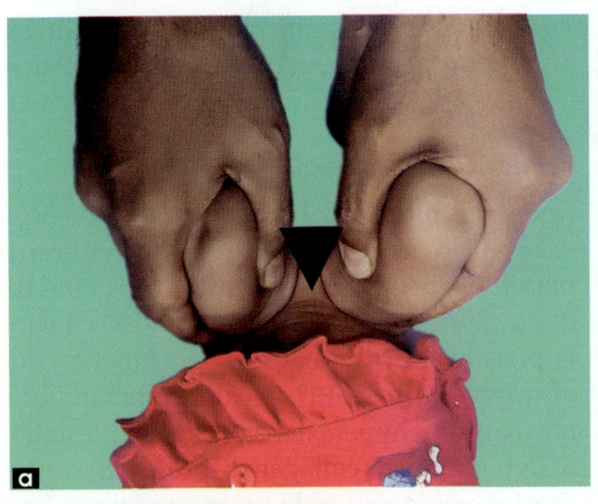

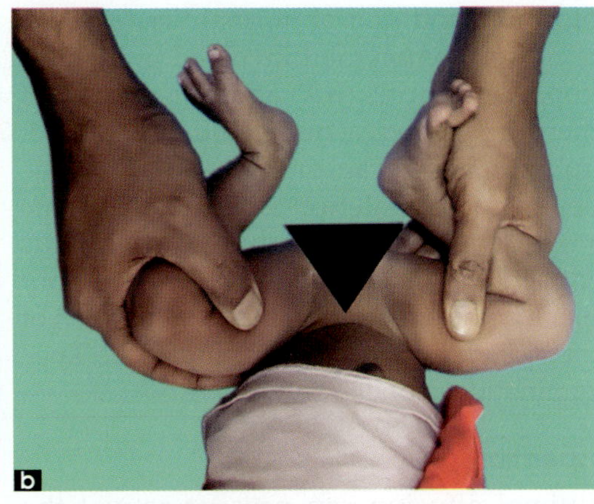

Fig. 15.36: Barlow's (a) Gentle posterior pressure over the knee in line with femur with adduction at hip is given and either a clunk (dislocatable) or a sensation of sliding (subluxatable hip) is felt in the region of greater trochanter. Ortolani test; (b) both limbs are held with hips and knees in flexion and the examiner keeps his thumb on the medial aspect of thigh and fingers posterolaterally over the greater trochanter. Attempt to reduce a dislocated hip is made by gentle traction, abduction and pushing anteriorly with the fingers.

are held with hips and knees in flexion and the examiner keeps his thumb on the medial aspect of thigh and fingers posterolaterally over the greater trochanter. Attempt to reduce a dislocated hip is made by gentle traction, abduction and pushing anteriorly with the fingers. A clunk is felt when the femoral head reduces and sits in the acetabular socket.

Barlow's maneuver: For a femoral head that is reduced but is dislocatable or subluxable, Barlow's maneuver is described. Gentle posterior pressure over the knee in line with femur with adduction at hip is given and either a clunk (dislocatable) or a sensation of sliding (subluxatable hip) is felt in the region of greater trochanter. Positive test warrants ultrasound evaluation and a detailed clinical examination preferably by a pediatric orthopedist.

Specific Conditions

Knowledge of characteristic presentation and age distribution, followed by a detailed history are prerequisites to any hip examination.

- Complain of decreased movements of the hip with a history of critical care admission and fever in a neonate, should raise a suspicion of septic arthritis of the hip.
- A click sound felt by parents while changing the diaper in infancy or painless limp when the child starts to walk could be a feature of developmental dysplasia of hip (DDH).
- In 4–8 years of age group, Perthes' disease is a possibility.
- Slipped upper femoral epiphysis (SUFE) is more common in pre-pubertal age (12–15 years in boys, 11–13 years in girls) usually during the 2nd growth spurt. It could be associated with some endocrinopathy or metabolic bone disease.

Developmental Dysplasia of Hip (DDH)

It occurs in 0.5 to 1% of all newborn babies with frank dislocation seen in around 0.1% infants. DDH represents a spectrum of hip abnormalities, ranging from a mildly dysplastic hip to one that is completely dislocated. If diagnosed early, DDH can often be managed non-operatively using brace treatment, which allows the hip joint to mature normally. However, undetected or late diagnosed DDH often requires more invasive surgical treatments. Asymmetrical thigh creases, unequal knee levels due to limb shortening and limited hip abduction of the affected side may be detected. In a neonate and young infant, special tests (Ortolani and Barlow's test) may be elicited. In a walking child, a positive Trendelenburg sign and a limp are detectable.

15.9 EXAMINATION OF THE KNEE JOINT

Common presenting symptoms can be pain, swelling, limitation of movements, deformity, and gait abnormalities. Knee is the most common joint involved in juvenile idiopathic arthritis (JIA) and thus history of other joint involvements should be enquired. Hip pathologies can present as pain in the knee region or anterior aspect of thigh due to overlapping nerve supply. An equinus contracture at ankle can lead to a compensatory flexion at the knee joint. Thus, examination of other joints of the limb precludes the knee examination proper.

Inspection

Minimal effusion can present as just the obliteration of groves by the side of patellar ligament. Localized swellings could be an abscess or of subcutaneous origin. Position of patella is noticed and compared to other side. Wasting of distal quadriceps/ vastus medialis is observed.

Palpation

- Palpation starts with feeling the temperature with back of hand and comparing with the other side.
- Bony landmarks and joint line are looked for point tenderness. The dip between the tibial and femoral condylar prominence on both sides are the medial and lateral joint lines. These are in continuation of the depression on either side of the patellar ligament and can be confirmed by some movement of the joint. Tenderness can be due to injury to a meniscus, collateral ligament or an arthritic joint. Tenderness should also be elicited over medial femoral condyle (osteochondritis dissecans), lateral and medial tibial condyles (synovitis/ meniscus tears), fibular head and tibial tuberosity (Osgood-Schlatter's disease) (Fig. 15.37).
- Palpate for any lump/localised swelling in the popliteal region (popliteal aneurysm or Baker's cyst).

Range of Movements

Knee is a modified hinge joint and flexion–extension are the primary movements possible. Thigh and leg in a straight line is the neutral position and around 140–150° flexion is possible till the back of leg touches that of thigh. Up to 5–10° of extension can occur normally but hyperextension is a manifestation of hyperlaxity or collagen disorders like Ehler-Danlos syndrome and Larsen syndrome. Both passive and active range of movements are assessed and documented. Lack of active full extension that can be corrected passively is usually caused by quadriceps weakness. This is referred to as extension lag or quadriceps lag.

Special Tests

Grinding or friction test is performed by pressing the patella against the femur and moving it from side-to-side. Painful grating is present in patella-femoral arthritis or chondromalacia patellae.

Patellar tap test. In cases of moderate effusion, when patella is pushed down by a tap from fingertip, it strikes the femoral surface and bounces back. This is also called patellar ballottement (Fig. 15.38).

Anterior drawer test: Knee is subject to rotational strains, especially in contact sports. There are chances of injury to the cruciate ligaments. Anterior drawer test is performed by flexing the knee to 90° with foot resting on couch. Proximal end of tibia is grabbed by

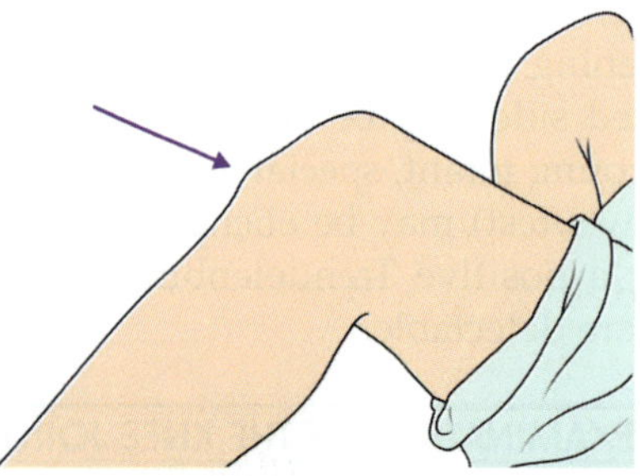

Fig. 15.37: Osgood-Schlatter disease is a condition that causes pain and swelling over tibial tuberosity.

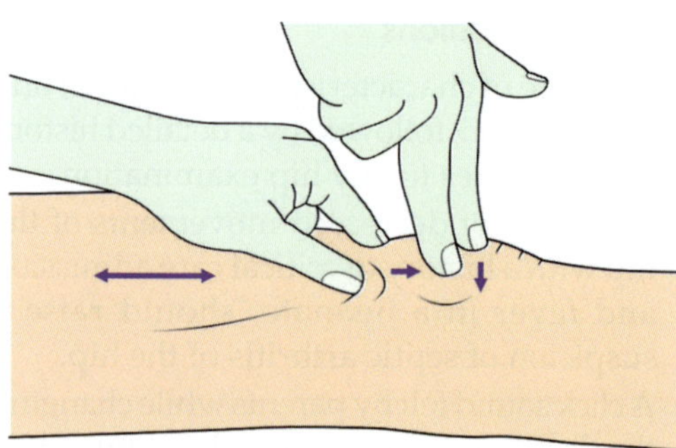

Fig. 15.38: Patellar ballottement or patellar tap test is performed for moderate effusions.

both hands and a forward thrust is applied. Forward migration of tibia with respect to femur occurs in case of anterior cruciate ligament injuries.

Posterior drawer test: Similarly, posterior translation of tibia on posterior thrust is due to posterior cruciate ligament insufficiency (*posterior drawer test*) (Fig. 15.39).

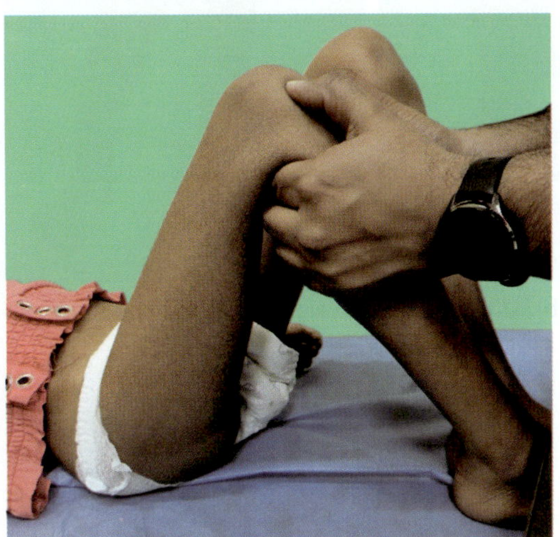

Fig. 15.39: Knee is kept in 90 degrees flexed position and feet firmly stabilized to perform anterior and posterior drawer tests.

Knee instability test: In 30° knee flexion, knee is held with one hand and varus/valgus stress is given with the other hand (Fig. 15.40). Any opening or pain on lateral/medial side of knee might suggest an injury to the lateral/medial collateral ligaments.

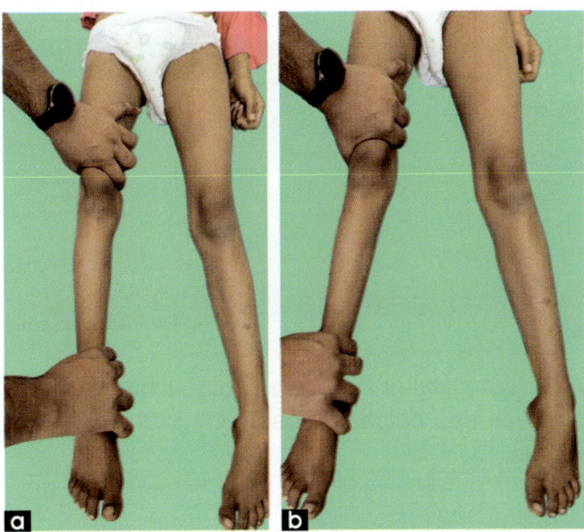

Fig. 15.40: Varus (a) and valgus (b) stress tests for knee instability.

While extending the flexed knee, normally the patella moves in a straight line or slight medially initially and then centers again in full extension. Excessive gliding or deviation to one side should be observed. Examiner also tries to subluxate the patella laterally with his fingers and sudden pain indicates a positive patellar apprehension test, indicating *patellar instability* (Fig. 15.41).

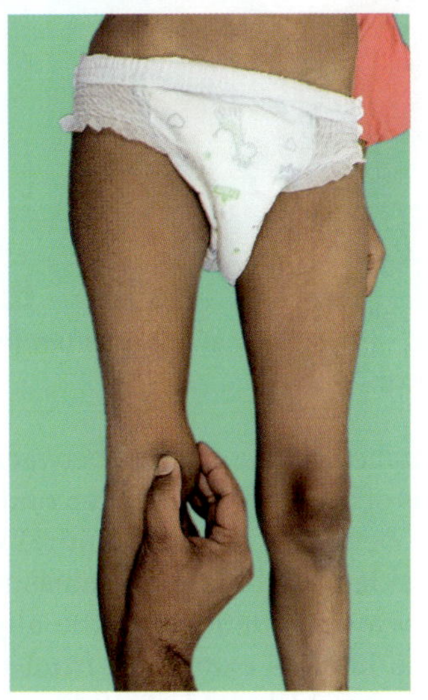

Fig. 15.41: Patellar apprehension test.

Specific Conditions

Genu Varum, Valgum and Recurvatum

For any joint, valgus is when the part distal to the joint points away from the midline and varus is when the distal part points towards the midline. Normal alignment at the knee joint keeps changing as the child grows. There is an increasing varus alignment peaking at around 1–1.5 years of age. As the child grows, this varus alignment decreases gradually and converts into valgus alignment which keeps increasing with maximum valgus at around 3–4 years of age. This physiological valgus slowly corrects and reaches the adult alignment by the age of 7 years. Normal adult alignment is that of slight (5–10°) valgus. These physiological variations (Fig. 15.42) should always be kept in mind before labelling the alignment as a deformity. Nevertheless, any varus/ valgus beyond physiological limits and any unilateral/asymmetrical deformity should be thoroughly evaluated for a pathological cause.

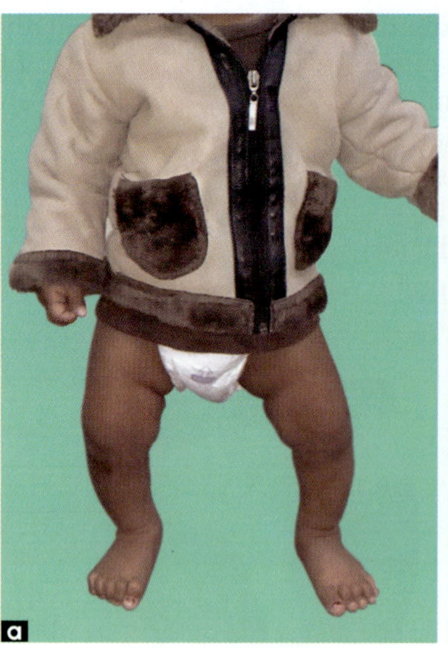

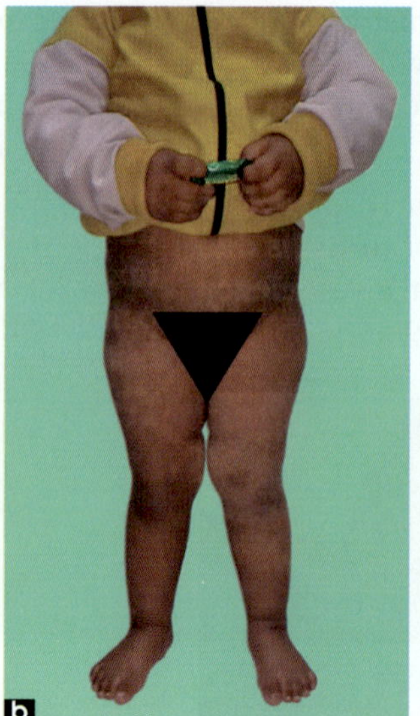

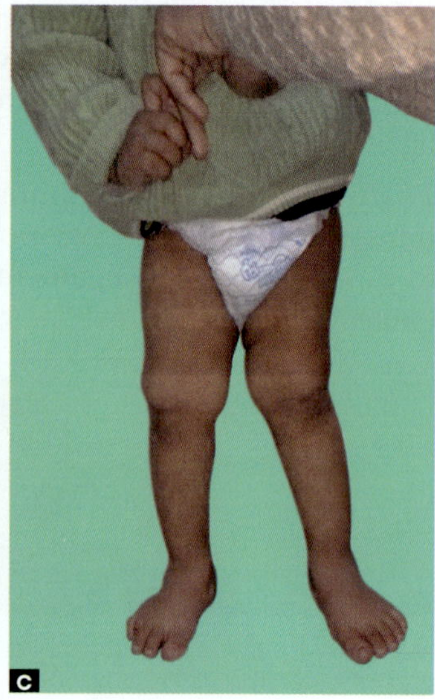

Fig. 15.42: Physiological genu varum (a), valgum (b). Unilateral genu valgum left side and therefore pathological.

Intermalleolar (the distance between medial malleolus of both sides) and intercondylar (the distance between medial femoral condyle of both sides) distances are measured and are one way of quantifying the alignment. When the knee is examined from the side, the child should be able to fully straighten the knee. A few degrees of hyperextension can be normal, especially in children with generalized ligamentous laxity, but more than 10° of hyperextension indicates *genu recurvatum* (back knees) characteristic of hypermobility syndrome. Inability to achieve full extension or a fixed flexion deformity is always pathological.

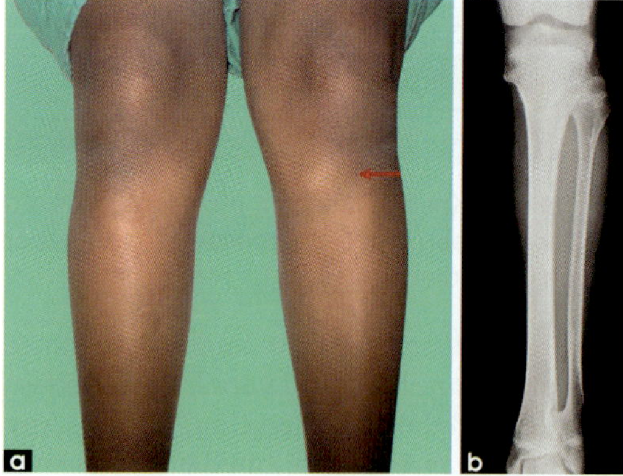

Fig. 15.43: Osteochondroma over proximal tibia left side (a), corresponding radiographs (b).

Osteochondroma of the Knee Region

Osteochondromas are common over distal femur and proximal tibia **(Fig. 15.43)**. They are usually asymptomatic and present with cosmetic complaints. If the location is posterior or lateral, neurovascular structures may be at risk of stretching. Sometimes, large osteochondromas are responsible for muscle stretching and pain.

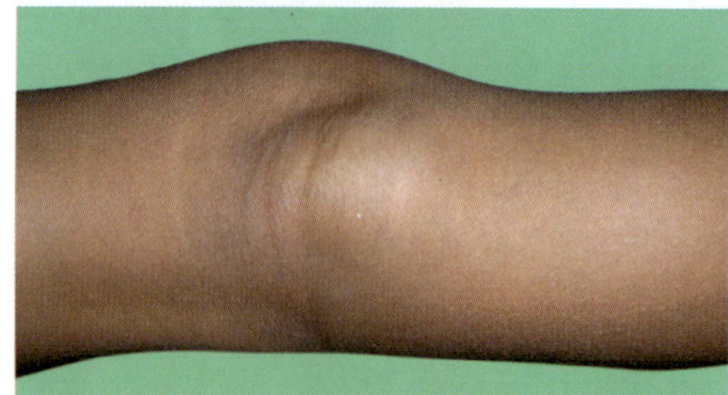

Fig. 15.44: Baker's cyst is an outpouching from the synovial sac palpable posteriorly in the popliteal region.

Baker's Cyst **(Fig. 15.44)**

The area at the back of the knee is called the 'popliteal space', so a Baker's cyst is also called a 'popliteal cyst'. Baker's cysts occur more commonly in boys between 4–8 years old. They present as a painless lump behind the knee more obvious while knee is extended. They have tendency to resolve spontaneously. Parental concerns are mainly cosmetic.

15.10. EXAMINATION OF THE ANKLE AND FOOT

The usual presenting symptoms in the ankle and foot can be pain, deformity, swelling, or restriction of movements. Apart from 'idiopathic' causes, foot deformities can be secondary to neuromuscular disease (cerebral palsy/syringomyelia/myelomeningocele) or syndromic affections (arthrogryposis multiplex congenita). Thus, examination of spine, other joints and facies becomes important in examination of this region. Also, always consider the child's age, developmental stage, and individual variations in the interpretation of the examination findings.

Inspection

Observe for any obvious deformity in both resting and standing positions.

Note ankle/foot movements and position during walking. Position of heel with respect to calf (eversion/inversion) is observed. A 5–10° eversion (valgus) of heel in standing position can be considered normal but any valgus beyond that or any varus (inversion) should warrant further evaluation.

Equinus and calcaneus refer to angulation of the ankle in plantar flexion and dorsiflexion, respectively. On standing, lowering of longitudinal arch (pes planus/flat feet) or a high arch (pes cavus) may be observed from medial aspect (Fig. 15.45).

Palpation

Tenderness is palpated at various bony landmarks like medial and lateral malleolus, heel, tendoachilles, various small joints and bones in the foot. Anterior joint line is palpated just distal to the lower end of tibia and any effusion may cause bulges in this region.

Range of Movements

When viewed from side, foot at the right angle to the leg is considered a neutral position. Movements at the ankle joint (tibio-talar joint) causing foot to move towards leg is called dorsiflexion (normal range, 15–25°) and opposite is plantar flexion (normal range, 40–50°) (Fig. 15.46). To assess subtalar movements, patient is made to lie prone and ankle is held in neutral or slightly dorsiflexed position. With one hand supporting the distal leg, calcaneum is grasped with other hand and turned inward (inversion) to 30° and outward (eversion) to 20°. Newborns may keep their ankle and foot in some specific posture due to *in utero* positioning and may be confused with a deformity. Gentle tickling on all sides of foot may reveal active range but a good passive range comparable on both sides should help the clinician in ruling out a deformity.

Specific Conditions

Flat Foot

Lowering of medial longitudinal arch is referred to as *flat foot (pes planus)*. Toddlers have a fat pad in the region of arch which obliterates the arch and gives and appearance of flat foot. This disappears usually resolves between 2–5 years of age. Flat foot can again be flexible and rigid. Heel raise test and *Jack's toe raise test* are used to differentiate between the two (Fig. 15.47). A mild-to-moderate flexible flat foot should be considered a variant of normal foot and does not require treatment until symptomatic. A rigid flat foot has an underlying bony pathology like tarsal coalition or a congenital vertical talus **(rocker bottom foot)** (Fig. 15.48).

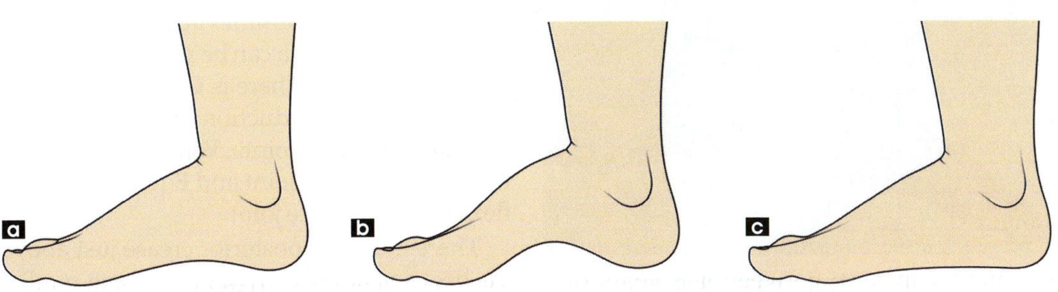

Fig. 15.45: Normal arch (a), high arch (b) and flat arch (c).

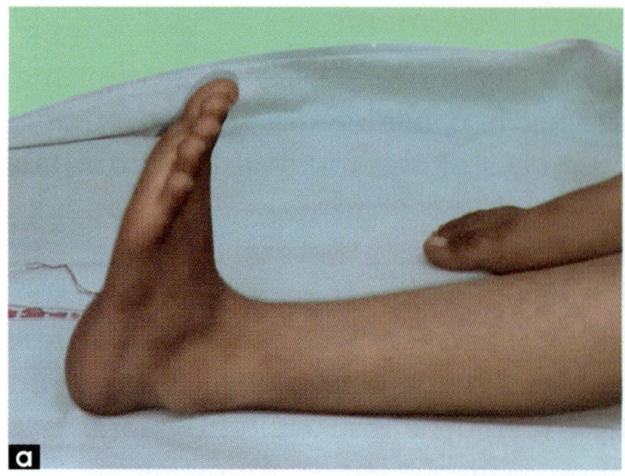

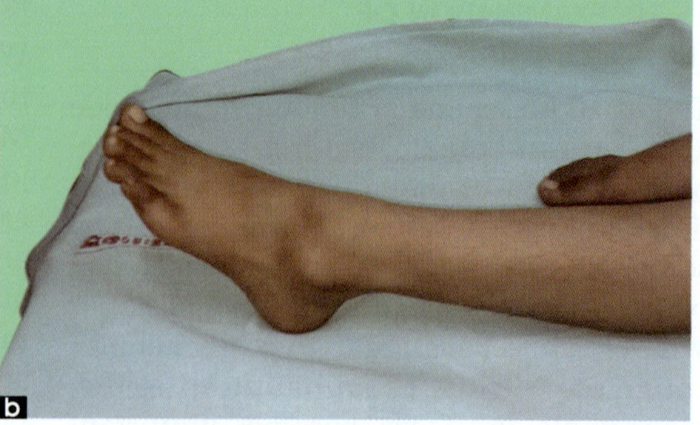

Fig. 15.46: Ankle dorsiflexion (a) and plantar flexion (b).

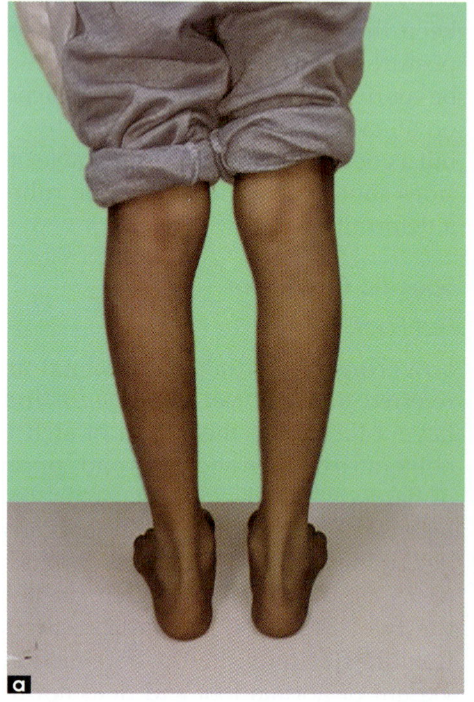

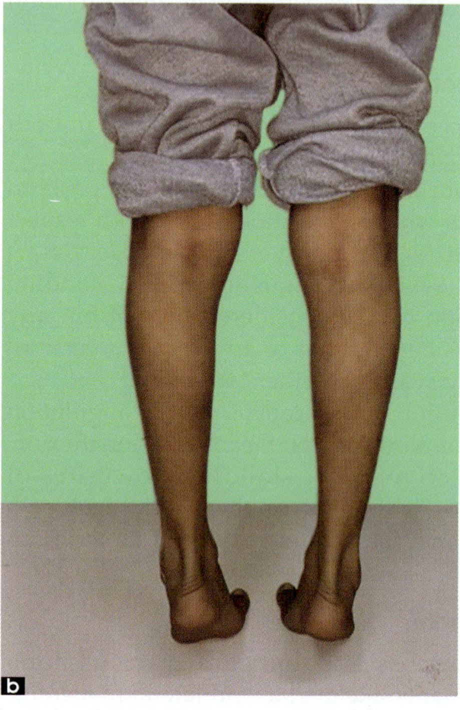

Fig. 15.47: There was flexible flat foot in this child (a). Arches became apparent with heel raise test (b).

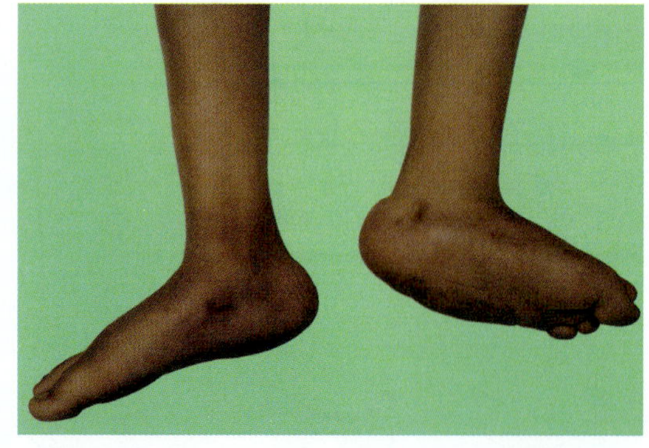

Fig. 15.48: Rigid flat foot in congenital vertical talus (left side).

Congenital Talipes Equino Varus (CTEV)

CTEV is one of the most common congenital anomalies of the feet **(Fig. 15.49)**. It is a combination of deformities at various joints of foot and ankle which can be remembered by a mnemonic CAVE. There is **C**avus (high arch) at the mid-foot, **A**dduction of the forefoot at the tarsometatarsal joints, **V**arus (inversion) at the heel or subtalar joint and **E**quinus (plantar flexion) at the ankle joint.

There is a deep posterior crease just above the heel and another one arising from medial border of foot. The lateral border of foot is

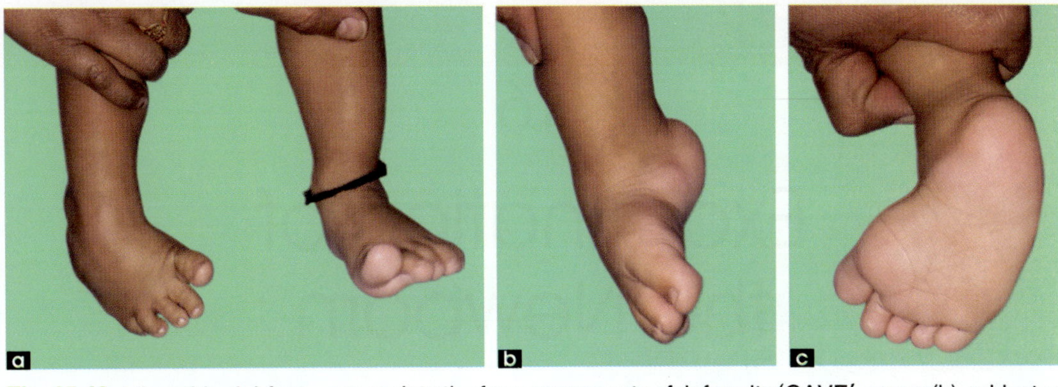

Fig. 15.49: Idiopathic clubfoot—appreciate the four components of deformity 'CAVE'- cavus (b), adductus (a, c), varus (c) and equinus (b).

long and curved and may have callosities in a walking child. The lateral head of the talus is palpable as a bony swelling over the dorsolateral aspect of foot. The heel is small, rotated and pulled up with an 'empty' feel on palpation. The calf may be thinner.

Metatarsus Adductus

Also known as metatarsus varus, is a common foot deformity that causes the forefoot to turn inward resulting in bean-shaped appearance (Fig. 15.50). There is no accompanying equinus and ankle dorsiflexion is full. It is thought to occur as a result of the infant's position inside the uterus.

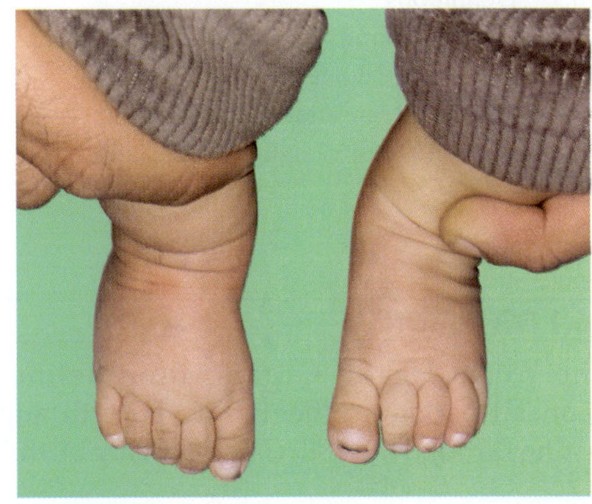

Fig. 15.50: Forefoot is turned inwards in metatarsus adductus.

Chapter

16

Examination of the Newborn

○ Ruchi Rai ○ Piyush Gupta

Structure

16.1 DEFINITIONS

The World Health Organization defines neonatal period as "beginning at birth and lasting through the 28th day following birth."

1. Categorization by Gestational Age

Neonates are classified as term, preterm, or post-term on basis of gestational age. Gestational age is estimated based on best obstetric estimate derived from last menstrual period (LMP) and first trimester sonography, rather than LMP alone **(Key Box 1)**. First trimester sonography is the most accurate method to confirm gestational age. If ultrasound dating before $14^{0/7}$ weeks differs by more than 7 days from LMP dating, the gestational age should be changed to correspond with the ultrasound dating.

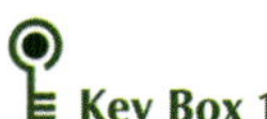

Key Box 1

Definitions of Newborn

1. *Neonate/newborn:* The infant from birth to four weeks (28 days)
2. *Early neonatal period:* First week (7 days) of life
3. *Late neonatal period:* From 7th to less than 28th day of life
4. *Newly born:* Infant in the first minutes to few hours after birth
5. *Stillbirth:* A fetal death at a gestational age of 28 weeks or more or weighing more than 1000 grams (WHO)
6. *Perinatal period:* From 28 weeks of gestation, to 7 completed days after birth

Gestational age is expressed as completed weeks. For example, a 32-week, 6-day fetus is considered a 32-week fetus. If pregnancy was achieved using assisted reproductive technology (ART), ART-derived gestational age should be used considering the age of the embryo and the date of transfer. This can be calculated by adding age of embryo and 2 weeks to the date of embryo transfer.

Chronological age (days, weeks, months, or years): Age since birth.

Postmenstrual age (weeks): Gestational age plus chronological age.

Corrected age (weeks or months): Chronological age reduced by the number of weeks born before 40 weeks of gestation. This term should be used only for children up to 3 years of age who were born preterm.

During the initial period of neonatal hospital stay, 'postmenstrual age' is preferred to describe the age of preterm infants. After the perinatal period, 'postmenstrual or corrected

Key Box 2

Newborn	Classification
Term	$37^{0/7}$–$41^{6/7}$ weeks gestation (early term: $37^{0/7}$–$38^{6/7}$ weeks; full term: $39^{0/7}$–$40^{6/7}$ weeks; late term: $41^{0/7}$–$41^{6/7}$ weeks)
Preterm	Less than 37 weeks gestation (late preterm: $34^{0/7}$–$36^{6/7}$ weeks; moderate preterm: $32^{0/7}$–$33^{6/7}$ weeks; very preterm: $28^{0/7}$–$31^{6/7}$ weeks; extremely preterm: <28 weeks)
Post-term	42 weeks gestation or more
LBW	Birth weight less than 2500 g
VLBW	Birth weight less than 1500 g
ELBW	Birth weight less than 1000 g
AGA	Birth weight between 10th and 90th percentile for gestational age
SGA	Birth weight below 10th percentile for gestational age
LGA	Birth weight greater than 90th percentile for gestational age

age' is the preferred term. 'Conceptional age,' 'postconceptional age,' 'conceptual age,' and 'postconceptual age' should not be used. A *term infant* is one whose birth occurs from 37 to less than 42 weeks of gestation. A *preterm* is one whose birth has occurred before 37 weeks of gestation, while a post-term infant is one who is delivered at or after 42 completed weeks **(Key Box 2)**.

2. Categorization by Birth Weight

Neonates are also classified according to birth weight. Low birth weight (LBW) neonates are defined as those having a birth weight of less than 2500 grams. Very low birth weight infants (VLBW) are those weighing less than 1500 grams at birth, while extremely low birth weight (ELBW) infants have a birth weight less than 1000 grams.

These classifications help in establishing the risk level for neonatal mortality, morbidity, and long-term developmental problems.

3. Categorization by Weight for Gestational Age

According to weight for gestational age, neonates are classified as small for gestational age (SGA), appropriate for gestational age (AGA), and large for gestational age (LGA).

SGA babies are defined as those having birth weight less than 10th percentile for a particular gestational age, while LGA babies have a birth weight greater than 90th percentile for that gestational age. AGA babies have birth weight between 10th and 90th percentile for their gestational age.

16.2 HISTORY-TAKING

The mother is the most reliable person to give information about her baby. A detailed maternal history is very important in evaluating a newborn baby. The maternal records should be screened thoroughly and this gives a lot of information which the mother may not be able to tell. The records must be checked for the pre-pregnancy weight, weight gain during pregnancy, mother blood group or any abnormal findings documented by the obstetrician. Components of neonatal history are summarized in **Key Box 3**.

A. Family and Maternal History

Family History

History of neonatal deaths in the extended family can point towards genetic disorders like inborn errors of metabolism. Details about the other siblings like the gender, age, medical illnesses (if any) and growth and development are important. Also inquire about family history of genetic disorders, tuberculosis or any other chronic or congenital problems.

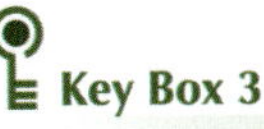

Key Box 3

Components of Neonatal History

1. Maternal, paternal and family history
2. History of antenatal events
3. Details of birth
4. History of immediate postnatal events
5. History of feeding, activity, and weight gain
6. Specific complaints, if any

Pre-pregnancy

Obtain history about any maternal illness before pregnancy. Ask about maternal diabetes, hypertension, thyroid disorders, any other chronic illness, and drug intake as these can affect the fetus and the newborn. Also, ask about the consanguinity of marriage, especially in suspected genetic illness.

Obstetric History

A detailed obstetric history will give you information about the gravidity, parity, or any abortions. Ask about any previous pregnancy-related complications, any birth-related complications, stillbirths, neonatal deaths or NICU admissions in previous births. Any such history will have an implication for this baby as it may be at high risk of developing a similar complication. The history of jaundice requiring phototherapy or exchange transfusion in a previous baby can be a clue for Rh/ABO incompatibility or genetic causes of neonatal hyperbilirubinemia.

B. Antenatal History

Ask whether the conception was spontaneous or assisted. An accurate gestational age can be calculated, if the mother is sure of the date of the 1st day of last menstrual period (LMP). We must know whether it was a singleton pregnancy or multiple gestation. Screen medical records of the mother. Obtain hemoglobin, blood group, HIV status from records. Record detailed trimester-wise history **(Key Box 4)**.

First trimester: The history of fever, rash, radiation exposure, drug intake may have an impact on the growing fetus. As the first trimester is the phase of organogenesis, any illness like intrauterine infections (toxoplasma, rubella, cytomegalovirus, herpes simplex, etc.) or drug exposure (including smoking and alcohol intake) can have teratogenic effect on the fetus.

2nd and 3rd trimesters: Details of antenatal checkups must be asked, like the number of antenatal visits, iron and folic acid supplementation, ultrasound scans and tetanus vaccination (Td). History of gestational diabetes, gestational hypertension, eclampsia, thyroid disorders, tuberculosis, anemia, blood transfusion or any other illness and medications, alcohol intake and smoking should be taken. History of polyhydramnios may point towards congenital anomalies, like esophageal atresia or duodenal atresia, and oligohydramnios may be due to fetal growth restriction, renal dysgenesis, or agenesis. If the mother is Rh-negative, you should ask about the administration of anti-D in pregnancy. Maternal HIV and hepatitis B status should be enquired. History of varicella, malaria, tuberculosis, and syphilis should also be taken, the baby can acquire these infections from the mother before, during or after birth.

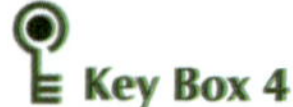

Key Box 4

Relevant Obstetric History

- *1st trimester:* Fever, skin rash, lymphadenopathy, exposure to any drug or radiation and history of folic acid intake during pre-conceptional period.
- *2nd and 3rd trimesters:* Antenatal care taken, iron and folate supplementation, receipt of two doses of tetanus toxoid, pregnancy-induced hypertension (PIH), gestational diabetes, anemia, infection, antepartum hemorrhage, leaking per vaginum, multiple pregnancy, fetal distress, bradycardia, or tachycardia, cervical incompetence, trauma, poly-hydramnios/oligohydramnios; peripartum fever, uterine tenderness, leucocytosis, glucocorticoids administration in case of preterm delivery before 34 weeks.
- Reports of physical and laboratory examination of the mother—findings of obstetric assessments done during pregnancy, blood pressure, blood sugar, complete blood count, blood grouping (ABO and Rh), HBsAg, TORCH screen, VDRL test, ELISA for HIV, etc.
- Assessment of fetal growth and condition.
- *Fetal testing:* Ultrasound examination, fetal monitoring, anti-D titer, amniocentesis, biophysical profile, Doppler velocimetry, genetic testing.
- Details of treatment received.
- Assessment of gestational age from LMP, and first trimester ultrasound.

C. Birth and Postnatal History

A detailed birth history becomes extremely important for babies presenting within first week of life. Record the age of the newborn (in hours in first 3 days) and thereafter in completed days.

Birth Details

Ask about onset and duration of labor, mode of delivery, abnormal presentation like breech, leaking per vaginum, bleeding per vaginum, foul smelling liquor, maternal fever during labor, and meconium-stained liquor. These might have implications for the immediate postnatal period. Ask whether the onset of labor was spontaneous or induced and in cases of Cesarean section, whether it was done as an emergency procedure or elective. An emergency cesarean section is usually done due to fetal compromise, therefore, the babies born are more at risk of complications. Bleeding per vaginum may cause anemia immediately after birth. Ask for the history or screen the maternal documents for administration of antenatal steroids in preterm deliveries.

Immediate Postnatal Details

Detailed history about the relevant events in the delivery room and timing of cry is important and is helpful in assessing the baby. History of delayed cry, Apgar score of the baby and details of resuscitation are other relevant information, that must be sought.

Risk of early onset sepsis (presenting <72 hours of birth)

- Leaking per vaginum >24 hours before birth
- Foul smelling liqor/discharge
- Confirmed or suspected intrauterine inflammation
- Prolonged labor >24 hours duration
- Severe perinatal asphyxia (Apgar score ≤3 at 1 min)
- Spontaneous preterm labor in absence of premature rupture of membranes

Preterm premature rupture of membranes (PPROM) is spontaneous rupture of membranes before 37 weeks of gestation before the onset of labor.

Feeding History

Ask the mother whether she is exclusively breastfeeding her baby. Ask about the frequency and duration of breastfeeds, whether the baby is being given night feeds or not. Ask the mother about any difficulty in feeding the baby. Breastfeeding may be painful for the mother during the initial days and may prevent the mother from exclusively breastfeeding the baby. She may have sore nipples or engorged breasts, which will need attention. If top milk is being given, then ask the mother the reason for giving it. Ask about the type of top milk being given, method of preparation and method of feeding.

Feeding pattern: A newborn demands breastfeeds every one and a half to two hours, as the mother's milk is easy to digest and the stomach gets empty very fast. The mother, therefore, develops a false belief that the baby is constantly crying, and her milk output is less.

Regurgitation: The tone of the lower esophageal sphincter is poor in newborns; therefore, they tend to regurgitate after feeds. The baby spits out the swallowed milk in the process. While feeding, the baby also swallows some air along with the milk. When the baby burps, this swallowed air is taken out by the baby. Along with air, some amount of milk is also taken out. This is a normal physiological phenomenon. This decreases as the baby grows older and the tone of the sphincter increases. A baby with physiological regurgitation grows well, is alert, healthy looking and gains good weight.

Vomiting: Be careful before labeling vomiting as physiological. Vomiting is pathological, if it is bile-stained, associated with abdominal distension or constipation, poor weight gain, or weight loss. Some congenital anomalies of the stomach and intestines may present with vomiting like, ileal or duodenal atresia and pyloric atresia/stenosis. Vomiting can also be due to many other non-abdominal causes like sepsis, raised intracranial tension, renal anomalies, and inborn errors of metabolism.

D. Bowel and Bladder History

Meconium: In the first 2–3 days of life, the newborn passes dark green sticky stools known as meconium (Fig. 16.1). Normally, a term newborn should pass meconium once within the first 24 hours of birth. If a healthy, term baby does not pass meconium on the first day of life, this could be due to hypothyroidism, imperforate anus, or Hirschsprung disease. The stools after 3–4 days then become thin, watery, and yellowish to greenish yellow.

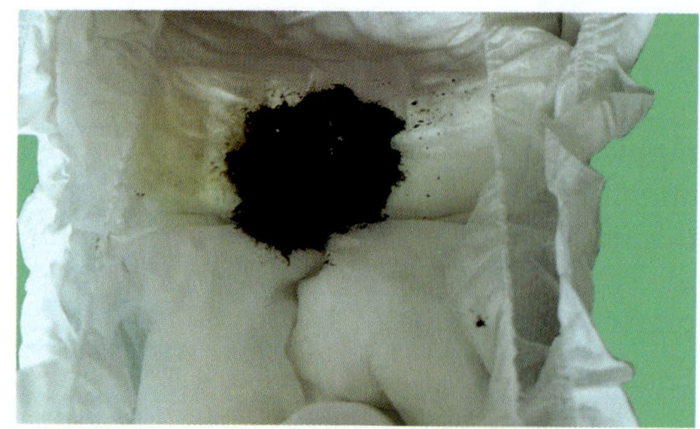

Fig. 16.1: Meconium.

Stools: Usually, a normal breastfed baby may pass stools which may vary in frequency from 1 per day to 12–15 per day. The gastrocolic reflex in newborns leads to passage of stools every time the baby feeds. This should not be considered as 'loose motions' or diarrhea. On the other hand, a breastfed baby may pass stool once in 4–5 days. This is not constipation; the stool is soft, and the baby has no discomfort in passing stools. There is no associated abdominal distension or vomiting.

A constipated baby passes hard stools which may be associated with blood and the baby has difficulty in passing stools. Also, there may be associated abdominal distension and vomiting. Constipation may be due to feeding with animal milk, hypothyroidism or Hirschsprung disease. This needs to be properly evaluated.

Urine: A newborn baby must pass urine within 48 hours of birth. Thereafter, the baby should pass urine at least 5–6 times in 24 hours. It is normal for newborns to cry just before and after passing urine or stool. It should not be mistaken for difficulty in passage of urine or stool.

Vaginal bleeding and discharge: Female newborns may have vaginal bleeding by the end of the first week of life. This is a normal hormonal withdrawal response, and the bleeding stops in 4–5 days without any treatment. Whitish thick vaginal discharge may occur in female babies from day 2–3 of life and subsides in a week.

E. Time Specific History

1. History-taking on Day 1

Ask whether the baby has started breast-feeding. Ask whether the newborn has passed urine and meconium. This has been discussed in the earlier text. A normal baby should pass meconium within 24 hours. Intestinal obstruction and Hirschsprung disease are two important causes for delayed passage of meconium. A few babies pass meconium *in utero*, in response to fetal distress; always check the records before sending investigations. *In-utero* passage of meconium in breech presentation may be normal.

Look for any pallor, jaundice, cyanosis, etc. Any jaundice within the first 24 hours of life must be considered pathological. Ask for any abnormal movements, head swelling, bleeding, respiratory difficulty, abdominal distension, and vomiting.

2. History-taking between 24 and 48 Hours

Ask for feeding difficulties. Look for correct signs of positioning and attachment. As the ductus closes, congenital heart diseases (duct-dependent cyanotic heart diseases) may manifest. Ask for cyanosis, respiratory distress, and feeding difficulty. Assess the extent of jaundice.

Most newborns pass urine in 48 hours. Also, ask for the character of stream of urine. A poor stream in a male newborn may be due to posterior urethral valve.

3. History-taking between 48 Hours and 7 Days

Ask whether the baby is feeding and sleeping well. Ask and look for danger signs, such as lethargy, refusal to feed, respiratory distress, cyanosis, yellow discoloration of body including palms and soles, abnormal movements, hematemesis, melena, vomiting, and abdominal distension. A healthy breastfed baby should pass light-colored urine at least 6 times a day after 48 hours of life.

4. History-taking between 1 and 4 Weeks

This should focus on symptoms such as lethargy, refusal to feed, diarrhea, vomiting, respiratory distress, abnormal movements/ seizures. Enquire also about the stool color and diaper staining of urine, which could be a pointer towards neonatal cholestasis.

Key Box 5 summarizes the various points to be ascertained while obtaining neonatal history.

Key Box 5

History of the Neonate

- Age of baby
- Birth weight; gestational age; any abnormalities detected
- Whether delayed cord clamping (>one minute) and immediate skin-to-skin contact done.
- Whether the baby was kept in observation or shifted to neonatal unit, if yes, then why?
- Whether vitamin K injection given after birth.
- *Feeds given:* Details of breastfeeding, e.g. at what time after birth first feed was given, whether colostrum was given, how many times mother is feeding now including night feeds
- Time of passing urine and meconium.

Any clinical problems, e.g. hypothermia, respiratory distress, lethargy, refusal to feed, persistent vomiting, diarrhea, abdominal distension, bleeding from any site, jaundice, abnormal movements, etc.

16.3 WHEN TO EVALUATE?

In the clinical practice of neonatology, there are at least 5 occasions of neonatal examination, which are summarized in **Key Box 6**. Although, there are many overlaps in these examinations, each has a different purpose or requirement.

1. First Assessment at Birth

The first examination of the baby immediately after birth is the most important examination. Immediately after the baby is born, a quick assessment of the gestational age, breathing/crying and tone must be done. Based on this examination, the further steps of resuscitation are done as per the neonatal resuscitation guidelines.

After initial steps of resuscitation have been done, the baby has been stabilized, it should be evaluated in detail for the temperature, respiration, color, activity, any birth injury, and congenital malformations.

Key Box 6

Five Occasions of Newborn Assessment

1. Assessment at birth to identify the need for resuscitation
2. Assessment after one hour as the newborn completes immediate skin-to-skin contact
3. Assessment at 24 to 48 hours of age and before discharge
4. Well baby examination in follow-up/ office visits
5. Evaluation of the sick neonate

Gender should be assigned immediately after birth. In case of ambiguous genitalia, the parents and family must be informed, and further evaluation should be initiated. Proper documentation of all the examination findings, whether normal or abnormal must be done.

Apgar Score

Named after Dr Virginia Apgar, it comprises of 5 parameters **(Table. 16.1)**. The score is used to assess the severity of asphyxia suffered the baby. It is done at 1 and 5 minutes of birth. If the score at 5 minutes ≤6, then it is noted at every 5 minutes till at least 20 minutes. We must note that the steps of neonatal resuscitation are not guided by the Apgar score. It is good score to represent the baby's condition in the labor room and useful for prediction of long-term neurodevelopmental outcome. One minute Apgar score does not correlate with the neonatal outcomes. A score <5 at 5 or 10 min of birth is associated with high mortality in the neonatal period and risk of cerebral palsy in the survivors.

2. Early Newborn Examination

This should be done after one-hour period of immediate skin-to-skin contact is over. Take care not to expose the infant to inappropriate cold stress. Note the following:

Table 16.1: Apgar score

Parameter	0	1	2
Color	Pale/cyanosis	Acrocyanosis	Pink
Heart rate	Absent	<100/min	≥100/min
Respiration	Absent	Weak cry, hypoventilation	Good, cry vigorous
Tone	Limp	Some flexion	Active motion
Reflex irritability	No response	Grimace	Cry or withdrawal

- *Appropriate signs of successful transition to the extrauterine environment,* by noting all vital signs and observing for general alertness, color, signs of respiratory distress, heart rate, rhythm, and ability to suck, swallow, and handle secretions.
- *Correct sex determination:* Delay sex assignment if any ambiguity is noted.
- *Anthropometrical parameters:* Weight, length, and head circumference.

Examination for Congenital Anomalies

Key Box 7 lists several conditions where a congenital anomaly should be suspected. Examine accordingly.

- Examine the cut end of umbilical cord for the presence of two arteries and one vein. Single umbilical artery occurs in approximately 1–2% of births and is associated with chromosomal and other congenital anomalies.
- Examine for any gross congenital anomaly, such as cleft lip (Fig. 16.2a), cleft palate (Fig. 16.2b), neural tube defects (Fig. 16.3), omphalocele (Fig. 16.4), congenital talipoequinovarus (CTEV) (Fig. 16.5), and polydactyly (Fig. 16.6).
- Suspect diaphragmatic hernia if the neonate has respiratory distress and a scaphoid abdomen. Apex beat is shifted and bowel sounds may be heard in chest.
- Rule out imperforate anus by inspecting the anal opening at the normal place. Routine

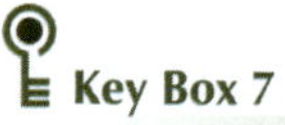

Key Box 7

When to Anticipate a Congenital Abnormality?

1. If there is a family history of congenital abnormalities
2. Maternal illness (fever, rash) in the first trimester, e.g. TORCH infections
3. Maternal diabetes poorly controlled during the first trimester
4. Consumption of alcohol during pregnancy or substance abuse
5. Teratogenic drug intake during pregnancy, e.g. warfarin or anticonvulsants
6. Maternal age 35 years or above
7. Polyhydramnios (esophageal/duodenal atresia)
8. Oligohydramnios (renal abnormalities)
9. Abnormal antenatal scans/investigations
10. Twins, especially, if they are identical

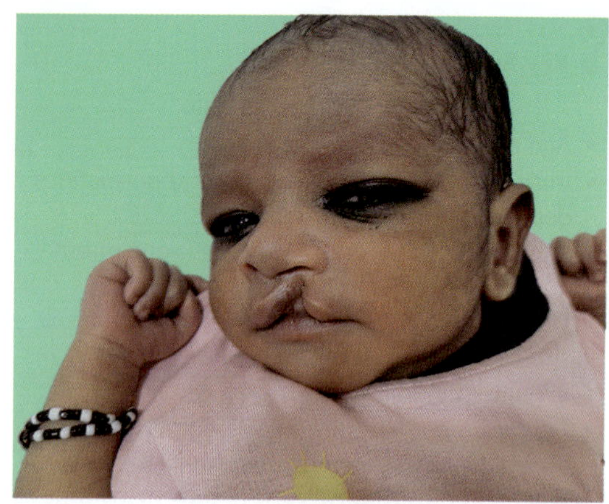

Fig. 16.2a: Cleft lip.

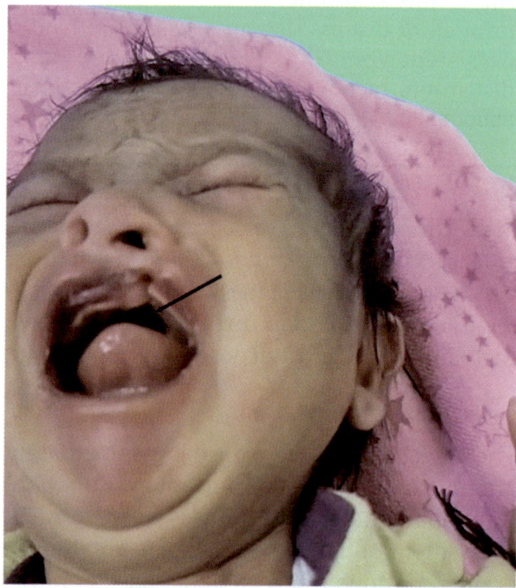

Fig. 16.2b: Cleft palate.

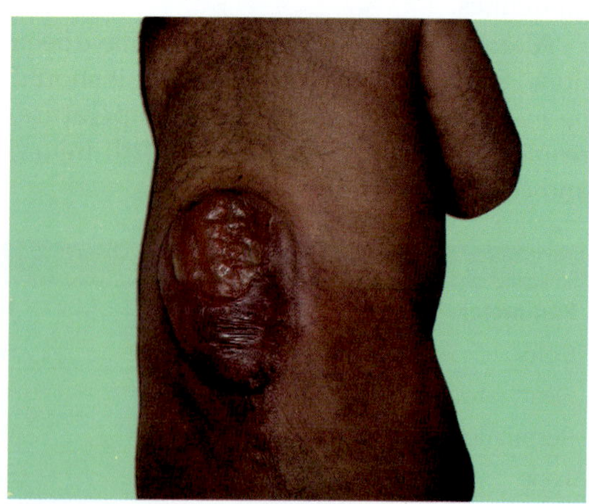

Fig. 16.3: Meningomyelocele.

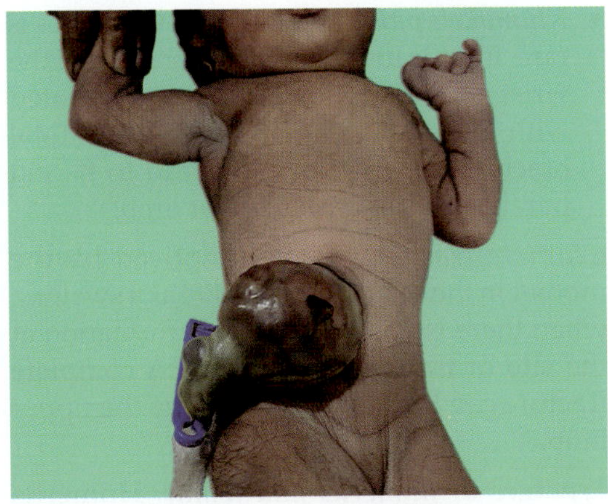

Fig. 16.4: Omphalocele.

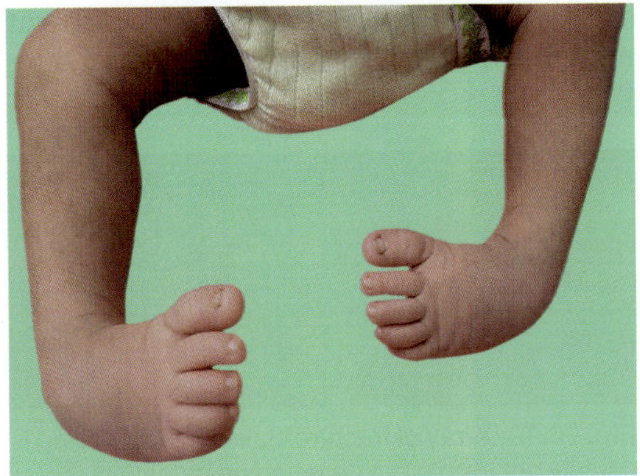

Fig. 16.5: Congenital talipes equinovarus deformity.

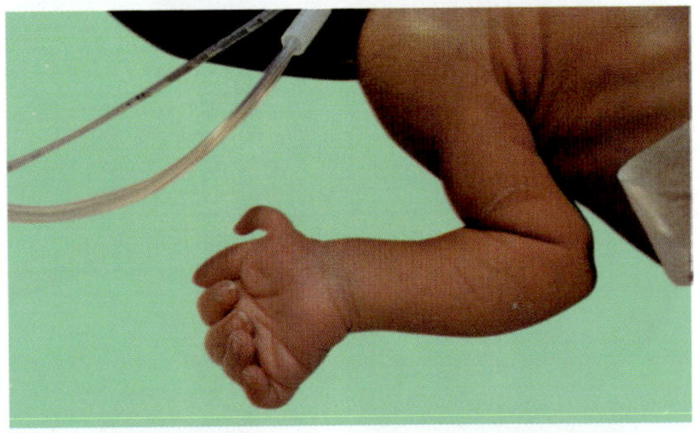

Fig. 16.6: Polydactyly.

testing of anal patency by inserting a catheter is NOT recommended. Sometimes, there is no opening but just a dimple at the site (Fig 16.7).

- Some malformations like esophageal atresia, congenital diaphragmatic hernia, congenital heart disease and renal anomalies etc. are not evident from physical examination. Esophageal atresia with

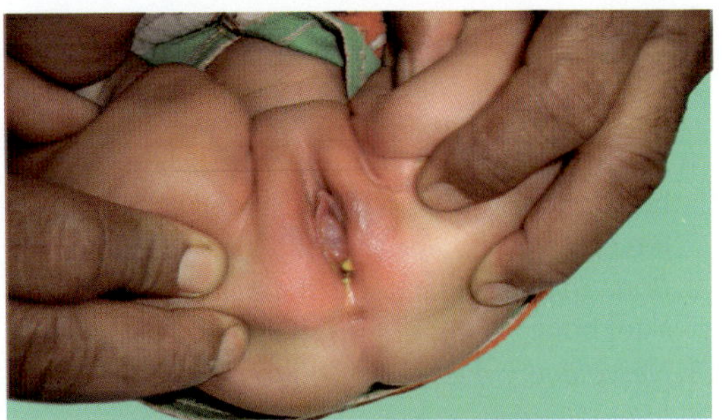

Fig. 16.7: Absent anal opening.

trachea-esophageal fistula will present on the first day of life with history of excessive frothing and salivation from mouth, vomiting and respiratory difficulty. It can be suspected, when you are unable to insert feeding tube (8Fr or 10 Fr) beyond a few centimeters. Checking the patency of the esophagus is not required for all babies. It should be done in high-risk babies, such as history of polyhydramnios, and SGA baby or presentation with symptoms.
- Suspect bilateral choanal atresia if infant has respiratory distress that resolves with crying due to opening of mouth. It can be easily confirmed by the inability to pass a catheter through nostrils.
- Record any abnormal facial features, microtia, or anotia.

Examination for Birth Injuries

Birth injuries are often signified by lack of motion or asymmetries of movement of the limbs or face. There may be obvious pain when an extremity or clavicle is palpated, and bruising may be apparent after a few hours of life. Birth injuries occur with greater frequency in LGA babies, breech deliveries and other abnormal presentations. The most common birth injuries are listed in **Key Box 8**.

Facial nerve palsy: Seen mostly following forceps application. This is the most common cranial nerve injury and is lower motor neuron type (Fig. 16.8).

Brachial plexus injury

- ***Duchenne erb palsy:*** Is the most common type involving C5 and C6. The hand is held in the "waiter's tip" posture with the upper limb held at adduction at shoulder, extension at elbow and internal rotation of the wrist (Fig. 16.9). The grasp is usually intact.

Key Box 8

Common Birth Injuries

1. *Scalp:* Cephalohematoma and subgaleal hematoma, injury from fetal scalp electrode or forceps
2. *Bone injuries:* Fractures of clavicle, humerus, skull bone
3. *Nerve injury:* Facial palsy, Erb palsy
4. *Internal organs:* Liver and spleen injury
5. Testicular trauma
6. Lacerations or scalpel injury

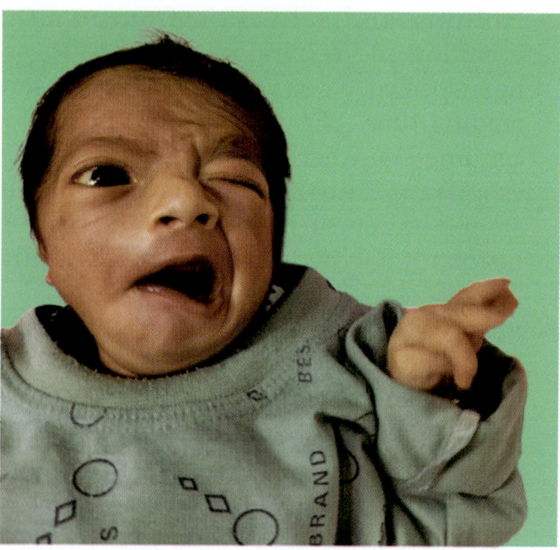

Fig. 16.8: Facial nerve palsy.

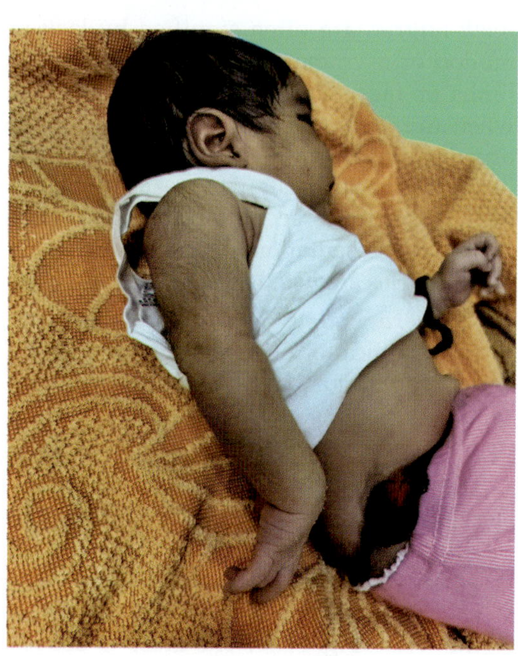

Fig. 16.9: Erb's palsy.

- ***Klumpke's palsy*** involving C7, C8 and T1 is rare. It leads to weakness or paralysis of the wrist and hand muscles and is associated with ipsilateral Horner's syndrome. Total brachial plexus injury will lead to flaccid paralysis of the whole upper limb.

Clavicle fracture: Usually noticed by the mother in the second week of life as a swelling when there is onset of a callous formation at the site of fracture **(Fig. 16.10)**. A complete fracture can lead inability to move the upper limb.

Fracture of humerus and femur: Humerus fracture can lead to asymmetric Moro's reflex and lack of movement of the arm with a swelling. Fracture of femur presents as absent movement of the lower limb and swelling **(Fig. 16.11)**.

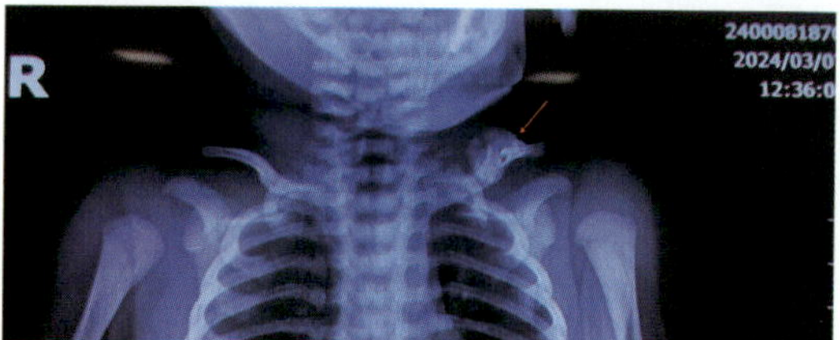

Fig. 16.10: X-ray of fracture clavicle: the swelling is usually not visible but detected on palpation.

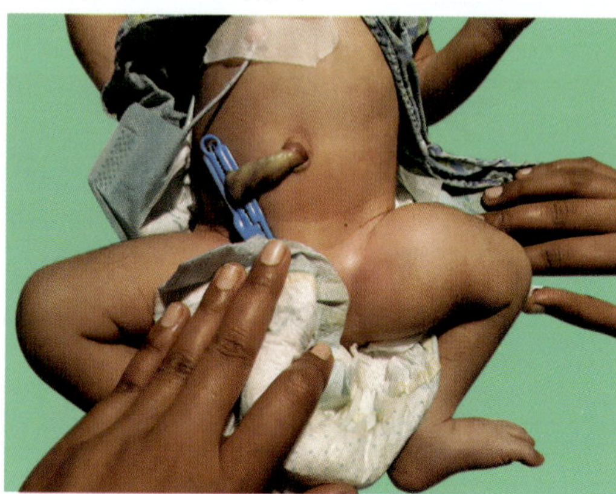

Fig. 16.11: Swelling of the left thigh due to fracture femur.

3. General Health Assessment

The newborn is assessed at 24–48 hours after birth for the following:

- Vital signs, temperature stability
- *Cardiopulmonary system:* Heart rate, respiratory rate, perfusion (capillary refill time), murmur, bilateral femoral pulses

- Ability and success of breastfeeding (weight loss since birth, duration of breastfeeding, effective suckling, proper attachment and positioning, urine output)
- Normal color (rule out cyanosis, pallor, plethora, jaundice)
- Hip stability (rule out developmental dysplasia of hip)
- Anterior fontanel size
- Normal behavioral stage
- Before discharge from the hospital, pulse oximetry newborn screening for congenital heart defects should be done. It helps to identify a newborn with critical congenital heart disease, such as coarctation of the aorta, double outlet right ventricle, Ebstein anomaly, hypoplastic left heart syndrome, interrupted aortic arch, pulmonary atresia, single ventricle, tetralogy of Fallot, total anomalous pulmonary venous return, d-transposition of the great arteries, tricuspid atresia, and truncus arteriosus, before signs or symptoms are evident.

The algorithm recommended by American Academy of Pediatrics is shown in Flowchart 16.1.

4. Well-Baby Examination in Follow-up Office Visits

A follow-up brief examination should be performed later in the first week (which may be in a setting other than hospital). The focus should be on care issues, breastfeeding, cardiac examination (left to right shunts may manifest with reducing pulmonary vascular resistance), and assessment of jaundice.

Flowchart 16.1: AAP algorithm on newborn screening by pulse oximetry.

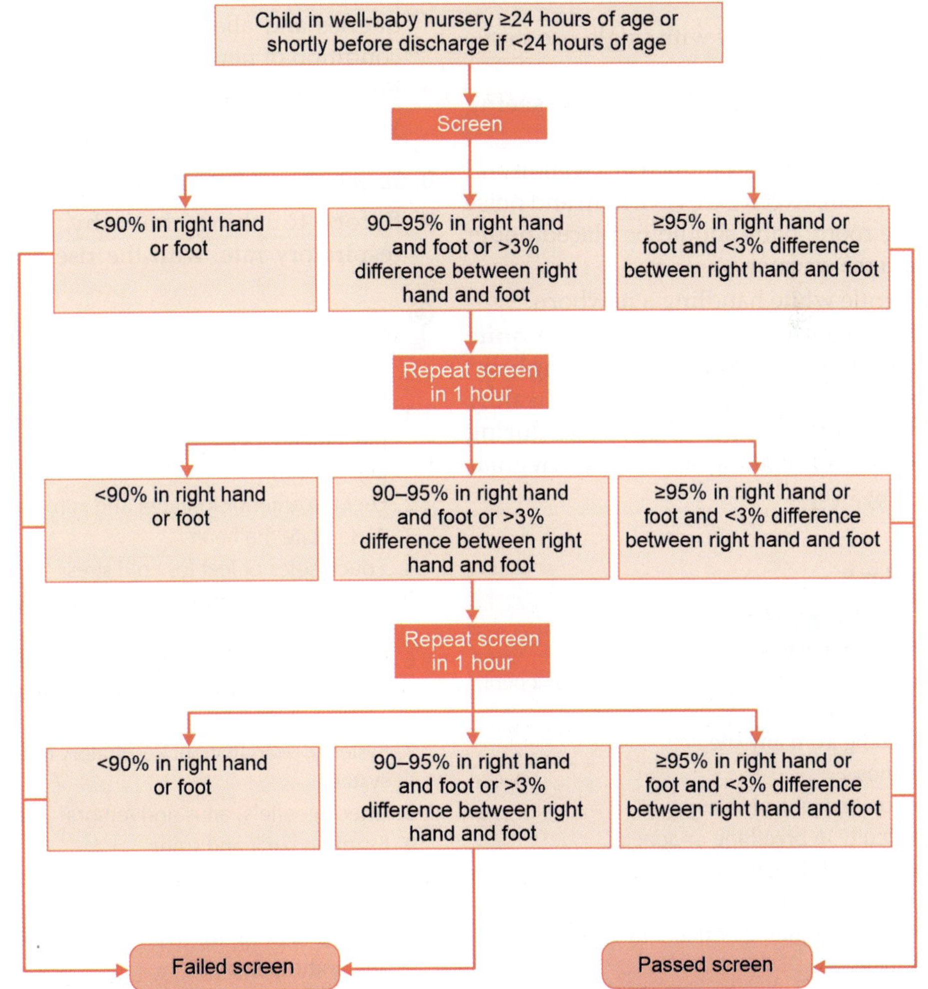

Weight gain and immunization status must be checked. Areas that may have been relatively inaccessible during the first examination, such as eyes and neuromotor evaluation must also be evaluated.

5. Differentiating between a Healthy and Sick Newborn

A neonate who (1) is active, (2) cries vigorously, (3) has good reflexes, (4) feeds well on the breast and (5) has warm and pink palms and soles is essentially a healthy baby. If any of the danger signs **(Key Box 9)** is present, the baby needs immediate attention.

16.4 ASSESSMENT OF VITAL SIGNS

A. Preparation for Examination

- Begin the examination with a brief introduction with mother. Tell your name and designation and convey what you are going to do.
- Wash hands and dry with single-use sterile towel/tissue.
- Use hand-sanitizer in between seeing babies.
- A baby should be examined in a well-lit and quiet room. Avoid excessive light and noise in the room. Baby should be placed under a radiant warmer.
- Be gentle while handling a newborn.
- A newborn is best examined in a quite awake state. Do not disturb a sleeping baby. Wait for him/her to wake up. A healthy newborn may appear hypotonic during sleep state. Breathing is also quite irregular during sleep.

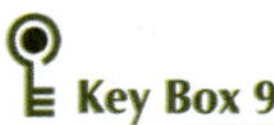

Danger signs in a newborn

1. Hypothermia/fever
2. Lethargy, excessive crying, inability to accept breastfeed
3. Bleeding from any site
4. Cyanosis
5. Yellow palms and soles
6. Difficulty in breathing or apnea
7. Abdominal distention
8. Bilious vomiting
9. Persistent vomiting or diarrhea
10. Convulsions

- Avoid handling a newborn soon after feeding due to risk of vomiting.
- If a newborn begins crying during examination, withhold examination for a few minutes until he/she settles down.
- Some useful information may still be gained while examining a crying baby, such as facial asymmetry and extremity movements. Even the intensity and duration of cry and ease of consolability may provide valuable information about the condition of a newborn.
- Document examination findings and keep records in a secure manner. Always mention the date and time, and age of newborn when examined.
- Do not leave baby unclothed at the end of examination. Help mother in dressing the baby.
- Communicate examination findings to parents in an easy language. Answer their queries and allay their anxiety about the condition of newborns.
- Finally say thanks to the parents before you leave.

B. Sequence of Examination (Key Box 10)

- Before touching the baby, assess the respiratory rate, with the rise and fall of

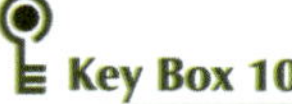

Sequence of Examination

1. Before touching, observe color, spontaneous movements, eye opening and respiratory rate and rhythm
2. Feel the anterior fontanel and sutures
3. Auscultate the heart
4. Touch soles of feet for cold stress
5. Palpate abdomen for liver, spleen and any mass
6. Undress the baby and do head-to-toe examination for congenital abnormality and general physical examination
7. Systemic examination: Respiratory and cardiac system
8. Check genitals, anus and femoral pulses
9. Examine back and spine
10. Neurological assessment
11. Moro reflex, hip assessment for DDH, New Ballard Scoring for assessment of gestation, and anthropometry

chest. Look for color, activity, and abnormal movements.

- Feel the anterior fontanel, skull, and sutures, look at the facies and eyes, auscultate the heart for any abnormal sound or murmur and gently palpate the abdomen.
- Now, undress the baby for head-to-toe examination. Remove the nappy and examine the genitalia, anus and femoral pulses. Turn to prone position and check the back and spine. Again, turn to supine position and assess the neurologic status.
- Neonatal reflexes, hip assessment for developmental dysplasia, New Ballard scoring for assessment of gestation and anthropometry should be left for the end.

C. Holding the Baby

Support the head in the palm of your left hand with fingers and thumb curled around. The baby's back rests on your right hand with the rest of his weight supported by your right forearm. It is wise to encircle the baby's upper left arm in your right thumb and index finger, to safeguard against accidental slipping of the baby.

D. Differentiating between a Healthy and Sick Newborn

Decide whether the baby is sick or well by observing the following:

- *Ask:* Is he normally active? Is the cry normal? Is the baby accepting feeds well?
- *Look:* Jaundice on palms and soles, fast or shallow breathing, groaning, chest retractions or cyanosis, bleeding from any site, cold to touch, delayed capillary filling time, bulging fontanel or signs of dehydration, abdominal distension, umbilical discharge or skin rashes/pustules.

E. Classify as Term or Preterm

You can differentiate between preterm and term babies based on certain physical features. Presence of following suggests a preterm baby (<37 weeks):

- *Deep sole creases* are absent or are limited to the anterior one-third of sole.
- *Genitalia:* Testes are at the external ring. Scrotum is small with few rugosities. Labia in female are widely separated exposing labia minora and clitoris.
- *Breast nodule* is less than 5 mm in diameter.
- *Ear cartilage* is deficient and has poor elastic recoil.

F. Vital Signs

These include temperature, heart rate, respiratory rate, color, capillary refill time (CRT), blood pressure, and oxygen saturation. Normal values are given in **Key Box 11**.

1. Temperature

Temperature should be measured in the axilla of a newborn. The digital thermometer is placed in the axillary pit against the roof and the baby's arm is then held close to its body **(Fig. 16.12)**. The temperature should be read when the thermometer gives a beep.

The normal axillary temperature of a newborn is 36.5–37.5°C. Temperature below 36.5°C is known as hypothermia. Temperature >37.5°C is known as hyperthermia **(Table 16.2)**. A quick evaluation of temperature can be done by touching the abdomen and extremities of the baby with the dorsum of hand. Baby has normal temperature if both the extremities and the abdomen are warm to touch **(Table 16.3)**. This is an easy and useful method of assessment of temperature at home by the mother, especially by those who cannot read a thermometer.

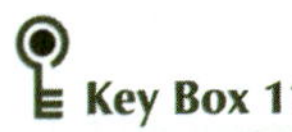
Key Box 11

Normal Vital Signs in a Newborn

1. Temperature	36.5 to 37.5°C axillary
2. Heart rate	120–160 beats per minute (as low as 80–100 during sleeping; as high as 180 during crying)
3. Respiration	40–60 breaths/min
4. Oxygen saturation	Above 95% in room air
5. Capillary refill time	<3 sec

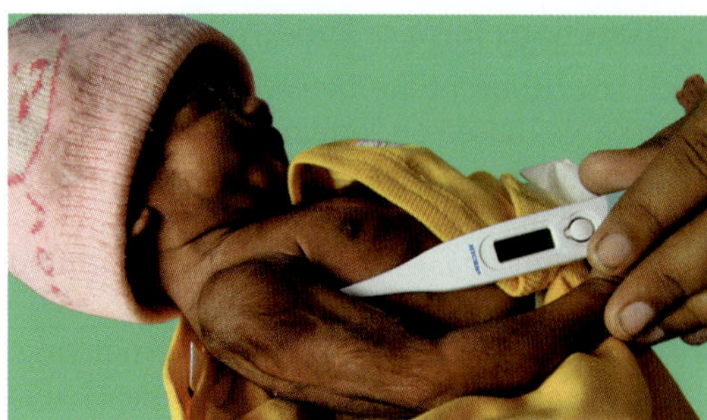

Fig. 16.12: Axillary temperature measurement.

Table 16.2: Grading of temperature in a newborn

Classification	Axillary temperature (°C)/(°F)
Normal temperature	36.5–37.5/97.7–99.5
Cold stress/mild hypothermia	36.0–36.4/96.8–97.5
Moderate hypothermia	32.0–35.9/89.6–96.6
Severe hypothermia	<32.0/89.6
Hyperthermia	>37.5/99.5

Table 16.3: Classification of hypothermia by touch

Classification	Peripheries/feet	Abdomen
Normal	Warm	Warm
Cold stress	Cold	Warm
Hypothermia	Cold	Cold

2. Respiratory Rate

The normal respiratory rate (RR) of a newborn is 40–60/min. They breathe at a faster rate than older children and adults. The RR should be counted for one minute. Newborns may have periodic breathing in which they have brief periods of rapid breathing followed by slow breathing or no breathing at all. If the rates are not counted for one minute, it may sometimes lead to a wrong count. If the respiratory rate is ≥60/min, it should be counted again. If the RR is still ≥60/min, then it is taken as tachypnea. It is also important to observe whether there is any respiratory distress (look for any suprasternal, intercostal, or subcostal retractions). Note any apnea or periodic breathing.

3. Heart Rate

The heart rate (HR) of a newborn is also more than that of older children and adults, i.e., 120–160/min. Pulse rate should not be taken as a surrogate for HR. All peripheral pulses should be palpated; they are weak/absent in case of hypothermia, shock, or coarctation of aorta.

4. Color **(Key Box 12)**

The color of the baby should be pink, there may be acrocyanosis (cyanosis of peripheries) within first few hours after birth, which is normal. The baby must be examined for pallor, cyanosis, especially central cyanosis and icterus (jaundice). Pallor should be examined on the palm or face. Some babies may appear to be excessively red in color. This may be due to polycythemia, usually seen in small for gestational age babies. Cyanosis present on the tongue and lips indicates central cyanosis, which is a grave sign and is seen in significant cardiac or respiratory disease.

Assessment of jaundice

- Jaundice is seen as yellowish discoloration of the skin in newborns. We do not look for jaundice in the conjunctiva of a newborn as we do in older people. The newborn keeps the eye closed most of the time and it is difficult to visualize the conjunctiva.
- It is easily seen on the skin by pressing on the skin with the index finger (to blanch the skin) at a bony prominence for around 3–5 seconds and then the finger is lifted **(Figs 16.13a, b)**. The yellowish discoloration of the skin is easily seen once the skin is blanched. Examination for jaundice must be done in natural light to avoid any errors. Examination under artificial light may give

Key Box 12

Color Guide for Newborn

1. *Red (plethora):* Polycythemia; (send PCV)
2. *Blue (cyanosis):*
   i. Hands and feet only—peripheral cyanosis (check temperature)
   ii. Lips and mucous membranes—central cyanosis (respiratory/cardiac cause)
3. *Pale (anemia):* Anemia or hypovolemia, (check for bleeding)
4. *Gray (circulatory shock):* Asphyxia, septicemia
5. *Yellow (jaundice):* Hyperbilirubinemia, (check by transcutaneous bilirubinometer or send serum bilirubin)

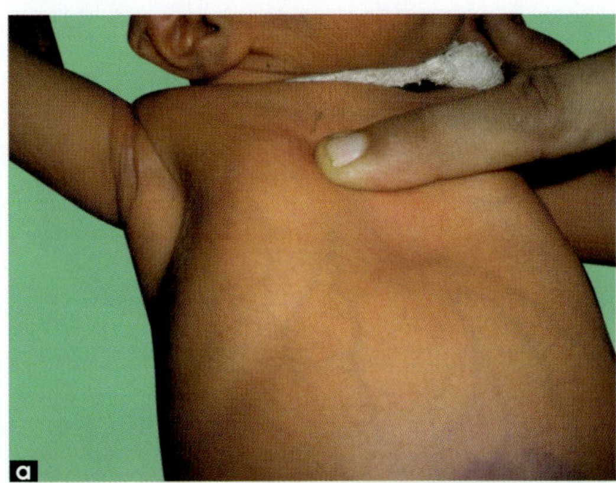

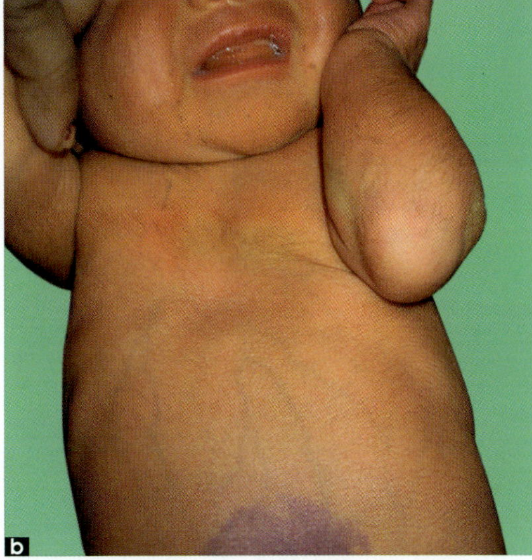

Figs 16.13a, b: Examination for jaundice.

a false impression of no jaundice or the baby may appear more icteric when examined under yellow light.

- Jaundice first appears first on the face and then progresses caudally as the levels of bilirubin rise.
- Any visible jaundice within the first 24 hours of life and persisting after 2 weeks in a term baby must be evaluated. A term newborn may have icterus up to chest or upper abdomen by day 4 or 5, (in physiological jaundice). Icterus on or below the thighs, or yellowish discoloration of the palms and soles present at any time are always pathological.
- Clinical examination of jaundice can give an approximate idea of the serum bilirubin by using the Kramer's scale **(Fig. 16.14)**. Whenever in doubt, a serum bilirubin estimation must be done.
- Once phototherapy has been started, the visual examination of jaundice is not reliable.

Physiological jaundice: Majority of newborns develop jaundice by day 3 of life. The serum bilirubin increases for next 3–4 days and then decreases such that jaundice is not visible by day 10 in most babies. In preterm babies, the jaundice may persist longer.

Pathological jaundice: The jaundice is pathological, if:

- It appears within 24 hours of birth
- Persists beyond 14 days
- Palms and soles are stained yellow at any time
- Associated with passage of clay-colored stools and/or high-colored urine

Key Box 13 summarizes a few important features to be asked for or looked for in a child with jaundice.

5. Capillary Refill Time (CRT)

Capillary refill time is seen to assess the circulation of the baby. CRT in newborns is

Modified Kramer's scale		
Dermal zone	**Area of body**	**Level of bilirubin**
1	Face	4–6 mg/dL
2	Chest, upper abdomen	8–10 mg/dL
3	Lower abdomen, thighs	11–14 mg/dL
4	Arms, lower legs	15–18 mg/dL
5	Palms, soles	15–20 mg/dL

Fig. 16.14: Kramer's scale for assessment of jaundice.

Key Box 13

History and Examination—
Features Relevant to Jaundice

- Is the infant unwell? (*sepsis and GIT obstruction can cause jaundice*)
- Is there dehydration or poor weight gain? (*both exacerbate jaundice*)
- *Gestation:* The incidence of hyperbilirubinemia increases with prematurity
- Jaundice before 24 hrs of age (*suggests hemolysis*)
- Jaundice persisting after 14 days of age (*more likely to be pathological*)
- Birth trauma, such as cephalohematoma, significant bruising (*will cause breakdown of heme*)
- Maternal history (*blood group, anti-Rh antibody injection, viral serology*)
- History of jaundice in previous siblings (*ABO/Rh incompatibility*)
- Family history of hemolytic disease (*ABO/G6PD, spherocytosis*)
- Dark urine or pale stools or staining of diapers (*suggest biliary obstruction*)
- Level of icterus in terms of cephalocaudal progression
- Pallor (*indicating hemolysis or blood loss*)
- Plethora (*may suggest polycythemia*)
- *Signs of bilirubin encephalopathy*, e.g. lethargy, hypotonia, seizure, opisthotonus, high-pitched cry
- Pallor, plethora, cephalohematoma, subaponeurotic hemorrhage
- *Signs of intrauterine infection* or metabolic problems, e.g. petechiae, hepatosplenomegaly

always assessed over the sternum. The skin over the sternum is pressed with the index finger for around 5 seconds to blanch the skin and empty the capillaries and then released. The time for the capillaries to refill, i.e. for the skin color to return to normal over the blanched area is noted **(Fig 16.15)**. The time can be noted by counting "one thousand one, one thousand two, one thousand three,....". A capillary refill time <3 seconds is the normal for a newborn. A CRT ≥3 seconds, is prolonged, which may be a sign of shock.

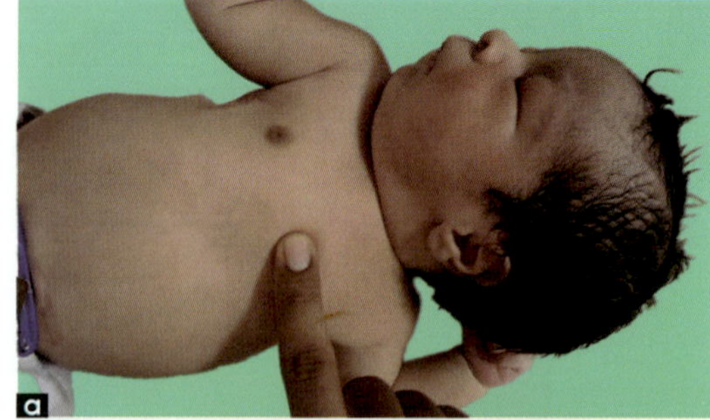

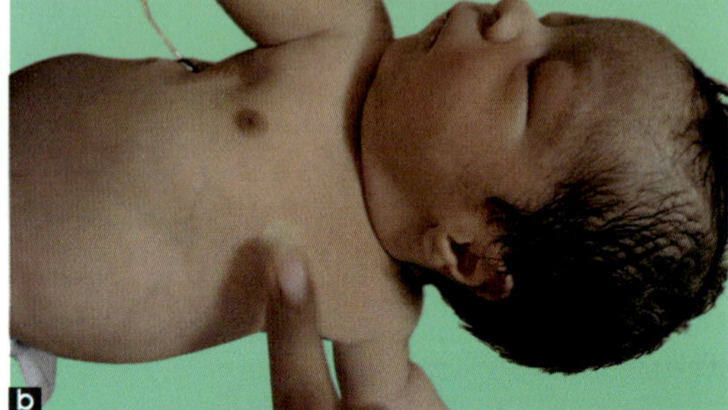

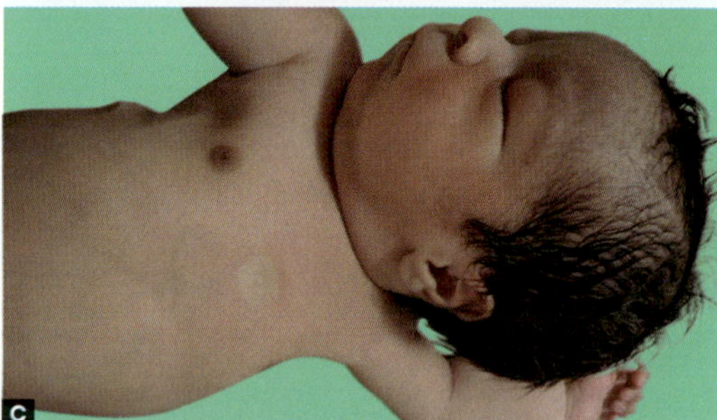

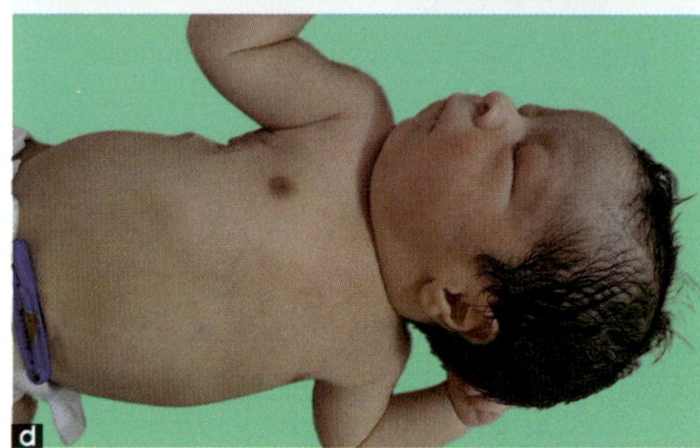

Fig. 16.15: Demonstration of capillary refill time (a) Pressing on sternum; (b) remove finger after 5 sec; (c) blanched area immediately after releasing pressure; (d) blanched area becomes pink within 2 seconds.

6. Blood Pressure

Blood pressure is not routinely measured in healthy newborns. It should be measured in all sick neonates by using an appropriate-sized neonatal cuff. There are 5 sizes of cuffs available for neonates. To choose an appropriately sized cuffs, use a cuff with bladder length encircling at least 80% of the arm and the cuff width should be half of the arm circumference.

Oscillometric method of blood pressure estimation is used in which the cuff is attached to the monitor through a cable and the BP is displayed. *Sphygmomanometric* method is not reliable in neonates and is therefore not used. There are reference charts available for the blood pressure in neonates based on the gestational age, postmenstrual age, and birth weight.

7. SpO_2 Monitoring

Monitoring of percentage of saturated hemoglobin is a good screening tool to evaluate the respiratory and cardiac status of the baby. The probe is attached to the wrist or feet and connected to the pulse oximeter and the reading is displayed on the monitor. The saturation in a newborn must be seen in the right upper limb in first 48–72 hours of life. A saturation <90% indicates hypoxia. A pre- and post-ductal saturation difference of >3% may indicate a right to left shunting through the ductus arteriosus. It is also used to screen for critical congenital heart diseases (*see* **Flowchart 16.1**).

16.5 ASSESSMENT OF WEIGHT AND GESTATION

A. Anthropometry

1. Weight

Weight should be measured in grams for greatest accuracy. You should measure it by putting the naked baby on the weighing scale, after resetting it to zero **(Fig. 16.16)**.

Depending on the size, newborns may be classified as appropriate for gestational age (AGA; birth weight between 10th and 90th percentile), small for gestational age (SGA; birth weight below 10th percentile) and large for gestational age (LGA; birth weight above 90th percentile) **(Fig. 16.17)**. SGA babies have a malnourished look with less subcutaneous fat and wrinkled skin **(Figs 16.18a, b)**.

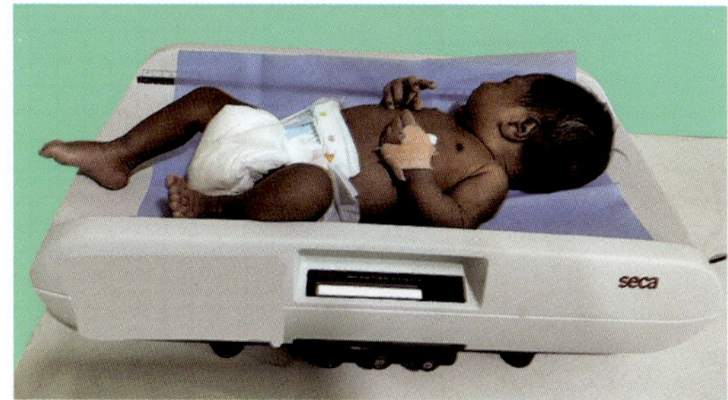

Fig. 16.16: Weighing a baby.

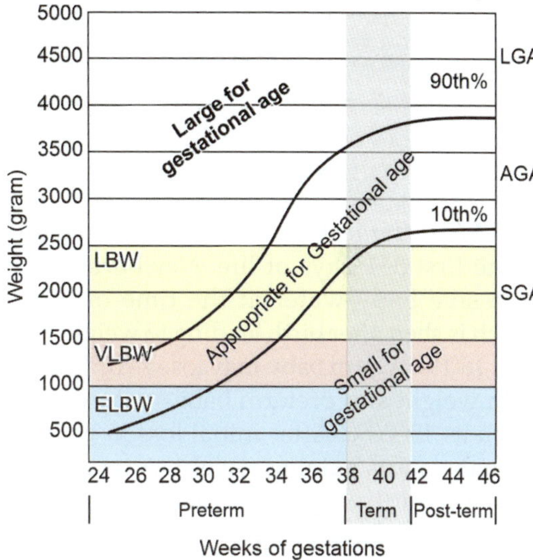

Fig. 16.17: Classification of a baby according to birth weight and gestational age.

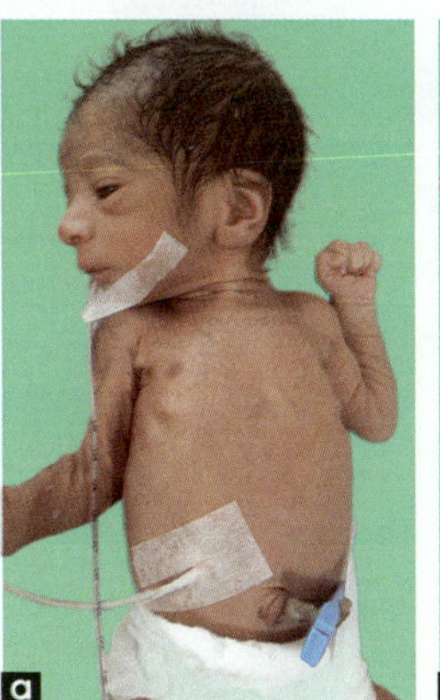

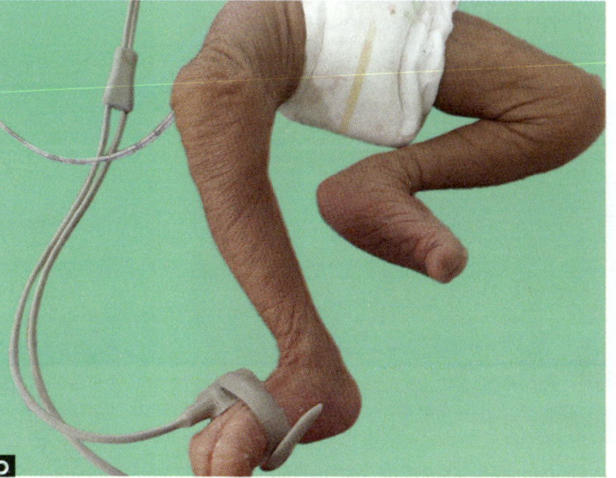

Figs 16.18a, b: Small for gestational age baby.

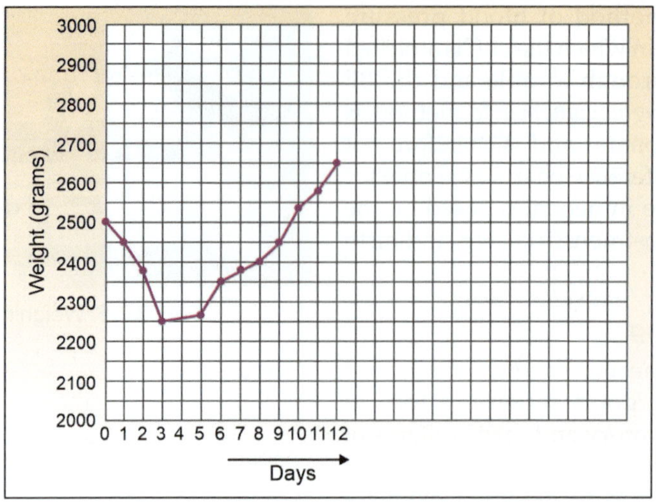

Fig. 16.19: Weight pattern of a term baby in first 10 days of life.

Weight pattern: All newborns lose weight in the first 3–4 days of life. Newborns have excessive body water at the time of birth, which is shed after birth leading to weight loss **(Fig. 16.19)**. A term baby may lose 7–10% of the birth weight and preterm babies may lose as much as 15–20%. After initial loss in weight, the baby starts gaining weight. A term baby regains its birth weight by 10 days and preterm babies by 14 days. After this, the baby starts gaining weight by 20–30 g/day.

2. Length

The length of the baby is measured using an infantometer **(Fig. 16.20)**. Two people are needed to measure the length of the newborn. The head-end of the infantometer is fixed and the foot-end can be adjusted, so that it touches the soles of the feet. The baby is made to lie on the infantometer. The head of the baby is stabilized at the head-end and the body is straightened and the knees are pressed down, the feet are held at 90° to the base such that the toes point upward. The length is then noted in cm. The length of a term baby is around 50 cm.

Fig. 16.20: Measuring length of a baby using an infantometer.

3. Ponderal Index

Ponderal index (PI) is calculated in SGA babies, by the following formula:

$$\text{Ponderal index (PI)} = \frac{\text{Birth weight (g)}}{[\text{Length (cm)}]^3}$$

A ponderal index helps differentiating between symmetrical (PI >2) and asymmetrical SGA (PI <2).

4. Head Circumference

The head circumference should be taken after 24 hours of birth **(Fig. 16.21)**. The baby may

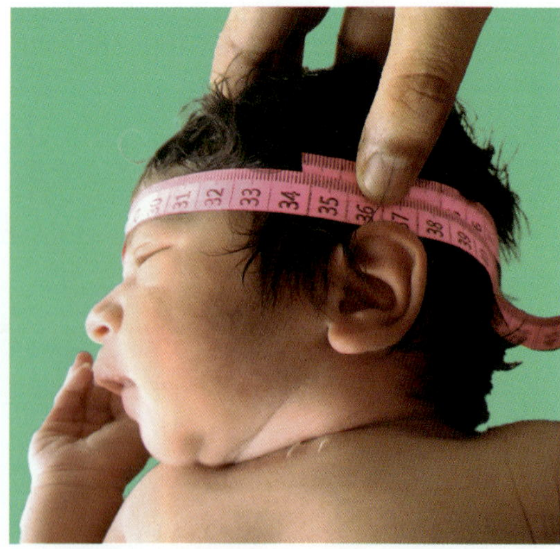

Fig. 16.21: Measuring head circumference.

have a caput succedaneum at birth due to which the head circumference will be falsely increased. Molding of skull during delivery may lead to falsely low circumference if the measurement is done within 24 hours. The normal head circumference of a term baby is 33–35 cm. An abnormally small **(Fig. 16.22)** or large **(Fig. 16.23)** head is due to an underlying central nervous system disorder and must be evaluated thoroughly.

5. Upper and Lower Segment Ratio

This is not routinely measured in newborns, this may be important for genetic disorders, especially skeletal dysplasia. Short limb dwarfism is typically seen in achondroplasia.

- Proximal limb shortening (humerus or femur) is known as *rhizomelia* as is seen in achondroplasia.
- Middle limb shortening (forearm or lower leg) known as *mesomelia* is seen in other rare forms of skeletal dysplasia like Ellis-van Creveld syndrome.
- Distal limb shortening (hands) is known as *acromelia* in which there are short hands and feet.

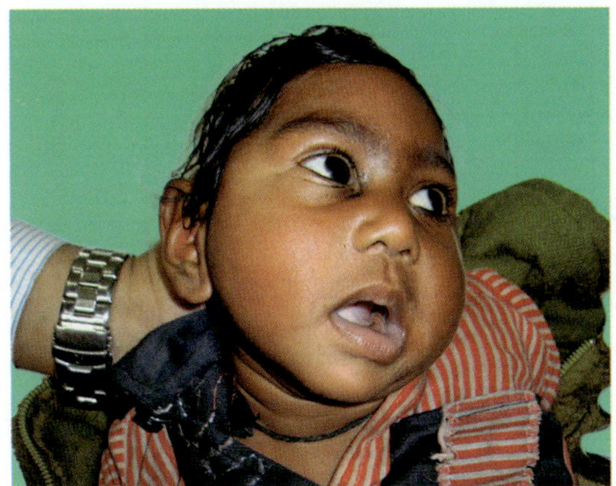

Fig. 16.22: Microcephaly.

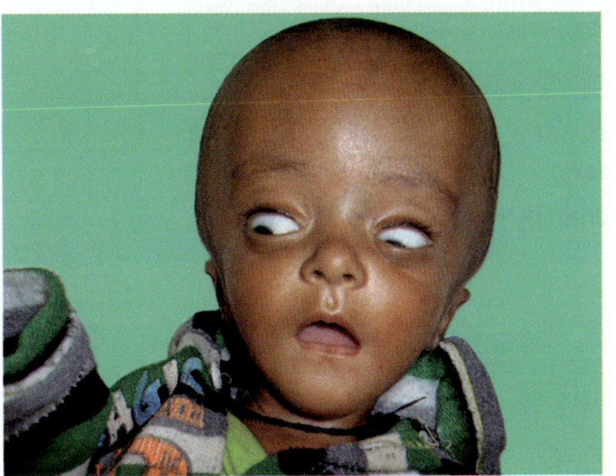

Fig. 16.23: Macrocephaly.

6. Growth Charts

The infant's weight, length and head circumference should be monitored using various available growth charts, which are gender specific. Fenton intrauterine growth charts **(Figs 16.24a, b)** allow a comparison of an infant's growth, first with the fetus as early as 22 weeks and then with the term infants to 10 weeks. Intergrowth 21 Standards provide standards for monitoring the size at birth **(Figs 16.25a, b)**. It also provides standards for monitoring postnatal growth of preterm infants **(Figs 16.25c, d)**. Once the babies become 40 weeks of postmenstrual age then the WHO MGRS charts can be used.

B. Gestational Age Estimation

The first aim is to establish if the baby is term or preterm. The next aim should be to assess the exact gestational age in weeks of completed gestation.

Last Menstrual Period

Estimated date of term delivery (EDD) is calculated by adding 9 calendar months and 7 days to the 1st day of mother's last menstrual period (LMP). This calculation is known as Naegele's rule. Alternatively, EDD is 280 days after the first day of LMP. These approaches assume a regular menstrual cycle of 28 days, with ovulation taking place on the 14th day after the beginning of menstrual cycle. However, these assumptions may not be true due to inaccurate recall of LMP, irregularities in cycle length, or variability in ovulation timing. Only 50% of women accurately recall their LMP. Currently, best obstetric estimate, a combination of LMP and first trimester sonography, is used to calculate gestational age and EDD during pregnancy.

Physical and Neurological Characteristics

These characteristics together can reliably provide an estimate of gestational age after the child is born. Also, gestational age that matches the 50th percentile for the child's

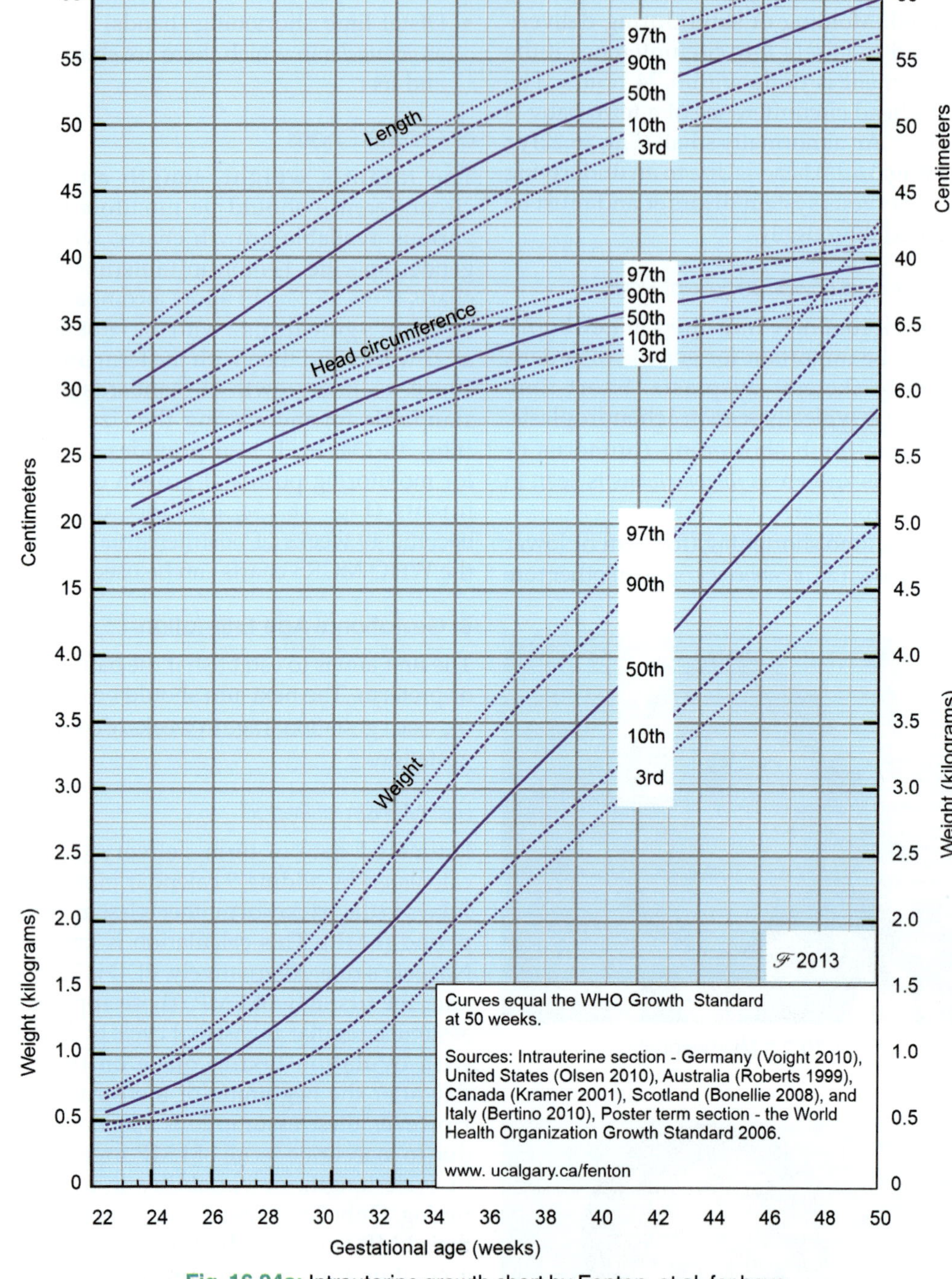

Fig. 16.24a: Intrauterine growth chart by Fenton, et al. for boys.

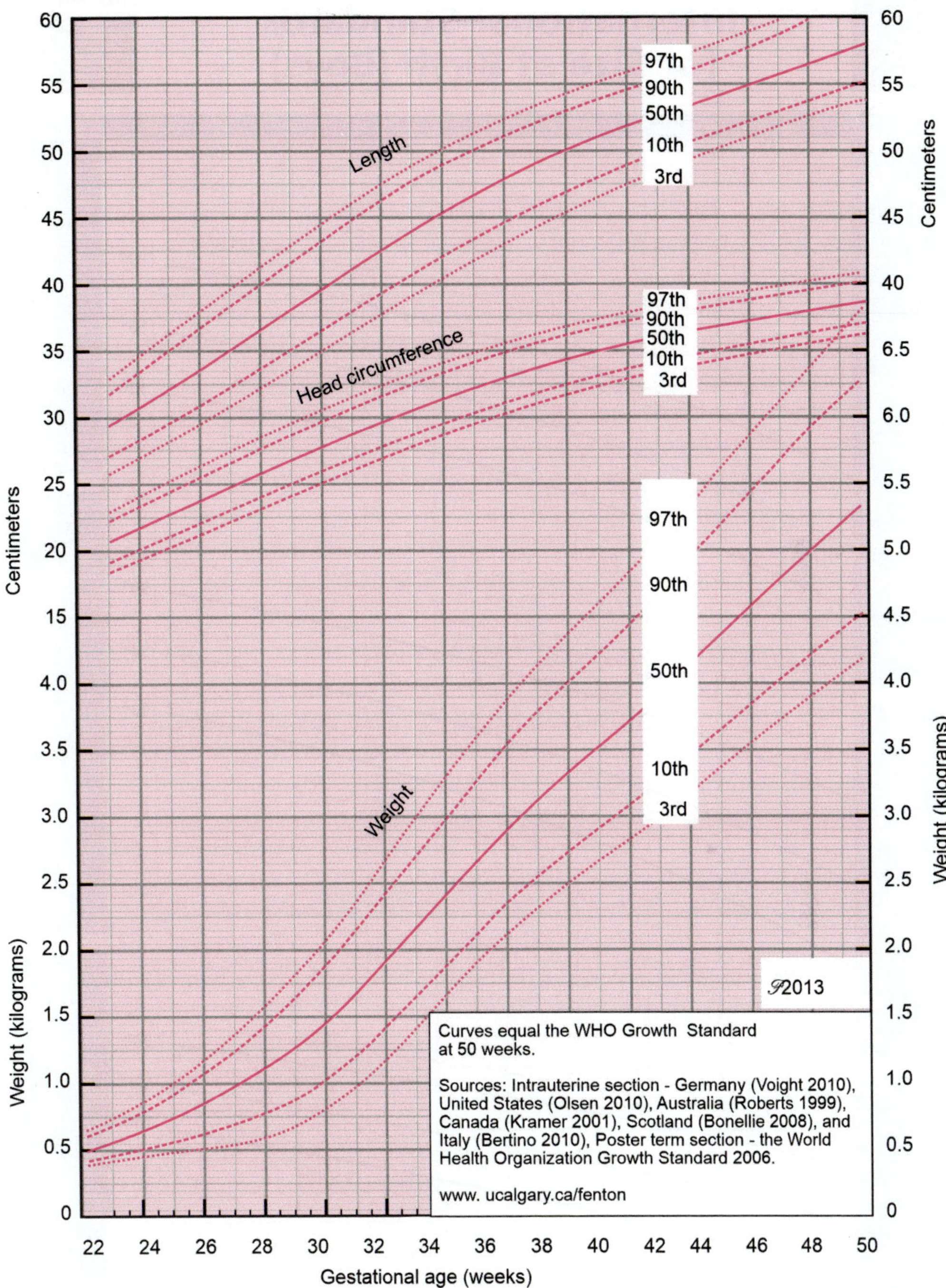

Fig. 16.24b: Intrauterine growth chart by Fenton, et al. for girls.

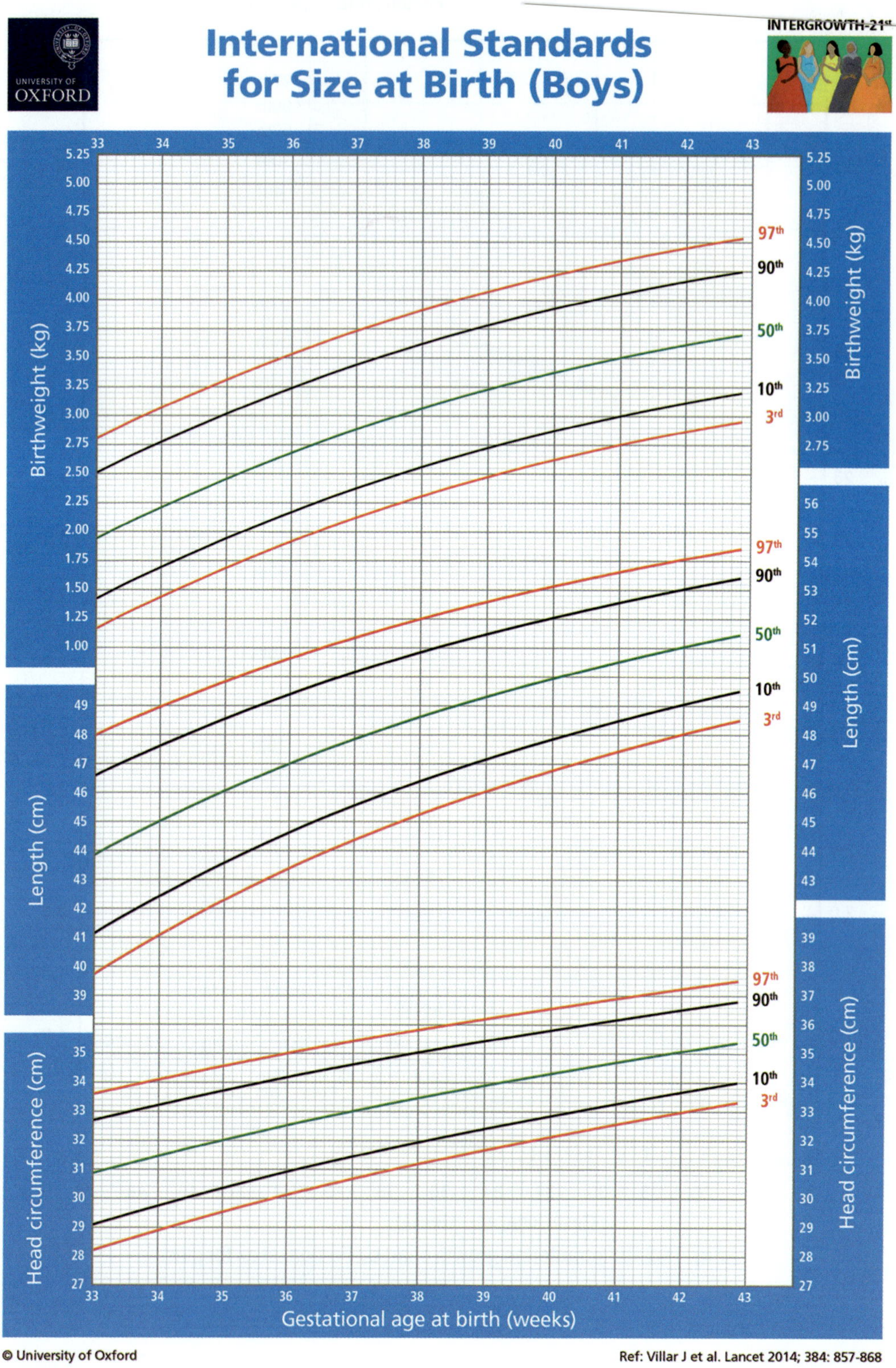

International Standards for Size at Birth (Boys)

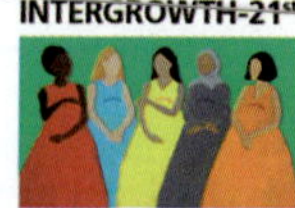

Birthweight (kg): 1.00, 1.25, 1.50, 1.75, 2.00, 2.25, 2.50, 2.75, 3.00, 3.25, 3.50, 3.75, 4.00, 4.25, 4.50, 4.75, 5.00, 5.25

Length (cm): 39, 40, 41, 42, 43, 44, 45, 46, 47, 48, 49, 50, 51, 52, 53, 54, 55, 56

Head circumference (cm): 27, 28, 29, 30, 31, 32, 33, 34, 35, 36, 37, 38, 39

97th, 90th, 50th, 10th, 3rd

Gestational age at birth (weeks): 33, 34, 35, 36, 37, 38, 39, 40, 41, 42, 43

Ref: Villar J et al. Lancet 2014; 384: 857-868

Fig. 16.25a: International (Intergrowth 21st) Standards for Size at Birth (Boys). Reprinted with the permission of the INTERGROWTH-21st Consortium, Oxford.

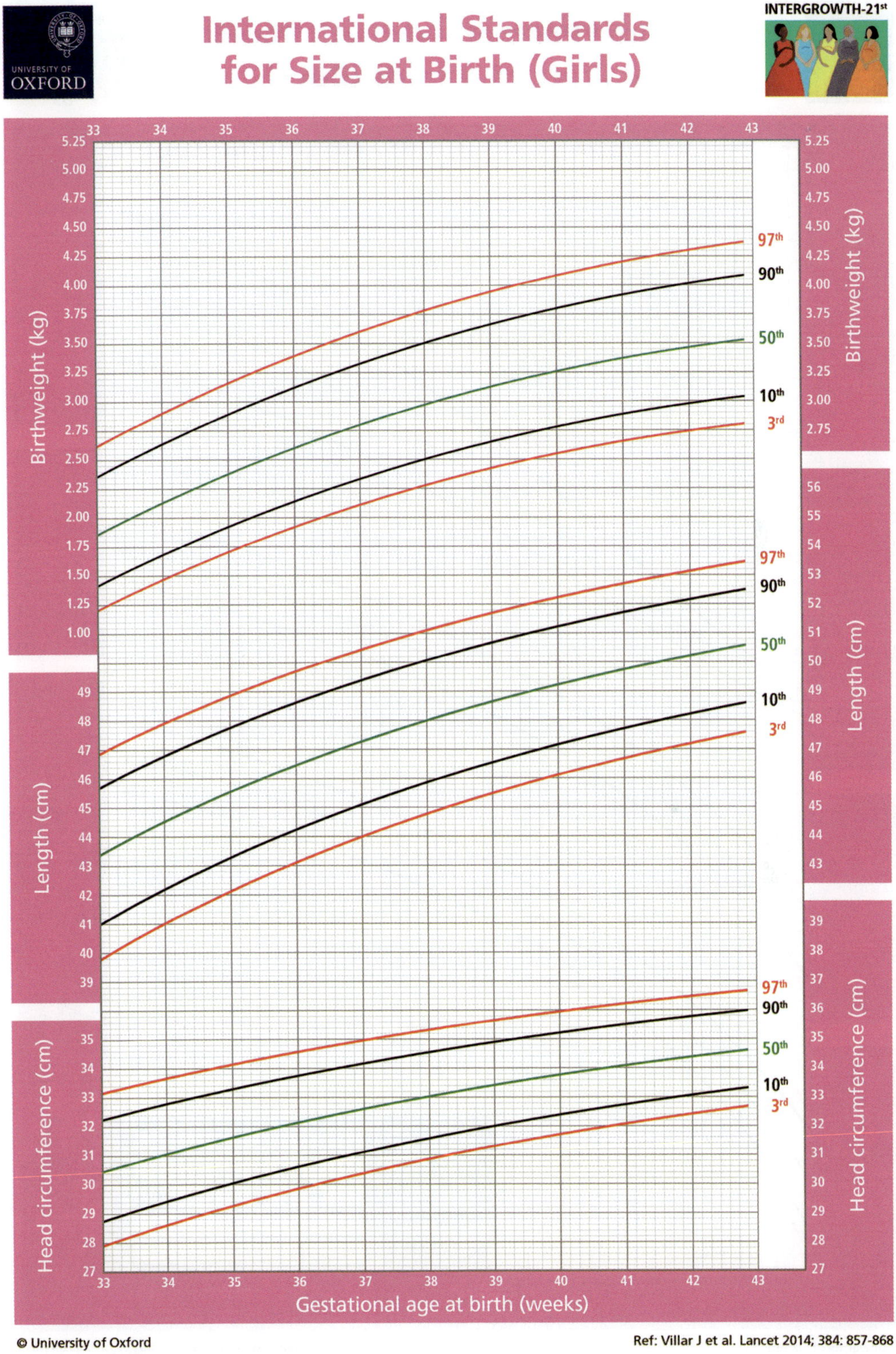

International Standards for Size at Birth (Girls)

Birthweight (kg)

5.25 5.00 4.75 4.50 4.25 4.00 3.75 3.50 3.25 3.00 2.75 2.50 2.25 2.00 1.75 1.50 1.25 1.00

97th 90th 50th 10th 3rd

Length (cm)

56 55 54 53 52 51 50 49 48 47 46 45 44 43 42 41 40 39

97th 90th 50th 10th 3rd

Head circumference (cm)

39 38 37 36 35 34 33 32 31 30 29 28 27

97th 90th 50th 10th 3rd

33 34 35 36 37 38 39 40 41 42 43

Gestational age at birth (weeks)

Ref: Villar J et al. Lancet 2014; 384: 857-868

Fig 16.25b: International (Intergrowth 21st) Standards for Size at Birth (Girls). Reprinted with the permission of the INTERGROWTH-21st Consortium, Oxford.

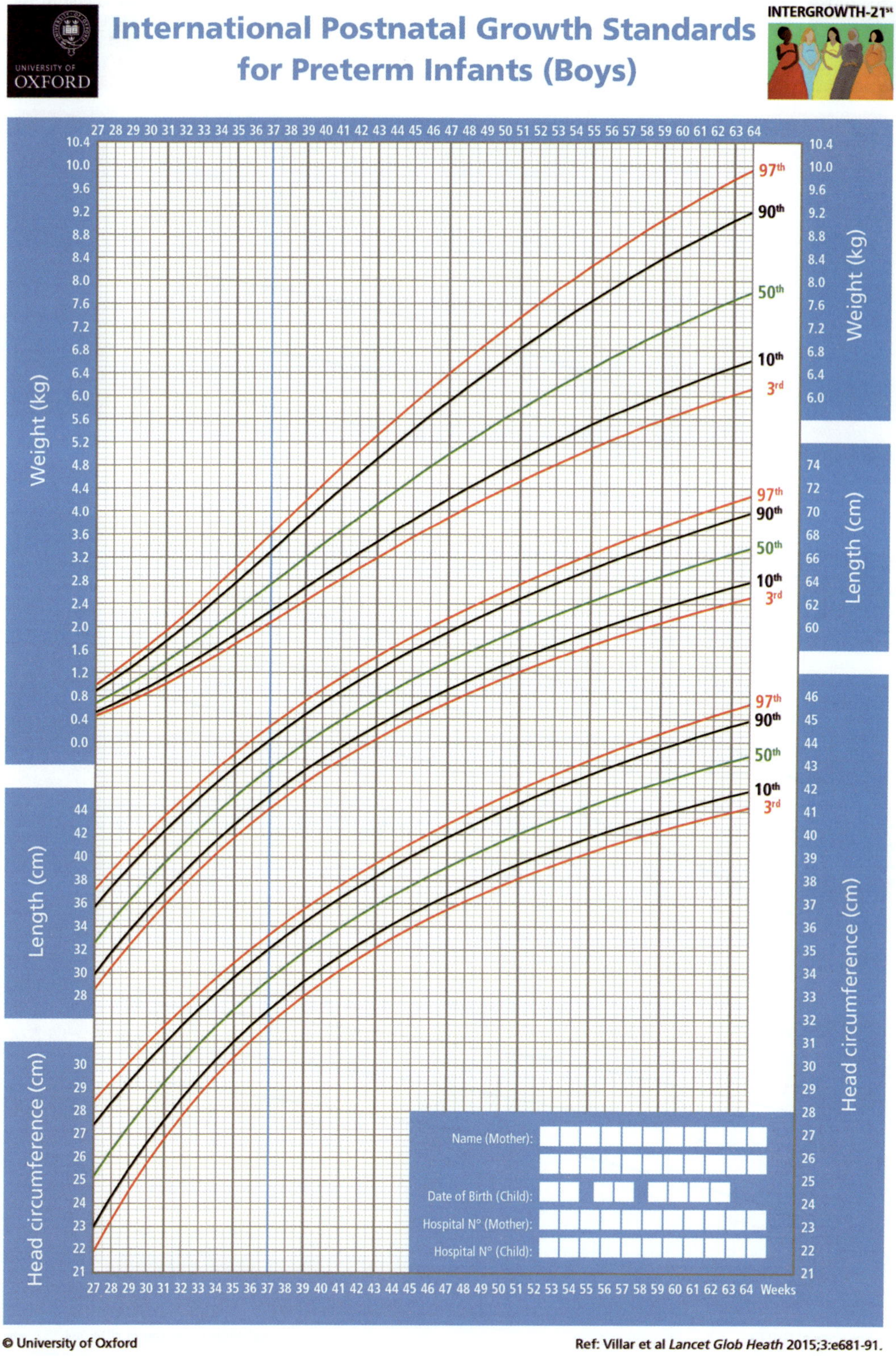

International Postnatal Growth Standards for Preterm Infants (Boys)

Ref: Villar et al *Lancet Glob Heath* 2015;3:e681-91.

Fig. 16.25c: International (Intergrowth 21st) Postnatal Growth Standards for Preterm Infants (Boys). Reprinted with the permission of the INTERGROWTH-21st Consortium, Oxford.

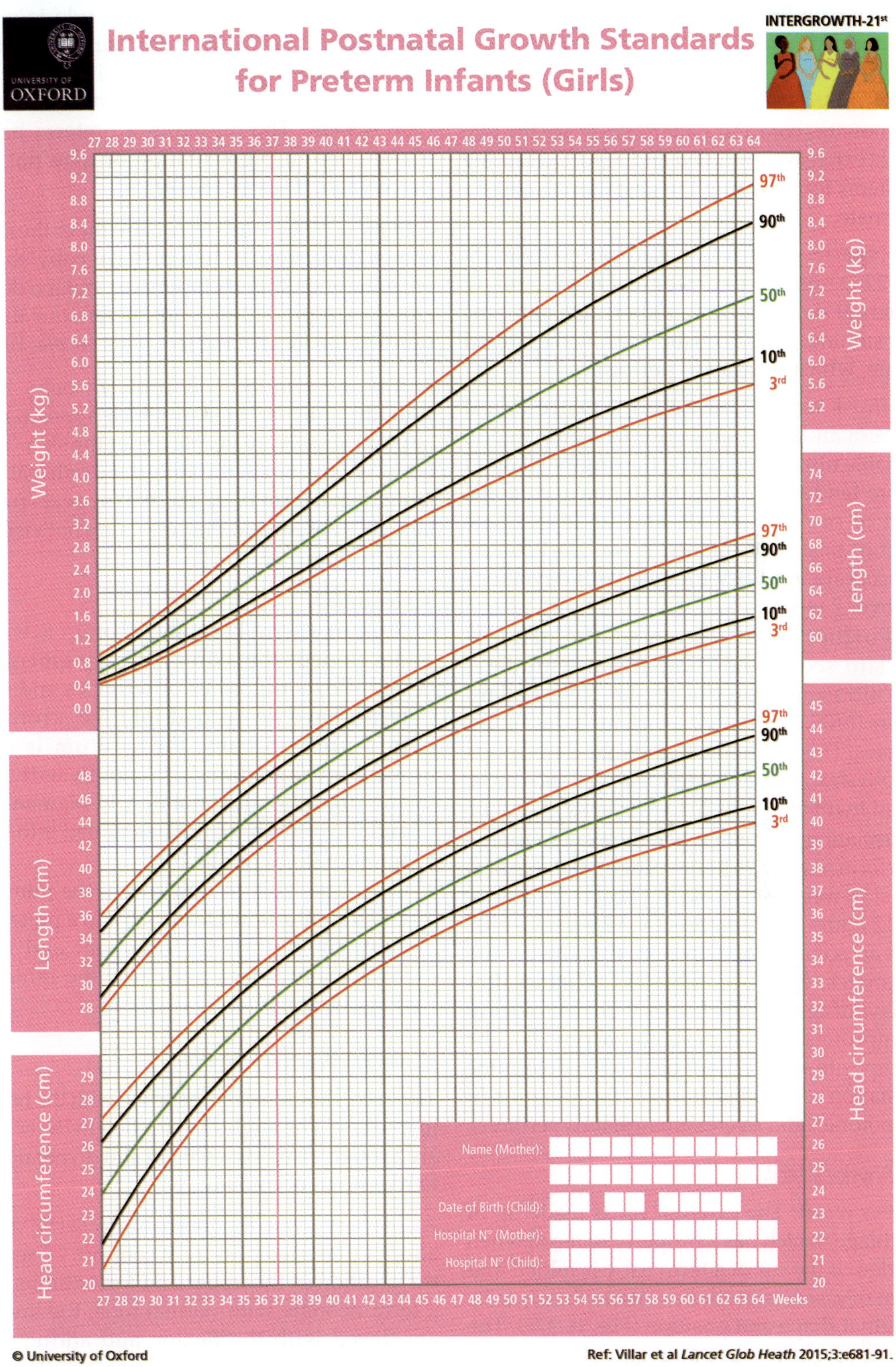

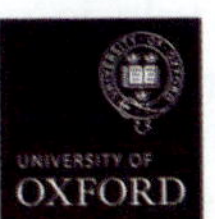

International Postnatal Growth Standards for Preterm Infants (Girls)

Weight (kg)

Length (cm)

Head circumference (cm)

97th 90th 50th 10th 3rd

27 28 29 30 31 32 33 34 35 36 37 38 39 40 41 42 43 44 45 46 47 48 49 50 51 52 53 54 55 56 57 58 59 60 61 62 63 64 Weeks

Name (Mother):

Date of Birth (Child):

Hospital N° (Mother):

Hospital N° (Child):

Ref: Villar et al *Lancet Glob Heath* 2015;3:e681-91.

Fig. 16.25d: International (Intergrowth 21st) Postnatal Growth Standards for Preterm Infants (Girls). Reprinted with the permission of the INTERGROWTH-21st Consortium, Oxford.

head circumference, length, and weight gives an approximate idea.

Scoring Systems

Dubowitz score and Ballard score are the two most extensively studied and reported scoring systems for assessing the gestational age of a neonate.

Dubowitz score was based on assessment of 22 items (10 neurological signs and 12 external signs). It was cumbersome and time consuming. It has been replaced by the Ballard score, which is easier to perform.

Ballard score is based on 6 neurological criteria and 6 physical criteria. Compared to reliable ultrasound dates, the original Ballard score tended to overestimate the gestational age of preterm infants and underestimate that of post-term infants. It was particularly inaccurate in ELBW infants, with deviations of over 2 weeks.

Further modification of the original Ballard scores and comparison with dates by ultrasound produced the New Ballard score (NBS, Fig. 16.26), which includes ELBW babies. This method expands the description of physical and neurologic features and can be used in infants from 20 to 44 weeks gestation. Correlation is similar when the examination is performed up to 96 hours of age in infants of at least 26 weeks gestation but best if done prior to 12 hours in infants less than 26 weeks. NBS has an accuracy of ±2 weeks. In more mature neonates, NBS becomes less reliable after 7 days of age. Also, in babies with neurological compromise (as in perinatal asphyxia), the composite score cannot be used to determine gestation as it underestimates the gestation (if hypotonic) and overestimates, if hypertonic.

I. Physical Maturity

1. Ear recoil: The external ear is made up of cartilage, which has a property to recoil when folded. If the ear of a term baby is folded and then released, it recoils back immediately to its original shape and position **(Fig. 16.27a)**. The ear also feels firm in a term baby. In a preterm baby, the ear recoils back slowly and does not feel firm **(Fig. 16.27b)**.

2. Breast nodule: The breast bud or nodule is palpated between the index finger and the thumb. In a term baby, the nodule is well palpable and measures more than 0.5 cm and the nipple is deeply pigmented. In a preterm, the nodule may not be felt at all or is less than 0.5 cm. The nipple in a preterm baby is not deep in pigmentation or may not be perceivable **(Figs 16.28a, b)**.

3. Plantar creases: In a term baby, the entire sole shows deep creases. In a preterm baby, there are numerous superficial creases, but the deep creases are present only in the anterior third (toward the toes) of the feet **(Figs 16.29a, b)**.

4. Lanugo and skin: A preterm baby has smooth, transparent skin which appears red or pink. Vessels are visible under the skin. The body is covered with abundant hair called lanugo. In a term baby, the skin appears pale, lanugo is absent and the vessels are not visible **(Figs 16.30a, b)**.

5. Genitalia:

- *Boys:* In a term baby, the scrotum is well-developed, the skin is hyperpigmented and shows rugosities or wrinkles and the testes have descended into the scrotum. In a preterm baby, the scrotum is not well-developed and is smooth without any rugosities. It is not deeply pigmented and the testes have not descended into the scrotum **(Figs 16.31a, b)**.
- *Girls:* The labia majora covers the minora and the clitoris in a term baby. In a preterm baby, the clitoris is prominent and the labia majora does not cover the minora **(Figs 16.32a, b)**.

II. Neuromuscular Maturity

The baby should be lying supine with the head in midline. The angles mentioned in the score are a rough visual assessment and do not need to measured accurately.

1. Posture: Wait for the baby to settle and adopt a preferred posture of comfort. Observe the position of the upper and lower limbs. In a term neonate with normal tone, the knees are flexed with the flexion and adduction of hip **(Fig. 16.33a)** and flexion of elbows. Flexed knees with abduction give a "frog like posture" which denotes hypotonia **(Fig. 16.33b)**. A preterm baby will also be hypotonic compared to a term baby.

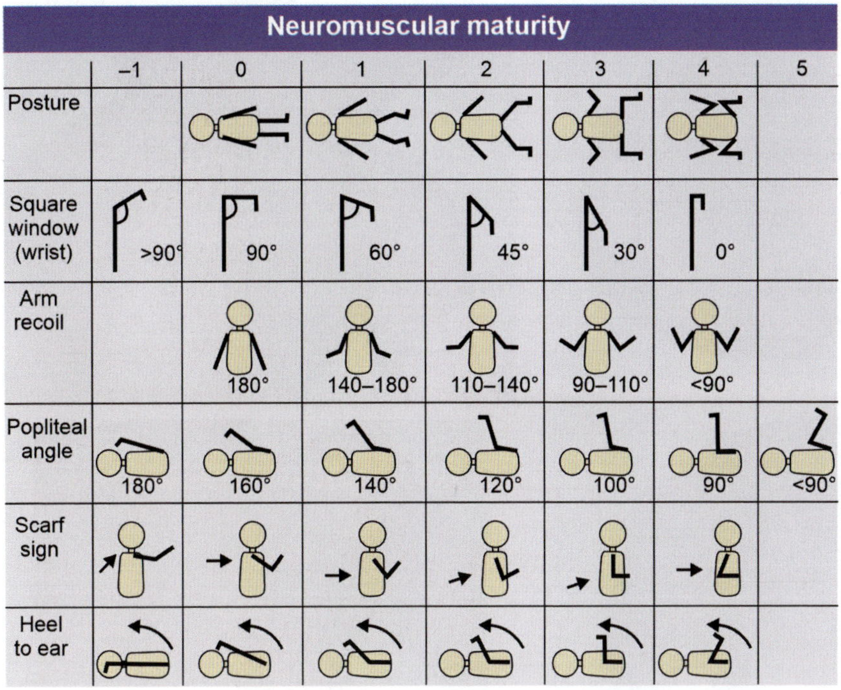

Neuromuscular maturity							
	–1	0	1	2	3	4	5
Posture							
Square window (wrist)	>90°	90°	60°	45°	30°	0°	
Arm recoil		180°	140–180°	110–140°	90–110°	<90°	
Popliteal angle	180°	160°	140°	120°	100°	90°	<90°
Scarf sign							
Heel to ear							

Maturity rating	
Score	Weeks
–10	20
–5	22
0	24
5	26
10	28
15	30
20	32
25	34
30	36
35	38
40	40
45	42
50	44

Physical Maturity

Score	–1	0	1	2	3	4	5
Skin	Sticky, friable, transparent	Gelatinous, red translucent	Smooth pink, visible veins	Superficial peeting &/ or rash, few veins	Cracking, pale areas, rare veins	Parchment, deep cracking, no vessels	Leathery, cracked wrinkled
Lanugo	None	Sparse	Abundant	Thinning	Bald areas	Mostly bald	
Plantar surface	Heel-toe 40–50 mm; –1 <40 mm; –2	>50 mm no crease	Faint red marks	Anterior transverse crease only	Crease ant. 2/3	Crease over entire sole	
Breast	Imperceptable	Barely perceptable	Flat areola no bud	Stipped areola 1–2 mm bud	Raised areola 3–4 mm bud	Full areola 5–10 mm bud	
Eye/ear	Lids fused Loosely: –1 Tightly: –2	Lids open Pinna flat Stays folded	Sl. curved pinna; soft; slow recoil	Well-curved pinna; soft but ready recoil	Formed & firm instant recoil	Thick cartilage ear stiff	
Genitals (male)	Scrotum flat, smooth	Scrotum empty, faint rugae	Tastes in upper canal, rare rugae	Testes descending few rugae	Testes down, goods rugae	Testes pendulous, deep rugae	
Genitals (female)	Clitoris prominent, labia flat	Prominent clitoris & small minora	Prominent clitoris & enlarging minora	Majora & minora equally prominent	Majora large, minora small	Majora cover clitoris & minora	

Fig. 16.26: The New Ballard score.

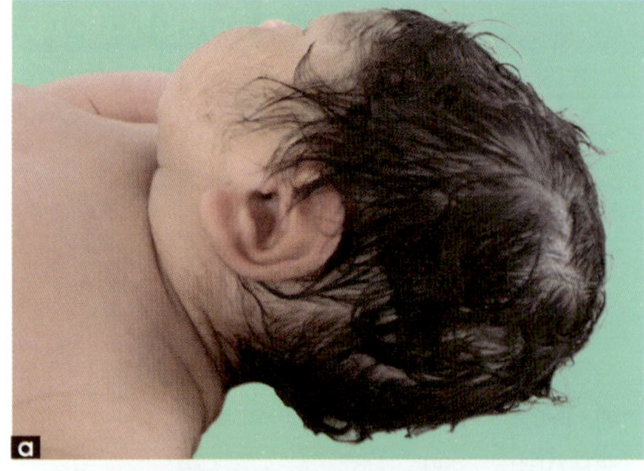

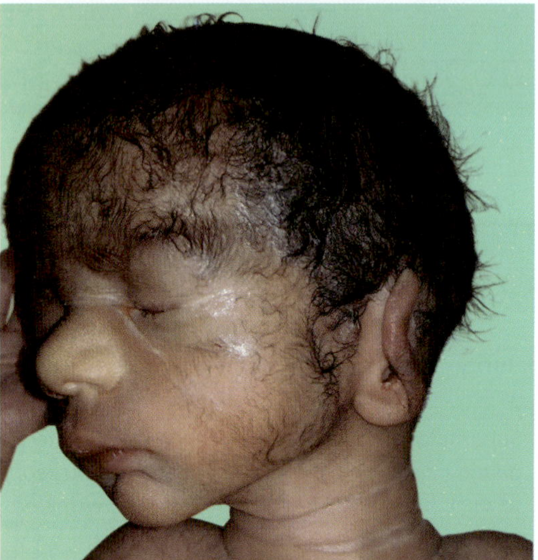

Fig. 16.27: Ear cartilage: (a) Term; (b) preterm with delayed recoil.

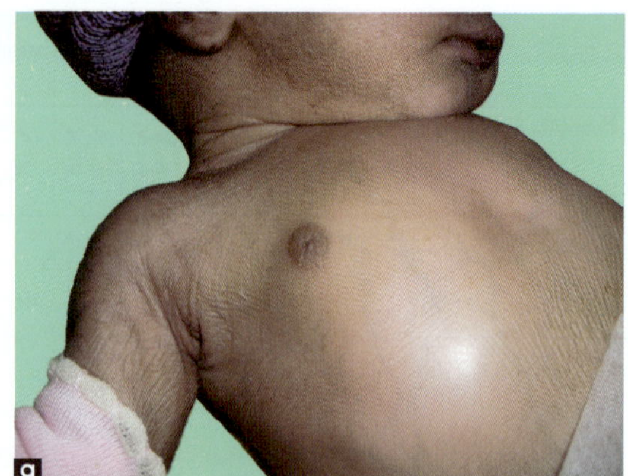

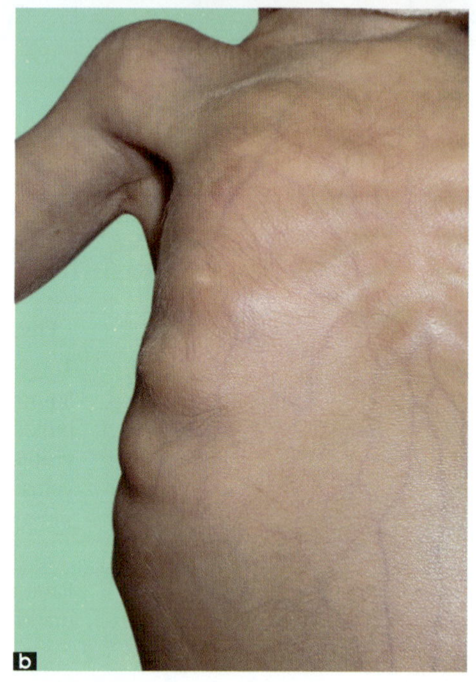

Fig. 16.28: Breast nodule: (a) Term; (b) preterm.

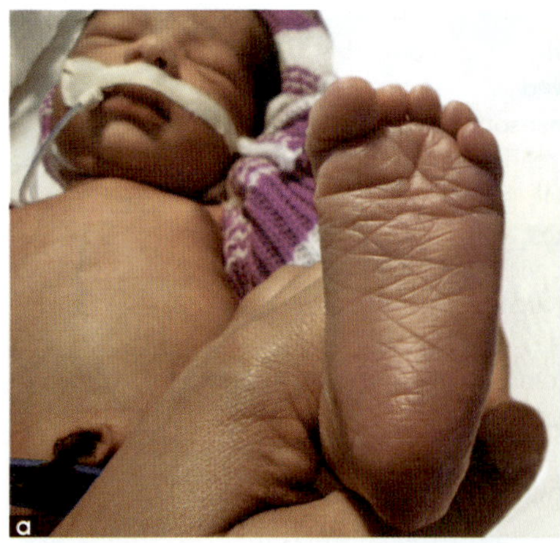

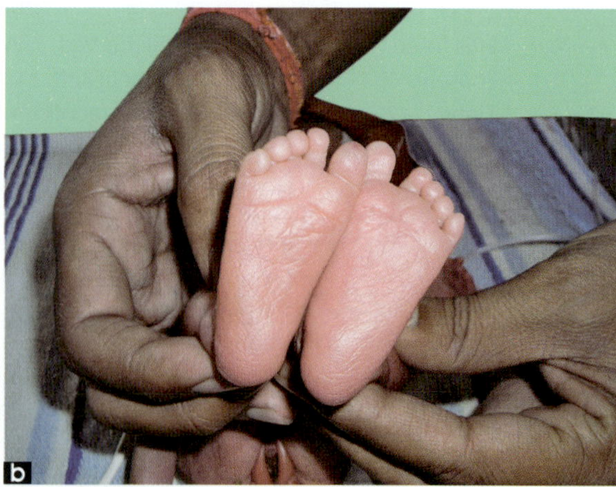

Fig. 16.29: Plantar creases: (a) Term; (b) preterm.

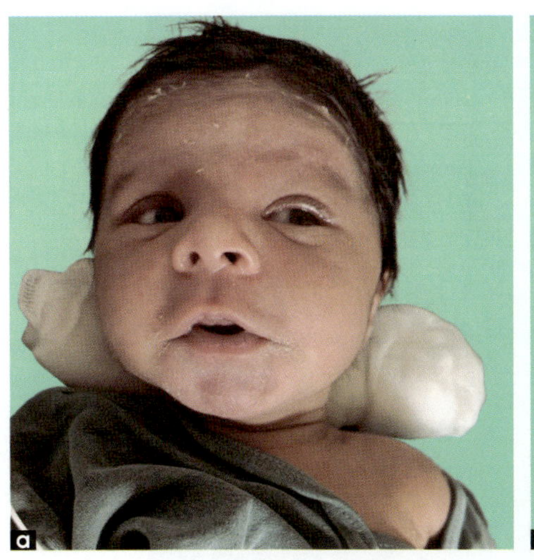
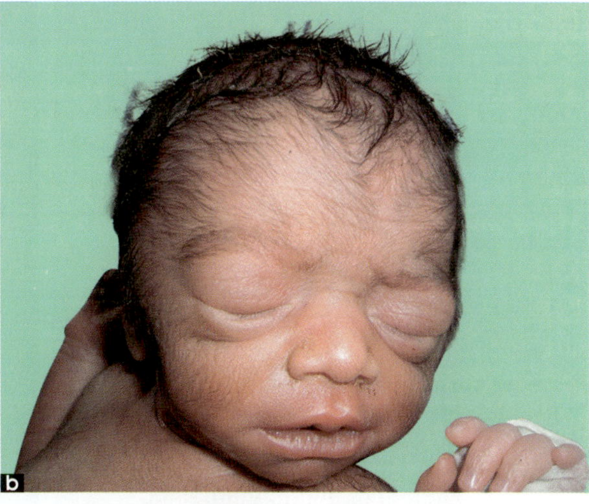

Fig. 16.30: Skin: (a) Term; (b) preterm.

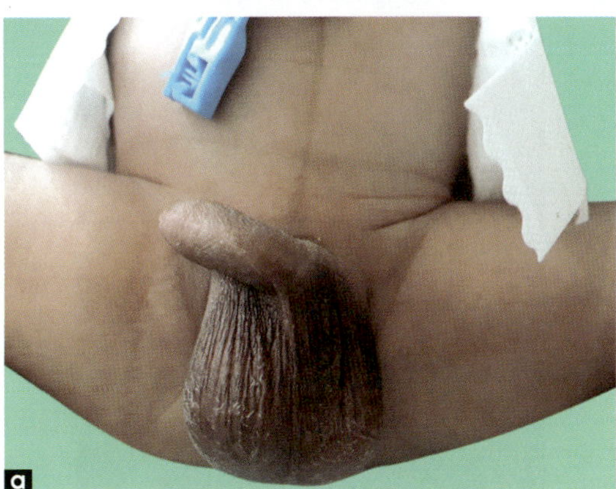
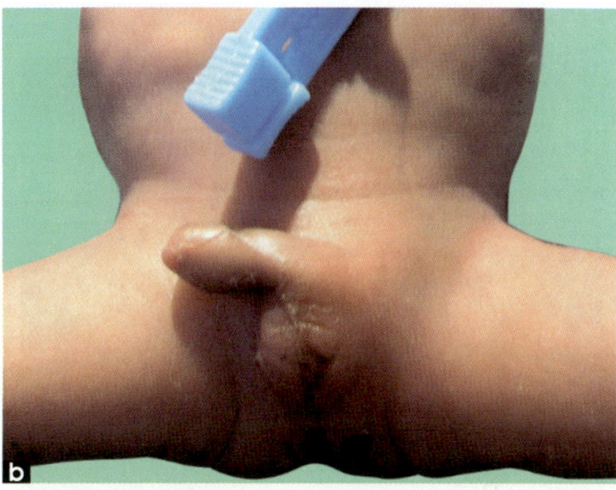

Fig. 16.31: Male genitalia: (a) Term; (b) preterm.

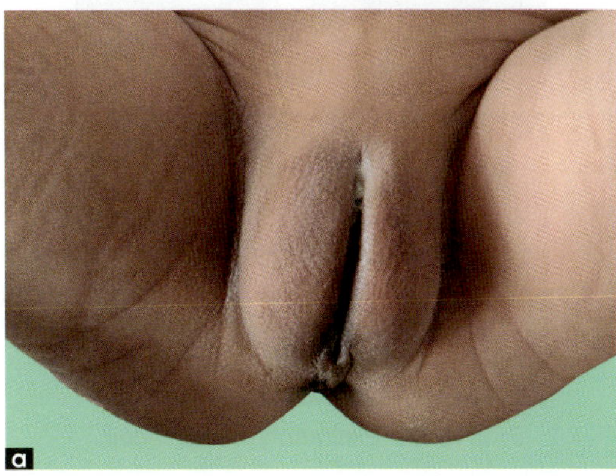
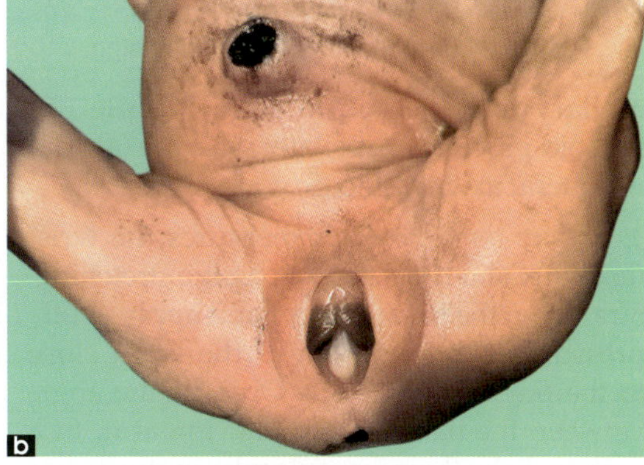

Fig. 16.32: Female genitalia: (a) Term; (b) preterm.

2. Scarf sign: This sign tests the passive flexor tone of the flexors of the shoulder joint. Pull the infants hand across the chest towards the opposite side and support it with your hand (Fig. 16.34). With the thumb of other hand, try to gently push the elbow of the baby across the chest. Note the position of the baby's elbow on its chest when you feel resistance. The score is given according to the position of the elbow; at the level of the neck (–1), contralateral

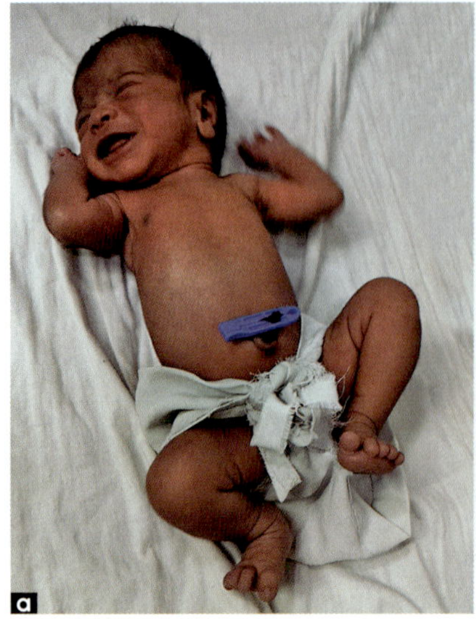

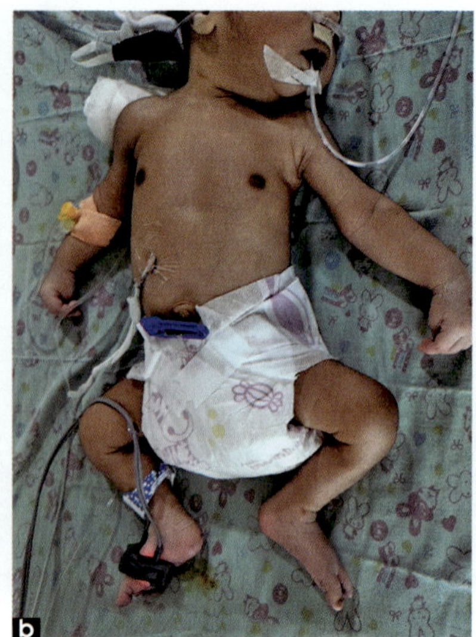

Fig. 16.33: (a) Normal posture of a term baby; (b) posture suggestive of hypotonia.

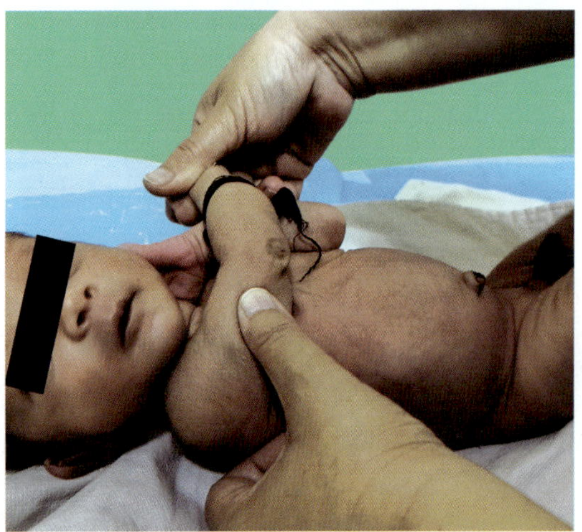

Fig. 16.34: Method for eliciting scarf sign.

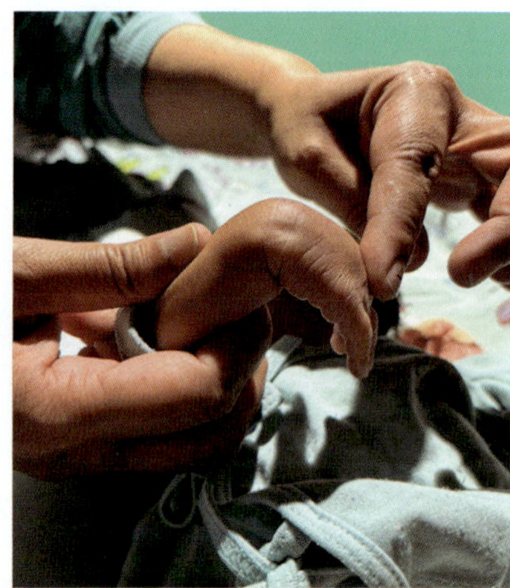

Fig. 16.35: Elicitation of square window sign.

axillary line (1), contralateral nipple (2), xiphoid process (3), ipsilateral nipple (4), and ipsilateral axillary line (5).

3. Square window: This measures the wrist flexibility and resistance to passive stretching. Straighten the baby's finger and apply gentle pressure on the dorsum of the hand close to the fingers (Fig 16.35). Observe the angle between the baby's hand and forearm. In a preterm baby the neuromuscular maturity has not been achieved and the ligaments cannot be stretched fully. Therefore, the angle is more in preterms, the angle decreases as the term gestation is reached.

4. Arm recoil: This maneuver measures the passive tone of the biceps in response to brief extension of the elbows. Hold the infant's hands and flex the elbows, then momentarily extend them, and release the hand. Observe for recoil of the forearm and angle made between the forearm and arm (Fig 16.36). The recoil is brisk in term babies and the angle decreases with progression of gestation.

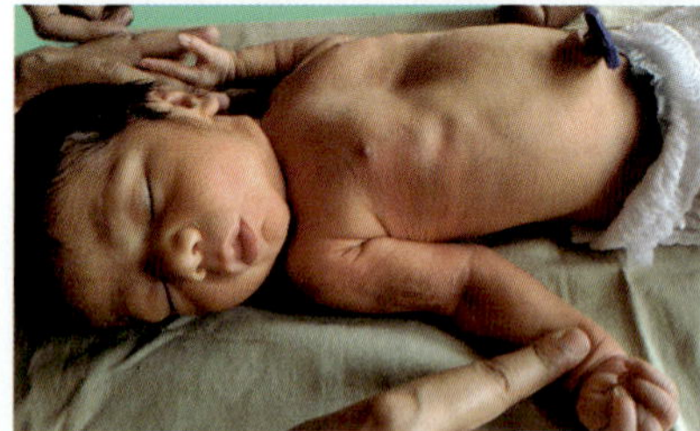

Fig. 16.36: Elicitation of arm recoil.

5. Popliteal angle: This assesses the maturation of passive flexor tone. Remove the diaper of the baby before performing the maneuver. Stabilise the thigh of the baby over the abdomen and flex the knee. Support the thigh with one hand, then hold the foot of the baby with other hand and try to extend the knee till some resistance is felt. The angle formed between the upper and lower leg at the knee is observed **(Fig. 16.37)**.

6. Heel to ear: This maneuver measures the passive flexor tone of the posterior hip flexor muscles. The infant is placed supine and the flexed lower extremity is brought to rest on the cot. The examiner supports the infant's thigh laterally alongside the body with the palm of one hand. The other hand is used to grasp the infant's foot at the sides and to pull it toward the ipsilateral ear. The examiner feels for the resistance to extension of the posterior pelvic girdle flexors and notes the location of the heel where significant resistance is appreciated **(Fig. 16.38)**.

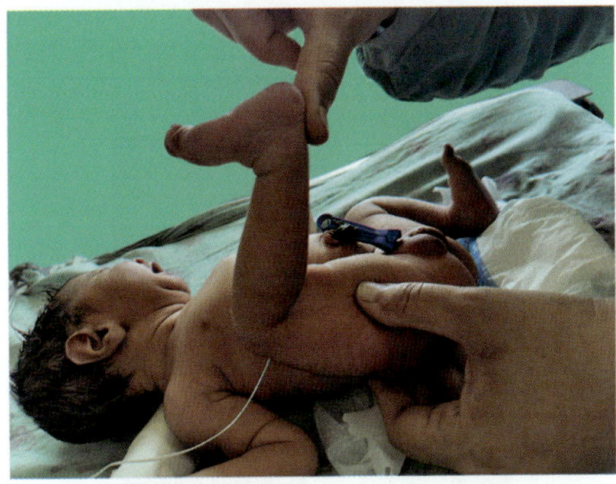

Fig. 16.37: Method of measuring popliteal angle.

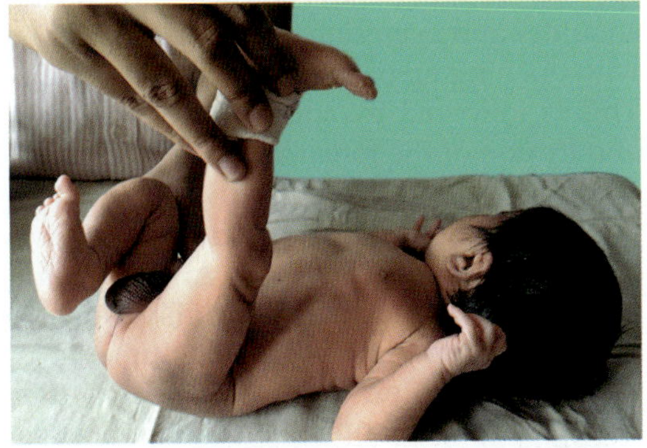

Fig. 16.38: Elicitation of heel to ear maneuver.

16.6 GENERAL EXAMINATION

Observe for the cry, body movements, and elicit neonatal reflexes.

A. Cry

The cry of a baby tells a lot about the condition of the baby.

- A healthy cry is loud and consolable, accompanied by active movements of the limbs.
- A CNS insult may lead to a *shrill, high-pitched cry* which is inconsolable.
- A baby with hypothyroidism may have a *hoarse cry*.
- Newborns with asphyxia or septicemia may have a *feeble cry* or may not cry at all.

B. Body Movements

A healthy baby shows writhing body movements involving the upper and lower limbs and the trunk. The movements show complexity and variability and are present continuously in an awake baby. There is extension and flexion with superimposed rotation making the movements smooth with low-to-moderate amplitude and speed. When the movements lose their complexity and diversity they are divided into poor repertoire, cramped synchronous, chaotic general body movements. These movements lack smoothness and are monotonous and repetitive. They may be involving the same limb with no alteration with the trunk and other limbs. Babies with CNS insult can have these abnormal movements which maybe predictive of cerebral palsy. A dull or a lethargic baby will have decreased or no spontaneous movements.

C. Neonatal Reflexes

Several primitive neonatal reflexes can be elicited in healthy term neonate. Their absence indicates illness.

1. Rooting and Sucking Reflexes

Rooting reflex: Touch a finger to the neonate's cheek or the corner of mouth. Alternatively, bring the mother's nipple into contact with infant's cheek. The baby turns the head toward the stimulus, opens the mouth and searches for the stimulus/nipple **(Fig. 16.39)**.

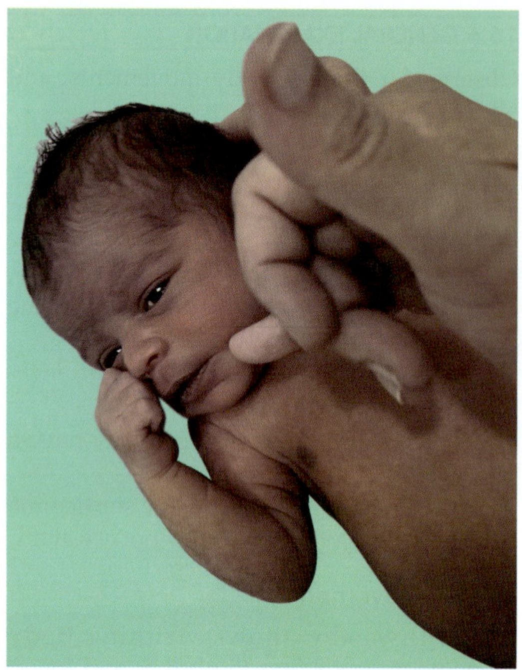

Fig. 16.39: Rooting reflex.

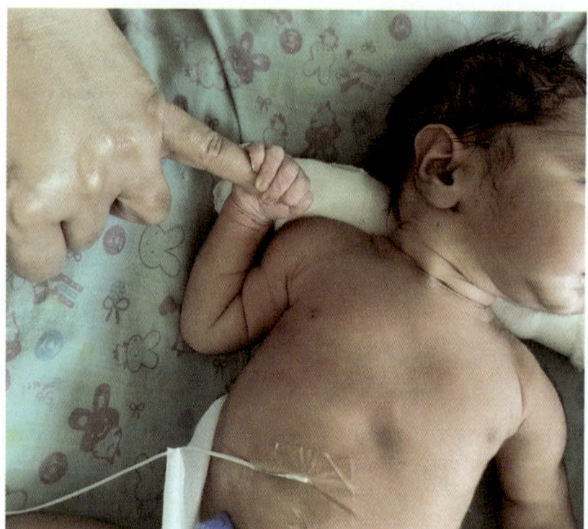

Fig. 16.40: Grasp reflex.

Sucking reflex: Stimulation of the upper and lower lips produces movement of the lip and tongue in the direction of the stimulus (sucking reflex). Sucking reflex is feeble in the sick and preterm infants. The observer evaluates the reflex by introducing a clean gloved finger into the infant's mouth and noting the strength and rhythm of sucking. The reflex is strong and well-synchronized with swallowing at 34 weeks.

2. Grasp Reflex

Stroke the baby's palm with your index finger. The baby's fingers will grasp your index fingers. Now, if you lift your index finger, the flexor muscles of the infant's forearm will become tight **(Fig. 16.40)**. Similarly, the toes turn inwards when the sole is stroked (plantar reflex) **(Fig. 16.41)**.

The grasp reflex usually disappears by the age of 12 weeks. Persistence of the reflex beyond this age should arouse suspicion of brain damage.

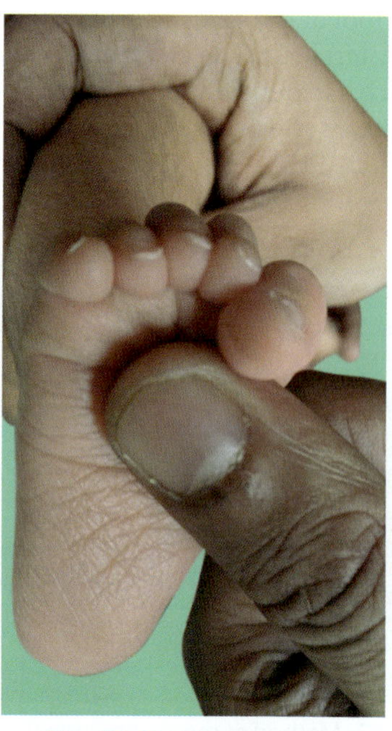

Fig. 16.41: Plantar grasp.

3. Moro Reflex

For eliciting Moro reflex, hold baby at an angle of 45° from the bed and then suddenly let the head fall back a few centimeters while still supporting it with hand. A positive response consists of sudden abduction of the arms at the shoulder and extension of arms at the elbow, with opening up of hand and curved fingers. This is followed by adduction of the arms and flexion of the forearm (i.e. an 'embrace') **(Figs 16.42a, b)**.

Infants with cerebral damage have exaggerated or absent response. An asymmetric response is seen in Erb's palsy, spastic hemiplegia, and fracture of the humerus or clavicle. The reflex usually disappears after the age of 4–5 months. Persistence beyond 6 months of age is considered pathological.

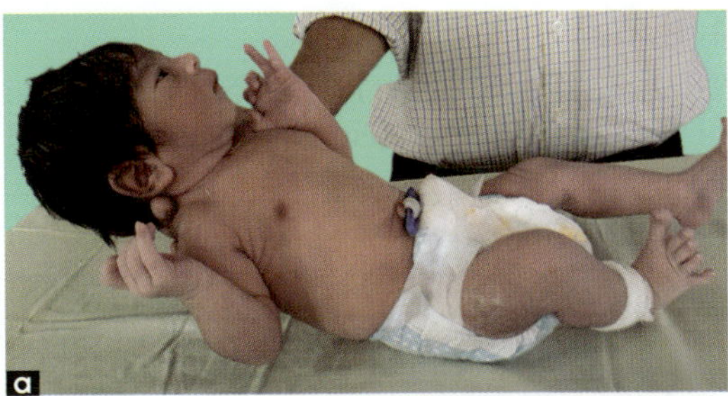

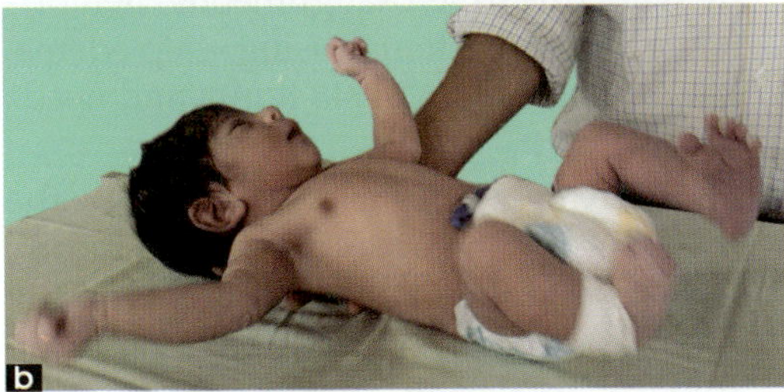

Fig. 16.42: (a) Elicitation of Moro reflex; (b) abduction of arms and flexion of forearms.

4. Glabellar Tap

Gently tap the glabella (junction between the nose and forehead) with your finger. Both eyelids of the neonate will blink.

5. Crossed Extension

Stroke the foot while the leg is held extended at knee. There is rapid flexion, adduction, and then extension of the opposite leg.

6. Tonic Neck Reflex

Turn the supine infant's head suddenly to one side. The arm and leg on the same side extend, while the opposite limbs go into flexion (Fig. 16.43). Persistence of the reflex beyond the age of 6 months or a constant tonic neck posture is abnormal, and usually indicates spastic cerebral palsy.

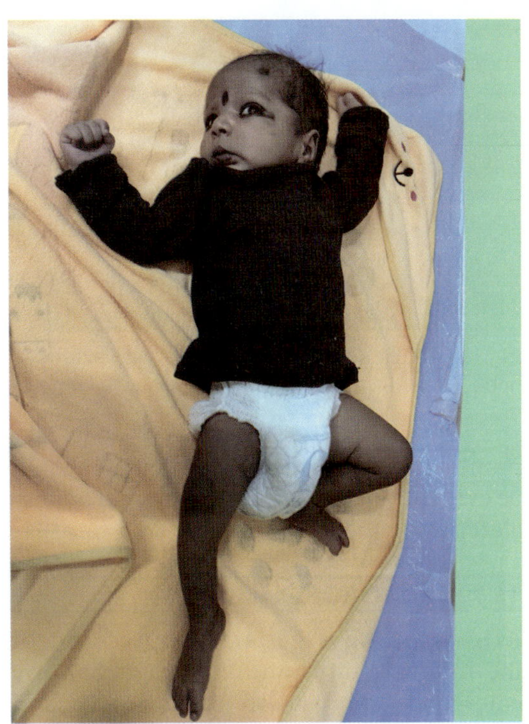

Fig. 16.43: Asymmetric tonic neck reflex.

D. Posture and Muscle Tone

Observing the infant is the most important aspect of the physical examination. It is best performed with the infant quiet and unclothed. Observe the state of alertness, the muscle tone, the activity, obvious anomalies or injuries, respiratory pattern, and the skin during inspection. The infant may appear sick or well, responsive, or lethargic.

A normal newborn lies with hip and knee flexed. In hypotonia, there is frog-like posture. Hypertonia is characterized by fisting, cortical thumb (Fig. 16.44), and hyperextended neck (Fig. 16.45). Also observe for any asymmetry of arms and legs. Scissoring of the lower limb and opisthotonos also indicate extensor hypertonia.

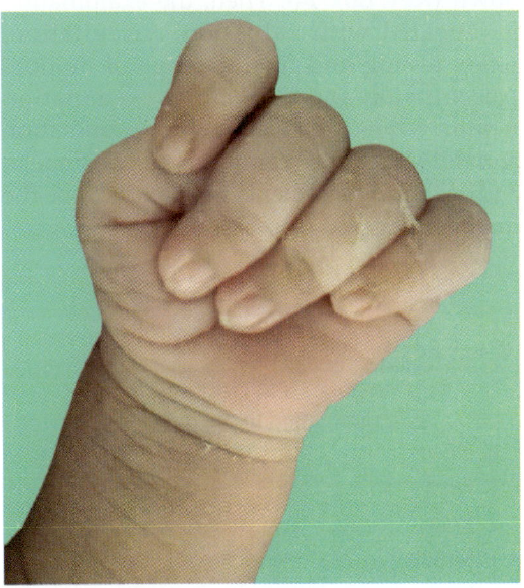

Fig. 16.44: Cortical thumb.

The muscle tone in a term infant should be sufficient for the hips, knees, and elbows to be flexed while the infant is lying supine or

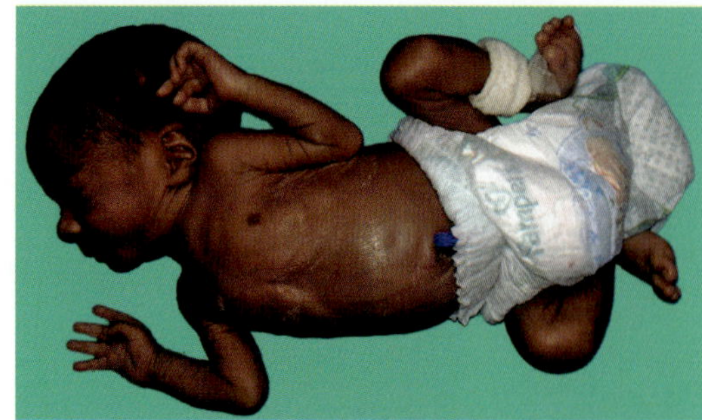

Fig. 16.45: Generalized hypertonia with extended neck.

prone. A few spontaneous movements should be evident, and the well infant should appear alert during the examination.

16.7 HEAD-TO-TOE EXAMINATION

After gaining a general impression of the infants' status and ensuring that any emergency intervention is not needed and vitals are stable, continue to observe the infant, usually starting at the head and working down **(Key Box 14)**. Then, the examination is repeated with palpation, auscultation, reflex testing and finally, range of motion. Auscultation and abdominal examination require a quiet infant. The hip examination and the Moro reflex testing should be done in end as these assessments frequently leave the infant crying and displeased.

Key Box 14

Components of Head-to-Toe Examination in Neonates

1. Head
2. Face
3. Eyes
4. Mouth
5. Ears
6. Nose
7. Neck
8. Skin
9. Chest
10. Umbilicus
11. Anus and genitalia
12. Spine and limbs
13. Hip joint

1. Head

The head should be examined for any swelling or abnormal shape. Also feel for sutures and fontanels.

- ***Caput succedaneum*** is a diffuse swelling over the scalp which is present at birth or may appear just after birth **(Fig. 16.46)**. It is normally seen after a difficult vaginal delivery due to serosanguineous/hemorrhagic fluid collection causing scalp edema. It subsides in next 24–48 hours and needs no treatment.
- ***Cephalohematoma*** is a swelling on the scalp due to subperiosteal bleeding mostly in cases of difficult delivery. It is typically not present at or immediately after birth. It starts appearing after the first day of life and may increase in size for next 2–3 days. It is usually present on one of the parietal bones and never crosses the suture lines **(Fig. 16.47)**. They are unilateral or bilateral, firm and fluctuant swellings over the scalp. Cephalohematoma does not need any intervention and may take 2–3 months to resolve. This may contribute to prolongation of jaundice in a newborn.
- Encephalocele and occipital meningocele are other swellings that may be present on the scalp **(Fig. 16.48)**.

Subgaleal Hemorrhage

The hemorrhage is under the aponeurosis of the scalp but above the periosteum.

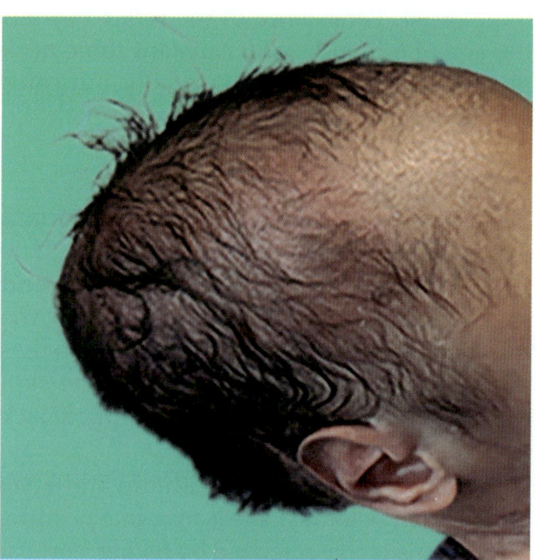

Fig. 16.46: Caput succedaneum.

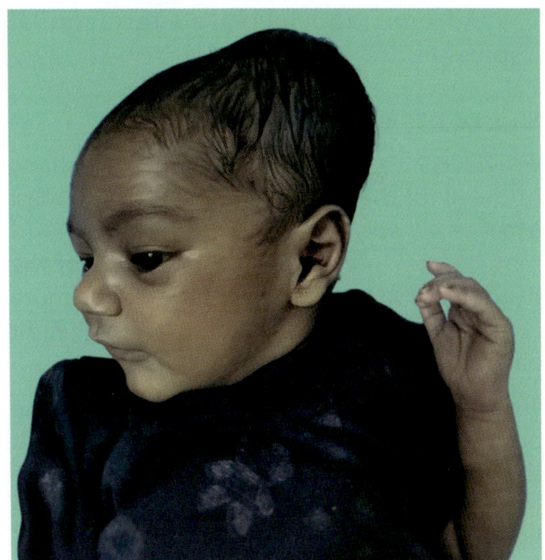
Fig. 16.47: Cephalohematoma.

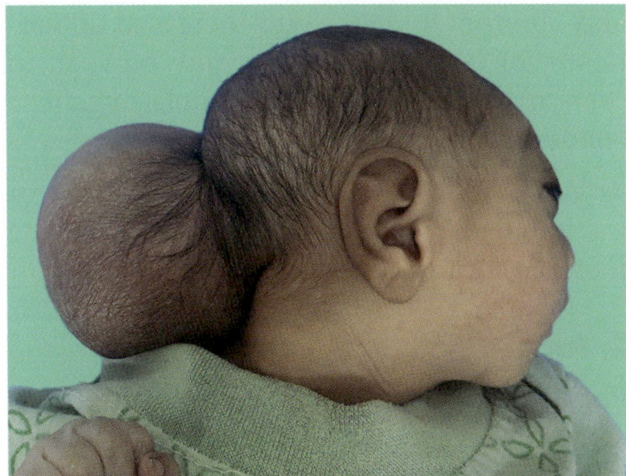
Fig. 16.48: Encephalocele.

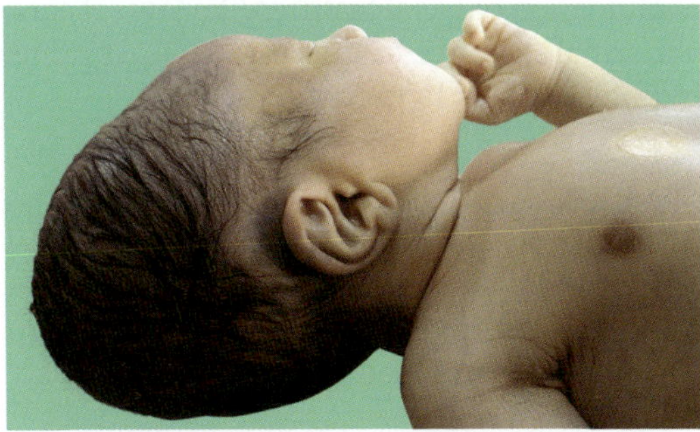
Fig. 16.49: Subgaleal hematoma.

The swelling is boggy, crosses suture lines (Fig. 16.49). The hemorrhage can extend into the neck and displace the ear. Watch for development of pallor, shock, and jaundice.

Fontanels and Sutures

The newborn infant's skull is composed of bony plates separated by sutures to accommodate transient skull distortion during birth and permit future growth of the brain. There are four major sutures: The metopic, coronal, sagittal, and lambdoid. Three additional sutures that contribute to calvarial development are considered minor: The frontonasal, temporosquamosal, and frontosphenoidal. The sagittal, coronal, and metopic sutures meet at the anterior part of the skull to form the anterior fontanel, palpable just behind the forehead in the midline. The posterior fontanel is formed by the intersection of the sagittal and lambdoid sutures (Fig. 16.50). While the metopic suture typically closes at 2 years of age, all remaining patent sutures close in adulthood following completion of craniofacial growth.

Fontanels

Including anterior and posterior fontanels, there are a total of 6 fontanels. There are two pairs of lateral fontanels known as the sphenoidal or anterolateral fontanels and the mastoid or posterolateral fontanels. The four lateral fontanels generally fuse in infancy and are clinically less significant. Fontanel and suture closure occur in a specific pattern.

- Fibrous closure of posterior fontanel is usually present at birth and it does not allow more than a fingertip to palpate. Complete closure of the posterior fontanel occurs at 2 months of age.
- Anterior fontanel closes by 9–24 months.

Anterior fontanel: It is a soft diamond shaped area between the frontal and the parietal skull

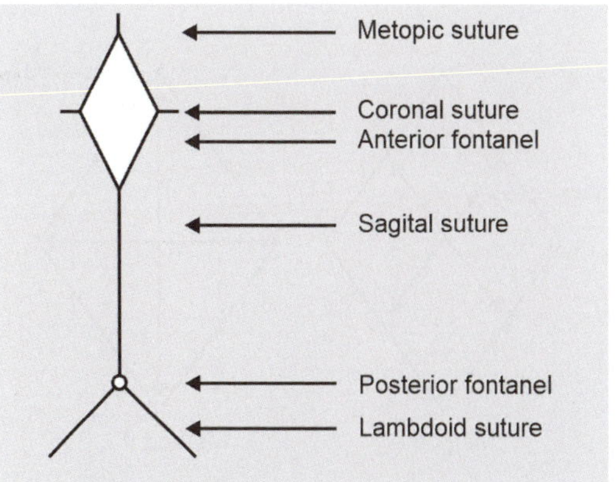

Fig. 16.50: Location of fontanels.

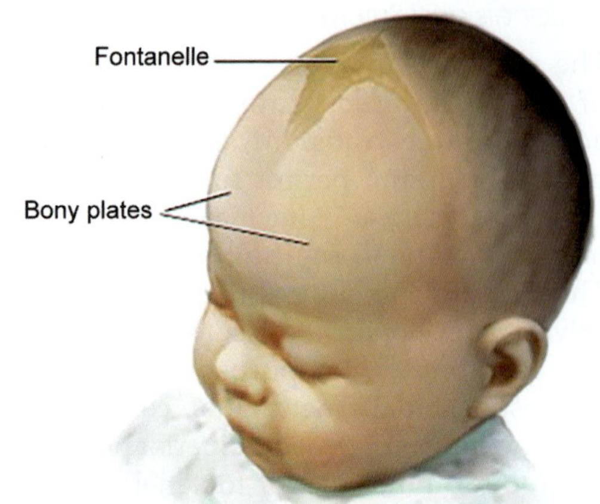

Fig. 16.51: Anterior fontanel.

bones (Fig. 16.51). It should be soft and at the level of the skull bones. A tense or a bulging anterior fontanel is a grave sign indicating raised intracranial pressure, which may be indicative of asphyxia, intracranial bleed, meningitis, or hydrocephalus. Sutures may be separated or splayed in cases of raised intracranial pressure.

Size: Size of anterior fontanel can be measured from edge of the wall to opposite wall or from corner to corner (Fig. 16.52).

- Fontanel size is influenced by brain growth due to its stimulation of skull bone growth, suture development, and subsequent osteogenesis.
- On the first day of life, the average anterior fontanel size varies from 0.6 to 3 cm.
- Premature neonates tend to have larger fontanels.
- Many disorders are associated with an abnormally large fontanel, e.g. congenital hypothyroidism, achondroplasia, Down syndrome, and increased intracranial pressure.

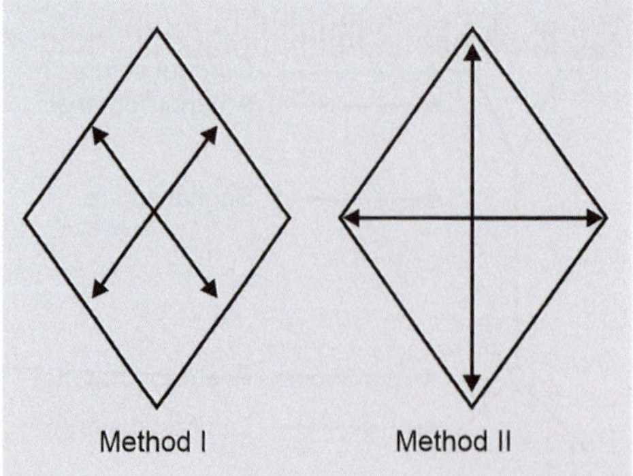

Fig. 16.52: Measurement of anterior fontanel.

Shapes of the Skull (Fig. 16.53)

Plagiocephaly: This is the asymmetrical shape of the skull due to flattening of skull bones. Most cases seen are sporadic in nature and may be due to prolonged positioning of the head in the same position (supine). It is more commonly seen in preterm or low birth weight babies.

Brachycephaly: There is flattening of the occipital bone leading to a short skull with decreased anterio-posterior dimension. The most common cause is positional, when the baby lies in the supine position for prolonged periods. It may be due to craniosynostosis in some cases.

Dolicocephaly: The skull becomes narrow and abnormally long with increased antero-posterior dimension. This may be seen in preterm babies or in some metabolic or genetic conditions.

Trigonocephaly: This is triangular shape of the forehead due to premature closure of the metopic suture.

2. Face

Facial features must be closely observed. Abnormal looking facies or facial dysmorphism is the presence of facial features which are abnormal and usually associated with a chromosomal abnormality like Down syndrome (Fig. 16.54). This may be a combination of facial features like low set ears, abnormal slant of eye, depressed nasal bridge, hypotelorism or hypertelorism, etc.

3. Eyes

- The eyes may show subconjunctival hemorrhage (Fig. 16.55), which may be a normal finding especially in babies born vaginally. The bleed resorbs spontaneously in 2 to 8 weeks.
- The eyes may show redness and purulent discharge. There may be watering from one or both eyes due to epiphora.
- An abnormal appearance of the eye may be seen in facial dysmorphism and will need a detailed evaluation.

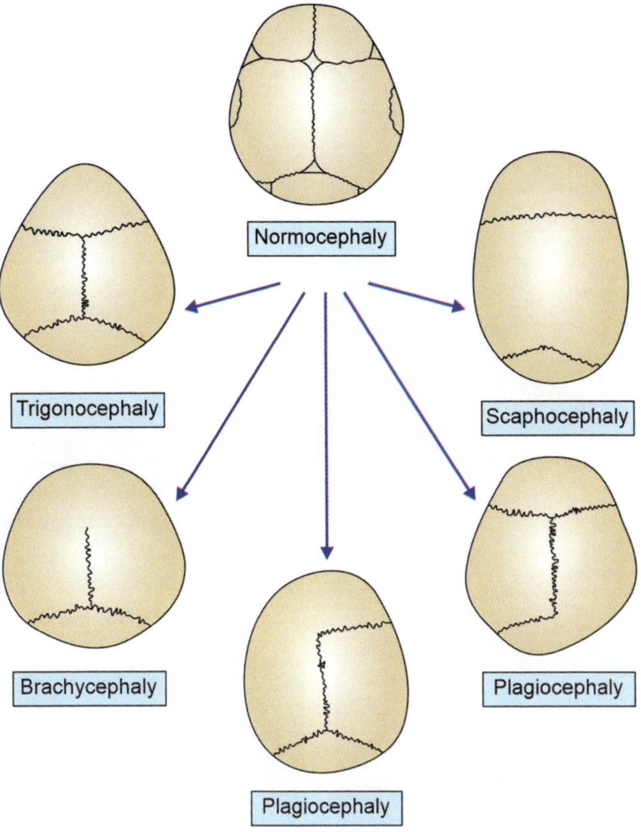

Fig. 16.53: Shapes of skull.

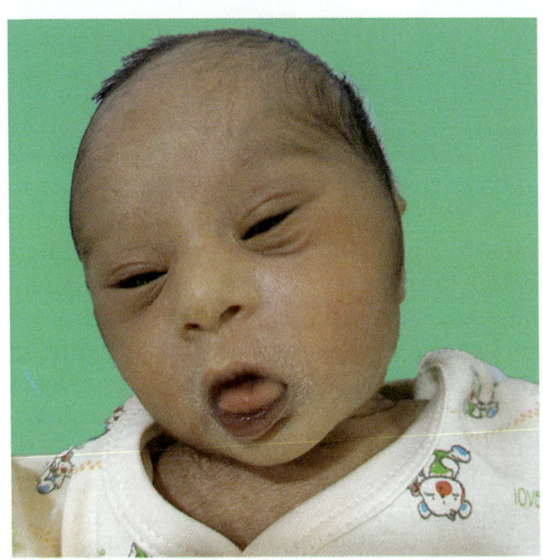

Fig. 16.54: Down syndrome.

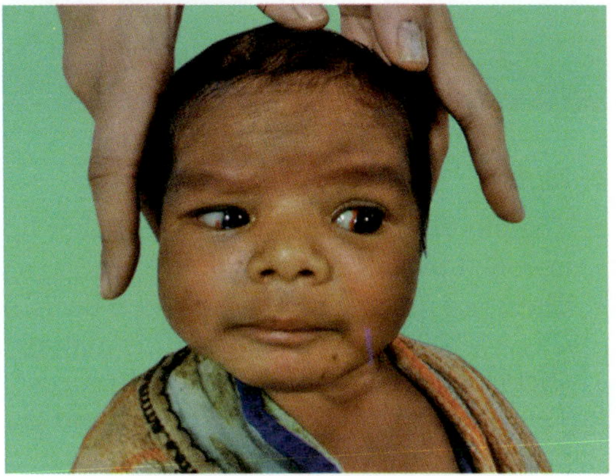

Fig. 16.55: Subconjunctival hemorrhage.

- ***Red eye reflex:*** This is seen by a direct ophthalmoscopic examination of both eyes. Both eyes should show a red reflex on examination, which should be symmetrical. Absence of red eye reflex or appearance of white reflex should be immediately evaluated for cataract or retinoblastoma.
- ***Nasolacrimal duct:*** It may be obstructed in the first few months of life in some babies. This leads to constant watering from eyes causing periocular crusting and discharge.
- Raised intracranial tension may give rise to *sun set sign* with a constant downward gaze (Fig. 16.56).

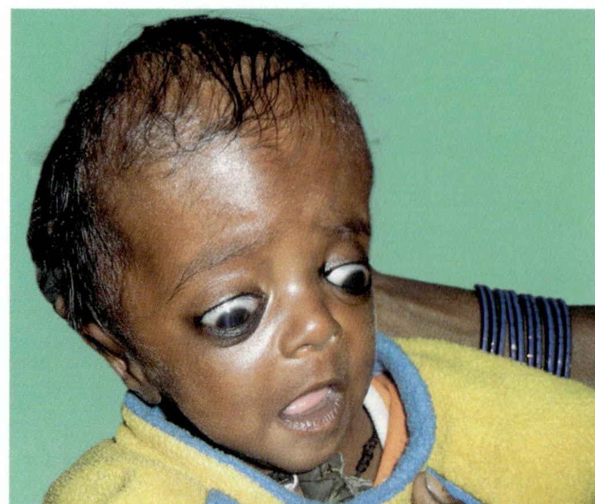

Fig. 16.56: Sunset sign.

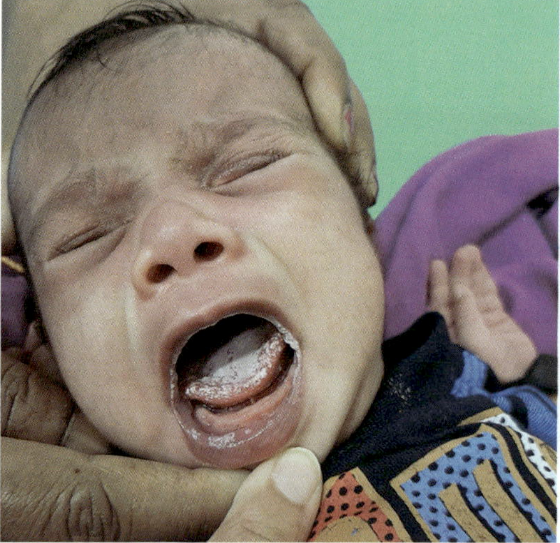

Fig. 16.57: Oral thrush.

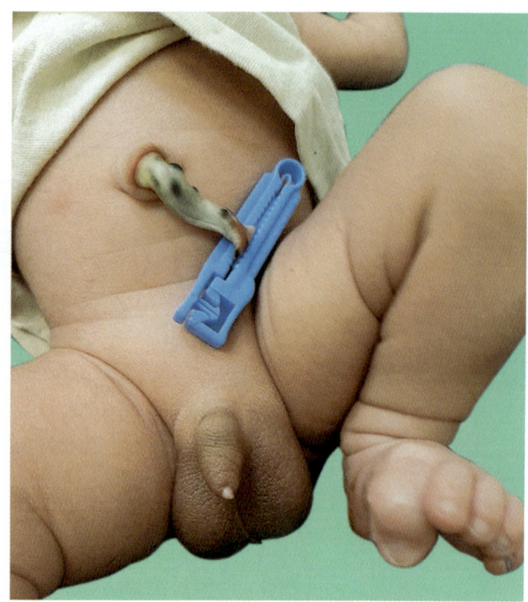

Fig. 16.58: Penile ebstein pearl.

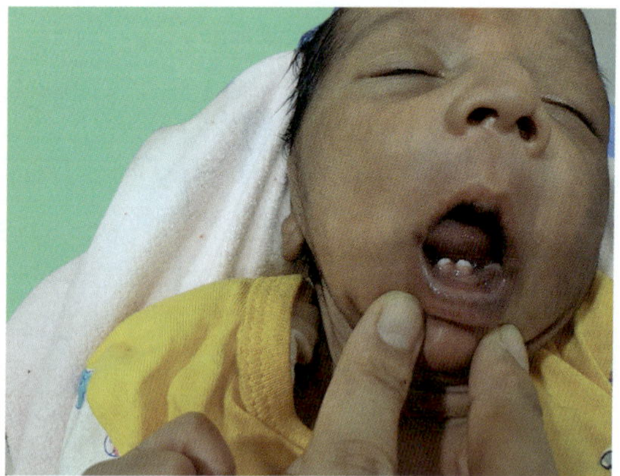

Fig. 16.59: Prenatal teeth.

4. Mouth

- The mouth must be examined for cleft lip and cleft palate.
- There may be oral candidiasis (oral thrush) (Fig. 16.57), which is a white curdy material sticking to the tongue and oral mucosa. This generally needs no treatment, and the parents need to be reassured.

Ebstein Pearl

These retention cysts appear as whitish cystic lesion on the hard palate and prepuce (Fig. 16.58) and do not require any treatment. These are sometimes present on the prepuce too.

Predeciduous Teeth

These are also called natal teeth and present at birth in the lower incisor position (mandibular) (Fig. 16.59), which normally shed before the primary dentition. Natal teeth may be associated with a variety of syndromes including chondroectodermal dysplasia (Ellis-van Creveld syndrome), pachyonychia congenita, Sotos syndrome, and Hallermann-Streiff syndrome. Extraction of natal teeth should be considered only if they cause feeding difficulties for the infant or mother. Excessive natal tooth mobility is considered a risk for aspiration. However, aspiration rarely occurs.

Tongue Anomalies

Congenital lesions of the tongue include cysts, mucoceles, macroglossia, ankyloglossia, lingual thyroid, and median rhomboid glossitis. Macroglossia is a true enlargement of the tongue, in contrast to glossoptosis, in which a normal-sized tongue fills a small oral cavity.

Macroglossia can be generalized or focal. Generalized macroglossia is seen in Beckwith-Wiedemann syndrome and hypothyroidism. Focal enlargement of the tongue usually is caused by congenital tumors, particularly lymphangioma, hemangiomas, or multiple endocrine neoplasia type 2B. When tongue enlargement is caused by lymphangiomas, the surface of the tongue is pebbly with multiple vesicle-like blebs by superficial dilated lymphatic channels.

Tongue-tie (Ankyloglossia)

Ankyloglossia occurs due to short lingual frenulum that may restrict tongue movements and impact breastfeeding. It has a male predominance. True ankyloglossia is rare. It usually does not delay speech and language development. Most infants with ankyloglossia have no feeding difficulty. Generally, no treatment is required.

5. Ears

The ears are examined for placement and deformation.

Low set ears: Draw an imaginary line backward from outer corner of eye towards the pinna. If more than 90% of the ear is below this line, it is said to be a low set ear. Small, abnormally-shaped, or low set ears often point to underlying chromosomal, renal, or cardiac anomalies.

Pre-auricular pit is a small sinus, seen just anterior to the auricle. It is commoner in girl and is of no significance. Pre-auricular tags (Fig. 16.60) situated anterior to auricle may be associated with renal anomaly.

6. Nose

Neonates are obligatory nose breathers. Patency of nares can be checked by holding a wisp of cotton at the orifice while occluding the other nares with the mouth closed. In bilateral choanal atresia, respiratory distress improves when the child cries due to opening of mouth. It can be diagnosed by passing a catheter through nostrils.

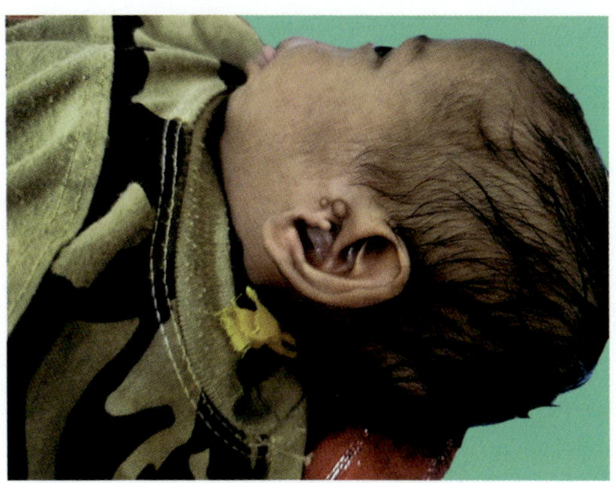

Fig. 16.60: Preauricular tag.

7. Neck

- *Congenital muscle (sternocleidomastoid) torticollis:* This presents as a swelling on either side of neck visible after the first week of life (Fig. 16.61). It is associated with limited movement of the neck to the side of the swelling. The swelling may be due to abnormal *in utero* position or stretching of the neck during delivery. No active intervention is needed in most babies.
- A very short, webbed neck may be associated with Klippel-Feil or Turner syndrome.
- The neck is palpated for cysts or masses. A thyroglossal duct cyst is usually palpable in the midline and retracts with tongue protrusion.
- Cystic hygromas are soft fluctuant swellings in neck, usually unilateral.

8. Skin

Evaluate the texture of the skin for scaliness, elasticity, thickness, and local or generalized edema. Jaundice is assessed by pressing the

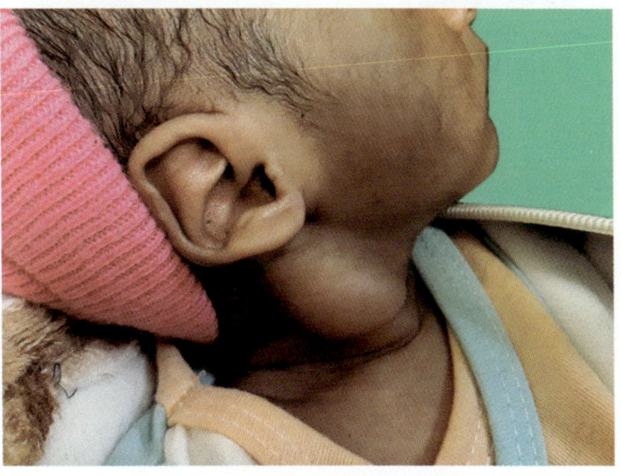

Fig. 16.61: Sternocleidomastoid tumor.

skin by fingers and looking at the color of tissue underneath.

- Look for hemangiomas (Fig 16.62), nevi, urticarial, pustular, vesicular, or nodular rashes.
- Skin is usually covered by vernix in the skinfolds of the axillas, neck, and groin at birth. Post-term infants have little vernix, and their skin is dry, cracked, and wrinkled (Fig. 16.63).
- Preterm infants may have fine downy hair (lanugo) over the shoulders, back, thighs, forehead, and ears. The lanugo regresses as they mature over weeks.
- Notice any ecchymoses or petechiae. Generalized and recurring petechiae, especially those not on the head and necklace region, may signify serious infectious or hematologic problems. Babies born by breech presentation may have bruised and extended lower limbs.
- Common benign findings:
  a. *Milia:* These are whitish papules 1–2 mm size on nose and face, which disappear spontaneously. These are caused by retention of keratin and sebum in the pilosebaceous follicle (Fig. 16.64).
  b. *Miliaria:* Miliaria is common in newborns during summer months. It is caused by accumulation of sweat beneath eccrine sweat ducts that are obstructed by keratin at the level of the stratum corneum. It is characteristically distributed on the face, scalp, and intertriginous areas.
  c. *Erythema toxicum:* These are discrete flat reddish lesions with a central vesicle (Fig. 16.65) which are most observed on the second or third day of life. These rashes usually disappear within 2–5 days.

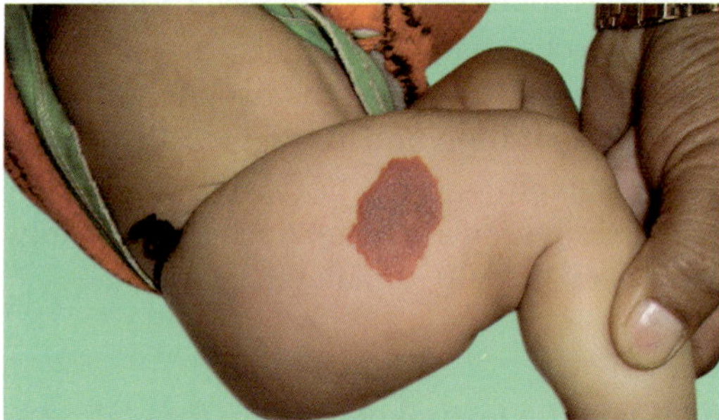

Fig. 16.62: Hemangioma.

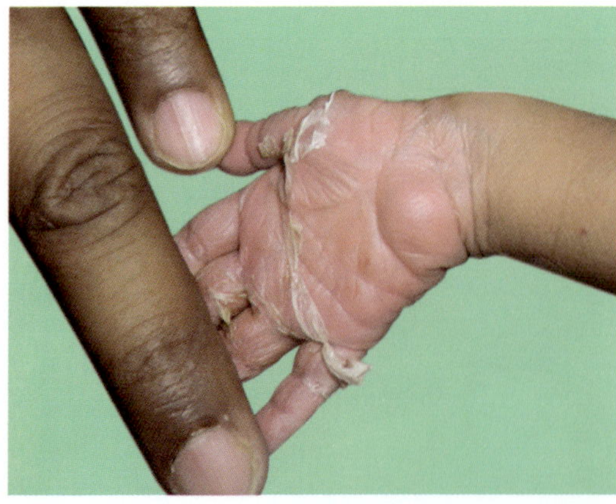

Fig. 16.63: Parchment like skin of a post-term baby.

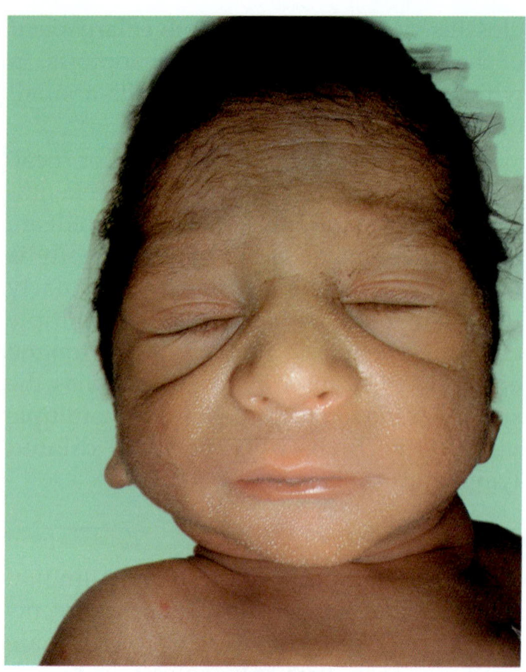

Fig. 16.64: Milia.

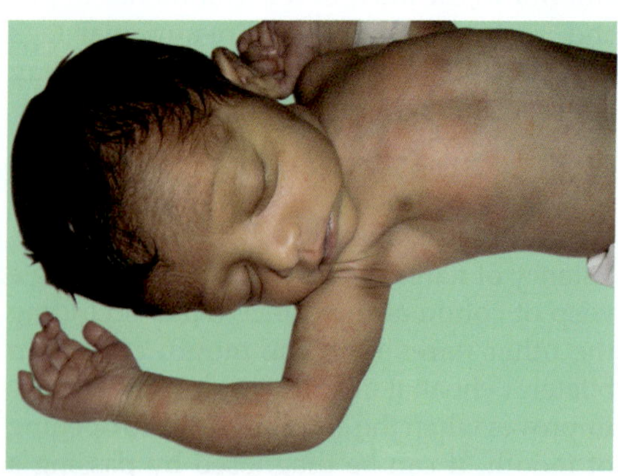

Fig. 16.65: Erythema toxicum.

d. *Café au lait macules* are non-raised pale brown patches with distinct edges. They are of no significance and are considered birthmarks. However, if there are more than five patches greater than 0.5 cm, a diagnosis of neurofibromatosis must be excluded.

e. *Mongolian spots:* These are bluish, well-demarcated spots over back and buttock. They become less obvious by one year of age **(Fig. 16.66)**.

f. *Vascular lesions:* These are pink macular areas (non-raised) that tend to redden when baby cries. They are also known as salmon patches and are present over forehead, upper eyelid and back of neck.

g. *Delivery marks:* Bruises may occur on any part of the body where pressure was applied during delivery. Forceps marks usually occur over the cheeks and ears.

- Pustules over the skin are commonly seen in newborns **(Fig. 16.67)**. Staphylococcal scalded skin syndrome is an extensive infection of skin in newborns **(Fig. 16.68)**.

9. Chest

Chest should be examined for shape, symmetry, or any deformity.

- The chest may appear barrel-shaped, i.e. increased antero-posterior diameter in meconium aspiration syndrome due to trapping of air.

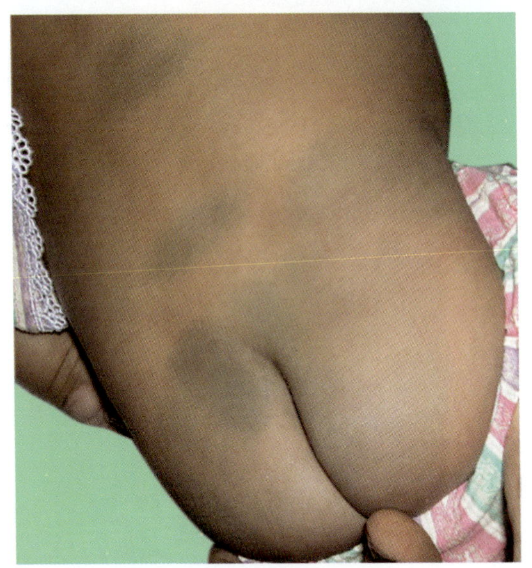

Fig. 16.66: Mongolian spots.

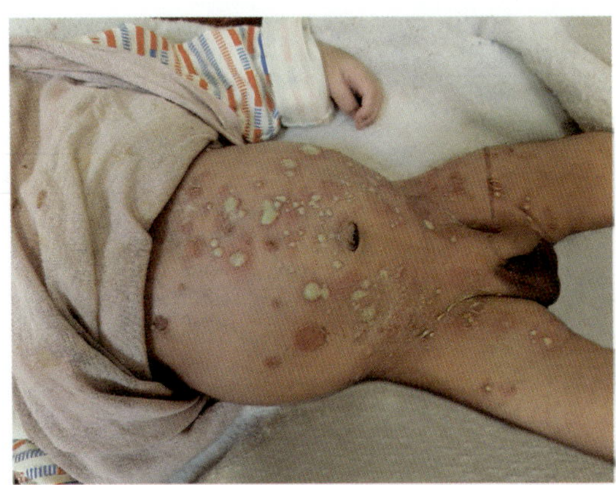

Fig. 16.67: Pustules over skin.

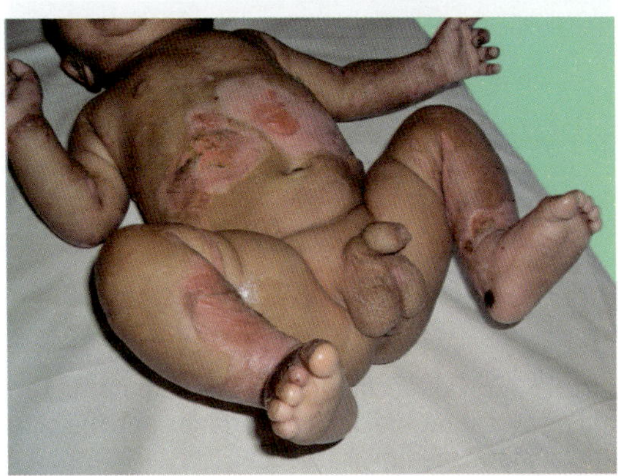

Fig. 16.68: Staphylococcal scalded skin syndrome.

- Unilateral absence or hypoplasia of the pectoralis major muscle suggests the diagnosis of Poland syndrome (rib defects, hypoplasia of the upper extremities, and syndactyly).
- Widely spaced nipples, excessive nuchal skin, and lymphedema are findings associated with Turner syndrome.
- A small bell-shaped thorax suggests pulmonary hypoplasia.
- *Mastitis neonatorum:* Engorgement of both breasts is a normal physiologic phenomenon in babies of both sexes due to maternal progesterone and estrogen transferred from the mother. There is swelling of the breast **(Fig. 16.69)** and there may be milk discharge, especially on squeezing. This needs no treatment and subsides within a week or two on its own.

10. Umbilicus

The umbilical cord maintains vascular flow between the fetus and the placenta *in utero*. The

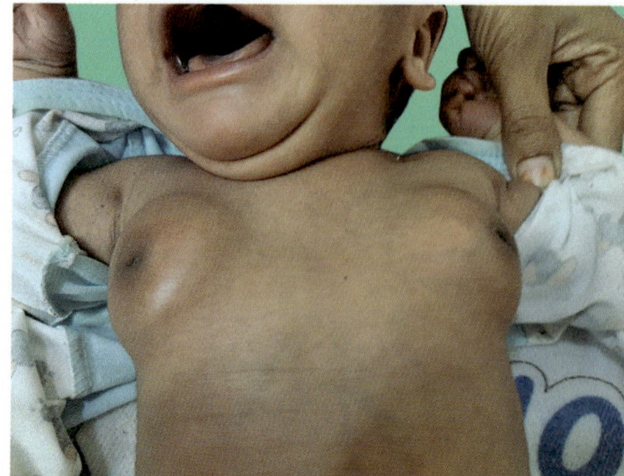

Fig. 16.69: Mastitis neonatorum.

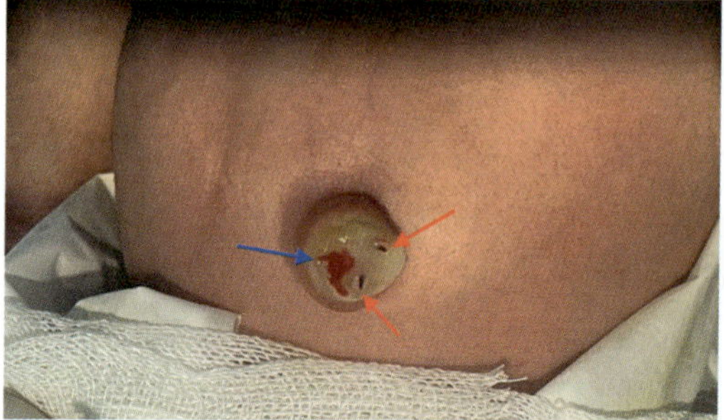

Fig. 16.70: Cut section of an umbilical cord. The red arrows show the umbilical arteries and the blue arrow shows the umbilical vein.

umbilical cord contains two arteries at 4 and 7 o'clock positions and one vein at 12 o'clock position, which are surrounded and supported by gelatinous tissue called Wharton jelly (Fig. 16.70). Umbilical arteries are thick-walled, and white in appearance while umbilical vein is thin-walled, patulous and mild oozing of blood can be seen. If only a single artery is present, look for other congenital abnormalities; the most affected organs being the kidneys, heart, gastrointestinal tract, and the central nervous system.

Delayed separation of the cord: Separation of the umbilical cord usually occurs one week after birth and is initiated by thrombosis and contraction of the umbilical vessels followed by phagocyte-mediated tissue breakdown and epithelialization of the cord stump. Bacterial colonization of umbilical stump plays an important role in cord separation. Cord should be kept dry, and no antiseptics should be applied. Any cord that persists after 4 weeks represents delayed cord separation. Delayed cord separation can be associated with underlying immunodeficiency (leucocyte adhesion deficiency), infection, or urachal abnormality.

Umbilical granuloma: Umbilical granuloma is detected after the cord has separated as a soft, moist, pink, pedunculated, friable lesion of granulation tissue of size 3 to 10 mm (Fig. 16.71). There is a history of persistent drainage of serous or serosanguinous fluid from the umbilicus. Granuloma formation is more likely to occur when there is inflammation of the umbilical cord usually due to infection, which also delays cord separation.

Umbilical polyp: Umbilical polyps are firm masses comprised of intestinal epithelium or uroepithelium, which are omphalomesenteric, ductal or urachal embryologic remnants. Umbilical polyps are rare and often larger than granulomas.

Omphalitis: Omphalitis is an infection of the umbilicus and/or surrounding tissues. It is characterized by purulent discharge from the umbilical cord stump with surrounding induration, erythema, and tenderness (Fig. 16.72). Umbilical stump bleeding may

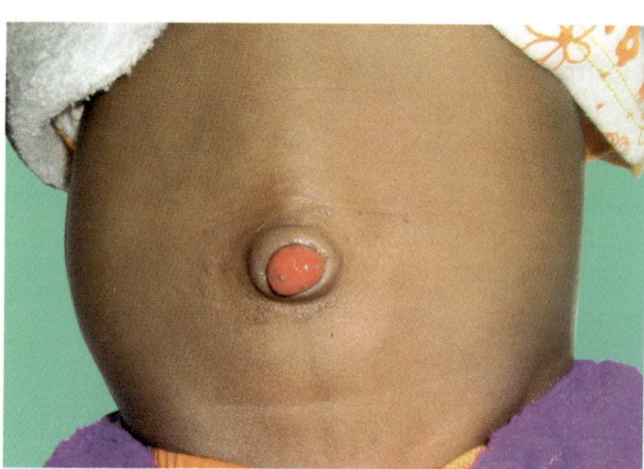

Fig. 16.71: Umbilical granuloma.

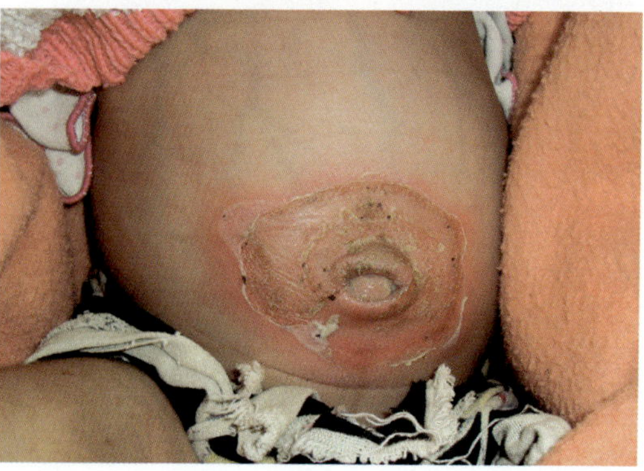

Fig. 16.72: Omphalitis.

also occur with omphalitis because of delayed obliteration of the umbilical vessels.

Omphalomesenteric duct anomalies: Partial or complete failure of involution of the omphalomesenteric duct can lead to a spectrum of anomalies like intestinal drainage from the umbilicus, persistent tissue at the umbilicus with no intestinal connection resulting in an umbilical polyp, Meckel diverticulum, omphalomesenteric duct cyst, and fibrous band between the umbilicus and terminal ileum, leading to small bowel obstruction.

Urachal anomalies: Urachus normally involutes, resulting in a fibrous cord between the umbilicus and the bladder. Disruption of this process can lead to a spectrum of rare anomalies like patent urachus with free communication between the bladder leading to persistently wet or draining umbilicus, umbilical polyp, bladder diverticulum, and urachal cyst.

Umbilical hernia: The umbilical scar fails to heal at birth leading to herniation of intestines through umbilical ring known as umbilical hernia. Umbilical hernias are detected as soft protrusion through abdominal ring, particularly when there is increased intra-abdominal pressure from crying (Fig. 16.73). Umbilical hernias are easily reduced even if they are quite large, and the borders of the fascial defects can be palpated through the skin. Most of the umbilical hernias close in the first 12 to 18 months of life. Umbilical hernias are frequently seen in patients with hypothyroidism, Ehlers-Danlos syndrome, Beckwith-Wiedemann syndrome, Down syndrome, mucopolysaccharidoses, and trisomy 18.

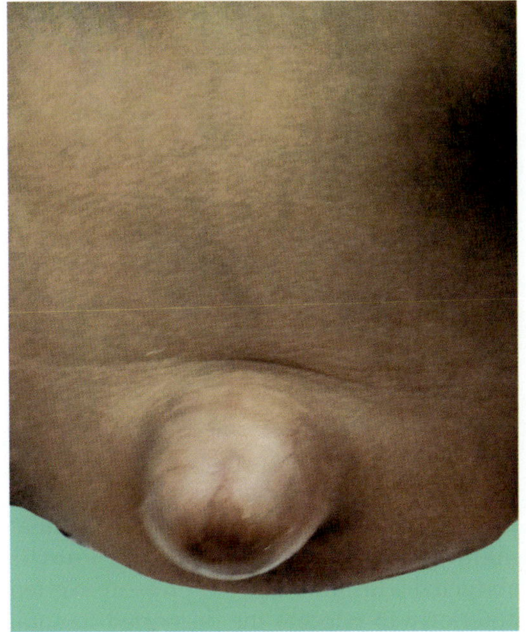

Fig. 16.73: Umbilical hernia.

11. Anus and Genitalia

- Check the position and patency of anus.
- Palpate the testis. Both testes should be descended in the scrotum in the term male baby. If they are not felt in the scrotum, the testes may just be present above the scrotum in the inguinal region. If testes are not palpable in a term baby (Fig. 16.74), it must be evaluated further. In a preterm male baby, the testes may not have descended into the scrotum. They usually descend by 34 weeks of gestational age.
- *Hydrocele* is a swelling of the scrotum due to accumulation of peritoneal fluid. This usually requires no intervention and resolves with time.
- It is also normal for newborns to have *phimosis*, i.e. the prepuce or the foreskin on the penis cannot be retracted. This causes a lot of anxiety in the parents. They should be advised not to forcefully retract the foreskin. It just needs reassurance as the phimosis will resolve as the foreskin becomes retractile with time.
- *Penile length:* The stretched penile length of a term baby should be >2.5 cm.
- *Hypospadias and chordee:* The urethral opening should be inspected for its position.

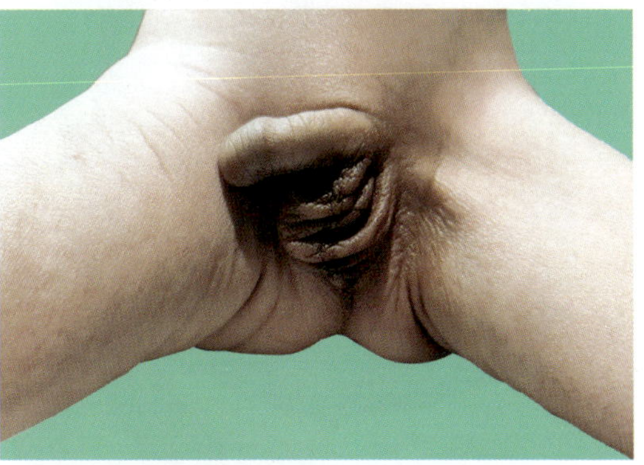

Fig. 16.74: Empty scrotum sac in undescended testes.

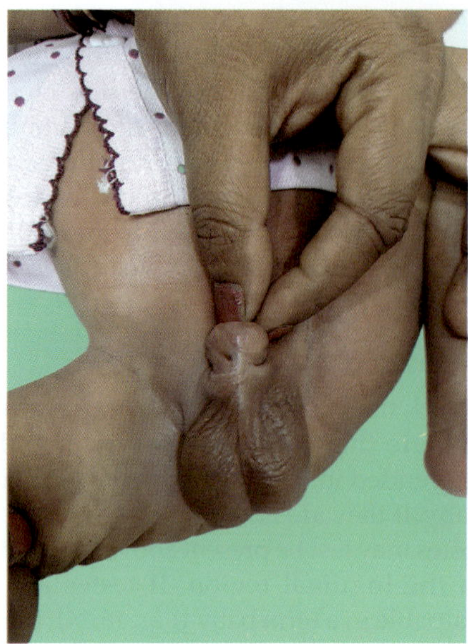

Fig. 16.75: Hypospadias.

It may be abnormally located on the ventral aspect of the penis (hypospadias) (Fig. 16.75) or rarely the dorsal aspect (epispadias). Hypospadias may be associated with abnormal curvature of the penis known as chordee.

12. Spine and Limbs

Examine the back for the presence of neural tube defect like meningocele. A dimple or tuft of hair over the lower back may indicate a hidden spinal deformity (Fig. 16.76). The curvature of the spine must also be checked for any abnormality.

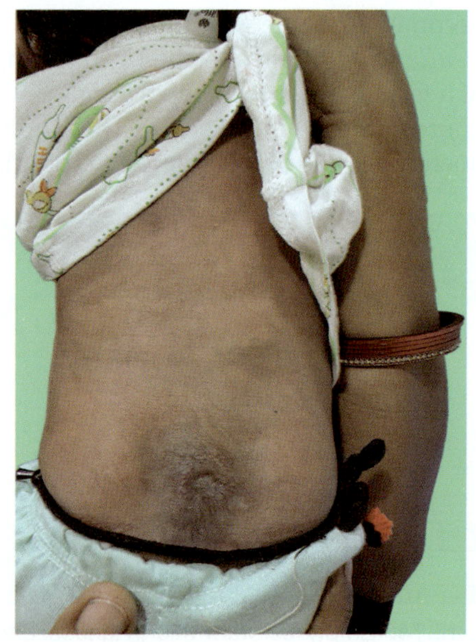

Fig. 16.76: Tuft of hair on the lower lumbar region.

All four limbs should be examined for range of movement at all joints. Decreased movement of the upper limbs can be due to fracture of the humerus during delivery. The abnormal position of the upper limb can be due to brachial plexus injury during delivery, most common being Erb's palsy.

Examine the digits for polydactyly (more than 5 digits), syndactyly (fused digits), edema, unusual skin ridge, whorls and creases, nail growth, and unusual digit placement or contractures.

13. Hip Joint

Newborns should be screened for developmental dysplasia of hip (earlier known as congenital dislocation of the hip). The most common presentation of DDH in neonates is hip instability, examined by the Ortolani and Barlow maneuvers. Each hip should be examined individually for instability.

The infant should be on a stable surface in the supine position, with the hip flexed to 90° and in neutral rotation. The examination should occur when the infant is calm and not crying. The hips are best examined with all clothing and diapers removed.

Barlow Maneuver

Flex the hip and knee at 90° angle and hold the thigh of the baby near the hip joint firmly, with your thumb on the inner thigh and your index and middle fingers on the greater trochanter. Try to dislocate the hip joint by adducting the joint and exerting simultaneous posterior pressure. The femoral head will be pushed out of the joint in case of an unstable joint, the test is positive if the femoral head can be popped out of the socket. Tests for both the hip joints can be performed simultaneously (Fig. 16.77).

Ortolani Maneuver

Ortolani's test is performed to confirm the dislocation of the hip joint after Barlow's maneuver has been performed. The test is performed by holding the thigh in a similar manner to Barlow test. The hip joint is abducted with simultaneous pressure exerted anteriorly to relocate the dislocated femoral head back into the socket. The test is positive

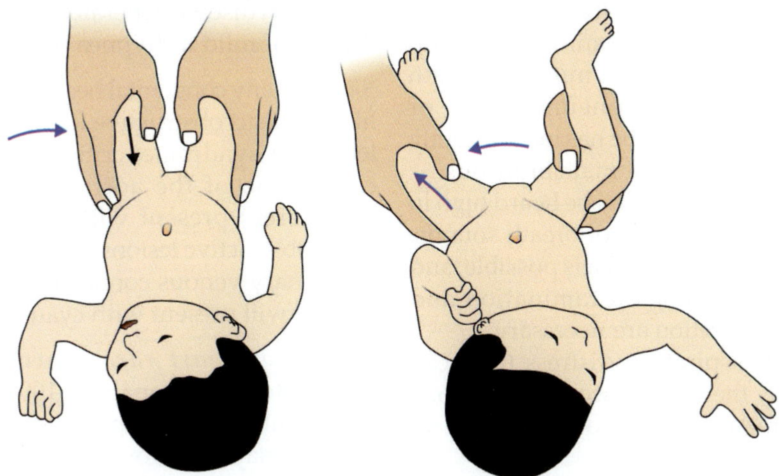

Fig. 16.77: Screening for developmental dysplasia of hip.

if the dislocated hip is reduced, and a 'clunk' is heard.

16.8 SYSTEMIC EXAMINATION

A. Respiratory System

Most of the neonates with disease involving the respiratory system will present with respiratory distress. The clinical presentation of respiratory distress in the newborn includes tachypnea, cyanosis, grunting, stridor, nasal flaring, intercostal and subcostal retractions, head nodding, and difficulty in feeding. In extreme cases, there may be gasping or apnea.

- *Tachypnea:* Respiratory rate ≥60/minute.
- *Grunt:* This sound is produced by partial closure of glottis during exhalation (attempt to maintain functional residual capacity and allow for adequate gas exchange).
- *Suprasternal retractions/tracheal tug:* Suggests upper airway obstruction.
- *Nasal flaring/intercostals or subcostal retractions:* These indicate increased work of breathing. Flaring occurs when the alae nasi start working and the newborn attempts to bring more air into the lungs. Intercostal or xiphoid retractions (*see* Fig. 15.31) may occur and have the appearance of a strong tug at the area of the xiphoid. Retractions may be mild, moderate, or marked.
- *Cyanosis:* Indicates hypoxia.

Inspectionv

Symmetry: The chest must be inspected for symmetry. Asymmetry of the chest may indicate tension pneumothorax, or mass lesions. Also look for labored breathing, meconium staining (meconium aspiration syndrome), excessive frothing (tracheoesophageal fistula), and scaphoid abdomen (diaphragmatic hernia).

Shape of the chest: A small chest in an infant manifesting with respiratory distress or failure may indicate pulmonary hypoplasia or, in a more severe form, asphyxiating thoracic dystrophy. Inspection of the chest may show a protruding xiphisternum (*pectus carinatum*), which is usually a normal variant. In contrast, a *pectus excavatum* deformity (which produces concave or sunken appearance of chest) may be present at birth. Mild subcostal retractions and indrawing of xiphisternum is normal in a preterm neonate.

Palpation

Localize the apex beat to identify if it is displaced. Palpate for any crepitus (suggestive of subcutaneous emphysema).

Percussion

Generally, not advised in newborns. Sometimes, pneumothorax may be detected by hyperresonance on the affected side. However, diagnosis of pneumothorax can be quickly made by transillumination of the chest wall.

Auscultation

- Inspiratory stridor implies large airway obstruction, and expiratory prolongation indicates small airway obstruction.

- Listening alternately in the right and left axillae may indicate diminished breath sounds on one side. Asymmetric breath sounds may indicate pneumothorax or that an endotracheal tube has inadvertently advanced into the right main bronchus.
- Rarely, bowel sounds may be heard high in the chest in the absence of breath sounds. If so, diaphragmatic hernia is possible, and emergency radiologic examination and surgical consultation are necessary.

Severity of respiratory distress (RD) can be assessed by the Downe score **(Table 16.4)** or Silverman-Anderson score for preterm neonates **(Table 16.5)**.

B. Cardiovascular System

The most common findings for an infant with heart disease in the newborn period are tachypnea, cyanosis, asymmetric pulses, hepatomegaly, and shock with an increased oxygen requirement.

Cyanosis: Cyanosis is an important sign of CHD, but mild desaturation may be difficult to appreciate visually. Pulse oximetry is helpful to detect mild desaturation. Cyanosis has been discussed earlier in detail. Remember that respiratory disease is more likely in cyanotic newborns who are tachypneic and using accessory muscles of respiration. Newborns with heart disease generally breathe normally, except for mild tachypnea or hyperpnea.

Shock: Many congenital heart diseases (CHD), like left heart obstructive lesions (hypoplastic left heart syndrome, critical aortic stenosis, coarctation of the aorta, and interrupted aortic arch) present with shock and right-sided obstructive lesions (e.g. total anomalous pulmonary venous connection and tricuspid atresia) will present with cyanosis.

Abnormal heart rate: Normal range of heart rate in a neonate is 100 to 160 beats per minute. Sleeping pulse rate in a healthy neonate may be as low as 80/min. Causes of abnormal neonatal heart rate include sinus or supraventricular tachycardia, large left-to-right shunts, heart failure, and myocarditis. In congenital heart block, heart rate is unusually slow.

Peripheral pulses: Assessment of bilateral symmetric femoral pulses is an essential part of the neonatal evaluation. The diagnosis of coarctation of the aorta (COA) or other aortic arch obstruction is strongly suggested in the infant with decreased or absent femoral pulses. A hyperdynamic pulse may suggest patent ductus arteriosus. A weak pulse may occur in shock or be associated with a congenital cardiac anomaly.

Table 16.4: Respiratory score (Downe score)

Score	0	1	2
Respiratory rate	40 to 60/minute	60 to 80/minute	>80/minute
Oxygen requirement	None	<40%	≥40%
Retractions	None	Mild-to-moderate	Severe
Grunting	None	Audible with stethoscope	Audible without stethoscope
Breath sounds	Normal	Decreased	Barely heard

A score of <5 indicates mild RD, a score of 5 to 8 moderate RD, and a score of >8 severe RD.

Table 16.5: Silverman-Anderson score for respiratory distress in preterm neonates

	Upper chest movement	Lower chest retraction	Xiphoid retraction	Dilatation of nares	Expiratory grunt
Score 0	Synchronized respiration	None	None	None	None
Score 1	Lag on inspiration	Just visible	Just visible	Minimal	Heard with stethoscope
Score 2	See-saw movements	Marked	Marked	Marked	Heard with naked ear

Score 10 = Severe respiratory distress; Score ≥7 = Impending respiratory failure; Score 0 = No respiratory distress

16

Clinical Methods in Pediatrics

Localization of the apex beat: Precordial palpation ascertains whether the heart is normally located on the left side of the chest. Isolated dextrocardia is often associated with complex CHD. Sometimes, it is difficult to locate the apex beat because of the small size of the thorax and transmission of vibration.

Auscultation: A single second heart sound (though difficult to appreciate) occurs in pulmonary hypertension, TGA, aortic and pulmonary atresia, and truncus arteriosus.

Murmur: Timing of the onset of murmurs is important. Frequently, murmurs that depend on pulmonary vascular pressure (e.g. left-to-right shunt through a patent ductus arteriosus) are not heard until pulmonary vascular resistance has decreased on the second to third day of life. Murmur of a large VSD becomes audible by the end of first week of age. The murmur of tricuspid insufficiency may be audible on first day.

Other characteristics that are important to note are the site where the murmur is heard best, the timing of the murmur regarding systole and diastole, the quality, and the loudness.

In newborns, the presence of a murmur does not always indicate a heart disease. Similarly, absence of murmur does not always exclude heart disease.

Do not forget to listen for cardiovascular problems in 'non-cardiac' areas, such as the axilla (peripheral pulmonic stenosis), the neck (aortic stenosis), and the head and liver (arterio-venous malformations).

C. Abdomen

Inspect abdomen for any distension **(Fig. 16.78)**, visible peristalsis, umbilical discharge, periumbilical redness, and prominent veins in flanks. Loops of intestine may be normally visible through abdomen in preterm babies. Palpate for organomegaly, masses, inflammation, and distention.

- Look for congenital malformations in the anterior abdominal wall, such as gastroschisis, omphalocele, umbilical hernia, and paraumbilical hernias.
- Unusual flatness or a scaphoid shape to the abdomen may be associated with congenital diaphragmatic hernia **(Fig 16.79)**.

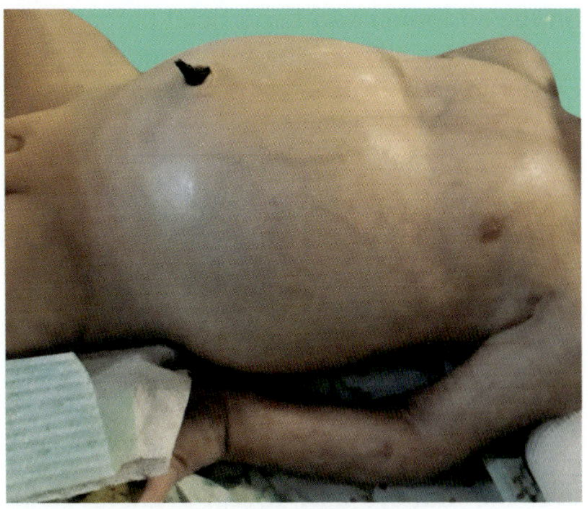

Fig. 16.78: Abdominal distention.

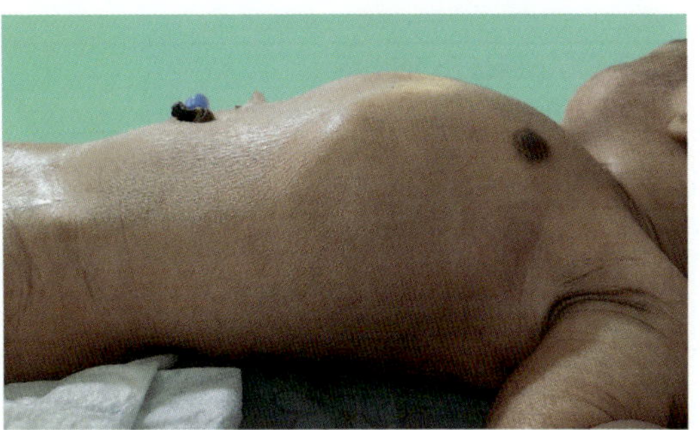

Fig. 16.79: Scaphoid abdomen.

- Normally, you can palpate a 1 to 2 cm liver edge below the right costal margin, a spleen tip overlying the stomach and the lower pole of the left kidney.
- Look for dilated veins on the abdominal wall indicating venous distention.
- Visible gastric or bowel patterns may be considered a certain sign of ileus or other obstruction.

Gastroschisis: The infant's intestines protrude through a defect in the abdominal wall usually on the right side. Intestine loops or other abdominal contents that protrude outside the body are not covered with any membranes and are clearly visible.

Omphalocele: In contrast to gastroschisis, the abdominal contents herniate in the abdominal midline through the umbilicus and are covered by a very thin layer of tissue.

Palpation: Palpation of the abdomen is best performed by approaching from the right-hand side of the baby. Hand should be clean and warm. The right hand is gently placed on the abdomen and superficial palpation is performed in all four quadrants and centrally. Once the baby is used to this, palpation may be attempted for the liver, spleen, and kidneys in usual manner.

Percussion: Percussion of the abdomen is generally not helpful in newborns.

Auscultation: Auscultate for bowel sound. The normal frequency should be 3–4/min. Bowel sounds may be sluggish or absent in hypokalemia, paralytic ileus due to sepsis, intestinal obstruction in late stage (adynamic phase), and NEC. Auscultation over the kidneys may reveal bruits in renal artery stenosis. Bruits over the liver indicate arteriovenous fistula.

16.9 EXAMINATION OF THE NEUROLOGICAL SYSTEM

A detailed neurological assessment is required in infants suspected of having neurological deficit, as in perinatal asphyxia or congenital muscular abnormalities. It should be assessed about 1–2 hours after feeding, when the newborn is sufficiently alert and not yet fretful (due to hunger)! Examine in the sequence given in **Key Box 15**.

While evaluating the neurological findings, always must consider the baby's birth weight, gestational age, medications the baby is getting and age of the baby. Findings normal for a preterm baby may be abnormal for a term baby. Similarly, neurological findings may change from the first day of life to the third or fourth week of life.

The examination of the skull, fontanelles, sutures, head circumference, dysmorphic facies, and spine also form a part of the central nervous examination. These have been discussed in other sections of the chapter.

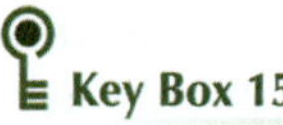

Key Box 15

The 7 Components of Neurological Examination of the Newborn

1. Consciousness/alertness
2. Cry and habituation
3. Cranial nerves
4. Motor functions including tone
5. Neonatal reflexes
6. Vision
7. Hearing

A. Level of Consciousness

Prechtl devised a scale for state of consciousness for healthy term infants, which is detailed in **Key Box 16**. Examination of the baby should be done in State III or IV of wakefulness. In State I and II, a baby could be unduly hypotonic; similarly in State V, the baby could be hypertonic.

Inability to provoke at least facial grimacing and movement of the extremities is abnormal and considered evidence for states of decreased consciousness.

Abnormal Level of Alertness

An abnormal level of alertness is one of the most observed neurologic deficits in the neonate. An altered level of alertness is defined as a diminished or absent response to arousal maneuvers (i.e. handling, perioral stimulation, shining a light, or ringing a bell). The following classification of altered alertness states for infants greater than 28 and 30 weeks gestation.

- ***Normal:*** The infant appears awake, and has normal arousal and noxious stimuli responses.
- ***Lethargic:*** The infant appears sleepy with slightly diminished arousal and noxious stimuli responses.
- ***Coma:*** The infant is unresponsive with absent arousal and noxious stimuli.

B. Cry and Habituation

1. Cry

As you perform various parts of the newborn examination, listen for the characteristics of cry.

- Is it husky, loud and sustained or is it shrill and high-pitched, indicating a possible

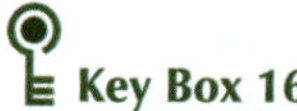

Key Box 16

Prechtl Scale for State of Consciousness

State I	Deep or quite sleep: Eyes closed with regular respiration and no movements
State II	Light or rapid eye movement sleep: Eyes closed with irregular respiration and no gross movements
State III	Awake, eyes open, no gross movements
State IV	Alert: Eyes open, gross movements, no crying
State V	Crying

central nervous system abnormality? High-pitched and incessant cry is marker of cerebral irritability [hypoxic ischemic encephalopathy (HIE), stage I].

- A weak cry/whimper may indicate overwhelming sepsis or neuromuscular disease.
- Inspiratory stridor indicates extrathoracic tracheal obstruction may be heard only when the infant is crying.
- Complete aphonia usually indicates bilateral vocal cord injury or paralysis.
- If the infant is crying, is it appropriate, i.e. in response to pain or hunger, and if he is consolable (quietens on talking or cuddling).

2. Habituation

Habituation to a repetitive stimulus should be tested. For example, repeatedly eliciting glabellar tap will fail to elicit a response after 3–4 attempts. Babies with neurological abnormality will not habituate even after repeated stimuli.

C. Cranial Nerves

- *Olfactory (I):* The baby does recognize the smell of the mother and her breastmilk but it is difficult to test and usually not tested.
- *Optic (II):* A baby ≥28 weeks, blinks when light is shone in the visual field. Fundus examination can also be done for optic nerve examination. Babies ≥34 weeks of gestation can fix and follow an object to some extent.
- *Oculomotor, Trochlear and Abducens (III, IV and VI):*
  - Pupillary reaction can be elicited in babies ≥30 weeks of gestation.
  - Do not attempt to force the eyes open, as they can be opened by stimulating sucking or rocking. Evaluate the size and reaction of pupils by introducing pencil-torch from lateral to medial. Normal pupillary size is 2–3 mm, reaction to light is present after 30 weeks.
    - ❑ *Bilateral large pupils:* HIE, intraventricular hemorrhage (IVH)
    - ❑ *Unilateral large pupil:* Intracranial hemorrhage, HIE, congenital 3rd nerve palsy
    - ❑ *Bilateral small pupils:* HIE
    - ❑ *Unilateral small pupil:* Horner syndrome
    - ❑ *Horizontal gaze palsy:* HIE
    - ❑ *Upward gaze palsy:* Hydrocephalus, posterior fossa hemorrhage, HIE, IVH
    - ❑ *Opsoclonus (rapid irregular, multidirectional, conjugate jerking of eyes):* Inborn error of metabolism (IEM), posterior fossa hemorrhage

    The pupillary reflex is consistently present after 31 weeks gestation, but is technically difficult to assess because of the *dazzle reflex*, in which a bright light causes immediate and sustained closure of the eyes for as long as the light is present.
  - Vestibulo-ocular reflex (Doll's eye maneuver) is positive in newborns. The eyes of the baby will deviate in the direction opposite to the direction of the head.
- *Trigeminal (V):* If rooting and sucking reflex are present, it ensures a normal functioning of the trigeminal nerve. Rooting and sucking reflexes test V, VII, and XII Cranial nerves.
- *Facial (VII):* Deviation of the angle of the mouth to the opposite side, absent nasolabial furrow and inability to completely close the eye is seen in facial nerve palsy.
- *Acoustic (VIII):* The baby startles on a loud sound in case the nerve is intact.
- *Glossopharyngeal and Vagus (IX, X):* Presence of a good swallowing reflex will test the normal functioning of these nerves. Sucking–swallowing coordination develops at ≥34 weeks of gestation. Weak swallowing is suggested by constant drooling of saliva.
- *Spinal (XI):* Spinal nerve can be tested by gently turning the head from side to side. The head should move easily without any limitation. This is not usually tested in newborns.
- *Hypoglossal (XII):* See for the symmetry of the tongue and presence of any fasciculation. This is also not usually tested in neonates.

> If a baby is sucking and swallowing well at the mother's breast, the cranial nerves V, VII, IX, X, XI and XII are likely to be normal.

D. Motor Function

1. Resting Posture

Resting posture indicates tone at rest and is one of the more important clues to neurological health. Resting tone increases with gestational age and follows a caudo-cephalic progression.

- A normal term newborn when lying supine keeps the hips abducted and partially flexed and knees and arms flexed.
- *Frog leg posture:* A hypotonic baby will have complete abduction of hip and partial flexion of the knee so that the lateral surfaces of the thigh and leg touch the couch. There is flexion at the elbow with upward facing palms besides the head.
- *Hypertonia:* A persistently tightly fisted hand, with the thumb constantly enclosed by the other fingers and not opening spontaneously (*fisting*), is abnormal and is sometimes a precursor of spasticity. Extension of both lower limbs in a manner that both legs cross each other (*scissoring*) is suggestive of hypertonia. Arching of back and neck (*opisthotonos*) also indicates hypertonia.

Common causes include hypoxic-ischemic encephalopathy and kernicterus; intermittent hypertonia and opisthotonos may suggest tetanus.

2. Tone

Tone is the resistance of muscle to stretch. The quality and quantity of spontaneous movements are the best indicators of neuromuscular function and are assessed by inspection. Decreased tone may be one of the first detectable abnormalities in a full-term infant with sepsis. Tone is gestation and illness dependent, with smaller and sick infants having decreased tone. Tone may also vary in different muscle groups. It can be assessed as passive and active tone.

Passive tone: It is defined as resistance of limbs to movement. It is assessed by observing the passive resistance applied by the muscle being tested. We can test the passive tone by maneuvers like popliteal angle, arm traction and leg traction.

- **Popliteal angle** is tested by stabilizing the thigh of the baby over the abdomen by flexing the knee and gently trying to extend the knee by one finger behind the heel till resistance is felt. In a term baby, the popliteal angle formed between the thigh and the leg is around 90 degrees. We must be careful not to apply too little or too much pressure. In hypotonia, the angle will be more, and it will be less in case of hypertonia.
- **Arm and leg traction:** Gently hold the wrist/ankle of the baby and try to pull up vertically. We feel the resistance while the limb lifts with flexion at the elbow/knee and the shoulder/hip lifts from the couch (Fig. 16.80). In a term neonate, the elbow/knee remain flexed as the shoulder/hip lifts from the couch. In cases of hypotonia, the shoulder/hip will lift with no/little flexion at the elbow/knee.
- Decreased resistance to passive extension is a non-specific finding encountered in newborns with cerebral depression, spinal injuries, disorders of the motor unit, and systemic illness. In newborns, signs of spasticity are more subtle and expressed as persistent fisting with the thumb inside the fist, resistance to passive movement, and sustained clonus.

Active tone: This refers to tone observed when infant makes an active movement in reaction to certain situations. Active tone of a baby can be tested by performing horizontal suspension, vertical suspension and pull to sit. These maneuvers involve active participation of the baby.

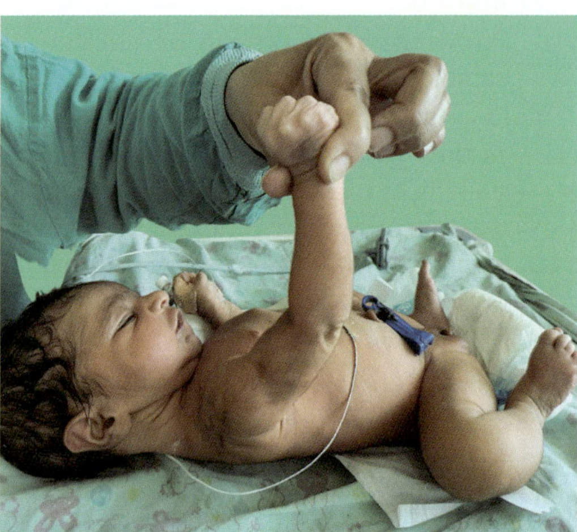

Fig. 16.80: Arm traction.

- **Pull to sit:** The baby is gently pulled up by holding both wrists from lying position, with slight support to the head. A term neonate with normal tone will be able to lift the head momentarily in line with the rest of the body. Hypotonia is suspected if the head always lags behind the body. If the head remains ahead of the body, this indicates hypertonia.
- **Horizontal suspension:** Hold the baby in prone and suspended position **(Fig. 16.81)**. A normal term baby will be able to keep the body in a straight line, lift the head to the level of the body and the limbs are kept in flexed position. In axial hypotonia, the back is rounded, and the limbs and head hang down.
- **Vertical suspension:** Hold the baby straight by holding at the baby under the arms **(Fig. 16.82)**. A baby with normal tone will be able to hold the head in midline and the baby does not feel like slipping between your hands. In a hypotonic baby, the head will fall forwards or backwards and the baby will slip through your hands unless you hold firmly.

3. Deep Tendon Reflexes (DTR)

Eliciting deep tendon reflexes in neonates is challenging. The method of elicitation is the same as in older children. We can use two fingers **(Fig. 16.83)** or a reflex hammer instead of the usual hammer to demonstrate the reflexes. Repeated stimulation may diminish the tendon reflexes which is known as habituation.

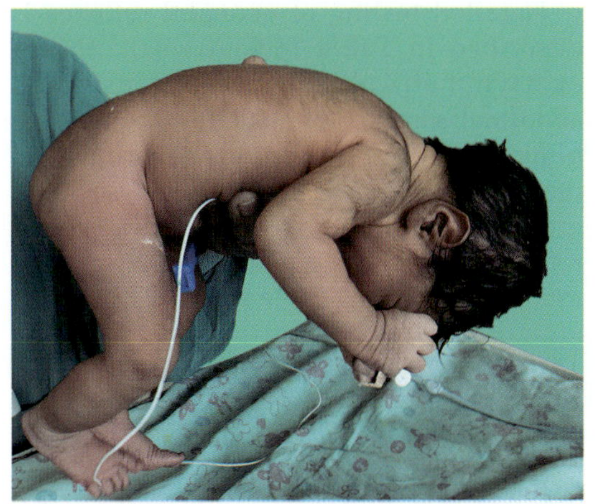

Fig. 16.81: Horizontal suspension.

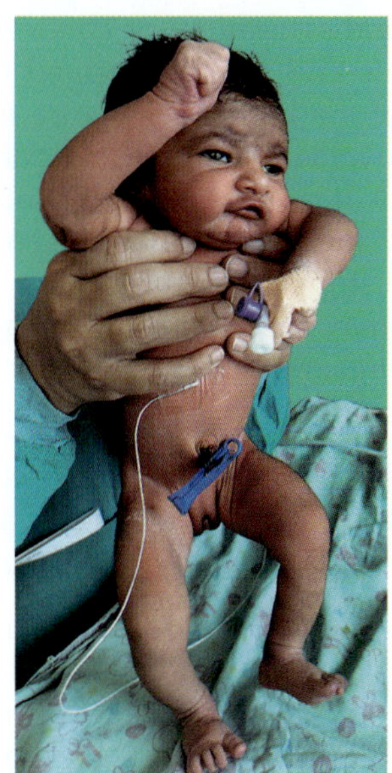

Fig. 16.82: Vertical suspension.

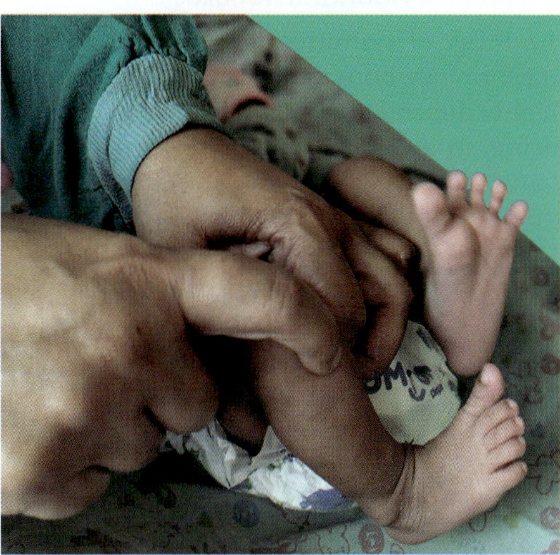

Fig. 16.83: Deep tendon reflexes testing with finger.

An ankle clonus can be seen in a normal newborn and is not a feature of upper motor neuron disease unless it is asymmetrical and associated with other abnormal neurological signs.

4. Other Findings

Jitteriness: These are non-epileptic, rapid involuntary movements usually involving the forearm and hand. They are rapid and rhythmic movements with equal amplitude. Jittery movements are usually precipitated by a stimulus, are not associated with autonomic phenomenon (like changes in heart rate, blood pressure and saturation) or abnormal ocular movements and can be stopped by gentle restraint of the limb. The seizure is a clonic jerking movement that has a fast and a slow component. It is associated with autonomous instability, abnormal ocular movements and cannot be stopped by restraining the limb. Jitteriness may be secondary to hypoglycemia, hypocalcemia, perinatal asphyxia or may be benign in nature.

Cortical thumb: A persistently closed fist with the thumb in constant flexion and adduction is a sign of upper motor *neuron lesion.*

Plantar reflex: A positive Babinski sign, i.e. extensor plantar reflex is normally seen in newborns. It can remain positive in the first year of life due to incomplete myelination and is not a sign of lesion of corticospinal tract.

E. Primitive Neonatal Reflexes

An array of primitive reflexes is present in the term newborn infant, but its expression is highly dependent on state—the most optimal being an awake alert state. Preterm infants have diminished responses with decreasing gestational age. Most common reflexes (Moro's, Grasp, Crossed extension, Tonic neck) have already been described in this chapter. Others are described below.

1. Traction Response

The traction response is sometimes referred to as the second component of palmar grasp reflex. After the baby grasps the finger, gently draw the finger upwards. The full-term baby will show progressive tensing of muscles from wrist to shoulder, until he hangs from the finger. It disappears by 2 to 3 months of life. With palmar pressure, the infant may open the mouth and yawn (palmar–mental reflex).

2. Placing and Stepping Reflex

When you stimulate the dorsum of the foot at the undersurface of the table, the infant lifts the stimulated foot and places it on the surface (*placing reaction*) **(Fig. 16.84)**.

When the examiner allows the plantar surface of the other foot to a table top, the infant makes crude sequential walking movements (*stepping reflex*).

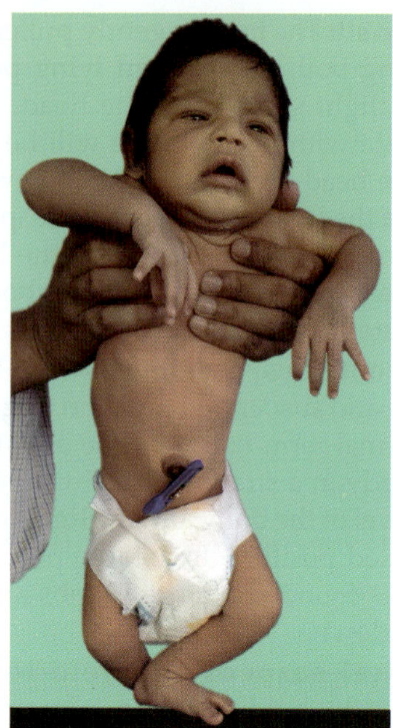

Fig. 16.64: Placing reflex.

3. Gallant and Perez Reflex

When the infant is supported prone by the examiner's hand, tickling the area of the lateral spine causes the buttocks to swing to the side of stimulation (truck incurvation reflex or *Gallant reflex*).

Holding the infant in the same position and running a finger from the base of the spine toward the neck elicits spinal extension. The child also passes urine, if the bladder is full, (*Perez reflex*).

4. Magnet Reflex

Apply light pressure with your finger to the sole of the foot which causes the legs to extend.

Detailed testing of neonatal reflexes is described in **Table 16.6**. A weak, absent or asymmetrical response is considered abnormal; some reflexes (such as the pupillary blink and gag reflexes) persist throughout life: Others (including the doll's eye, sucking, grasp, Babinski, Moro, Fencing, and Gallant reflexes) normally disappear a few weeks or months after birth **(Table 16.7)**.

16.10 THE 7-POINT RAPID NEWBORN ASSESSMENT

1. Record the vital signs, such as temperature, respiratory rate, heart rate, color, oxygen saturation and capillary filling time.

Table 16.6: Neonatal reflexes: How to test?

Reflex	Testing method	Normal responses
Sucking	Place a clean finger in the neonate's mouth (the mother's nipple also should trigger this reflex).	Sucks on the finger (or nipple) forcefully and rhythmically, sucking is coordinated with swallowing. Onset: 28 weeks; disappears: 4 mo (awake) and 7 mo (asleep)
Rooting	Touch a finger to the neonate's cheek or the corner of mouth (the mother's nipple also should trigger this reflex.)	Turns the head toward the stimulus, opens the mouth and searches for the stimulus. Onset: 28 wk; Disappears: 3–4 months
Pupillary (light)	Darken the room and shine a penlight directly into the neonate's eye for several seconds.	Pupils constrict equally bilaterally.
Doll's eye	With neonate supine, slowly turn the neonate's head to either side.	The eyes remain stationary and appear to move in opposite direction.
Moro	Suddenly but gently drop the neonate's head backward	Extends and abducts upper extremities bilaterally, symmetrically; and then adducts and flexes the extremities.
Startle	Make a loud noise near the neonate.	Cries and flexes all extremities.
Grasp	*Palmar reflex:* Place a finger in the neonate's palm. *Plantar reflex:* Place a finger against the base of the neonate's toe.	Grasps the finger. The toes curl downward and grasp the finger.
Stepping (automatic walking)	Hold the neonate in an upright position, and touch one foot lightly to a flat surface (such as the bed).	He makes walking motions with both feet.
Crossed extension	Position the neonate supine with head in midline; extend one leg and stimulate the sole with a light pinprick or finger flick.	Swiftly flexes, adducts and extends the opposite leg as though trying to push the stimulus away from the other foot.
Babinski (plantar)	Use drag of a thumbnail along the lateral margin of sole. Do not touch the area just below the toes. It may elicit plantar reflex.	Neonate hyperextends the toes. Dorsiflexes the great toe and fans the toes outward.

Table 16.7: Timing of appearance and disappearance of neonatal reflexes

Reflex	Appears	Well established	Disappears (postnatal age)
Palmar grasp	28 weeks	32 weeks	2–3 months
Rooting	32 weeks	36 weeks	2–3 months
Sucking	26–28 weeks	34 weeks	10–12 months
Moro	28–32 weeks	37 weeks	5–6 months
Tonic neck	35 weeks	1 months postnatal	6–7 months
Parachute	7–8 months postnatal	10–11 months postnatal	Persists throughout life

2. Record the weight, length, and head circumference.
3. Classify as term, preterm or post-term.
4. Examine from head to toe for congenital anomalies.
5. Assess for overall well-being, ascertain presence of danger signs.
6. Assess movements for quality, quantity and symmetry, posture, and muscle tone.
7. Examine the neonatal reflexes. Some common physical findings of clinical significance in a neonate are given in **Key Box 17**. Findings of little clinical significance are summarized in **Key Box 18**.

Key Box 17

Common Physical Findings of Clinical Significance

1. **Respiratory system:** Apnea, tachypnea, grunting, cyanosis, decreased breath sounds
2. **Cardiac system:** Tachypnea, tachycardia, hepatomegaly, asymmetrical pulses, gallop rhythm, murmur
3. **General:** Hypotonia, organomegaly, jaundice on 1st day or jaundice below knees, purpura, pallor, petechiae
4. **Congenital anomalies**
5. **Nervous system;** Hypotonia, hypertonia, seizures, cortical thumb, dissociation between gestation assessment by physical and neurological criteria

Key Box 18

Common Findings of Little Clinical Significance

Head	Caput succedaneum, asymmetry of posterior cranium, bony protrusions, molding
Ears	Skin tags
Eyes	Conjunctival hemorrhage
Nose	Asymmetric nares
Mouth	Ranula, sucking callocities, epulis, frenulum, natal teeth, Epstein pearls
Face	Unusual features not consistent with known syndromes
Skin	Sparse petechiae, erythema toxicum, mongolian spot, nevi, inclusion cysts, bruises, prominent lanugo or vernix, milia, miliaria, dark pigmentation over genital skin, peeling of skin, skin tags
Chest	Nipple spacing, extra nipples along the 'milk line', mastitis neonatorum
Umbilicus	Umbilicus cutis, umbilical hernia after separation of the cord
Abdomen	Just palpable liver and spleen
Heart	Evanescent murmurs
Genitalia	Prominent labia, mucoid secretions, hymenal tags, transient vaginal bleeding, non-retractile prepuce
Extremities	Syndactyly, polydactyly, hips tight to abduction, extended neck or extremities after breech delivery
Neurologic	Transient tone asymmetries, jitteriness, benign sleep myoclonus

A checklist for physical assessment of the newborn is provided in **Key Box 19**.

Key Box 19

Neonatal Assessment Checklist

Vital Signs
- Temperature:
- Respiratory rate:
- SpO_2:
- Heart rate:
- Capillary refill time:
- Non-invasive blood pressure:

Anthropometry
- Weight:
- Length:
- Head circumference:

Gestation
- Appropriate/small/large for date:

Skin
- Color: Pink/Pallor/Plethora/Jaundice/Cyanosis:
- Texture:
- Turgor:
- Rash/pigmentation:

Head
- Shape:
- Fontanel:
- Cephalhematoma:
- Hair:

Face
- Eyes and pupils:
- Nose and mouth:
- Ears:
- Dysmorphic features:

Neck
- Swelling:

Chest
- Chest retractions/grunt:
- Clavicle:
- Breasts:
- Bilateral air entry:

Heart
- Bilateral femoral pulses:
- S1, S2
- Murmurs:

Abdomen
- Shape and umbilicus:
- Genitalia and anal dimple:
- Organomegaly:

Back
- Spine: Meningocele/meningomylocele
- Sacral area: Tuft of hair/dimple/pigmentation

Upper limbs
- Position:
- Tone:
- Joints:
- Hands and nails:

Lower limbs
- Position:
- Tone:
- Hips: (rule out DDH)
- Legs and feet:

Higher Mental Functions
- Wakefulness: Alert/Response to voice/Response to pain only/Unresponsive

Motor Function
- Posture:
- Tone:
- Spontaneous movements:
- Pull to sit:
- Ventral suspension:
- Scarf sign:
- Adductor angle:
- Reflexes: Babinski/Deep tendon reflexes/ Superficial reflexes

Cranial nerves
- Papillary reflexes:
- Spontaneous eye movements:
- Facial symmetry:
- Breastfeeding:

Neonatal reflexes
- Moro's
- Rooting and sucking:
- Palmar and Planter grasp:
- Stepping:
- Tonic neck:

Chapter

17

Clinical Approach to Common Cases

○ Piyush Gupta ○ Swati Kalra ○ Dheeraj Shah

Structure

17.1 CHILD WITH FEVER

A. Definition and Classification

1. Fever of short duration (less than 14 days)

Fever (temperature ≥38°C or ≥100.4°F of less than 2 weeks duration is called a *short-duration fever*. It is usually infectious in origin, and due to viruses, bacteria or protozoa. Localizing symptoms and signs can give a clue to the etiology of fever.

2. Fever of prolonged duration (more than 14 days)

Fever lasting for more than 2 weeks is considered *prolonged fever*. Infections remain the most important cause of prolonged fever. However, it can also be caused by non-infectious illnesses such as vasculitis, collagen vascular disease, malignancies, and certain endocrine, hematological, and neurological disorders.

3. Fever without focus

Fever not presenting with any other symptom complex is referred to as *fever without focus*. It is further categorized into "fever without localizing signs" or "fever without source (FWS)" and "fever of unknown origin (FUO)".

a. ***Fever without localizing signs:*** Refers to short duration fever (<7 days), having no symptoms or signs that could indicate involvement of a particular system or a probable etiology.
b. ***Fever of unknown origin (FUO):*** Defined as fever (rectal temperature ≥38°C) documented by a health care provider, for which no cause is identifiable after 3 weeks of outpatient evaluation, at more than 2 hospital visits, and after 1 week of inpatient evaluation including a careful history, examination, and initial investigations.

Now, we will discuss the history, approach to diagnosis and differential diagnoses of the most common clinical scenarios where the major presenting illness is fever.

B. Fever of Short Duration (Less than 14 Days)

Common clinical scenarios in children presenting with short duration fever are listed as follows:

1. Fever less than 14 days without any major association
2. Fever with cough
3. Fever with cough with breathlessness/ fast breathing
4. Fever with rash
5. Fever with jaundice
6. Fever with pain in abdomen
7. Fever with burning micturition
8. Fever with abnormal movements and/or altered sensorium

9. Fever with skin boils
10. Fever with joint pains

1. Fever <14 days, no other major symptoms

History: The following should be included in the history of present illness to rule out specific systemic involvement:

- Any history of cough, cold or ear discharge (suggesting upper respiratory tract infection)
- Any history of breathing difficulty or noisy breathing (*suggesting lower respiratory tract illness*)
- Any history of rash over body (*suggesting viral exanthematous illness*)
- Any history of significant loose stool, vomiting or pain abdomen (*suggesting gastrointestinal involvement*)
- Any history of yellowish discoloration of eyes or urine (*suggesting hepatobiliary involvement*)
- Any history of pain abdomen, urinary urgency, frequency or burning micturition (*suggesting urinary tract infections*)
- Any history of abnormal movements or altered sensorium (*suggesting CNS involvement*)
- Any history of boils or abscess (*suggesting skin and soft tissue infection*)
- Any history of joint pain or joint swelling (*suggesting arthritis*)

Approach to diagnosis: Possible diagnoses with explanation are tabulated in **Table 17.1**.

2. Fever with cough (without breathlessness)

Duration and character of cough can give important clues towards underlying etiology. Ask about onset, aggravating/relieving factors, postural variation, paroxysmal nature, and presence of sputum. Also ask about noisy breathing, diurnal variation, family history, and any symptom of breathing difficulty. History of fast breathing, breathing difficulty, cyanosis, refusal to feed, head nodding, altered sensorium, noisy breathing (stridor/wheeze) suggests possible lower respiratory tract infection and is dealt within next section. Refer to Section 7.2 for more details on cough.

Onset and duration: It is mostly *acute* in onset (viral infections, pneumonia, aspiration, congestive heart failure) but can be *recurrent* (underlying congenital heart disease, asthma, immune deficiency disorders).

Aggravating and relieving factors: Aggravation with exercise, dust, cold and seasonal variation may point towards underlying allergic disorders that can get trigerred with a viral infection. Relieving factors like nebulization with bronchodilators can determine asthma as an underlying cause of cough.

Nature of cough: Paroxysmal nature may point towards pertussis. Nocturnal cough may suggest asthma.

Table 17.1: Possible diagnosis of fever <14 days with no other major symptoms

Possible diagnosis	Type of fever	Clinical presentation	Features suggesting severity
Malaria	Usually intermittent, may be continuous	High grade fever with chills and rigors occurring at regular intervals	Altered sensorium, seizures, severe anemia, renal failure, jaundice, breathlessness, bleeding
Dengue/ Chikungunya	Usually biphasic	High grade fever (with or without rash)/or non-specific symptoms like myalgia, bodyache, malaise, joint pain, loss of appetite, vomiting, and pain abdomen. Respiratory symptoms are usually absent	Shock, severe bleeding, hepatic failure, renal failure, myocarditis, encephalo-pathy
Typhoid fever	Usually continuous, may be intermittent	Moderate to high grade fever with loss of appetite, occasional vomiting, abdominal pain, constipation or diarrhea	Shock, encephalopathy, coma, painful abdominal distension with constipation suggestive of intestinal perforation, gastrointestinal bleeding

Approach to diagnosis: Possible diagnoses for a child with fever and cough (without breathlessness) are presented in **Table 17.2**.

3. Fever with cough and breathlessness

Fast breathing/Tachypnea: Age 0–2 months: RR >60/min, 2 mo–1 yr: RR >50/min; 1–5 yr: RR >40/min.

Lower chest indrawing: Visible inward movement of lower part of the chest wall with inspiration. It is suggestive of involvement of lower respiratory tract. It increases as the severity of illness increases.

Stridor: Harsh high-pitched breathing sound predominantly heard during inspiration suggests stridor which occurs due to narrowing in the upper airway at the level of supraglottis, glottis, subglottis or trachea.

Wheezing: Musical high-pitched breathing sound predominantly heard during expiration suggests wheeze which is characteristic of narrowing of lower airways.

Crackles: These are auscultatory sounds produced when air passes through an air-fluid interface. These are characteristically heard in pneumonia, pulmonary edema, etc.

History: History of bluish discoloration of lips (central cyanosis), lethargy, refusal to feed, altered sensorium convulsions, head nodding, audible grunt in a child with fever, cough, and breathing problem indicates hypoxia due to *severe disease* that may require oxygenation and other supportive measures.

Approach to diagnosis: Follow the clues from history and clinial presentation to arrive at a possible diagnosis in a child presenting with fever, cough, and breathlessness **(Table 17.3)**.

4. Fever with rash

The child may present with any of the following scenarios:

- Fever, cough, coryza and reddish maculo-papular rash
- Fever and a vesicular rash
- Fever >5–7 days and generalized erythematous rash all over the body

In each of these scenarios, ask for the following:

i. Day of onset of rash
ii. Type and pattern of rash (area of involvement, change in appearance of rash)
iii. Other characteristics

Table 17.2: Approach to diagnosis of fever with cough

	Clinical presentation	Possible diagnosis	Common etiology
Elicit history of following symptoms to get a clue to the underlying etiology: 1. Rhinorrhea 2. Ear discharge 3. Throat pain or/and difficulty in swallowing 4. Hoarseness of voice 5. Neck swelling *Also, ask about rash.* Presence of rash suggests associated viral exanthematous illness. Approach to a child with fever and rash is discussed further in this section.	Runny nose, congested eyes, sneezing	**Common cold**	Rhinoviruses, influenza and parainfluenza viruses, coronaviruses
	Ear discharge	**Acute otitis media**	Streptococcus pneumoniae, *H. influenzae*
	Headache, post nasal drip, nasal stuffiness	**Acute sinusitis**	Streptococcus, Moraxella, *H. influenzae, Coronavirus*
	Sore throat, difficulty in swallowing	**Acute pharyngo-tonsillitis, Acute pharyngitis**	Group A β-hemolytic streptococci (*Strep. pyogenes*), or viruses (influenza, para-influenza, corona viruses, Adeno-viruses, coxsackievirus)
	Hoarse voice	**Acute laryngitis**	Adenovirus
	Neck swelling in an unimmunized child	**Diphtheria**	Corynebacterium diphtheriae
		Cervical lymphadenitis, Ludwig angina	*Streptococcus, Staphylococcus aureus,* Anaerobes

Table 17.3: Approach to diagnosis of fever with cough and breathlessness

	Clinical presentation	Possible diagnosis	Common etiology
Elicit the history of following symptoms 1. Noisy breathing 2. Lower chest indrawing 3. Bluish discoloration of lips (central cyanosis) 4. Altered sensorium 5. Lethargy 6. Chest pain 7. Feed intolerance 8. Suck-rest-suck cycle 9. Feeding diaphoresis, failure to thrive 10. Recurrent episodes in past	Hoarse voice, noisy breathing during inspiration	**Laryngotracheobronchitis/ croup**	Parainfluenza type A/B, influenza type A/B
		Acute epiglottitis	*H. influenzae* type B
		Diphtheria with obstruction	*Corynebacterium diphtheriae*
	Cough, fast breathing/ difficult breathing, examination reveals crepitations over lungs	**Pneumonia** *Young age (<5 yr) with acute onset illness favors bronchopneumonia* While older age >5 years favors lobar pneumonia	**Age up to 2 months:** Gram negative organisms, *Strept. pyogenes*, Chlamydia **Age 2 mo–5 yrs:** *H. influenzae*, *Streptococcus pneumoniae*, *Staphylococcus aureus*, *Strept. pyogenes*, Viruses, including Covid-19, *Mycoplasma* **Age >5 yrs:** *Streptococcus pneumoniae*, *Staphylococcus aureus*, Viruses, *Mycoplasma pneumoniae*
	First episode of wheeze in a child below 2 years of age, preceded by rhinorrhea, cold, sneezing, fever, red eyes.	**Bronchiolitis**	Respiratory syncytial virus Adenovirus
	Wheezy child. History of similar episodes in past, history of nebulization in past, age less than 5 years	**Wheezy RTI** OR **multitrigger wheeze**	Can be secondary to any viral or bacterial infection of the respiratory tract
	Chest pain (indicates pleural involvement)	**Empyema** OR **Lobar pneumonia** with **synpneumonic effusion**	*Staphylococcus aureus*, *Streptococcus pneumoniae*, *Streptococcus pyogenes*
	Feed intolerance, suck-rest-suck cycle, feeding diaphoresis, failure to thrive, and history of recurrent episodes	**Congestive heart failure**	Congenital heart disease leading to increased blood flow to lungs: • VSD, PDA—acyanotic heart disease • TGA—cyanotic heart disease

Table 17.4 provides an approach to diagnosis for a child presenting with fever and rash, based on the day of onset of rash, type of rash, and clinical presentation.

5. Fever with jaundice

Table 17.5 provides an approach to diagnosis for a child presenting with fever and jaundice, based on the history and clinical presentation.

6. Fever with pain in abdomen

In the absence of jaundice, follow the differential diagnoses approach given in **Table 17.6**.

7. Fever with burning micturition

Table 17.7 provides an approach to diagnosis and probable etiology of fever with burning micturition in an older child.

8. Fever with abnormal movements and/or altered sensorium

Elicit the following history to assess the area of brain involvement:

- Focal seizures (suggests unilateral involvement of brain parenchyma)
- Altered sensorium (suggests encephalitis or encephalopathy)
- Tonic posturing (suggests cerebral edema due to raised intracranial pressure)
- Cranial nerve deficit (suggests brainstem involvement)
- Limb weakness (suggests motor system involvement)
- Paresthesias, tingling, numbness (suggests sensory system involvement)
- Ataxia, nystagmus (suggests cerebellar involvement)

Table 17.4: Approach to diagnosis of a child with fever and rash

Day of onset of rash	Type of rash	Clinical presentation	Possible diagnosis
Day 1–2 of fever	Maculopapular to vesicular rash, lesions present in multiple stages	Typically begins within 24 hours of onset of fever, spares palms and soles	**Chickenpox**
Day 3–4 of fever	Maculopapular rash beginning from face or neck, spreading centrifugally. Usually leaves dark pigmentation	Koplik spots in oral mucosa associated with conjunctival congestion, coryza.	**Measles**
Day 1–5 of fever	Generalized erythematous rash over extremities and face which blanches on pressure	Palmoplantar erythema, itching, not usually associated with cough/cold	**Dengue or Chikungunya**
Day 1–5 of fever	Maculopapular rash beginning from face/forehead and spreading towards trunk and disappearing in the same manner	Forchheimer sign: Petechiae over soft palate Associated with painful posterior auricular lymphadenopathy	**Rubella**
Day 4–5 of fever	Malar rash with slapped cheek appearance followed by erythematous macular—morbilliform rash over extremities	Typical slapped cheek appearance	**Erythema infectiosum** (fifth disease) caused by Parvovirus B19
Day 6–7 of fever	Salmon colored, blanchable, maculopapular rashes over trunk (Rose spots)	Pain abdomen, poor appetite, vomiting	**Typhoid fever**
	Maculopapular rash with generalized erythematous skin with periungal desquamation and edema of hands and feet	Strawberry tongue, red/cracked lips, unilateral conjunctivitis and cervical lymphadenopathy	**Kawasaki disease**
Rash appearing after some drug intake	Maculopapular rash occurring within 3–5 days of certain drugs	No prodromal symptoms Drug history present	**Drug rash**

Table 17.5: Approach to diagnosis of fever with jaundice

History	Clinical presentation	Possible diagnosis	Common etiology
Elicit the following history to get a clue to the underlying etiology: 1. Exposure to persons with similar illness 2. Travel to endemic area or similar cases in neighbourhood 3. Blood transfusion or sexual contact or I/V drug abuse 4. Family history of jaundice or neurological illness Presence of altered sensorium, hematemesis, malena, ecchymosis suggests acute liver failure	Prodromal phase of low-to-moderate grade fever, headache, malaise followed by jaundice. It may be associated with mild vomiting, anorexia and pain in upper abdomen. There may be history of similar cases in neighborhood	**Acute viral hepatitis** (feco-oral transmission)	Hepatitis A virus Hepatitis E virus
	Prodromal phase (as above) followed by jaundice. This may be associated with arthralgia or arthritis along with a maculopapular rash. There may be a history of blood transfusion or sexual contact or I/V drug abuse	**Acute viral hepatitis** (blood-borne)	Hepatitis B virus Hepatitis C virus
	Moderate to high grade fever for >5–7 days with toxic look. Jaundice is mild	**Typhoid fever** **Scrub typhus**	*Salmonella typhi* *Rickettsia (Orientia tsutsugamushi)*
	High grade fever with chills and rigors	**Severe malaria,** or **Severe dengue**	*Plasmodium* sp. Dengue virus
	Decreased urine output	**Leptospirosis/Severe malaria**	*Leptospira, Plasmodium* sp.
	Abdominal pain Chills and rigors	**Cholangitis**	*E. coli, Salmonella,* Anaerobes

Table 17.6: Approach to diagnosis of a child with fever and pain abdomen (without jaundice)

Points in history	Clinical presentation	Possible diagnosis	Common etiology
Elicit the history of the following symptoms: 1. Loose stools mixed with blood 2. Preceding trauma or viral illness like mumps 3. History of cough, cold, or fast breathing	Loose stools mixed with blood Crampy abdominal pain	**Dysentery**	*Shigella*, EHEC, EIEC
	Abdominal lump, red currant jelly stools	**Intussusception**	
	High grade fever with chills, along with severe pain on right side of the upper abdomen	**Liver abscess**	*Staphylococcus aureus* *Entamoeba histolytica*
	Fever with lower abdominal pain on right side with rebound tenderness	**Acute appendicitis**	Gram negative infections, Amoebic infections
	Fever with chills and rigors, associated with flank pain, vomiting, urinary complaints, etc. May find abdominal mass on palpation	**Pyelonephritis**	Gram-negative organisms including *E. coli (80%), Klebsiella, Enterobacter.* Gram-positive organisms including *Staph. aureus,* and *Enterococcus*
	Preceding history of preauricular swelling (mumps) OR trauma	**Acute pancreatitis**	Drugs (antiretroviral, L-asparaginase)
	Cough/cold/fast breathing Pain in upper abdomen	**Acute tonsillitis, Pneumonia**	*Straptococcus pneumoniae* viruses

Table 17.7: Approach to diagnosis of a child with fever and burning micturition

Points in history*	Clinical presentation	Diagnosis	Common etiology
Elicit the history of following symptoms to get a clue to the underlying etiology: 1. Dysuria, urgency, frequency 2. Lower abdominal pain 3. Itching, foul smelling discharge per vaginum	Dysuria, urgency, frequency, suprapubic pain, urinary incontinence	**Cystitis**	Gram-negative organisms including *E. coli* (80%), *Klebsiella, Enterobacter,* Gram-positive organisms including *Staph. aureus* and *Enterococcus*
	Dysuria, itching, foul smelling discharge, bleeding at the beginning of micturition	**Urethritis**	• Infections: *E. coli, Chlamydia trachomatis* • Bladder stones, ureterocele

*Suspect pyelonephritis, if fever is high along with chills and rigor.

- Abnormal movements like chorea, athetosis, tremors (suggests basal ganglia involvement)
- Urinary or fecal retention/incontinence (suggests bladder/bowel involvement)

An approach to clinical and etiological diagnosis, based on history and clinical presentation in a child with fever and seizures and/or altered sensorium is provided in **Table 17.8**.

9. Fever <2 weeks with miscellaneous signs/symptoms

Presentation	Clinical diagnosis
Fever with skin boils	Abscess, pustules, impetigo, cellulitis
Fever with joint pain and/or swelling	Chikungunya, Septic arthritis, Rheumatic fever
Fever with lymphadenopathy	Suppurative lymphadenitis (bacterial, usually associated with pharyngitis, tonsillitis, dental infections, scalp infections), Kawasaki disease, Infectious mononucleosis

C. Fever of Prolonged Duration

Fever lasting for more than 2 weeks is considered prolonged fever. Infections remain the most important cause of prolonged fever. Inflammatory (collagen vascular) disorders and malignancies are the other common causes of prolonged fever. Certain endocrine, hematological, and neurological disorders may also cause prolonged duration fever **(Table 17.9)**.

History

The following history should be included in history of present illness for any clue towards the specific systemic involvement in fever >2 weeks:

- History of cough with sputum/fast breathing (respiratory system)
- History of abdominal distension, jaundice, hematemesis, malena (hepatobiliary system)
- History of persistent diarrhea, chronic diarrhea, malena, hematochezia (gastrointestinal system)
- History of paleness of body, bleeding spots over skin/mucosa, nodular swellings (reticuloendothelial system, malignancies)
- History of flank pain, dysuria, urgency, frequency, foul smelling urine (genitourinary system)
- History of rash over face/body, joint pain or joint swelling with restriction of movement (collagen vascular disorders)
- History of abnormal movements, altered sensorium, focal neurological deficit (CNS)
- History of recurrent boils, significant weight loss, loss of appetite (immune deficiency state)

Examination findings that may help to differentiate between various causes of prolonged fever include presence of lymphadenopathy, rash, arthritis, and hepatosplenomegaly **(Table 17.10)**.

Table 17.8: Approach to clinical diagnosis of a child with fever and seizure

	Clinical presentation	Possible diagnosis	Common etiology
Elicit the following history to get a clue to the underlying etiology: 1. Age of the child 2. Altered sensorium 3. Focal neurological deficit 4. Headache, vomiting, photophobia 5. Neck rigidity 6. History of preceding viral illness 7. Family history of similar illness	• Age 6 months–5 years • Seizure at the peak of fever • No altered sensorium • No neurological deficit • No neck rigidity • Past history of similar episode	**Febrile seizure**	Upper respiratory tract infections, viral fevers, urinary tract infections, gastrointestinal infections
	• Acute onset febrile illness • Presence of headache, vomiting, photophobia • Bulging fontanelle in infants • Neck rigidity in age >1–2 years • Altered sensorium or behavior • Presence of a typical rash indicates meningococcal meningitis.	**Acute pyogenic meningitis**	**Age <1 month:** *E. coli*, Group B streptococci, *Listeria monocytogenes* **Age 1 month–2 years:** *Hemophilus influenzae, Streptococcus pneumoniae, Neisseria meningitidis, E. coli* **Age >2 years:** *N. meningitidis, S. pneumoniae*
	• Acute onset febrile illness • Altered sensorium or behavior • Headache, vomiting • Focal neurological deficit and meningeal signs usually absent • Feature of raised intracranial pressure (ICP) frequently present	**Acute febrile encephalopathy**	Viral encephalitis (arboviruses, herpes viruses, enteroviruses, measles, mumps, adenovirus), cerebral malaria, enteric encephalopathy
	• Fever >5 days • Altered sensorium and/or unconsciousness • Headache, vomiting • Meningeal signs • Focal neurological deficit • Cranial nerve involvement • Features of raised ICP	**Tubercular meningitis**	*Mycobacterium tuberculosis*
	• Acute onset illness • Focal seizures • Focal neurological deficit • Features of raised ICP	**Brain abscess**	*Staphylococcus aureus*, Streptococci, Anaerobes, Gramnegative organisms like *Proteus, Pseudomonas, Citrobacter* and *Hemophilus influenzae*

Table 17.9: History of present illness and differential diagnosis of fever persisting more than 2 weeks

Nature of illness	Clinical presentation	Etiology
Infections	• History of cough with sputum/fast breathing • Flank pain, dysuria, urgency, frequency, foul smelling urine • History of abdominal pain, constipation or diarrhea, toxic look, splenomegaly • Recurrent infections, significant weight loss, loss of appetite	• Tuberculosis • Urinary tract infections • Typhoid fever • HIV infection, systemic fungal infections
Inflammatory disorders	• Joint pain or joint swelling with restriction of movement • Rash over face/body • Nodular swellings over body	• Juvenile idiopathic arthritis, systemic lupus erythematosus, Kawasaki disease, other connective tissue disorders
Malignancies	• Paleness of body, bleeding spots over skin or mucosa • Nodular swellings over body • Abdominal distension or lump • Bony pains	• Lymphoma, leukemia, brain tumors, neuroblastoma, • Wilms' tumor
Endocrine causes	• Excessive sweating, palpitations, proptosis • Polyuria, polydipsia	• Thyrotoxicosis • Diabetes insipidus
Hematological disorders	• Paleness of body • Lump abdomen or abdominal distension • Recurrent infections	• Agranulocytosis, hemolytic anemia, disorders of T and B cells, immune deficiency disorders, malignancy
Neurological disorders	• Excessive sweating	• Familial dysautonomia, anhidrotic ectodermal dysplasia, hypothalamic and third ventricular lesions
Miscellaneous causes	• No major associations except for history of drugs	• Drug fever, factitious fever

17.2 CHILD WITH LOOSE STOOLS

A. Definitions

Diarrhea: Increase in frequency and change in consistency of stools, i.e. passage of loose or watery stools three or more times a day.

Dysentery: Loose stools with blood.

Persistent diarrhea: Loose stools with acute onset but lasting for >14 days, usually infective in origin.

Chronic diarrhea: Loose stools >14 days with insidious onset, usually non-infective, may be due to malabsorption. It is usually associated with failure to thrive.

B. History

Elicit the history of following symptoms in a child with suspected diarrheal illness:

- *Duration* (to differentiate between acute watery diarrhea and persistent diarrhea)
- *Consistency* and frequency of stools (rice watery stools suggest cholera)
- Presence of *blood in stools* (to differentiate between diarrhea and dysentery)
- Symptoms suggestive of *some dehydration*: Increased thirst, irritability, passing lesser amount of urine
- Symptoms suggestive of *severe dehydration*: Lethargy, decreased oral acceptance and not passing urine
- Symptoms suggesting *dyselectrolytemia*: Seizures, altered sensorium, abdominal distension
- Symptoms suggesting *systemic involvement*: High grade fever, altered sensorium, persistent vomiting, cough, urinary complaints, neck rigidity

Table 17.10: Examination findings and differential diagnosis of fever

Physical finding	Duration of fever	
Hepatomegaly	*Less than 2 weeks*	*More than 2 weeks*
	Infections: Acute viral hepatitis, liver abscess, enteric fever, dengue, scrub typhus	Chronic hepatitis, amebic liver abscess, enteric fever, scrub typhus
	Hematological: Sickle cell anemia with crisis	Acute leukemia
	Malignancy: Acute leukemia	Acute leukemia, lymphoma, hepatoblastoma
Splenomegaly	*Infections:* Malaria, infective endocarditis, enteric fever	Kala-azar, chronic malaria, infective endocarditis
	Malignancy: Acute leukemia	Acute leukemia, Chronic myeloid leukemia, non-Hodgkin lymphoma
Hepatosplenomegaly	*Infections:* Malaria, enteric fever, infectious mononucleosis, rickettsial infections	Tuberculosis, kala-azar, brucellosis, infectious mononucleosis
	Malignancy: Acute leukemia	Acute leukemia, lymphoma, histiocytosis
	Connective tissue diseases	SLE, JIA
Lymphadenopathy	Suppurative lymphadenitis, Kawasaki disease	Tuberculosis, HIV, lymphoma, ALL, systemic onset JIA
Hepatosplenomegaly with lymphadenopathy	Acute leukemia, infectious mononucleosis	Tuberculosis, HIV, lymphoma, ALL
Rash	Infections: Dengue, measles, varicella, meningococcemia	Lupus vulgaris (tuberculosis)
	Connective tissue diseases/vasculitis: Kawasaki disease, Henoch-Schönlein purpura (HSP)	Systemic onset JIA, SLE
Arthritis	Septic arthritis, Kawasaki disease, HSP, rheumatic fever, chikungunya	Juvenile idiopathic arthritis, SLE, acute rheumatic fever, dermatomyositis, polymyositis, reactive arthritis, tubercular arthritis

C. Clinical Scenarios and Differential Diagnosis

Table 17.11 presents several different clinical scenarios in a child with loose stools, to differentiate between acute watery diarrhea, dysentery, cholera, persistent diarrhea, chronic diarrhea, etc. based on the history of presenting illness. Causes of common complications (seizures, altered sensorium, abdominal distension, etc.) are also discussed.

D. Examination Findings

Vitals

- ***Consciousness:*** Irritable and restless in some dehydration, lethargic or unconscious in severe dehydration
- ***Pulse:*** Tachycardia and low volume pulse in severe dehydration
- ***Respiratory rate:*** Fast and deep breathing in acidosis
- ***Blood pressure:*** Hypotension in severe dehydration and/or shock

Table 17.11: Approach to clinical and etiological diagnosis of a child with loose stools, based on presenting illness

Chief complaint	Associated complaints	Probable diagnosis	Explanation and etiology
Loose, watery stools, 8–10 times/day × 3 days	Non-bilious, non-projectile vomiting, 1–2 episodes Fever	**Acute watery diarrhea**	• Loose watery stools >3 times/day, without blood suggests acute diarrhea. • Rotavirus is the most common cause followed by enterotoxigenic *E. coli* • Fever also may not always indicate a systemic involvement. It can be a part of acute diarrheal illness
Loose stools with *mucus*, 5–8 times/day × 4 days	No specific associations	**Acute watery diarrhea**	• Presence of mucus does not always indicate dysentery
Loose, watery stools 20–25 *times per day* × 1–2 days	Ask for rice watery character of stools, especially in children >2 years	**Cholera**	*Vibrio cholerae*
Loose stools with blood, 5–6 times/day × 3 days	May be associated with cramps or pain abdomen	**Dysentery**	• Gross blood in stools is the most reliable sign of dysentery. • Most common organisms: *Shigella, E. coli* • E. histolytica is not a common cause in children <5 years.
Loose stools 6–8 times/day × 15 days	Starts as an episode of acute watery diarrhea.	**Persistent diarrhea**	• Acute diarrhea persisting for more than 14 days is known as persistent diarrhea. • More common in malnourished children and children <2 years • Occurs either due to delayed clearance of infection or transient lactose intolerance
Loose, semi-formed stools, 4–5 times/day × 2 *months* on and off	Stools are bulky, frothy and sticky. There is intermittent abdominal distension especially after meals.	**Chronic diarrhea**	• Diarrhea with "abnormal stools" which continue or recur over several months. • Malabsorption disorders are the most common cause. • Usually associated with failure to thrive anemia and vitamin deficiencies
Loose stools with altered sensorium	History of giving ORS in inappropriate dilution.	**Acute diarrhea with dyselectrolytemia**	Hyponatremia Hypernatremia Hypoglycemia
	History of persistent vomiting	**Encephalopathy** OR **Viral encephalitis**	Enteroviral diarrhea, *Shigella* encephalopathy

Contd...

Table 17.11: Approach to clinical and etiological diagnosis of a child with loose stools, based on presenting illness (*Contd...*)

Chief complaint	Associated complaints	Probable diagnosis	Explanation and etiology
Loose stools with seizures	High grade fever	**Febrile seizure**	There may be co-existing systemic infection
	Altered sensorium	**Hyponatremia**	Serum sodium <125 mEq/L
		Hypernatremia	Serum sodium >150 mEq/L
		Hypoglycemia	Blood sugar <50 mg/dL
	Clonic seizure or tetany	**Hypocalcemia**	Serum calcium <7 mg/dL
		Hypomagnesemia	Serum magnesium <1.5 mg/dL
	Neck rigidity, excessive crying, irritability, bulging fontanelle	**Meningitis**	*Streptococcus pneumoniae* (all ages) *Meningococcus* (>2 yr) Gram –ve bacilli (<2 yr)
Loose stools with *abdominal distension*	Neck flop or hypotonia	**Hypokalemia**	Increased losses, especially in already malnourished child
	Sick looking child, not feeding well	**Paralytic ileus**	Septicemia or hypokalemia

Anthropometry

- Wasting in acute diarrhea
- Severe wasting in persistent diarrhea
- Moderate or severe stunting in chronic diarrhea

General Physical Examination

- *Signs of dehydration:* Sunken eyes, skin pinch goes back slowly, consciousness, eagerness to drink
- *Pallor:* In chronic diarrhea/malabsorption
- *Signs of vitamin deficiency:* Features suggestive of vitamin A or vitamin D deficiency are common in (a) malabsorption disorders presenting as chronic diarrhea; and (b) severe acute malnutrition presenting with persistent diarrhea.

Systemic Examination

- *Chest:* Look for signs of coexisting pneumonia
- *Abdomen:* Abdominal distension with absent bowel sounds suggests paralytic ileus due to hypokalemia or sepsis.
- *Central nervous system:*
  - Altered sensorium may be seen in severe dehydration, meningitis, encephalopathy, hyponatremia, hypernatremia, or cortical venous thrombosis.
  - Neck flop, absent deep tendon reflexes, and hypotonia suggest hypokalemia.
  - Presence of meningeal signs indicates meningitis.
  - Presence of focal neurological deficit indicates thrombosis secondary to dehydration.

17.3 CHILD WITH EDEMA

Edema

It refers to the presence of excess fluid in the interstitial space of the body. It can be localized or generalized. Systemic disorders result in generalized edema. Edema usually occurs due to one of the three mechanisms: (i) reduced oncotic pressure, (ii) increased intravascular volume, and (iii) increased capillary permeability. The causes of edema are listed in **Table 17.12**.

A. Differential Diagnosis of Childhood Edema

Characteristics of edema, and presence of associated features can provide some useful clues to the etiopathogenesis of edema. An approach is presented in **Table 17.13**.

B. Renal Causes of Edema

The most common renal causes of edema in children are nephrotic syndrome and nephritic syndrome. Nephrotic syndrome is mainly minimal change disease type; while poststreptococcal glomerulonephritis is the

Table 17.12: Causes of childhood edema
1. *Reduced oncotic pressure (due to hypoproteinemia)* • Nephrotic syndrome • Chronic liver disease • Malnutrition • Protein losing enteropathy • Severe burns
2. *Increased intravascular volume (due to cardiovascular or renal diseases)* • Congestive heart failure • High-output heart failure due to hyperthyroidism, anemia, or beriberi • Acute glomerulonephritis • Renal failure • Arteriovenous fistula
3. *Increased capillary permeability* • *Allergic diseases:* Angioneurotic edema, aeroallergens, food allergy • *Vasculitis:* Anaphylactoid purpura, systemic lupus erythematosus, dermatomyositis, polyarteritis nodosa, scleroderma, Kawasaki disease

most common cause of nephritic syndrome. Distinguishing features of the two entities are compared in **Table 17.14**.

Typical Scenarios

Nephrotic syndrome: A 3-year-old boy presenting with first episode of gradually progressing generalized body swelling starting from face for last 15 days along with decreased urine output for 4–5 days, without history of hematuria, fever, drug intake, or any systemic complaints.

On examination, child is hemodynamically stable with normal blood pressure except for generalized edema (anasarca) involving face, abdomen, scrotum, and limbs. Abdomen is grossly distended with no periumbilical redness or caput medusae. Shifting dullness is present. Breath sounds are diminished in the right infra-axillary region.

Nephritic syndrome: A 6-year-old girl presenting with painless hematuria with typically cola-colored urine, decreased urine

Table 17.13: Approach to etiological diagnosis of edema

Characteristics of edema	Associated features	Probable pathology	Common causes
Edema starting from dependent areas (feet), more during evening	Tachycardia, fast breathing or dyspnea, fatigue, raised JVP, cardiomegaly, hepatomegaly	**Congestive heart failure**	• Congenital heart disease: VSD, PDA, TGA • Valvular heart diseases • Pericardial effusion • Anemia • Myocarditis • Severe anemia
Edema starting from abdomen, going down to feet and later on involving face	Jaundice, ascites, spider nevi, failure to thrive, hematemesis malena	**Liver disease**	• Acute viral hepatitis • Autoimmune hepatitis • Chronic liver disease • Drug-induced hepatitis
Edema starting from periorbital region, and is maximum during morning hours. Finally, it progresses to generalized edema (anasarca)	Decreased urine output There may be associated hematuria and hypertension	**Nephrotic syndrome** **Glomerulonephritis** **Renal failure**	• Minimal change Nephrotic syndrome • Post-streptococcal glomerulonephritis • Rapidly progressive glomerulonephritis • Focal segmental glomerulosclerosis
Dependent edema	Weight for length/height <–2 SD, psychomotor changes, dermatosis, hypopigmented hair	**Kwashiorkor** OR **Nutritional edema**	• Hypoproteinemia • Free radical mediated dysadaptation

Table 17.14: Differentiating features of nephrotic syndrome and nephritic syndrome

	Nephrotic syndrome	Nephritic syndrome
Edema	Gross (++++)	Mild-to-moderate (+ to ++)
Oliguria	May/may not be present	Always present
Hypertension	Absent/minimal	Common
Hematuria	Absent/microscopic	Marked/gross (cola-colored urine)
Proteinuria	Gross (4^+ or nephrotic range)	Moderate
Serum cholesterol	Elevated	Normal/mildly elevated
Glomerular filteration rate	Normal	Decreased
Common causes	• Minimal change disease (idiopathic) • Focal segmental glomerulosclerosis • Mesangioproliferative glomerulonephritis • Secondary nephrotic syndrome due to SLE, malignancies, infections, drugs, etc.	• Post-streptococcal glomerulonephritis • Membranoproliferative glomerulonephritis • Henoch-Schönlein purpura • Wegener granulomatosis

output, and facial puffiness for last 4 days. This was preceded by a sore throat around 10 days ago. There is no associated complaint of abdominal pain, jaundice, or trauma.

On examination, child has mild tachypnea, tachycardia, and hypertension (blood pressure: 150/100 mm Hg). Periorbital puffiness is present along with pedal edema. There is no edema on abdomen and genitalia; and no anemia, jaundice, or rash. Systemic examination reveals bilateral basal crepts. There is no tenderness, mass, or distension of the abdomen.

C. Approach to a Child with Nephrotic Syndrome

Approach to history-taking in a child with nephrotic syndome is depicted in **Table 17.15**.

Definitions

Nephrotic syndrome: Glomerular disease characterized by all of the following criteria.

1. Generalized edema
2. Proteinuria (>40 mg/m^2/hour)
3. Hypoalbuminemia (Serum albumin <2.5 g/dL)
4. Hyperlipidemia (Serum cholesterol >200 mg/ dL)

Infrequently relapsing nephrotic syndrome: Less than 2 relapses in 6 months of initial response or <4 relapses within any 12-month period.

Frequently relapsing nephrotic syndrome: Two or more relapses in 6 months of initial response or 4 relapses within any 12-month period.

Examination

First impression: Conscious and alert child with generalized anasarca, looks puffy with distended abdomen.

Vitals: Usually normal. Check blood pressure. Hypertension indicates a significant glomerular lesion. Increased respiratory rate with shallow respiration indicates possibility of pleural effusion or pulmonary edema. Tachycardia may occur secondary to a systemic infection or heart failure due to fluid overload.

Anthropometry: Usually normal. Weight for height is likely to be high because of edema. Growth retardation may occur in children on long-term steroid therapy.

General physical examination

- Check edema over face (periorbital), abdominal wall, genitalia, and pedal edema.
- Look for pallor, icterus to rule out secondary causes of nephrotic syndrome.
- Palpate for lymphadenopathy to rule out possibility of tuberculosis, HIV.

Abdomen examination

Inspection: May be grossly distended with shiny skin due to ascitis. Look for periumbilical erythema. Check genitalia.

Table 17.15: Approach to history-taking in a child with nephrotic syndrome

	History	Explanation
Typical scenario A 4-yr-old child presenting with chief complaints of swelling all over the body × 15 days and decreased urine output × 4–5 days **Elicit the history of following symptoms to get a clue to the underlying etiology and complications:** History of red-colored urine, burning micturition, dysuria, jaundice/black-colored stools, insect bite, skin rash, joint pain, joint swelling, drug intake, fast breathing, palpitations headache, blurring of vision	Any history of red-colored urine	• Significant glomerular involvement and acute nephritic syndrome less likely in absence of hematuria
	Any history of fever, burning micturition, dysuria	• For associated systemic infections, and urinary tract infections
	Any history of jaundice/black-colored stools	• For any hepatic causes of edema
	History of insect bite	• For angioedema
	Any history of skin rash, joint pain, joint swelling, drug intake, nodular swelling over body	• For secondary causes of nephrotic syndrome such as: SLE, HIV, hepatitis B, Hodgkin lymphoma, and drug-induced secondary to NSAIDs, gold, d-penicillamine
	Any history of redness or pain over abdomen	• For any possibility of spontaneous bacterial peritonitis (mainly caused by *Streptococcus pneumoniae* or *E. coli*)
	Any history of fast breathing, palpitations, headache	• For complications of nephrotic syndrome, i.e. left ventricular failure, pleural effusion, hypertension
	History of headache, blurring of vision	• Suggests hypertension. Common with FSGS or mesangioproliferative glomerulonephritis

Palpation: Dipping method preferred due to edema. Check for guarding, tenderness, rigidity (to rule out peritonitis). Look for hepatomegaly, and renal angle tenderness (possibility of UTI).

Chest examination: Check for signs of pleural effusion, mediastinal shift, and features suggestive of pleural effusion (dullness on percussion and diminished breath sounds on auscultation). CVS is usually normal. Rarely, signs of pericardial effusion (soft or distant heart sounds, pericardial rub) may be present.

Nervous system: Usually normal unless thrombotic complications or hypertensive emergency set in.

17.4 CHILD WITH PALLOR

A. Pallor and Anemia

Any condition that decreases the concentration of hemoglobin or alters the distribution of blood away from the body's surface may present as pallor. Clinically, pallor caused by anemia usually can be appreciated when the hemoglobin concentration is below 8 to 9 g/dL, although the complexion of the child and the rapidity of onset may influence this value.

Hematological Causes of Pallor

I. Decreased RBC production

a. *Deficiency of essential nutrients:* Iron deficiency, vitamin B_{12} deficiency, folic acid deficiency, vitamin B_6 deficiency
b. *Reduced erythropoiesis:* Aplastic anemia, chronic infections, chronic inflammatory diseases, bone marrow infiltration (leukemia, lymphoma), thyroxine deficiency

II. Increased destruction of RBC

a. *Intracorpuscular defects:* Thalassemia, red cell enzyme deficiency, RBC membrane defects (spherocytosis, elliptocytosis, lead toxicity)

b. *Extracorpuscular defects:* Immune hemolytic anemia, hypersplenism, disseminated intravascular coagulation, hemolytic uremic syndrome

III. Blood loss

a. Acute
b. Chronic

B. History-taking in Anemia

Elicit the history as detailed in **Table 17.16** to get a clue to the underlying etiology.

C. Examination of a Child with Anemia

Look for the physical findings as detailed in **Table 17.17** as a clue to the cause of anemia.

D. Common Clinical Scenarios of Anemia after Newborn Period

Several clues help in arriving at the etiological diagnosis of anemia. These include the age at onset of symptoms, presenting complaints and findings on physical examination. An approach to diagnosis of anemia, based on these parameters is detailed in **Table 17.18**.

Table 17.16: History-taking in a child presenting with anemia/pallor and its interpretation

	History	Probable etiology (common)
Age of the child	Neonatal period (up to 1 month)	Placental abruption, twin-to-twin transfusion, intracranial hemorrhage, G6PD deficiency, isoimmunization, anemia of prematurity
	1–6 months	Anemia of prematurity, Diamond-Blackfan anemia, congenital aplastic anemia like Fanconi anemia
	6 months to 3 years	Nutritional anemia due to deficiency of iron, vitamin B_{12}, or folate, thalassemia, sickle cell anemia, leukemia
	Above 3 years	Nutritional anemia, acquired hemolytic anemia (autoimmune hemolytic anemia, drug-induced hemolysis, infection-induced hemolysis), aplastic anemia, leukemia, lymphoma, anemia due to hookworm infestation
	Adolescent girl	Menstrual blood loss (excessive), puberty
	Any age	Acute blood loss
Sex	Common in boys (X-linked disorders)	G6PD deficiency Pyruvate kinase deficiency
Race	Parsees	G6PD deficiency
	Sindhis, Punjabis, Lohanas, Gaud community (in India)	Thalassemia
	Gonds, Bhils (MP) tribes of Maharashtra, Gujarat, Tamil Nadu and Nilgiri region	Sickle cell anemia
Severity of symptoms	Mild-to-moderate (pallor, fatigue, weakness, lethargy)	Iron deficiency anemia, beta thalassemia minor, chronic gastrointestinal blood loss due to parasitic infestations, cow milk protein allergy
	Moderate-to-severe (dyspnea, drowsiness, shock)	Thalassemia major, sickle cell anemia, leukemia, aplastic anemia, acute severe blood loss

(Contd...)

17

Clinical Approach to Common Cases

Table 17.16: History-taking in a child presenting with anemia/pallor and its interpretation (*Contd.*)

	History	Probable etiology (common)
Dietary history	History of pica, geophagia, pagophagia	Iron deficiency anemia
	Inadequate complementary feeding with predominant milk based diet	Iron deficiency anemia
	Vegetarian diet lacking in fruit/ vegetables, with goat milk intake	Megaloblastic anemia
History of bleeding	Superficial bleeds (petechiae, purpura)	Aplastic anemia, leukemia, hemophilia, idiopathic thrombocytopenic purpura, disseminated intravascular coagulation
	Deep bleeds (hematemesis, malena, intracranial bleed, hemoglobinuria)	Hemophilia, severe thrombocytopenia
History of fever	May be associated with hemoglobinuria	Malaria
	May have petechiae or purpura	Infectious mononucleosis, typhoid fever, infective endocarditis, Kala-azar, leukemia, lymphoma
Past infections	Viral hepatitis	Aplastic anemia
	Parvovirus B19 infection	Red cell aplasia
Systemic symptoms	Chronic diarrhea	Megaloblastic anemia, anemia of malabsorption syndromes (celiac disease)
	Worm infestation	Iron deficiency anemia
	Jaundice (mild)	Thalassemia, hereditary spherocytosis, sickle cell amemia, autoimmune hemolytic anemia
	High-colored urine (hemoglobinuria)	Hemolytic anemia (G6PD deficiency, auto-immune hemolytic anemia, PNH), consider malaria if associated with fever
	History of nodular swellings, bony pains, weight loss, anorexia	Leukemia, lymphoma
	Neurological symptoms like cognitive impairment, loss of vibration sense, and/ or joint position	Vitamin B_{12} deficiency Pyridoxine deficiency may present with anemia and seizures
	Failure to thrive and not growing well	Celiac disease, chronic renal disease
	Abnormal facies or other skeletal anomalies	Fanconi anemia, dyskeratosis congenita Diamond-Blackfan anemia
Family history	Family history of anemia, jaundice, gallstones, splenomegaly	Thalassemia, hereditary spherocytosis, sickle cell anemia
History of drug intake	Phenytoin, phenobarbitone, purine and pyrimidine analogues	Megaloblastic anemia
	Primaquine, sulfamethoxazole, and nitrofurantion like oxidant drugs, dapsone, PAS, chloramphenicol, quinolones like nalidixic acid	G6PD deficiency-induced hemolytic anemia

Table 17.17: Approach to etiological diagnosis of anemia, based on physical examination findings

System	Clinical finding	Possible etiology
Skin	Generalized hyperpigmentation with hypopigmented patches	Fanconi anemia
	Hyperpigmentation of the knuckles	Megaloblastic anemia due to vitamin B_{12} deficiency
	Petechiae, purpura	Aplastic anemia, leukemia, autoimmune hemolytic anemia with thrombocytopenia, megaloblastic anemia, thrombocytopenia with excessive blood loss
	Jaundice (mild)	Acute and chronic hemolytic anemia, aplastic anemia
	Cavernous hemangioma	Microangiopathic hemolytic anemia
	Leg ulcers	Sickle cell anemia, thalassemia intermedia
General physical examination	Edema	Congestive heart failure due to severe anemia
	Clubbing	Malabsorption disorder
	Lymphadenopathy	Leukemia, lymphoma, infectious mononucleosis, collagen vascular/infiltrative disorder, malignancy *Presence of significant lymphadenopathy usually rules out aplastic anemia*
	Marked wasting or gross emaciation	Anemia of malnutrition because of multiple micronutrient deficiency
	Tongue—glossitis	Megaloblastic anemia
	Bald tongue	Iron deficiency anemia
	Mouth—angular cheilosis	Malabsorption
Facies	Hemolytic facies—large head, depressed nasal bridge, frontal and parietal bossing, malar prominence, anterior over-riding of maxillary teeth	Chronic hemolytic anemia (thalassemia major, sickle cell anemia, hereditary spherocytosis)
Eyes	Microcornea	Fanconi anemia
	Microaneurysms of retinal vessels	Sickle cell anemia
	Blindness	Osteopetrosis
	Xerophthalmia	Malabsorption
Hands	Triphalangeal thumb	Red cell aplasia (Diamond-Blackfan syndrome)
	Hypoplasia of thenar eminences, absent/abnormal thumb	Fanconi anemia
	Koilonychia, platynychia	Iron deficiency anemia
Chest	Shield chest	Diamond-Blackfan syndrome
	Basal crepts	Congestive cardiac failure due to severe anemia
Abdomen	Hepatosplenomegaly	Hemolytic anemia (thalassemia, G6PD) deficiency, hereditary spherocytosis *Infiltrative disorder:* Leukemia, lymphoma *Presence of hepatosplenomegaly usually rules out aplastic anemia*
Cardiovascular system	S3, gallop rhythm, ejection systolic murmur	Congestive cardiac failure due to severe anemia

Table 17.18: Approach to diagnosis of anemia, based on age at onset, presenting history and physical examination

Age (median)	Presenting illness	Important history	Clinical findings	Diagnosis
6 months–4 years (18–24 months)	Progressive paleness with irritability, easy fatiguability, and decreased appetite	Predominantly milk-based diet with inadequate complementary feeding, history of pica and/or worm infestation, repeated infections, and dyspnea on exertion	*Present:* Moderate pallor, koilonychia or platynychia, glossitis, angular stomatitis. Presence of tachycardia, cardiomegaly, ejection systolic murmur (due to hyperdynamic circulation) *Absent:* Lymphadenopathy, bleeding spots, splenomegaly	**Iron deficiency anemia** (nutritional)
6 months–5 years (18–24 months)	Progressive pallor with irritability and decreased appetite	Predominantly vegetarian or milk-based diet; there may be history of intake of goat milk. There may be history of mucosal bleeds and/or developmental delay	*Present:* Pallor, hyperpigmentation of knuckles, petechiae, glossitis, and mild splenomegaly Tremors, peripheral neuropathy, and hypotonia may be observed in vitamin B_{12} deficiency *Absent:* Significant bleeding, lymphadenopathy	**Megaloblastic anemia** (*nutritional deficiency of vitamin* B_{12})
6 months to 3 years (9–18 months)	Progressive paleness of body with irritability, poor appetite and abdominal distension	Failure to thrive, mild jaundice, history of repeated blood transfusion. There may be family history of transfusions, death due to severe anemia, or gallstones	*Present:* Moderate or severe pallor, mild jaundice, hemolytic facies, and hepatosplenomegaly *Absent:* Lymphadenopathy and petechiae	**Thalassemia major**
Above 3 years (6–8 years)	Fever, anemia, bleeding spots or epistaxis/malena	Insidious onset of anemia, bleeding	*Present:* Moderate-to-severe pallor, petechiae *Absent:* Lymphadenopathy, hepatosplenomegaly	**Aplastic anemia**
		Skeletal defects or gross congenital anomalies Previous episode of bleeding (superficial/deep)	Short stature, absent radius, abnormal thumb, facial dysmorphism, café au lait spots	**Congenital Inherited aplastic anemia**
		Preceding history of viral or bacterial illness or drug intake 2–3 months back	Moderate-to-severe pallor, petechiae, fever, no skeletal abnormalities No lymphadenopathy, jaundice, or hepatosplenomegaly	**Acquired aplastic anemia**

(Contd...)

Table 17.18: Approach to diagnosis of anemia, based on age at onset, presenting history and physical examination (*Contd...*)

Age (median)	Presenting illness	Important history	Clinical findings	Diagnosis
Above 6 months (2–6 years)	Fever, paleness of body with easy fatiguability, bleeding spots over body for 15 days	Bony pains, nodular swellings over body	Moderate-to-severe pallor, petechiae, purpura, generalised lymphadenopathy, sternal tenderness, and hepatosplenomegaly	**Leukemia**
4–12 years	Progressive paleness with irritability, easy fatiguability, pain abdomen off and on poor scholastic performance, and decreased appetite	Passage of worms in stool, chronic diarrhea, abdominal distension, there may be history of pica or itching in perianal region especially during night time *There may be a history of defecation in open and walking barefoot in fields*	*Present:* Moderate pallor, platynychia or koilonychias. Spleen may be palpable in 30% cases *Absent:* Lymphadenopathy, petechiae, marked hepatosplenomegaly, short stature	**Iron deficiency anemia** *(due to hookworm infestation)*
Adolescent girl	Easy fatiguability, decreased appetite, history of excessive menstrual blood loss	Headache, palpitations, dyspnea on exertion, pain abdomen	Moderate-to-severe anemia, tachycardia	**Iron deficiency anemia** *(due to excessive menstrual blood loss and pubertal growth spurt)*
Any age	Sudden onset paleness of body with red-colored urine in a boy	Mild jaundice, history of intake of drugs like NSAIDs or antimalarials or fava beans intake Family history of similar episodes in maternal uncle History of recent infection	Moderate pallor, jaundice, No lymphadenopathy or petechiae splenomegaly	**G6PD deficiency-induced hemolysis or Autoimmune hemolytic anemia**
Any age	Easy fatiguability, paleness of body, yellow eyes, abdominal distension	There may be family history of transfusions, death due to severe anemia, or gall stones	Mild-to-moderate splenomegaly with jaundice No lymphadenopathy, no petechiae	**Hereditary spherocytosis**
Any age	Chronic diarrhea, abdominal distension and insidious onset paleness of body	No gastrointestinal bleeding, no history of worm infestation	Mild-to-moderate pallor, inadequate response to iron therapy, and **short stature**	**Celiac disease**

17.5 CHILD WITH CONGENITAL HEART DISEASE (CHD)

Model Case Scenario 1: Acyanotic CHD—Left to Right Shunt

Chief Complaints

A 2-year-old girl was brought to pediatric emergency room with following complaints:

1. Frequent episodes of cough, fever and fast breathing since 3 months of age
2. Not growing well for last 18 months
3. Marked breathlessness with fever, cough, and chest retractions for 3 days
4. Refusal to take feeds for 1 day

History of Presenting Illness

The child was born at term gestation to G4P3 mother with birth weight of 2.8 kg with uneventful perinatal period. She was discharged on 4th day without any immediate neonatal problems. Child was apparently well till 3 months of age when she started having frequent episodes of cough, fast breathing, and fever. These episodes used to occur every 2–3 months and lasted for 5–7 days. Thrice in the last one year she had to be admitted for episodes of acute severe cough, fever, breathing difficulty for 10–15 days every time and was treated with antibiotics. In the current episode, she was again admitted with marked breathlessness with chest retractions, cough, and refusal to feed.

The mother also noticed that child was not growing well. On probing, she recalls that the baby used to have some feeding problems in infancy. At 2 months of age, she noticed that the child used to stop feeding after sucking for some time at the breast, and restart sucking after some time. This cycle used to be repeated several times during a feed. Mother had also noticed increased rate of breathing during these periods and excessive sweating over the forehead and over the back of the head. The child was started on complementary feeding only after 8 months of life and is presently having a significant lag in calorie and protein intake.

There is no history of bluish discoloration of oral cavity, body, or extremities during crying or otherwise. There is also no history suggestive of squatting episodes or lying in knee-chest posture. There is no history of abnormal movements, altered sensorium, bleeding from any site, neurological deficit, or significant developmental delay. There is no history of prolonged fever. There is no history of maternal fever with rash, irradiation, drug or alcohol intake, or diabetes during the antenatal period. There is no family history of congenital heart disease.

Clinical Examination

General Physical Examination

- Poorly nourished child, conscious but lethargic, dyspneic with marked intercostal and subcostal retractions.
- HR—172/min, RR—76/min, SpO_2—94% in all four extremities, BP—82/56 mmHg in right arm and 90/56 in right leg.
- Peripheries are cool and pulse volume is low.
- Prominent visible neck venous pulsations with significant sweating over forehead, minimal periorbital puffiness with significant pedal edema although no cyanosis, clubbing
- No dysmorphic features

Anthropometry

Weight, height and head circumference are below –2 SD for age.

Cardiovascular Examination

- ***Inspection:*** Left precordial bulge with bilateral Harrison sulcus on lower chest with prominent left parasternal pulsations and apical thrust.
- ***Palpation:*** Diffuse systolic pulsations felt in left lower parasternal region; and ill sustained hyperdynamic apical impulse in 6th left intercostal space was felt.
- ***Auscultation:*** S1 was normal. P2 was loud. S3 was heard. There was a grade 3/6 early systolic murmur from third left intercostal space down to the xiphisternum. There was another ejection systolic murmur in pulmonary area along with a flow mid-diastolic murmur over the mitral area.

Lungs

Bilateral crepitations.

Abdomen

Liver 5 cm below right costal margin in midclavicular line with 11 cm span, and spleen felt below costal margin.

Clinical Diagnosis

Congenital acyanotic heart disease with left to right shunt, possibly a moderate-to-large ventricular septal defect (VSD) with hyperkinetic pulmonary arterial hypertension *in* sinus rhythm *with* congestive heart failure *with* acute lower respiratory tract infection, *and* failure to thrive.

Points favoring diagnosis	
Heart disease	Suggested by • History of fatigability during feeding • Precordial bulge • Grade 3/6 systolic murmur • Diastolic murmur
Acyanotic nature	Absence of cyanosis
Congenital heart disease	Early age of onset, parasternal murmurs
Increased pulmonary blood flow	Recurrent lower respiratory tract infection
Congestive heart failure	Feeding difficulties, cardiomegaly, tachycardia, tachypnea, hepatomegaly, failure to thrive abnormal S3
Ventricular septal defect	Age of onset—8 weeks Location and character of murmur
Large size of VSD	• Pulmonary arterial hypertension • S3 and mid-diastolic murmur

Model Case Scenario 2: Cyanotic CHD—Right to Left Shunt

Cyanotic CHD—Decreased Pulmonary Blood Flow (Tetralogy of Fallot)

Chief complaints: A 1-year-old boy was brought to pediatric emergency room with following complaints:

1. Bluishness of the body since 3 months of age
2. Periodic episodes of exaggerated intensity of bluishness since 3 months of age
3. Not moving right upper and lower limb for 2 days

History of Present Illness

The child was born at term gestation with birth weight of 2.8 kg. There were no significant antenatal, natal or immediate postnatal problems. Child was exclusively breastfed and was thriving well till 3 months of age when the mother noticed bluishness of the body which has persisted till now, more so on lips, tongue, finger, nails, and toes. From 3 months of life, the child also started having periodic episodes of increased intensity of bluishness, brought about by crying, straining while passing stools, needing periodic hospitalizations. These episodes used to be treated by administration of intravenous fluids, drugs, and oxygen, and the condition improved in 4–5 days each time. In between the episodes, the child otherwise remained well, except that he was not gaining weight adequately. The child was reported to prefer to lie in prone position.

There was no history of episodes of fever, cough, swelling of feet, or puffiness of eyelids. There was no history of suck-rest-suck cycles and/or sweating while feeding. Parents were told of the child's heart condition and were advised to go to a tertiary care center for investigations and surgical correction. They could not do so because of economic status.

Two days ago, parents noticed sudden onset of weakness of the right upper and lower limb. There is no history of seizures, altered sensorium, facial asymmetry, drooling of saliva, or inability to close the eye. Two days prior to the onset of weakness of right arm and leg, he had mild fever, running nose, mild cough and occasional vomiting. There is no history of ear discharge.

During this febrile period, child was fussy, irritable, and crying incessantly. During such intense crying spells, parents noticed child turning intensely blue in the face, lips and limbs.

Clinical examination

General physical examination

- Central cyanosis and clubbing of fingers and toes, no abnormal facies or external malformations.

- Sensorium was normal, feeding actively and moving the left upper limb and lower limb but not the right upper and lower limb.
- *Vitals:* RR—36/minute, HR—86/min; all peripheral pulses were felt, CFT—normal; peripheries were warm to touch; BP—80/60 mmHg; SpO_2—70% on room air.
- No puffiness of face, eyelids or pedal edema.

Cardiovascular examination

- ***Inspection:*** Chest was symmetrical and precordium was unremarkable. Apical impulse was not visible. Few pulsations were visible in the left lower fourth and fifth parasternal region.
- ***Palpation:*** There was grade 1 parasternal heave. Apical impulse was diffusely felt in left 3rd and 4th intercostal space medial to midclavicular line. Epigastric pulsations were felt.
- ***Auscultation:*** S1 was normal. S2 was single. There was grade 3/6 ejection systolic murmur in the pulmonary area. No other murmurs were heard. No continuous murmur at back.

Neurological examination

- Sensorium, interaction with parents, and cranial nerve examination (except mild ipsilateral upper motor neuron type facial nerve weakness) were normal. Optic fundi: normal.
- ***Motor system:*** Right upper and lower limbs were flaccid with power grade 2/5 in the upper limb muscle groups and 3/5 in the lower limb muscle groups. DTR were exaggerated on the right side. There was ill sustained ankle clonus in the right ankle joint. Right abdominal reflexes were absent. Right plantar was extensor while left was flexor in response.

Abdomen and lungs: Other systems were normal.

Clinical diagnosis

Congenital cyanotic heart disease: Right to left shunt lesion *with* decreased pulmonary blood flow—tetralogy of Fallot or Fallot's variant (double outlet right ventricle with VSD with PS, or single ventricle with VSD with PS, or transposition of great arteries with VSD with PS, or tricuspid atresia with VSD with PS) *with* acute stroke presenting *with* right sided hemiplegia.

Points favoring diagnosis	
Heart disease	Presence of cyanosis, clubbing, and grade 3 systolic murmur
Cyanotic nature Decreased pulmonary blood flow	Central cyanosis • Cyanotic spells • Squatting episodes (preference for prone positioning) • No history of recurrent chest infections • Absence of CHF (No feeding difficulties, No tachypnea, No hepatomegaly, No cardiomegaly)
Tetralogy of Fallot OR Fallot physiology	• Most common cyanotic heart disease with decreased pulmonary blood flow • CVS findings suggestive of right ventricular hypertrophy and pulmonary stenosis
Acute stroke	• Sudden onset right hemiparesis • Caused by thrombus formation because of hyper viscosity/polycythemia secondary to hypoxia caused by pulmonary stenosis and pulmonary oligemia • Brain abscess due to infected embolus from endocarditis unlikely a cause of hemiparesis because of a relatively stable child with no significant features of raised ICT or high fever

17.6 CHILD WITH SEIZURES

A. Definition

A seizure is a transient occurrence of signs and/or symptoms resulting from abnormal excessive or synchronous neuronal activity in the brain. It is defined as a paroxysmal involuntary disturbance of brain function that may manifest as an impairment or loss of consciousness, abnormal motor activity, behavioral abnormality, sensory disturbances, or autonomic dysfunction.

Seizures can be provoked or unprovoked. Provoked seizures occur following—fever;

electrolyte imbalance; structural, inflammatory or metabolic disorders of brain; infections such as meningitis, encephalitis; or stroke. It is essential to recognize that provoked seizures often improve with treatment of underlying etiology and they do not require long-term antiepileptic drugs.

Epilepsy is defined as 2 or more unprovoked seizures occurring more than 24 hours apart. This definition excludes single cluster occurring within 24 hours, single episode of status epilepticus, febrile seizures, neonatal seizures, and acute symptomatic/provoked seizures.

B. Common Causes

Causes of seizures can be categorized as per the age of the child. Common causes at various ages and their clinical presentations are described below. Ask the age of the child and history of provocative factors, frequency of seizures, events before, during and after seizure, semiology of seizure. Ask for birth and neonatal details (history of asphyxia, seizures) and attainment of milestones to ascertain whether the development is normal or delayed. Elicit family history of epilepsy and febrile seizures. These details can help in getting a clue to the underlying etiology as shown in **Table 17.19**.

C. History of Seizure Episode (emphasize on video recording of event, if available)

It is important to get a detailed account of the event or spell from a witness in order to get the answer of three most important questions:

1. Is it a seizure? (could it be a "non-epileptic paroxysmal event")
2. What is the type of seizure?
3. What is the etiology of seizure?

Preictal Phase (Aura)

- History of preictal events like abdominal discomfort, fear or any other unpleasant sensations before the spell.
- Presence of aura is often only described by older children.
- Presence of aura is indicative of focal seizure.

Ictal Phase

Classify into motor manifestation(tonic, clonic, tonic-clonic, myoclonic), sensory manifestation, autonomic features (urinary or fecal incontinence), etc.

- Ask for history of impairment of consciousness, repetitive behavior
- Record duration of each episode, number of episodes, and frequency of such episodes

Post-ictal Phase

History of duration of post-ictal phase, transient paralysis (Todd palsy), headache, vomiting, persistent neurological deficit (for more than 48 hours).

A description of a few common types of seizures is given in **Key Box 1**.

D. Clinical Scenarios

I. Newborn with Seizure

Case scenario 1: Presence of subtle or mutifocal clonic seizure within 24 hours of life with or without encephalopathy in background of delayed cry, prolonged labor, or meconium stained liquor, or maternal risk factors (maternal hypertension, diabetes) at birth points to perinatal asphyxia as a possible cause.

Think of hypoxic ischemic encephalopathy.

Case scenario 2: Clonic seizures in a jittery newborn who is accepting feeds well with no evidence of encephalopathy often points to metabolic cause especially in background of prematurity, maternal diabetes, or perinatal asphyxia.

Think of hypocalcemia or hypoglycemia.

Case scenario 3: Multifocal clonic seizures in a preterm newborn suggests intracranial bleed (preterm infants are prone to intraventricular bleed, especially when anterior fontanelle is tense and bulging) or neurological dysfunction.

Think of intraventricular hemorrhage, or major brain damage.

Case scenario 4: Seizures in a lethargic, sick, febrile, or hypothermic newborn indicates CNS infection. There may be a history of prolonged leaking per vaginum or maternal chorioamnionitis.

Think of sepsis with meningitis and/or dyselectrolytemia.

Case scenario 5: Presence of multifocal or myoclonic seizure in a newborn with encephalopathy, hypertonia, and tense bulging

Table 17.19: Approach to diagnosis of a child with seizure

Age; presence of provocative factors; and significant birth, developmental, and family history	What to think first?
Neonatal period (birth to 28 days)	
History of prolonged labor, meconium-stained liquor, perinatal asphyxia, delayed cry, prolonged ventilation, instrumental delivery	Birth asphyxia, hypoxic–ischemic injury, intracranial bleed
History of prematurity, maternal diabetes, birth asphyxia	Metabolic disorders like hypocalcemia, hypoglycemia
History of pathological jaundice	Bilirubin encephalopathy (Kernicterus)
History of consanguinity, pregnancy loss, repeated abortions, abnormal odor of urine, unexplained lethargy, worsening following initiation of feeds	Inherited disorders of metabolism like urea cycle disorders, aminoacidurias, organic acidurias
Small head or abnormal looking facial features, other congenital anomalies	CNS malformations
History of excessive lethargy, fever, refusal to feed, fast breathing, poor feeding	Sepsis, meningitis
1 month–1 year	
Cow's milk intake with high phosphate load, delayed initiation of complementary feeding, poor sunlight exposure, history of liver disease, renal disease, facial dysmorphism	Hypocalcemic seizures
History of developmental arrest or regression with onset of epileptic spasms	West syndrome
6 months to 5 years	
History of high grade fever with preceding viral prodrome in a developmentally normal child	Febrile seizure
More than 5 years	
Unprovoked focal seizure in developmentally normal child	Focal lesions like neurocysticercosis, tuberculoma
Contact with patient of tuberculosis	Tuberculoma
All ages	
History of fever, headache, neck rigidity	Meningitis, systemic sepsis
History of head trauma, drug ingestion	Trauma-induced seizure, toxic brain
History of repeated vomiting, severe headache, deviation of eyes (6th CN palsy) [older children], persistent irritability, vomiting and head banging [infants] (features of raised intracranial pressure)	Intracranial tumor or focal lesions with perilesional edema like large tuberculoma or brain abscess
History of cognitive regression with history of myoclonic seizures	Progressive myoclonic epilepsy seen among children with neurodegenerative disease (gray matter disease) like sub-acute sclerosing panencephalitis (SSPE)
History of delayed attainment of milestones	Child with global developmental delay like cerebral palsy
History of sudden onset of weakness of one-half of body or face in the background of history of bleeding diathesis, congenital heart disease can make us think in terms of vascular insult (stroke)	Stroke
Family history of seizure, febrile seizure, epilepsy, neuro-cutaneous syndromes	Febrile seizures, tuberous sclerosis, Sturge-Weber syndrome, neurofibromatosis

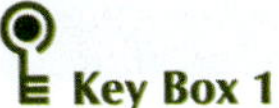

Key Box 1

Description of Various Types of Seizures

Subtle	Comprise 50% of neonatal seizures and include eye phenomenon like sustained eye opening with apparent visual fixation or orobuccolingual movements like chewing, sucking or lip smacking or alternating limb movements like pedaling, boxing, rowing or swimming movements or autonomic phenomenon like sudden change in skin color associated with tachycardia. Typically observed in newborns with birth asphyxia and HIE
Tonic	Continuous stiffening of extremities
Clonic	Rhythmic alternating contraction and relaxation of muscles. Usually caused by metabolic derangements (hypoglycemia, hypocalcemia)
Tonic clonic	Seizure activity starting with tonic stiffening followed by clonic phase of rhythmic jerks
Absence	Brief staring spells (3–30 seconds) accompanied by a cessation of activity, classically precipitated by hyperventilation
Myoclonic	Brief body jerks (electric shock like) often occurring in irregular flurries. Typical of progressive myoclonic epilepsy and Juvenile myoclonic epilepsy
Epileptic spasm	Sudden flexion or extension of body (salaam attack) associated with cry occurring in clusters and more on awakening from the sleep are characteristics of epileptic spasm in West syndrome

Focal seizures: Arise focally in one hemisphere, limited to one part or one side of body and may lead to impairment of consciousness. It may start with aura (e.g. abdominal rising pain) followed by motor manifestations (like clonic jerks involving one-half of face and/or body) or automatism (lip smacking, fumbling of hands) or version of eyes or head (forced twisting or turning, eye deviation or eye fluttering). Most commonly observed in stroke, ring enhancing lesions (neurocysticercosis, tuberculoma), and intracranial tumors.

anterior fontanel points to possibility of intracranial bleed.

Think of vitamin K deficiency.

Case scenario 6: Focal clonic seizures in a newborn associated with hemiparesis and/or apnea suggests a vascular cause. There may be a history of trauma, coagulation disorders, congenital heart disease, maternal diabetes, cocaine exposure; placental abruption, chorioamnionitis; polycythemia, or DIC.

Think of neonatal stroke.

II. Seizure Beyond Neonatal Period

Some typical case scenarios of children presenting with seizures are described in **Table 17.20**, along with their most probable diagnosis.

17.7 CHILD WITH HEMIPLEGIA

A. Definition and Etiology

The term Hemiplegia means paralysis of the one side of body (including both upper and lower limb on the same side) with or without facial involvement. Hemiparesis refers to weakness of one side of the body that may not amount to a complete paralysis. In a typical hemiparesis upper limb is involved more than the lower limb. Common causes are listed in **Key Box 2**.

B. Chief Complaints

A 5-year-old boy was brought with following complaints:

1. Sudden weakness of right half of body with deviation of mouth to left side × 3 days
2. Inability to speak × 3 days

C. History of Present Illness

Child was apparently well three days back. He was sitting in room and was asked to go out and play. When he stood up, he fell on the ground. The child could not move the right leg or hand. He was also unable to stand. He could sit with some support but more or less, he was bed ridden. The child was unable to hold things in his right hand noticed in the form of clumsiness in holding the objects offered to him. He could not raise the right arm above the shoulder while attempting to

Table 17.20: Typical case scenarios of various conditions presenting with seizures

Case description	What to think of?
Seizures in a febrile, developmentally normal child aged 6 months–5 years in absence of encephalopathy and no signs/symptoms of meningeal irritation. Past history of similar episodes may be present. Family history of febrile seizures/epilepsy may be present.	Febrile seizure
Seizures with fever, headache, vomiting, altered sensorium, loose motions, rash, neurological deficit, and/or features of raised ICT	CNS infection (Meningitis, encephalitis, brain abscess, cerebral malaria), enteric encephalopathy, *Shigella* encephalopathy, Reye syndrome, etc.
Multiple episodes of focal clonic seizures with normal interictal period in an afebrile infant, otherwise neurologically and developmentally normal, predominantly fed on cow milk	Hypocalcemic seizure
Generalized/focal seizures in a previously well, afebrile child without any specific provocating factor, in an older child	Epilepsy secondary to ring enhancing lesions like neurocysticercosis or tuberculoma
Generalized/focal seizures with altered sensorium, in a previously well, afebrile child	Drug intake, toxin ingestion, trauma, poisoning
Focal seizure with headache, vomiting, features of raised intracranial tension, personality changes, cranial nerve involvement	Brain tumor
History of multiple episodes of epileptic spasms with developmental regression or arrest especially when there is history of perinatal insult	West syndrome
Seizures with global developmental delay with tone abnormalities; there may be history of prematurity, perinatal asphyxia, intracranial hemorrhage, neonatal hypoglycemia, neonatal hyperbilirubinemia. May be associated with a small head	Cerebral palsy with seizure disorder; may be associated with microcephaly

change his clothes. While lying in the bed, he could not move his legs and was unable to lift his leg above the couch or move his right feet on command. His movements on left side of body were normal. He could turn on bed from left to right side but not the reverse. He could lift head off the bed. According to mother, the weakness appeared equal in both the upper and lower limbs. Weakness was maximum at the onset, over next 3 days, there has been gradual improvement in weakness and now on day 3 of illness, he could flicker his fingers and could lift the right upper and lower limb minimally (*describes the onset, progression and duration of illness*); also *indicates the recovering nature of illness, typical of a vascular etiology, i.e. stroke.*

Simultaneously, parents noticed deviation of angle of mouth towards left side. There was no drooling of saliva. Child was keeping the eyes shut during sleep (*indicates that only lower part of right face was involved, probably due to a upper motor neuron facial palsy*).

On day 1 of illness, the child was not able to speak anything, though he understands and obeys instructions by non-verbal gestures like nodding his head or indicating using his left hand. The child has been fully conscious and recognizing the mother for these three days of illness.

- There is *no history of* loss of vision, double vision, deviation of eyeball, drooping of eyelids, numbness of face, difficulty in chewing, impaired hearing, nasal regurgitation of fluids, neck flop, choking or gagging, or deviation of tongue (*no features suggestive of other cranial nerve involvement*).

Key Box 2

Causes of Hemiplegia in Children

A. Arterial Ischemic stroke

- *Cardiac:* Congenital heart disease, endocarditis, Kawasaki disease, arrhythmias, cardiomyopathy
- *Hematological:* Iron deficiency anemia, hemoglobinopathies especially sickle cell anemia, leukemia, lymphoma, procoagulant states
- *Inflammatory:* CNS infections and vasculitides following varicella, bacterial meningitis, tuberculosis
- *Metabolic:* Homocysteinemia, Fabry disease, mitochondrial disease, organic acidemias, urea cycle defects
- *Vasculopathies:* Moyamoya disease, transient arteriopathy, arterial dissections, and fibromuscular dysplasia
- *Miscellaneous:* Trauma, child abuse

B. Cerebral venous thrombotic stroke

- *Infections:* Bacterial, fungal, viral, syphilis, leptospira
- *Collagen vascular disease:* SLE, rheumatoid arthritis, scleroderma
- *Necrotizing vasculitis:* Polyarteritis nodosa, Wegener granulomatosis
- *Systemic diseases:* Ulcerative colitis
- *Miscellaneous:* Drugs, malignancy, irradiation

C. Hemorrhagic stroke

- *Vascular anomalies:* Arteriovenous malformations, venous angiomas, cavernous malformation, aneurysm, drugs
- *Vasculopathies:* Ehlers-Danlos syndrome, pseudoxanthoma elasticum, Moyamoya disease
- *Intravascular:* Hemophilia, ITP, vitamin K deficiency bleeding disorder, hypertension, vasculitides, hemolytic uremic syndrome, acute liver failure
- *Trauma:* Middle meningeal artery injury, subarachnoid hemorrhage, hemorrhagic contusion, iatrogenic

- There is *no history of* loss of consciousness, seizure or abnormal movements, vomiting, headache, stiffness of neck, excessive crying, irregular or fast respiration (*no features suggestive of encephalitis, meningitis, raised intracranial pressure*).
- There is *no history of* tightness of limbs although mother feels right upper and lower limb are floppy and soft when compared to left side (*to look for evolution of spasticity*).
- There is *no history of* abnormal twisting posture, flowing abnormal movement, distal writhing movement (*to look for extrapyramidal involvement*)
- There is *no history of* loss of perception of touch, hot or cold fluids, or painful stimulus on left half of body (*no features suggestive of sensory involvement*).
- There is *no history of* bladder and bowel involvement or urinary or fecal incontinence or retention (*no features of autonomic spinal involvement*).
- There is *no history of* trauma to head or neck, no history to suggest intraoral trauma (*to rule out traumatic dissection of internal carotid artery*)
- There is *no history of* fluid filled skin lesions over the body (*varicella*) in the recent past
- There is *no history of* preceding fever, vaccination, cough, respiratory distress, ear discharge, vomiting, loose motions, burning micturition, rash, or a chronic discharging sinus (*for any post-infectious demyelination*)
- There is *no history of* fever, ear discharge (*no history suggestive of chronic suppurative otitis media leading to brain abscess*)
- There is *no history of* perception of heartbeat or breath sounds, bluish discoloration of tongue or lips, mouth, or nails on crying, increased sweating, or easy fatigability (*for any underlying cardiovascular lesion*).
- There is *no history of* pain in abdomen, pallor, jaundice, pain in feet or hands, rash, bone pains, swelling in body, or blood

transfusion (*no feature suggestive of hemolytic anemia, and sickle cell anemia as underlying cause*).

- There is *no history of* photosensitivity, joint pains, abnormality in gait, episodes of vomiting, confusion (*for vasculitis secondary to SLE or other collagen disorder*).
- There is *no history of* abnormal urinary or body odor, whitish opacity in eyes, yellow/black deposits in eyes, elbow, or back, hypo- or hyperpigmented or erythematous lesion, spinal deformity, or increased mobility of joints (*no feature suggestive of metabolic causes as underlying causes*).
- There is *no history of* previous similar episode (*recurrence is typical of certain lesions*).
- There is *no family history of* mental subnormality, seizures, cardiac defects, hearing or vision abnormality, bleeding disorder, malignancy, anemia, premature death, or storage disorder.

Summary of the history: A 5-year-old, developmentally normal boy presented with sudden and non-progressive weakness of right half of the body, 7th cranial nerve involvement on the same side and aphasia of three-day duration, with relatively preserved sensorium, no features of raised intracranial pressure, with no other cranial nerve involvement, without autonomic or bowel and bladder involvement. Child has shown significant improvement over last 2 days after its onset.

D. Physical Examination Findings

- Lying comfortably in bed with intravenous cannula in left arm
- Spontaneous eye opening with meaningful contact present
- Crying on painful stimulus.
- Moving left side of body but right upper and lower limbs lying limp, extended and externally rotated with minimal movements

Vitals

Temp 98°F, all peripheral pulses palpable, HR—100/min, RR—20/min, BP—100/80 mmHg.

General Examination

- No pallor, cyanosis, clubbing, icterus, lymphadenopathy, petechiae, pedal edema, or raised JVP
- No abnormal hyper or hypopigmented lesions, port wine stain, xanthomas, or other neurocutaneous markers
- No signs of vitamin deficiencies
- Skin, mouth, throat are normal
- Musculoskeletal system, spine, and genitalia are normal

CNS Examination

Higher functions: The child is alert, conscious with spontaneous eye opening. He is obeying motor command on left side, with intact nonverbal gestural communication. Other parts of higher mental functions including orientation, memory, attention span, perception, insight, calculation and individual lobe function assessment could not be tested owing to limited verbal output.

Speech: Verbal output markedly decreased although comprehension, naming and writing is preserved. Fluency, articulation, reading and articulation could not be assessed owing to paucity of verbal output.

Cranial nerves

- 1st—not tested
- 2nd—visual acuity: Able to read his comics, pupillary reflex present, color vision and field of vision could not be tested owing to lack of cooperation. Fundus was normal.
- 3rd/4th/6th—normal extraocular movements, no squint, no ptosis.
- 5th—muscles of mastication are intact, sensory function is normal, jaw jerk and corneal reflexes normally present.
- 7th—right side upper motor neuron type of facial palsy.
- 8th—responds to sound normally, no nystagmus.
- 9th, 10th, 11th—uvula is central, palato-pharyngeal reflex is intact, no regurgitation, nasal twang, or nasal cry.
- 12th—no deviation of tongue on protruding it.

Motor system

- ***Posture:*** Child is bedridden lying supine with paucity of movement of right upper and lower limbs. Right lower limb is lying flail, externally rotated, extended with lateral border of foot touching bed suggestive of right-sided hemiparesis
- ***Bulk:*** Bilateral symmetrical
- ***Tone:*** Rt side N to ↑
- ***Power:*** Decreased in RUL (1/5) and RLL (3/5) as compared to 5/5 on left side
- ***Deep tendon reflexes:*** Normal on left side; Brisk on right side, both in upper and lower limbs.
- ***Ankle clonus:*** Present on right side
- ***Superficial reflexes:*** Abdominal and cremasteric reflex absent, plantar extensor response on right side (positive Babinski sign)
- ***Sensory evaluation:*** Normal pain and touch sensations
- No meningeal signs, no cerebellar signs
- ***Spine:*** Normal

Systemic examination: Chest, CVS, abdomen—normal

E. Interpretation of History and Examination

Site of Lesion

The boy has acute onset right-sided hemiparesis with right-sided UMN facial nerve palsy. This presentation can be caused by a left-sided lesion in cortex, corona radiata, internal capsule or brainstem. Consider **Table 17.21** and **Fig 17.1**, while making the anatomical diagnosis. Presence of aphasia in this child points towards cortical lesion; however, for a cortical lesion to cause paresis of entire right side, the lesion has to be a large one.

Why this is unlikely to be a lesion of internal capsule? Can there be aphasia in internal capsule lesion?

Internal capsule has corticospinal, corticobulbar and sensory fibres all densely packed. Aphasia is purely cortical in origin and does not have representation in fibers in internal capsule. Presence of aphasia always points to cortical lesion. By and large, aphasia is uncommon in pediatrics and occurs only in extensive lesions. Dysarthria (both spastic and extrapyramidal) are rather more common in children.

Table 17.21: Making an anatomical diagnosis in a child with hemiplegia

Site of lesion	Effect of lesion	
	Same side	*Opposite side*
Cortex	Normal	Monoparesis (common), hemiparesis (uncommon), aphasia, cortical signs and convulsions
	Motor aphasia, sensory aphasia (if dominant lobe involved)	
Corona radiata	Normal	Unequal hemiparesis, 7th cranial nerve UMN palsy
Internal capsule	Normal	Uniform hemiplegia, 7th cranial nerve UMN palsy, hemianesthesia
Midbrain*	Paralysis of 3rd (suggested by ptosis) and 4th cranial nerves	Hemiparesis, 7th cranial nerve UMN palsy
Pons**	LMN involvement of 6th, 7th cranial nerves	Hemiparesis
Medulla (bulbar)	Involvement of 9,10,11 cranial nerves, dysphagia, dysarthria, nasal regurgitation	Hemiparesis
Spinal cord	Hemiparesis + bladder/bowel involvement	Normal

*Weber syndrome—unilateral 3rd nerve paralysis with contralateral hemiplegia

* *Millard-Gubler syndrome—unilateral, 6th and 7th nerve palsy with contralateral hemiplegia

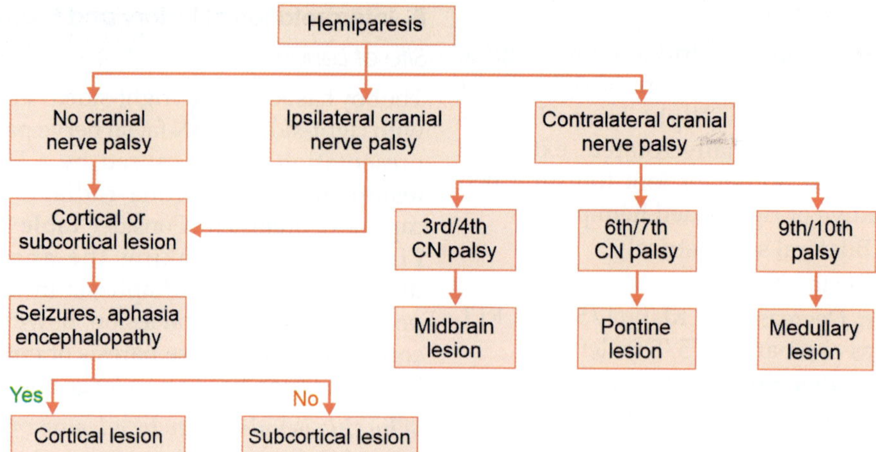

Fig. 17.1: Approach to anatomical diagnosis in acute hemiphlegia.

Pathophysiology of Lesion

Presence of focal neurological deficit of cortical origin which was sudden in onset and non-progressive in nature suggests a **Stroke**. It could be present in both arterial ischemic stroke as well as venous or hemorrhagic stroke. However, absence of encephalopathy and seizure in this case, point towards *arterial ischemic stroke* rather than hemorrhagic stroke or venous stroke. Among the thrombotic and thromboembolic types of arterial ischemic stroke, sudden onset favors thromboembolic over thrombotic cause, but both are possible. It is believed that venous strokes often have more of encephalopathy and seizure as compared to arterial ischemic strokes. Hemorrhagic stroke and thromboembolic stroke often have hyperacute presentation.

Etiology

Since there is no fever, infections are unlikely. Also, cardiac causes are less likely in view of absence of history of cyanosis, cyanotic spells, and a normal CVS examination. Metabolic strokes are unlikely considering prior normal development but still a possibility.

Inflammatory causes are also less likely in absence of any suggestive symptomatology (fever, rash, joint pains, systemic involvement) but still possible. Demyelinating illnesses and intracranial space occupying illnesses are also less likely (no raised intracranial tension, absence of seizures) but still can be considered in the differential diagnoses.

The etiological possibility could be as follows:

1. ***Vasculopathy:*** Transient cerebral arteriopathy, moyamoya disease
2. ***Hematological causes:*** Hypercoagulable stage including deficiency of protein C, protein S, or antithrombin; prothrombin gene mutation
3. ***Metabolic causes:*** Strokes are unlikely considering prior normal development but still a possibility
4. ***Inflammatory cause:*** CNS vasculitis
5. ***Others less likely causes:*** Demyelinating illnesses and intracranial space occupying lesions.

F. Final Diagnosis

Diagnosis: Acute onset right hemiparesis with right upper motor neuron 7th nerve palsy with motor aphasia

Lesion: Cerebral cortex (left side)

Pathophysiology: Thromboembolic phenomenon (stroke), arterial in nature, involving circulation of left distal internal carotid artery or middle cerebral artery

Causes: Vascular, haematological, metabolic, inflammatory, ICSOL.

Chapter 18

Practical Procedures

❍ Piyush Gupta ❍ Nidhi Bedi ❍ Lokesh Guglani

Structure

18.1 INFORMED CONSENT

A. Definitionss

Informed Consent

Informed consent is a communication process that is ethically required before initiation of any treatment or procedure. It is the process of providing the patient or in case of a minor, the custodial parent or legal guardian with relevant information regarding the diagnosis and treatment needs so that an educated decision regarding the intervention can be made by them.

Informed Assent

Informed assent implies child's agreement to medical procedures in circumstances where he or she is not legally authorized or lacks sufficient understanding for giving consent competently. It consists of very basic explanation of the procedure or treatment and ensures child's voluntary participation. The assent empowers the child to the extent of their capacity, involving them in discussions about their health care for a better physician–patient relationship. Assent demonstrates the respect for the child and his developing autonomy. It also reinforces the child's trust with the parents.

B. Essential Elements of Disclosure

The healthcare provider must include all of the following elements about the illness and desired procedure so that parents can provide an informed consent:

- Diagnosis of illness;
- Nature of procedure;
- Purpose of the procedure;
- Methodology of the procedure;
- Discussion of the risks/hazards or benefits involved in the procedure;
- Available alternative means of diagnosis; and
- Prognosis and further course of action, if parents do not consent to the procedure.

C. Who Should Obtain the Consent?

Ideally the healthcare provider performing the desired procedure is in the best position to obtain the informed consent. However, the task may be accomplished by another healthcare provider like a resident working under the guidance of the attending physician. When the care is delivered in a hospital or other institutional setting, one might be held liable for any failure to obtain an informed consent.

D. Who Can Give Consent?

A child below 12 years (minor) cannot give consent, although a child between 12 and 18 years can give consent only for medical examination but not for any procedure. Parents or the legal guardian can consent as legal representative in the best interest of their child. However, in case of emergencies, a local caretaker like school teacher or principal can consent to treatment (loco parentis). Minors can consent to a procedure only if the court has declared them as emancipated, i.e. living away from home, being economically independent, is married/pregnant/parent or is a member of armed forces.

E. Principles for Obtaining Informed Consent

- Respect parental competency and emotional status while obtaining the consent.
- Emergency exceptions to informed consent exist when delay in treatment or obtaining informed consent could be detrimental to patient health.
- The decision of the parents must be fully informed and must be made free of coercion or any undue influence.
- Provision of the information in patient's understandable language and not including too many medical terms.
- Consent form must be comprehensive with short and simple sentences. It should be signed by parents as well as the attending physician with mention of time and date.
- Assessment of parental understanding of the information that has been provided and that their queries have been answered to their satisfaction.
- A note must be made in the patient record regarding the content of disclosure and the persons who witnessed and signed the consent procedure.
- When the consent cannot be obtained in person, it may be obtained by telephone and a copy of consent form be signed by the witness who heard the disclosure and the consent being given.

F. Parental Refusal to Consent

Parental refusal to consent (dissent) may be based on their unique personal, religious and cultural beliefs. This might pose a legal and ethical responsibility of the attending healthcare provider to render competent medical care based on what patient needs, not what someone else expresses. Parental dissent needs to be acknowledged especially when the desired procedure is not essential to the child's welfare or can be deferred without substantial risk. However, parental refusal to consent to life-saving treatment for their children may have to bear the best interest of the child in mind. In case of persistent refusal, a case of medical negligence amounting to child abuse can be conducted in the court of law against the parents.

G. Waiver of Consent

The parents/legal guardians are entitled not to have such information when they would be unduly distressed by it or would simply prefer to let the physician make the necessary treatment decision. Such an attitude of the parents or the guardian is called *waiver of consent*, and it must be documented in the medical records.

18.2 UNIVERSAL PRECAUTION AND ASEPSIS ROUTINES

A. Elements of Universal Precaution

For all procedures and examinations that involve contact with body fluids or have the potential for transmission of disease, a set of precautions called 'Universal precautions' must be strictly followed for the safety of all healthcare providers. We shall discuss these under four sections:

a. Maintain hand hygiene
b. Using adequate personal protective equipment (PPE)
c. Proper disposal of bio-medical wastes
d. Ensuring appropriate management of accidental spillage

B. Maintain Hand Hygiene

Hand hygiene means cleaning your hands by using either handwashing (washing hands with soap and water), antiseptic hand wash, antiseptic hand rub (i.e. alcohol-based hand sanitizer including foam or gel), or surgical hand antisepsis.

Hand washing is the single most important, cost-effective and economic measure of maintaining asepsis and preventing nosocomial infection. Details of the technique are described in Fig. 18.1 and Table 18.1.

Indications for Hand Washing

1. Before and after any direct patient contact and between patients, whether or not gloves are worn.
2. Immediately after gloves are removed.
3. Before handling an invasive device.
4. After touching blood, body fluids, secretions, excretions, non-intact skin, and contaminated items, even if gloves are worn.
5. During patient care, when moving from a contaminated to a clean body site of the patient.
6. After contact with inanimate objects in the immediate vicinity of the patient.

Antiseptic Agent

An antimicrobial substance which reduces or inhibits the growth of microorganisms on living tissues. These agents include alcohols, chlorhexidine gluconate, chlorine derivatives, iodine, chloroxylenol, quaternary ammonium compounds, and triclosan. Of these, the most common ones used in hand hygiene are alcohol and chlorhexidine.

Alcohol: Alcohol-based (hand) rub contains either ethanol, isopropanol or n-propanol, or a combination of two of these products concentrations of which is expressed as percentage of volume, weight or weight/volume. The antimicrobial activity of alcohols results from their ability to denature proteins. Alcohol solution containing 60–80% alcohol is most effective, with higher concentrations being less potent. CDC recommends 60% ethanol and 70% isopropyl alcohol as the active ingredients in alcohol-based hand sanitizers. Sanitisers are not effective when hands are visibly soiled, greased, or contaminated with blood.

Chlorhexidine: This has significant residual activity and is preferred as an addition in low concentration (0.5–1%) to alcohol-based preparations. The antimicrobial activity of chlorhexidine is not much affected by presence of organic material including blood.

When using an alcohol-based sanitizer, put an adequate amount on hands and rub together to cover all surfaces as mentioned in hand washing. Hands should be rubbed till they feel dry, taking around 20 seconds.

C. Personal Protective Equipment (PPE)

Personal protective equipment (PPE) is used to protect health care workers from getting infected and also to prevent the spread of cross-infection other patients. The type of

Table 18.1: Hand washing routine

Action	Rationale
1. A minimum of two minutes of hand washing to be done after removing watches, bangles, rings, etc. and rolling up sleeves above elbows.	• To ensure removal of any pathogens carried from other sources. • These articles may harbor potentially infective organisms.
2. Using water and soap, **six important areas** are to be scrubbed in the following order: Palms, fingers and web-spaces, back of hands, fingers and knuckles, thumbs, fingertips, wrist and forearm up to elbow.	• To ensure that no areas are missed in hand washing and a uniform procedure is followed every time.
3. About 15 seconds of hand washing to be done before and after touching every baby in the Nursery.	• To avoid cross-contamination and prevent the spread of nosocomial infections.
4. Never keep long/polished nails.	• Potential sources of infection as they could harbor dirt and pathogens.

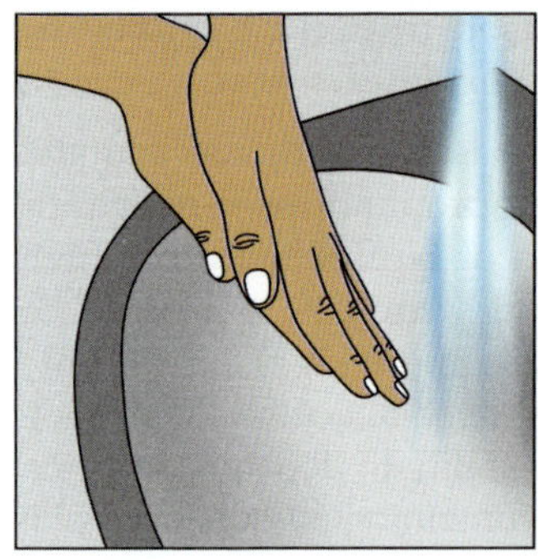

Step 1
Rub palm to palm 5 times

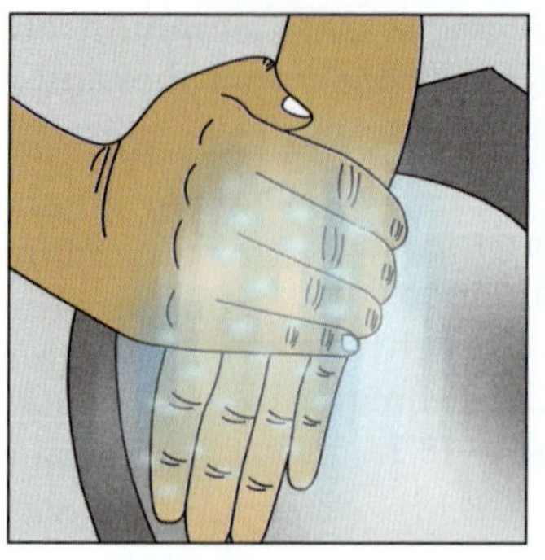

Step 2
Rub right palm over the back of the left hand up to wrist 5 times. Do the same with the other hand.

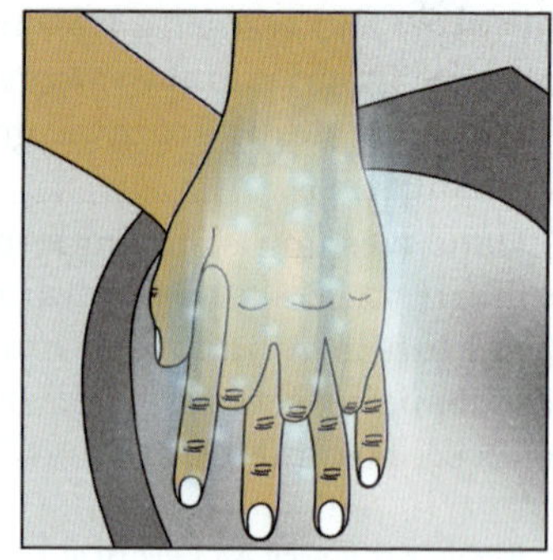

Step 3
With right hand over back of left hand, rub fingers 5 times. Do same with other hand.

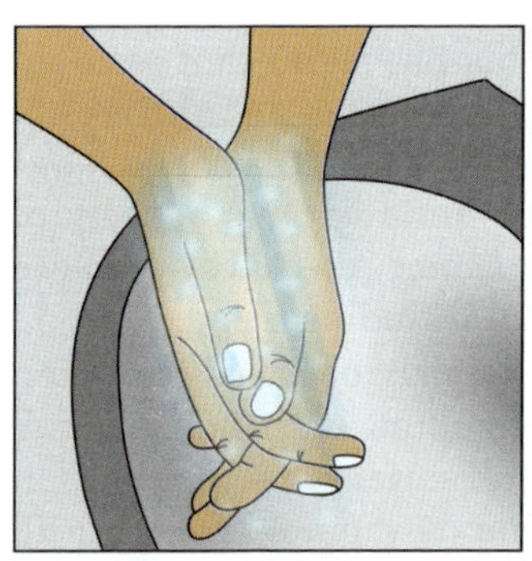

Step 4
Rub palm to palm with the fingers interfaced.

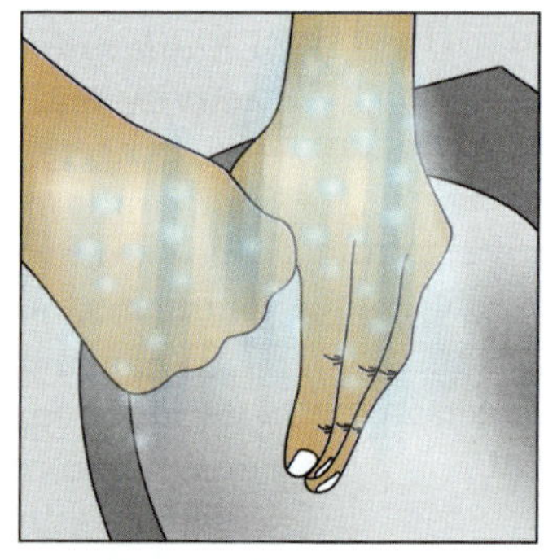

Step 5
Wash thumbs of each hand separately using a rotatory movement.

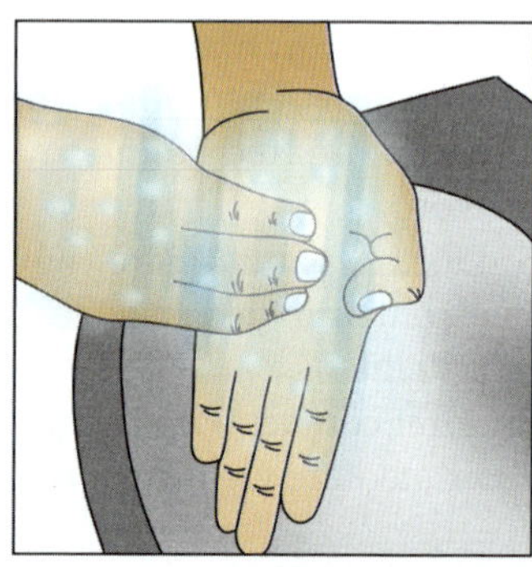

Step 6
Rub the tips of the fingers against the opposite palm using a circular motion. Also ensure nail beds are washed.

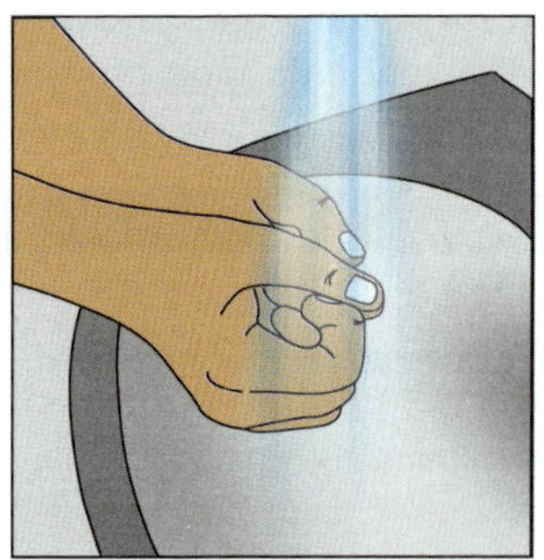

Step 7
Rinse hands thoroughly under water to remove all traces of soap.

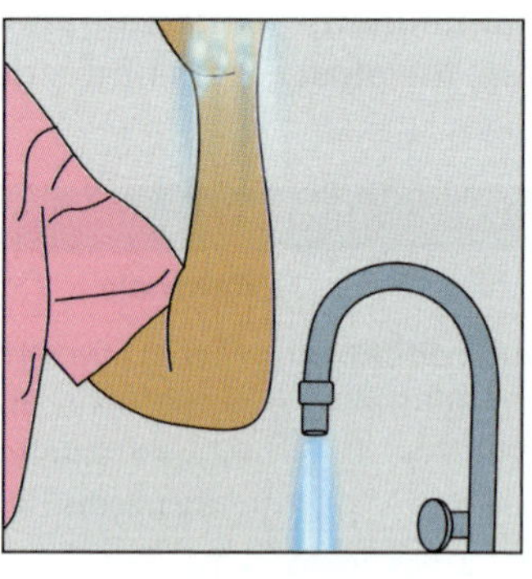

Step 8
Turn off taps using elbows.

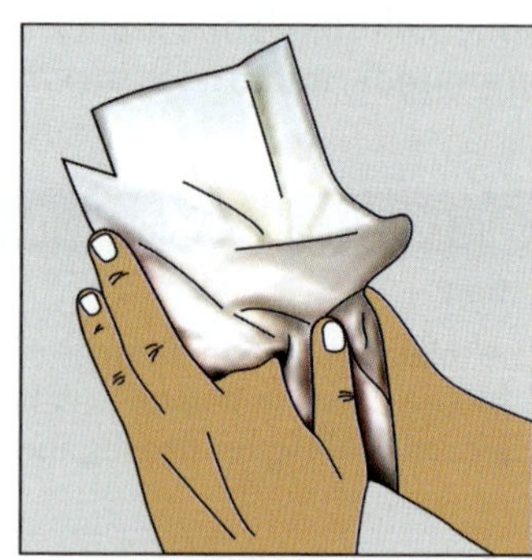

Step 9
Dry hands completely using a disposable towel.

Fig. 18.1 Steps of hand washing.

PPE used depends on the mechanism of transmission of the disease and the type of exposure in the procedure being conducted.

- A disease which is spread by contact alone like viral diarrhea or viral hepatitis requires fluid proof gown and gloves only.

- Conditions like COVID-19 may need complete PPE including face shield, gown, eye cover, gloves, and shoe covers. In terms of procedure, a person handling a multi-drug resistant patient on ventilator may need complete PPE.
- A healthcare worker managing a blood sample only may suffice with gloves, gown, and shoes cover.

One should also ensure that the PPE are well fitted. Loose or tight fitting may lead to unwanted manipulation and spread of contamination. Components of PPE are discussed below.

Face Shield and Goggles

Face shield should cover forehead, extend below chin and wrap around side of face. It protects the contamination of mucous membrane of face, nose, mouth, and eyes by droplets, during aerosol generating procedures and touching of contaminated hand. The goggles should provide good seal with the skin of the face, adequately cover the eyes, and accommodate refractive errors, if any. Optical glasses are not a replacement for the goggles.

Masks

Masks protect the respiratory tract from the infections spread from droplets and aerosols or from contaminated hands. The two most common type of masks recommended for medical personnel are (a) triple layer medical mask; and (b) N-95 respirator mask.

Triple layer medical mask: This is a three-layered disposable mask with two outer layers (one white and one colored) and a middle layer which acts as filter. The filter is resistant to fluids, thereby protecting from aerosols generated while coughing, sneezing, or talking. The colored side should face outwards while wearing a mask.

N-95 respirator mask: These are duckbill shaped or non-collapsible cup-shaped with a high filtration efficiency to airborne particles. They are designed to provide close seal around the face. The masks are fluid resistant and have good breathability (preferably with an expiratory valve). If correctly worn, the filtration capacity of these masks exceeds those of triple layer medical masks.

Masks should never be touched from the outer aspect during the procedure or while removing, to minimize contact with infected surface.

Gloves

Gloves should be worn to prevent infection to be transmitted to patients and the health personnel. While performing any sterile procedure sterile disposable gloves should be used to maintain asepsis, whereas clean disposable gloves can be used if handling infected patients or objects/surface potentially contaminated by them. Nitrile gloves resist chemicals and hence are preferred over latex gloves which have high rate of latex allergy. Nonpowdered gloves are preferred to powdered gloves. Gloves are not a substitute for hand hygiene. Gloves should be changed if they get damaged, visibly soiled, or when changing over to next patient. Gloves should be removed in glove-in-glove pattern and discarded in right place to avoid contamination.

Coverall/Gowns

Coverall/gowns reduce the contact and droplet exposure by forming a barrier between the patient and health personnel. They are designed to cover the whole body, back, legs and if required head and feet. They are provided with tapes or threads which are easy to open with minimum touch.

Shoe Covers and Head Covers

Shoe covers are made of impermeable material to prevent any seepage of spills or contaminated fluids. Head covers are often used with gowns not having head covers. All hair and extensions are ensured to be fit inside the head cover.

Putting on (Donning) and Taking-off (Doffing) of PPE

Donning of PPE

Follow a fixed sequence for donning of PPE to get the best protection. The gown should be donned first, followed by mask or respirator. Ensure that the mask or respirator is well fitted. The next to don are goggles and face shield. Gloves should be worn at the end **(Table 18.2) (Fig. 18.2)**.

Table 18.2: Sequence of donning (putting on) personal protective equipment (PPE)

Action	Rationale
Wash hands or perform hand hygiene	To remove contamination from hands before putting on PPE
Put on a gown and tie it at the back of neck and waist area.	To reduce the chances on contamination of personal clothing with pathogens
Put on an appropriate mask	To prevent the inhalation of pathogens from the patient during the patient encounter
Wear safety goggles and/or face shield • For airborne-droplet precautions • Where splashing of body fluids • Aerosol generating procedure	To prevent the aerosol/droplets/secretions into eyes or mucous membranes of mouth/nose of healthcare worker.
Wear gloves • Choose correct size and type • Cover gown cuffs with gloves	To prevent the contamination of healthcare workers' hands after coming into contact with patient
Additional precautions • Keep hands away from your face • Limit the touching of surfaces inside the patient room • Change gloves if torn/visibly soiled • Avoid touching or adjusting PPE	

Source: Centers for Disease Control and Prevention (CDC), USA

18

Doffing of PPE

It is important to understand what is considered *clean* and *contaminated* in a worn PPE. Outside of gloves are the most contaminated. Irrespective of visible soiling whether present or not, the outside front and sleeves of the isolation gown, outside front of the goggles, mask, respirator and face shield are all considered contaminated. Rest of the areas which are inside and back of the gown, ties, elastic of the mask, inside of the goggles and face shield are relatively clean and should be touched while doffing of PPE. If the contaminated part gets accidently touched anytime during doffing, immediate hand hygiene should be followed.

The first to remove in PPE are the gloves, next is goggles and face shield, followed by gown, and lastly the mask or respirator. Mask or respirator should be removed outside the patient room once the door is closed. The last step of doffing is the same as first step of donning, i.e. hand washing (**Table 18.3** and **Fig. 18.3**). An alternate technique is shown in **Fig. 18.4**. Each part of PPE should be discarded immediately into the correct waste bin before proceeding for next step of removal of PPE.

D. Disposal of Biomedical Wastes

Waste disposal should be done in appropriate bags or bins as per standard guidelines.

Yellow bins: These are nonchlorinated yellow plastic bags which undergo incineration, plasma pyrolysis, or deep burial. The wastes to be included in this bin are human anatomical waste, animal anatomical waste, soiled waste, expired or discarded medicines and cytotoxic drugs along with glass or plastic ampoules and vials, chemical waste, micro, clinical laboratory waste, discarded linen, mattresses, beddings contaminated with blood or body fluids, and routine mask and gown.

Red bins: These are nonchlorinated plastic bags which undergo autoclaving, microwaving, or hydroclaving and then sent for recycling. The wastes included in this category are recyclable contaminated waste vacutainers, tubing, bottles, intravenous tubes and sets, catheters, urine bags, syringes (without needles), and gloves.

Black bins: These are nonchlorinated plastic bags or containers for discarding general wastes.

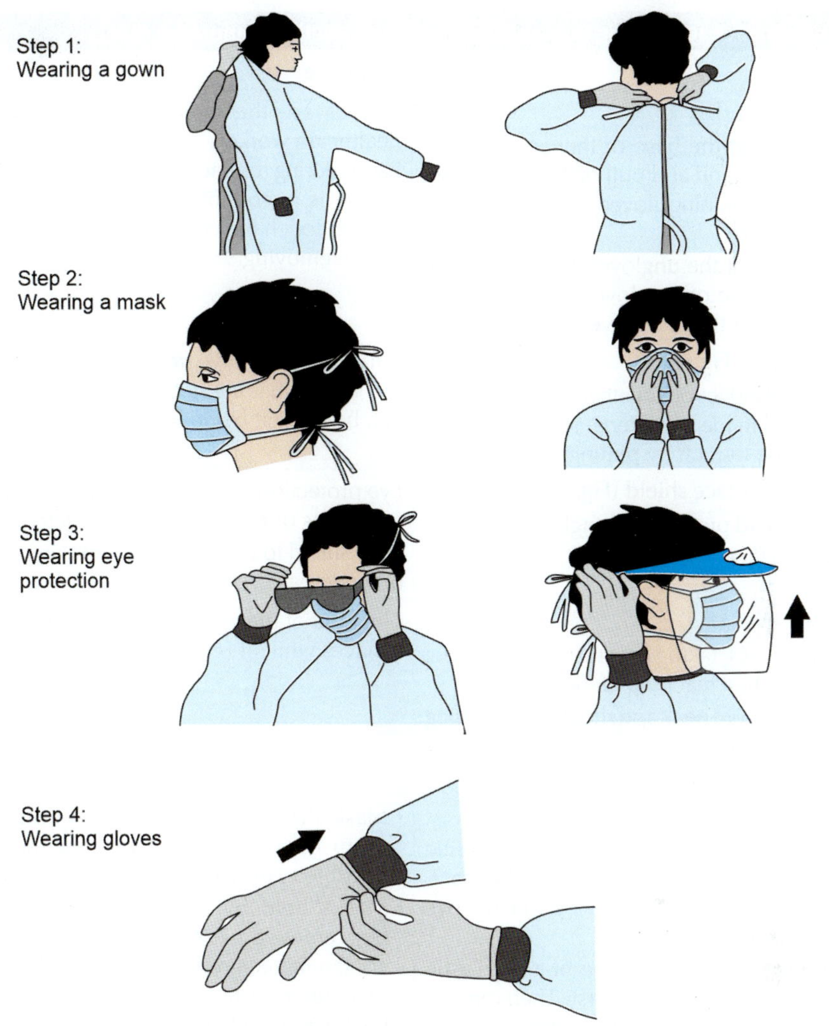

Fig. 18.2: Steps involved in putting on (donning) personal protective equipment (PPE) after perfoming hand washing. *Source:* CDC. Available at https://www.cdc.gov/hai/pdfs/ppe/ppe-sequence.pdf

White containers: These are puncture leak and tamper-proof containers which are subjected to auto or dry heat sterilization followed by shredding or mutilation or encapsulation. Waste sharps to be put include metal sharps—needles, syringes with fixed needles, needles from needle tip cutter/burner, scalpels, and blades.

Blue boxes: These are cardboard boxes with blue colored marking. They are puncture proof and leak proof boxes or containers with blue colored marking which undergo disinfection or autoclaving, microwaving, hydroclaving and then sent for recycling. Metallic body implants and broken/discarded glass medicine vials and ampoules except those contaminated with cytotoxic wastes are discarded in blue box.

E. Management of Accidental Spillage of Body Fluids

The first thing for any spill is to confine the area. All spillage should be managed wearing PPE. Spills should be cleaned up before the area is cleaned as adding cleaning liquids increase the size of spill. Aerosol generation during spillage should be avoided. All sharps involved should be picked by forceps and discarded in a puncture resistant container.

All contaminated material should be discarded in correct waste bin.

Table 18.3: Sequence for doffing (taking off) personal protective equipment (PPE)

Action	Rationale
Take off gloves first **(Fig. 18.3)** • Pinch the palm at the base of thenar eminence with one gloved hand and pull off the glove from that hand. The remaining gloved hand should hold the removed glove • Slide the fingers of the ungloved hand under the wrist portion of the other glove and peel off the second glove over the first glove OR	Gloves are the most contaminated part since healthcare workers are touching patients with their hands during routine care. They should be discarded first. It is important to not allow uncontaminated parts to touch the contaminated parts of the gloves while removing.
Take off gown first **(Fig. 18.4)** • Take gown and gloves off together if the gowns are disposable and made of material such that ties at the back can be torn off by pulling.	This is an alternative strategy that can be used when the gowns that are not made of cloth and the ties can be torn off by pulling.
Remove goggles or face shield **(Fig. 18.3)** • Grasp ear or head pieces with ungloved hands • Lift away from face	Eye protection is essential when splashes of secretions or body fluids are expected. Face shield to be worn for aerosol generating procedures.
Remove gown **(Fig. 18.3)** • Unfasten gown ties, taking care that sleeves do not contact body when reaching for ties. • Pull gown away from neck and shoulders, touching inside of gown only. • Turn gown inside out and discard	The front of the gown should not touch any other surfaces while it is being removed.
Remove mask **(Fig. 18.3)** • Grasp bottom ties or elastics of the mask and untie them or pass them over your head to the front. Then untie/remove the ones at the top, and remove mask without touching the front • For a particulate respirator: The bottom elastic should be lifted over the head first. Then remove the top elastic. This should be done slowly to prevent the respirator from "snapping" off the face.	• Mask should be removed outside the patient's room or as further away from the patient as possible to prevent exposure. • Masks held by ties or elastic bands should be removed carefully to avoid the potentially contaminated areas from coming in contact with other unprotected parts of the face or hands of the healthcare worker.
Wash hands or use an alcohol-based sanitizer immediately after removal of PPE	To prevent the contamination of other surfaces or or your own clothing and before going to see the next patient.

Small Spill

Up to 10 mL of spill is labelled as small spill. The spill should be covered and mopped with hypochlorite moistened paper (1% dilution containing minimum 500 ppm chlorine) and discard in appropriate bin. The area should again be mopped with a cloth moistened with 1% hypochlorite solution and let it dry naturally.

Large Spill

Spills more than 10 ml are considered large volume spills. The spill should be covered with cloth or paper to avoid further spread and further discarded as infected waste. The area should then be covered with hypochlorite solution till spill and cloth gets completely covered and left for 5 minutes. The process should be repeated until all area is cleaned and all waste to be disposed appropriately. The area should be wiped with a cloth mop moistened with 1% hypochlorite solution and allow it to dry naturally.

18.3 INTRAVASCULAR ACCESS

Intravascular access is essential for administering medications and fluids directly into the intravascular compartment. Intravenous

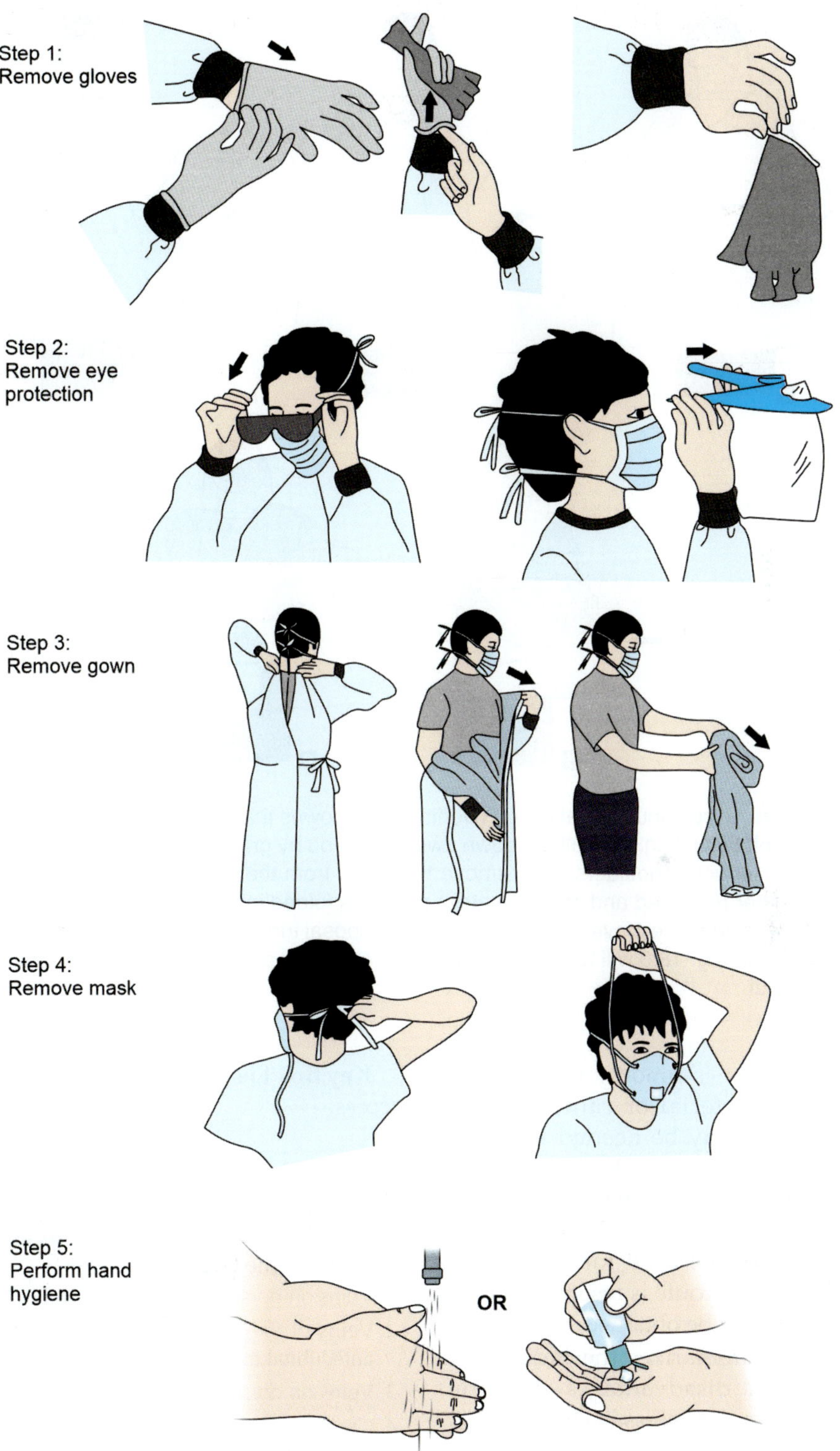

Fig. 18.3 Steps involved in taking off (doffing) personal protective equipment (PPE). *Source:* CDC. Available at https://www.cdc.gov/hai/pdfs/ppe/ppe-sequence.pdf

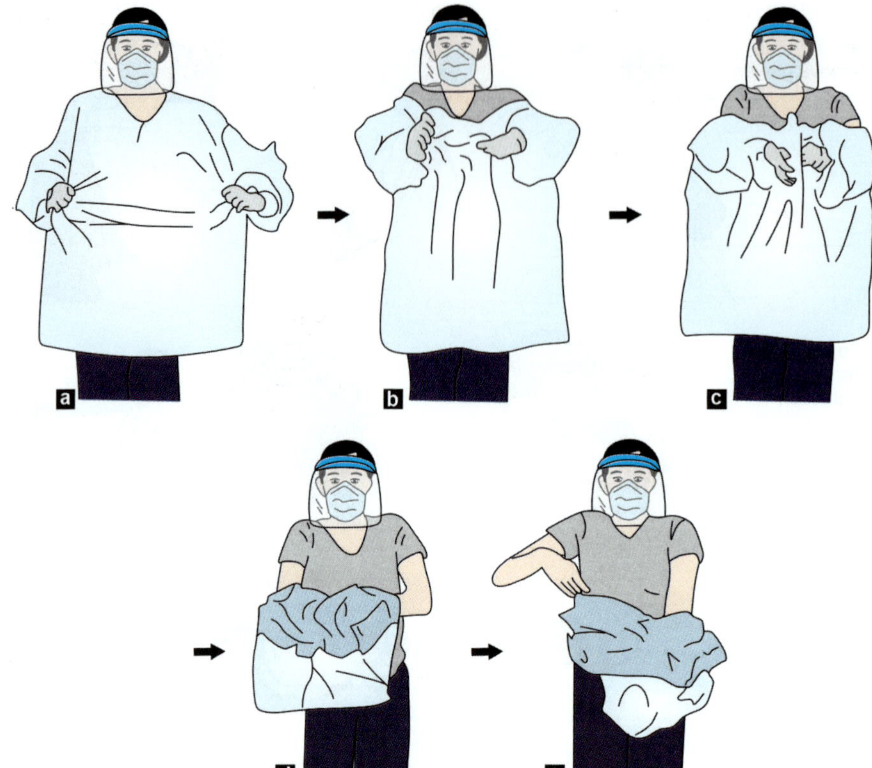

Fig. 18.4 Alternative technique for taking off (Doffing) with gowns that are not made of cloth and whose ties can be torn off by pulling. (a) Pull the gown away from you by grasping the front part. (b) Pull down the gown from over your shoulders. (c) Remove the gown from the arms, one at a time. (d) Fold the gown that the outer (exposed and contaminated) part gets folded inwards. (e) Remove of hands from each glove while leaving the glove inside the gown for disposal together. After this, the rest of the steps 2, 4 and 5 shown in Fig. 18.3 will follow. *Source:* CDC. Available at https://www.cdc.gov/hai/pdfs/ppe/ppe-sequence.pdf

access is the most commonly used method although intra-arterial or catheterization of central veins may be needed in certain situations. Over-the-needle catheters are preferred, their size depending upon the age of the child and caliber of veins. Butterfly/scalp vein needles may be used for cannulating scalp veins but this route is resorted to when other access cannot be obtained.

Table 18.4 summarizes the indications, advantages, and disadvantages of various methods for vascular access in children.

A. Peripheral Venous Access

1. Indication

Intravenous access is achieved to provide drugs, fluids, nutrition when administration via gastrointestinal tract is not possible.

Key Box 1 lists the various sites used for IV access.

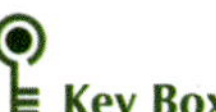

Key Box 1

Sites of Intravenous Access in the Order of Preference

1. Veins on dorsum of hand
2. Veins of the forearm, median cubital vein in antecubital fossa
3. Veins on dorsum of feet
4. Great saphenous vein at ankle
5. Vein in the center of volar aspect of wrist
6. Scalp veins
7. Proximal great saphenous vein

Table 18.4: Indications, advantages, and disadvantages of various methods for vascular access in pediatric patients

Methods	Indications	Advantages	Disadvantages
Peripheral	Short-term	Easy to insert, low cost	Easily dislodged, high rate of occlusion, tissue injury with extravasation of irritants
Intraosseous	Emergency or short-term	Rapid and easy to insert, relatively safe	Not suitable for long-term use, tendency to leak at site
Polyethylene central catheter	Long-term	Percutaneous insertion, safe with hypertonic solutions	Altered body image, bacterial colonization of tunnel
Silastic central catheter	Long-term	More pliable, less thrombogenic, decreased infection rate	High cost, risk of bacteremia, trauma to major vessels, thrombus formation
PICC* lines	Intermediate-term, patients with access problems	Excellent for neonates with access problems	Easily occluded, can be difficult to advance into central vein
Venous cut-down	Long-term or emergency	Direct exposure of vein in patients with difficult access	High rate of dislodgement and infection, incision required
Central ports	Long-term access	Low visibility, reliable, lowest rate of infection	Higher cost, requires expertise

*May require general anesthesia. PICC = Peripheral intravenous central catheter.

Avoid vessels across the joints as immobilization becomes difficult.

2. Procedure for Peripheral Venous Access

For all attempts at gaining an intravenous access, the skin at the point of entry should be prepared meticulously so as to prevent entry of harmful micro-organisms into the bloodstream. Materials required include gloves, spirit and iodine, and sterile swabs. Details of the procedure are depicted in **Table 18.5**. The usual sites of IV access include antecubital veins, veins on the dorsum of hands, ankle, and scalp **(Fig. 18.5)**. Once the skin has been prepared, over-the-needle cannula can be inserted at the selected site as detailed in **Table 18.6**.

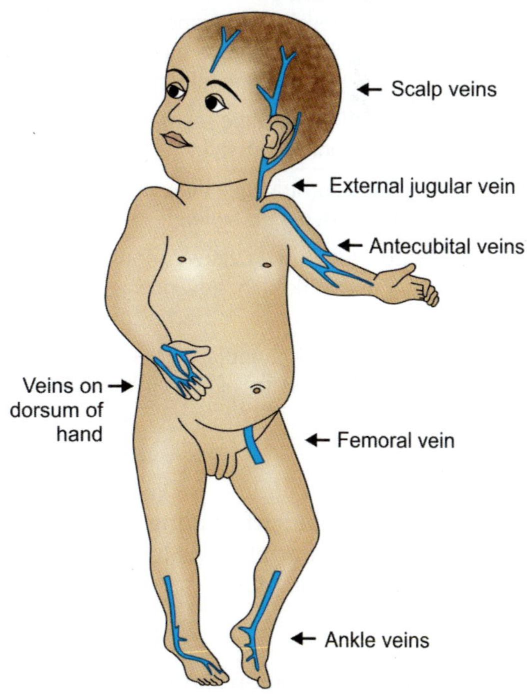

Fig. 18.5: Sites for peripheral venous access.

3. Intravenous Cannula (Intracath)

Intracath is a polyethylene cannula **(Fig. 18.6)** riding a metal needle that is introduced into the vein; needle is withdrawn leaving the polyethylene cannula in the vein.

Procedure: Stretch the overlying skin using one hand to secure the position of vein while inserting the intracath. With another hand, grasp the intracath between the thumb and first finger and insert the cannula along the length of the vein **(Fig. 18.7)**. After obtaining venous access, anchor the intracath with

Table 18.5: Preparing skin for intravenous cannulation

Action	Rationale
1. Wash hands and wear gloves.	To maintain asepsis and follow universal precautions.
2. Position child and limb, place tourniquet/human restraint if necessary (rubber band may be used around infant's head for locating a scalp vein).	For ensuring immobilization and proper visualization of the veins.
3. Select appropriate skin site (dorsal venous network in hands and feet, veins in arms or legs, scalp veins).	Avoid using foot veins in children who walk and the dominant hand in older children.
4. Swab with alcohol first, using an outward circular motion and let it dry.	To avoid contamination from peripheral areas.
5. Swab with iodine on the same site with same technique and let it dry.	To ensure adequate antiseptic action.
6. Swab with alcohol again and let it dry.	To remove excess iodine and allow adequate visualization.

Table 18.6: Insertion of intravenous cannula

Action	Rationale
1. Puncture the skin with the bevel of the needle facing upwards and the needle at 30-degree angle to the skin surface. The point of entry should be 0.5 cm distal to the vein with needle aimed at the course of the vein in its direction of blood flow.	To avoid excess trauma to the skin and blockage of the cannula at the time of entry.
2. As soon as the skin is punctured, reduce the angle to almost skin level and advance needle slowly till the needle is felt to have pierced the vessel wall (a slight 'pop' may be felt).	A small subcutaneous portion gives better stability to the cannula and reduces cross-puncturing of the vessel wall.
3. Backflow of blood into the set may be seen. If not, gently withdraw the stylet.	A good maintained backflow indicates that the cannula is inserted properly inside the vein.
4. As blood appears, advance the cannula into the vein while removing the stylet.	This ensures that the cannula remains in vein throughout the insertion.
5. If no blood return is seen, draw cannula back and keeping it under the skin, advance again slowly to attempt reinsertion.	Repeated removal of the cannula will create multiple puncture sites and increase the risk of contamination.
6. Flush the inserted cannula with some normal saline to confirm patency of the vein and cannula.	To ensure that the vein has not been cross-punctured. In case swelling appears just proximal to the site of cannula insertion on flushing, remove the cannula, and do not reattempt cannulation in the same vein.

adhesive tapes to the surrounding skin. Secure the site with use of armboards to restrain the limb if required (Fig. 18.8).

4. Care of IV Line

The site of IV cannulation should be checked frequently for timely detection of any extravasation, infection, or blocking of the cannula. The site of the cannulation should be observed carefully for the following:

- Any diffuse swelling, either proximal or distal to the site (*extravasation*).
- Tenderness, redness and undue prominence of vein (*thrombophlebitis*).
- Slowing of rate or stopping of infusion (*blockage of cannula*), air within the line, or any problem with the infusion pump.
- Raised local skin temperature with tenderness, redness, and edema (*cellulitis*).

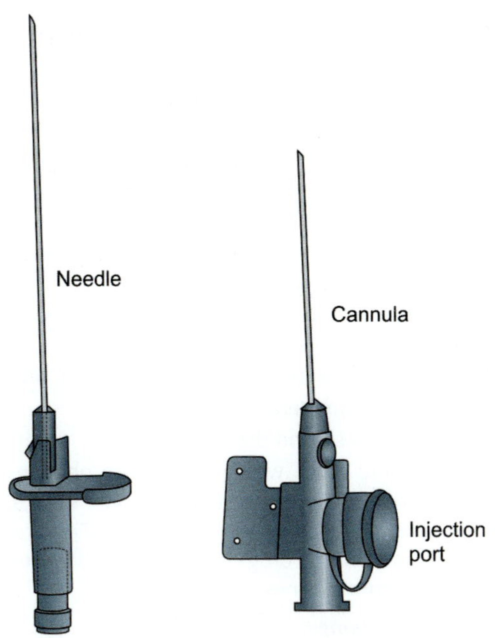

Fig. 18.6: Intravenous cannula.

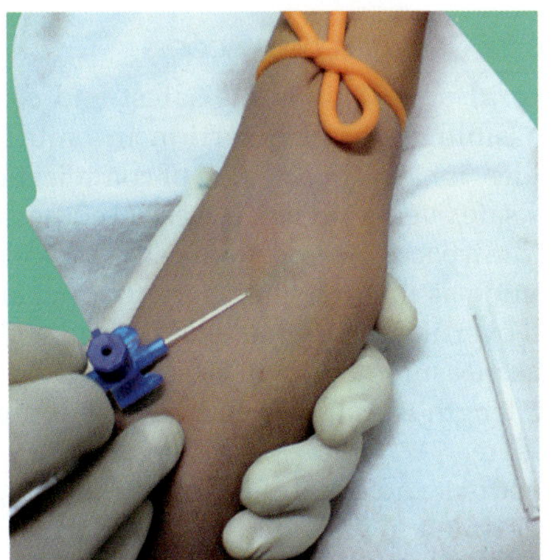

Fig. 18.7: Inserting intravenous cannula.

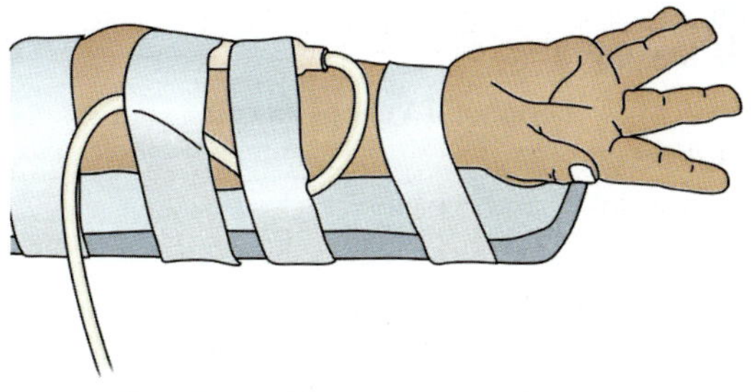

Fig. 18.8: Splinted arm for IV infusion.

- Bleeding from IV puncture site (current or old) may be seen with disseminated intravascular coagulation (DIC).
- *Absence of distal pulsations or blanching at the site:* Cannula may be accidentally placed intra-arterially.

Most of these conditions warrant change of the site of IV cannulation (except when there is DIC). For removing air within the line, disconnect the infusion line and let the IV fluid flow out of the line till the air bubbles are out of the tubing and then reconnect. Blanching of the nearby skin site may normally be seen, if the infusion contains vasoconstrictor drugs, like dopamine or dobutamine; removal is not required in this situation alone. For blockage, gentle flushing with saline may be tried initially but if it persists, the site should be changed taking full precautions while removing the cannula. Steps for removal of IV cannula are provided in **Table 18.7**. Advantage and disadvantages of peripheral, intravenous access are summarized in **Key Box 2**.

Table 18.7: Steps to remove IV cannula

Action	Rationale
1. Stop flow of IV fluid and disconnect tubing.	To avoid wastage.
2. Wash hands, and wear gloves.	Asepsis and universal precautions.
3. Holding the cannula, remove the adhesive tape. Press the point of entry with a sterile cotton swab and gently remove the cannula.	To avoid oozing of blood.
4. If there was any discharge or cellulitis/ thrombophlebitis at the site, send swab or catheter tip for culture.	To document infection, identify the causative organism and treat according to its sensitivity pattern.
5. Once removed, use disinfectant and seal the puncture site.	To avoid the puncture site from becoming a point of entry for infection.

Key Box 2

Peripheral Venous Access

Advantage

Easy to insert and cheap.

Disadvantages

1. Not suitable for central venous pressure monitoring and regular blood sampling.
2. A peripheral cannula can be placed only for 48–72 hours.
3. It can get easily dislodged.
4. High rates of occlusion.
5. Risk of tissue injury with use of irritants.

In case no other access is available, and it is imperative to administer drugs or fluids in an emergency situation, the following may be tried:

- Cannulation of a central vein.
- Intraosseus infusion.
- Insertion of a central vein catheter
- Venous cut-down.

5. Complications

These include hematoma formation, venospasm, thrombophlebitis and embolism, and infiltration of subcutaneous tissue.

Management of extravasation injury: Remove the intravenous cannula, stop the intravenous fluids, and elevate the limb to reduce edema. In extensive tissue necrosis and swelling, some authors recommend multiple punctures of edematous area to allow free drainage and prevent further tissue injury.

Extravasated fluid can be dissolved by using hyaluronidase within 2 hours of extravasation injury. It is especially useful in injury secondary to use of antibiotics, calcium, and parenteral nutrition through the site. Phentolamine and topical nitroglycerine can also be used in extravasation injury secondary to use of dopamine infusions. Keep the area clean, and do daily dressing with application of silver sulfadiazine. Time to heal ranges between 7 days to 3 months.

B. Central Venous Access

For children requiring long-term intravenous medications, central venous access is preferred over venous cut-down. Indications are listed in **Key Box 3**.

Key Box 3

Central Venous Access

Indications

1. Central venous monitoring: For continuous assessment of intravascular volume or cardiac function
2. Long-term intravenous medication administration
3. Aggressive fluid resuscitation, if a good peripheral access is not possible
4. Conditions requiring repeated blood sampling
5. Long-term parenteral nutrition
6. Plasmapheresis and dialysis
7. Hypertonic drugs which may cause phlebitis in peripheral lines, such as hypertonic salines, dextrose at higher concentrations (>10%); and a few vasopressor drugs which cannot be given from peripheral lines

Contraindications

1. Uncorrected bleeding diathesis
2. Skin infection at the local site

Sites for Central Venous Access

Femoral vein: This is the safest and easily accessible route of insertion in children. Besides, it has very low rate of complications so is safe even with less experienced person. The drawbacks include more risk of secondary infection as the route lies close to groin area. Moreover, it is not a good line to monitor CVP as the measurements will be affected from the long length of catheter and intra-abdominal pressure.

Abduct and externally rotate the thigh. Sometimes a roll may be needed to be kept under the thigh. Locate the femoral artery pulsations 1–2 cm below the inguinal ligament. Insert the needle about 1–2 cm medial to these pulsations. Enter the skin at around 10–20° angle.

Internal jugular vein: The next most common site is internal jugular vein. Internal jugular vein can be accessed from three locations:

1. The apex of a triangle bounded by the sternal and clavicular heads of sternocleidomastoid and clavicle;
2. A point midway along the anterior boundary of sternocleidomastoid towards ipsilateral nipple, with the needle tipped 30 to 40 anteriorly and the carotid artery displaced medially; and

3. Beneath the sternocleidomastoid from a point along one-third of the length of the muscle from its clavicular insertion towards the suprasternal notch. This site is more suitable for measuring CVP and also carries lower risk of infections but the risk of potentially serious complications is more than with femoral line.

Subclavian vein: The next common site is subclavian vein. It is more commonly accessed through an infraclavicular approach, guiding the needle posteriorly to the clavicle from a point just inferior and lateral to the midclavicular bend, towards the suprasternal notching. Due to larger diameter and absence of valves this site has lesser chances of thrombosis and catheter related infections.

Procedure

1. Clean and drape the area. Anesthetize the skin using EMLA (eutectic mixture of local anesthetics) cream, if available.
2. Position patient as per the route of insertion.
3. Introduce the needle attached with a syringe at the particular site as per the route of insertion decided. Gently aspirate as the needle is moved in.

   Once there is a free flow of venous blood into the syringe, remove the syringe and insert the J wire through the needle, introducing the wire from the curved J side.
4. Withdraw the needle over J wire, taking care that the wire does not come out.
5. Thread the dilator in the vein by passing over the guidewire in a twisting motion but without applying too much of force. Gradually, remove the dilator over the wire ensuring that the wire does not come out. Pass the central venous catheter over the J wire till the wire comes out from the other end of the catheter lumen. Hold the wire from the other end and advance the catheter into the vein.
6. Make sure that the line is patent and blood can be withdrawn freely. Secure the line with sutures and sterile dressing.
7. Verify the position of central line by radiograph. The line should be flushed with heparinized 0.9% saline.

Complications: Arterial puncture, bleeding, injury to nerves, cardiac arrhythmias, and pneumothorax. Thrombosis and infection are late complications.

Types of Central Venous Catheters

Two types of central venous catheters are currently in use:

1. ***Polyurethane (or polytetrafluoroethylene) and polyethylene catheters:*** These are the preferred catheters for short-term use and for monitoring. Of the two, polyurethane or polytetrafluoroethylene also known as teflon catheters are preferred over polyethylene catheters as they are associated with lesser infection rates **(Fig. 18.9)**.
2. ***Silastic central venous catheters:*** These are soft catheters, preferred for long-term use. These are associated with lower rates of infection and thrombus formation. These are placed into subclavian, internal jugular, or femoral veins and advanced with fluoroscopy into the distal superior vena cava, if intended for long-term use.

C. Venesection or Venous Cut-down

When peripheral veins are not available for giving an intravenous infusion in an emergency situation, it may be necessary to perform a cut-down.

1. A site anterior to the medial malleolus is usually selected **(Fig. 18.10)**.
2. After the usual antiseptic precautions and draping, local anesthetic (1% xylocaine) is infiltrated into the skin and a full thickness skin incision is made at right angles to the vein. Using blunt mosquito forceps, the vein is exposed.

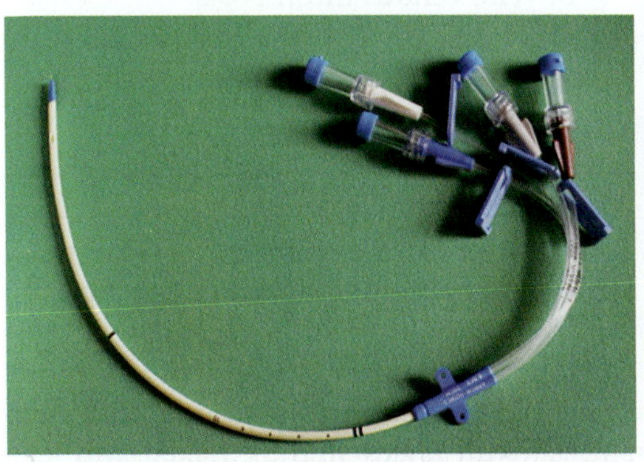

Fig. 18.9: Central venous catheter.

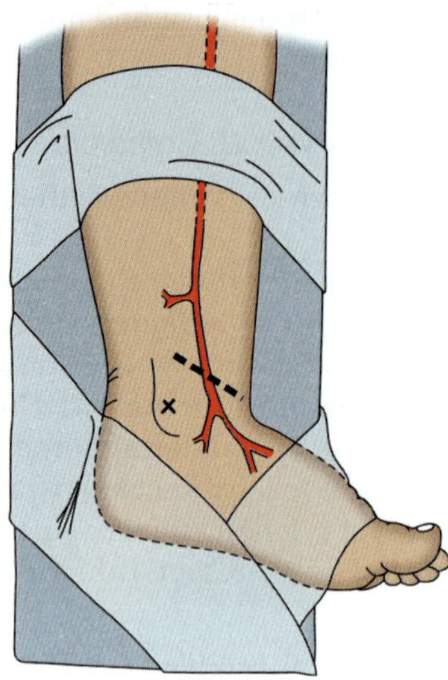

Fig. 18.10: Site for cut-down.

3. Using the forceps, two silk sutures are looped around the vein; the distal one may be used to ligate the vein.
4. Using a fine dissecting forceps, a small incision is made on the vein below the proximal loop of the thread.
5. Slowly guide the catheter up the vein through this incision as the tension on the vein wall by the thread is released simultaneously.
6. As the blood starts flowing through the catheter, it is tied with catgut or thread loop to prevent seepage of blood around the catheter.
7. The skin wound is closed with silk sutures.
8. The catheter is looped around the area under dressing to prevent its slipping by inadvertent traction on the catheter.
9. ***Complications:*** Cellulitis, phlebitis, hematoma, perforation of posterior wall of vein, venous thrombosis.
10. Over the time, intraosseous therapy has overtaken venesection in acute emergencies.

18.4 INTRAOSSEOUS ACCESS

Indications and contraindications for intraosseous access are listed in **Key Box 4**.

A. Position of Patient

The child is made to lie supine on a firm surface with knees slightly flexed and legs positioned with slight external rotation.

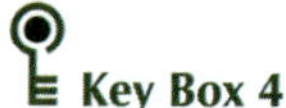

Key Box 4

Intraosseous Access

Indications

1. Effective method of vascular access in critically ill or injured child in shock for administration of medications and fluids

Contraindications

1. Previous attempts at the same site
2. Fractures and crush injuries at or near the site
3. Condition in which bones are fragile like osteogenesis imperfecta
4. Infection in the overlying tissue

B. Sites of Access

1. Most common site is proximal tibia just below the growth plate in a triangular area at the proximal end of medial surface of tibia just distal to the tibial tuberosity. It can be located 1–3 cm below and medial to tibial tuberosity.

   It is important to move from distal to proximal site, in case previous attempt fails. The fluid will start leaking from previous attempt site if you move distal to it (instead of proximal).
2. Distal femur.
3. Anterior superior iliac spine.

C. Procedure

1. Identify the site and clean the desired area with spirit, povidone iodine, followed by spirit.
2. Stabilize the leg on a firm surface. Be careful not to hold your hand behind the desired site.
3. Use a standard intraosseous needle for the access. In case of non-availability, a bone marrow aspiration needle can be used. Alternatively, a thick 18 gauge spinal needle with stylet can be used in emergency.
4. Insert the needle perpendicular to the skin. Drill the needle into the bone using a twisting motion (Fig. 18.11). Insert the needle through the cortical bone till there is a sudden loss of resistance once the marrow is entered. Correct spacing of the needle is indicated by firm placement without any support.

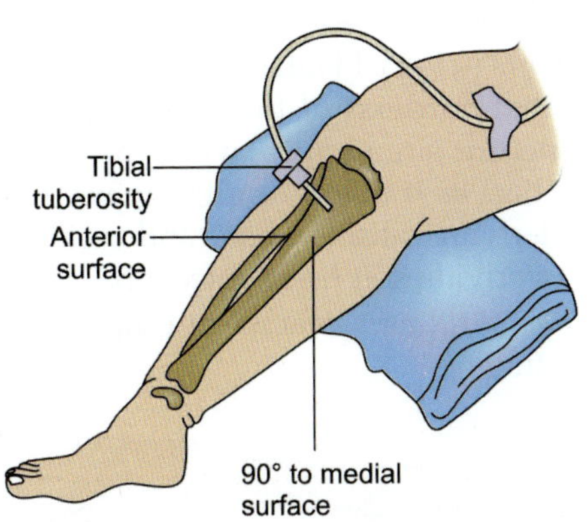

Fig. 18.11: Method of intraosseous access.

5. Remove the stylet, and attach a syringe. Aspiration of the bone marrow particles and blood reconfirms the correct placement. The aspirated content may be sent to laboratory for analysis, if required.
6. Remove the syringe, and infuse a small amount of saline; and observe for swelling in the insertion site or posteriorly opposite the site.
7. Stabilize the needle using tapes, and connect the needle to intravenous tubing; and give the desired fluids and medications. All medications which can be given by intravenous route can be given by intraosseous route.
8. Check regularly for development of swelling and try to establish an intravenous access as fast as possible as intraosseous access should not ideally be used for more than 24 hours.

D. Complications

Fractures can be caused by excessive force. Incorrect placement can result in fluid extravasations into subcutaneous, subperiosteal or into the surrounding soft tissue.

18.5 SAMPLING PROCEDURES

A set of procedures designed to withdraw blood sample for laboratory analysis is called sampling procedures. The blood can be withdrawn from vein, artery, or capillary bed. The universal precautions apply to all sampling procedures. The sample withdrawn must be labeled and sent to laboratory with complete patient details.

A. Venipuncture (Key Box 5)

Procedure of Venipuncture

1. Select veins so as to spare larger vessels for intravenous cannulation or failed attempts at venesection.
2. *The following choice of veins is suggested in the order of preference:* Dorsum of hand, antecubital fossa, dorsum of feet, great saphenous vein at ankle, vein in the center of volar aspect of wrist, scalp, proximal great saphenous vein, then finally neck veins, if all of the above fail to obtain blood sample.
3. Locate the desired vein, warm the extremity, apply an EMLA (eutectic mixture of local anesthetic) cream if available, and prepare the area with antiseptics.
4. Apply a tourniquet proximal to the vein to enhance the visualization of the vein by venous distension. The tourniquet is secured by a knot, ensuring that the knot is not very tight and the one which be removed immediately.
5. A 23 gauge needle is considered best as 24–26 gauge needles (smaller bore) might result in clotting and 21–22 gauge needles (wide bore) might result in prolonged bleeding following sampling.

Key Box 5

Venipuncture

Indications

1. To withdraw blood sample for laboratory studies
2. For administration of drugs

Contraindications

1. Venesection of deep veins in known cases of coagulation disorders
2. Local infection/gangrene at the site of venesection

Precautions

1. Avoid femoral vein for sampling. Femoral venesection can result in reflex femoral arterial spasm resulting in gangrene of extremity, septic arthritis of hip, and penetration of peritoneal cavity. In coagulation disorders, it may lead to a large hematoma
2. Avoid internal jugular vein for the fear of laceration of adjacent carotid artery, and risk of pneumothorax/subcutaneous emphysema
3. Avoid neck veins in infants with intracranial bleed/raised intracranial pressure

6. The needle is inserted at 25–40° angle with bevel turned upward. The needle must be inserted along the direction of blood flow.
7. Sample can be collected by the "drip method", i.e. collecting drops of blood flowing through the needle in desired vials. Alternatively, a syringe can be attached to the needle prior to insertion and blood withdrawn by negative suction. This method is not very useful in infants and where larger amounts of blood need to be withdrawn as the veins are easily collapsible. Vacutainer-needle can also be used alternatively.
8. Remove the tourniquet before removing the needle after the sampling is done to avoid massive bleed from the venipuncture site.
9. Always apply local pressure with dry gauze to achieve hemostasis.

Precautions for Venipuncture

1. Take universal precautions while sampling.
2. Remember to palpate for a pulse in scalp venipuncture to avoid inadvertent arterial puncture.
3. Sites of venous bifurcation must be preferred as compared to puncturing along the length of the vein. This avoids rolling back of the vein in the latter case.
4. Long veins must be preserved for intravenous cannulation rather than for sampling.
5. Remove the tourniquet, if applied for prolonged period, prior to insertion of needle, to allow blood to return, before reapplying for a next attempt.
6. Avoid using alcohol-soaked swab for hemostasis as they impair the hemostasis and are often painful.
7. Avoid more than 2 attempts, seek some help from a colleague.
8. Avoid puncturing nearby arteries like radial artery while doing venesection.

B. Capillary Puncture

Indications

Capillary puncture is a convenient method for collection of small amount of blood for estimation of glucose, hemoglobin, packed cell volume, bilirubin, and for making a peripheral blood smear.

Sites of Capillary Puncture

- *Infants* (<1 yr): Plantar surface (lateral and medial borders) of the foot **(Fig. 18.12)**. Puncture site should avoid the pulp of the heel as it might result in injury to the underlying calcaneal bone and predispose to overlying soft tissue infection.
- *Older children:* Great toe or pulp of 3rd or 4th finger.

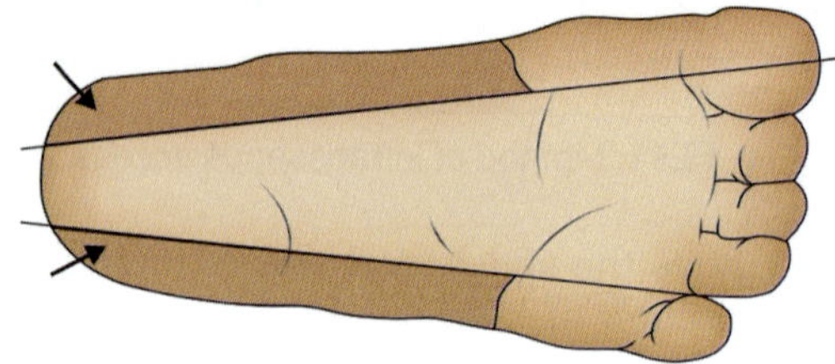

Fig. 18.12: Correct area (shaded) for collection of capillary sample from heel.

Procedure of Capillary Puncture

1. Warm the heel or pulp of fingers prior to puncture to improve the local circulation.
2. Clean the desired area (heel of the foot/finger pulp) with antiseptic. Allow the area to dry prior to puncture.
3. Blood lancet is used for capillary puncture. The depth of puncture should not exceed 2 mm to avoid injury to underlying bone. The puncture is performed perpendicular to the skin to ensure free flow of blood.
4. The first drop of the blood is wiped off.
5. Gently squeeze the lower leg and ankle/fingers for collection of sample. Do not squeeze firmly as it might dilute the sample and give faulty results.
6. Apply firm pressure bandage to achieve hemostasis.

C. Arterial Puncture

Indications for arterial puncture are listed in **Key Box 6**.

Procedure of Arterial Puncture

1. Decide on the site of arterial puncture. Most common site is radial artery, if the ulnar collaterals are intact. Other sites include dorsalis pedis, posterior tibial, and brachial arteries.
2. *Position the limb:* Extend the wrist with the elbow supinated for radial artery puncture.

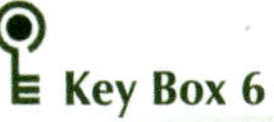

Key Box 6

Arterial Puncture

Indications

1. Arterial blood gas analysis
2. Blood sampling when venous or capillary access was unsuccessful

Contraindications

1. Uncorrected coagulation disorder/thrombocytopenia
2. Gangrene of the extremity

Precaution

1. Avoid use of femoral artery because of the risk of arterial spasm, gangrene, and injury to femoral nerve

3. *Perform the Allen's test for testing ulnar collaterals* for radial arterial puncture: Occlude both radial and ulnar arteries, massage the palm towards wrist, release occlusion of ulnar artery only. Return of color of the palm within 10 seconds indicates adequate collateral supply.
4. Palpate the arterial pulse. The artery can also be localized with the help of transillumination using cold light source.
5. Choose the smallest possible needle (23–26 gauge) to minimize trauma to vessel.
6. Use aseptic precautions and clean the desired site with antiseptic.
7. The needle is inserted at an angle of 40° with the bevel of the needle directed upward. Insert the needle slowly till a gush of blood is noted in the syringe attached to the inserting needle. Failure to obtain blood warrants a slight manipulation of the needle till the sampling is achieved. Remember to sterilize the overlying skin before every attempt.
8. Compress the site for a minimum of 5 minutes or till satisfactory hemostasis has been achieved.
9. For arterial blood gas analysis, use a heparinized syringe, bend the needle after the sampling, and remove any residual air bubbles in the syringe, store the sample in ice-pack and transport to the laboratory as soon as possible.

Complications

Arterial puncture can cause hemorrhage, hematoma, or thrombus formation. Other known complications include formation of aneurysm or arteriovenous fistula, distal ischemia and gangrene formation, and posterior tibial or femoral nerve injury. Compartment syndrome may occur in forearm following radial artery puncture.

D. Arterial Line Placement

Indications

- Invasive blood pressure monitoring in critically sick children
- Frequent blood sampling
- Repeated blood gas analysis specially in ventilated children

Contraindication: Bleeding diathesis.

Sites: Radial artery, dorsalis pedis, posterior tibial, femoral. Prior to its insertion, one must perform Allen's test as explained previously. For insertion of radial artery, hyperextend and restrain the hand over a small roll.

Procedure

Palpate the arterial pulse. The two commonly used methods to place the radial arterial line are 'over the wire' and 'over the needle' technique.

- *Over the wire approach:* The needle should be entered as for arterial puncture. The needle should be advanced a few millimeters farther through the vessel. The wire should be kept ready and the needle slowly withdrawn until pulsatile blood flow is seen. Now, the wire should be advanced into the vessel. The needle can be removed and the catheter is advanced over the wire. Once the catheter is in place it should be secured with firm pressure and wire be removed. The catheter should then be sutured at the site.
- *Over-the-needle technique:* The initial steps are same. Once pulsatile blood return is seen in the catheter, the catheter should be advanced slightly ahead and then the catheter angle is slightly lowered so that the catheter is advanced over the needle into the vessel. The needle can then be removed and catheter secured.

18.6 ADMINISTRATION OF MEDICATIONS

A number of medications that are to be given to children require different routes of administration and once the physician gives the drug and dosage to be given, it is the duty of the nurse to ensure that it is given properly while observing the '*Five Rights*' of medication administration.

1. Five Rights of Medication Administration

i. ***Right medication:*** Check and compare the medication sheet with the label on the medicine vial. Know the mechanism of action and potential side effects of the drug
ii. ***Right patient:*** Verify the child's name and registration number
iii. ***Right time***
iv. ***Right route of administration***
v. ***Right dose:*** Calculate the dose as per the child's weight. Check with pharmacy and question order, if the dose written is outside the recommended amounts

2. Oral Medications

For liquid medications, measure the right amount and place along the side of the mouth with dropper or syringe and wait for the infant to swallow before giving more. For tablets, crush and mix with sugar syrup or juice, if child is not able to swallow.

3. Per-rectally Administered Medications

This route is utilized for administering suppositories or other irritant medications that cannot be given orally. This route can also be used when the patient is having recurrent vomiting or uncontrollable seizures and it is difficult to get IV access.

Place the child in lateral decubitus position, open the buttocks, visualize the anal opening and insert the medication; hold the buttocks tightly for 2–3 min to avoid immediate expulsion of drug.

Diazepam or paraldehyde can be given via a nasogastric tube inserted per rectally beyond the sphincter and injecting the medication through it followed by flushing with 2–3 mL normal saline.

4. Intramuscular Injections

The preferred site for the infant is the vastus lateralis muscle, along the lateral aspect of thigh **(Fig. 18.13)**. After the child has been walking for 1 year, dorsogluteal muscles may be used. In older children, ventrogluteal site or deltoid is preferred. The site of injection is decided by the following factors:

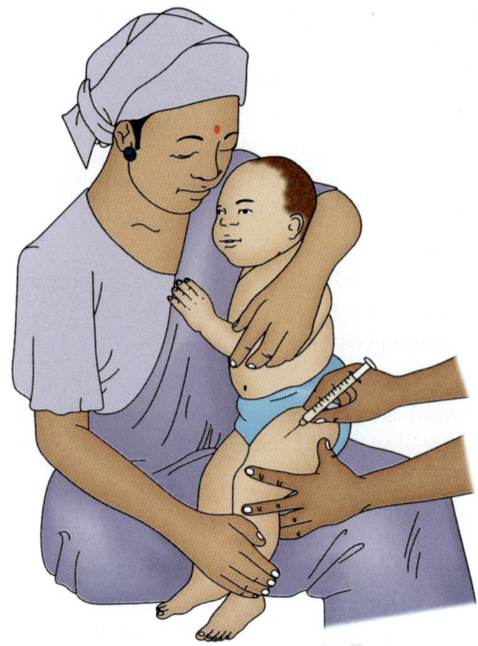

Fig. 18.13: Intramuscular injection.

- Age of child
- Amount of muscle mass
- Density and total volume of medication to be administered.

Infants should not be given more than 0.5 mL at a single site at a time, whereas small children may be given up to 1 mL at a time. The recommended size of the needle to be used is 22 to 25 gauge with a length of at least 0.5 to 1 inch for infants. The procedure to be followed is the same **(Table 18.8)** and knowledge of the anatomy of vessels and nerves of the site selected is a must.

5. Subcutaneous Injection

This is another route, which may be used for certain medications like vaccines (e.g. measles) or drugs (e.g. adrenaline). The recommended size of the needle is 25 or 26 gauge with a length just enough to penetrate the subcutaneous tissue (below skin and fat and above muscle). The usual sites are dorsum of upper arm or anterior aspect of thigh **(Fig. 18.14)** for newborns, infants, and toddlers. The procedure is described in **Table 18.9**.

Table 18.8: Intramuscular administration of drugs

Action	Rationale
1. Use appropriate restraint.	To avoid movement of the child during the procedure.
2. Locate site and clean with spirit swab and let it dry.	
3. Grasp the chosen muscle between thumb and index finger of left hand.	To obtain a good grip and inject in the correct site.
4. Uncap the syringe prefilled with the right dose of the right medication and insert in one smooth motion at a 90° angle to the skin surface.	
5. Pull back the plunger to see if any blood is aspirated. If none, push the plunger and while withdrawing the needle cover the site with gauze.	In case blood is aspirated, withdraw the needle as a vessel has been reached and give the injection at a different site.
6. Do not recap needle and discard in puncture-proof container.	As per the universal precautions.
7. Document it and ask patient to report immediately, if swelling/redness appears.	

Table 18.9: Subcutaneous injection—procedure

Action	Rationale
1. Use appropriate restraint.	
2. Locate site, clean it with spirit swab, and let it dry.	
3. Pinch the skin with your thumb and index finger.	So that the needle may be inserted in the subcutaneous plane above the muscle.
4. Uncap the syringe and insert the needle at 45° angle to the skin, release the skin pinch, and pull back the plunger.	
5. If no blood is aspirated, inject the medication and withdraw the needle at the same angle. Cover the area with gauze.	Do not put alcohol swab, as it will sting.
6. Do not recap the needle, discard in a puncture-proof container.	As per the universal precautions.

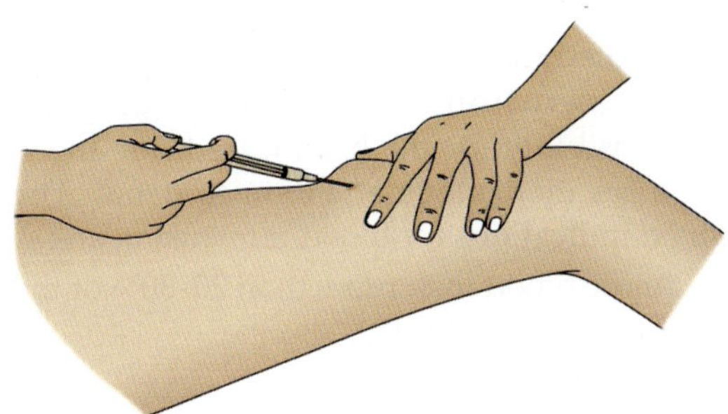

Fig. 18.14: Subcutaneous injection.

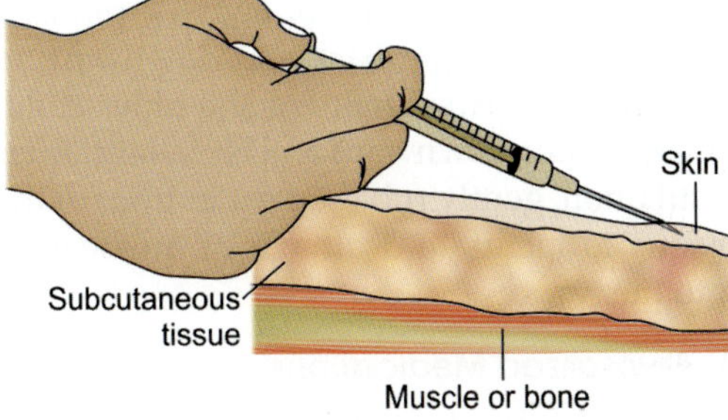

Fig. 18.15: Intradermal injection.

6. Intradermal Injections (Fig. 18.15)

These may be needed for giving the Mantoux test and the BCG vaccine. Injecting in the right plane is very crucial as it must be restricted to the dermis (just below the epidermis and above the subcutaneous fat). The usual site is volar aspect of the left forearm for the Mantoux test and skin over the left upper arm for the BCG vaccine. A 1 mL tuberculin syringe with a 26-gauge needle is used to administer

Table 18.10: Technique of intradermal injection

Action	Rationale
1. Use appropriate restraint.	
2. *Do not* apply spirit swab to the site.	Alcohol can denature the proteins in the injected material.
3. After locating the site, stretch the skin between the thumb and the index finger and insert the needle with the bevel facing upwards and needle almost parallel to the skin surface.	To allow for a very superficial entry of the needle, into the dermis.
4. The needle should not be advanced too far or too deep under the skin surface and while the medication is being injected, the thin overlying skin becomes raised with an orange peel appearance.	In case a wheal with an orange peel appearance is not formed, the dose has been given inappropriately.
5. Remove the needle after injecting the entire amount and do not apply anything on the skin surface.	Also instruct the patient not to rub the site or scratch it. This may spread the material and give erroneous results.
6. Ask patient to report back after 48 hours in case of a Mantoux test for reading the results.	The level of induration (not redness) is measured after 48–72 hours using the pen method in the transverse plane of arm.
7. For BCG, a small bleb that breaks down to form an ulcer that heals on its own in 6–8 weeks, is the normal response.	This is due to the response of the immune system to the administered attenuated tubercular organisms.

these. The right technique will raise a 0.5 cm wheal with a peau d'orange (orange peel) appearance **(Table 18.10)**.

7. Medications in the Eye and Ear

Optic medications should be administered in lower conjunctival sac after appropriate restraint and pulling down the lower eyelid with the non-dominant hand.

Eardrops: While giving otic medication in a child less than 3 years of age, the pinna is to be pulled straight back and downward to straighten the ear canal. For the older child, pull the pinna downward and backward. After instillation, gently rub the area in front of the tragus to facilitate drainage of medication into the ear.

8. Aerosolized Medications

This route is used to administer medications, like bronchodilators, steroid, and antibiotics directly into the airways. The medication is delivered as a fine mist, which reaches up to the most peripheral parts of the lungs and due to rapid absorption over a wide surface area, has a relatively rapid onset of action. The medicine is placed in the cup of the mask or aerosol kit and administered over a period of 10 minutes at an oxygen flow rate of 5 L/min. Other modes of administration of these medications include metered dose inhalers, rotahalers, spinhalers, and spacer devices.

Table 18.11 describes the dose forms, advantages, and disadvantages of various modes of drug administration.

9. Blood Transfusion

Administration of blood or blood products via transfusion is a procedure of great responsibility for the healthcare team and it requires meticulous attention to detail. The main indications for blood transfusion are:

- Acute blood loss, more than 20–30% of the total blood volume;
- Severe anemia;
- Septic shock; and
- To provide platelets in thrombocytopenia, and plasma for clotting factors.

Once, the order to set up a blood transfusion has been received and the blood/blood product arranged from the blood bank, the following steps need to be taken to ensure a safe blood transfusion **(Table 18.12)**.

Table 18.11: Routes of drug administration

Route	Dose form	Advantages	Disadvantages
Oral	Mixture, syrup, tablet, powder, capsule	Convenient, cheap	Uncertain absorption, gradual effect, low peak values, gastric irritation
Sublingual	Tablets, aerosol	Act rapidly	Difficult to handle, problem of overdosing
Rectal/vaginal	Suppositories, enema, tablet, ovule, cream	Convenient in patients with swallowing problems	Local irritation, uncertain absorption, needs trained administrator, poor patient acceptability
Inhalation	Gases, vapors, aerosol, powders	Fast effect, less systemic side effects	Local irritation, need handling by trained staff
Injections	Subcutaneous (SC), intramuscular (IM), intravenous (IV), intradermal (ID) infusion	Fast effect, accurate dose possible	Painful, need skilled staff, more costly, overdose possible
Local	Skin (ointment, cream, lotion, paste), eye, ear and nose drops	High concentrations possible, limited systemic penetration	Sensitization possible, may be difficult to handle

Do's and Don'ts of Blood Transfusion

- Always ensure that there is a genuine reason for transfusion. Blood transfusion carries its own risks and may even be fatal.
- Always inform the relatives/patient about the risks and benefits of transfusion.
- Ensure that the blood is transported from the blood bank to the required place at right temperature for that particular type of blood.
- Whole blood and red cells should be transfused within 30 minutes of removal from refrigeration. Transfusion should get completed preferably over next 4 hours.
- Warming of blood is only needed, if infusion rates are faster than 15 mL/kg/hour. If needed, warm only in blood warmers or else their is a risk of hemolysis.
- Platelets and fresh frozen plasma infusion should be started immediately/as early as possible after release and preferably be given over a period of 20 minutes.
- Do not transfuse blood, if the blood bag shows any signs of discoloration or leakage.
- Any blood bag showing clotted blood should be returned back to blood bank.

18.7 FLUID THERAPY

A. Calculation of Fluid Requirements

Most sick, hospitalized children, and neonates require intravenous (IV) fluids for meeting the fluid and caloric requirements for their basal metabolic processes while they are recovering from illnesses and cannot be fed enterally. These intravenous fluids are composed of water, glucose, sodium, and potassium and help to (i) maintain hydration; and (ii) prevent electrolyte imbalances, starvation ketoacidosis, and protein catabolism. They cannot be substituted for nutrition over long periods of time and most patients on maintenance intravenous fluids can lose up to 0.5–1% of their body weight per day. The following discussion pertains to normal fluid requirements.

1. Amount of Maintenance Fluid

Holliday and Segar showed that the basal caloric requirements for children are as follows:

Body weight 0 to 10 kg	100 kcal/kg/day
Between 10 and 20 kg	1000 kcal + 50 kcal/ kg/day/for each kg
More than 20 kg	1500 kcal + 20 kcal/ kg/day/for each kg

Table 18.12: Process for setting up a blood transfusion

Action	Rationale
1. Identify the blood bag and compare the following with the requisition slip: – Child's name, age, sex and hospital registration number. – Blood bag number – Blood group and Rh type of blood in the bag and that of patient – Date of collection and expiry After checking, sign on the requisition slip with another nurse.	Checking all these parameters will ensure that the right child gets the transfusion with the right blood group and Rh type in the right amount.
2. Check the blood bag for any bubbles, dark areas or sediments.	To detect any clots or sediments of lysed cells.
3. Ask the child/family for any history of previous transfusions and any documented allergic/ transfusion reactions.	If positive, the child will need to be premedicated and transfusion performed with readiness for resuscitation.
4. Estimate the volume to be transfused and determine the rate of infusion.	To give the right amount of blood over adequate time. Too rapid infusion can cause congestive heart failure.
5. Take the baseline vital signs.	To have a reference for the measurements made during transfusion.
6. Connect the tubing to the bag and flush the line completely with blood ensuring no air is present in the line.	Presence of air could block the progression of the transfusion.
7. Flush the iv cannula with saline and ensure its patency.	Same as above.
8. Connect the tubing to the cannula and slowly start open the clamp—on switch, adjusting the flow with the roller.	Ensure the distal end of the tubing remains sterile till it is connected with the cannula.
9. The initial flow rate should be low and later increased, if no reaction occurs.	Most immediate transfusion reactions occur within the first 20 minutes, so it is essential to be watchful in this period.
10. Vital signs should be taken every 5 minutes for the first 15 minutes, every 15 minutes for the first hour and then hourly till the transfusion ends.	In case a transfusion reaction develops, stop the blood transfusion, switch to normal saline infusion and immediately inform the physician.
11. A mid-transfusion diuretic to be given, if ordered.	To reduce the possibility of fluid overload.
12. Document all vital signs, responses and interventions.	To ensure records for future reference.
13. Continue monitoring even after the transfusion is over.	Late transfusion reactions may occur up to 3 days after the transfusion.

For children with normal renal function and under basal metabolic conditions, provision of 50 mL for every 100 kcal consumed per day will replace the normal insensible water losses (IWL), and 66.7 mL per 100 kcal consumed per day will replace the average urinary losses. This adds up to 116.7 mL per 100 kcal consumed per day as maintenance fluids, if we ignore the minimal losses through stool. But, 16.7 mL of water is produced as water of oxidation for every 100 kcal metabolized by the body. So, the net requirement comes to 100 mL/100 kcal per day to replace the renal and extrarenal losses. Using the weight-based calculations for caloric requirements as described above, the total maintenance fluid requirements can thus be calculated as shown in **Table 18.13a**.

2. Composition of Maintenance Fluid

The composition of the maintenance fluids should be such that its osmolality is close to the normal plasma osmolality of 285–295 mOsm/kg. Also the body needs 3 mEq/kg of sodium, 2 mEq/kg of potassium and 2 mEq/kg of chloride per day for maintenance of normal homeostasis.

The composition of various intravenous fluids commonly used in pediatric practice is depicted in **Table 18.13b**.

In general, Isolyte-P is the fluid of choice for newborns till one month of age, and dextrose normal saline (DNS) in children between 1 month and 18 years.

3. Neonatal Fluid Requirements

Neonates have a shift of fluid from intracellular to extracellular fluid compartment after birth, which leads to postnatal diuresis and physiologic weight loss in the first week of life (up to 10% of body weight in term neonates and up to 15% in preterm neonates). In addition, neonatal kidneys have limited capacity for solute and water load handling, which leads to the salt and water diuresis in the first 48–72 hours.

Therefore, the fluids for neonates for the first 48 hours are without any electrolytes (10% dextrose only for the initial 48 hours). Total fluids administered are increased on a daily basis by 10–15 mL/kg/day increments, up to a maximum of 150 mL/kg/day by the end of 1 week of life **(Table 18.14)**. Sodium and potassium are added in intravenous fluids from day 3 of life.

For babies with prematurity, intrauterine growth retardation, and for those who are born to diabetic mothers, it may be necessary to add calcium gluconate (10% solution: 8 mL/kg/day) to initial intravenous fluids since they are at risk for developing hypocalcemia.

B. Fluid Requirements in Special Circumstances

1. Fever

Increased body temperature results in increased insensible water loss. In children with fever, 12.5% extra fluid should be added

Table 18.13a: Estimation of maintenance fluid requirements

Body weight	Fluid	Infusion rate
Less than 10 kg	100 mL/kg/day	4 mL/kg/hr
10–20 kg	1000 + 50 mL/kg/day × (wt–10)	40 mL/hr + 2 mL/kg/hr × (wt–10)
20–30 kg	1000 + 500 + 20 mL/kg/day × (wt–20)	60 mL/hr + 1 mL/kg/hr × (wt–20)
Maximum	2400 mL per day	100 mL/hr

For obese children, calculate the fluid requirements according to the ideal body weight and not the actual weight.

Table 18.13b: Composition of various IV fluids

Fluid type	Sodium (mEq/L)	Potassium (mEq/L)	Chloride (mEq/L)	Dextrose (g/L)	Others
Normal saline	154	—	154	—	—
Dextrose normal saline	154	—	154	50	—
Isolyte P	25	20	22	50	Acetate: 23 Phosphate: 3 Magnesium: 3
Ringer lactate	131	5	111	—	Lactate 28 Calcium 3
Half normal saline	77	—	77	—	—
Hypertonic 3% saline	512	—	512	—	—

18

Practical Procedures

Table 18.14: Daily fluid requirements in the first week of life (mL/kg)

Age (days)	<1000 g	1000–1500 g	>1500 g
1	80	80	60
2	100	95	75
3	120	110	90
4	130	120	105
5	140	130	120
6	150	140	135
7	160	150	150

for every degree centigrade rise in temperature above 38°C.

2. Neonates under Warmers or Phototherapy

20 mL/kg/day needs to be added to the maintenance fluid requirements.

3. Dehydration

In children with acute gastroenteritis (diarrhea/vomiting) with dehydration, fluid therapy depends on the degree of dehydration (mild, moderate, and severe).

Amount of fluid per day = Deficit + Maintenance + Ongoing losses

Deficit: Amount of fluid deficit depends on degree of dehydration **(Key Box 7)**.

Maintenance: Amount of maintenance fluid is calculated as described above.

Ongoing loss: Amount of fluid being lost in stools/vomits (15–20 mL/kg for large stool/vomit and 8–10 mL/kg for small stool/vomit).

Key Box 7

Degree of Dehydration and the Estimated Fluid Deficit

Degree of dehydration (% weight loss)	*Amount of fluid deficit*
Mild dehydration (5% in <1 y; 3% in >1 y)	50 mL/kg
Moderate dehydration (10% in <1 y; 6% in >1 y)	100 mL/kg
Severe dehydration (15% in <1y; 9% in >1y)	150 mL/kg

Example: *Fluid requirement in diarrhea*

A 5-year-old child (wt 15 kg) with acute gastroenteritis presents with severe dehydration passing 10 large stools per day.

The amount of fluid to be given

= Deficit + Maintenance + Ongoing losses

= (90 mL/kg × 15 kg) + (1000 mL + 50 ml/kg × 5 kg) + (20 mL/kg × 10)

= 1350 + 1250 + 200 = 2800 mL/day

Half of this fluid is given over first 8 hrs and rest half over next 16 hrs. The most appropriate fluid for replacement of diarrheal losses is Ringer's lactate.

4. Shock

Shock is a state of circulatory failure resulting in inadequate oxygenation and perfusion to tissues. American Heart Association (pediatric advanced life-support—PALS) has laid down guidelines for management of shock as outlined in **Fig. 18.16**.

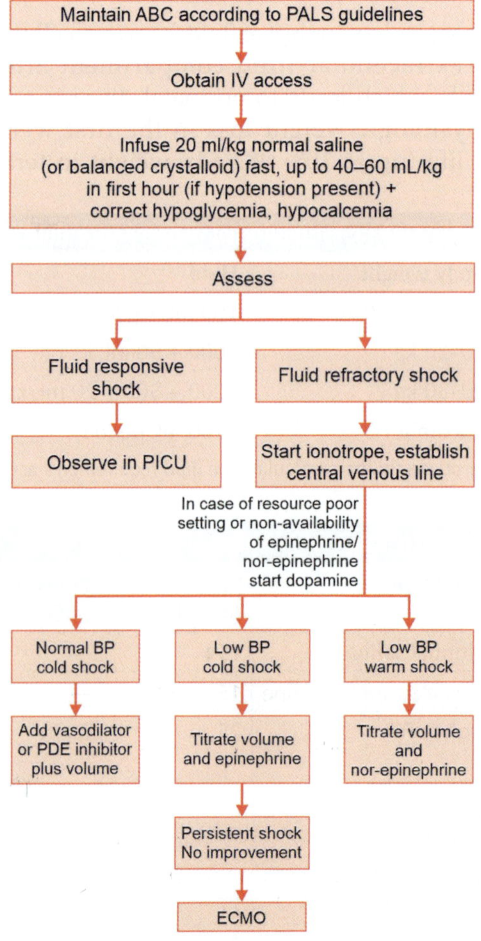

Fig. 18.16: Management of shock.

5. Acute Renal Failure

These children are not passing adequate urine. Thus, the maintenance fluid will consist of only the insensible losses and the volume of fluid lost as urine. Insensible losses (300–400 mL/m^2 of body surface area per day) are replaced volume for volume every 6 hours by 10% dextrose; while urine output is replaced by half NS (N/2 saline).

Correct the hyperkalemia (by administering calcium gluconate, insulin-glucose drip, sodium bicarbonate, or nebulized salbutamol), hyponatremia (fluid restriction, 3% saline), hyperphosphatemia (phosphate binders, dietary phosphate restriction) and hypocalcemia (reduce phosphate).

Child presenting with oliguria (urinary output <0.5 mL/kg/h) is initially resuscitated with a fluid challenge of 20 mL/kg of normal saline over 30 minutes. If the child does not pass urine, then think of intrinsic renal or postrenal failure and give a single shot of furosemide 2–4 mg/kg. If there is no response despite both these measures and with rising blood urea levels, restrict the intravenous fluids and shift to acute renal failure regimen.

Example: *Fluids in acute renal failure*
Total amount of fluids
= Amount of insensible fluid losses (300–400 mL/m^2/day) + Urine output + Extrarenal losses
Insensible losses are replaced with 10% dextrose and renal losses with N/2 normal saline.

6. Congestive Heart Failure

Restrict the maintenance fluid to two-thirds of the normal maintenance with an isotonic crystalloid fluid, like normal saline or DNS. Maintenance potassium may be added, if needed.

7. Chemotherapy

Newly diagnosed patients with lymphoreticular malignancies who are being started on induction chemotherapy regimen for the treatment of their malignancy are at risk for *tumor lysis syndrome*. This results from rapid cell death induced by chemotherapeutic agents. This puts the patients at risk for various metabolic complications, including hyperkalemia, hyperphosphatemia, hyperuricemia, and hypocalcemia.

To prevent the occurrence of these complications, these children are given extra fluids, usually 3 L/m^2 body surface area, with sodium bicarbonate (instead of normal saline in the fluid) to alkalinize the urine for facilitating the excretion of excess uric acid while at the same time limiting the total amount of sodium delivered to 3 mEq/kg/day.

8. Meningitis

Isotonic crystalloid fluids should be used as maintenance fluids in these children. Restriction of fluid because of risk for **S**yndrome of **i**nappropriate **a**nti-**d**iuretic **h**ormone (SIADH) secretion is now debatable and not routinely followed. Studies have shown that most of the cases have high **a**nti-**d**iuretic **h**ormone (ADH) because of underlying hypovolemia. Hence it is important to first ensure that there is euvolemic state. If serum sodium persists to be low even after the underlying volume status is adequate, one should consider fluid restriction. One should avoid overhydration as well.

9. SIADH

Fluid restriction to 1000 mL/m^2/day (500 mL/m^2/day urinary losses + 500 mL/m^2/day non-urinary losses).

10. Raised Intracranial Tension

Only isotonic crystalloids, like NS or DNS, should be used as maintenance fluids. Hypotonic solutions (e.g. isolyte-P) can worsen the cerebral edema. 3% saline and mannitol are also used as anti-edema measures.

C. Preparing Different Strengths of IV Fluids

1. Standard IV Fluid Preparations

The composition of the commercially available standard intravenous fluid solutions should be known before we can prepare any unconventional fluid preparations. The following fluids are available:

Dextrose solutions: *5%, 10%, 25% and 50%.* A 5% solution means 5 g of dextrose dissolved in 100 mL of distilled water.

Saline solutions: *Normal saline (NS).* Normal saline contains 0.9 g of sodium chloride in 100 mL of distilled water. One liter of NS contains 9 g of sodium chloride or 154 mEq/L of sodium. The half-normal saline would have half that strength, i.e. 77 mEq/L of sodium.

Dextrose with saline: Normal saline with 5% dextrose (DNS). 100 mL of this solution will have 5 g of dextrose and 0.9 g of sodium chloride (154 mEq/L).

Ringer's lactate: This is commonly used for IV rehydration; it contains 131 mEq/L of sodium, 4 mEq/L of potassium, 3 mEq/L of calcium, and 28 mEq/L of lactate.

Isolyte P: It contains 5% dextrose, 25 mEq/L of sodium, and 20 mEq/L of potassium.

Although these standard preparations suffice for most patients for everyday use, there may be certain situations where solutions of different strengths may be required.

2. Calculation of Glucose Infusion Rate (GIR)

High glucose infusion rates (beyond the standard 4–6 mg/kg/min) may be required in neonates with hypoglycemia. Use the following formula for calculation

GIR (glucose infusion rate in mg/kg/min)

$$= \frac{\text{concentration of infusion (\%)} \times \text{fluid infusion rate (mL/kg/d)}}{144}$$

3. How to Prepare?

The solutions are prepared in sterile conditions, ideally under laminar flow. It is necessary to calculate the exact proportion of each ingredient before beginning the preparation process. A few examples are discussed on the next page.

The calculations should always be re-checked as any error in calculation may result in electrolyte imbalance.

Example 1: *Prepare 100 mL of 7.5% dextrose*

What is needed?

7.5% dextrose, i.e. 7.5 g of dextrose in 100 mL of solution.

What we have?

i. 5% dextrose, i.e. 5 g of dextrose in 100 mL of solution; and
ii. 10% dextrose, i.e. 10 g of dextrose in 100 mL of solution.

What to do?

We can prepare a solution of 7.5% dextrose by mixing 5% and 10% dextrose, since 7.5 is a number between 5 and 10. However, we need to know how much of 5% and 10% dextrose should be mixed together to make 100 mL of 7.5% dextrose solution.

We start the calculation by assuming that the number of mL of 5% dextrose in the 100 mL of 7.5% solution is x mL. The number of mL of the 10% dextrose will be 100–x. Therefore, we can derive this equation:

$$5(x) + 10\,(100 - x) = 7.5\,(100)$$

where figures in brackets indicate the amount of solution.

Solving this equation, we get x = 50 mL.

Answer

Thus for preparation of 100 mL of 7.5% dextrose, we will mix 50 mL of 5% dextrose solution with 50 mL of 10% dextrose.

Example 2: *Prepare 1000 mL of 9% dextrose*

Using the method described above, we get the following equation, with x being the number of mL of 5% solution:

$$5(x) + 10\,(1000 - x) = 9\,(1000)$$

where figures in brackets indicate the amount of solution.

Solving this equation, we get x = 200 mL.

Answer

Therefore, 9% dextrose will be made up by mixing 200 mL of 5% dextrose with 800 mL of 10% dextrose.

D. Fluid Administration with Infusion Pump

Infusion pumps help to administer specific amounts of medications and fluids over specified time periods at predetermined rates and avoid the need to monitor drip rates and also prevent dosing errors. For smaller amounts of medications and infusions, syringe infusion pumps are used, but for maintenance fluids, in-line infusion pumps are used.

1. Syringe Infusion Pumps

Syringe infusion pumps **(Fig. 18.17)** are good for delivering small amounts of medication at steady rates. The method for use is detailed in **Table 18.15**.

- Syringe infusion pumps may be prone to electromagnetic interference from cell phones.

Example 3: *Prepare 1000 mL of 15% dextrose*

We can prepare a solution of 15% dextrose by mixing 10% dextrose and 25% dextrose, since 15 is a number between 10 and 25. Using the method described above, we get the following equation, with *x* being the number of mL of 10% solution.

$$10(x) + 25\,(1000 - x) = 15\,(1000)$$

where figures in brackets indicate the amount of solution.

Solving this equation, we get $x = 666.7$ mL.

Answer

Therefore, 1000 mL of 15% dextrose will be made up by 666.7 mL of 10% dextrose and 333.3 mL of 25% dextrose.

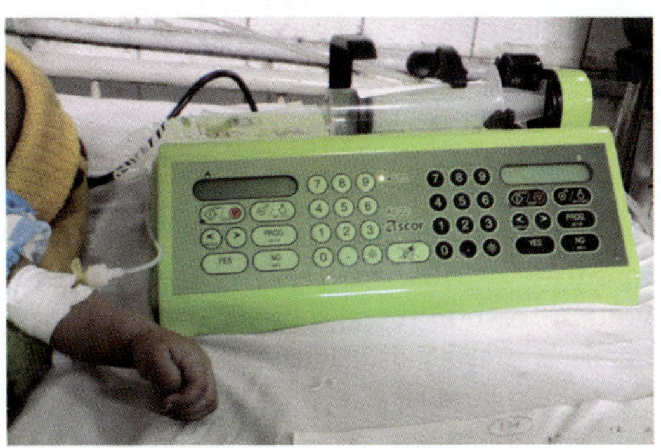

Fig. 18.17 Syringe infusion pump.

Example 4: *Prepare 100 mL of N/3 solution*

We can prepare N/3 solution by diluting normal saline to one-third of its concentration. A simple way is to mix 1 part of normal saline (33.3 mL) with 2 parts of distilled water (66.7 mL). Similarly, if 1000 mL of N/5 saline is to be prepared, mix 1 part of NS (200 mL) with 4 parts (800 mL) of distilled water.

- If there is an occlusion alarm, stop the infusion, and then rectify the problem. Never try to push the medication into the patient as a bolus in an attempt to flush the occlusion.
- Never ignore the low battery warning as it may make the infusion stop all of a sudden.

2. In-line Infusion Pumps

In-line infusion pumps (Fig. 18.18) are useful for delivering large volumes over shorter periods of time at higher flow rates, with intravenous fluid bottles. The method for use is detailed in **Table 18.16**.

18.8 OXYGEN THERAPY

A. Indication

Documented or suspected hypoxemia with PaO_2 <60 mmHg and SaO_2 <94% in room air.

Table 18.15: Fluid administration by syringe infusion pump

Action	Rationale
1. Prepare and draw the medication or fluid to be administered in the right size of syringe (10 mL, 20 mL or 50 mL) in appropriate concentration and connect the tubing to the syringe.	Different syringe sizes may be selected based on the quantity of the infusate and the duration of infusion.
2. Check the medication or fluid order to determine the rate of infusion.	This will be the rate which needs to be set in the infusion pump before initiating the infusion.
3. Switch the power on after setting up the infusion pump at the patient's bedside. Make sure the battery is fully charged, if running on battery.	Battery back up is important to ensure continuous delivery of medications in the event of power failure.
4. Load the pre-filled syringe on to the pump and set the clamp and plunger in appropriate position with a proper fit.	It is important to ensure that the syringe is properly fixed to enable uninterrupted delivery of the drug.
5. Connect the distal end of the tubing to the intravenous access site after ensuring the patency of the intravenous line.	It is important to always check the patency of the IV line prior to starting the infusion by flushing some saline through it.
6. Set the desired infusion rate and start the infusion. Monitor for any changes at the iv site and for any possible reactions to medication (if applicable).	Always re-check the calculation of the infusion rate to avoid overlooking of dosing errors.

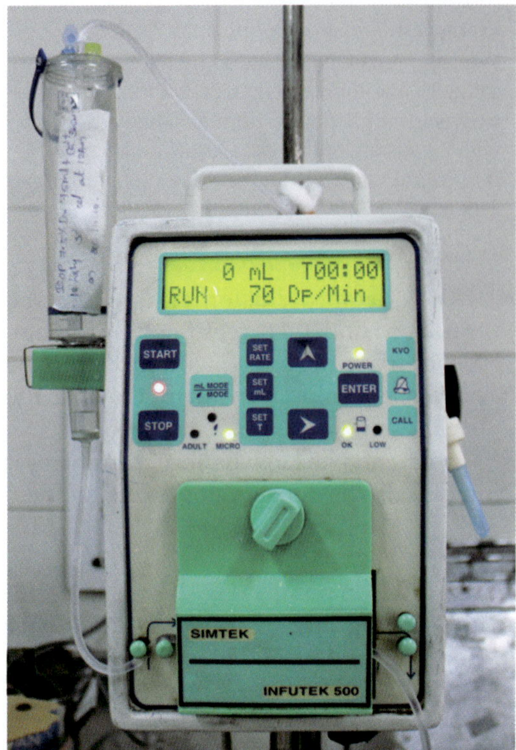

Fig. 18.18: Volumetric infusion pump.

B. Benefits of Oxygen Therapy

1. It increases the oxygenation at tissue level maintaining aerobic metabolism.
2. It decreases the work of breathing by improving the ventilation.
3. It decreases the workload on myocardium by improving the cardiac output.
4. It improves the oxygen supply to myocardium and respiratory muscles.
5. It results in pulmonary vasodilation hence decreasing the afterload on right ventricle.

C. Aim of Oxygen Therapy

To maintain minimum SaO_2 >94–99% and PaO_2 >60–74 mmHg.

D. Oxygen Delivery Devices

There are two types of oxygen delivery devices: Variable performance device or low-flow system and fixed performance device or high-flow system.

1. Variable Performance Device or Low-flow System

These devices provides only a part of patient's inspiratory flow needs or patient's tidal volume, rest of the patient's inspiratory flow needs is met by dilution with room air. The oxygen flow rate is usually less than 10 L/min. The rate of oxygen flow in these devices is less than the patient's inspiratory flow resulting in mixing of oxygen with room air.

Table 18.16: Fluid administration by in-line infusion pump

Action	Rationale
1. Prepare the solution for administration and connect the tubing to the bottle/IV fluid container while maintaining asepsis. Flush the tubing so that it is ready to flow.	Preparation of the solution should be done under laminar flow and with thorough asepsis precautions.
2. Switch on the in-line infusion pump by the patient's bedside and hang the IV fluid in container on the pole.	It is important to ensure that the back-up battery is fully charged to ensure continuity of infusion case of power failure.
3. Insert the tubing in the infusion pump as per the manufacturer's specifications.	Different models of infusion pumps have different methods of fixing the tubing.
4. Connect the distal end of the tubing to the patient's intravenous access site after ensuring that there are no air bubbles in the hub/tubing.	This will prevent chances of air embolism.
5. Set the desired rate of infusion based on the infusion quantity of the infusate and the planned duration of the infusion.	It is important to re-check the calculations of the rate to avoid dosage errors.
6. Start the infusion and observe the iv access site for any extravasation.	It is important to observe the site of infusion for at least 5 minutes to observe for early signs of extravasation.

These devices deliver a variable FiO_2 (range 23–50%) (hence called variable performance device) and the delivered FiO_2 depends upon patient's inspiratory flow rate and the oxygen flow rate of the device. These devices are suitable for patients requiring low to moderate FiO_2 (0.3–0.6) and having stable breathing pattern. Nasal cannula and simple oxygen mask are examples of low-flow system.

Table 18.17 depicts the devices included in low-flow system.

2. Fixed Performance Device or High-flow System

These devices provide all of the patient's inspiratory flow needs and tidal volume.

High-flow system can reliably deliver either low or high inspired oxygen concentration (FiO_2). High-flow system should be used in emergency settings to reliably deliver a high inspired oxygen concentration (up to 100%) to a child with hypoxia.

The oxygen flow rate is usually more than 15 L/min. These devices deliver a constant FiO_2 which does not get affected by patient's inspiratory pattern. It is usually suitable for patients requiring consistent FiO_2 or those requiring high FiO_2 (>0.7) or those having varying breathing pattern. These devices are listed in **Key Box 8**.

3. Oxygen Delivery Systems

Some of the commonly used oxygen delivery systems are discussed below:

***Nasal cannula* (Fig. 18.19):** This is a low-flow oxygen delivery system which is well tolerated by children requiring minimal oxygen support. Oxygen flow up to 4 liters/min can be delivered. An average FiO_2 provided with 1 liter/min is 24%. With every increase of 1 liter/min of oxygen up to 4 liters/min, FiO_2 rises by 4%.

Table 18.17: Low-flow or variable performance oxygen delivery devices

Device without rebreathing	Device with rebreathing
Nasal cannula	Nasal cannula with reservoir
Nasal catheter	Simple oxygen mask
Nasal mask	Partial rebreathing mask
Transtracheal catheter	Non-rebreathing mask

Key Box 8

Fixed Performance Device or High-flow System

1. Air entrainment mask (AEM) like venturi mask, ventimask, or HAFOE system
2. Air entrainment nebulizer (AEN)
3. Partial rebreathing mask with reservoir and non-rebreathing mask with reservoir
4. Oxygen hood
5. Oxygen tent
6. Face tent

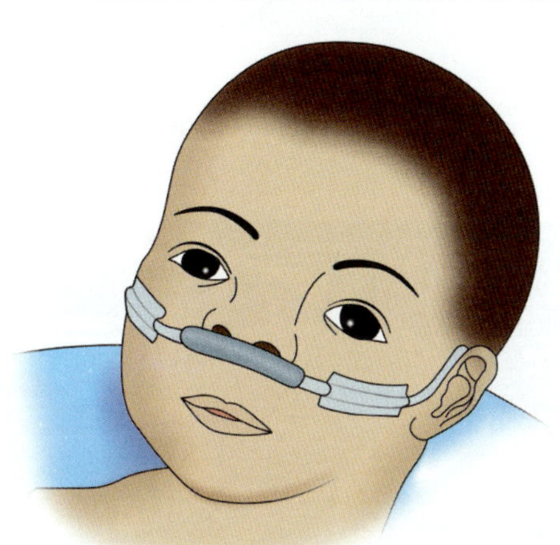

Fig. 18.19: Nasal cannula.

High-flow oxygen by nasal cannula causes irritation and dryness of nasopharynx as humidification is not possible with this method. For neonates and infants, not more than 2 liters/min oxygen flow should be used.

***Simple oxygen mask* (Fig. 18.20a):** It is a low-flow oxygen device that provides 35–60% FiO_2 at oxygen flow of 6–10 liters/min. With each liter increase in oxygen, FiO_2 increases by nearly 10%. Flow less than 5 liters/min should not be used as it can cause carbon dioxide retention and rebreathing of retained CO_2.

***Partial rebreathing mask* (Fig. 18.20b):** The partial rebreathing mask provides 35–70% FiO_2 at oxygen flow rates of 6–15 liters/min. It is similar to a facemask but has an extra oxygen reservoir and side ports. The oxygen flow should be maintained to a level such that only one-third of reservoir gets empty during inspiration. During expiration, first one-third

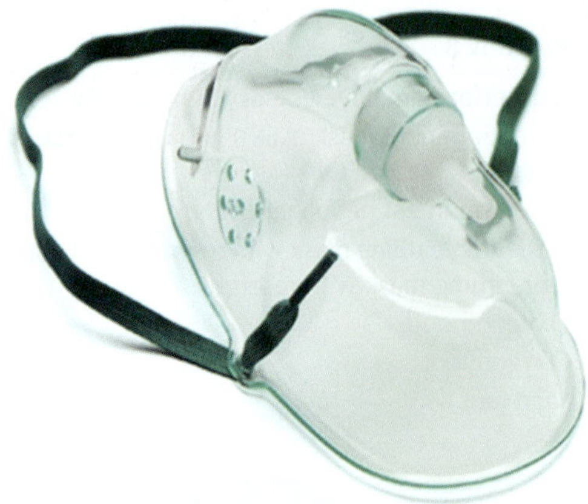

Fig. 18.20a: Simple oxygen mask.

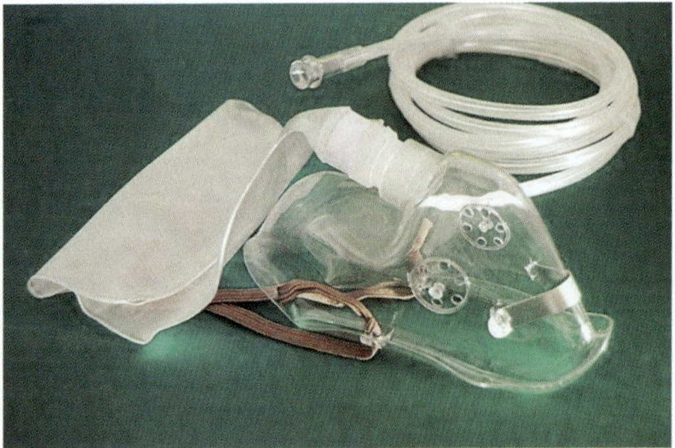

Fig. 18.20b: Partial rebreathing mask.

of the exhaled air enters the reservoir. This predominantly comes from the anatomic dead space and hence is still rich in oxygen as well as humidified. The reservoir bag should be filled with oxygen by occluding the outlet before placing on the patient.

Non-rebreathing mask (Fig. 18.20c): It provides an FiO_2 of 80–100% at oxygen flow rate of 8–15 L/min. It is similar to non-rebreathing mask other than a one-way valve between the mask and reservoir as well as over exhalational ports of the mask. In expiration, port valves open and reservoir valve closes. During inspiration, port valves close and reservoir valve opens and hence is able to provide high concentration of FiO_2.

Venturi mask (Fig. 18.20d): It combines oxygen with room air to give a high flow oxygen concentration at a fixed and constant FiO_2. Color-coded jets are attached to the mask to deliver the required amount of oxygen. It can

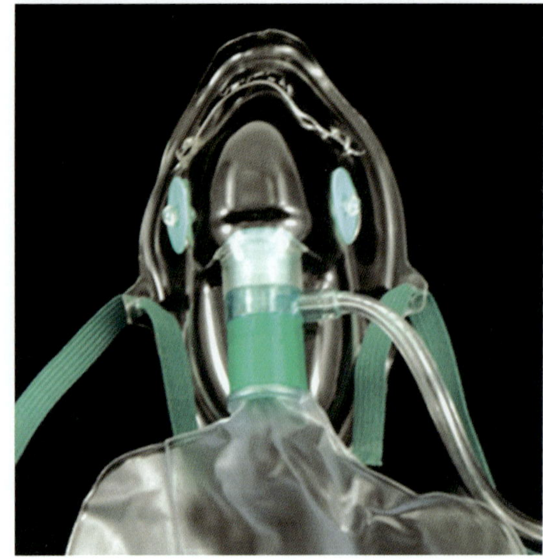

Fig. 18.20c: Non-rebreathing mask.

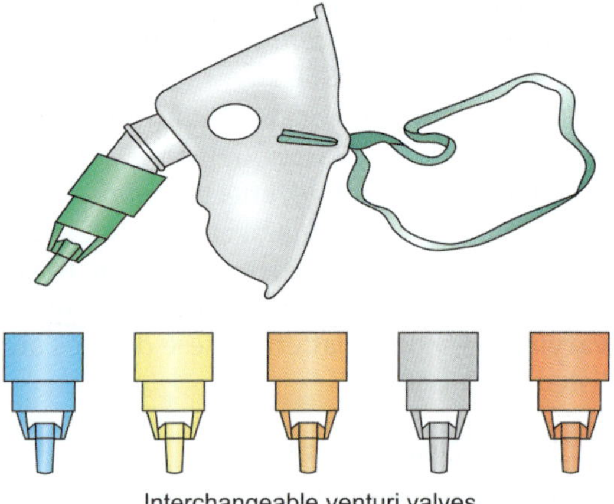

Fig. 18.20d: Venturi mask.

deliver an FiO_2 ranging from 24–50%. The recommended flow rate is 12–15 L/min.

Oxygen hood: It is well-tolerated by infants less than 1 year of age. Almost 80–90% oxygen can be delivered at oxygen flow rate of 10–15 L/min. Both the oxygen delivery and humidification can be provided in controlled manner. For neonates and infants, a minimum flow of 6 liters/min and 15 liters/min, respectively is required. Low flow carries the risk of carbon dioxide retention.

E. Hazards of Oxygen Therapy

These include hypoventilation, absorption atelectasis, retrolental fibroplasia of prematurity, oxygen toxicity, and fire hazards.

18.9 NASOGASTRIC TUBE INSERTION

Indications, contraindications and precautionary measures for nasogastric tube insertion are detailed in **Key Box 9**. Before inserting, select the appropriate size of the tube as per **Table 18.18**.

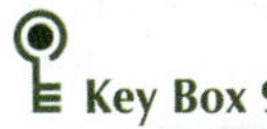

Key Box 9

Nasogastric Tube Insertion

Indications

1. Feeding sick and premature infants
2. Feeding an unconscious child
3. For gastric decompression in cases of intestinal obstruction, paralytic ileus
4. To administer medications
5. Gastric lavage in cases of poisoning
6. For diagnosis of tracheoesophageal fistula

Contraindications

1. Facial trauma
2. Base of skull fracture
3. Recent esophageal perforation/repair

Precautions

1. Stop the insertion immediately, if the child has bouts of cough or develops respiratory distress. This often indicates wrong insertion into airway instead of esophagus
2. While removing the nasogastric tube, always pinch the outer end to avoid emptying the contents into pharynx

Table 18.18: Selection of appropriate size nasogastric tube

Age	NG tube size (Fr)
<1 m	6–8
1–6 m	8–10
1–3 yr	10–12
3–6 yr	12
6–8 yr	12–14
>8 yr	14–16

Process

The detailed process of insertion of a nasogastric tube is given in **Table 18.19**. The process has its risks that include apnea or bradycardia; oxygen desaturation; irritation of nasal mucosa leading to bleed or ulceration; and perforation of esophagus/stomach. The tube may get misplaced on insertion: It might get coiled up in oropharynx or esophagus or it might be inserted into trachea. The tube can also get displaced due to inappropriate fixation or length.

Table 18.19: Procedure for inserting a nasogastric tube

Action	Rationale
1. Use adequate restraint. Explain the procedure to the older child.	As this procedure causes a lot of discomfort.
2. Child should be lying supine with head end elevated.	
3. Measure the length of tube to be inserted: From the tip of the nose to the tragus and then to the xiphoid process **(Fig. 18.21)**.	Corresponds to the distance from lip to upper end of stomach.
4. Apply lubricant at distal end of the tube.	To facilitate easy passage.
5. With the neck slightly flexed, pass the tube into the nose along the floor of the nose straight backwards. If the child gags when the tube goes beyond oropharynx, flex the neck and have him/her take sips of water, if possible.	• Extension of neck increases the likelihood of tube entering the esophagus. • Giving sips of water will suppress gag reflex.
6. Advance the tube till mark is reached, and then check its position by pushing air into the tube and simultaneously auscultating over the abdomen to listen for the rush of air.	This ensures that the tube has reached the stomach and is not coiled up in esophagus (as in esophageal atresia or fistula) or in the trachea.
7. Secure the tube to the nose with adhesive tape.	So that it remains in place.

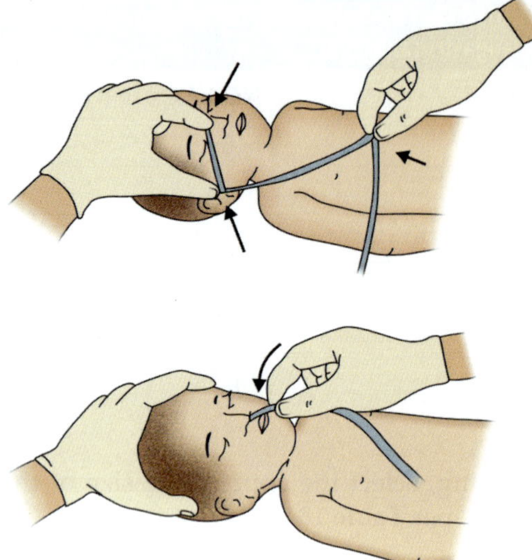

Fig. 18.21: Nasogastric tube insertion.

18

Checking Tube Position

- Push air into the tube and simultaneously auscultate over the abdomen to listen for the rush of air.
- Aspirate the secretions from the nasogastric tube and check the pH. Gastric pH should be less than 5.5. It may not be so if the patient is on proton pump inhibitors.
- Chest X-ray can help to confirm the position at the time of X-ray.

The tube position should be checked at initial placement; before administering each feed; before giving medication; following vomiting, retching and coughing; and if there is any evidence of tube migration (loose tapes, more tube outside).

Precautions

- Stop the insertion immediately, if the child has bouts of cough or develops respiratory distress. This often indicates wrong insertion into airway instead of esophagus.
- While removing the nasogastric tube, always pinch the outer end to avoid emptying the contents into pharynx.

Orogastric Tube

An orogastric tube is used in the following circumstances:

- Suspected base of skull fracture
- Baby with choanal atresia
- Craniofacial anomalies where airway may get compromised on inserting nasogastric tube.

The technique of insertion remains same as nasogastric tube except that the length of tube to be put in should be measured from lips to xiphisternum. The tube has to be directly passed from the mouth.

18.10 NEONATAL RESUSCITATION

American Heart Association and American Academy of Pediatrics in 2020 laid down new guidelines for resuscitating newborn that need to be followed for a smooth transition from intrauterine to extrauterine life. Subsequently Indian Academy of Pediatrics (IAP) along with National Neonatology Forum (NNF) in 2023, modified the guidelines based on Indian settings. The steps of revised neonatal resuscitation protocol for India are summarized in Fig. 18.22.

A. Principles of Successful Resuscitation

A successful resuscitation depends on (i) adequate preparation; (ii) anticipation and immediately recognizing the infant in need of resuscitation; (iii) initiating the procedure promptly; and (iv) performing the procedure skilfully.

1. Communication

Adequate preparation for an anticipated high-risk delivery requires communication between the persons caring for the mother and those responsible for resuscitation of the newly born. Details of antepartum and intrapartum maternal medical conditions and treatment as well as specific indicators of fetal conditions (fetal heart rate, lung maturity, ultrasonography) should be known. To assess risk for neonatal resuscitation, three questions need to be known predelivery:

1. What is the expected gestational age?
2. Is there a single or multiple fetuses?
3. Are there any other risk factors?

Table 18.20 lists important antepartum and intrapartum factors associated with delivery of high-risk babies. The team leader should try to meet and introduce self to the parents before proceeding for delivery. Any

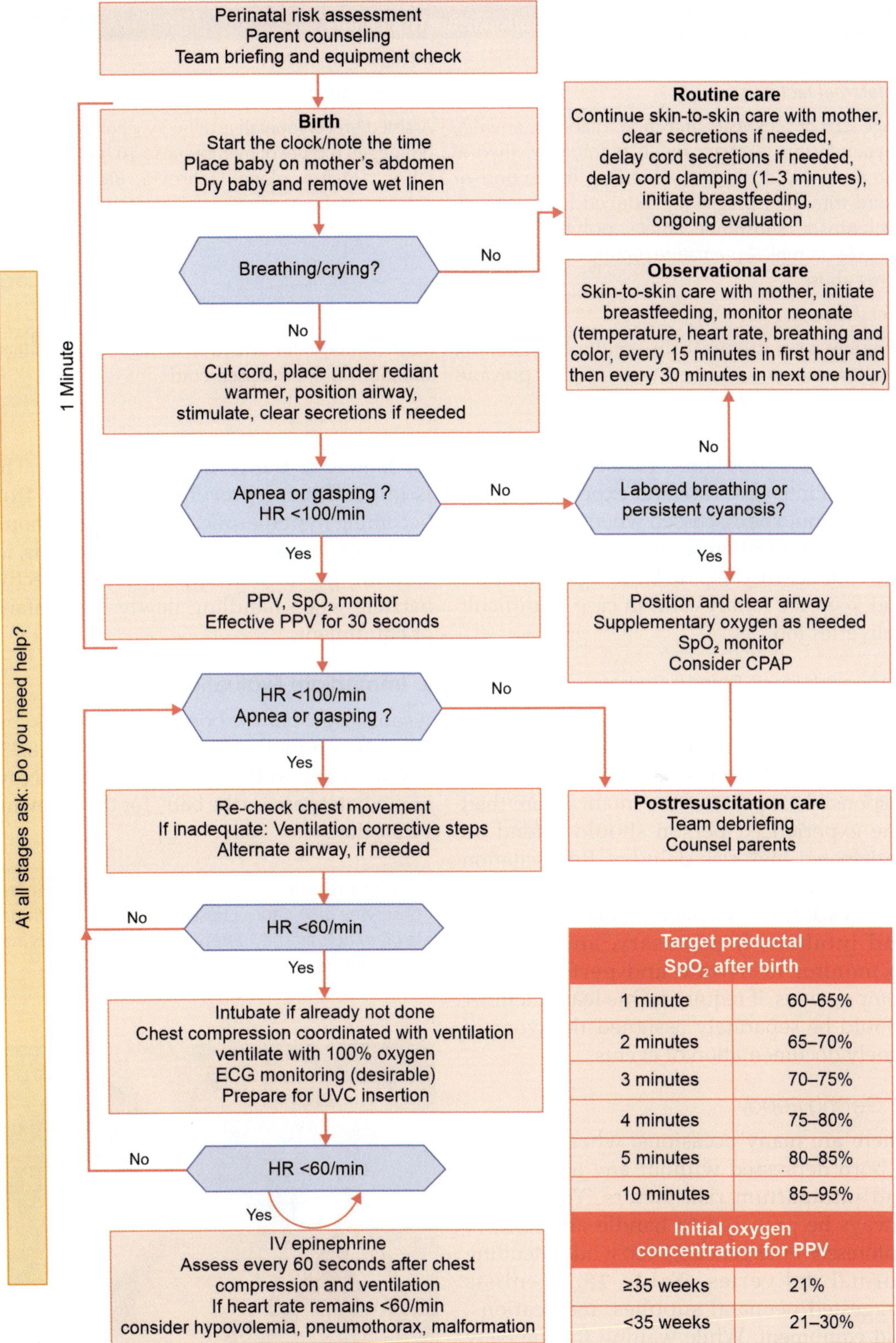

Target preductal SpO_2 after birth	
1 minute	60–65%
2 minutes	65–70%
3 minutes	70–75%
4 minutes	75–80%
5 minutes	80–85%
10 minutes	85–95%
Initial oxygen concentration for PPV	
≥35 weeks	21%
<35 weeks	21–30%

Fig. 18.22: Steps of neonatal resuscitation (*Source:* IAP-NNF Textbook of Neonatal Resuscitation, 2023).

Table 18.20: Important antepartum and intrapartum risk factors

Antepartum factors	Intrapartum factors
Maternal factors	*Maternal factors*
Age <16 or >35 years, infection, diabetes, anemia, hypertension, cardiac, renal, pulmonary, thyroid or neurologic disease, bleeding in second or third trimester, pregnancy-induced hypertension, eclampsia, substance abuse, polyhydramnios, oligohydramnios, premature rupture of membranes, drug abuse	Assisted/breech/operative delivery, chorioamnionitis, prolonged rupture of membranes >18 hrs, prolonged labor >24 hrs, placenta previa, uterine tetany, antepartum hemorrhage
Fetal factors	*Fetal factors*
Preterm or post-term baby, multiple gestation, malformation, diminished fetal activity, previous fetal or neonatal death.	Bradycardia, fetal arrhythmia, meconium-stained amniotic fluid, prolapsed cord

anticipated problems, possible need for neonatal intensive care and expected plan of action should be discussed whenever feasible. The communication should be precise, clear, and concise. This helps to build a good rapport and keep the family calm in case of difficult deliveries too.

2. Availability of Trained Personnel

A person (doctor or a nurse) capable of initiating resuscitation should attend every delivery; at least one such person should be responsible for care of the infant. More than one experienced person should attend an anticipated high-risk delivery. Resuscitation of a severely depressed newly born infant requires at least two persons, one to ventilate and intubate, if necessary, and another to monitor heart rate and perform chest compressions, if required. One team member should be separately assigned the work of timely documentation of events.

3. Getting Ready

There are many occasions, when the baby is born depressed without any antepartum and intrapartum risk factors. You should always be prepared to handle any kind of unforeseen emergencies, even while attending normal deliveries. **Table 18.21** enlists suggested neonatal supplies, medications, and equipment. While waiting for the baby to arrive, set up the resuscitation trolley, and check that all equipment are working and you have everything you might need. Go around and close all the doors and windows and turn off fans near the resuscitation trolley. This is important for preventing the baby from becoming hypothermic. All personnel should follow universal or standard precautions, i.e. wearing gloves and appropriate protective barriers when handling newly born infants or equipment.

B. Immediate Evaluation: 1 Question

A soon as the baby is born, start the clock, put the baby on mother's abdomen **(Fig. 18.23)**, dry the baby and remove wet linen. Now, immediately assess the baby for the following 1 question:

> Is the baby is breathing or crying. This is done by observing the infant's chest movements. Breathing is classified as spontaneous if the baby is crying or having regular effective respiration.

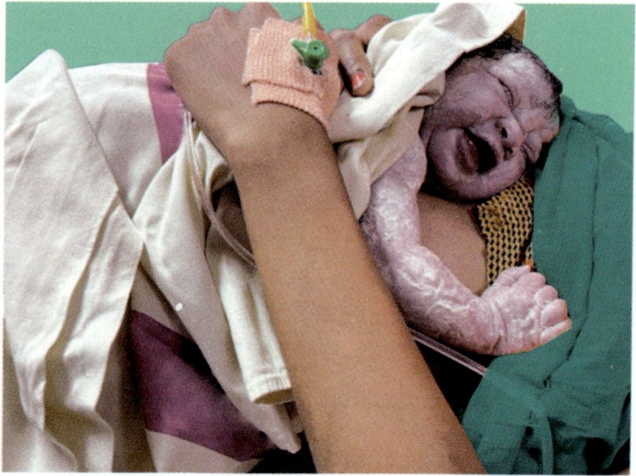

Fig. 18.23: Placing the baby on mother's abdomen. (*Source:* IAP-NNF Textbook of Neonatal Resuscitation 2023).

Table 18.21: A 10-point check-list of neonatal supplies, medications and equipment

1. Turned on *radiant warmer* with prewarmed clean sheets, thermometer (room, digital), plastic wrap for preterms <32 weeks
2. *Flow meter* (up to at least 10 L/min) • *Oxygen source* • *Oxygen blender*/oxygen-air mix (set to 21–30% in preterm, 21% in term).
3. *Airway:* Secretion clearance—suction—turn it on and check that it is producing adequate pressure. Ensure that a suction catheter, size 10 or 12 F is connected. Set the suction pressure at 80–100 mmHg. It is better to have additional manual suction trap/mucus extractor available. To maintain patency—oropharyngeal airway (00,0,1), shoulder roll
4. *Ventilation:* T-piece resuscitator or self-inflating bag along with face mask. Bag and mask equipment consists of a soft self-inflating bag with (i) a blow off pressure valve; (ii) oxygen reservoir/corrugated tube; (iii) facemasks: Soft cushioned for both preterm (size 0 or 00) and term (size 1 or 2) babies; and (iv) oxygen source with flowmeter (up to 10 L/min atleast) and tubing.
5. *Laryngoscope:* A straight blade (size 00, 0, 1) should be fitted; ensure that it works, and the bulb is bright enough. Have a spare bulb and batteries.
6. *Endotracheal tubes* of various sizes (2.5, 3.0, 3.5 and 4.0) should be available. It is better to use blue line neonatal portex tube attached with adaptors. Also ensure that adaptor fits into the bag.
7. *Other tubes:* Infant feeding tube (size 5, 6, 8 F), umbilical catheterization set including umbilical catheter of size 3.5, 4, 5 F.
8. *Drugs:* Adrenaline (1 in 10,000 concentration), normal saline, Ringer lactate.
9. *Syringes* (1, 2, 5, 10, 20, 50 mL), needles, scissors, sterile gauze, and adhesive tapes should be available.
10. *Others:* Cardiac monitor, ECG leads, stopwatch/timer, stethoscope, three-way stopcock, alcohol sponges, povidone iodine, gloves, scalpel blade, forceps, oropharyngeal airway, pulse oximeter with neonatal probe, cord clamp tie, measuring tape, transport incubator, extra batteries, laryngeal mask, if available, end-tidal CO_2 detector, if available

If the Answer is Yes (i.e. baby is crying or having spontaneous respiration)

The baby is good and does not need further steps of resuscitation. This child should be further nursed with the mother by continuing skin-to-skin care by placing the baby prone on mother's abdomen and face-to-one side. Cover the mother and baby with another warm, dry, clean linen. Clear secretions, only if any visible as unnecessary suction can lead to trauma and bradycardia. Conduct a delayed cord clamping (1–3 minutes), cut the cord, and continue ongoing evaluation.

> Delayed cord clamping for at least a minute has been found to have many advantages (improved survival, cardiovascular stability, less risk of anaemia) and hence should be practiced in all vigorous newborns who do not need any resuscitation. Cord milking, however, should be avoided.

- The baby is then shifted between the two breasts and skin-to-skin care continued for at least an hour.
- The mother should be encouraged to breastfeed the baby within this time, as soon as possible.
- An identification tag containing all the required details should be placed on baby's wrist.
- Other things like weighing the baby and giving vitamin K can be done after the first hour.
- *Suction of these babies is not necessary and may produce trauma or bradycardia.*
- Vitamin K is administered 1 mg intramuscularly.

If Answer to the Question is No (i.e. the baby is not breathing or crying)

Proceed to the initial steps of resuscitation; detailed as follows.

C. Initial Steps of Resuscitation

1. Provide Warmth

Receive the baby in a pre-warmed towel in slight Trendelenburg position. DO NOT hang the baby upside down. Place the infant under radiant heat source on a prewarmed mattress (Fig. 18.24). Remove the wet towel or sheet. Maintaining temperature between 36.5°C and 37.4°C in the newly born is vital. Avoid hyper- or hypothermia.

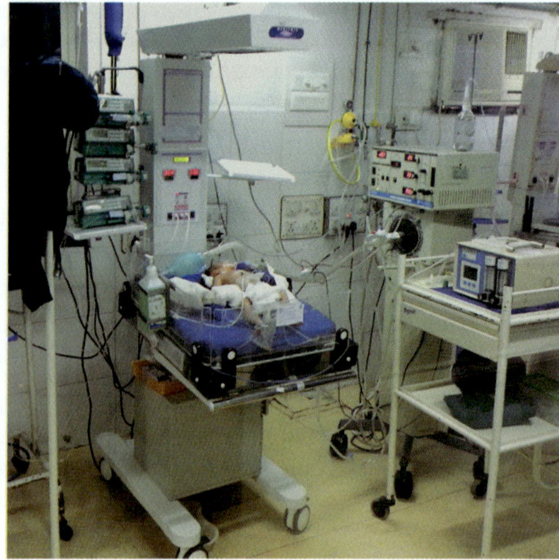

Fig. 18.24: Radiant warmer for placing a newborn.

2. Positioning

Place the newborn supine on a flat surface with neck slightly extended. You can place a shoulder roll (made up of a rolled blanket or towel 3/4–1 inch thick) under the shoulders (Fig. 18.25). If the infant has copious secretions in mouth, then his head may be turned to one side. Do not hang the baby upside down.

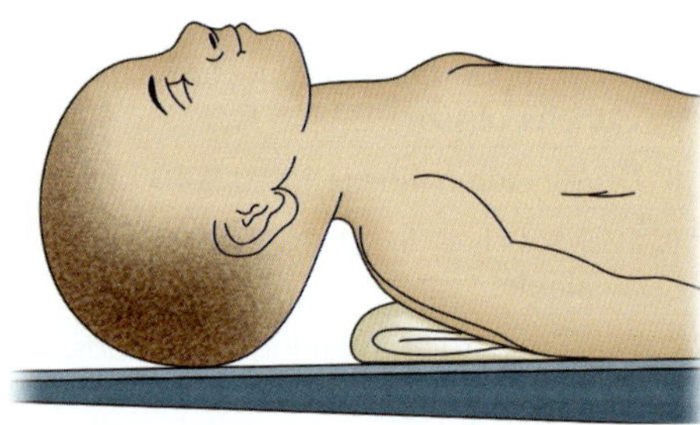

Fig. 18.25: Rolled towel under the shoulders.

3. Providing Tactile Stimulation

Usually drying produces enough stimulation to induce respiration in the newly born. However, if the baby does not have adequate respiration, additional tactile stimulation may be provided by (i) flicking or slapping the soles of feet; or (ii) rubbing the infant's back, trunk, or extremity (Fig. 18.26). Only one or two flicks or rubbing the back once or twice, can initiate breathing.

Caution: Do not keep on providing continuous tactile stimulation after one or two attempts, as you might be losing valuable time. DO NOT employ the following methods of stimulation: Slapping the back, squeezing the ribcage, forcing thighs on abdomen, dilating anal sphincter, or sprinkling hot/cold water on the baby.

4. Clear Airways

Routine suctioning is not needed. Suction should be reserved for babies who have obvious obstruction to spontaneous breathing or who might require positive pressure ventilation

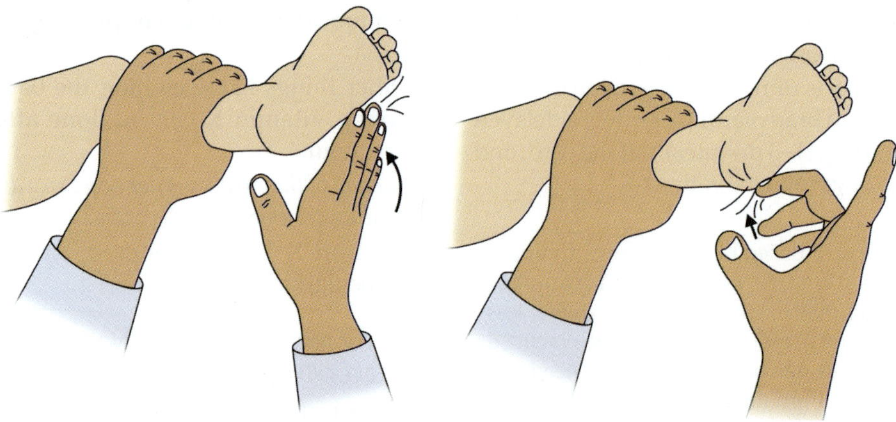

Fig. 18.26: Flicking the sole and heel.

Key Box 10

TABC of Neonatal Resuscitation

T–Maintenance of temperature
1. Provision of radiant heat source
2. Drying the baby
3. Removing wet linen

A–Establish an open airway
1. Position the infant to open the airway
2. Suction the mouth and nose, if required
3. If necessary, insert an ET tube to ensure an open airway

B–Initiate breathing
1. Tactile stimulation to initiate respiration
2. PPV when necessary, using either bag and mask or bag and ET tube

C–Maintain circulation
1. Stimulate and maintain the circulation of blood with:
2. Chest compressions and/or medications

(PPV). It is mandatory that mouth should always be suctioned first followed by nose. Use a suction catheter (size 8 or 10 French) attached to a suction device or use a bulb syringe or DeLee suction trap. Suction should be done gently as stimulation of posterior pharyngeal wall might lead to bradycardia and/or apnea. The negative pressure should not exceed 100 mmHg.

D. Assessment after Initial Steps

Further assessment of the newly born infant is based on heart rate and respiration.

1. Respiration

Check the baby's breathing by watching at the chest movements. If the baby is still not breathing or gasping, start PPV (positive pressure ventilation) with a bag and mask.

2. Heart Rate (HR)

Auscultate the heart or palpate the umbilical pulsations for 6 seconds. Auscultation of the heart at the precordium is the preferred method. Whatever the number of beats, multiply by 10 to obtain heart rate/min (e.g. a count of 11 in 6 seconds is HR of 110/min). If heart rate is less than 100/min, initiate positive pressure ventilation (PPV).

Special scenarios

1. *Meconium in Amniotic Fluid*

Approximately, 10% babies are born with meconium in the amniotic fluid. There is no difference in the steps of neonatal resuscitation for meconium-stained babies, whether vigorous or non-vigorous. Removal of residual meconium in the hypopharynx by suctioning under direct vision using a laryngoscope is NO longer recommended.

2. *Baby is breathing with heart rate>100 beats/minute but cyanosed*

Such babies should be immediately assessed for oxygen saturation. If the oxygen saturation is less than the target range (*see* **Fig 18.22**), the baby should be provided with free flow of oxygen with a mask, T-piece, or flow-inflating device. Humidified oxygen should preferably be given via a blender at a flow rate of 10 L/minute to control the delivered FiO_2. The initiating FiO_2 should be 30%, which may be increased slowly if oxygen saturation of baby remains belong the specified targets. DO NOT USE self-inflating bag to provide free flow oxygen.

3. *Baby has laboured breathing with heart rate >100 beats/minute*

These babies should be supported with continuous positive airway pressure (CPAP), using blended oxygen, delivered via flow-inflating bag or a T-piece resuscitator device.

E. Bag and Mask Ventilation

1. Indications

Bag and mask ventilation is indicated if after tactile stimulation: (i) baby is apneic or gasping or (ii) if the heart rate is below 100 beats/minute. **Figure 18.27** shows parts of a self-inflating bag. **Figure 18.28** shows correct placement of mask over the face.

2. Procedure

- Always use the bag with oxygen reservoir, so as to provide the exact oxygen concentration as titrated.
- Initial inflation pressure of 20 cm H_2O is effective, some babies may require 30–40 cm pressure to open up.
- Place the little and ring fingers of your left hand under baby's chin and with gentle traction slightly extend the neck. This prevents the head from moving around and maintains an open airway.

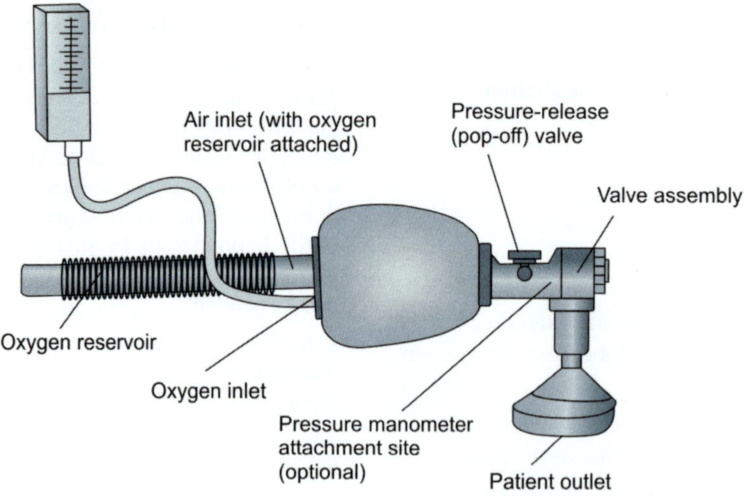

Fig. 18.27: Parts of a self-inflating bag.

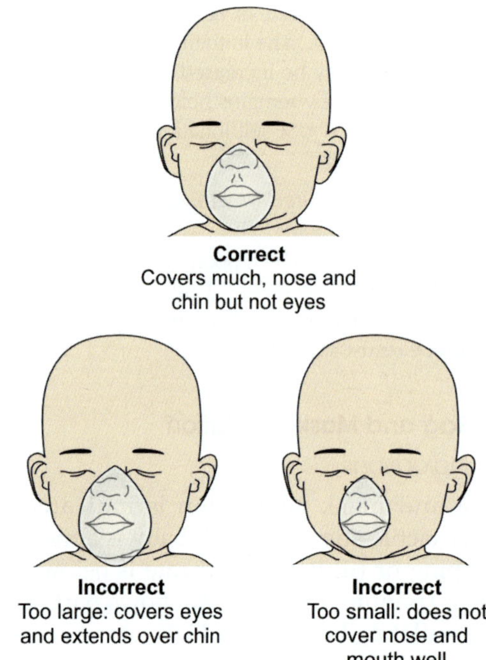

Fig. 18.28: Correct (top) and incorrect (bottom) mask sizes.

- With other fingers and thumb, apply the mask firmly to the baby's face to ensure tight seal. Tight seal is confirmed by when you squeeze the bag and there is a characteristic rasping noise as the valve opens. If the seal is inadequate, the valve makes no noise and you will not feel any resistance when squeezing the bag. This can be practiced with the mask against the palm of your hand.
- Use only thumb and two fingers, rather than whole hand, to squeeze the bag. Do not empty the bag but gently depress it to few centimeters only. The smaller the baby, the gentler you must be.
- The rate should be maintained at 40–60 per minute. Follow a squeeze, one, two-squeeze sequence. The best guide to adequate pressure during bag and mask ventilation is an easy rise and fall of chest with each breath.
- If chest does not rise then reapply mask, reposition infant's head. Check for secretions, check that bag is not leaking. **Figure 18.29** and **Key Box 11** show correct position for giving bag and mask ventilation.
- Once PPV is started, ensure simultaneous assessment of heart rate, respiration, and SpO_2.
- If the bag and mask ventilation is used for more than 2 minutes, insert a nasogastric tube in the stomach and aspirate with a syringe, and leave the end open to decompress so that respiration is not compromised due to distension of stomach.

3. Other Devices for PPV

T-piece resuscitator: It comes either as in-built with the warmer **(Fig. 18.30a)** or as a separate device **(Fig. 18.30b)**. It uses compressed gas for inflation. The cap of the T-piece has an opening which is regulated by the operator to produce inflation, done by intermittently occluding the

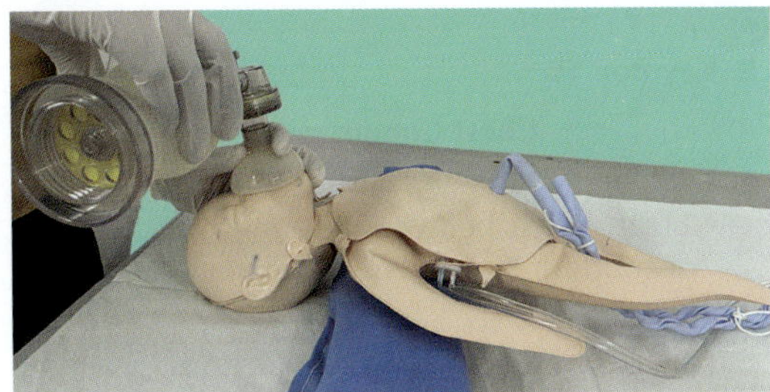

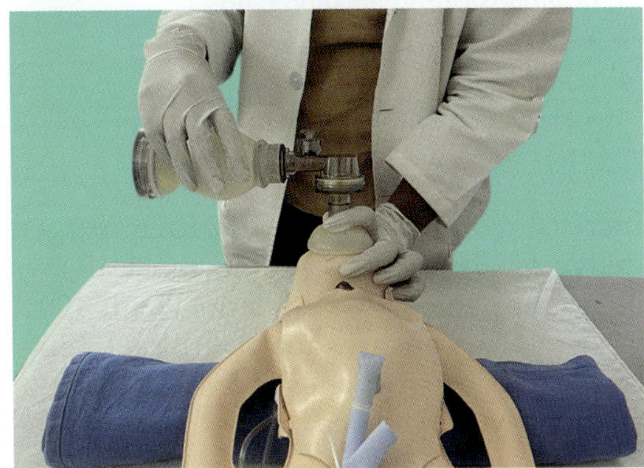

Fig. 18.29: Giving bag and mask ventilation.

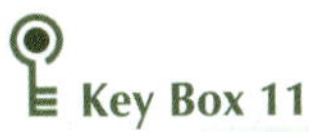

Key Box 11

Bag and Mask Ventilation

When to begin

1. Baby is apneic or gasping
2. Heart rate is below 100 /min

Rate

1. 40–60 per minute, when given alone

When to stop

1. Baby is having spontaneous respiration
2. Heart rate is more than 100/min

opening. Peak inspiratory pressure (PIP) and positive end-expiratory pressure (PEEP) can be delivered by this method.

Flow-inflating bag: This device also works when attached to a source of compressed gas. The pressure delivery can be controlled by the operator with the help of an attached manometer. This device can also provide PEEP (Fig. 18.31).

4. Oxygenation

As per the latest IAP and NNF guidelines 2023, positive pressure ventilation need not be started at 100% oxygen for all children.

For term and late preterm babies (≥35 weeks), start resuscitation at room air.

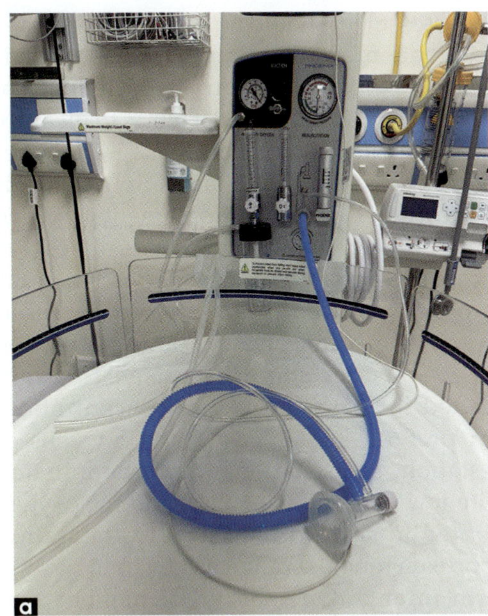

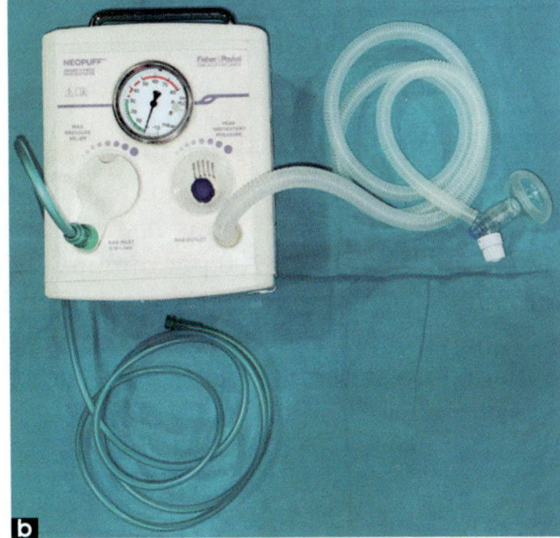

Fig. 18.30: T-piece resuscitator with oxygen blender (a) and T-piece resuscitator (b). *Courtesy:* Sweta Kumari, Piyush Gupta

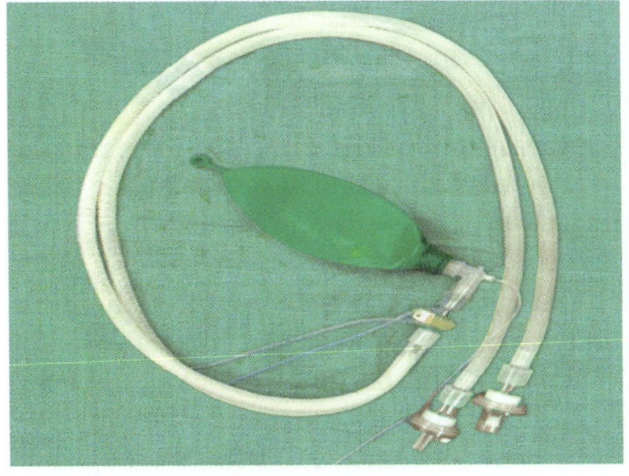

Fig. 18.31: Flow inflating bag. (*Source:* IAP-NNF Textbook of Neonatal Resuscitation 2023)

The assessment should be based on heart rate, oxygenation, and respiration. Oxygenation is assessed by pulse oximetry. Attach neonatal probe to right hand or wrist (so as to measure pre-ductal saturation). It may take 1–2 minutes for tracing to come. The target SpO_2 range is as shown in Fig. 18.22. Supplemental oxygen should be started after 30 seconds of positive pressure ventilation resuscitation. Increase in oxygen concentration should be based on pulse oximetry and the target saturation range. Blender should be used to attain graded increase in oxygen concentration. For preterm babies less than 35 weeks of gestation, resuscitation should be initiated with low oxygen (21 to 30%) and the oxygen titrated to achieve preductal O_2 saturation approximating the range achieved in healthy term infants. One should remember that pulse oximetry should not be a replacement to clinical assessment.

5. Evaluation

After the infant has received 30 seconds of ventilation, check the spontaneous respiration and heart rate. If spontaneous respiration is present and heart rate >100 per minute, PPV is discontinued. If spontaneous respiration is inadequate or heart rate is <100 bpm, assisted ventilation must continue. *If heart rate is <60 bpm, continue positive pressure ventilation and begin chest compression.*

> Effectiveness of resuscitation can be assessed by: 1. Heart rate; 2.Pulse oximetry; and 3. Respiration. Increase in heart rate is the most sensitive indicator of resuscitation efficacy.

F. Chest Compression (Key Box 12)

Chest compressions consist of rhythmic compressions of the sternum pressing the heart against the spine. It results in rise of the intrathoracic pressure and circulation of blood to the vital body organs.

The heart circulates blood throughout the body and delivers oxygen to vital organs. When an infant becomes hypoxic, the heart rate slows and myocardial contractility decreases. As a result, there is a diminished flow of blood and oxygen to the vital organs. Chest compressions are used to temporarily increase circulation and improve oxygen delivery. Chest compressions must always be accompanied by ventilation with 100% oxygen. This ensures that the blood being circulated during chest compressions is adequately oxygenated.

Key Box 12

Chest Compression

1. *When to begin*
   - Heart rate is below 60 beat/min after 15–30 seconds of bag and mask ventilation.
2. *Rate*
   - 90 per minute, with 30 ventilations
3. *Compression:* Ventilation ratio
   - 3:1.
4. *When to stop*
   - Heart rate is more than 60/min.

1. Indications

Chest compression is indicated, if the heart rate is below 60 bpm or absent, even after 30 seconds of PPV. Use 100% oxygen, for PPV whenever chest compressions are provided. Endotracheal intubation should be done at this stage, if expertise is available. Once the heart rate is more than 60 beats/min, stop chest compression.

2. Procedure

There are two techniques of chest compression: (a) thumb technique and (b) two-finger technique.

- With the *thumb technique*, the two thumbs are used to depress the sternum, with hand encircling the chest and fingers supporting the back (Fig. 18.32). Thumb technique achieves higher perfusion pressure and is now the recommended method, preferred over two-finger technique.
- With the *two-finger technique*, the tips of the middle finger and either the index finger or ring finger of one hand are used to compress the sternum. This is **no longer recommended.**
- The pressure is applied to the lower third of the sternum (just below an imaginary horizontal line joining two nipples).
- With the finger placed on sternum, there should be enough pressure to depress

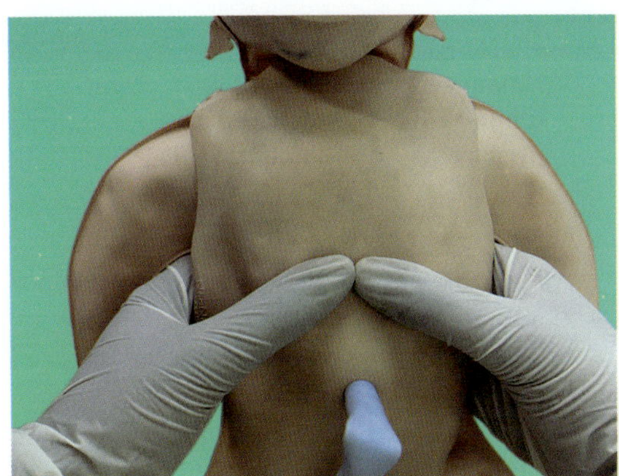

Fig. 18.32: Cardiac compressions

the sternum by one-third of the anterior-posterior diameter of the chest.

3. Rate

Compression is done at the rate of 90 per minute. One ventilation should follow every third chest compression. Thus, in one minute, 90 chest compressions and 30 positive pressure breaths are administered, in a ratio of 3:1.

- Do not remove your thumb or fingers off the chest wall in-between compressions.

Caution: Improper chest compressions may result in broken ribs, lacerations of liver and pneumothorax.

4. Evaluation

Check the heart rate again after 60 seconds of chest compressions. Heart rate response to cardiac compressions should preferably monitored with ECG whenever possible. The heart rate can be less or more than 60 per minute.

If HR is more than 60 per min: Discontinue chest compression, but continue ventilation, till the heart rate is above 100/min and infant is breathing spontaneously.

If HR below 60 per min: Continue chest compression and positive pressure ventilation with bag and mask or bag and tube ventilation with 100% oxygen. In addition, start medications as follows.

G. Medications

Medications are rarely needed for neonatal resuscitation. Medications useful in resuscitation are—epinephrine (adrenaline) and volume expanders (normal saline or Ringer's lactate). Medications like sodium bicarbonate, atropine, dexamethasone, calcium, mannitol, and dextrose are not indicated for resuscitation in the delivery area.

1. Indications

- Initiate drugs, if the heart rate remains below 60 despite adequate ventilation with 100% oxygen and chest compression.
- *Adrenaline* is the first drug to be used preferably via intravenous route. It can be repeated every 5 minutes till the heart rate rises above 100/min. If the response is not adequate, consider *volume expanders*.
- *Volume expanders* are indicated, if child is pale or has signs of hypovolemia, such as poor pulses or a capillary filling time of more than 3 seconds, or if the heart rate is not responding to other measures. The dose can be repeated twice.
- *Naloxone* is no more indicated in labor room. The focus should be on effective ventilation.
- *Sodium bicarbonate:* There is no evidence to recommend sodium bicarbonate routinely for treatment of post resuscitation metabolic acidosis in newborns. This may worsen the acidosis, if ventilation is not established. Sodium bicarbonate may improve the pH but interferes with other acid buffer systems in the body. Intraventricular hemorrhage is a potential complication if sodium bicarbonate is administered rapidly.

Dosages of different medications are given in **Table 18.22**.

2. Route of Medication

Umbilical vein is the preferred route for intravenous administration. For umbilical venous catheterization, 4 or 5 Fr umbilical catheter (or a feeding tube) is inserted into the umbilical vein, such that the tip is just inside skin surface, and there is free flow of blood. There is lack of evidence for endotracheal administration of adrenaline. It can be tried (0.1 mg per kg) till IV access is achieved.

H. Endotracheal (ET) Intubation

ET intubation is required in only a few cases. The indications are:

Table 18.22: Dosages of medications used in neonatal resuscitation

Medication	Available form	Concentration to be administered	Route	Amount to dilute and prepare	Dose of the prepared solution	Rate
Adrenaline	1 : 1000	1 : 10000 (i.e. diluted × 10)	IV, IT, SC	0.5 mL in 5 mL	0.1 mL/kg to 0.3 mL/kg	Rapid
Volume expanders	Normal saline, Ringer's lactate, or whole blood		IV	40 mL in infusion set or multiple syringes	10 mL/kg	5–10 min

IV: intravenous, IT: intratracheal, IM: intramuscular, SC: subcutaneous.

1. When bag and mask ventilation is ineffective or prolonged.
2. When chest compressions are performed.
3. When diaphragmatic hernia is suspected.

A laryngeal mask may be considered as an alternative to tracheal intubation, if tracheal intubation is not feasible or not successful. Laryngeal mask airway can also be considered when there is problem in placement of mask as in orofacial anomalies. The device is preferred in babies > 34 weeks. Spontaneously breathing preterm infants with respiratory distress may be supported with CPAP initially, rather than routine intubation for PPV.

The tube should be of non-irritating material, of uniform diameter, have vocal cord guide and centimeter markings. The size of tube varies according to weight and gestational age of the baby as shown below:

Tube size (mm)	Weight (g)	Gestational age (wks)
2.5	<1000	<28
3.0	1000–2000	28–34
3.5	2000–3000	34–38
4.0	>3000	>38

A neonatal laryngoscope is required. Straight blades of sizes '0' (pre-term) and '1' (term) should be available. Intubation is not difficult, if you understand the process (Fig. 18.33).

Indicators of correct placement of endotracheal tube include condensation in ET tube, chest movement, and presence of breath sounds bilaterally. Exhaled CO_2 detection is recommended for confimation of ET tube placement.

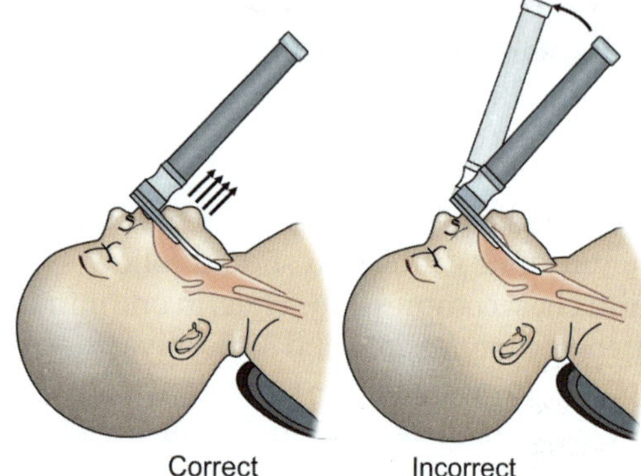

Fig. 18.33: Direction of pull on the laryngoscope.

If done forcefully, you might injure the soft tissues or sometimes reflex bradycardia may be induced. Remember that during the intubation the infant is not getting any oxygen, so if you have difficulty, stop after 20 seconds, give oxygen by bag and mask for 30 seconds, and then try to reintubate.

18.11 PEDIATRIC BASIC LIFE SUPPORT (BLS)

A. Aims of Basic Life Support

Pediatric basic life support aims at understanding the basic steps of cardiopulmonary resuscitation (CPR) (**Key Box 13**). Pediatric advanced life support aims at prevention of pediatric injury and avoidance of pediatric cardiac arrest through early recognition and prompt appropriate treatment of respiratory failure or shock.

Pediatric chain of survival illustrates a sequence of critical interventions to prevent death of children. It consists of four main series of links:

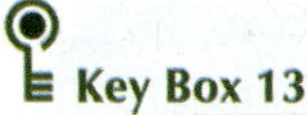

Key Box 13

ABCD of Basic Life Support

1. Airway
2. Breathing
3. Circulation
4. Defibrillation

1. Prevention of injury or cardiac arrest.
2. Early recognition of cardiac arrest and effective high quality CPR.
3. Early activation of emergency medical services (EMS).
4. Prompt pediatric advanced life support including stabilization, transport, and post-resuscitation care.

B. Steps of Basic Life Support (BLS) for Healthcare Providers

1. Check for Response

Assess the victim for a response by tapping the shoulder of victim and shout "are you all right?" If there is no response, check for breathing. The evaluation should take at least 5 seconds but not more than 10 seconds. If there is no response and no breathing or gasping, shout for help. Send someone to activate the EMS and get the defibrillator/AED.

2. Check for Pulse

If the child is not breathing or gasping, check for pulse. This should take not more than 10 seconds. In infants, check the brachial pulse; and carotid pulse in children.

3. Inadequate Breathing with Pulse

If there is a palpable pulse ≥60/min, start rescue breaths at 12–20 breaths per minute (1 breath every 3–5 seconds). Continue ventilation till spontaneous breathing resumes. Check pulse every two minutes (not taking more than 10 seconds).

4. No Pulse or Bradycardia with Poor Perfusion

If there is no pulse or pulse is less than 60 per minute with poor perfusion, begin chest compressions with high quality CPR.

5. Chest Compression

The 2015 AHA guidelines for CPR recommend a change in the CPR sequence from A-B-C to C-A-B. For a lone rescuer, begin 30 compressions and 2 breaths. For 2 rescuers, give 15 compressions and 2 breaths. The rescuer should ensure that high quality CPR is given. This includes:

- ***Correct comppression finger placement:*** For a child, the fingers should be placed correctly over lower half of the sternum. In infants, place the fingers just below the intermammary line. Do not compress on the ribs or xiphoid process.
- ***Adequate rate:*** At least 100/min (deliver each set of 30 compressions in less than 18 seconds). Push hard and push fast.
- ***Adequate depth:*** Deliver compressions at least one-third of the depth of the sternum (i.e. approximately 4 cm in infants and 5 cm in children).
- ***Complete recoil:*** Allow complete chest recoil after each compression, but ensure not to lift the fingers at any time.
- ***Minimize interruptions:*** Minimize interruptions in between chest compressions. Give 2 breaths in less than 10 seconds. After 2 minutes of CPR with two rescuers, the rescuers should change position, not taking more than 5 seconds.

6. Ventilation

After 30 compressions (15 compressions by two rescuers), open the airway to give 2 breaths. The airway is opened with a head tilt-chin lift maneuver. In cases of cervical spine injury, the above maneuver is avoided and jaw-thrust maneuver is used.

i. ***Head tilt-chin lift:*** The neck is slightly extended and the head is tilted to place it into a neutral position by placing one hand on to the child's forehead. Index finger of the other hand (NOT THUMB) is placed under the chin to lift the mandible up and outward **(Fig. 18.34)**.

ii. ***Jaw thrust:*** It is used for victims of neck injury and can be accomplished without extending the neck. Fingers of each hand are placed under the sides of lower jaw to lift it up and outward **(Fig. 18.35)**.

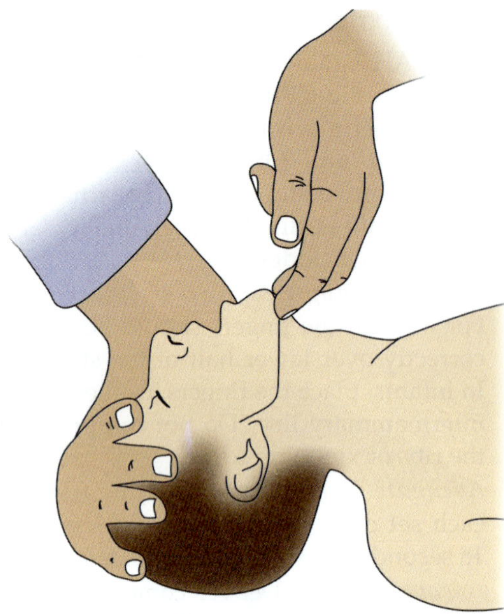

Fig. 18.34: Head tilt-chin lift maneuver.

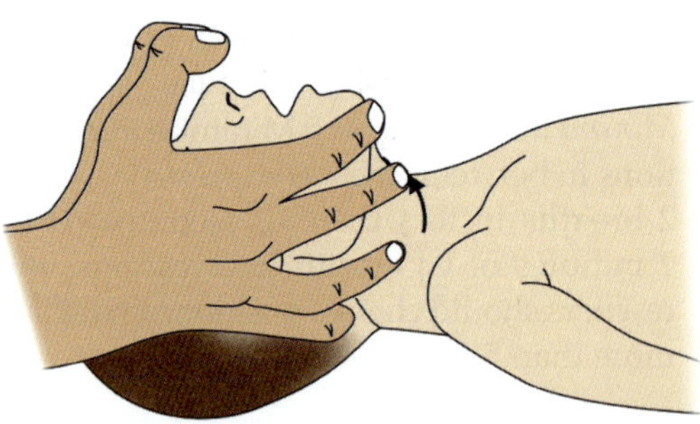

Fig. 18.35: Jaw-thrust maneuver.

Remove any vomitus or foreign body, if visible. Do not close the mouth.

The breaths can be given by mouth-to-mouth breathing, mouth to barrier device breathing, mouth to mask breathing, or bag and mask breathing.

Mouth-to-mouth ventilation: Place your mouth over the mouth and nose (in case of an infant) and over the mouth only in an older child. Create a seal. Pinch the nose in case of an older child. Give two breaths (1 second per breath) (Fig. 18.36).

The correct volume for breath is assessed by adequacy of chest rise. If rescue breathing fails to produce chest expansion despite attempts at opening of the airway, suspect a foreign body airway obstruction.

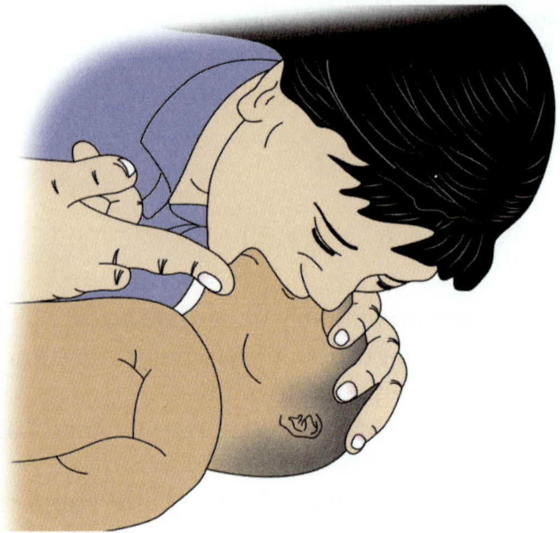

Fig. 18.36: Mouth-to-mouth breathing.

7. Defibrillation/Automated Electrical Defibrillator (AED)

After 5 cycles of compression and ventilation, if defibrillator has arrived, attach the defibrillator and check the rhythm, if it is shockable or not. In a pulseless child, ventricular fibrillation and ventricular tachycardia without pulse are the two shockable rhythms. If a manual defibrillator is used, 2 J/kg is the recommended first energy dose. The second energy dose is 4 J/kg. If a manual defibrillator is not available, an AED equipped with pediatric attenuator is preferred in children <8 years of age. If that is not available, an AED without a dose attenuator may be used. If shockable, give one shock and resume the CPR immediately. Check the rhythm and pulse after every 5 cycles and continue till advanced life support providers take over or the victim starts moving.

Figure 18.37 summarizes the American Heart Association guideline algorithm on pediatric basic life support.

18.12 REMOVAL OF FOREIGN BODY

A. Recognition of Airway Obstruction

Early recognition of airway obstruction is essential for initiation of active intervention and successful outcome. American Heart Association (AHA) has laid down guidelines for health care professionals for identification and management of foreign body obstruction in infants and children.

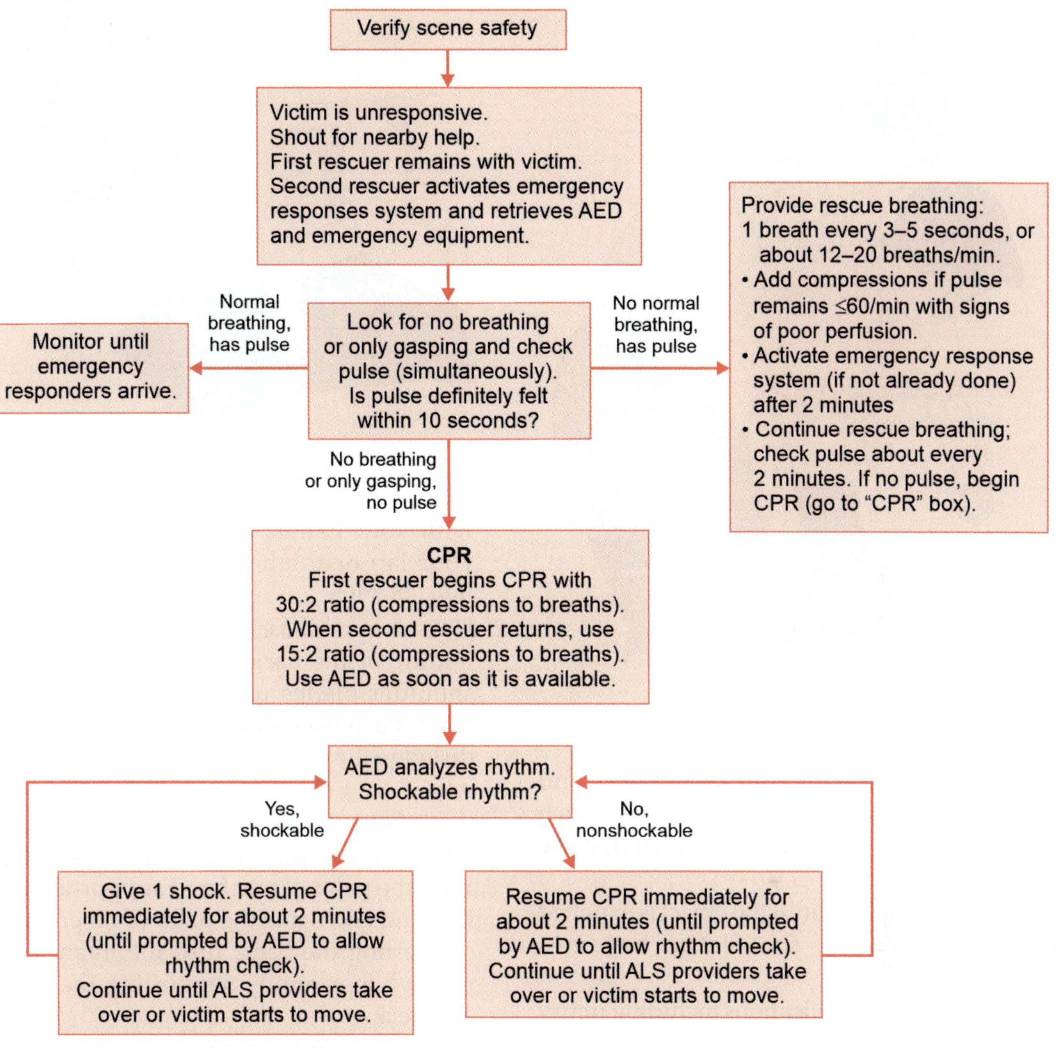

Fig. 18.37: American Heart Association algorithm for pediatric basic life support (BLS) with two rescuers.

The airway obstruction can be *mild* or *severe*.

1. Mild Obstruction

A child who is responsive and could cough forcefully, with a good air entry and occasional wheeze between the cough is apparently having *mild airway obstruction*.

2. Severe Obstruction

A child with *severe airway obstruction* would present with weak and ineffective cough, inability to speak, high-pitched noise, respiratory distress, possible cyanosis, poor or no air exchange. A choking child can indicate his symptoms by clutching the neck with thumbs and fingers making *universal choking sign*.

Heimlich maneuver is used for relief of obstruction, if foreign body is witnessed or strongly suspected and the child presents with *severe airway obstruction*. Do not attempt Heimlich maneuver in children with mild airway obstruction.

B. Heimlich Maneuver

1. This maneuver consists of abdominal thrust delivered to relieve choking in responsive and conscious adults and children.
2. Stand behind the victim and wrap your arms around the victim's waist.
3. Make a fist with one hand with the thumb side of your fist against the victim's abdomen. It must be placed between the xiphisternum and umbilicus (Fig. 18.38).

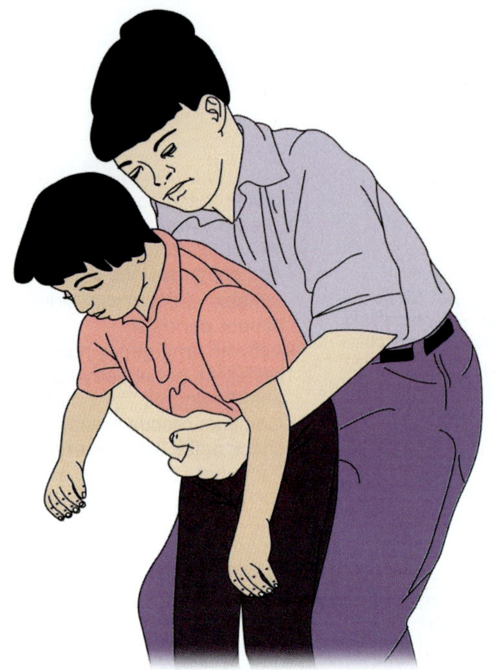
Fig. 18.38: Heimlich maneuver.

4. Grasp the fist with your other hand, and press upwards and inwards quickly. Each thrust must be intended to dislodge the foreign body.
5. Repeat the thrust until the object is expelled from airway or the victim becomes unresponsive.
6. Examine for complications including injury to abdominal organs.
7. If the victim is unresponsive, activate the emergency medical services (EMS), and open the mouth and look and remove the foreign body, if visible. Do not blindly sweep the finger inside the mouth as it might push the body further inside.
8. Initiate the cardiopulmonary resuscitation (CPR) as described in the previous section. After every 5 cycles of CPR, open the airway and look for the foreign body.

Attempt to give 2 breaths and continue with cycles of chest compressions and ventilation till the foreign body is expelled.

C. Relief of Choking in Infants: Back Slaps and Chest Thrusts

1. In responsive infants, hold the infant along the length of your forearm in prone position with infant's head and jaw being supported with your hands. Rest your forearm on your lap or thigh to support the infant (Fig. 18.39).

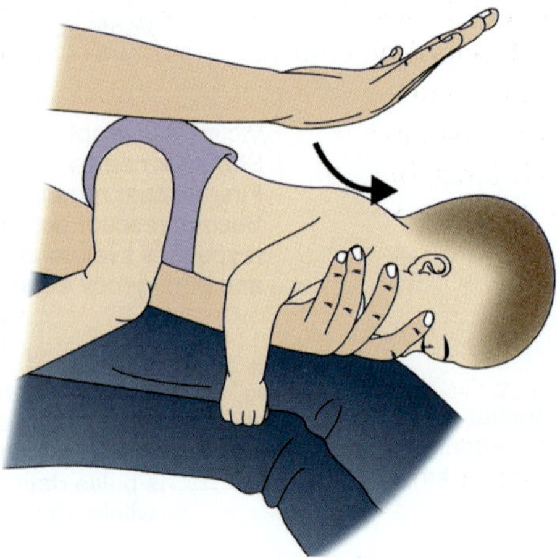
Fig. 18.39: Back blows.

2. Deliver up to 5 *back slaps* forcefully in the middle of the back between the infant's shoulder blades using the heel of your hand. Each back slap must be intended to dislodge the foreign body.
3. After 5 back slaps, place your free hand on the infant's back, supporting the back of infant's head with the palm of your hand. With the palm of one hand supporting the face and jaw while the palm of other hand supporting the back, turn the infant as a unit while carefully supporting the head and neck.
4. Keep the infant's head lower than chest. Give up to 5 quick *chest thrusts* with your hand just below the nipple line at a rate of 1 per second. Each chest thrust must intend to dislodge the foreign body (Fig. 18.40).

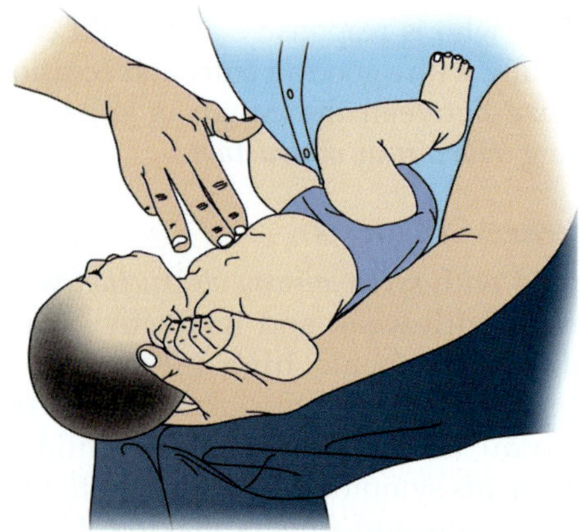
Fig. 18.40: Chest thrusts.

5. Repeat 5 back slaps and 5 chest thrusts till the foreign bodies are expelled or the victim becomes unconscious.
6. In unresponsive infants, perform CPR as in infants, but at the end of every 5 cycles of CPR, open the airway and look for the foreign body and remove it.

18.13 URINARY PROCEDURES

A. Urine Collection

Urine collection for microscopy, culture, and a variety of other tests is done by urine bag collection in small children (vide supra) and by clean-catch collection in older children. The latter method can only be used in toilet trained children who can understand and follow the instructions regarding collection of a midstream sample, otherwise the parents may be instructed to do the collection. The procedure is described in **Table 18.23**. The urine sample should be immediately transported to the laboratory. Cultures of samples collected from urine bag are less reliable. In young infants, suprapubic aspiration may be done to collect urine samples without any contamination from the urinary tract.

B. Bladder Catheterization

Prepare the instruments: Foley's catheter **(Table 18.24)**, lignocaine jelly, gloves, syringe

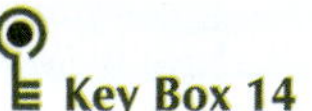

Key Box 14

Indications of Urinary Bladder Catheterization

1. Drainage of bladder in case of retention of urine secondary to obstruction.
2. Drainage of bladder following major pelvic or rectal surgeries.
3. To document urinary output in critically ill children.
4. To obtain urine sample for culture examination.

with water to inflate the balloon and urinary bag for collection.

Explain the procedure to the parents and the child. Indications are listed in **Key Box 14**.

For Male Catheterization

1. Make the child lie straight on his back.
2. Under all aseptic precautions, gently retract the foreskin with a sterile swab with the non-dominant hand. Using the dominant hand, clean the glans with povidone iodine.
3. Lubricate the end of urinary catheter with lignocaine jelly to facilitate its entry.
4. If required, anesthetic gel can be instilled into the urethra and penis squeezed for 3–5 minutes. Hold the penis firmly at the base and gently insert the lubricated end of the catheter in a sterile manner. Keep on inserting the catheter till some resistance is

Table 18.23: Collecting urine sample for culture

Action	Rationale
For Male Child	
1. Instruct child to pull back foreskin and clean the meatus 3 times using different gauze each time.	To ensure that there is no contamination with normal flora of the meatus.
2. Ask the child to pass some urine into the toilet, stop the flow, and then pass some into the sterile container, which should be then capped immediately.	To ensure that a midstream sample is collected as the initial part of the sample may be contaminated.
For Female Child	
1. Ask child to sit on the toilet seat with legs as far apart as possible. Instruct child to spread labia with fingers and wipe each side with separate gauze using a front-to-back stroke. The third wipe should be to clean the meatus with same front-to-back motion.	To reduce contamination. The front-to-back stroke is applied to avoid contamination with perianal flora.
2. Ask child to pass some urine into the toilet, stop the flow, and then pass some into the container, which should be capped immediately.	To ensure that a midstream sample is collected.

Table 18.24: Appropriate size of urinary catheter

Age group	Males	Females
Infant (<1 yr)	8–10 Fr	5–8 Fr
1–3 yr	10–12 Fr	8–10 Fr
3–12 yrs	12–14 Fr	10–12 Fr

felt. This is the site of bladder neck. Rotate the catheter slightly between fingers and thumbs till the sphincter relaxes and the catheter moves in freely ahead. Urine starts flowing out of the catheter outlet which should be connected to urinary drainage bag.

5. Once catheterization is completed, pull back the foreskin.

For Female Catheterization

1. Make the child lie down on her back with legs far apart.
2. Separate labia firmly with non-dominant hand and locate the urethral meatus.
3. Clean the urethral meatus by downward stroke only.
4. Lubricate the catheter with lignocaine gel and gently insert the catheter till urine starts flowing into the catheter bag.

Both for Male and Female Catheterization

1. Continue inserting the catheter till it reaches the Y junction.
2. Inflate the balloon of the catheter with 2–3 mL sterile water and gently pull the bulb till the bladder neck. Ensure that the balloon is not inflated when the catheter is in urethra; it might result in urethral rupture.
3. Secure the catheter and maintain local asepsis by cleaning the catheter and surroundings by soap and water or by povidone iodine.
4. Empty the drainage bag regularly at least every 24 hrs. Place the urine bag below the level of bladder but nerver touching the floor.
5. Replace the catheter, if visibly dirty or clogged, or there is a peritubal leakage.
6. While removing the catheter, deflate the balloon and then gently remove the catheter to avoid any urethral injury.
7. Beware of the complications which include urinary infection, urethral injury and subsequent stricture formation, hematuria, bladder stones, or blockage resulting in urinary retention and latex allergy.

C. Suprapubic Bladder Aspiration

Suprapubic bladder aspiration is the most reliable method for obtaining urine for culture in a newborn and children less than 2 years, as the bladder is primarily intra-abdominal in this age group.

1. The child is placed supine and restrained with help of an assistant.
2. Site of aspiration is 1–2 cm above the symphysis pubis in the midline.
3. Ensure that the bladder is full by checking that infant's diaper has been dry for last 1 hour. The fullness of bladder can also be confirmed by palpating or percussing the bladder.
4. Clean the area with spirit, povidone iodine, followed by spirit. Drape with sterile linen.
5. Under sterile aspesis, palpate the symphysis pubis and insert the needle 1–2 cm above the symphysis in the midline. The needle is inserted perpendicular to skin angling 10–20° cephalad and advancing it through the skin under negative pressure throughout.
6. Entry into bladder is indicated by return of urine in the syringe. If no urine is obtained, angle the needle more perpendicular but avoid excessive poking.
7. Do not insert beyond 2.5 cm. If still there is no urine, try it after sometime or try other method, like catheterization.

Complications include abdominal wall abscess, persistent hematuria, and intestinal perforation/peritonitis.

18.14 LUMBAR PUNCTURE

Indications of lumbar puncture are listed in **Key Box 15**.

A. Positioning

The child should be placed in a lateral recumbent posture with the neck flexed, knees drawn upward towards the abdomen (*fetal posture*), and the back placed to the edge of the table as shown in **Fig. 18.41**.

An alternative position is with child sitting and bending forward as shown in **Fig. 18.42**.

Key Box 15

Lumbar Puncture: Indications

Indications

1. To diagnose CNS infection (meningitis, encephalitis)
2. To monitor the efficacy of treatment in presence of CNS infection
3. To diagnose subarachnoid hemorrhage
4. To diagnose CNS involvement in leukemia
5. Evaluation of demyelinating, degenerative, and collagen vascular diseases
6. To inject chemotherapeutic agent (methotrexate, cytarabine) and immunoglobulins (tetanus immunoglobulin)
7. To instill contrast material for myelography

Contraindications

1. Uncorrected bleeding diathesis
2. Moribund sick patient with cardiovascular instability
3. Gross lumbosacral anomaly
4. Infection in the skin or underlying tissue at the puncture site
5. Glasgow Coma Scale <8
6. Unequal pupils, tonic posturing, abnormal breathing pattern. All of them may be the initial manifestation of impending cerebral herniation
7. Thrombocytopenia
8. Uncontrolled seizures
9. Focal neurological signs
10. Papilledema in fundus

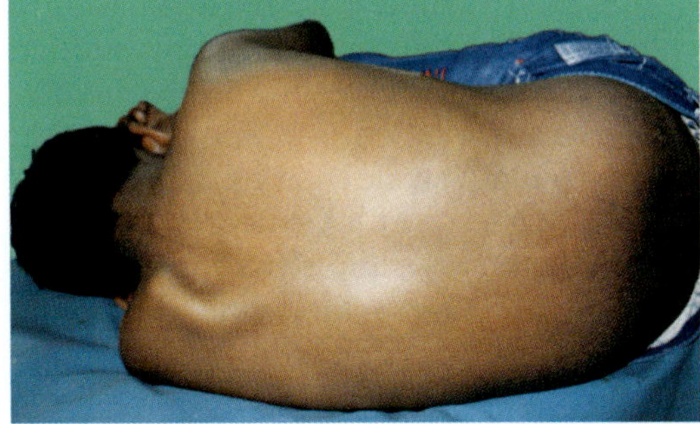

Fig. 18.41: Lateral positioning for lumbar puncture.

This method is recommended in case of suspected cervical spine fracture where the former posture could not be adopted.

B. Site of Lumbar Puncture

Lumbar puncture is done at the intersection of an imaginary line drawn joining the superior

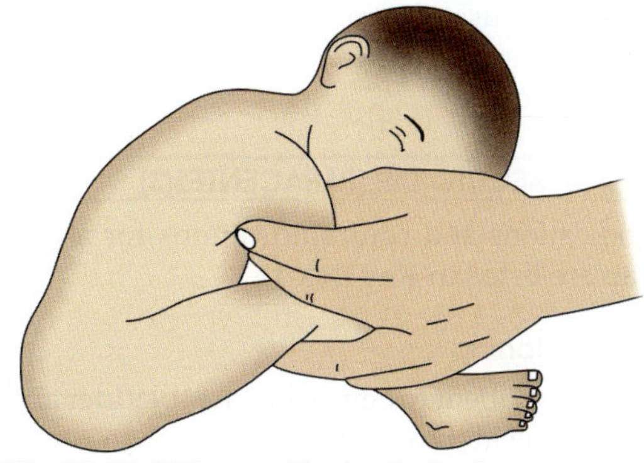

Fig. 18.42: Sitting positioning for lumbar puncture.

portion of iliac crest with the spinous process (L4). It is usually done at the level of L3–L4 or L4–L5 interspace.

C. Procedure

1. Perform a fundus examination to rule out features of raised intracranial pressure. Neuroimaging should be done prior to lumbar puncture.
2. Identify the desired site of lumbar puncture; clean the area with spirit, povidone-iodine followed by spirit. Drape the area with sterile linen.
3. Skin and underlying tissue may be anesthetized with a local anesthetic.
4. The spinal needle (22 G needle, 1–2 inch long with stylet) is introduced gently perpendicular to back aimed towards umbilicus and directed slightly cephalad. A sudden loss of resistance or *give in* will be felt as the needle penetrates the dura mater.
5. Stylet is removed to check and collect CSF for estimation of protein, sugar, cell count, Gram staining, and culture.
6. Instruct the parents to keep the child in horizontal position, to avoid post-lumbar puncture headache.

D. Complications

These include cardiorespiratory arrest, if the child is held very tight with subsequent respiratory arrest and impaired venous return. Raised intracranial tension may cause transtentorial or cerebellar herniation. Other complications include post-lumbar puncture headache, introduction of infection during the procedure, and spinal cord hematoma. Intraspinal dermoid formation is reported following use of spinal needle without stylet as it tends to introduce the epidermis into the spinal canal.

18.15 ASCITIC TAP (PARACENTESIS)

Indications and contraindications for ascitic tap are listed in **Key Box 16**.

A. Positioning

Ask the patient to empty his/her bladder and lie supine in the couch.

B. Site of Aspiration

Ascitic tap can be done in 2 positions:

- Child with large ascites can lie supine with head end elevated to 30–45°.
- Those children with less ascites are preferred to lie in lateral decubitus position.

The site of insertion also varies.

Enter 2 cm below the umbilicus in midline where the fascia of the rectus abdominis join the linea alba to become avascular, thin, and fibrous. If the fluid is less, this method is not preferred. At some places, it is avoided to decrease the risk of bowel and bladder injury. Sometimes the region may not be avascular as expected and can lead to bleeding by injuring the vessels extending down.

The other site is lateral to rectus sheath of muscles, to prevent injury to epigastric vessels, midway between anterior superior iliac spine and umbilicus (Fig. 18.43). In this, the needle is inserted in mild lateral decubitus position on the dependent side.

An ultrasound scan, if available, should be done before and the point for paracentesis should be marked. Besides, it helps to know the distance between the skin and the fluid which is generally 1 cm and also the distance to the mid-point of the collection which is usually 3 cm.

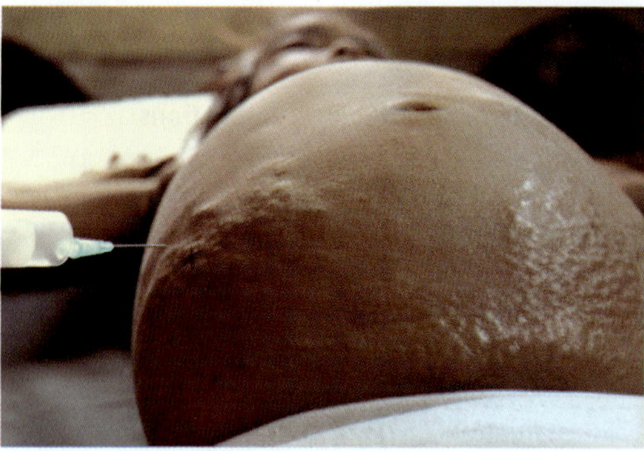

Fig. 18.43: Ascitic tap.

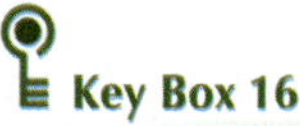

Key Box 16

Ascitic Tap

Indications

1. Diagnosis of ascites of undetermined etiology.
2. Evaluation for possible peritonitis.
3. Relief of abdominal pain or dyspnea by tense ascites (therapeutic indication).

Contraindications

1. Bleeding disorder.
2. Thrombocytopenia.
3. Severe jaundice with impending hepatic coma.
4. Infection/scar at site of needle entry.
5. Acute abdomen.

C. Procedure

1. Prepare the area with spirit, povidone iodine followed by spirit. Drape the area with sterile linen.
2. Anesthetize the skin with 1–2% lignocaine.
3. Use a 18 to 20 G needle attached to a 3-way stopcock with one end attached to a 30 mL syringe and the other end attached to a tubing for collection in case of therapeutic drainage of massive tense ascites.
4. A long needle is selected and is gently inserted using a "Z" technique, i.e. the needle is initially inserted along the direction of skin in subcutaneous plane and then turned perpendicularly into peritoneal cavity evidenced by sudden loss of resistance or feeling of 'give in'. The alternative method is to retract the skin 2 cm caudally while entering the abdomen. It is not released till the needle enters the peritoneum and fluid starts coming.
5. Gently aspirate the fluid while advancing the needle. Do not enter further as soon as fluid starts flowing. Stabilize the needle and aspirate the fluid. Following the procedure, remove the needle slowly. In case of therapeutic tap, leave the plastic sheath/cannula in place and remove the needle. Drain the required amount of fluid by connecting the plastic cannula to a 3-way attached to the tubing.
6. Apply tincture benzoin to seal the site of aspiration and pressure dressing.

7. Subject the collected sample of ascitic fluid for LDH, glucose, protein, cell count, Gram staining, culture, and other relevant investigations based on clinical suspicion.

Also, calculate the albumin gradient of the ascitic fluid **(Table 18.25)**. This will help in identifying the etiology of the ascites.

D. Complications

These include (i) acute liver cell failure and precipitation of hepatic coma; (ii) massive drainage leading to hypotension; (iii) bleeding into peritoneal fluid; (iv) perforation of bowel; and (v) peritonitis.

18.16 PLEURAL ASPIRATION (THORACOCENTESIS)

Indications for pleural aspiration are listed in **Key Box 17**.

A. Positioning

Patient sits comfortably in a chair leaning forward with arms and head supported on an adjustable table **(Fig. 18.44)**. Too much leaning forward can increase the risk of injury to liver/spleen. In small infants and very sick children who cannot sit, the child can lie supine with the lateral chest wall of the affected side brought to the edge of the table. Supine posture is preferred for decompression of tension pneumothorax.

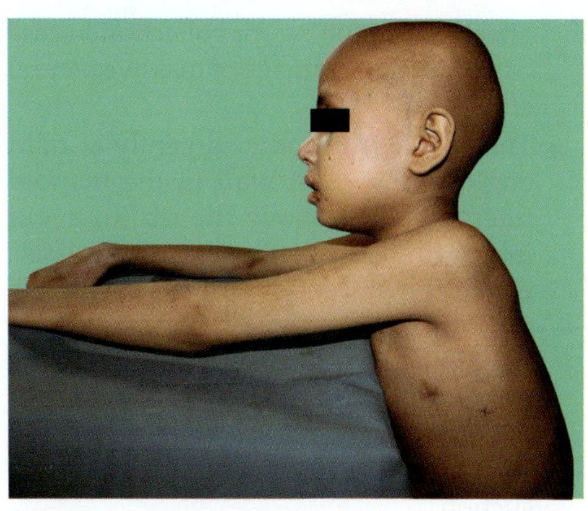

Fig. 18.44: Position of the child and site of pleural tap.

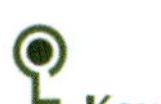

Key Box 17

Pleural Aspiration

Indications

1. Therapeutic aspiration in massive pleural effusion
2. Diagnostic aspiration in case of pleural effusion of unknown cause
3. Emergency management of tension pneumothorax

Contraindications

1. Bleeding diathesis or anticoagulant therapy
2. Thrombocytopenia

B. Site of Aspiration

- *Pleural effusion:* Site of maximum dullness (lowest part of fluid collection), usually corresponds to 7th–9th intercostal spaces in posterior axillary line.
- *Pneumothorax* (decompression of tension pneumothorax): 2nd or 3rd intercostal space in the midclavicular line.

C. Procedure

1. Confirm the site of aspiration with percussion note, auscultation, and chest X-ray and mark it.
2. Monitor the vital signs.
3. Clean the area with spirit, povidone-iodine (betadine) followed by spirit. Drape the site with sterile linen.
4. Anesthetize the skin, subcutaneous tissue and parietal pleura with 1% lignocaine.
5. Use an 18 to 20 G needle attached to a 3-way stopcock with one end attached to a 30 mL syringe and the other end

Table 18.25: Causes of high and low serum ascitic albumin gradient

Serum ascitic albumin gradient >1.1 g/dL	Serum ascitic albumin gradient <1.1 g/dL
1. Cirrhosis/ chronic liver failure	1. Peritoneal tuberculosis
2. Congestive heart failure	2. Biliary/pancreatic ascites
3. Liver metastasis	3. Nephrotic syndrome
4. Budd-Chiari syndrome	4. Bowel obstruction

Serum ascitic albumin gradient (SAAG) = Serum albumin – Ascitic fluid albumin attached to a tubing for collection in case of therapeutic drainage of massive pleural effusion.

6. The needle is introduced gently at right angle to the chest wall in the marked interspace just above the rib (to avoid injury to intercostal nerves and vessels which run at inferior end of rib). Slowly advance the needle and gently aspirate while advancing. Insert slowly till we puncture the parietal pleura which is felt by sudden decrease in the resistance. Withdraw the pleural fluid by gentle suction.
7. Stop the aspiration immediately, if the child complains of severe tightness in chest, intractable cough with thin frothy blood-stained sputum, or if the child develops cardiorespiratory compromise.
8. Do not aspirate more than 10 mL/kg at one time as it precipitates pulmonary edema.
9. Collect the pleural fluid for estimation of protein, LDH, glucose, cell count, Gram stain and culture and other desired analysis as per the clinical suspicion.
10. Emergency decompression of tension pneumothorax requires the needle to be attached to a underwater seal drainage. The needle is inserted slowly perpendicular to the chest wall till a gush of air is appreciated in the underwater seal.

Criteria to differentiate a transudate from exudate in pleural/peritoneal fluid are tabulated in **Table 18.26**.

D. Complications

These incude vasovagal episode, injury to lung leading to hemothorax or pneumothorax causing tightness of chest and severe pain, injury to liver or splenic puncture; and subcutaneous emphysema and air embolism. Sudden expansion of underlying collapsed lung can lead to pulmonary edema resulting in intractable cough with thin frothy blood-stained sputum.

18.17 BONE MARROW ASPIRATION AND BIOPSY

Indications for bone marrow aspiration and bipsy are listed in **Key Box 18**.

A. Positioning

Position of the patient depends on the site of aspiration. The infant is placed supine for tibial aspiration. For aspiration from posterior superior iliac spine, the child is placed in prone posture.

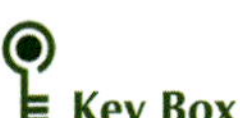

Key Box 18

Bone Marrow Aspiration and Biopsy

Indications

1. Evaluation of hematological disorders: severe anemia, pancytopenia, megaloblastic anemia, refractory anemia or suspected leukemia
2. Severe neutropenia (<500/μL) persisting for >3 days or unresponsive to G-CSF
3. Severe thrombocytopenia (<50000/μL) persisting for >7days
4. Evaluation of suspected storage disease, e.g. Gaucher disease
5. Staging of lymphoma and other solid tumors
6. Evaluation of pyrexia of unknown origin.
7. Unexplained splenomegaly

Contraindications

1. Severe bleeding diathesis/coagulation disorder
2. Local skin infection or underlying osteomyelitis

Table 18.26: Criteria for differentiation between exudate and transudate

Parameter	Exudate	Transudate
Color	Cloudy	Clear
Specific gravity	<1.016	>1.016
Protein	>3 g/dL	<3 g/dL
LDH	>200	<200
Pleural fluid/serum protein	>0.5	<0.5
Pleural fluid/serum LDH	>0.6	<0.6
Pleural fluid glucose	Less than serum glucose	More than serum glucose

B. Site of Aspiration

At birth, hematopoietic marrow is found in all bones of body. By early childhood, fat cells begin to replace bone marrow hematopoietic cells in peripheral skeleton. In adults, hematopoiesis is limited to axial skeleton and proximal portions of extremities. Thus, the most common site of aspiration in children is posterior superior iliac spine (PSIS).

In infants (<1 yr), preferred site is a triangular area at the proximal end of medial surface of tibia just distal to the tibial tuberosity. Other sites of aspiration include sternum, anterior superior iliac spine, and greater trochanter. The marrow is just 1 cm thick at sternum at the level of 2nd intercostal space. Hence, a deeper aspirate might injure heart and great vessels. Anterior superior iliac spine is preferred only when the PSIS is infected, irradiated, or a surgery has been done at the site.

C. Procedure

1. Position the child prone and examine the site (PSIS) for any evidence of infection and mark the area.
2. Clean the desired area with spirit, povidone–iodine followed by spirit. Drape the area with sterile linen.
3. Prepare the bone marrow aspiration needle (Fig. 18.45) and arrange clean glass slides for making smears of the aspirate.
4. Anesthetize the skin, subcutaneous tissue till periosteum with 1–2% lignocaine using a 23 gauge needle and wait for 2–3 minutes.
5. Make a small incision of 3–5 mm in the skin to facilitate the entry of needle especially when a biopsy is planned along with aspiration. Sedate, if the child is uncooperative.
6. Stabilize and restrain the child for proper positioning.
7. Ensure the trocar is completely inserted inside the needle.
8. Hold the bone marrow needle between the thumb and forefinger, and introduce the needle at 90° angle and advance into marrow cavity with a slow, twisting motion (Fig. 18.46). A feel of sudden loss of resistance or 'give in' is felt once the needle enters the cavity. The correct insertion into cavity is confirmed once the needle is fixed to underlying bone.
9. Remove the trocar from the needle and attach a 10–20 mL syringe to the needle and aspirate forcefully until a small drop of marrow appears in the syringe hub. Suction should be stopped as soon as 0.2–2 mL of marrow is obtained since excessive suction will dilute the sample with peripheral blood. Aspiration might cause a brief sharp pain. If no marrow is obtained, advance the needle further and rotate and try aspirating again.
10. Remove the syringe immediately from the needle, and place the drop of marrow in 5–6 slides and prepare them immediately with the help of an assistant. Presence of grossly visible bony spicules indicates suitable specimen.
11. Remove the needle using twisting motion, and apply pressure dressing over the site to avoid bleed from the site of aspiration.
12. If *bone biopsy* is necessary, prepare the biopsy needle (Jamshidi needle) and advance it into the cortical bone with

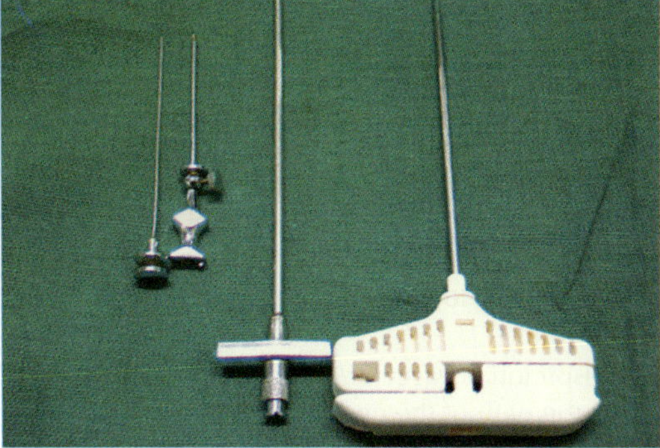

Fig. 18.45: Bone marrow aspiration (left) and bone marrow biopsy (right) needles.

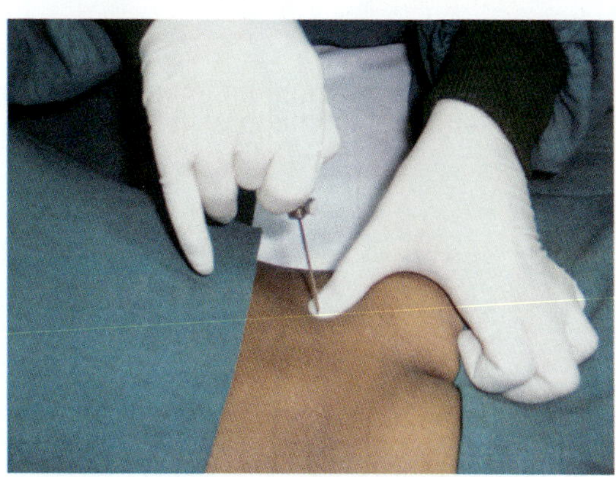

Fig. 18.46: Bone marrow aspiration needle insertion.

steady rotating movement until it is firmly lodged into the bone (Fig. 18.47). Then, remove the stylet and with rotating motion advance the needle another 5–15 mm, the needle tip is redirected, the trocar removed and advanced 2 cm and rotated 360° to obtain the specimen (Fig. 18.48).

Remove the needle by twisting motion and apply pressure dressing. A blunt obturator is used to push the specimen out of needle. Prepare a bone marrow imprint smear on glass slide and preserve the specimen in formalin and send for histopathological examination.

D. Complications

These include subperiosteal bleeding, cellulitis or osteomyelitis, limb fracture, and injury to blood vessels and heart in case of sternal puncture.

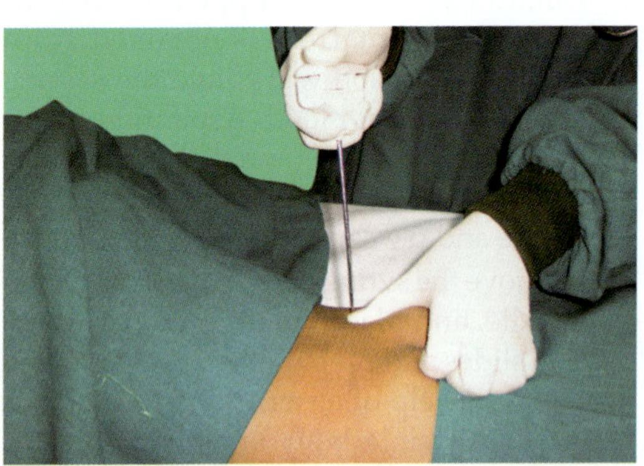

Fig. 18.47: Bone biopsy needle insertion.

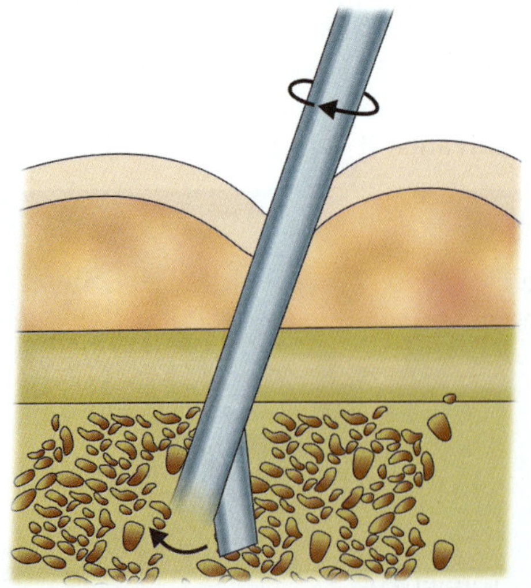

Fig. 18.48: Rotating the bone biopsy needle to obtain the specimen.

18.18 LIVER BIOPSY

Key Box 19 lists the indications and contraindications for liver biopsy.

A. Positioning

The infant or the child is placed in supine posture after appropriate sedation. A rolled towel is placed under the right upper back to push the liver forward and stabilize the position.

B. Route of Biopsy

Transcutaneous: In the transcutaneous route, biopsy can be performed by intercostal or subcostal approach. It can be done in a blind manner or under ultrasonographic guidance. In intercostal approach, biopsy is done at the level of 8th or 9th intercostal space in mid-axillary line. However, when the liver is enlarged the biopsy can be performed below the costal margin in mid-axillary line (subcostal approach).

Transvenous: This method is recommended in patients with deranged coagulation profile where liver biopsy is essential. It is done either by transjugular approach or femoral approach.

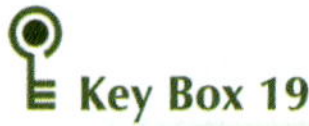

Liver Biopsy

Indications

1. Neonatal cholestasis
2. Diagnosis of chronic active hepatitis and metabolic liver disease
3. Suspected malignancy (primary or secondary)
4. Diagnosis of congenital hepatic fibrosis
5. Unexplained liver disease or persistently abnormal liver function tests
6. To detect inborn errors of metabolism for enzyme analysis
7. Analysis of stored material-like iron (hemosiderosis) and copper (Wilson disease)
8. Monitoring the liver following a liver transplant

Contraindications

1. Prolonged prothrombin time (PT) with test >3 seconds over the control (INR >1.6)
2. Thrombocytopenia (platelet count <50,000 per cu mm)
3. Suspicion of vascular/cystic or infectious lesion in the path of the needle
4. Severe tense ascites
5. Grossly dilated bile ducts

Laparoscopy: This may sometimes be used during laparoscopic surgeries.

C. Procedure

1. All medications that increase the risk of bleeding, like aspirin or non-steroidal anti-inflammatory agents, must be stopped 5–7 days prior to the procedure.
2. The child is kept nil per oral for 5 hrs prior to the procedure.
3. Bleeding time, clotting time, prothrombin time and platelet count should be measured prior to the procedure.
4. Place an intravenous access for appropriate sedation and analgesia.
5. Desired area is cleaned with spirit, povidone–iodine followed by spirit and draped with sterile linen.
6. The skin, subcutaneous tissue, intercostal muscles are anesthetized with 1–2% lignocaine.
7. A small incision in the skin can be made to facilitate the entry of biopsy needle.
8. The patient is asked to hold his breath at end expiration.
9. Tru-cut biopsy needle (23 gauge) **(Fig. 18.49)** is inserted perpendicular to the skin at the marked site till a sudden feel of resistance is felt once the needle enters the liver. The position of the needle is confirmed by the movement of the needle with respiration.
10. The outer sheath of the needle is held firmly, the cutting needle is inserted quickly. The outer sheath is advanced rapidly over the cutting needle and thereafter the entire device is withdrawn **(Fig. 18.50)**.
11. The biopsy specimen is placed in 10% neutral buffered formalin for histopathological examination. An ideal sample is 10–20 mm long. In suspected Reye syndrome, the sample needs to be frozen immediately (liquid nitrogen).

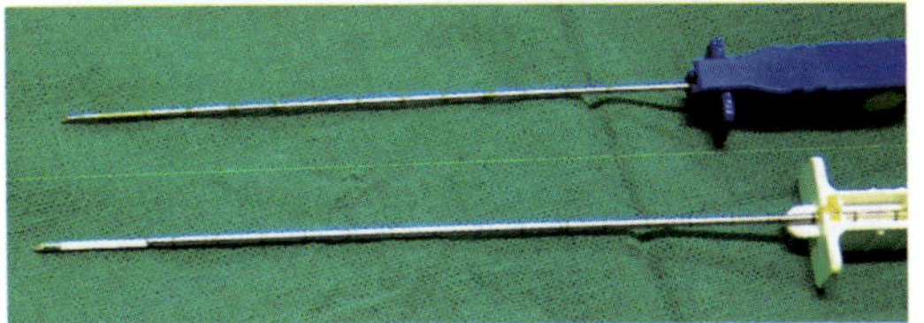

Fig. 18.49: Tru-cut biopsy needle: Outer sheath (above) and cutting needle (below).

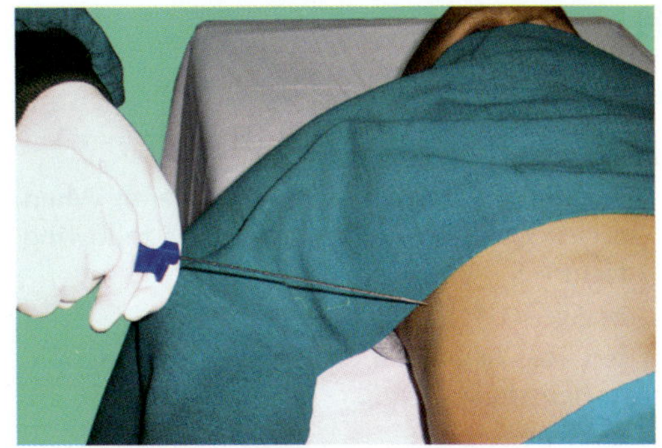

Fig. 18.50: Liver biopsy: Holding and advancing the needle.

12. Local pressure is applied for few minutes and pressure dressing is done.
13. Monitor the vital signs and watch for bleeding for next 24 hours.

Many centers are now using biopsy gun which is a modified version of tru-cut needle, where the cutting needle works by spring mechanism. This is faster and less painful.

D. Complications

These include hemorrhage, hematoma formation, creation of arteriovenous fistula, and pneumothorax or bile peritonitis.

18.19 KIDNEY BIOPSY

Indications and contraindications for kindney biopsy are listed in **Key Box 20**.

A. Positioning

The child lies prone with the head turned to one side, arms abducted, and forearm besides his head. A towel can be rolled up and placed under lower ribs and epigastrium so that kidneys are pushed posteriorly and stabilize their position.

B. Site of Biopsy

Percutaneous kidney biopsy is done at the angle between the lower end of 12th rib and lateral border of sacrospinalis muscle.

C. Procedure

1. Patient should be fasting for 3–4 hours. The biopsy can be performed blindly or under the guidance of ultrasound (preferred).
2. Bleeding time, clotting time, prothrombin time, and platelet count should be

Key Box 20

Kidney Biopsy

Indications

1. Nephrotic syndrome (steroid resistant): When a case of nephrotic syndrome has following features:
   a. Age <1 yr or >8 yrs
   b. Gross hematuria or persistent microscopic hematuria
   c. Hypertension
   d. Low C3 levels (hypocomplementemia)
   e. Features of renal failure not attributable to hypovolemia
   f. Suspected secondary causes of nephritic syndrome
   g. Proteinuria persisting despite 4 weeks of daily steroid therapy
   h. Before initiation of treatment with cyclosporine A or tacrolimus
2. Renal failure of unknown cause
3. Rapidly progressive renal failure/rapidly progressive glomerulonephritis (RPGN)
4. Systemic disease with renal involvement (lupus nephritis, systemic vasculitis)
5. Inherited nephropathies
6. Unexplained or persistent hematuria/proteinuria

Contraindications

1. Uncontrolled hypertension
2. Uncontrolled bleeding disorder
3. Uncooperative patient
4. Single functioning kidney
5. Polycystic kidney
6. Obstructed kidney
7. Untreated uremia
8. Shrunken, small kidneys

measured prior to the procedure. A normal blood pressure and correction of azotemia with dialysis should be ensured.

3. Sedation is often required in children and infants for renal biopsy.
4. Clean and drape the desired area.
5. The biopsy site is marked and anesthetized locally with 1–2% lignocaine in the skin, subcutaneous tissue till renal capsule.
6. Tru-cut biopsy needle (23 gauge) is inserted perpendicular to the skin at the marked site till a sudden feel of resistance is felt once the needle enters the kidney after piercing the renal capsule (Fig. 18.51). The position of the needle is

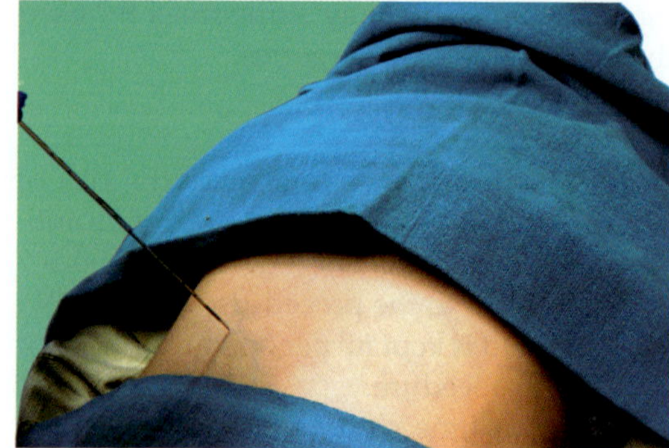

Fig. 18.51: Kidney biopsy: Insert the needle vertically.

confirmed by the movement of the needle with respiration.

7. The outer sheath of the needle is held firmly, the cutting needle is inserted quickly. The outer sheath is advanced rapidly over the cutting needle and thereafter the entire device is withdrawn.
8. Two tissues are required for histopathological examination with one fixed in buffered formalin and the other in saline for immunofluorescence. For electron microscopy, the tissue is fixed in glutaraldehyde. An adequate sample should have at least 8–10 glomeruli.
9. Local pressure is applied for a few minutes and pressure dressing is done.
10. Monitor the pulse rate, blood pressure, and urine output for every 15 minutes for first 2 hours, and then 1 hourly for next 24 hours.
11. Measure hemoglobin 2–4 and 6–12 hours after biopsy. Repeat ultrasonography after 24 hours to rule out perirenal hematoma.

Look for RBC in urine for gross or microscopic hematuria. Repeat hemoglobin can be done after few hours to monitor for blood loss. Hypotension, tachycardia, or severe abdominal or back pain demands urgent assessment.

D. Complications

Gross hematuria may persist for initial 24 hours but rarely beyond. Blood replacement and conservative management is usually sufficient. Inadvertent injury to adjacent organs, perinephric hematoma, transient hypertension, and infection at biopsy site are the other potential complications. AV fistula is a late complication.

Index

B

D

E

Q

R

T

U

V

W

X

Y

Z